HANDBOOK OF
PERSONALITY DISORDERS

Handbook of
Personality
Disorders

Theory, Research, and Treatment

Edited by

W. John Livesley

The Guilford Press
NEW YORK   LONDON

© 2001 The Guilford Press
A Division of Guilford Publications, Inc.
72 Spring Street, New York, NY 10012
www.guilford.com

Printed in the United States of America

This book is printed on acid-free paper.

Last digit is print number: 9 8 7 6 5 4 3 2 1

Library of Congress Cataloging-in-Publication Data

Handbook of personality disorders : theory, research, and treatment
        p. ; cm.
    Includes bibliographical references and indexes.
    ISBN 1-57230-629-7 (hardcover : alk. paper); aa05 01-22-01
    1. Personality disorders—Handbooks, manuals, etc.   I. Livesley, W. John.
    [DNLM: 1. Personality Disorders—therapy.   2. Personality Disorders—etiology. WM
190 H23697 2001]
    RC554 .H36 2001
    616.85′8—dc21

                                                                    2001016208

About the Editor

W. John Livesley, MD, PhD, is Professor and former Head of the Department of Psychiatry, University of British Columbia, Vancouver, British Columbia, Canada. He is also Editor of the *Journal of Personality Disorders* and has contributed extensively to the literature on personality disorder. His research focuses on the classification, assessment, and origins of personality disorder, and his clinical interests center on an integrated approach to treatment based on current empirical knowledge about personality disorder and its treatment.

Contributors

Hassan F. Azim, MD, Department of Psychiatry, University of British Columbia, Vancouver, British Columbia, Canada

Kim Bartholomew, PhD, Department of Psychology, Simon Fraser University, Burnaby, British Columbia, Canada

Lorna Smith Benjamin, PhD, Department of Psychology, University of Utah, Salt Lake City, Utah

Ivy-Marie Blackburn, PhD, Professor of Psychology, Cognitive and Behavioral Therapies Centre, University of Newcastle, Newcastle-upon-Tyne, United Kingdom

Lee Anna Clark, PhD, Department of Psychology, University of Iowa, Iowa City, Iowa

Emil F. Coccaro, MD, Department of Psychiatry, Pritzker School of Medicine, University of Chicago, Chicago, Illinois

Jean Cottraux, MD, PhD, Unité de Traitement de l'Anxiété, Université Lyon, Lyon, France

Richard A. Depue, PhD, Department of Human Development, Cornell University, Ithaca, New York

Regina T. Dolan-Sewell, PhD, Division of Mental Disorders, Behavioral Research, and AIDS, National Institute of Mental Health, Bethesda, Maryland

Glen O. Gabbard, MD, Karl Menninger School of Psychiatry and Mental Health Sciences, Menninger Clinic, Topeka, Kansas, and University of Kansas School of Medicine, Wichita, Kansas

Seth D. Grossman, MA, Institute for Advanced Studies in Personology and Psychopathology, Miami, Florida

John G. Gunderson, MD, Department of Psychiatry, Harvard Medical School at McLean Hospital, Cambridge, Massachusetts

Julie A. Harrison, PhD, Department of Psychiatry, Indiana University School of Medicine, Indianapolis, Indiana

Stephen D. Hart, PhD, Department of Psychology, Simon Fraser University, Burnaby, British Columbia, Canada

Todd F. Heatherton, PhD, Department of Psychological and Brain Sciences, Dartmouth College, Hanover, New Hampshire

Andre M. Ivanoff, PhD, School of Social Welfare, Columbia University, New York, New York

Robert F. Krueger, PhD, Department of Psychology, University of Minnesota, Minneapolis, Minnesota

Marilyn J. Kwong, PhD, Department of Psychology, Simon Fraser University, Burnaby, British Columbia, Canada

Kerry L. Jang, PhD, Department of Psychiatry, University of British Columbia, Vancouver, British Columbia, Canada

Anthony S. Joyce, PhD, Department of Psychiatry, University of Alberta, Edmonton, Alberta, Canada

Mark F. Lenzenweger, PhD, Department of Psychology, Harvard University, Cambridge, Massachusetts

Marsha M. Linehan, PhD, Department of Psychology, University of Washington, Seattle, Washington

W. John Livesley, MD, PhD, Department of Psychiatry, University of British Columbia, Vancouver, British Columbia, Canada

K. Roy MacKenzie, MD, Department of Psychiatry, University of British Columbia, Vancouver, British Columbia, Canada

Paul Markovitz, MD, PhD, Mood and Anxiety Research Center, Fresno, California

Jill I. Mattia, PhD, Department of Psychiatry and Human Behavior, Brown University, Providence, Rhode Island

Sarah E. Meagher MS, Institute for Advanced Studies in Personology and Psychopathology, Miami, Florida

Theodore Millon, PhD, DSc, Institute for Advanced Studies in Personology and Psychopathology, Miami, Florida

J. Christopher Muran, PhD, Department of Psychiatry, Beth Israel Medical Center, New York, New York, and Albert Einstein College of Medicine, Bronx, New York

Joel Paris, MD, Department of Psychiatry, McGill University, Montreal, Quebec, Canada

Paul A. Pilkonis, PhD, Department of Psychiatry, Western Psychiatric Institute and Clinic, University of Pittsburgh School of Medicine, Pittsburgh, Pennsylvania

William E. Piper, PhD, Department of Psychiatry, University of British Columbia, Vancouver, British Columbia, Canada

Christie Pugh, PhD, Department of Psychology, University of Utah, Salt Lake City, Utah

Clive J. Robins, PhD, Department of Psychiatry and Behavioral Sciences, Duke University Medical Center, Durham, North Carolina

Richard N. Rosenthal, MD, Department of Psychiatry, Beth Israel Medical Center, New York, New York, and Albert Einstein College of Medicine, Bronx, New York

Ana M. Ruiz-Sancho, MD, Department of Psychiatry, McLean Hospital, Belmont, Massachusetts, and Apartado de Correos, Cadiz, Spain

Anthony Ryle, DM, FRCPsych, Kings College, Combined Psychological Treatment Services, Munro Centre, Guys Hospital, London, United Kingdom

M. Tracie Shea, PhD, Department of Psychiatry, Brown University, Providence, Rhode Island

George W. Smith, MSW, Department of Psychiatry, McLean Hospital, Belmont Massachusetts

Michael H. Stone, MD, Columbia University College of Physicians and Surgeons, New York, New York

Jennifer J. Tickle, BA, Department of Psychological and Brain Sciences, Dartmouth College, Hanover, New Hampshire

Philip A. Vernon, PhD, Department of Psychology, University of Western Ontario, London, Ontario, Canada

Thomas A. Widiger, PhD, Department of Psychology, University of Kentucky, Lexington, Kentucky

Arnold Winston, MD, Department of Psychiatry, Beth Israel Medical Center, New York, New York, and Albert Einstein College of Medicine, Bronx, New York

Lauren G. Wittenberg, PhD, Office of Management and Budget—OIRA Branch, Washington, DC

Mark Zimmerman, MD, Department of Psychiatry, Rhode Island University, Providence, Rhode Island

Preface

For much of its history, personality disorder was a relatively neglected domain of psychopathology. Knowledge consisted almost entirely of theoretical speculations based on observations made in the course of clinical practice and the in-depth treatment of small numbers of patients. Recently, however, this situation has changed: Over the last two decades, the field has become an active arena of empirical inquiry, with issues that were originally settled by reference to one school of thought or another, or by appeal to tradition, now more likely to be subjected to empirical scrutiny. Diverse theoretical approaches and multiple disciplines are contributing different perspectives that challenge previous ideas. These developments are beginning to forge a new understanding of the nature, origins, and treatment of personality disorder. Current approaches to classification are being challenged by empirical evaluations that offer minimal support for traditional diagnostic formulations but rather point in new directions and indicate the need for new nosological systems. Ideas about the structure of personality disorder and its relationship to other clinical syndromes are changing. Far from being fundamentally distinct entities, it appears that personality disorder and a variety of other mental disorders have at least some common origins. As these etiological links are identified, the distinction between Axis I and Axis II in the DSM system is becoming increasingly blurred.

Similar changes are occurring at the interface between normal and disordered personality. In the past, personality disorder was studied independently of studies of normal personality and little cross-fertilization of ideas occurred. Over the last few years, these distinctions have begun to break down, raising fundamental questions about the nature and definition of disorder and the way it may be differentiated from normality. Empirical and conceptual analyses fail to support categorical distinctions between normal and disordered personality. Instead, many aspects of personality disorder appear to represent the extremes of normal variation—an idea with major implications for classification and research.

In tandem with these developments, a new understanding of the etiology and development of personality disorder is emerging from work in behavior genetics and developmental psychology, and as a result of the cognitive revolution in psychology, that differs substantially from older explanations based on clinical reconstruction. Accounts of the development of personality disorder based on psychosocial factors are being supplemented by an understanding of biological and developmental mechanisms. Even our understanding of the environment is changing with recognition that individuals seek out and create environments that are consistent with their genetic predispositions and emerging personality patterns. Such developments not only challenge traditional theories about the origins of personality disorder but also question the assumptions of many treatments that have neglected the biological underpinnings of personality. At the same time, new treatment approaches are being developed to supplement and sometimes replace traditional methods.

Given these developments, it is timely to provide a handbook that documents the current state of knowledge. The surge of progress that has brought personality disorders into greater prominence has also created a sense of flux as the field seeks to assimilate new findings. Looking backward, it is easy to see the changes that have occurred and the progress that has been made. Looking forward, however, it is difficult to discern the directions that the field is likely to take. That change is occurring and that our ideas need to accommodate new findings is not in question. It is not clear, however, exactly what accommodations are required or the form that they will take. Progress toward theoretical integration lags substantially behind empirical research, creating uncertainty about the meaning and significance of new findings and their relationship to previous theories and models.

The field needs a new theoretical framework to organize evolving knowledge. Unfortunately, it is probably premature to contemplate theoretical integration. While it is apparent that new findings call into question the grand, broad theories that have dominated thinking about personality disorder for so long, and that monolithic positions have begun to break down, it is also apparent that our understanding remains fragmented and that knowledge has not progressed to the point where a new integration is possible. Nevertheless, sufficient empirical and conceptual progress has occurred to merit an in-depth survey and appraisal of the contemporary situation. This handbook is intended to fulfill this function by providing an overview and evaluation of current ideas. The field seems to be at the point where it would be worthwhile to produce a handbook that emphasizes empirical research and conceptual issues. The hope is that systematic accounts of the major empirical findings and succinct statements of the core issues as they pertain to the various topics central to understanding personality disorders will lay the foundation for theoretical integration in the future.

Although the intention is to be comprehensive, it is not possible to include every topic. The field is too fragmented and a systematic body of knowledge does not exist that would allow a comprehensive account. This meant that substantial selectivity had to be exercised concerning topics to be included and the way the topic of personality disorder should be approached. When considering these questions, the decision was made to give greatest weight to empirical research and that the primary objective was to produce a volume that would provide the practicing clinician with an up-to-date understanding about personality disorder that would be relevant to clinical practice.

These considerations had major implications for the content and structure of the volume. Because the focus is on empirical knowledge and the implications it has for theory and practice, the grand theories of personality disorder that have dominated the field in the past and which have tended to dominate the literature on treatment are not given prominence. Despite the impact that theories such as classical psychoanalysis, object relations theory, and self psychology have had on clinical practice, they have not been effective in stimulating systematic empirical research. For this reason, they are not given the attention that many would consider appropriate. The problem is not that these theories are wrong but rather that they are incomplete and do not incorporate important developments elucidating the structure and origins of personality disorder. A new and different kind of synthesis is required for the field to progress.

For somewhat related reasons, the decision was made to organize the volume around such topics as theoretical and conceptual issues, etiology, diagnosis and assessment, and treatment, rather than specific disorders as listed in the *Diagnostic and Statistical Manual of Mental Disorders* (DSM-IV) or the *International Classification of Diseases* (ICD-10). This reflects the belief that current classifications are arbitrary and temporary systems that have heuristic value in stimulating and guiding research and in organizing clinical observations, rather than definitive statements of the way that personality pathology should be organized. Empirical support for these systems is limited and the validity of most diagnostic concepts is not yet established. Indeed, the evidence for these models is not as strong as the evidence against them. For these reasons, it was decided to organize the volume around key topics rather than to allow contemporary models to impose a structure that is not justified by the evidence available. Overall, the intention is to provide a systematic account of empirical knowledge that is as little constrained as possible by the unsubstantiated assumptions of traditional models and theories, while recognizing the importance of theory generally.

Concern with clinical relevance led to a volume that was compiled with the clinician in mind. Emphasis is placed on the clinical implications of current research, while also seeking to provide critical overviews to stimulate further development. Major themes, such as classification, etiology, stability and change, and assessment, are important theoretical issues that have a direct bearing on clinical practice. Emphasis is also placed on treatment because ideas about treatment are changing and the clinician is faced with a wide and almost confusing array of treatment options. Few texts bring together succinct accounts of the range of options available along with evidence of efficacy that allows the clinician to compare different models and select what best suits his or her needs.

The initial idea for a handbook of personality disorders came from Seymour Weingarten, Editor-in-Chief at The Guilford Press, who kindly invited me to assume the role of editor. This provided an interesting and rewarding opportunity for which I am grateful. I also appreciate the support and encouragement that he and his colleagues at Guilford provided through what proved to be a long and at times arduous editorial process. As editor, I am also indebted to the advice and comments received from various reviewers during the early stages of the project and to the many contributors who accepted the invitation to participate and worked so diligently to complete their chapters.

My hope is that this volume will help to disseminate existing knowledge about personality disorder in a way that also encourages readers to question the most fundamental assumptions of traditional ideas and theorics as well as to contemplate new approaches to studying and theorizing about personality disorders. Perhaps even more important, it is hoped that this handbook will also contribute toward the development of improved treatments as well as a better and more tolerant understanding of a comparatively neglected, distressing and painful, and often misunderstood disorder.

Contents

———⟫◆⟪———

PART IV. TREATMENT

PART V. TREATMENT MODALITIES AND SPECIAL ISSUES

PART I

THEORETICAL AND NOSOLOGICAL ISSUES

CHAPTER 1

※◆◆※

Conceptual and
Taxonomic Issues

W. JOHN LIVESLEY

It has been said that each generation of mental health professionals has to discover for itself the importance of personality disorder. Although personality disorder often seems elusive and to defy systematization, the diagnosis seems to be clinically indispensable. This certainly appears to be true of the current generation. Since the publication of DSM-III in 1980 interest in the topic has grown almost exponentially, and personality disorder has come to occupy a more central role in the diagnostic process. The significance of the condition as an important clinical problem with substantial public health and social implications is now widely recognized. Historically, personality disorder has been considered separate from other forms of mental disorder. Recently, however, the field increasingly recognizes that not only is personality disorder an important source of morbidity in itself but also it has major implications for understanding and treating other mental disorders. These clinical developments have been paralleled by similar progress in research that has transformed the field from one that was dominated by clinical observation and impression into an active arena for empirical analysis.

Despite this progress, major problems still confront the field, and our understanding of the nature and origins of personality disorder remains disjointed and piecemeal. These problems are conceptual as much as they are empir-

ical. Multiple models and theories have been created to explain various the various phenomena of personality pathology, but none offer a comprehensive account or provide the coherence required of a satisfactory theory. The result is a complex and confusing array of poorly coordinated theories and concepts. Theory and classification are somewhat unrelated and contemporary taxonomies are increasingly recognized as inadequate and poorly supported by empirical research. Basic questions remain unresolved. What is the relationship been such concepts as personality, personality disorder, temperament, and character? What are the defining features of personality disorder? What is its relationship to other mental disorders? Does the diagnosis warrant the special status of a separate axis? What taxonomic principles and concepts are most applicable to classifying personality pathology? What are the essential components of individual differences in personality pathology? These are just some of the questions that we must begin to answer to establish a solid body of knowledge and develop a valid classification.

HISTORY

It is worth understanding something of the history of contemporary conceptions of personality disorder because historical themes continue to influence contemporary thought even though the field has changed greatly over the last half century. Terms such as "personality," "personality disorder," "temperament," "character," and "psychopathy" that are commonly applied to this form of psychopathology have changed meanings considerably over the last two centuries adding to the confusion that still besets the field. Although interest in patterns of behavior that are similar to modern categories of personality disorder dates to antiquity, and concepts such as psychological types and temperament can be traced at least to ancient Greece, the concept of personality disorder as used today did not take shape until early in the 20th century. According to Berrios (1993), it was only with the work of Schneider (1923/1950) that the contemporary concept truly emerged. Nevertheless, several developments during the 19th century helped to structure current ideas.

The term "character" was widely used during that time to describe the stable and unchangeable features of a person's behavior. Writings on the topic also used of the concept of type, and Berrios noted that "character" became the preferred term to refer to psychological types. The term "type" was used as it is today to describe discrete patterns of behavior. It is interesting to note that the term "personality" was also used although with a very different meaning from present usage. The word is derived from the Greek term for mask, and prior to the 19th century it referred to the mode of appearance of the person (Berrios, 1993). Gradually, however, the term took on a more psychological meaning when it was used to refer to the subjective aspects of the self. Hence 19th century writings about the disorders of personality referred to mechanisms of self-awareness and disorders of consciousness and not to behavior patterns that we would now recognize as personality disorder. It was only in the early 20th century that personality began to be used in its present sense.

The term "temperament" was also used as it had been in Greek medicine to refer to the biological basis of the enduring characteristics that defined the person's character. Descriptions of temperament continued to rely on typal concepts of behavior. This work was important because it established the idea that personality patterns have a biological basis. It also contributed to the development of types of the kind that underlie the categorical diagnoses of contemporary classifications such as DSM-IV.

Work on moral insanity by Pritchard (1835) and others during the 19th century was particularly important for the evolution of the concept of personality disorder. Although this term is often regarded as the predecessor of psychopathy, there is little resemblance between Pritchard's description and Cleckley's (1976) concept or DSM antisocial personality disorder (Whitlock, 1967, 1982). Instead, Pritchard was concerned with describing forms of insanity that did not include delusions. The predominant understanding of the time was that delusions were an inherent component of insanity, an idea developed by Locke. The term "moral insanity" was used to describe diverse disorders, including mood disorders, that had in common the absence of delusions. Berrios suggested that Pritchard encouraged the development of a descriptive psychopathology of mood disorders that promoted the differentiation of these disorders and related conditions. He also helped to differentiate personality from mental disorder by distinguishing between more transient symptomatic states and those that are related to more enduring characteristics. This was an important distinction that contributed to the emergence of personality disorder as a separate diagnostic grouping.

Moral insanity continued to receive attention throughout the 19th century. Maudsley (1874) developed Pritchard's concept further noting that some individuals seem to lack a moral sense, thereby differentiating what was to become the concept of psychopathy in the more modern sense. In 1891, Koch proposed the term "psychopathic" as an alternative to moral insanity to refer to these individuals. At about the same time the concept of degeneration, taken from French psychiatry, was introduced to explain this behavior.

The significance of these developments was that the idea of psychopathy as distinct from other mental disorders began to gain acceptance. This set the stage for Schneider's concept of psychopathic personalities as a distinct nosological group. Before this occurred, however, Kraepelin (1907) introduced a different perspective by suggesting that personality disturbances were attenuated forms (*formes frustes*) of the major psychoses. Thus Kraepelin did not distinguish between mental state disorders and personality disorders but conceived of them as a continuity. Kretschmer (1925) took this idea further by positing a continuum from schizothyme through schizoid to schizophrenia—an idea that anticipated current thinking about schizophrenia spectrum disorders. The notion of personality disorders as part of a continuum with mental state disorders and the idea that they are distinct nosological entities are themes that continue to influence current conceptions of personality disorder.

Despite the frequent resurgence of the idea that personality disorders and mental disorders are linked, the overriding assumption of psychiatric classification for much of the last century has been that the two are distinct. This idea was given a theoretical rationale by Jaspers (1923/1963), who distinguished between personality developments and disease processes. The former are assumed to lead to changes that can be understood from the individual's previous personality, whereas disease processes lead to changes that are not predictable from the individual's premorbid status.

These ideas led to the proposal that different forms of psychopathology require different methods of classification. Jaspers suggested that conditions arising from disease processes could be conceptualized as either present or absent and hence classified as discrete categories. These categories could be defined by a necessary and sufficient set of attributes (monothetic categories) or by a larger number of attributes of which only a smaller number need be present to confirm the diagnosis (polythetic categories). According to Jaspers, personality disorders (and neuroses) should be classified as ideal types. The argument that different classificatory concepts are required to encompass the range of psychopathology embraced by classifications of mental disorders has not been accepted by official systems. DSM-IV uses polythetic categories throughout. Recently, however, the idea that personality disorder requires a different nosological approach has been revived with suggestions that a dimensional (Cloninger, 2000; Costa & Widiger, 1994; Livesley, 1991; Livesley, Schroeder, Jackson, & Jang, 1994; Widiger, 1993, 2000) or prototype approach (Westen & Shedler, 2000) should be adopted.

Schneider's volume *Psychopathic Personalities* originally published in 1923 had a considerable impact. Berrios suggested that by adopting the term "personality," Schneider made concepts such as temperament and character redundant. Unfortunately, this clarity was not widely accepted and the terms continue to be used. Schneider also made the conceptually important distinction between abnormal and disordered personality. Abnormal personality was defined as "deviating from the average." Thus, abnormal personality is merely an extreme variant of normal personality. However, Schneider recognized that this was not an adequate definition of pathology. Not all forms of abnormal personality are necessarily associated with disability or dysfunction. The subgroup of abnormal personalities that are dysfunctional was referred to as psychopathic personalities. These were defined as "abnormal personalities who either suffer personally because of their abnormality or make a community suffer because of it" (p. 3). Schneider did not discuss abnormal personality in detail. Instead, he concentrated on describing 10 varieties of psychopathic personality: hyperthymic, depressive, insecure (sensitives and anankasts), fanatical, attention seeking, labile, explosive, affectionless, weakwilled, and asthenic. Within German psychiatry, psychopathic personality did not have the narrow definition ascribed by British or American psychiatry, but rather the term embraced all forms of personality disorder and neurosis. Schneider noted in the preface to the ninth edition, written in 1950, that the term "psychopath" was not well understood and that his work was not the study of asocial or delinquent personality. He added that "some psychopathic personalities may act in an antisocial manner but . . . this is secondary to the psychopathy" (p. x). Thus, he avoided the tautology inherent in conceptions of antisocial personality that are defined in term of social deviance whereupon the diagnosis is then used to explain deviant behavior.

Although psychopathic personalities were portrayed as types, it is important to note that Jaspers's and Schneider's concept of ideal type is not a simple diagnostic category in the DSM sense. Rather, ideal types are descriptions of patterns of being as opposed to diagnoses. According to Jaspers, an ideal typology consists of polar opposites such as dependency and independence or introversion and extraversion. The diagnostic process is not one of simply ascribing a typal diagnosis. Instead, individuals are compared with contrasting poles to illuminate clinically important aspects of their behavior and personality. The typology provides a framework to guide clinical inquiry and organize an understanding of individual cases. Moreover, ideal types are not stable in the sense that DSM diagnoses are assumed to be stable. Instead, some are episodic and reactive. Schneider also disagreed with Kraepelin's idea that personality disorders are systematically related to major psychoses, although he assumed that personality type has a pathoplastic effect on the form that a psychosis takes. Schneider clearly anticipated current ideas derived from dimensional models that personality disorders represent extremes of normal variation, although he added criteria to differentiate pathological from nonpathological variation. Schneider's position is not without problems, particularly in regard to the definition of suffering. Nevertheless, he introduced into classification a conceptual clarity that has rarely been matched.

Within British and American psychiatry, the concepts of psychopathy and psychopathic personality came to have dissimilar meanings to those proposed by Schneider. Psychopathy was defined more narrowly to describe what we now call antisocial personality disorder, although the two are not synonymous. Descriptions of psychopathy and, later, descriptions of personality disorders, were largely based on clinical observation. Theoretical factors that influenced Jaspers and Schneider played little part in the development of classifications. Diverse definitions emerged as individual clinicians emphasized different facets of these disorders and different aspects of the overall class.

Incorporation of psychoanalytic concepts into classification increased diagnostic and descriptive confusion. These ideas have enriched our understanding of psychopathology, but they have not led to diagnostic or classificatory clarity. Although Freud was not primarily interested in articulating an account of personality disorder, his theory of psychosexual development led to descriptions of character types associated with each stage (Abraham, 1921/1927) that were used to delineate forms of character disorder. Subsequently, the concept of character was formulated more clearly by Reich (1933/1949), who discussed the way that psychosexual conflicts lead to relatively fixed patterns that he characterized as character armor. Reich's interest in the application of psychoanalysis to the treatment of these conditions led to the description of individuals who were neither psychotic nor neurotic that paved the way for modern concepts of borderline personality disorder.

The confusion created for psychiatric classification by diverse concepts led ultimately to DSM-III and the decision to classify personality disorder on a separate axis distinct from other mental disorders and to provide precise descriptions of each diagnosis using diagnostic criteria. Subsequently, diagnostic reliability was found to be poor (Mellsop, Varghese, Joshua, & Hicks, 1982; Spitzer, Forman, & Nee, 1979), leading to the introduction of more specific behavioral criteria in DSM-III-R. The changes wrought by DSM-III led to an expanded clinical and research focus that resulted in a substantial increase in publications on personality disorder over the last decade (Blashfield & McElroy, 1987).

An overview of the field suggests that three phases to the study of personality disorder can be identified (Livesley, 2000). The *pre-DSM-III phase* that dates from the 19th century and earlier was largely one of clinical description that led to the gradual emergence of the concept through the pioneering work of Kraepelin, Kretschmer, Jaspers, and Schneider. Subsequently, psychoanalytic thinkers began to formulate concepts of character disorder based initially on a conception of psychosexual development. The 1960s and 1970s saw the first empirical investigations with pioneering work of Roy Grinker, Werble, and Drye (1968), followed quickly in Europe by studies by Henry Walton and Presly (1973). These early attempts at empirical analysis were rapidly consolidated following the publication of DSM-III in 1980, an event that ushered in what might be referred to as the *DSM-III phase*. Placement on a separate axis and the development of diagnostic criteria ensured both clinical attention and empirical investigation. Much of this empirical work was dominated by DSM concepts. Structured interviews were developed to assess DSM criteria. These stimulated studies of diagnostic reliability, diagnostic overlap, relationships with Axis I disorders, and so on. At the same time, treatments were increasingly directed toward specific DSM diagnoses. Now, the study of personality disorder seems to be evolving into a third stage—the *post-DSM-III/IV era*. Despite the progress of the last 20 years, problems with the DSM model are all too obvious. The approach has limited clinical utility. Diagnostic overlap is a major problem, and there is limited evidence that current categories predict response to treatment. In sum, the construct validity of the system has yet to be established. Problems are equally apparent from a research perspective. DSM diagnoses are too broad and heterogeneous to use in investigations of biological and psychological mechanisms forcing investigators to use alternative constructs and measures (Siever & Davis, 1991). Many of the issues with which past generations of clinicians struggled remain unresolved.

PERSONALITY AND RELATED TERMS

The previous discussion showed how several of the concepts applied to personality disturbance have changed over time and how ideas gradually consolidated into the current conception of personality disorder. Yet the field continues to use a confusing variety of terms to describe personality pathology, and these terms influence contemporary thinking. Given the centrality of the term "personality" it may be helpful to consider the meaning of the term and how it relates to such concepts as character and temperament classifications. As will be seen, an analysis of the term helps to clarify essential features of personality disorder and to set an agenda for research.

Personality

Although the term "personality" is widely used in psychiatry surprisingly little attention has been paid to its definition. The situation is different in psychology. As long ago as 1937, Gordon Allport listed more than 50 definitions. Since then definitions have continued to proliferate. Initially this diversity may appear to constitute an obstacle to developing an understanding of the relationship between normal and disordered personality. However, a consensus exists about the essential elements of personality and an understanding of these elements clarifies our ideas about personality disorder. First, the term refers to regularities and consistencies in behavior and forms of experience (Bromley, 1977). It does not pertain to occasional behaviors but, rather, to behaviors that recur across situations and occasions. Personality also refers to consistencies in thinking, perceiving, and feeling. This is also how we think about personality disorder. DSM-IV, for example, defines personality disorder as "an enduring pattern of inner experience and behavior" (American Psychiatric Association, 1994, p. 633). Second, most approaches emphasize the integrated and organized nature of personality (Hall & Lindzey, 1957). As McAdams (1997) pointed out, all major theorists emphasize the "consis-

tency and coherence of normal personality and view the individual organism as an organized and complexly structured whole" (p. 12). Allport (1961), for example, defined personality as "the dynamic organization within the individual of those psychophysical systems that determine . . . characteristic behavior and thought" (p. 28). In other words, personality is not merely of a collection of traits or other attributes; it also includes the configuration and organization of the different qualities that make up the person. Thus, a central theme of the field is to understand the coherence of personality (Cervone & Shoda, 1999).

These twin themes of personality study also apply to personality disorder. Just as personality assessment and trait psychology have been concerned with identifying and assessing behavioral regularities (usually conceptualized in terms of traits), psychiatric nosology has also been concerned with identifying stable and clinically important regularities in personality pathology. However, controversy surrounds the best way to represent these regularities. Should they be described by the categorical constructs used to describe other mental disorders? Should a different approach be used such as the ideal type approach of Jaspers and Schneider? Or, should we adopt the model of individual differences used in personality assessment and trait psychology and use dimensions that are continuous with normal personality variation?

Similarly, the task of understanding how people establish organized and coherent lives, and how they forge a coherent sense of self from the diversity of their experiences that gives direction and meaning to their lives, is matched in clinical psychiatry by attempts to understand the cohesiveness of the self and identity and the consistency of personality attributes; both are impaired in personality disorder. Thus an important task for the study of personality disorder is to understand how and why integrative processes fail and to develop methods to help patients to construct a more coherent and authentic sense of self that gives stability to their behavior and experience and more control over their lives. The importance of impaired integration is recognized by clinical contributors with diverse theoretical views. Kernberg (1975, 1984), for example, emphasized the importance of identity problems in borderline personality organization, a broad concept that embraces many DSM personality diagnoses. Important aspects of the concept are poorly integrated concepts of self and others and problems integrating diverse and apparently incompatible traits (Akhtar, 1992). Similarly, Kohut (1971) described impaired cohesiveness of the self observed in narcissistic conditions. Like the concept of borderline personality organization, Kohut's concept of narcissism applies to several DSM disorders rather than to a single diagnosis.

In its modern usage, "personality" is an all-encompassing concept that describes a field of study and a set of phenomena. This is the way Schneider used the term when describing psychopathic personalities. As Berrios (1993) noted, the term apparently makes other terms unnecessary. However, terms such as "temperament" and "character" continue to be used and it is important to understand how they relate to this central construct.

Temperament

Temperament has traditionally been used to refer to the biological substratum of personality. It continues to be used in this way. However, behavior–genetic studies showing that all individual differences in personality are heritable (Plomin, Chipeur, & Loehlin, 1990) leave the distinction between personality and temperament unclear. If it were possible to separate genetically determined personality traits from environmentally determined traits, the term "temperament" would have a clearly defined meaning. Although twin studies show that genetic and environmental factors make similar contributions to phenotypical variability, they do not give rise to separate traits. Instead, each trait arises from the interaction of genetic and environmental factors. Hence, all individual differences in behavior are heritable (Turkheimer, 1998), and the heritability of so-called temperament traits is not different from that of other traits. Thus it is not clear that an additional term is required to describe the biological aspects of personality.

Although a case could be made for simply using the general term "personality," the concept of temperament has a long tradition. Usually the term is used to describe the simple, stylistic features of personality that are present in infancy, as opposed to the more complex, substantive, goal-directed, or motivational aspects of personality (Rutter, 1987). With this usage, emotional reactivity and activity are considered temperament but dependency and compulsivity are not. This is the meaning of the term as used by Thomas

and Chess (Chess & Thomas, 1984; Thomas, Birch, Hertzig, & Korn, 1963; Thomas & Chess, 1977). In this sense, the term is convenient, although it should be noted that the distinction between temperament and other personality traits is imprecise.

Character

Traditionally, character referred to enduring traits and behavior patterns. Within the psychological literature in the last century the term fell into disuse, being replaced by the more general term "personality." Allport (1961) noted, however, that the term was often used interchangeably with personality and that European psychologists seemed to prefer the term "character" whereas North American psychologists seemed to prefer "personality". Allport opted for "personality" noting that in everyday usage character usually involved an evaluation as in phrases such as "good character." He suggested that character was essentially personality evaluated. The psychoanalytic literature continued to use the term as in character neurosis probably because of its European origins—Freud usually referred to character rather than personality—although the term "character disorder" was often used as if synonymous with "personality disorder."

Recently confusion surrounding the term has increased because it is not always used with its traditional meaning. Instead, it is used to refer to aspects of personality that are assumed to be the product of learning and interaction with the environment. In this usage, character is usually contrasted with temperament which refers to genetically determined traits. The idea is appealing for the way it assigns roles to environmental and genetic determinants of personality disorder that lead to defined roles for biological and psychotherapeutic interventions. Unfortunately, however, the distinction between temperament traits and character traits is not so clear-cut. Given behavior–genetic data that all personality traits appear to be heritable, it would perhaps be best to follow Allport's advice and abandon the term "character" as a scientific concept.

CONCEPTS AND DEFINITIONS OF PERSONALITY DISORDER

Current classifications incorporate diagnostic concepts drawn from diverse theoretical systems such as classical phenomenology, traditional psychoanalytic theory, object relations theory, self psychology, and social learning theory. Besides this eclectic array of diagnoses, contemporary ideas also embrace a variety of concepts of personality disorder. These include the following:

1. Personality disorder as a *forme fruste* of major mental state disorders as proposed by Kraepelin and Kretschmer. Within DSM-IV, this concept is represented by schizotypal personality disorder that appears to be part of the schizophrenia spectrum.
2. Personality disorder as the failure to develop important components of personality, as illustrated by Cleckley's (1976) concept of psychopathy as the failure to learn from experience and to show remorse. Similarly, psychoanalytic theories postulate defective superego development individuals with this condition. Deficit models of borderline pathology also assume the failure to acquire specific structures and processes.
3. Personality disorder as a particular form of personality structure or organization is illustrated by Kernberg's (1984) concept of borderline personality organization which is defined in terms of identity diffusion, primitive defenses, and reality testing.
4. Social deviance concepts of personality disorder are represented by Robins's (1966) concept of sociopathic personality as the failure of socialization.
5. Personality disorder as abnormal personality (in the statistical sense) is represented by models of personality disorder derived from normal personality structure. These models conceptualize disorder as extremes of normal variation. This is the approach proposed by Schneider although, as noted earlier, he distinguished between abnormal and disordered personality.

Several of these concepts are not fully developed theoretical formulations; thus it is not always clear whether they represent different theoretical positions or alternative descriptions of the same dysfunction. For example, social deviance and deficit models of psychopathy may not necessary be inconsistent. With the exception of personality disorder as extreme variation, none of these concepts provides a systematic definition of the type that is required for classification.

A critical issue for the classification of personality disorder raised by these concepts is whether these disorders are systematically related to major Axis I disorders as suggested by the *form fruste* conception, or whether they are distinct entities. If personality disorders are variants of Axis I disorders they could be spread throughout the classification by incorporating them into various diagnostic spectra. If, however, they are distinct diagnostic entities, classification becomes a pertinent issue. Given the importance of this issue, it is fortunate that empirical evidence on the relationship between personality disorders and other mental disorders is clear. As Rutter (1987) noted, some personality disorders have traditionally been viewed as variants of such conditions as affective disorders, autism, and schizophrenia; however, beyond these conditions remains a substantial range of conditions characterized by chronic interpersonal problems. The only condition considered a personality disorder by DSM-IV that has consistently been shown to bear an etiological or spectrum relationship to a major Axis I disorder is schizotypal. Family studies suggest that schizotypal personality disorder is related to the schizophrenia spectrum (Nigg & Goldsmith, 1994). The evidence that other Cluster A diagnoses are also part of the spectrum is less convincing especially for schizoid personality disorder. It has also been suggested that borderline personality disorder is part a variant of mood disorder, although this assertion is not supported by the evidence (Nigg & Goldsmith, 1994).

It appears that apart from schizotypal personality disorder, all DSM-IV personality diagnoses form a separate class of disorders that are not systematically related to other mental disorders. This means that a systematic definition of personality disorder is required as the first step toward constructing a classification. The following sections consider five approaches to definition: (1) clinical concepts of personality disorder, (2) the DSM-IV definition, (3) ideas based on normal personality variation, (4) definitions that conceptualize personality disorder as extreme positions on specific traits, and (5) the idea of personality disorder as adaptive failure that involves a "harmful dysfunction" (Wakefield, 1992) of the normal adaptive functions of personality. When considering these definitions it is useful to bear in mind that a satisfactory definition should explicate the defining features of the disorder, specify the ways personality disorder differs from other mental disorders, show how the concept is derived from normal personality, and specify how disordered and normal personality differ.

Clinical Concepts

Although the clinical literature does not always provide systematic definitions of personality disorder, it contains several assumptions about the central features. It is convenient to begin a critical appraisal of definitions by examining these ideas because they represent clinical wisdom distilled over the years. If a classification is to have clinical utility it should be consistent with these ideas.

Clinical descriptions typically emphasize two features: chronic interpersonal difficulties and problems with self or identify. Rutter (1987) concluded that personality disorder is "characterized by a persistent, pervasive abnormality in social relationships and social functioning generally" (p. 454). Similarly, Vallaint and Perry (1980) noted that personality disorder is inevitably manifested in social situations. They also suggested that personality disorder involves "the tendency to create a vicious cycle in which already precarious interpersonal relationships are made worse by the person's mode of adaptation" (p. 1563). The idea of cyclical maladaptive interpersonal relationships is developed further by interpersonal approaches to personality that conceptualize personality disorder as repetitive maladaptive patterns of thoughts, feelings, and actions that occur in relationship to significant others (Benjamin, 1993, 1996, see also Chapter 20, this volume; Carson, 1982; Kiesler, 1986; McLemore & Brokaw, 1987; Pincus & Wiggins, 1990).

A second aspect of clinical description focuses on the significance of self-pathology. "Identity diffusion," a term originally coined by Erikson (1950) to describe the failure to establish an integrated sense of identity during adolescence, is a central element in Kernberg's (1984) concept of borderline personality organization. Identity diffusion is "represented by a poorly integrated concept of the self and of significant others . . . reflected in the subjective experience of chronic emptiness, contradictory self-perceptions, contradictory behavior that cannot be integrated in an emotionally meaningful way, and shallow, flat, impoverished perceptions of others" (Kernberg, 1984, p. 12). Similarly, Kohut (1971) and the self psychology school described the failure to develop a cohesive sense of self in narcissistic conditions. From a different perspective, cognitive therapists have described the self-pathology that characterizes most personality disorders in terms of thoughts, beliefs, and schemas used to process information about the self and to construct self-images. The DSM-IV general criteria also make reference to disturbances of the self.

Putting aside differences in terminology and theoretical explanations, there appears to be a measure of agreement that self problems and chronic interpersonal dysfunction are the core features of personality disorder. Cloninger, Svrakic, and Przybeck (1993) recognized this combination when they defined personality disorder as low self-directedness and low cooperativeness.

Official Definitions: The DSM Definition

DSM-III and subsequent editions defined personality disorders as clusters of personality traits that are "inflexible and maladaptive and cause either significant functional impairment or subjective distress." The definition makes *traits* the major conceptual unit for describing and analyzing personality disorder (Berrios, 1993). This idea is significant because it differs from other conceptions that emphasize that personality disorder involves structural problems as, for example, the concept of borderline personality organization (Kernberg, 1984). More important, the emphasis on traits established, at least in principle, the possibility of a conceptual continuity between normal and disordered personality because for many personologists, personality is best described using trait constructs. The definition also implies that personality disorders are combinations or constellations of traits. This definition is also consistent with trait theories that conceptualize personality as a hierarchical structure consisting of a large number of lower-order traits that are organized into fewer higher-order dimensions such as neuroticism and extraversion. Despite this similarity, DSM radically departs from normative personality theories when it adopts a categorical approach that is consistent with the neo-Kraepelian assumptions about mental disorder (Klerman, 1978). Jaspers and Schneider's arguments that personality disorders (along with the neuroses) are not psychiatric illnesses and hence require a different classificatory approach are ignored.

The other feature about the definition that is important is the distinction made between traits and disorder. Extreme levels of a trait are not sufficient for diagnosis. It is only when these traits are inflexible or maladaptive or cause significant functional impairment or subjective distress that disorder is diagnosed. This is similar to Schneider's approach.

DSM-IV took definition a stage further by providing criteria for general personality disorder as well as criteria sets for each diagnosis. This provision separated the diagnosis of personality disorder as a distinct nosological entity from the diagnosis or assessment of individual differences in personality disorder (Livesley et al., 1994). Cloninger (2000) proposed a similar distinction. This change in DSM was an important taxonomic development and one that should probably be a feature of future systems (Livesley, 1998). The actual criteria proposed to diagnose personality disorder, however, are problematic. The criteria set lists four features: (1) ways of perceiving and interpreting the self, other people, and events; (2) the range, intensity, lability, and appropriateness of emotional response; (3) interpersonal functioning; and (4) impulse control. Although these criteria are clinically based and probably acceptable to most clinicians, they are too vaguely worded to translate into reliable measures. They also lack a rationale based on an understanding of the functions of normal personality. Instead, they merely catalogue features that characterize a wide range of psychopathology.

Extremes of Normal Variation

Accumulating evidence that the features of personality disorder are continuously distributed has led to suggestions that these conditions could be understood to represent extremes of normal variation. The assumption that personality disorder involves either too much or too little of a given characteristic is part of the interpersonal circumplex model of psychopathology (Kiesler, 1986; Leary, 1957; Wiggins & Pincus, 1989) and trait approaches to personality disorder (Eysenck, 1987). The problem with defining disorder in terms of extremity alone is that statistical deviance is neither a necessary nor sufficient criterion for disorder (Wakefield, 1992). An extreme score on dimensions such as conscientiousness, extraversion, or agreeableness is not necessarily pathological. Some additional factor needs be present to jus-

tify the diagnosis. Unfortunately, current descriptions of personality disorder often confound extreme scores on a personality trait with disordered functioning (Parker & Barrett, 2000).

Widiger (1994), proposing a classification based on the five-factor model of personality, suggested that personality disorders could be diagnosed at that point along the continuum of personality functioning that is associated with clinically significant impairment. This could presumably be achieved by developing general criteria for assessing clinical significance such as those proposed by DSM or by specifying maladaptive expressions of each trait. In the latter case, it would be important to explicate the rationale for features selected to ensure that the assumptions underlying the approach are explicit and therefore testable. Widiger and colleagues (Widiger & Sankis, 2000; Widiger & Trull, 1991) suggested that clinical significance could be understood as dyscontrolled impairment or maladaptivity in psychological functioning. This suggestion was made with reference to a general definition of mental disorder and hence should apply to personality disorder. The challenge for this approach is to construct criteria to assess "dyscontrolled malapativity" reliably. The problem with the approach is that it seems to embrace an ideal concept of normality because as Widiger (1994) noted, everyone shows some degree of a maladaptive expression of basic traits. Hence the distinction between normality and clinically significant impairment would be even more blurred than at present.

Extremes of Specific Dimensions

Although an extreme level of any trait is insufficient to diagnose disorder, it may be possible to identify a trait or cluster of traits for which an extreme score is indicative of personality disorder. Cloninger et al. (1993) suggested that personality traits could be divided into temperament traits (harm avoidance, reward dependence, persistence, and novelty seeking) and character traits (self-directedness, cooperativeness, and self-transcendence). They suggested that low scores on certain character traits define personality disorder. For example, all categories of personality disorder are characterized by low self-directedness as measured with the Temperament and Character Inventory (Cloninger et al., 1993; Svrakic, Whitehead,

Przybeck, & Cloninger, 1993). Mulder, Joyce, Sullivan, Bulik, and Carter (1999) also found an association between measures of personality disorder and low self-directedness. Although many of the correlations between self-directedness and personality disorder assessed using the SCID-II (Structured Clinical Interview for DSM-III-R, Axis II) were significant, the magnitude was low ranging from a statistically nonsignificant value of –.15 for adult antisocial and schizoid personality disorders to –.46 for borderline personality disorder. This suggests that low self-directedness alone may not be sufficient to diagnose personality disorder. The correlations of the other "character" dimensions of cooperativeness and self-transcendence with specific personality disorders ranged from –.01 to –0.32 and from zero to –.24 for cooperativeness and self-transcendence respectively.

Further development of the approach led Cloninger (2000) to define personality disorder as low scores on self-directedness, cooperativeness, affective stability, and self-transcendence. With this framework, two of the four features would be required for diagnosis. More than two features would indicate greater severity. An interesting feature of the proposal is that the order in which the four foregoing features were listed offers efficient screening because the most consistent feature of personality disorder is low self-directedness. Low self-transcendence is listed last because it is associated only with severe personality disorder (Cloninger, 2000).

This approach moves the classification of personality disorder away from a concern with only individual differences in patterns of personality disorder by placing priority on establishing the presence of personality disorder as the first step in the diagnostic process. Once the presence of personality disorder is confirmed, the next step in the diagnostic process is to describe personality along other dimensions. An appealing feature of the proposal is the extent to which it is grounded in empirical research showing that personality disorder diagnoses are most closely associated with the dimensions listed. Diagnosis is also based on a small number of items for each dimension that are clearly defined unlike general criteria proposed in DSM-IV. By including low affective stability in the definition of personality disorder, Cloninger seems to have moved away from conceptualizing personality disorder only in

terms of character dimensions that were assumed to have low heritability. This is a useful development given problems identifying nonheritable traits. Affective instability is clearly a temperament dimension in the sense discussed earlier; that is, it is a stylistic feature that is usually apparent in infancy (Buss & Plomin, 1984). The approach is also consistent with DSM-IV. As Cloninger (2000) noted, the four dimensions correspond reasonably well to the DSM general criteria. This does, however, raise the concern expressed about the DSM criteria that they are more a catalogue of features associated with personality disorder than a systematic definition based on an understanding of the functions of normal personality and the way that these functions are disturbed in personality disorder.

Adaptive Failure

An alternative approach is to derive a definition of personality disorder from an understanding of the functions of normal personality. This would ground the concept firmly in a general conception of personality structure and functions rather than a somewhat arbitrary array of tenuously related traits and other features. A theoretical framework of this type would bring coherence to what is currently a patchwork of diverse theoretical and descriptive concepts. Such a unified approach could be achieved only through the development of a systematic theory of personality that articulates a universal conception of the functions of personality. Although this seems an unrealizable objective given current knowledge, it may be possible to move toward this goal by developing a theoretical framework to organize our understanding of the adaptive functions of personality. Perhaps the most obvious general model that could be used for this purpose is evolutionary theory (Livesley et al., 1994; Millon, 1990; Millon, with Davis, 1996). Millon, with Davis (1996) suggested that "personality could be conceived as representing the more-or-less *distinctive style of adaptive functioning* that an organism . . . exhibits as it relates to its typical range of environments" (p. 70). Within this framework, personality disorder would "represent particular *styles of maladaptive functioning* that can be traced to deficiencies, imbalances, or conflicts in a species' capacity to relate to the environment it faces" (Millon, with Davis, 1996, pp. 70–71).

Millon's seminal contributions set the stage for a systematic approach that anchors the concept of personality disorder in an understanding of the way the adaptive functions of personality become disrupted. Evolutionary processes are concerned with the selection of mechanisms that enable the individual to adapt to their environment and thereby reproduce. Although evolutionary perspectives on human behavior and personality are at preliminary stage of development we can discern some fundamental principles about the nature of personality that may aid in defining personality disorder.

Adaptive Functions of Personality

More than 50 years ago Allport (1937) stated that "personality *is* something and personality *does* something" (p. 48). Most accounts of personality, including DSM, are concerned with what personality *is*—that is, they concentrate on describing the traits and other structures that characterize personality (Cantor, 1990). Less attention has been paid to the functional aspects of personality and the dysfunctions associated with personality disorder (Livesley, 1995). Yet personality systems serve an adaptive purpose. To understand personality disorder, we need to understand the functional aspects of personality and the way these functions become disturbed.

Starting with Allport's statement, Cantor (1990) proposed that what personality *does* is best understood in terms of the solution of major life tasks. These are the tasks or adaptive problems that the person must solve to adapt effectively. Life tasks may be described in various ways. Some are personal tasks that individuals impose upon themselves. Others are cultural tasks that everyone living in that culture must address. Other tasks are universal problems that affect all humans because they derive from a common human nature. Especially important from our perspective are universal tasks imposed by the environment in which our remote ancestors lived as hunter–gatherers. Life tasks that have evolutionary significance are particularly relevant to the definition of personality disorder because they offer the possibility of developing a definition that is applicable to all cultures (Livesley et al., 1994).

Plutchik (1980) described four universal tasks that are basic to adaptation: identity, hierarchy (issues of dominance and submissiveness), territoriality (belongingness), and temporality (problems of loss and separation).

Adaptive solutions to these tasks were critical to effective functioning and survival in the ancestral environment. They are probably equally relevant to adaptation in contemporary society. Solutions to these tasks form core components of personality, and the failure to achieve adaptive solutions to one or more of these tasks represents some of the core dysfunctions of personality disorder.

It is of interest that the universal tasks proposed by Plutchik resemble the clinical concepts of personality disorder discussed earlier. Both emphasize the development of a sense of self or identity and the capacity to develop effective interpersonal relationships. This similarity offers the possibility of developing a definition that captures both clinical ideas and concepts derived from evolutionary psychology and personality theory.

If evolutionary life tasks are restated in clinical language, personality disorder could be said to be present when "the structure of personality prevents the person from achieving adaptive solutions to universal life tasks" (Livesley, 1998, p. 141). This is a deficit definition in that personality disorder is considered a "harmful dysfunction" due to the failure to acquire the structures required to function effectively in these realms (Wakefield, 1992). Three separate but interrelated realms of functioning may be identified: self-system, familial or kinship relationships, and societal or group relationships. These dysfunctions could be specified as (1) failure to establish stable and integrated representations of self and others; (2) interpersonal dysfunction as indicated by the failure to develop the capacity for intimacy, to function adaptively as an attachment figure, and/or to establish the capacity for affiliative relationships; (3) failure to function adaptively in the social group as indicated by the failure to develop the capacity for prosocial behavior and/or cooperative relationships. To complete this definition it is necessary to add that these deficits are enduring failures that can be traced to adolescence or at least early adulthood, and that they do not arise from a pervasive and chronic Axis I disorder such as a cognitive or schizophrenic disorder.

To translate this definition into reliable diagnostic items requires a more detailed description self and interpersonal pathology. Oldham and Skodol (2000) acknowledge that this definition establishes conceptual continuity between personality and personality disorder but question the extent to which it is possible to develop items to assess all components of the definition reliably. They cite in particular problems that may be encountered in developing items for self-pathology. These are understandable concerns. Although the clinical literature contains many references to self or identity problems, operational definitions have not been developed and considerable conceptual and empirical work is required to construct appropriate criteria. However, if the construct validation approach described by Loevinger (1957) is used this appears feasible (Livesley, 1998). This approach requires a systematic definition of a construct and its components that are to generate assessment items. These components are then subjected to an iterative process of data collection and item analysis to develop a homogeneous set of items that measure the same underlying construct (Jackson, 1971).

Using this process, the failure to develop a coherent sense of self and integrated representations of other were systematically defined. The coherence of the self was understood to arise from the interrelationships that exist in the person's knowledge of the self and from the connections that exist among the individual's images of self and others. Thus the self is conceptualized as a system that consists of elements (qualities, constructs, ideas, and beliefs attributed to the self) and organization (the relationships or connections among these attributes). Self-pathology observed in personality disorder consists of dysfunctional elements (maladaptive cognitions about the self) and failure to integrate different aspects of self knowledge into a coherent and integrated structure. The latter could be defined in terms of six dimensions of self-pathology: diffuse self-boundaries, lack of self-clarity or certainty, labile self-concept, inconsistency and fragmentation, lack of autonomy and agency, and defective sense of self. The resulting description based on a cognitive model of the self is similar to clinical descriptions of identify diffusion (Akhtar, 1992; Kernberg, 1984). Preliminary empirical studies suggest that these dimensions may be defined sufficiently precisely to be used to compile a set of reliable diagnostic items (Livesley, 1998). This approach to definition appears to meet the requirement of integrating clinical concepts with normative personality theory while meeting the requirement for reliable assessment. Subsequent empirical analyses may well show that not all parts

of the definition are required to yield reliable and valid diagnoses of personality disorder

CLASSIFICATION: CATEGORICAL MODELS

Although it is recognized that personality disorders are fuzzy concepts, classifications of personality disorder have traditionally employed categorical diagnoses. The category concept used, however, varies across systems. Official classifications such as DSM and ICD tend to use either monothetic and polythetic categories. Other approaches have adopted ideal types as proposed by Jaspers and prototypical categorization (Cantor, Smith, French, & Mezzich, 1980).

Monothetic and Polythetic Categories

Monothetic categories are defined by a set of attributes or diagnostic criteria that are considered necessary and sufficient for category membership. These categories were used for some personality disorder diagnoses in DSM-III. However, personality disorders do not lend themselves to such an approach, and DSM-III-R and DSM-IV adopted polythetic categories. These categories are defined using a set of criteria none of which are necessary or sufficient for diagnosis. Polythetic categories as used in traditional biological classification are defined by a large number of features, and each member of the category possesses many of these attributes (Beckner, 1959). As a result, most members of the category have a large number of features in common. The polythetic categories used in DSM depart from this approach in several ways. First, categories of personality disorder are defined by a small number of features (typically seven to nine) of which a fewer number (usually about five) need to be present to confirm the diagnosis. These rules lead to considerable heterogeneity in category membership because some members may have few features in common. As a result, groups of subjects selected on the basis of DSM diagnosis can show considerable intragroup variability. Second, the use of a cutting score to specify category membership based on a specified number of criteria creates the impression that there is a clear distinction between normality and pathology. However, cutting scores are purely arbitrary (Widiger & Corbitt, 1994) and it is not apparent that individuals with one fewer criteria than are required to meet a diagnosis are substantially different from those with the required number of criteria.

The polythetic categories of biological classifications based on a set theory model, are organized into a hierarchy. Classifications of mental disorders are also hierarchically organized. The superordinate category of personality disorder divides into three clusters. Unfortunately, the rationale for this arrangement is not specified, so it is unclear whether the arrangement is merely one of convenience—10 categories are easier to use if grouped into three clusters—or whether it reflects fundamental features in the ways personality pathology is organized. Given the lack of clarity, the cluster structure seems to have been assigned more substance than is warranted and several studies have explored the extent to which personality disorders are organized in this way (Hyler & Lyons, 1988; Kass, Skodol, Charles, Spitzer, & Williams, 1985). Regardless of the problems with the DSM system, however, the idea that personality disorder constructs are hierarchically arranged is a convenient heuristic for organizing a classification.

Ideal Types and Prototypes

Alternative category concepts that have been proposed for personality disorder are ideal types (Jaspers, 1923/1963; Schneider, 1923/1950; Schwartz, Wiggins, & Norko, 1989) and prototypes (Livesley, 1985; Weston & Shedler, 2000). Earlier, reference was made to Jaspers's suggestion that ideal types be used to classify neuroses and personality disorders. An ideal type is a hypothetic construct "denoting a configuration of characteristics which on the basis of theory and observations, are assumed to be interrelated" (Wood, 1969, p. 227). A type describes ideal or prototypical cases: Actual cases that match the ideal type in all particulars are rare. In psychiatry, ideal types are idealized descriptions that offer a particular perspective on a condition (Schwartz et al., 1989) and thereby impose conceptual clarity on cases that by their nature are fuzzy and imprecise. In the process, the relationship among the features that describe the ideal case are clarified and understood.

A related categorical concept is the prototype. Prototypical categories are organized around prototypical cases (the best examples of the concept) with less prototypical cases forming a continuum away from prototypical cases (Rosch, 1978). Psychiatric diagnoses show many of the features of prototypical categorization being inherently fuzzy in nature without clear boundaries between categories (Cantor et al., 1980; Livesley, 1985). This structure appears to be especially pertinent to classifying personality disorder because clinicians seem to use prototypical categorization intuitively in everyday discussion when they describe patients as "typical borderline personality disorder" or "classical histrionic personality" (Livesley, 1985). Clinicians also show high levels of agreement on the prototypal features of DSM diagnoses (Livesley, 1986). Prototypes readily accommodate the fuzziness of personality disorders by establishing gradients of category membership so that category membership is not an all-or-none matter as it is with monothetic or polythetic categories but rather a graded quality. Although prototypes resemble ideal types there are important differences (Schwartz et al., 1989). Prototypes are merely lists of features that define a concept or diagnosis that are not organized in any way except in terms of the degree to which each feature is prototypical of the diagnosis. Ideal types, however, are theoretical constructs that incorporate an account for the relationship among these features.

Westen and Shedler (2000) suggested that the classification of personality disorder would be substantially improved by explicitly adopting a prototype approach based on empirically derived prototypes. They developed descriptions of prototypes using Q-sort methodology (Westen & Shedler, 1999a, 1999b). Clinicians (N = 496) were asked to evaluate one patient using 200 descriptive statements developed to represent clinical concepts. Statements are sorted into eight categories according to the degree to which they are descriptive of the person. Q-factor analysis was used to identify clusters or groupings of patients. Q-factor analysis is a type of inverse factor analysis in which explores the relationship among subjects rather than descriptive items or traits as in standard factor analysis. Seven clusters were identified that were labeled dysphoric (consisting of five subtypes), schizoid, antisocial, obsessional, paranoid, histrionic, and narcissistic. Prototypes of each cluster were then constructed based on the most highly rated items. Westen and Shedler (2000) proposed a prototype matching procedure to diagnose personality disorder in which clinicians are asked to rate the degree to which a patient matches a given prototype. They justify this approach by arguing that clinicians are good at making observations and drawing inferences, and that they are better at picking up subtle features that are not readily identified using structured tests. They suggest that their procedure capitalizes on the things clinicians do well and minimizes the use of things they do badly such as aggregating and combining data. The proposal certainly capitalizes on the way in which clinicians appear to make decisions. The evidence suggests that they do not combine information about personality disorder as required by DSM (Morey & Ochoa, 1989) but rather form opinions based on the degree to which patients resemble clinicians' conceptions of the disorder. For this reason, a prototype matching approach to diagnosis is likely to be easy to use and user-friendly. Unfortunately, it is not clear whether prototypes represent the way personality is organized (i.e., describe patterns of behavior in patients) or whether they merely represent information processing structures and heuristics that clinicians use to organize information about their patients. The method seems to be a useful way to study clinical decision making. It is not clear, however, that it is a useful way to study personality.

Limitations of Contemporary Categorical Models

Although official classifications will be discussed in detail in Chapter 3 (this volume), it is useful to consider the limitations of such systems here because they form a context for examining other approaches. A consensus seems to be emerging among clinicians and researchers that there are fundamental problems with the DSM classification of personality disorders that require radical change (Westen & Shedler, 2000). Problems cover (1) the formal features of the system including an underdeveloped theoretical structure, unclear differentiation of personality disorders from other mental disorders, and the use of a categorical approach; (2) inadequate psychometric properties including reliability and validity; and (3) substantive problems relating to the conceptualization of specific diagnoses and criteria sets.

Atheoretical Approach

Although the DSM system deliberately sought to be atheoretical with respect to etiology be-

cause of the limited evidence to support etiological speculations, it is also atheoretical in the sense that it fails to provide an explicit theoretical or empirical rationale for selecting diagnoses or criteria. Diagnoses are arbitrary selections drawn from diverse sources. Diagnoses such as histrionic personality disorder originate in both classical psychoanalytic models of psychosexual development and classical phenomenology. Others like schizotypal personality disorder, although new to DSM-III, can be traced to Kraepelin's formulation of *formes frustes* conditions. Borderline and narcissistic personality disorders stem from more recent psychoanalytic thinking. Avoidant personality disorder originated in the social learning conception of Millon (1969). This is an uneasy combination of concepts derived from conceptual models that are not always consistent with each other. Under these circumstances it is not surprising that the operating characteristics of the system in terms of diagnostic overlap, coverage, and reliability are poor.

At a more fundamental level there is also lack of clarity about the theoretical assumptions that led to the system having its current structure. What are the principles that led to the decision to separate personality disorders from all other mental disorders? What led to the assumption that personality disorder is organized into discrete categories? What is the rationale for proposing three clusters of disorders? What principles and concepts were used to select diagnoses and criteria? The failure to explicate these issues means that it is difficult to test the system empirically and to evaluate the consistency with which underlying taxonomic assumptions were applied.

Diagnostic Concepts

A major problem with current diagnostic concepts that is often neglected is their limited empirical support. Multivariate studies consistently fail to generate DSM diagnostic categories whether the personality disorder is described using diagnostic criteria (Austin & Deary, 2000; Ekselius, Lindstrom, von Knorring, Bodlund, & Kullgren, 1994; Kass et al., 1985), personality disorder traits (Clark, 1990; Livesley, Jackson, & Schroeder, 1989, 1992), or behaviors prototypical of personality diagnoses (Livesley & Jackson, 1986). These findings cannot be attributed to the assessment methods used because they are consistent across studies using different methods of measurement including structured interview, personality questionnaires, and behavioral self-ratings.

Psychometric Limitations

Current classifications have poor psychometric properties (Blais & Norman, 1997). Although diagnostic reliability improved considerably with DSM-III due to the development of diagnostic criteria and fixed rules for applying them, demonstrations of improved reliability rely largely on structured interviews. Few studies have investigated the reliability of clinical assessment. Even when structured interviews are used diagnostic agreement remains a problem (Zimmerman, 1994) and agreement across different interviews is modest (O'Boyle & Self, 1990).

The validity of most diagnoses has not yet been established. Of the various forms of validity that are applied to psychiatric diagnoses, construct validity is the one the most pertinent to personality disorder (Livesley & Jackson, 1991, 1992). When applied to psychiatric diagnoses, construct validity can be divided into internal and external components (Skinner, 1981). Internal validity refers to the extent to which diagnostic criteria form homogeneous clusters. External validity refers to the extent to which diagnostic concepts are distinct from each other and the degree to which they predict important external criteria such as etiology and prognosis. The evidence suggests that internal validity is limited. Internal validity begins with content validity. As Blashfield (1989) pointed out, a satisfactory classification should capture diagnostic concepts that clinicians consider important. However, this does not seem to have been achieved with recent editions of DSM. Clinicians have difficulty matching criteria to disorders (Blashfield & Breen, 1989; Blashfield & Haymaker, 1990), and criteria sets do not always include features that clinicians consider prototypical of the diagnosis (Livesley, Reiffer, Sheldon, & West, 1987). Moreover, there is little evidence to suggest that criteria were systematically selected to sample all aspects of each diagnosis.

There are also problems with other aspects of internal validity. Although many studies were based on earlier versions of DSM there is no reason to believe that they do not apply to DSM-IV, which was developed in a similar way to its predecessors. Criteria sets show limited internal consistency and some criteria correlate higher with other diagnoses than with the one for which they were proposed (Blais & Norman, 1997; Morey, 1988). As Blais and Norman (1997) noted, of the 21 DSM-III-R criteria that were more strongly correlated with other diagnoses than the one for which the were proposed, 9 were retained in the DSM-IV. Retention of such items means that diagnostic overlap is inevitable. Internal consistency improved with DSM-IV although coefficient alpha falls below the usual criterion level of .7 recommended by Nunnally and Bornstein (1994) for histrionic, dependent, and schizotypal personality disorders (Blais & Norman, 1997).

Problems with external validity are even greater. External validity has two components: convergent and discriminant validity and external validity. Convergent–discriminant analyses are critical tests of a classification. Convergent validity requires that different measures of the same diagnosis lead to the same diagnosis; that is, different measures should converge with each other. Discriminant validity is based on evidence that diagnoses are distinct from each other and that this distinction holds across different measures. Evidence of convergence is variable—different measures of the same diagnosis show modest levels of agreement (O'Boyle & Self, 1990). Discriminant validity is an even greater problem. As studies of diagnostic overlap show, multiple diagnoses are the norm (Oldham et al., 1992; Pilkonis et al., 1995; Widiger et al., 1991). This suggests that DSM contains too many diagnoses (Rutter, 1987; Tyrer, 1988). The poor discriminant properties of the system also arise from the use of criteria that correlate strongly with diagnoses other than the one for which they are proposed leading to considerable covariation among diagnoses. For diagnoses such as narcissistic and histrionic personality disorders and avoidant and dependent personality disorders criterion discrimination is so poor that it is difficult to differentiate between them (Blais & Norman, 1997). At a more fundamental level, overlap probably arises from the failure to define diagnoses that are conceptually distinct. In terms of external validity, there is limited evidence that diagnoses predict important external variables related to etiology and outcome.

Exclusiveness and Exhaustiveness

A basic requirement of any classification is that it contains categories that are mutually exclusive—categories do not overlap—and exhaustive—all cases can be classified (Simpson, 1961). As the previous discussion indicated, there are problems in both areas. Substantial evidence of the lack of exclusiveness is provided by studies of diagnostic overlap mentioned previously. Overlap is often misleadingly referred to as comorbidity. However, comorbidity refers to the co-occurrence of distinct diagnoses and there is no evidence that personality disorder diagnoses are distinct in this sense. When applied to personality disorder, the term "comorbidity" simply obscures a fundamental flaw in the system. For some diagnoses, such as paranoid personality disorder, overlap with other personality diagnoses occurs in almost all cases, and even with the most distinctive category, obsessive–compulsive personality disorder, overlap occurs in approximately 70% of cases (Widiger et al., 1991). The usual response to this problem is to change criteria to improve the discriminant properties of the classification. The problem, however, is more fundamental and unlikely to be solved by minor changes to criteria or even by adding or subtracting diagnoses.

Exhaustiveness is also a problem. DSM-IV achieves exhaustiveness through the use of the "wastebasket" category "personality disorder not otherwise specified." Such categories are justified when used infrequently, but this is not the case with Axis II. The prevalence of this diagnosis indicates that the system does not have diagnostic constructs to cover many of the conditions that clinicians think lie within the scope of the classification. Further evidence of inadequate coverage is provided by Weston and Arkowitz-Westen (1998), who found that approximately 60% of patients receiving treatment for personality pathology defined as enduring maladaptive patterns of thought, feeling, motivation, and behavior that lead to dysfunction or distress could not be diagnosed on Axis II. It is possible that these were cases of limited personality disturbance rather than personality disorder; nevertheless, this study raises serious doubts about the clinical relevance of Axis II.

Clinical Utility

Most diagnoses have limited clinical utility. They often fail to help the clinician to predict outcome and to plan treatment. As Sanderson and Clarkin (1994) noted, categorical diagnoses are often too heterogeneous and global for treatment planning. Psychosocial and pharmacological interventions are usually organized around specific features or clusters of related features rather than diagnostic categories. Moreover, most diagnoses consist of several traits (Shea, 1995) that may differ in terms of etiology and response to treatment. Hence more specific information about salient personality features is required in clinical practice than is provided by global diagnoses. As a result, clinicians and investigators are beginning to use alternative diagnostic concepts. For example, investigators exploring the biological correlates and pharmacological treatments focus on dimensions such as affective instability, impulsivity, cognitive disorganization, and anxiousness (Siever & Davis, 1991; Soloff, 1998, 2000).

The Categorical Approach

Many of the problems noted with current classifications arise primarily from an attempt to impose categories upon behavior that is continuously distributed. The categorical model requires discontinuities, or at least points of rarity (Kendell, 1975, 1986), in the distribution of clinical features. Such discontinuities have been difficult to demonstrate for most forms of mental disorder. The problem is even more apparent with personality disorder. Problems such as overlap, high usage of the personality disorder not otherwise specified diagnosis, low reliability, and limited evidence of validity can be attributed to failure to adopt a dimensional model.

The evidence suggests that whenever the category versus dimension distinction has been subjected to empirical evaluation, the results almost invariably support a dimensional representation of personality pathology (Clark, Livesley, & Morey, 1997; Livesley et al., 1994; Widiger, 1993). Yet the debate about which model should be used continues and it is likely to be a major issue when DSM-V is developed. Resolution is difficult because DSM is not clear about the nature of the categorical distinctions that are proposed. At least four models are possible (Livesley et al., 1994). First, the distributions of phenotypical features are discontinuous or show points of rarity. The evidence suggests, however, that the features of personality disorder whether described using diagnostic criteria or traits in patient or nonpatient samples are continuous, and that it is not possible to identify a discontinuity in the distributions of the kind that would support categorical diagnoses (Frances, Clarkin, Gilmore, Hurt, & Brown, 1984; Kass et al., 1985; Livesley et al., 1992; Nestadt et al., 1990; Widiger, Sanderson, & Warner, 1986; Zimmerman & Coryell, 1990). Second, a categorical distinction between personality disorder and normality could be supported if there was evidence that disability only occurred when a given threshold was reached in terms of the number of features present. Nestadt et al. (1990) showed that risk of anxiety and alcohol use disorders increased when the number of criteria of obsessive–compulsive and antisocial personality disorders increased. Similarly, Nakao et al. (1992) reported that impairment assessed using the Global Assessment of Functioning Scale associated with personality disorder was continuously distributed.

A third model states that although the traits delineating personality disorder may be continuously distributed, the structural relationships among these traits differ in personality-disordered and nonpersonality-disordered subjects. Eysenck (1987) noted that this was a critical test of the category model. Several studies have shown that the factorial structure of traits is the same across samples differing in the presence of personality disorder (Livesley et al., 1992; Livesley, Jang, & Vernon, 1998; Tyrer & Alexander, 1979). Evidence of continuity between normal and disordered personality traits is not dependent on the statistical method used. Pukrop, Herpertz, Sass, and Steinmeyer (1998) reported similar finding using facet theoretical analysis.

Finally, the latent structures underlying continuous phenotypical characteristics may be discontinuous. In other words, a discrete taxon may underlie phenotypical continuity. The evidence related to this model is less consistent. Trull, Widiger, and Guthrie (1990) assessed the occurrence of a discrete taxon underlying borderline personality disorder criteria using the maximum covariance analysis method proposed by Meehl (1992; Meehl & Golden, 1982). Their results did not support the existence of a taxon. However, Harris, Rice, and Quinsey (1994) reported a possible taxon underlying extreme scores on a measure of psychopathy. Similar results have not been reported for other traits and the current evidence suggests that most personality disorder traits are continuously distributed.

Overall the evidence provides overwhelming support for a dimensional model of personality disorder traits. For these reasons, and because of the other difficulties noted with current categorical classifications, the argument is frequently made that an evidence-based approach to personality disorder must incorporate a dimensional scheme to represent individual differences.

CLASSIFICATION: DIMENSIONAL MODELS

There is little doubt that the adoption of a dimensional model would solve many of the problems noted with DSM-IV. Nevertheless, such proposals do not gain ready acceptance. Objections are usually based on the assumption that categorical diagnoses are easier to use, more in keeping with medical diagnoses, and easier to translate into clinical decisions. There is little convincing evidence to support these assumptions. Physicians do not apparently have difficulty managing dimensional information about physical disorders whether in the form of laboratory reports or clinical observations such as blood pressure, nor do they have difficulty translating this information into treatment decisions. Usually they rely on a cutting score that has been shown to be clinically significant. It is difficult to understand why mental health professionals should be less adept at managing dimensional information about personality disorder. A dimensional system with empirically derived cutting points would in many ways be simpler to use than classifications that force patients into categories that poorly resemble their personalities.

Research Strategies

Investigations of the dimensions underlying personality disorder diagnoses typically use one of four strategies. One approach is to identify the dimensions underlying diagnostic categories by examining the covariation among diagnoses using either factor analysis (Hyler & Lyons, 1988; Kass et al., 1985) or multidimensional scaling (Blashfield, Sprock, Pinkson, & Hodgkin, 1985; Widiger, Trull, Hurt, Clarkin, & Frances, 1987). These studies were usually designed to test the DSM proposal that diagnoses fall into three separate clusters. The results suggest that a few higher-order dimensions underlie personality disorder diagnoses:

typically two to four dimensions are identified. Unfortunately, these results do not help to identify a dimensions model of personality disorder because differences in instruments and procedures lead to different dimensions being identified. It is also difficult to label these dimensions. Personality diagnoses are multidimensional (Shea, 1995) and hence it is unclear which features account for the observed covariation.

A second approach is to relate personality disorder diagnoses to a taxonomy of normal personality traits such as those developed by Eysenck (1987) or the five-factor approach (Costa & Widiger, 1994). A third approach is to explore the dimensional structure underlying the terms clinicians use to describe personality disorders. This traditional way of investigating the structure of normal personality traits has been used less frequently to investigate the structure of personality disorder traits. Independently of each other, Livesley (Livesley et al., 1989, 1992), Clark (1990), and Harkness (1992) investigated the lower-order traits delineating personality disorders. Although these investigators used different starting points and different procedures, the resulting structures showed substantial similarity (Clark & Livesley, 1994; Clark, Livesley, Schroeder, & Irish, 1996; Harkness, 1992). The fourth approach is to develop a theoretical model of personality that is then evaluated empirically. This is the approach that Cloninger (1987; Cloninger et al., 1993) used to identify temperament traits based on hypothesized relationships with neurotransmitter systems (Cloninger, 2000).

Models Based on Normal Personality Structure

Although a wide range of models of normal personality are available that could conceivably be used to classify individual differences in personality disorder, attention has concentrated on the two-dimensional structure of the interpersonal circumplex and three- and five-factor descriptions of trait structure. Trait models in particular have received attention because of DSM's emphasis on traits in the definition of personality disorder.

Interpersonal Circumplex

Circumplex models of interpersonal behavior derived from the interpersonal approach of Harry Stack Sullivan were first developed by Leary and colleagues (Freedman, Leary, Ossorio, & Coffey, 1951; Leary, 1957). They suggested that two orthogonal dimensions dominance–submission and hostility–affection (also labeled communion, love–hate, and hostile–friendly in different versions) underlie interpersonal behavior. When interpersonal behaviors are plotted on these axes the result is an interpersonal circle (see Chapter 20, this volume). Leary suggested that the quadrants of the circumplex represent the four humors or temperaments of ancient Greek medicine. More detailed division of the circumplex into octants define classes of interpersonal actions that represent various combinations of the two components. Dependent, for example, involves equal contributions from submission and affection. Within the circumplex, distance from the center is a measure of severity or intensity.

In Kiesler's (1982) version of the circumplex, the two axes are labeled dominant–submission and hostile–friendly and the circle is divided into 16 segments. Each segment is divided into three levels. The inner circle designates the range of interpersonal behavior using 16 labels such as dominant, exhibitionistic, friendly, trusting, and submissive. The next circle represents the mild–moderate or more normal level of the segment. At this level the labels are changed—dominant becomes controlling, exhibitionistic becomes spontaneously demonstrative, friendly becomes helpfully cooperative, trusting becomes trusting and forgiving, and submissive becomes docile. In interpersonal theory, abnormal behavior is "defined as inappropriate or inadequate interpersonal communication. It consists of a rigid, constricted and extreme pattern of interpersonal behaviors by which the abnormal person, without any clear awareness, engages others who are important in his or her life" (Kiesler, 1986, p. 572). This is represented by the outer level. At this level, the labels change to dictatorial, histrionic, indulgent and devoted, merciful and gullible, and subservient, respectively. With this arrangement behaviors may involve blends of related or adjacent segments. It is also possible for the individual to show behaviors from opposing segments to create patterns that are conflicted.

The interpersonal circumplex has been proposed as an alternative way to represent the psychopathology including Axis II (Benjamin, 1993, 1996, see also Chapter 20, in this volume; Carson, 1982; Kiesler, 1986; McLemore & Brokaw, 1987; Pincus & Wiggins, 1990). With this approach , extreme, rigid, or conflicted patterns of interpersonal behavior are represented using circumplex constructs. The evidence shows that many personality disorder diagnoses form an approximately circumplex arrangement when plotted along two axes (Pincus & Wiggins, 1990; Plutchick & Platman, 1977; Romney & Brynner, 1989, Wiggins & Pincus, 1989). DSM-III diagnoses of avoidant, schizoid, dependent, narcissistic, histrionic, and antisocial personality disorders appear to be strongly related to the circumplex (Wiggins & Pincus, 1989), and in a subsequent study, paranoid personality disorder could also be accommodated within the structure (Pincus & Wiggins, 1990). However, the circumplex does not capture all personality disorders. A consistent finding across studies is that borderline, compulsive, and passive–aggressive diagnoses did not fit the structure. Given the clinical importance of these disorders, this is a major limitation of the model. It is interesting to note that when additional axes were added to the two dimensions of the circumplex to represent other dimensions of the five-factor approach a better fit was found for most diagnoses (Wiggins & Pincus, 1989).

The value of circumplex models is that they provide a coherent approach to classification that integrates research and theory. The major dimensions that form the basis for description and classification were not selected in an arbitrary way, nor are they the simple products of empirical enquiry. Instead, they represent an ordering of interpersonal behavior that derives from an underlying theoretical structure that has empirical support. The limitation of the approach is that it is a model of interpersonal behavior not personality psychopathology. Although interpersonal behavior is an important element to personality disorder it is not the total picture. Other features are also important, including cognitive styles, dysfunctional cognitive processes, and traits that are only indirectly related to interpersonal behavior. Also, another problem is that in the final analysis, the circumplex remains a two-dimensional model albeit a sophisticated one. The approach does, however, have a feature that personality disorder classification should emulate, namely, the strong theoretical component that defines the relationship between normality and pathology and provides a coherent set of descriptive patterns.

The Three-Factor Approach

One of the oldest factor models proposed as an alternative to Axis II is Eysenck's (1987) three-factor model. Like most trait theories, the model suggests that personality is a hierarchical structure in which a large number of specific traits are organized into three higher-order factors, extraversion (E), neuroticism (N), and psychoticism (P). The specific traits defining each factor (Eysenck & Eysenck, 1985) are as follows:

Extraversion: sociable, lively, active, assertive, sensation-seeking, carefree, dominant, surgent, venturesome
Neuroticism: anxious, depressed, guilt feelings, low self-esteem, tense, irrational, shy, moody, emotional
Psychoticism: aggressive, cold, egocentric, impersonal, impulsive, antisocial, unempathic, creative, and tough-minded.

The theory proposes that these dimensions have a genetic basis and speculates on the biological basis of each dimension. For example, autonomic reactivity is said to be related to neuroticism, and conditionability is hypothesized to be related to extraversion.

A long-standing proponent of a dimensional approach to the classification of psychiatric disorders, Eysenck (1987) maintained that unless a dimensional model is adopted "personality disorder might forever remain elusive" (p. 213). He hypothesized that "personality disorders of various kinds will be located in the octant of a three dimensional space defined by P, E, and N where high scores on all three personality dimensions are combined; that is, the space characterized by high P, high E, and high N" (p. 215). The model proposes that differences in behavior arise from a predominance of one of these dimensions over the others and the interaction among them.

The model is appealing for its parsimony and evidential support. The dimensions proposed have considerable generality, being identified repeatedly in factor-analytic studies. As will be seen later, statistical analyses of personality disorder traits also yield factors that resemble these factors, although they also identify additional components. The specific features of Eysenck's proposal are more problematic. The idea that all personality disorders are located in the space defined by high P, high E, and high N is not consistent with current clinical concepts. Key disorders such as schizoid, paranoid, and avoidant could not be located in this space. Nevertheless, the three dimensions describe important patterns of behavior that are likely to be important components of a satisfactory dimensional scheme.

The Five-Factor Approach

One of the interesting developments in recent personality research has been the emergence of the five-factor structure as the dominant account of the trait structure of personality (Digman, 1990, 1996). The structure arose from two different traditions, a lexical analysis of the natural language of personality (Goldberg, 1990) and psychometric analyses of personality measures that span nearly half a century. The currently popular version of the approach is Costa and McCrae's (1992) five-factor model of neuroticism, extraversion, openness to experience, agreeableness, and conscientiousness. According to this approach each domain is subdivided into six facets traits as follows:

Neuroticism: anxiety, hostility, depression, self-consciousness, impulsivity, vulnerability

Extraversion: warmth, gregariousness, assertiveness, activity, excitement seeking, positive emotions

Openness to experience: fantasy, aesthetics, feelings, actions, ideas, values

Agreeableness: trust, straightforwardness, altruism, compliance, modesty, tendermindedness

Conscientiousness: competence, order, dutifulness, achievement striving, self-discipline, deliberation

This five-factor model has been distinguished from the Big Five structure derived from lexical analyses (John & Robbins, 1993). The Big Five structure is considered a descriptive account of personality attributes, whereas the Costa and McCrae model claims to provide a theoretical explanation of behavior based on dispositions that are assumed to have a biological origin (Saucier & Goldberg, 1996). Both structures are remarkably stable across languages and cultures. There are, however, differences in the labels applied to the five domains. Agreement exists regarding extraversion, agreeableness, and conscientiousness and emotional stability or neuroticism. However, there

is disagreement on the interpretation of the remaining factor. Costa and McCrae refer to it as openness to experience whereas the lexical model conceptualizes it as intellect or imagination (Digman, 1990). This difference is important when evaluating the five-factor approach for clinical purposes because multivariate analyses of personality disorder traits fail to identify a factor corresponding to openness.

Saucier and Goldberg (1996) also pointed out that although the five domains are often presented as if they were equally replicable and important, this is not the case. They maintain that extraversion, agreeableness, and conscientiousness are more readily replicated than emotional stability or neuroticism and intellect (imagination) or openness. The latter being the least replicable. For this reason they consider assumptions that the domains are equally important, and that each domain has the same number of facets, to be questionable. If the domains differ in relative importance it is to be expected that they would also differ in number of facets. This is the case with factor analyses of personality disorder traits in which the first higher-order factor that resembles neuroticism is defined by many more specific traits than the remaining factors of dissocial behavior (equivalent to negative agreeableness), inhibitedness (introversion), and compulsivity (conscientiousness) (Livesley et al., 1998). One might also add that it is unusual for biological systems to be organized in such a consistent and symmetrical manner as each trait having an identical facet structure.

Models Based on Studies of Personality Disorder

Fewer attempts have been made to reduce the many descriptive terms used to describe personality disorder to fewer dimensions using multivariate statistical techniques than is the case with normal personality. One of the earliest investigations was by Walton and colleagues (Presly & Walton, 1973; Walton, Foulds, Littman, & Presly, 1970; Walton & Presly, 1973). In these studies, patients were rated on 45 personality descriptors. Multivariate analyses identified five factors: sociopathy, submissiveness, hysterical, obsessional, and schizoid (Walton, 1986).

Subsequently, Tyrer and Alexander (1979) extracted four factors from an analysis of 24 descriptive features assessed by structured interview. The factors, labeled sociopathic, passive–dependent, inhibited, and anankastic, show substantial resemblance to those described by Walton and colleagues. An interesting finding was that the factor structure was similar in patients with and without personality disorder. As Eysenck (1987) pointed out, this is strong evidence for a dimensional structure. Subsequent studies using larger samples and more systematic selection of descriptive features have largely replicated the factors identified by Walton and Tyrer. Two sets of investigations will be described that use different approaches and measurement instruments—the Dimensional Assessment of Personality Pathology (DAPP; Livesley & Jackson, in press) and the Structured Assessment of Normal and Abnormal Personality (SNAP; Clark, 1993).

Dimensional Assessment of Personality Pathology

Studies leading to the development of the DAPP structure of personality disorder traits began with an extensive content analysis of the clinical literature, including official classifications, to identify a large pool of terms describing personality disorder. These were grouped into the diagnoses listed in DSM-III. Systematic samples of clinical judges rated each item for prototypicality for their respective DSM diagnosis (Livesley, 1986) . These rating were used to organize descriptive items into 100 trait categories (Livesley, 1987). The approach could be considered to result in prototypical descriptions of DSM diagnoses. Self-report scales were constructed to assess each trait using the structured methods described by Jackson (1971). The factorial structure underlying the 100 traits was then evaluated by administering these scales to samples of general population subjects and patients with personality disorder (Livesley et al., 1989, 1992). Fifteen factors were identified and the structure was stable across clinical and nonclinical samples.

Although these studies were originally planned as an attempt to validate DSM diagnoses, the factors identified showed limited resemblance to DSM diagnostic concepts. The results were used to develop a self-report instrument, the Dimensional Assessment of Personality Pathology—Basic Questionnaire (DAPP-BQ), to assess 18 traits that provide a systematic representation of the domain of personality disorder. Eighteen scales were devel-

oped from the 15 factors because some factors were divided into several scales based on further psychometric studies. The 18 scales are Anxiousness, Affective Lability, Callousness, Cognitive Dysregulation, Compulsivity, Conduct Problems, Identity Problems, Insecure Attachment, Intimacy Avoidance, Narcissism, Oppositionality, Rejection, Restricted Expression, Self-Harm, Social Avoidance, Stimulus Seeking, Submissiveness, and Suspiciousness. Four higher-order factors underlie the 18 traits: emotional dysregulation, dissocial behavior, inhibitedness, and compulsivity (Livesley et al., 1998). Again this structure was stable across clinical and nonclinical samples. These factors show some resemblance to borderline, antisocial, schizoid–avoidant, and obsessive–compulsive personality disorders. The association between lower-order or basic traits and higher-order factors is as follows:

Emotional dysregulation: anxiousness, affective lability, submissiveness, identity problems, social avoidance, insecure attachment, cognitive dysregulation,

Dissocial behavior: callousness, rejection (angry-hostility), conduct problems, stimulus seeking, suspiciousness, narcissism.

Inhibitedness: intimacy problems, restricted expression of affects, insecure attachment (negative)

Compulsivity: compulsivity, oppositionality (negative)

The analyses on which this structure is based suggest that the different higher-order domains are not equally important and differ in breadth as Goldberg and Saucier suggested in their critique of the five-factor model. Behavior–genetic analyses indicated that all scales are heritable (Jang, Livesley, Vernon, & Jackson, 1996; Livesley, Jang, Jackson, & Vernon, 1993) and that four genetic factors underlie the 18 scales that closely resemble the higher-order phenotypical dimensions (Livesley et al., 1998). Thus, the phenotypical structure of personality disorder closely resembles the underlying genetic architecture.

Structured Assessment of Normal and Abnormal Personality

The initial set of descriptive features used to develop the SNAP was compiled primarily from DSM-III diagnostic criteria for personality and related disorders. A conceptual sorting task was used to identify 22 symptom clusters (Clark, 1990). Self-report scales were developed to assess each cluster and an iterative series of analyses resulted in 15 scales: Negative Temperament, Mistrust, Self-Harm, Eccentric Perceptions, Aggression, Manipulativeness, Entitlement, Exhibitionism, Positive Temperament, Detachment, Dependency, Disinhibition, Impulsivity, Workaholism, and Propriety.

Although the initial item set and procedures used by Clark differed from those used by Livesley and colleagues, conceptual comparisons of the two instruments indicated considerable similarity (Clark & Livesley, 1994). There are no scales without a counterpart in the other instrument. Differences in the number of scales in the two instruments are due to some constructs being divided into several scales. For example, the SNAP Dependency scale is represented in the DAPP Submissiveness and Insecure Attachment scales. Direct empirical comparison of the trait scales also indicated considerable convergence in the content and structure of the two systems (Clark et al., 1996). Of the 24 predicted convergent correlations, 22 were above .40, and the average convergent correlation was .53. The average discriminant correlation was .22. This degree of convergence is encouraging given differences in instrument development. It is also encouraging considering the problems noted with the convergent and discriminant properties of DSM. Similar convergence was observed between the higher-order structures for the two instruments. These factors also resemble the neuroticism, extraversion, agreeableness, and conscientiousness domains of the five-factor approach. Given this convergence, these results provide a starting point for developing a dimensional representation of personality disorder.

Application of Dimensional Models to Classification

Although the evidence supports a dimensional representation of personality disorder, it is important to consider the extent to which trait models provide a convenient and parsimonious account of the range of pathology that clinicians traditionally consider personality disorder. There are two issues: whether normative models can accommodate the full spectrum of personality diagnoses and whether they can ac-

count for all aspects of personality pathology including those features that are used to define personality disorder (Livesley, in press).

Both the three-factor (Eysenck, 1987) and the five-factor approaches (Costa & Widiger, 1994; Widiger, 2000) have been proposed as alternatives to classify personality disorder. Analyses of the relationship between normal trait theories and personality disorder have largely involved the five-factor approach as assessed using the NEO Personality Inventory—Revised (NEO-PI-R; Costa & McRae, 1992). Conceptual analysis suggests that the DSM personality disorder diagnoses can be adequately translated into the five-factor framework (Widiger, Trull, Clarkin, Sanderson, & Costa, 1994). For example, Widiger and colleagues suggested that borderline personality disorder could be represented by high scores on all the facets of neuroticism; the gregariousness, assertiveness; positive emotions facets of extraversion, and low scores on the agreeableness facets of straightforwardness and compliance; and the achievement striving scale of conscientiousness.

Empirical studies largely confirm conceptual analyses. Multiple studies provide convincing evidence that the DSM personality disorder diagnoses show a systematic relationship to the five factors and that all categorical diagnoses of DSM can be accommodated within the five-factor framework (Ball, Tennen, Poling, Krazler, & Rounsaville, 1997; Blais, 1997; Dyce & Connor, 1998; McCrae et al., in press; Reynolds & Clark, in press; Trull, Widiger, & Burr, in press). This differs from studies of the interpersonal circumplex that found that the model was not able to accommodate all disorders.

There is also evidence that the five-factor model may also be useful in clarifying the structure of some diagnoses. For example, Miller, Lynam, Widiger, and Leukfield (in press), showed that an analysis of psychopathy within the NEO-PI-R structure clarified the two-factor structure of psychopathy underlying the Psychopathy Checklist—Revised (Hare, 1991). The first factor is usually assumed to represent the interpersonal and affective component that is considered to be central to the construct and the second factor is assumed to represent a deviant lifestyle. When examined from the perspective of the five-factor model, the first factor is associated with low agreeableness and low neuroticism while the second factor involves a mixture of low agreeableness and conscientiousness, and high neuroticism.

Other studies have examined the structure underlying DSM personality disorders by factor-analyzing measures of personality disorder in association with normal personality scales. Studies using measures of Eysenck's personality dimensions tend to yield a three-factor structure consisting of a general distress factor associated with neuroticism, a factor associated with psychoticism and antisocial personality disorder, and a factor representing social avoidance characterized by a negative loading on extraversion (O'Boyle, 1995; O'Boyle & Holzer, 1992). Other studies report a four-factor structure consisting of the above factors and a compulsivity or conscientiousness factor (Austin & Deary, 2000; Deary, Peter, Austin, & Gibson, 1998; Livesley et al., 1998; Schroeder, Wormworth, & Livesley, 1992). Mulder and Joyce (1997) suggested that the four factors be labeled the four A's: asthenic, antisocial, asocial, and anankastic. Austin and Deary (2000) showed that an item-level analysis of DSM-IV criteria assessed with the SCID questionnaire produced three- and eight-factor solutions. The three-factor solution resembled Eysenck's dimensions. Higher-order analysis of the eight-factor solution yielded four factors consistent with the four A's. These studies provide strong evidence that four broad factors underlie the DSM-IV domain of personality disorder and that these factors are consistent with the major dimensions of normal personality.

The existence of systematic relationships between trait structures and personality disorder does not mean, however, that normal trait taxonomies are the best alternative to DSM-IV categorical diagnoses. Reynolds and Clark (in press) found that the lower-order facets of the NEO-PI-R led to enhanced prediction over the broader domain scores and that the SNAP first-order scales provided additional information beyond that conveyed by the NEO-PI-R. This finding has important implications for classification and clinical use of trait scales. It suggests that domain scores may not be sufficient for clinical purposes. The SNAP scales appear to have an advantage over the NEO-PI-R and the NEO-PI-R facet scales may not capture some clinically important behaviors. Further evidence of this point is provided by Schroeder et al. (1992), who reported that not all the content of the DAPP is adequately represented by the NEO-PI-R. Traits such as cognitive dysreg-

ulation and insecure attachment that are important features of many clinical presentations are poorly represented by the NEO-PI-R. It appears that scales designed specifically to assess personality disorder traits may offer some predictive advantage over those derived from studies of normal personality. This finding is not surprising because these scales were derived empirically from clinical concepts unlike the facet scales of the NEO-PI-R which were based largely on rational analyses.

Studies of the relationship between normal and disordered personality traits point to the following conclusions. First, the findings suggest caution in assuming that the five-factor approach can be directly translated into a diagnostic alternative to DSM (Livesley, in press). Second, the higher-order dimensions such as neuroticism (or the clinical equivalent of emotional dysregulation or asthenia), negative agreeableness (dissocial behavior or antisocial), introversion (inhibitedness or asocial), and conscientiousness (compulsivity or anankastic) appear to represent fundamental aspects of behavioral organization that should be part of an empirically based classification. These dimensions are useful for a range of clinical purposes including the broader aspects of treatment planning. For example, patients with high conscientiousness scores appear to respond better to structured interventions (Miller, 1991). However, for many purposes, especially the selection of specific interventions, these descriptions need to be augmented with detailed information about specific traits. Third, at this lower level further work is required to identify a facet structure that meets the needs of clinical practice. Studies are required that explore these domains using traits and behaviors based on both normal personality concepts and clinically relevant traits.

Although trait models potentially provide a more coherent representation of individual differences in personality disorder than categorical diagnoses, it is not clear that they can accommodate all aspects of personality disorder (Pincus & Wilson, in press). As noted earlier, personality disorder involves more than maladaptive traits (Livesley & Jang, 2000). To conceptualize it in these terms risks reducing the term to an idealized conception of normality and trivializing the disorder by creating a conception that would apply to a sizable proportion of the population. McAdams (1994) described three levels to personality: dispositional traits;

personal concerns which include motives, roles goals, and coping strategies; and the life narrative which provides an integrated account of past, present, and future. This framework draws attention to the integrating and organizing aspects of personality discussed earlier. Although trait theory has tended to neglect the coherence and organization of personality, it is important aspect of personality study (Cervone & Shoda, 1999). For this reason, trait descriptions are only one component of a classification. The other consists of the criteria for personality disorder discussed earlier.

FUTURE DIRECTIONS IN CLASSIFICATION

Dissatisfaction with the current classification of personality disorder for assessment and treatment planning and as a way to represent personality pathology for research purposes seems to be increasing. Although the problem of whether personality disorder should be classified using a dimensional or categorical model has received the most attention it is only one of the problems that future classifications must address. There is also the question whether personality disorders should be classified on a separate axis. This raises questions about its relationship to other mental disorders. Given the overwhelming clinical and research evidence that personality disorders merge with each other and with normal personality and hence individual variation in personality disorder is best represented by a dimensional system, this section begins to consider future directions by examining the reasons underlying the resistance to implementing such an approach. It then considers whether personality disorder should continue to be placed on a separate axis and finally considers the requirements for an empirically based classification.

On the Persistence of Categorical Models

An understanding of the factors responsible for the continued support for categorical approach despite the evidence may help to construct a classification that is both consistent with the evidence and generally acceptable. Five factors seem to be involved. First, there is a general reluctance to use an approach that seems to differ so markedly from the general diagnostic approach of medicine which relies largely on categorical diagnoses. Second, the categorical model has become an enshrined component of the neo-Kraepelian approach to psychiatry that forms the major conceptual foundation of DSM-III and subsequent editions. As Klerman (1978) noted, the neo-Kraepelian framework postulates that psychiatry is a branch of medicine, that a boundary exists between the normal and the sick, and that there are discrete mental illnesses. There seems to be a reluctance to question these assumptions and the extent to which they apply across the range of behaviors included in classifications of psychopathology. The categorical approach has to some extent become equated with the medical model and part of the assumptions of psychiatry as a discipline leading to considerable resistance to adopt of alternative structures.

Third, the approach is consistent with the way humans process information. The ubiquity of categorical concepts in classifications dealing with the natural world suggest that cognitive mechanisms evolved to handle such information in an economical manner (Atran, 1990; Blashfield & Livesley, 1999). This suggests that the ready acceptance of categories of personality disorder, and the tenacity with which they are retained, arises in part from the fact that they are consistent with cognitive heuristics that developed to process information about the natural world.

Fourth, it is often argued that the current approach is retained because there is little agreement on a dimensional alternative. The proponents of a categorical framework point to the lack of agreement on the nature and number of dimensions required to account for individual differences proposals ranging from the three dimensions favored by Eysenck through the five dimensions of the five-factor approach to the seven dimensions advocated by Cloninger (2000). There is some merit to this argument. However, as noted earlier, differences in the number of dimensions proposed obscures considerable agreement regarding some of the more important dimensions.

Finally, trait models are sometimes rejected because they are thought to be insufficient to represent the complexity and diversity of personality and because of assumed limitations of the factor analytic methods on which they are based. These models invariably result in between three and seven dimensions (Block, 1995). This parsimony is an advantageous feature of factor analysis but it raises the possibility that the structures identified are mere artifacts of the methodology. Although the number of factors may be explicable in terms of the parsimonious qualities of factor analysis, there are no compelling methodological reasons why the same factors, rather than the same number of factors, are identified. Indeed, the robustness of a few general factors such as neuroticism (emotional dysregulation), extraversion (inhibitedness), and psychoticism or negative agreeableness (dissocial behavior or psychopathy) suggests that they represent fundamental units of behavioral organization.

Common versus Separate Axes

The decision to place personality disorders on a separate axis in DSM-III was an innovation that appears to reflect pragmatic rather than theoretical or empirical considerations. Other multiaxial classifications had been proposed earlier (Ottosson & Perris, 1973; Rutter, Shaffer, & Shephard, 1975; Straus, 1975) but none suggested that mental disorders should be spread across several axes. The reason for this innovation was to draw clinicians' attention to personality disorder. In this sense, the change has been remarkably successful. This success has, however, incurred costs. The distinction is rather like that made in biological classification between vertebrates and invertebrates—it implies that personality disorder is fundamentally different from other mental disorders. This has encouraged a pejorative attitude toward those with personality disorder and created problems with access to care, at least in some jurisdictions. Given these problems and the pragmatic reasons for the decision, it is reasonable to reconsider the value of such a fundamental distinction among mental disorders. When considering this issue it is important to bear in mind that the issue is not whether personality disorder differs from other mental disorders but whether it is so fundamentally different from all other mental disorders that it warrants a special place in the classification.

Perhaps the clearest discussion of the relationship between personality disorder and other mental disorders or clinical syndromes is found in the work of Foulds (1965, 1976) who examined five possible forms of relationship:

1. Clinical syndromes and personality disorders are mutually exclusive so that the two cannot co-occur. This model is inconsistent with the evidence of considerable comorbidity (see Chapters 4 and 26, this volume).

2. All individuals with a clinical syndrome have a personality disorder but not all individuals with a personality disorder have a clinical syndrome. This model suggests that personality disorder is a prerequisite for a clinical syndrome. Again this does not fit the evidence.

3. The opposite model, that all individuals with a personality disorder have a clinical syndrome, is also inconsistent with the evidence.

4. The relationship between personality disorder and clinical syndromes is one of identity or degree. This is the *forme fruste* model advanced originally by Kraepelin that was noted earlier to apply only to limited forms of personality disorder.

5. Clinical syndromes and personality disorder are distinct entities that can co-occur. With the exception of spectrum disorders, this is the only model that fits current evidence. This forces us to consider the grounds for suggesting that personality disorder is sufficient different from all other forms of mental disorder to justify a major cleavage in two groups of disorder. Three possible grounds for making this assertion are phenomenology, etiology, and clinical course. None stand the test of empirical or conceptual analysis (Livesley et al., 1994).

Phenomenology

The idea that personality disorders are phenomenologically distinct from other mental disorders was expressed most clearly by Foulds (1965, 1976). He suggested that whereas other disorders are diagnosed by symptoms and signs, personality disorders are diagnosed by traits and attitudes. The significance of this distinction rests on the idea that the onset of symptoms and signs represents a discontinuity in development in that they occur suddenly, at least in developmental terms, and wax and wane over time. Traits and attitudes on the other hand are said to be relatively enduring and have their origin early in development. The distinction is similar to that made by Jaspers between disease processes and personality developments.

Although the idea introduces conceptual clarity it does not withstand careful examination. The proposal confuses personality with personality disorder and treats them as if they were the same concept. Personality clearly differs from psychopathology in the ways Foulds suggests. Personality disorder does not. Personality disorder not only consists of traits and attitudes but also other personality features such as beliefs and other cognitions many of which are not as stable as traits. Moreover, many attitudes also change over time. Personality disorder also includes symptoms such as dysphoria, impulsivity, and cognitive disorganization that are similar to Axis I symptomatology.

Even if it is accepted that the personality characteristics of personality disorders are stable, it is apparent that the clinical picture associated with the diagnosis fluctuates. The borderline patient, for example, is not in a constant state of crisis. Instead, for many patients, periods of instability are interspersed with periods of stability and reasonable levels of functioning. Even the presentation in a crisis may change within a given patient. On one occasion it may take the form of self-harming acts, on another the symptoms may resemble a mood disorder, and on another the presentation may be more like an anxiety disorder. The clinical presentations of such patients do not differ greatly from those of many cases of other mental disorders. Anxiety disorders, for example, can fluctuate in the same way and the form of the disorder may change across presentations.

Those arguing for a fundamental distinction would probably counter this contention with the proposal that the essential difference is that in personality disorder the underlying personality features remain between episodes. But is this specific to personality disorder? Neuroticism or trait anxiety is a predisposing factor for several Axis I disorders that remains after the Axis I symptoms have remitted (Clark, Watson, & Mineka, 1994; Rapee, 1991). As Slater and Roth (1969) pointed out "tachycardia, feelings of fear, insomnia, depression, faints, fugues, and all the other phenomena that we call neurotic symptoms, are easily thought of a manifestations of a given personality and constitution in circumstances favourable to their development. We could also consider tendencies to seek relief in alcohol, outbursts of temper, wandering, dereliction of duty, lying and thieving, and acts of ruthlessness and cruelty in the same light" (p. 62). It appears that stable vulnerabilities underlie Axis I disorders that do not differ greatly from the vulnerabilities underlying personality disorder.

Etiology

When DSM-III was first published there was a general assumption that Axis I disorders were largely biological in origin whereas Axis II disorders had a psychosocial etiology. Such a distinction would be sufficient to warrant a separate axes. In the case of Axis I disorders this assumption was never justified because it has long been apparent that psychosocial stressors play an important role in the causation and maintenance of many conditions. Over the last decade evidence has progressively accumulated that personality disorder has a complex etiology that includes psychosocial and biological factors (Siever & Davis, 1991). In particular, genetic studies suggest a substantial genetic contribution to personality disorders (McGuffin & Thapar, 1992; Nigg & Goldsmith, 1994) and that the major traits delineating personality disorder have a substantial heritable component (Jang et al., 1996; Livesley et al., 1993; Livesley et al., 1998). It appears therefore that etiology provides the least justifiable grounds for maintaining fundamental distinctions between the two axes.

Temporal Course

The most convincing reason for placing personality disorder on a separate axis is the argument that they are more stable and enduring than clinical syndromes which tend to have a more fluctuating course. In this sense personality disorder differs from episodic mental disorders. Temporal stability is a feature of personality which is usually defined in terms of enduring features that are stable across situations and time. However, the considerable evidence for the stability of personality traits (Heatherton & Weinberger, 1994) does not apply to all aspects of personality (see Chapter 11, this volume). Nor does it necessarily apply to all features of personality disorder. Indeed, there is considerable evidence of temporal instability in the features of personality disorder (Barasch, Frances, Hurt, Clarkin, & Cohen, 1985; Clark, 1992; Mann, Jenkins, Cutting, & Cowen, 1981). This seems to be a function of the effects of state factors on personality disorder diagnoses. As noted in the discussion of phenomenology, many forms of personality disorder show a fluctuating course at least in terms of acute symptomatic states and crises. Thus the distinction between personality disorder and forms of episodic disorder is not clear-cut. Arguments that personality disorder is more stable than other mental disorders often confuse the stability of personality with the stability of the disorder.

It should also be noted that any difference in temporal stability between personality disorder and other mental disorders applies only to episodic mental disorders and not to those that follow a more chronic course. Disorders such as dysthymic disorder, schizophrenia, and some cases of delusional disorder show levels of stability that are not appreciably different from those of personality disorder. Again it seems difficult to establish definite distinctions based on course.

Conclusions

There do not appear to be fundamental distinctions between personality disorder and *all* other mental disorders of the kind that would warrant a major distinction between them. This is not to say that they are not different. The difference, however, is similar to that observed among the 17 classes of disorder recognized in DSM-IV. Mood disorders are not the same as anxiety or somatization disorders. Moreover, it appears that the difference between personality disorder and such conditions as somatization, anxiety, and dysthymic disorders is substantially less than the difference between these disorders and such conditions as schizophrenia or cognitive disorders. If personality disorder is classified on a separate axis in future classifications it should be acknowledged that the decision was based on practical and conventional considerations rather than solid empirical or theoretical grounds, unless of course new evidence emerges to support the distinction. This may perhaps ameliorate some of the practical problems created by the distinction in terms of access to care.

Requirements for an Empirically Based Classification

When considering the possible organization and contents of future classifications it is useful to consider some general principles that should guide the construction of future classifications (Livesley & Jackson, 1992).

The classification should have an explicit structure that is specified in a testable way. This requires that the theoretical and conceptual principles on which the classification is based should be specified along with the principles used to select, evaluate, and revise diagnostic constructs. Throughout this chapter reference was made to the limitations of DSM is this regard. When underlying principles are implicit rather than explicit they are difficult to evaluate. It also leads to a structure that resists change because is not easy to test basic assumptions.

The conditions for validity should be incorporated from the outset. The ultimate goal of classification is to establish a system that has satisfactory construct validity (Skinner, 1981). This requires that the system is constructed from the outset to facilitate such an objective. Current approaches to classification seem to imply that validity is something that is established after a reliable system has been constructed. This is not the optimal way to develop a classification. The beginnings of construct validity should be built into the system by specifying the conceptual basis of each diagnosis and selecting criteria on the basis of these definitions taking care to ensure that all critical features of the diagnosis are represented in the criteria set. This simple requirement demands a more systematic approach to construction than has thereto been used with DSM.

The classification should be stated in ways that permit systematic evaluation and revision. Any classification that is likely to be formulated in the near future will be subject to change. It is important therefore that systems are constructed in ways that facilitate revision. This means that the process of developing a classification should be considered an iterative process in which the system is constructed to permit evaluation and systematic revision based on new findings. When deficiencies with diagnoses or specific criteria are identified in the present system it is often unclear what specific remedies should be adopted. If the construct validation approach were used in which criteria were selected to assess specific facets of a diagnosis, remedies would be more apparent. For example, if a given criterion was found to be a poor marker of a given trait an alternative could be developed. If all criteria for a given trait were found to be problematic, it would suggest problems with the way the trait was defined or that it was not a critical component of the diagnosis. In this way evaluation leads to systematic change rather than periodic revision, and the classification increasingly approximates a valid system.

The classification should be based on empirical evidence. This statement appears to be so obvious that it should not need to be stated. However, current classifications are not based on empirical fact as much as on clinical tradition. This is not a criticism of the considerable scholarship that contributed to recent editions of DSM or ICD-10 but rather a reflection of the field at the time and the diverse pressures that influence the development of official systems. It is clear, however, that contemporary classifications are at variance with empirical fact in terms of classificatory principles and diagnostic constructs. Yet an effort to change the system to accommodate the new understanding of personality disorder that is emerging from recent research is unlikely to be a straightforward task. Political and social factors tend to give rise to a conservative approach to changing psychiatric classifications that may be incompatible with the requirement for an evidence-based system.

The importance of developing a system that has clinical utility is often cited as a major issue. Clinical utility, however, has several components although it is often interpreted only as ease of use. There is little doubt that current categorical systems are easy to use although they do not have great utility in terms of organizing etiological information or predicting treatment response. Nevertheless, it will be a major challenge to develop a classification that captures the complexity of personality disorder as revealed by current empirical evidence that is as convenient to use as DSM-IV.

The classification should be theory based. The emphasis that recent editions of DSM placed on being atheoretical with respect to etiology may have been a necessary step to free the classification of mental disorders from unsubstantiated etiological assumptions. In the long run, however, this is an untenable position. As biology has shown, theory lies at the very heart of any classificatory system. Biological classification is often proposed as a model that psychiatry should emulate. Biology was so successful because classification is based on a powerful integrating theory: the theory of evolution. Hence, in the long run it is impossible to divorce the classification of personality disorder from a theory of personality disorder. Although such a theory is not available, current empirical knowledge, accumulated clinical experience, and concepts of normal personality provide a solid foundation for a classification

that should be an improvement on what is available and form the basis for further research.

The classification should be consistent with the general classification of psychopathology. The current distinction between Axes I and II lacks a coherent theoretical rationale and creates practical problems. The notion that personality disorder is a form of mental disorder has immediate implications for organizing a classification. Based on this idea it is proposed that the diagnosis of personality disorder (not personality disorders) be included with other mental disorders on Axis I and that an additional axis be used to code clinically significant personality traits (Livesley, 1998). Thus, the classification would explicitly distinguish between the diagnosis of personality disorder and the assessment of personality on clinically relevant dimensions.

The system should be consistent with conceptions of normal personality. As noted previously, the classification of personality disorder should be consistent with conceptions of the structure and functions of normal personality and with empirically based descriptions of normal personality variation. Such a development would provide the theoretical foundation that the classification of personality disorder currently lacks.

The system should be consistent with knowledge in related fields. Contemporary classifications seem to have been constructed with minimal attention to related fields of knowledge. The classification should, however, be consistent with knowledge in such related disciplines as personality theory, cognitive science, neuroscience, behavior genetics, and evolutionary psychology.

The classification should be based on the phenotypical structure of personality disorder. Although the classification should be consistent with biological thinking and behavior-genetic analyses may help to resolve persistent problems regarding basic dimensions, the diagnostic concepts incorporated in the classification should reflect personality phenotypes because it is the phenotype that we seek to explain and treat.

A STRUCTURE FOR AN EMPIRICALLY BASED CLASSIFICATION

The overview of concepts of personality disorder and approaches to definition indicate a modest consensus that the classification of personality disorder should have two components: (1) a definition of the disorder and associated criteria that permit reliable diagnosis and (2) a system for describing individual differences in personality pathology that are clinically significant. With this arrangement the diagnostic process would involve two steps: diagnosis of personality disorder and assessment of individual differences in personality. Although such a structure has only been explicitly proposed by Cloninger (2000) and Livesley and colleagues (Livesley, 1998; Livesley & Jang, 2000; Livesley et al., 1994), the idea is implicit in the DSM-IV listing of general criteria for personality disorder.

Definition

A systematic definition is required to differentiate personality disorder from other mental disorders on the one hand and normal personality on the other. This is required whether individual differences are represented by categories or dimensions. With a categorical approach, a definition is needed to differentiate personality disorder from other classes of mental disorder. This would help to correct the diagnostic confusion and overlap created by the failure of DSM-IV to specify how the different groups of disorder are distinguished. With a dimensional system, a definition is also required to determine when an extreme score is indicative of personality disorder. As discussed earlier, an extreme position is not in itself sufficient to diagnose disorder.

Although the requirements for a satisfactory definition can be specified, a consensus definition is not currently available. This is an important conceptual and empirical problem that needs to be solved for the next iteration in classification. The defining attributes or criteria are likely to be dimensional in nature. However, clinical practice probably requires that assessments of the defining features be converted into a categorical diagnosis. This could readily be achieved using empirically derived cutting scores.

System for Describing Individual Differences

The second component of the classification, a scheme to describe individual differences in personality, could adopt a categorical or dimensional framework. However, if the system is to be evidenced based, the classification needs to accommodate overwhelming empirical evidence that the phenotypical features of personality disorder are continuously distributed. This means that a dimensional framework needs to be incorporated into the system.

There appears to be a consensus that the best construct for conceptualizing individual differences is the trait. The use of traits in future classifications would establish conceptual continuity with DSM-IV, which defines personality disorders as clusters of maladaptive traits, and conceptions of normal personality. There also appears to be a consensus that traits are hierarchically organized with a larger number of lower-order traits combining to form fewer higher-order traits. There are good reasons to consider that both levels of the hierarchy are important for understanding and treating personality problems. Description based on a few higher-order traits offers a convenient and parsimonious way to communicate about personality, and these patterns appear to represent differences that have substantial implications for treatment. Specific treatment decisions, however, seem to require the detailed evaluation of personality provided by description of the lower-order traits.

Despite the consensus that this structure offers a convenient taxonomy of individual differences, it is not clear whether the lower-order traits are simply subcomponents of the higher-order traits or whether they are separate entities that co-occur to create the higher-order trait. Consider, for example, the higher-order trait of neuroticism which Costa and McCrae (1992) suggested consists of six facets: anxiety, hostility, depression, self-consciousness, impulsivity, and vulnerability. Are these facet traits simply ways to subdivide neuroticism for descriptive purposes, or are they distinct entities with independent etiologies that tend to co-occur? Although this question may appear esoteric and unrelated to clinical practice, it has important implications for classification and understanding personality developments.

Behavior–genetic analyses of twin study data are beginning to provide an answer to this question. Traits associated with normal and disordered personality have a substantial heritable component that typically ranges from 40% to 60% (Jang et al., 1996; Livesley et al., 1993; Plomin et al., 1990). This raises the question whether the heritability of lower-order traits such as anxiety and vulnerability is due to the fact that they are subcomponents of neuroticism or whether they are distinct entities with their own specific heritable component. Expressed differently, the issue is whether the genetic variation of a lower-order trait consists only of general variance due to the higher-order trait or whether is consists of general variance plus a specific component. Investigations of this issue have been limited, but recently it was shown that the specific facet traits of the five-factor model have substantial residual variance when the effects of the five higher-order dimensions are removed (Jang, McCrae, Angleitner, Riemann, & Livesley, 1998). In the case of the six facets of neuroticism, the heritability of the residual components ranged from 21% to 29%. Similar results are found for the specific traits of personality disorder (Livesley et al., 1998).

This finding suggests that personality phenotypes are based on of a large number of genetic building blocks that have relatively specific effects and a few factors with more widespread effects. This would explain the complex variation observed in the phenotypical structure of personality and personality disorder. It also implies that discrete categories of personality disorder as proposed in classifications such as DSM-IV and ICD-10 are unlikely. Instead, an almost infinite variety of configurations of personality traits are likely to occur as these building blocks are combined in multiple ways. For this reason, the most important level in the hierarchy for coding clinically relevant traits is the basic or lower-order level.

Although the evidence suggests that the lower-order traits are distinct entities, other aspects of the hierarchical structure are still unclear. Trait theories tend to assume that all lower-order traits are incorporated into a higher-order dimension. However, if each lower-order trait is a distinct etiological entity (i.e., each is based on a distinct genetic dimension), it is conceivable that some specific traits are not associated with any higher-order domain. In that case, the resulting hierarchy would be incomplete with some traits combining to define higher-order patterns and some remaining relatively distinct. This has led to the suggestion that some apparently higher-order factors (e.g., compulsivity) which are less pervasive than other higher-order traits (e.g., neuroticism or emotional dysregulation) should be considered lower-order traits within a classification of personality disorder (Livesley, 1998).

Which higher-order dimensions should be used to classify personality disorder is likely to be controversial, with proposals differing in respect to the nature and number of dimensions considered necessary. However, as noted earlier, the evidence suggests consensus on three higher-order dimensions: neuroticism or emotional dysregulation; introversion or inhibitedness; and psychoticism, negative agreeableness, or dissocial behavior. There is also substantial support for a dimension of conscientiousness or compulsivity although, as noted, there may be some dispute whether this should be considered a higher-order or lower-order dimension. No matter which additional higher-order dimensions are included, it is apparent that an evidenced based system needs to incorporate these dimensions or some variant of them.

Identification of a consensual set of lower-order traits awaits further research because studies of normal and disordered personality yield slightly different mappings of each higher-order domain. As noted, however, there is substantial agreement across studies of personality disorder on the lower-order traits defining the overall domain.

CONCLUSIONS

This overview reveals the changing understanding of personality disorder emerging from the growth of empirical research stimulated by DSM-III. The evidence points to the fact that personality disorder involves the extremes of normal personality variation and that clear distinctions between normality and pathology and different forms of personality disorder are unlikely. It is also apparent that there are few cogent reasons for assuming that personality disorders are so radically different from other mental disorders that they require a separate axis. Indeed, the evidence suggests that personality disorders and other disorders may have some vulnerabilities in common.

It is increasingly apparent that there are major conceptual and empirical problems to solve before a valid classification can be developed. The evidence points overwhelmingly to substantial and probably irremediable problems with the categorical approach adopted by DSM and ICD systems. Despite this evidence, the field seems reluctant to accept the need for new approaches. Part of the difficulty is that an alternative system is not readily available. There is also the problem that current empirical knowledge is somewhat fragmentary because it is derived from investigations informed by diverse perspectives and constructs. Consequently, progress in developing a more systematic understanding and classification has been slow. Nevertheless, a framework for an empirically based system that can be modified to accommodate new findings is beginning to emerge. Ultimately, however, progress depends on the development of a comprehensive theory that integrates the diverse empirical knowledge about personality and personality disorder and articulates a sound basis for classification.

REFERENCES

Abraham, K. (1927). *Selected papers on psychoanalysis.* London: Hogarth Press. (Original work published 1921)

Akhtar, S. (1992). *Broken structures: Severe personality disorders and their treatment.* Northvale, NJ: Jason Aronson.

Allport, G. W. (1937). *Personality: A psychological interpretation.* New York: Holt.

Allport, G. W. (1961). *Pattern and growth in personality: A psychological interpretation.* New York: Holt, Rinehart & Winston.

American Psychiatric Association. (1994). *Diagnostic and statistical manual of mental disorders* (4th ed.). Washington, DC: Author.

Atran, S. (1990). *Cognitive foundations of natural science.* Cambridge, UK: Cambridge University Press.

Austin, E. J., & Deary, I. J. (2000). The four As: A common framework for normal and abnormal personality? *Personality and Individual Differences, 28,* 977–995.

Ball, S. A. Tennen, H., Poling, J. C., Krazler, H. R., & Rounsaville, B. J. (1997). Personality, temperament, and character dimension and the DSM-IV personality disorders in substance abusers. *Journal of Abnormal Psychology, 106,* 545–553.

Barasch, A., Frances, A., Hurt, A. J., Clarkin, J. F., & Cohen, S. (1985). Stability and distinctiveness of borderline personality disorder. *American Journal of Psychiatry, 12,* 1484–1486.

Beckner, M. (1959). *The biological way of thought.* New York: Columbia University Press.

Benjamin, L. S. (1993). *Interpersonal diagnosis and treatment of personality disorders.* New York: Guilford Press.

Benjamin, L. S. (1996). *Interpersonal diagnosis and the treatment of personality disorders.* (2nd ed.). New York: Guilford Press.

Berrios, G. E. (1993). European views on personality disorders: A conceptual history. *Comprehensive Psychiatry, 34,* 14–30.

Blais, M. A. (1997). Clinician ratings of the five-factor model of personality and the DSM-IV personality disorders. *Journal of Nervous and Mental Disease, 185,* 388–393.

Blais, M. A., & Norman, D. K. (1997). A psychometric evaluation of the DSM-IV personality disorder criteria. *Journal of Personality Disorders, 11,* 168–176.

Blashfield, R. K. (1989). Alternative taxonomic models of psychiatric classification. In L. N. Robins & J. E. Barrett (Eds.), *The validity of psychiatric diagnosis.* New York: Raven.

Blashfield, R. K., & Breen, M. J. (1989). Face validity of the DSM-III-R personality disorders. *American Journal of Psychiatry, 146,* 1575–1579.

Blashfield R. K., & Haymaker, D. (1990). A prototype analysis of the diagnostic criteria for DSM-III-R personality disorders. *Journal of Personality Disorders, 2,* 272–280.

Blashfield R. K., & Livesley, W. J. (1999). Classification. In T. Millon, P. H. Blaney, & R. D. Davis (Eds.), *Oxford textbook of psychopathology.* Oxford, UK: Oxford University Press.

Blashfield, R. K., & McElroy, R. A. (1987). The 1985 journal literature on personality disorders. *Comprehensive Psychiatry, 28,* 536–546.

Blashfield R. K., Sprock, J., Pinkson, K., & Hodgkin, J. (1985). Exemplar prototypes of personality disorder diagnoses. *Comprehensive Psychiatry, 26,* 11–21.

Block, J. (1995). A contrarian view of the five-factor approach to personality description. *Psychological Bulletin, 117,* 187–215.

Bromley, D. B. (1977). *Personality description in ordinary language.* London: Wiley.

Buss, A. H., & Plomin, R. (1984). *Temperament: Early developing personality traits.* Hillsdale, NJ: Erlbaum.

Cantor, N. (1990). From thought to behavior: "Having" and "doing" in the study of personality and cognition. *American Psychologist, 45,* 735–750.

Cantor, N., Smith, E. E., French, R., & Mezzich, J. (1980). Psychiatric diagnosis as prototype classification. *Journal of Abnormal Psychology, 89,* 181–193.

Carson, R. C. (1982). Self-fulfilling prophecy, maladaptive behavior, and psychotherapy. In J. C. Anchin & D. J. Kiessler (Eds.), *Handbook of interpersonal psychotherapy.* Elsford, NY: Pergamon Press.

Cervone, D., & Shoda, Y. (1999). Social-cognitive theories and the coherence of personality. In D. Cervone and Y. Shoda (Eds.), *The coherence of personality* (pp. 3–33). New York: Guilford Press.

Chess, S., & Thomas, A. (1984). *The origins and evolution of behavior disorders.* New York: Brunner/Mazel.

Clark, L. A. (1990). Toward a consensual set of symptom clusters for assessment of personality disorder. In J. Butcher & C. Spielberger (Eds.), *Advances in personality assessment* (Vol. 8, pp. 243–266). Hillsdale, NJ: Erlbaum.

Clark, L. A. (1992). Resolving taxonomic issues in personality disorders. *Journal of Personality Disorders, 6,* 360–376.

Clark, L. A. (1993). *Manual for the Schedule for Nonadaptive and Adaptive Personality.* Minneapolis: University of Minnesota Press.

Clark, L. A., & Livesley, W. J. (1994) Two approaches to identifying the dimensions of personality disorder. In P. T. Costa & T. A. Widiger (Eds.), *Personality disor-*

ders and the five-factor model of personality (pp. 261–277). Washington, DC: American Psychological Association Press.

Clark, L. A., Livesley, W. J., & Morey, L. (1997). Personality disorder assessment: The challenge of construct validity. *Journal of Personality Disorders, 11,* 205–231.

Clark, L. A., Livesley, W. J., Schroeder, M. L., & Irish. S. L. (1996). Convergence of two systems for assessing personality disorder. *Psychological Assessment, 8,* 294–303.

Clark, L. A., Watson, D., & Mineka, S. (1994). Temperament, personality, and the mood and anxiety disorders. *Journal of Abnormal Psychology, 103,* 103–116.

Cleckley, H. (1976). *The mask of insanity* (5th ed.) St. Louis, MO: Mosby.

Cloninger, C. R. (1987). A systematic method for clinical description and classification of personality variants. *Archives of General Psychiatry, 44,* 573–588.

Cloninger, C. R. (2000). A practical way to diagnose personality disorder: A proposal. *Journal of Personality Disorders, 14,* 99–106.

Cloninger, C. R., Svrakic, D. M., & Przybeck, T. R. (1993). A psychobiological model of temperament and character. *Archives of General Psychiatry, 50,* 975–990.

Costa, P. T., & McCrae, R. R. (1992). *Revised NEO Personality Inventory (NEO-PI-R) and the NEO Five-Factor Inventory (NEO-FFI) professional manual.* Odessa, FL: Psychological Assessment Resources.

Costa, P. T., & Widiger, T. A. (Eds.). (1994). *Personality disorders and the five factor model of personality.* Washington DC: American Psychological Association.

Deary, I. J., Peter, A., Austin, E. J., & Gibson, G. J. (1998). Personality traits and personality disorders. *British Journal of Psychology, 89,* 647–662.

Digman, J. M. (1990). Personality structure: Emergence of the five-factor structure. *Annual Review of Psychology, 41,* 417–440.

Digman, J. M. (1996). The curious history of the five-factor model. In J. S. Wiggins (Ed.), *The five-factor model of personality* (pp. 1–20). New York: Guilford Press.

Dyce, J. A., & Connor, B. P. (1998). Personality disorders and the five-factor model: A test of facet-level predictions. *Journal of Personality Disorders, 12,* 31–45.

Ekselius, L., Lindstrom, E., von Knorring, L., Bodlund, O., & Kullgren, G. (1994). A principal component analysis of the DSM-III-R Axis II personality disorders. *Journal of Personality Disorders, 8,* 140–148.

Erikson, E. (1950). *Childhood and society.* New York: Norton.

Eysenck, H. J. (1987). The definition of personality disorders and the criteria appropriate to their definition. *Journal of Personality Disorders, 1,* 211–219.

Eysenck, H. J., & Eysenck, M. W. (1985). *Personality and individual differences: A natural science approach.* New York: Plenum.

Foulds, G. A. (1965). *Personality and personal illness.* London: Tavistock.

Foulds, G. A. (1976). *The hierarchical nature of personal illness.* London: Academic Press.

Frances, A. J., Clarkin, J., Gilmore, M., Hurt, S., & Brown, S. (1984). Reliability of criteria for borderline personality disorder: A comparison of DSM-III and the diagnostic interview for borderline patients. *American Journal of Psychiatry, 42,* 591–596.

Freedman, M. B., Leary, T. F., Ossorio, A. G., & Coffey, H. S. (1951). The interpersonal dimension of personality. *Journal of Personality, 20,* 143–161.

Goldberg, L. R., (1990). An alternative "Description of personality": The Big-Five factor structure. *Journal of Personality and Social Psychology, 59,* 1216–1229.

Grinker, R. R., Werble, B., & Drye, R. C. (1968). *The borderline syndrome.* New York: Basic Books.

Hall, C. S., & Lindzey, G. (1957). *Theories of personality.* New York: Wiley.

Hare, R. D. (1991). *Manual for the Hare Psychopathy Checklist—Revised.* Toronto: Multi-Health Systems.

Harkness, A. R. (1992). Fundamental topics in the personality disorders: Candidate trait dimensions from the lower regions of the hierarchy. *Psychological Assessment, 4,* 251–259.

Harris, G. T., Rice, M. E., & Quinsey, V. L. (1994). Psychology as a taxon: Evidence that psychopaths are a discrete class. *Journal of Consulting and Clinical Psychology, 62, 2,* 387–397.

Heatherton, T. F., & Weinberger, J. L. (Eds.). (1994). *Can personality change?* Washington, DC: American Psychological Association.

Hyler, S. E., & Lyons, M. (1988). Factor analysis of the DSM-III personality disorder clusters: A replication. *Comprehensive Psychiatry, 29,* 304–308.

Jackson, D. N. (1971). The dynamics of structured personality tests. *Psychological Review, 78,* 229–248.

Jang K. L., Livesley, W. J., Vernon, P. A., & Jackson, D. N. (1996). Heritability of personality disorder traits: A twin study. *Acta Psychiatrica Scandinavica, 94,* 438–444.

Jang, K. L., McCrae, R. R., Angleitner, A., Riemann, R., & Livesley, W. J. (1998). Heritability of facet-level traits in a cross-cultural twin study: Support for a hierarchical model of personality. *Journal of Personality and Social Psychology, 74,* 1556–1565.

Jaspers, K. (1923/1963). *General psychopathology* (J. Hoenig & M. W. Hamilton, Trans.). Chicago: University of Chicago Press. (Original work published 1925)

John, O. P., & Robbins, R. W. (1993). Gordon Allport: Father and critic of the five-factor model. In K. H. Craik, R. Hogan, & R. N. Wolfe (Eds.), *Fifty years of personality psychology* (pp. 215–236). New York: Plenum.

Kass, F., Skodol, A., Charles, E., Spitzer, R. L., & Williams, J. B. W. (1985). Scaled ratings of DSM-III personality disorders. *American Journal of Psychiatry, 142,* 627–630.

Kendell, R. E. (1975). *The role of diagnosis in psychiatry.* Oxford, UK: Basil Blackwell.

Kendell, R. E. (1986). What are mental disorders? In A. N. Freedman, R. Brotman, I. Silverman, & D. Hudson (Eds.), *Issues in psychiatric classification* (pp. 23–45). New York: Human Sciences Press.

Kernberg, O. F. (1975). *Borderline conditions and pathological narcissism.* New York: Jason Aronson.

Kernberg, O. (1984). *Severe personality disorders.* New Haven, CT: Yale University Press.

Kiesler, D. J. (1982). *The 1982 interpersonal circle: A taxonomy for complementarity in human transactions.* Richmond: Virginia Commonwealth University.

Kiesler, D. J. (1986). The 1982 interpersonal circle: An analysis of DSM-III personality disorders. In T. Millon & G. L. Klerman (Eds.), *Contemporary directions in psychopathology: Toward the DSM-IV* (pp. 571–597). New York: Guilford Press.

Klerman, G. L. (1978). The evolution of a scientific nosology. In J. C. Shershow (Ed.), *Schizophrenia: Science and practice.* Cambridge, MA: Harvard University Press.

Koch, J. L. A. (1891). *The psychopathic inferiorities.* Ravensburg, Germany: Dorn.

Kohut, H. (1971). *The analysis of the self.* New York: International Universities Press.

Kraepelin, E. (1907). *Clinical psychiatry* (A. R. Dienfendorf, Trans.). New York: Macmillan.

Kretschmer, E. (1925). *Physique and character.* New York: Harcourt Brace.

Leary, T. (1957). *Interpersonal diagnosis of personality: A functional theory and methodology for personality evaluation.* New York: Ronald Press.

Livesley, W. J. (1985). The classification of personality disorder: 1. The choice of category concept. *Canadian Journal of Psychiatry, 30,* 353–358.

Livesley, W. J. (1986). Trait and behavioral prototypes of personality disorder. *American Journal of Psychiatry, 143,* 728–732.

Livesley, W. J. (1987). A systematic approach to the delineation of personality disorder. *American Journal of Psychiatry, 144,* 772–777.

Livesley, W. J. (1991). Classifying personality disorders: Ideal types, prototypes, or dimensions? *Journal of Personality Disorders, 5,* 52–59.

Livesley, W. J. (1995). Past achievements and future directions. In W. J. Livesley (Ed.), *The DSM-IV personality disorders* (pp. 497–505). New York: Guilford Press.

Livesley, W. J. (1998). Suggestions for a framework for an empirically based classification of personality disorder. *Canadian Journal of Psychiatry, 43,* 137–147.

Livesley, W. J. (2000). Introduction to special feature: Critical issues in the classification of personality disorder, Part I. *Journal of Personality Disorders, 14,* 1–2.

Livesley, W. J. (in press). Commentary. *Journal of Personality.*

Livesley, W. J., & Jackson, D. N. (1986). The internal consistency and factorial structure of behaviours judged to be associated with DSM-III categories of personality disorders. *American Journal of Psychiatry, 143,* 1473–1474.

Livesley, W. J., Jackson, D. N. (1991). Construct validity and the classification of personality disorders. In J. Oldham (Ed.), *DSM-III-R Axis II: Perspectives on validity* (pp. 3–22). Washington DC: American Psychiatric Association.

Livesley, W. J., & Jackson, D. N. (1992). Guidelines for developing, evaluating, and revising the classification of personality disorders. *Journal of Nervous and Mental Disease, 180,* 609–618.

Livesley, W. J., & Jackson, D. N. (in press). *Manual for the dimensional assessment of personality pathology.* Port Huron, MI: Sigma Press.

Livesley, W. J., Jackson, D. N., & Schroeder, M. L. (1989). A study of the factorial structure of personality pathology. *Journal of Personality Disorders, 3,* 292–306.

Livesley, W. J., Jackson, D. N., & Schroeder, M. L. (1992). Factorial structure of traits delineating personality disorders in clinical and general population samples. *Journal of Abnormal Psychology, 101,* 432–440.

Livesley, W. J., & Jang, K. L. (2000). Toward an empirically based classification of personality disorder. *Journal of Personality Disorders, 14,* 137–151.

Livesley, W. J., Jang, K. L., Jackson, D. N., & Vernon, P. A. (1993). Genetic and environmental contributions to dimensions of personality disorder. *American Journal of Psychiatry, 150,* 1826–1831.

Livesley, W. J., Jang, K. L., & Vernon, P. A. (1998). The phenotypic and genetic architecture of traits delineating personality disorder. *Archives of General Psychiatry, 55,* 941–948.

Livesley, W. J., Reiffer, L. I., Sheldon, A. E. R., & West, M. (1987). Prototypicality of the DSM-III personality criteria. *Journal of Nervous and Mental Disease, 175,* 395–401.

Livesley, W. J., Schroeder, M. L., Jackson, D. N., & Jang, K. L. (1994). Categorical distinctions in the study of personality disorder: Implication for classification. *Journal of Abnormal Psychology, 103,* 6–17.

Loevinger, J. (1957). Objective tests as instruments of psychological theory *Psychological Reports, 3,* 635–694.

Mann, A., Jenkins, R., Cutting, J. C., & Cowen, P. J. (1981). The development and use of a standardized assessment of abnormal personality. *Psychological Medicine, 11,* 839–847.

Maudsley, H. (1874). *Responsibility in mental disease.* London: King.

McAdams, D. P. (1994). Can personality change? Levels of stability and growth in personality across the life span. In T. F. Heatherton & J. L. Weinberger (Eds.), *Can personality change?* (pp. 299–313). Washington, DC: American Psychological Association Press.

McAdams, D. P. (1997). A conceptual history of personality psychology. In R. Hogan, J. Johnson, & S. Briggs (Eds.), *Handbook of personality psychology* (pp. 3–39). San Diego, CA: Academic Press.

McCrae, R. R., Yiang, J., Costa, P. T., Dai, X., Yao, S., Cai, T., & Gao, B. (in press). Personality profiles and the prediction of categorical personality disorders. *Journal of Personality.*

McGuffin, P., & Thapar, A. (1992). The genetics of personality disorder. *British Journal of Psychiatry, 160,* 12–23.

McLemore, C. W., & Brokaw, D. W. (1987). Personality disorders as dysfunctional interpersonal behavior. *Journal of Personality Disorders, 1,* 270–285.

Meehl, P. E. (1992). Factors and taxa, traits and types,

differences of degree and differences of kind. *Journal of Personality, 60,* 117–174.

Meehl, P. E., & Golden, R. R. (1982). Taxometric methods. In J. N. Butcher & C. C. Kendall (Eds.), *The handbook of research methods in clinical psychology* (pp. 127–181). New York: Wiley.

Mellsop, G., Varghese, F., Joshua, S., & Hicks, A. (1982). The reliability of Axis II of DSM-III. *American Journal of Psychiatry, 139,* 1360–1361.

Miller, J. D., Lynam, D. R., Widiger, T. A., & Leukfield, C. (in press). Personality disorders as extreme variants of common personality dimensions: Can the five-factor model adequately represent psychopathy? *Journal of Personality.*

Miller, T. R. (1991). The psychotherapeutic utility of the five factor model of personality: A clinician's experience. *Journal of Personality Assessment, 57,* 415–433.

Millon, T. (1969). *Modern psychopathology: A biosocial approach to maladaptive learning and functioning.* Philadelphia: Saunders.

Millon, T. (1990). *Toward a new personology: An evolutionary model.* New York: Wiley.

Millon, T., with Davis, R. (1996). *Disorders of personality: DSM-IV and beyond.* New York: Wiley.

Morey, L. C. (1988). A psychometric analysis of the DSM-III-R personality disorder criteria. *Journal of Personality Disorders, 2,* 109–124.

Morey, L. C., & Ochoa, E. S. (1989). An investigation of adherence to diagnostic criteria: Clinical diagnosis and the DSM-III personality disorders. *Journal of Personality Disorders, 3,* 180–192.

Mulder, R. T., Joyce, P. R. (1997). Temperament and the structure of personality disorder symptoms. *Psychological Medicine, 27,* 1315–1325.

Mulder, R. T., Joyce, P. R., Sullivan, P. F., Bulik, C. M., & Carter, F. A. (1999). The relationship among three models of personality psychopathology: DSM-III-R personality disorder, TCI scores and DSQ defences. *Psychological Medicine, 29,* 943–951.

Nakao, F., Gunderson, J. D., Phillips, K. A., Tanaka, N., Yorifuji, K., Takaishi, J., & Nashimura, N. (1992). Functional impairment in personality disorders. *Journal of Personality Disorders, 6,* 24–33.

Nestadt, G., Romanoski, A., Chahal, R., Merchant, A., Folstein, M., Gruenberg, E., & McHugh, R. (1990). An epidemiological study of histrionic personality disorder. *Psychological Medicine, 20,* 413–422.

Nigg, J. T., & Goldsmith, H. H. (1994). Genetics of personality disorders: Perspectives from personality and psychopathology research. *Psychology Bulletin, 115,* 346–380.

Nunnally, J., & Bornstein, I. (1994). *Psychometric theory* (3rd ed.). New York: McGraw-Hill.

O'Boyle, M. (1995). DSM-III-R and Eysenck personality measures among patient in a substance abuse programme. *Personality and Individual Differences, 18,* 561–565.

O'Boyle, M., & Holzer, C. (1992). DSM-III-R personality disorders and Eysenck's personality dimensions. *Personality and Individual Differences, 13,* 1157–1159.

O'Boyle, M., & Self, P. (1990). A comparison of two interviews for DSM-III personality disorders. *Psychiatric Research, 32,* 283–285.

Oldham, J., & Skodol, A. (2000). Charting the future of Axis II. *Journal of Personality Disorders, 14,* 17–29.

Oldham, J., Skodol, A., Kellman, H., Hyler, S., Rosnick, L., & Davies, M. (1992). Diagnosis of DSM-III-R personality disorder by two semistructured interviews: Patterns of comorbidity. *American Journal of Psychiatry, 149,* 213–220.

Ottoson, J. O., & Perris, C. (1973). Multidimensional classification of mental disorders. *Psychological Medicine, 3,* 234.

Parker, G., & Barrett, E. (2000). Personality and personality disorder: Current issues and directions. *Psychological Medicine, 30,* 1–9.

Pilkonis, P., Heape, C., Proietti, J., Clark, S. W., McDavid, J., & Pitts, T. E. (1995). The reliability and validity of two structured interviews for personality disorders. *Archives of General Psychiatry, 52,* 1025–1033.

Pincus, A. L., & Wiggins, J. S. (1990). Interpersonal problems and conceptions of personality disorders. *Journal of Personality Disorders, 4,* 342–352.

Pincus, A. L., & Wilson, K. R. (in press). Interpersonal variegation in dependent personality. *Journal of Personality.*

Plomin, R., Chipeur, H. M., & Loehlin, J. C. (1990). Behavior genetics and personality. In L. A. Pervin (Ed.), *Handbook of personality: Theory and research* (pp. 225–243). New York: Guilford Press.

Plutchik, R. (1980). A general psychoevolutionary theory of emotion. In R. Plutchik & H. Kellerman (Eds.), *Emotion: Theory, research, and experience* (pp. 3–33). San Diego, CA: Academic Press.

Plutchik, R., & Platman, S. R. (1977). Personality connotations of psychiatric diagnosis: Implications for a similarity model. *Journal of Nervous and Mental Disease, 165,* 418–422.

Presly, A. J., & Walton, H. J. (1973). Dimensions of abnormal personality. *British Journal of Psychiatry, 122,* 269–276.

Pritchard, J. C. (1835). *Treatise on insanity.* London: Sherwood, Gilbert & Piper.

Pukrop, R., Herpertz, S., Sass, H., & Steinmeyer, E. M. (1998). Personality and personality disorders: A facet theoretical analysis of the similarity relationships. *Journal of Personality Disorders, 12,* 226–246.

Rapee, R. (1991). Generalized anxiety disorder: A review of clinical features and theoretical concepts. *Clinical Psychology Review, 11,* 419–440.

Reich, W. (1949). *Character analysis* (3rd ed.) New York: Farrar, Straus, & Giroux. (Original work published 1933)

Reynolds, S. K., & Clark, L. A. (in press). Predicting dimensions of personality disorder from domains and facets of the five-factor model. *Journal of Personality.*

Robins, L. (1966). *Deviant children grow up.* Baltimore: Williams & Wilkins.

Romney, D. M., & Brynner, J. M. (1989). Evaluation of a circumplex model of DSM-III personality disorders. *Journal of Research in Personality, 23,* 525–538.

Rosch, E. (1978). Principles of categorization. In E. Rosch & D. B. Lloyd (Eds.), *Cognition and categorization.* Hillsdale, NJ: Erlbaum.

Rutter, M. (1987). Temperament, personality and personality disorder. *British Journal of Psychiatry, 150,* 443–458.

Rutter, M., Shaffer, D., & Shephard, M. (1975). *Multiaxial classification of child psychiatric disorders.* Geneva: World Health Organization.

Sanderson, C., & Clarkin, J. F. (1994). Use of the NEO-PI personality dimensions in differential treatment planning. In P. T. Costa & T. A. Widiger (Eds.), *Personality disorders and the five-factor model of personality* (pp. 219–236). Washington, DC: American Psychological Association Press.

Saucier, G., & Goldberg, L. R., (1996). The language of personality: Lexical perspectives on the five-factor model. In J. S. Wiggins (Ed.), *The five-factor model of personality* (pp. 21–50). New York: Guilford Press.

Schneider, K. (1950). *Psychopathic personalities* (9th ed. English trans.). London: Cassell. (Original work published 1923)

Schroeder, M. L., Wormworth, J. A., & Livesley, W. J. (1992). Dimensions of personality disorder and their relationships to the big five dimensions of personality. *Psychological Assessment: A Journal of Consulting and Clinical Psychology, 4,* 47–53.

Schwartz, M. A., Wiggins, O. P., & Norko, M. A. (1989). Prototypes, ideal types, and personality disorders: The return to classical phenomenology. *Journal of Personality Disorders, 3,* 1–9.

Shea, M. T. (1995). Interrelationships among categories of personality disorders. In W. J. Livesley (Ed.), *The DSM-IV personality disorders* (pp. 397–406). New York: Guilford Press.

Siever, J., & Davis, K. L. (1991). A psychobiologic perspective on the personality disorders. *American Journal of Psychiatry, 148,* 1647–1658.

Simpson, C. G. (1961). *Principles of animal taxonomy.* New York: Columbia University Press.

Skinner, H. A. (1981). Toward an integration of classification theory and methods. *Journal of Abnormal Psychology, 90,* 68–87.

Slater, E., & Roth, M. (1969). *Clinical psychiatry* (3rd ed.). London: Bailliere, Tindall, & Cassell.

Soloff, P. H. (1998). Algorithms for pharmacological treatment of personality dimensions: Symptom specific treatments for cognitive–perceptual, affective, and impulsive-behavioral dysregulation. *Bulletin of the Menninger Clinic, 62,* 195–214.

Soloff, P. H. (2000). Psychopharmacology of borderline personality disorder. *Psychiatric Clinics of North America, 23,* 169–192.

Spitzer, R. L., Forman, J., & Nee, J. (1979). DSM-III field trials: I. Initial inter-rater reliability. *American Journal of Psychiatry, 136,* 815–817.

Strauss, J. S. (1975). A comprehensive approach to psychiatric diagnosis. *American Journal of Psychiatry, 132,* 1193–1197.

Svrakic, D. M., Whitehead, C., Przybeck, T. R., & Cloninger, C. R. (1993). Differential diagnosis of personality disorders by the seven-factor model of temperament and character. *Archives of General Psychiatry, 50,* 991–999.

Thomas, A., Birch, H., Hertzig, M., & Korn, S. (1963). *Behavioral individuality in early childhood.* New York: New York University Press.

Thomas, A., & Chess, S. (1977). *Temperament and development.* New York: Brunner/Mazel.

Trull, T. J., Widiger, T. A., & Burr, R. (in press). A structured interview for the assessment of the five-factor model of personality. *Journal of Personality.*

Trull, T. J., Widiger, T. A., & Guthrie, P. (1990). Categorical versus dimensional status of borderline personality disorder. *Journal of Abnormal Psychology, 99,* 40–48.

Turkheimer, E. (1998). Heritability and biological explanation. *Psychological Review, 105,* 782–791.

Tyrer, P. (1988). What's wrong with the DSM-III personality disorders? *Journal of Personality Disorders, 2,* 287–291.

Tyrer, P., & Alexander, M. S. (1979). Classification of personality disorder. *British Journal of Psychiatry, 135,* 163–167.

Vaillant, G. E., & Perry, J. C. (1980). Personality disorders. In H. Kaplan, A. M. Freedman, & B. Sadock (Eds.), *Comprehensive textbook of psychiatry/III* (pp. 1562–1590). Baltimore: Williams & Wilkins.

Wakefield, J. C. (1992). Disorder as harmful dysfunction: A conceptual critique of DSM-III-R's definition of mental disorder. *Psychological Review, 99,* 232–247.

Walton, H. J. (1986). The relationship between personality disorder and psychiatric illness. In T. Millon & G. L. Klerman (Eds.), *Contemporary directions in psychopathology: Toward the DSM-IV* (pp. 553–569). New York: Guilford Press.

Walton, H. J., Foulds, G. A., Littman, S. K., & Presly, A. S. (1970). Abnormal personality. *British Journal of Psychiatry, 116,* 497–510.

Walton, H. J., & Presly, A. S. (1973). Use of a category system in the diagnosis of abnormal personality. *British Journal of Psychiatry, 122,* 259–268.

Weston, D., & Arkowitz-Weston, L. (1998). Limitations of Axis II in diagnosing personality pathology in clinical practice. *American Journal of Psychiatry, 155,* 1767–1771.

Weston, D., & Shedler, J. (1999a). Revising and assessing Axis II: I. Developing a clinically and empirically valid method. *American Journal of Psychiatry, 156,* 258–272.

Weston, D., & Shedler, J. (1999b). Revising and assessing Axis II: II. Toward an empirically and clinically sensible taxonomy of personality disorders. *American Journal of Psychiatry, 156,* 273–285.

Weston, D., & Shedler, J. (2000). A prototype matching approach to diagnosing personality disorders: Toward the DSM-IV. *Journal of Personality Disorders, 14,* 109–126.

Whitlock, F. A. (1967). Pritchard and the concept of moral insanity. *Australian and New Zealand Journal of Psychiatry, 1,* 72–79.

Whitlock, F. A. (1982). A note on moral insanity and the psychopathic disorders. *Bulletin of the Royal College of Psychiatrists, 6,* 57–59.

Widiger, T. A. (1993). The DSM-III-R categorical personality disorder diagnoses: A critique and alternative. *Psychological Inquiry, 4,* 75–90.

Widiger, T. A. (1994). Conceptualizing a disorder of personality from the five-factor model. In P. T. Costa & T. A. Widiger (Eds.), *Personality disorders and the five-factor model of personality* (pp. 311–317).

Washington, DC: American Psychological Association Press.

Widiger, T. A. (2000). Personality disorder in the 21st century. *Journal of Personality Disorders, 14,* 3–16.

Widiger, T. A., & Corbitt, E. (1994). Normal versus abnormal personality from the perspective of the DSM. In S. Strack & M. Lorr (Eds.), *Differentiating normal and abnormal personality* (pp. 158–175). New York: Springer.

Widiger, T. A., Frances, A. J., Harris, M., Jacobsberg, L., Fyer, M., & Manning, D. (1991). Comorbidity among Axis II disorders. In J. Oldham (Ed.), *Personality disorders: New perspectives on diagnostic validity* (pp. 163–194). Washington, DC: American Psychiatric Press.

Widiger, T. A., Sanderson, C., & Warner, L. (1986). The MMPI prototypal typology ad borderline personality disorder. *Journal of Personality Assessment, 50,* 540–553.

Widiger, T. A., & Sankis, L. M. (2000). Adult psychopathology: Issues and controversies. *Annual Review of Psychology, 51,* 377–404.

Widiger, T. A., & Trull, T. J. (1991). Diagnosis and clinical assessment. *Annual Review of Psychology, 42,* 109–133.

Widiger, T. A., Trull, T. J., Clarkin, J. F., Sanderson, C., & Costa, P. T. (1994). A description of the DSM-III-R and DSM-IV personality disorders with the five-factor model of personality. In P. T. Costa & T. A. Widiger (Eds.), *Personality disorders and the five-factor model of personality* (pp. 41–56). Washington, DC: American Psychological Association Press.

Widiger, T. A., Trull, T. J., Hurt, Clarkin, J. F., & Frances, A. J. (1987). A multidimensional scaling of the DSM-III personality disorders. *Archives of General Psychiatry, 44,* 557–563.

Wiggins, J. S., & Pincus, A. L. (1989). Conceptions of personality disorder and dimensions of personality. *Psychological Assessment, 1,* 305–316.

Wood, A. L. (1969). Ideal and empirical typologies for research in deviance and control. *Sociology and Social Research, 53,* 227–241.

Zimmerman, M. (1994). Diagnosing personality disorders: A review of issues and research methods. *Archives of General Psychiatry, 51,* 225–242.

Zimmerman, M., & Coryell, W. (1990). Diagnosing personality disorder n the community: A comparison of self-report and interview measures. *Archives of General Psychiatry, 47,* 527–531.

CHAPTER 2

⬥

Theoretical Perspectives

THEODORE MILLON
SARAH E. MEAGHER
SETH D. GROSSMAN

The complex composition of personality and psychopathological disorders, and the diversity of practical approaches and frames of reference, call for a rigorous task of conceptualizing and organizing clinical data. Behaviorally, such disorders can be conceived and grouped as complex response patterns to environmental stimuli. Biophysically, they can be approached and analyzed as sequences of complex neural and chemical activity. Intrapsychically, they can be inferred and categorized as networks of entrenched unconscious processes that bind anxiety and conflict. Quite evidently, the complexity and intricacy of personological phenomena make it difficult not only to establish clear-cut relationships among phenomena but to find simple ways in which these phenomena can be classified or grouped. Should we artificially narrow our perspective to one data level to obtain at least a coherency of view? Or, should we trudge ahead with formulations which bridge domains but threaten to crumble by virtue of their complexity and potentially low internal consistency?

Psychologists still grapple with this intrinsically complex problem and have yet to manifest a completely satisfying approach to the vinculum of personality to psychopathology. In spite of a long history of brilliant cogitations, psychopathologic nosology still resembles Ptolemy's astronomy of over 2,000 years ago: Our diagnostic categories describe, but they do not

really explain. Like so many crystalline spheres, each lies in its own orbit, for the most part uncoordinated with the others. We do not know why the universe takes its ostensive form. There is no law of gravity which undergirds and binds our psychopathologic cosmos together. In fact, the word "cosmos" implies an intrinsic unity, a laudable ideal, which is not appropriate in its usage: Our "star charts," our DSMs, remain an aggregation of taxons, not a true taxonomy. Their reliability, but dubious validity, lends our field the illusion of science but not its substance. Such a state of affairs is simply unscientific.

Our most radical (albeit reactional) alternative would be to discard taxonomies altogether. This, of course, would be impossible, as a taxonomy serves indispensable clinical and scientific functions. Clinically, it provides a means of organizing pathological phenomena, the signs and symptoms or manifestations of mental disorder. By abstracting across persons, a taxonomy formalizes certain clinical commonalities and relieves the clinician of the burden of conceptualizing each patient *sui generis,* as an entity so existentially unique it has never been seen before nor ever will again. For psychopathology to be practiced at all, there cannot be as many groups as individuals. Even if the formal categories that constitute a taxonomy are but convenient fictions of dubious reality, some groups are better than no groups at all.

To be possessed of a fully comprehensive, scientific knowledge base about nature, it is crucial that a valid and reliable classification system represent it. We cannot be so presumptuous as to profess an ability to transcend the gulf between subject and object in a mutual absorption of mind and nature. Only the mystic might be able to make such a claim. Indeed, the very lure of mystical knowledge is that it is unmediated. Mysticism promises a direct mode of seeing, one that possesses an "absolute" quality difficult to argue with. Were such knowledge possible and readily available, science itself would be unnecessary. Mind and nature would be perfectly coordinated without need of intermediate representations and nomological linkages. In this sense, perhaps the most existentially disappointing aspect of religion is that there is more than one: The mystics have gone to the mountain and come back with different tales.

Despite any existential disenchantment, personological taxonomists may take a lesson from the mystic, both as a point of contrast and as a point of departure. This particular metaphor helps us realize and assert our goals: In short, we want what the mystic has (or says he has). We want a clear vision; we want freedom from confusion. Our greatest dream is one of almost mystical insight, wherein our representational blinders are removed and the inner essences of reality are revealed, for this chapter, the substantive structural and functional variables that comprise personology and its nexus with psychopathology.

Our scientific sensibilities, however, inform us that the actual mystical experience might not be all that we wish for. It almost invariably resists representation, perhaps actively so, proving ultimately too numinous and ineffable to articulate. Science, of course, cannot afford the luxury of being numinous and ineffable. Science depends on self-conscious knowledge. What is numinous to the mystic is vague to the scientist. Whereas the mystic comprehends nature in its totality as a radically open system of seamless unity, scientists must create artificially closed relational systems. We are wedded to representational systems, including taxonomies, so wedded in fact, that the abandonment of all representational schemas would be an abandonment of knowledge itself. In the best of all possible worlds, of course, we would have *both* the experience of true seeing *and* a representational system by which to articulate it. Such is the holy grail of a taxonomy of per-

sonality disorders, and only such a taxonomy "should be viewed as having objective existence in nature" (Hempel, 1965), as carving nature at its joints or affording a sense of communion that goes beyond intervening variables and construct systems, the only true validity, that which comes from an intuition of nature as it is. Scientifically borne thinking within such a taxonomy might never become conscious of the representational aspect; the taxonomy would be completely transparent. Whether such a taxonomy exists or whether it must remain an ideal that all actual taxonomies will fall short of in various degrees, only just such a taxonomy will prove ultimately scientifically satisfying for the personality disorders and ultimately satisfying to the researchers and clinicians who must work inside it.

We continue our theme of examining intentions throughout this chapter. Our assumptions about the nature of the world seem to prescribe our methods of investigation as well as what we ordain to be truth or fiction. We argue that only a theoretical approach is prepared to reveal the "essential entities" which have "objective existence" in nature called personality disorders. In one way or another, our discussion returns to the issue of the comorbidity of the personality disorders. Much of the research and commentary that been addressed to the problems of Axis II of late concerns comorbidity, so an investigation of the assumptions underlying this area of contention is potentially illuminating. The prevailing view is that comorbidity is a great evil, as if any at all were too much. This view is backed up by empirical research which shows that many patients are diagnosed with four or more personality disorders. More troublesome, as we lack the direct knowledge of the mystic, we cannot be sure whether this enigmatic state of affairs is an intrinsic feature of the personologic domain itself or whether it is a by-product of intervening variables. In any case, such a bounty of descriptors seems to undermine the validity of any one descriptor.

THE CHARACTERISTICS OF PERSONALITY CONCEPTS

How do we go about investigating personologic phenomena? Should we adhere to the time-tested rules of common sense, continuously and painstakingly refining our measures and methods until we are virtually infallible? Or should we explore innovative new concepts that will partition the personological realm in ways that are more theoretically and clinically fruitful? One option would be to anchor personological phenomena directly in the empirical world of observables in a one-to-one fashion, tying each attribute to only one indicator. Each attribute would then be its mode of measurement, possessing no information beyond that contained in the procedure itself, akin to *operational definitions* (Bridgeman, 1927).

Operational definitions are quite pleasingly precise but considerably limited in scope. Ultimate empirical precision can only be achieved if every defining feature that distinguishes a taxon is anchored to a single observable in the real world; that is, a different datum for every difference observed between personality syndromes. This goal is simply not feasible or desirable: The subject domain of personology is inherently more weakly organized than that of the so-called hard sciences. As one moves from physics and chemistry into biological and psychological arenas, unidirectional causal pathways give way to feedback and feedforward processes, which in turn give rise to emergent levels of description that are more inferential than the physical substrates that underlie them. Intrapsychic formulations, for example, require that the clinician transcend the level of the merely observable. Owing to their abstract and hypothetical character, these indeterminate and intervening concepts are known as *open concepts* (Pap, 1953).

The polar distinction between operational definitions (the paradigm of those who prefer to employ data derived from empirical–practical contexts) and open concepts (those whose ideas are derived from a more causal–theoretical stance) represents in part an epistemological continuum of conceptual specificity to conceptual openness (Millon, 1987). Each end of this polarity embraces a compromise between scope and precision. The virtue of each hides its vices. The advantage of operationism is obvious: Personality syndromes and the attributes of which they are composed are rendered unambiguous. Diagnostic identifications are directly translatable into measurement procedures, maximizing precision. However, the direct mapping of attributes to measurement procedures required ignores the biases incumbent to any one procedure, so that operationism is fatally deficient in scope.

The "open concept" model, likewise, has its own advantage: Open concepts acknowledge the desirability of multiple measurement procedures and encourage their user to move freely in more abstract and inferential realms. Each open concept can be embedded in a theoretical matrix or network from which its meaning is derived through its relations with other open concepts, with only indirect reference to explicit observables. The disadvantage is that open concepts may become so circuitous in their references that they become tautological and completely decoupled from observables. No doubt clarity gets muddled and deductions become tautological in statements such as "in the borderline the mechanisms of the ego disintegrate when libidinous energies overwhelm superego introjections." In such formulations, the scope of a theory overwhelms the testability of its empirical linkages, rendering precision zero.

Due to simple pragmatism, all scientific models, being simplifications of nature, must reach a compromise between scope and precision. We are not yet mystics at the beginning of a science: Unlike the individually borne thinking in a taxonomy which carves nature at its joints, we are acutely conscious that the relations among our naive representations are not those intrinsic to the subject domain itself. No one today would seriously put Hippocrates's humoral theory forward as a model of personality syndromes. Instead, such formulations resemble the more or less unrefined and often self-contradictory knowledge of common sense than the well-criticized and well-corroborated knowledge of science. As disputable as common sense is, it is nevertheless the point of departure for scientific knowledge (Pepper, 1942) and a source of commonsense taxonomies. Hempel (1965) framed this progression in terms of stages:

> The development of a scientific discipline may often be said to proceed from an initial "natural history" stage ... to more and more theoretical stages, in which increasing emphasis is placed upon the attainment of comprehensive theoretical accounts of the empirical subject matter under investigation. The vocabulary required in the early stages of this development will be largely observational: It will be chosen so as to permit the description of those aspects of the subject matter which are ascertainable fairly directly by observation. The shift toward systematization is marked by the introduction of new, "theoretical" terms, which refer to various theoretically postulated entities, their characteristics, and the processes in

which they are involved; all these are more or less removed from the level of directly observable things and events.

These terms have a distinct meaning and function only in the context of the corresponding theory. (pp. 139–140)

On an individual level, what distinguishes these two broad approaches? What does each individual scientist do to carry out his or her approach? Evidently, the theoretical approach is driven primarily by taking perspective on sense-near representations in order to discover underlying theoretic–causal relations from which a more coherent, internally corroborating system of constructs might be established. New constructs are generated, "more or less removed from the level of directly observable things and events." Some old ones are discarded, while others have their meaning sharpened or transformed as the system of relations is made more explicit. A process of reflection seems essential. Such representations are referred to as theoretical constructs, to reinforce their abstract origins in the mind of a reflective scientist.

Empiricism, however, tends to keep close to sense-near representations and holds theory as a dubious entity. The empiricist's vocabulary, then, remains "largely observational" (Hempel, 1965). As an ideal type, empirical preoccupations tend toward the progressive refinement of methods of observing of preexisting constructs, rather than the generation of new ones, toward ever greater agreement of man-with-man (interrater reliability), man-with-himself (reliability over occasions), and greater purity of observation (internal consistency).

Few members of the modern scientific community are naive empiricists, yet "no science embraced empiricism more wholeheartedly than psychology" (Kukla, 1989, p. 785). Moreover, some of the assumptions underlying empiricism are insidious and difficult to escape from, even when one ostensibly believes in the utility of theory. Foremost among criticisms is that the empiricism of common sense, naive realism, believes that the world it takes in is the world as it is. Commonsensical empiricism literally believes its constructs *are* the world. There is no reason to leave the security of immediate perception. Ultimately, this agenda rests on the assumption that theory-neutral data exist; that is, that one can know the world without transforming it. In the world view of radical empiricism, there are no mediating mental constructs to foul things up. If only it were so, then every act of observation would be an act of knowledge. Each small fact would present us with an objectivity, to be plucked from the world like fruit, collected as a hobby, or catalogued like microscope slides. Because naive empiricism remains unconscious of the potentially deceiving role of mental constructs, it believes itself to be carving nature at its joints just as it is. Naive empiricism, then, is really a false mysticism which breaches the gulf between subject and object by denying that any such gulf exists; it is a naive realism which believes that what you see is what you get.

THEORETICAL MODELS OF PERSONALITY DISORDER

Assuming one's temperament is oriented more toward theoretical explanation rather than empirical description, that is, that one's propensity runs more toward reflecting on the near-sense representations and propositions of common-sense as a means of refining them, how might one go about one's labors? Are there different kinds of theoretical approaches? If so, what are the potential benefits of each for producing a taxonomy of personality disorders? Is a synthesis possible, such that the strengths of each might be combined in coherent framework? How does each regard the comorbidity or codiagnosis of personality disorders?

Two kinds of theory must be distinguished. Again, the distinction is one concerning the scope of inquiry, whether a single or a few diagnostic categories are addressed, here referred to as a monotaxonic orientation, or whether the entire domain of personality pathology is parsed in its entirety, here referred to as a polytaxonic orientation. The former orientation is primarily concerned with a single taxonomic unit of analysis, whether categorical, dimensional, circumplical segment, or DSM hierarchic cluster; however, its core feature is that it does not attempt to bring order to the entire personality milieu but, rather, limits its aspirations.

The Monotaxonic Theoretical Model

The within-category theoretical orientation is probably what comes to mind when most people think about theory or testing a theory. Because it is limited in scope, it is primarily concerned with the essential elements that eventuate in and sustain a particular kind of personality pattern. In its most impressive longitudinal incarnation, models for personality pathology produced by this approach may be explicated through diagrams and flowcharts that detail the developmental history of the disorder, complete with the inputs of various factors that predispose or immunize against the disorder along the way. Alternately, it may develop as a stage model, with pathology representing the regression to earlier stages of development, as in the oral character, the anal character, and so on.

While this approach potentially leads to gains in precision, it tends to be somewhat deficient in scope. Because the intention is to understand the origins of pathology, it tends to accept whatever categories are given it and then account for the developmental origin of these pathologies. There is a tendency to parse the particular personality pattern in terms of a single-area clinical domain, whether behavioral, phenomenological, intrapsychic, or biophysical. The classical view of narcissism, for example, contends that it is the result of developmental arrests or regressions to earlier periods of fixation. An important elaborator of the narcissism construct is Kohut (1971). Kohut does not challenge the content as such but, rather, the sequence of libidinal maturation, which, he believed, has its own developmental line and sequence of continuity into adulthood. That is, it does not fade away by becoming transformed into object–libido, as contended by classical theorists, but unfolds into its own set of mature narcissistic processes and structures. Pathology occurs as a consequence of failures to integrate one of the two major spheres of self-maturation, the "grandiose self" and the "idealized parent imago." If they are disillusioned, are rejected, or experience cold and unempathic care at the earliest stages of self-development, serious pathology, such as psychotic or borderline states, will occur. Trauma or disappointment at a later phase will have somewhat different repercussions depending on whether the difficulty centered on the development of the grandiose self or the parental imago.

What is notable is that Kohut's is a developmental theory of self and not a personality characterization. Indeed, it is difficult to see how such developmental models could ever give rise to the kind of taxonomies of scope needed for the DSMs. Thus, while this kind of theoretical approach may illuminate the developmental origins of personality pathology, though almost certainly with some bias as to domains of content, the monotaxonic theoretical approach works best when it is not held to account for why certain individuals have been segregated into a particular pattern of disorders in the first place; it needs to be given its pathology to begin with; it is *nongenerative* with respect to categories of personality pathology.

Theories that bridge multiple clinical domains are far fewer, perhaps because any attempt to do so seeks the assimilation of elements which to some extent intrinsically resist unification—otherwise they could not be thought of as existing as domains at all. Accordingly, these models also tend to be reductionistic in the sense that while all these domains are of an integrated organism, only one area is focused on at a time. Relevant manifestations of pathology from other areas tend to be reduced to operations in that one. Often this kind of reductionism is passive rather than active—that is, other domains are passively ignored. As a result, the same diagnostic term, anchored exclusively to one domain, may acquire diverse connotations. Of course, organismic domains have been with us much longer than relatively well-developed taxonomies such as the DSMs. Sometimes these domains themselves are responsible, perhaps not for the very origin of terms but for elaborating them to such an extent that they have been recruited as diagnostic labels and thus have become potentially more multireferential in scope, taking on nuances of meaning far removed from that of their original elaborators.

The Polytaxonic Theoretical Model

The monotaxonic theoretical orientation seeks to explain the origins of personality pathology, but typically it must be given its raw material, the disorder of interest, first, and work backward from there. Can a complete science rest on such a foundation? Is it enough merely to accept some external consensus concerning which constellations of traits are problematic? While the periodic table is the unique province of chemistry, the problematic behaviors which are to be carved up into diagnostic categories are often given to psychopathologists by parties whose standards are extrinsic to psychopathology as a science. The polytaxonic approach, however, asks that categories of personality pathology account for themselves, by persistently asking, "Why these categories rather than others?"

Philosophers of science agree that the system of kinds undergirding any domain of inquiry must itself be answerable to the question that forms the very point of departure for the scientific enterprise: Why does nature take this particular form rather than some other? Accordingly, one cannot merely accept any list of kinds or dimensions as given, even if arrived at by committee consensus. Instead, a taxonomic scheme must be justified, and to be justified scientifically, it must be justified theoretically. Taxonomy and theory, then, are intimately linked. Quine (1977) makes a parallel case:

> One's sense of similarity or one's system of kinds develops and changes . . . as one matures. . . . And at length standards of similarity set in which are geared to theoretical science. The development is away from the immediate, subjective, animal sense of similarity to the remoter objectivity of a similarity determined by scientific hypotheses . . . and constructs. Things are similar in the later or theoretical sense to the degree that they are . . . revealed by science. (p. 171)

Is such a taxonomy possible? The stakes are nothing less than whether personology is to possess its own intrinsic taxonomy or remain a pseudo-science which services the larger society, establishing diagnostic standards according to extrinsic standards. Perhaps we live in a more enlightened age, but was it not so long ago that Sullivan proposed the "homosexual personality"? Or that the "masochistic personality" came under fire as being prejudicial against women? Although the DSM was deliberately and appropriately formulated atheoretically in order not to alienate special interest groups among psychological consumers, ultimately we require some way of culling the wheat from the chaff which depends on scientific necessity rather than decision by committee.

The deductive approach generates a true taxonomy to replace the primitive aggregation of taxons which preceded it. This generative power is what Hempel (1965) meant by the "systematic import" of a scientific classification. Meehl (1978) has noted that theoretical systems comprise related assertions, shared terms, and coordinated propositions that provide fertile grounds for deducing and deriving new

empirical and clinical observations. What is elaborated and refined in theory, then, is understanding, an ability to see relations more clearly, to conceptualize categories more accurately, and to create greater overall coherence in a subject, that is, to integrate its elements in a more logical, consistent, and intelligible fashion. Pretheoretical taxonomic boundaries that were set according to clinical intuition and empirical study can now be affirmed and refined according to their constitution along underlying polarities. These polarities lend the model a holistic, cohesive structure which facilitates the comparison and contrast of groups along fundamental axes, thus sharpening the meanings of the taxonomic constructs derived.

CATEGORICAL VERSUS DIMENSIONAL FRAMEWORKS

Strictly speaking, categories and dimensions are taxonomic constructs, not models of personality. Usually, the idea of a model conjures up the work of some theorist, along with arguments to the effect that their pet variables or organizing principles constitute the framework through which personality should be organized and discussed. Not surprisingly, psychiatry has favored the so-called medical model of mental disorders, wherein personality disorders (as described in DSM-IV) are assumed to be categories of mental illness, with discrete boundaries between normality and pathology and between one personality and another. Psychologists, however, have usually eschewed categories, instead preferring to think in terms of dimensions, which allow a continuous gradient between normality and abnormality. In contrast, the layperson switches easily between categorical and dimensional modes. To the average person, the statement "You're so narcissistic!" is almost identical in meaning to "You're such a narcissist!" The first statement, however, locates the individual at the upper end of a continuous distribution, whereas the second states that the individual is exemplary of a particular type. In their everyday work, even professionals who strongly believe in the dimensional model often lapse into an implicitly categorical framework. A subject whose test profile has schizoid and compulsive as the highest scales may thus be described as a "schizoid compulsive." Here, the entire personality profile is distilled into two words and rendered as a type, as if other scales were irrelevant.

Categorical Frameworks

The idea that personalities come in types is probably the most basic model of personality possible, the model of naive commonsense, as in "What personality type are you?" Essentially, it reflects the simple belief that there are things in the world, and that these things sort themselves into various kinds, extended to the realm of human beings. In this prescientific conception, personality is essentially a substance which fills the vessel of the person, static and internally undifferentiated. Were this model true, various "sections" of the mind would be homogeneous all the way through. There is no dynamism, no speculation about the relationships between various structures of the mind (i.e., no "topographic model," as Freud used the term). Moreover, anything can be considered a type; thus there are potentially as many types as there are individuals to be typed. In casual usage, a pensive type is just as plausible as a melancholy type. This gives the idea of types great currency, because kinds can be invented as needed and adapted to any individual person. Everyone can be classified. There are no residual cases. Modern classification systems, which inevitably include a "not otherwise specified" (NOS) category, cannot say as much. However, the scope of casual usage is exactly what makes it prescientific: No rational basis is set forward to constrain the number of types. The first order of business in graduating from the natural history stage of commonsense observation, then, is to ask which types are fundamental and which are spurious. Three directions have been pursued to answer this question.

First, a theory of personality can be advanced. If our budding scientist is asked why this particular constellation of types exists rather than some other, the reply is that these are preferred because they are anchored to a theory, and that the theory provides a means of understanding the relation of the types both to each other and in terms of the deeper principles on which the theory rests. Many famous figures in the history of psychology have followed this direction. Whatever its real merit, the idea of the oral, anal, phallic, and genital characters represents an effort to derive a system of types from a model of psychosexual development.

Likewise, Sheldon (Sheldon & Stevens, 1942) and Kretschmer (1922) developed the idea of the somatotype, classifying individuals in accordance with physical principles as ectomorphs, mesomorphs, or endomorphs. Such types assume a special status because of their link to theory, which ultimately underwrites their very reality. Unfortunately, establishing some constraint on the number of types also introduces another problem. No matter how compelling a particular system of types may be, some individuals are not readily described within the system. Such persons are a nagging reminder that all theories are but partial views and will not fruitfully apply to all instances.

Second, experts in a particular area can be brought together with the formal purpose of deciding among themselves which types the science will address. This is the direction pursued by DSM-IV, and it has its own advantages and shortcomings. On the one hand, the agreement of seasoned experts is to be preferred to naive common sense. Moreover, requiring consensus from a body of diverse experts ensures that no one theoretical statement can foreclose further speculation and investigation before a more complete, and presumably more valid, theory can be formulated. DSM has yet to officially endorse a set of principles that would relate the Axis II constructs to each other and allow them to be understood in terms of deeper principles. Because it is arbitrated by committee, not derived through a coherent theory or the systematic application of a methodology, DSM cannot completely free itself from its prescientific heritage. Committee consensus does forestall anarchy by putting the official constructs under oligarchical control, but consensus is a means of governing, not a scientific explanation. In the DSM-IV deliberations, for example, sadistic personality disorder was dropped in part because it was seldom diagnosed in most clinical settings (Fiester & Gay, 1991). We might ask, however, whether the composition of a taxonomy is to be decided by base rates, that is, by the frequency with which a disorder appears. Chemistry has its periodic table of elements, whereas physics has what is known as the standard model. Both recognize as fundamental taxa elements and particles which are never found in nature but only in the course of experimentation. Some of these exist only for exceedingly brief moments, perhaps less than a thousandth of a second. Yet, it is precisely the effort to account for these rare entities that has been instrumental in driving the science of particle physics forward. Apparently, physicists have yet to appreciate the utility of a category such as esoteric particles NOS.

The third and most sophisticated modern development in the categorical tradition is taxometrics (Meehl, 1995; Meehl & Golden, 1982). Taxometrics explores the ontological aspects of the concept of type; that is, how a type, should it exist, would be manifest, and what methods might be used to discover it and refine its detection. When it is suspected that a pathology may be categorical in nature, taxometrics is appropriate. The methodology was developed by Meehl, mainly in conjunction with his theory of schizophrenia and the identification of what are termed "schizotaxics," individuals who possess a genetic predisposition to the development of schizophrenia but may or may not remain compensated (Meehl, 1962), depending on environmental stressors. Meehl emphasized the heterogeneity of schizophrenia, the fact that interpersonal aversiveness, language abberations, and eye-tracking disturbances all occur together empirically but without a psychologically compelling reason to do so. Taxometrics is thus intended to evaluate taxonicity on the basis of multiple indicators that co-occur with poor face validity within a particular diagnostic class but remain largely uncorrelated in other persons. Cutting scores may be derived to classify subjects into catgories on the basis of available indicators, and other indicators may be added to bootstrap the classification system to successively higher levels of validity. Meehl (1995) thus argues that taxometrics solves a chronic problem in history of psychopathology, the absence of a reliable and valid diagnostic criterion. Potentially, its widespread use could replace the use of committees in determining diagnostic standards.

Dimensional Frameworks

Whereas the categorical model holds that there are discrete boundaries between normality and pathology, and between various personality types, the dimensional model holds instead that personality characteristics are expressed on a continuous gradient. At the prescientific level of common sense, the unit of analysis in the dimensional model is the personality trait, and there are literally thousands of personality traits. In contrast to terms used to describe psychological *states,* such as mad, happy, and angry, *traits* describe enduring characteristics of the person that are stable across time and situational context. Examples would include such terms as "gregarious," "arrogant," "thoughtless," or "helpful" (many terms are used to describe both states and traits, a source of ambiguity and confusion in our discipline). In addition, while types tend to be mutually exclusive, so that an individual cannot be classified within two personality types simultaneously, dimensions readily coexist. Taxonomy and person reverse priority, so that the classification system is literally put inside the person, who receives some score on each trait dimension of the system. Because everyone can be thus dimensionalized, there are no residual cases. Traits thus form a rich vocabulary through which any given person can be described. As before, the problem is to cull from an overwhelming multitude of traits only those that are psychologically fundamental and therefore might serve as a scientific basis for a taxonomy of personality and its disorders.

THEORY VERSUS METHODOLOGY

Theory and methodology form two fundamentally different ways of determining which personality contents are fundamental. Theoretical models usually seek principles that underlie an entire perspective, which is assumed to organize the contents of all other personality domains, which are then cast as peripheral or derivative. Interpersonal theorists, for example, see interpersonal conduct as basic to the development of personality. In contrast, cognitive theorists would argue that because internal cognitive structures always mediate perception, interpretation, and communication, cognitive theory is the best candidate for an integrative model. And herein lies a principal problem with theoretical approaches to personality: the tendency to reject essential aspects of experience or behavior.

In contrast, methodologically driven models resist making a priori theoretical commitments and so are free to address any domain of personality for which data are available. First, the universe of personality descriptors is sampled according to some definition of personality. Second, persons may be asked to rate themselves on the resulting of list of traits, called external ratings, or to somehow rate the degree to which different terms are similar to each other, called internal ratings. Third, factor analysis, a multivariate statistical technique which extracts from an observed pattern of correlations a much smaller number of dimensions, is applied in order to telescope hundreds of traits into a parsimonious handful of higher-order dimensions. The researcher may have no a priori notion about what dimensions will emerge. Such rationales can be generated at a later date. Structure and sufficiency are thus offered in compensation for lack of a compelling theory.

Factor models provide well-developed examples of an inductive–dimensional approach to personality and have a number of appealing and interrelated features that form a neat package. First, factor models assume there is no sharp division between normality and pathology, only a smooth unbroken gradation. In contrast, Axis II has been criticized as being archaically categorical (Widiger, 1993). Second, factor models are almost always sufficient, meaning that the model accounts for most of the variation in the data set from which it is developed. The correlation matrix of variables is factored until negligible "residual variance" remains, so that sufficiency is an automatic product of the methodology. Third, where the factors are extracted to be uncorrelated, cognitive economy is further maximized, as the majority of traits are linked to only one factor. DSM, in contrast, assumes that some disorders may have several traits in common, as evidenced by their overlapping criteria sets. Fourth, factor models are almost always parsimonious, extracting between three and seven factors regardless of the variables factored (Block, 1995). This leads to a fifth promise, the idea that a factor model might serve as a coherent taxonomy to which all personality psychology can be anchored, thus providing an organizing force for future research. Sixth, because factor models are explicitly constructed to telescope almost all the variance in a particular domain into a handful of dimensions, they necessarily maximize the possibility of finding statistically significant relationships between some measure of the resulting factors and variables in adjacent domains of study. In contrast, the DSM personality disorders constructs exist only within the realm of pathology, with no official endorsement of more normal variants that might encourage their application within related fields. And finally, factor models are explicitly mathematical and provide some assurance that the fuzzy domain of the social sciences can be quantified

like the harder sciences of chemistry and physics. For its appealing features, it has nevertheless proven extremely difficult within the factor tradition to specify exactly which dimensions should be considered fundamental. Many proponents have concluded that five dimensions are sufficient to account for personality but disagree about the substance of these five, particularly the nature of the fifth and slimmest factor. Goldberg (1993), for example, has sought to distinguish the Big Five model derived from the lexical tradition from the five-factor model of Costa and McCrae (1992). Interested readers are referred to John, Angleitner, and Ostendorf (1988), Digman (1990), John (1990), and Goldberg (1993) for a complete history of these approaches.

As Quine (1977) noted in his discussion of natural kinds, the basis on which a system of kinds is founded and explicated, our attachment to a taxonomy loosens in favor of the underlying principles. After all, it was these very underlying principles which allowed the deduction of the taxonomy in the first place. Those who are familiar with the deductive personologic taxonomy developed by Millon know, for example, that both the narcissistic and antisocial personalities are independent types in that both are oriented toward the self. What distinguishes them is primarily their orientation toward their ecological milieu. The narcissist is a passive–independent, the antisocial an active–independent type. Similarly, the dependent personality is a passive–dependent type, whereas the narcissist is a passive–independent type. What distinguishes them is primarily their orientation toward others versus an orientation toward self. Nevertheless, both narcissists and antisocials and narcissists and dependents share important characteristics.

In the deductive schema explicated by Millon (1981, 1990; Millon & Davis, 1996), the dependent, narcissistic, and antisocial types are deduced from underlying theoretical principles. Far from being orthogonal, then, measures which dimensionalize these types will be correlated *because* they reflect an intrinsic relationship predicted by the underlying principles. In fact, it is difficult to see how any set of categories which purports to lay claim to scientific necessity through a deductive framework might be dimensionalized and still remain orthogonal, as the deduced types will share common elements, whereas orthogonality is, by definition, the absence of relationship. The very generativity of a personological model which claims deductive scientific necessity is then encoded in the intercorrelations of measures of its derived categories. Accordingly, the task of personological science is to account for these intercorrelations, not to suppress them methodologically as done through factor analysis. Thus the antisocial type is often narcissistic, and the narcissist is also dependent.

Nor must these intercorrelations be confined to the personological domain. As noted, the multiaxial model has been structurally composed to require the explanation of the Axis I symptoms in the context of Axis II personality patterns. Explanation can only occur if some predictions are made. In other words, multiaxial explanation requires that the Axis I disorders will not be distributed randomly with respect to Axis II, because if distributed randomly, they would again be independent or orthogonal. If a theoretical model of personology is at all worth its salt, it should make some predictions about the way in which various personality styles dysfunction psychiatrically, or, in disease terms, make some predictions about the Axis I–Axis II comorbidity. Thus the generativity of a personological model with regard to Axis I symptoms will again be encoded in the intercorrelations of measures of Axis I disorders and Axis II personality patterns, often discussed as spectrum disorders when these intercorrelations are brought into the foreground.

Far from being a nuisance, then, correlations between diagnostic measures are highly desirable, if these correlations are expected clinically and can be explained theoretically. Significant correlations (dimensional framework) or dual diagnoses (categorical framework) between narcissistic and antisocial personality disorders, for example, should be expected. In fact, the absence of any such correlation would cause us to question the validity of the diagnostic system.

The disadvantage of this approach is that it requires a high degree of clinical and theoretical sophistication. Numerous questions must be answered at theoretical and statistical levels. Are the underlying principles from which the personological taxonomy derived cogent? Do they in fact allow one to understand clinical phenomena? Do they give a complete representation of the subject domain? Do they help explain why each personological type dysfunctions in some ways and not others? What degree of intercorrelation between the intervening variables which dimensionalize the theory-generated diagnostic types is desirable?

Given these complications and an empirical disposition, perhaps it is more pragmatic in the short run to work with statistically independent gauges extracted through a particular multivariate methodology, based on superficial similarities, such as the five-factor model. However, pragmatic virtues are not necessarily scientific, and only a theoretical approach can ultimately form a firm foundation for a science of clinical personology, one that explains rather than merely describes, one that explicates and gives logic to syndromal relationships rather than forcing them apart to meet archaic and undesirable goals.

THEORIES OF PERSONALITY DISORDER

Personality can be discussed from any number of perspectives. Major viewpoints include the psychodynamic, interpersonal, neurobiological, behavioral, and cognitive, but more esoteric conceptions could also be included, including the existential, phenomenological, cultural, and perhaps even religious. Even among the major perspectives, some offer only a particular set of concepts or principles, whereas others offer strongly structural models which generate entire taxonomies of personality and personality disorder constructs. Whatever their orientation, theorists within each perspective usually maintain that their content area is core or fundamental, drives the development of personality and its structure, and thus serves as the logical basis for the treatment of its disorders. In the earlier dogmatic era of historical systems, psychologists strongly wedded to a particular perspective would either assert that other points of view were peripheral to core processes or just ignore them. Behaviorists, for example, denied the existence of the mental constructs, including self and personality. In contrast, psychodynamic psychologists held that behavior is only useful as a means of inferring the properties and organization of various mental structures, namely the id, ego, and superego, and their "drive derivatives." Most authors probably take this stance for two reasons: First, history remembers only those who father or contribute significantly to the development of a particular point of view. There are no famous eclectics. Second, acknowledgments that other content areas might operate according to their own autonomous principles necessarily impugns the sufficiency of one's own approach. As a result, various perspectives have tended to develop to high states of internal consistency, the dogmatic schools of the history of psychology, and it is not at all clear how one model might falsify another or how two models might be put against one another experimentally.

Intrapsychically Based Theories

Before there were personality disorders, there were character pathologies. In colloquial usage, character refers to an individual's respect for moral or social conventions. In psychoanalytic usage, however, character refers to the "the habitual mode of bringing into harmony the tasks presented by internal demands and by the external world" by the ego (Fenichel, 1945, p. 467). Although Freud's writings focused mainly on the psychosexual roots of specific and narrowly circumscribed symptoms, such as compulsions or conversions, he did suggest that character classification might be based on the structural model of id, ego, and superego (Freud, 1915). In 1931 he sought to devise character types determined by which intrapsychic structure was dominant (Freud, 1931). The erotic type was governed by the instinctual demands of the id. The narcissistic type was dominated by the ego, so much so that neither other persons nor the id or superego could influence them. The compulsive type was regulated by a strict superego that dominated all other functions. Finally, Freud identified a series of mixed types, combinations in which two of the three intrapsychic structures outweighed the third.

The foundations for an analytic characterology were set forth by Karl Abraham (1921/1927; 1924/1927a; 1924/1927b) in accord with Freud's psychosexual stages of development. Certain personality traits are believed to be associated with frustrations or indulgences during these stages. For example, the oral period is differentiated into an oral-sucking phase and an oral-biting phase. An overly indulgent sucking stage yields an oral–dependent type, imperturbably optimistic and naively self-assured. Happy-go-lucky and emotionally immature, serious matters do not affect them. An ungratified sucking period yields excessive dependency and gullibility as deprived children learn to "swallow" anything just to ensure they receive something. Frustrations at the oral-biting stage yield aggressive oral tendencies such as sarcasm and verbal hostility in adulthood. These "oral–sadistic characters" are inclined to pessimistic distrust, cantankerousness, and petulance. In the anal stage, children learn control. Their increasing cognitive abilities allow them to comprehend parental expectancies, with the option of either pleasing or spoiling parental desires. "Anal characters" take quite different attitudes toward authority depending on whether resolution occurs during the anal-expulsive or anal-retentive period. The anal-expulsive period is associated with tendencies toward suspiciousness, extreme conceit and ambitiousness, self-assertion, disorderliness, and negativism. Difficulties that emerge in the late anal, or anal-retentive, phase are usually associated with frugality, obstinacy, and orderliness, a hairsplitting meticulousness, and rigid devotion to societal rules and regulations.

With the writings of Wilhelm Reich in 1933, the concept of character was expanded. Reich held that the neurotic solution of psychosexual conflicts was accomplished through a total restructuring of the defensive style, ultimately crystalizing into a "total formation" called character armor. The emergence of specific pathological symptoms now assumed secondary importance, because the impact of early instinctual vicissitudes was no longer limited to symptom formation but now included the genesis of character itself. Nevertheless, Reich's ideas remained firmly ensconced in the conflict model and did not specify nondefensive ways in which character traits or structures might develop. Character formations, according to Reich, have an exclusively defensive function, forming an inflexible armor against threats from the external and internal world. Reich extended Abraham's developments to the phallic and genital stages. In the phallic stage, libidinal impulses normally directed toward the opposite sex may become excessively self-oriented. Frustration leads to a striving for leadership, a need to stand out in a group, and poor reactions to even minor defeats. This "phallic narcissistic character" was depicted as vain, brash, arrogant, self-confident, vigorous, cold, reserved, and defensively aggressive.

Modern thinkers (e.g., Kernberg, 1996) regard the psychosexual types to be of value mainly for less severe personality disorders. More severe personality disorders effectively mix aspects from all stages of psychosexual development, thus limiting the heuristic value of any psychosexual characterology. For example, oral conflicts are valuable in understanding the depressive–masochistic personality, while anal conflicts are valuable in understanding the obsessive–compulsive personality. Neither of these personality disorders, however, is considered severe, and the translation of psychosexual conflict into personality type is fairly straightforward. In contrast, individuals functioning at what is termed the "borderline level of personality organization," which includes the paranoid, antisocial, and some narcissistic personalities, variously combine aspects from all psychosexual stages. Prior to the 1950s, such patients were variously labeled as suffering borderline states, or as being psychotic characters, or as ambulatory or pseudoneurotic schizophrenics. Eventually, the idea of a borderline personality was created to fill the gulf between the neuroses and psychoses, particularly schizophrenia.

Kernberg (1984, 1996) advocates classifying various personalities types, some from DSM and some from the psychoanalytic tradition, in terms of three levels of structural organization: psychotic, borderline, and neurotic. Understanding this framework requires some knowledge of the basic principles of contemporary psychoanalysis. The psychoanalytic conception of normality provides a useful point of departure (Kernberg, 1996). Normal personalities are characterized by a cohesive and integrated sense of self which psychoanalysts term "ego identity." Simply put, most of us know who we are, and our sense of self remains constant over time and situation. We know our likes and dislikes, are conscious of certain core values, and know how we are similar to, and yet different from, others. Ego identity is thus fundamental to self-esteem and to the pursuit and realization of long-term life goals and desires. We must know who we are to like ourselves, or to know what we want to become. Likewise, ego identity provides a foundation for intimacy, genuineness, commitment, empathy, and the ability to make valid social appraisals. We cannot know others, or know how others feel, unless we know how they compare and contrast with ourselves. Individuals with a well-integrated ego identity are said to possess ego strength, the ability of remain integrated in the face of pressures from internal drives and affects and external social forces. In addition, normal persons also possess an integrated and mature internalization of social or moral value systems, the

superego. Some pathological personalities, particularly the narcissistic and antisocial, exhibit a lack of superego development, whereas others exhibit an immature and all-condemning superego, reflecting the internalization of harsh parental discipline or abuse. In contrast, normal mature superego development features a stable value system which includes such features as personal responsibility and appropriate self-criticism. Finally, the ego integration and superego capacities of normal persons allow the management of the basic drives of the analytic perspective, sex and aggression, to be integrated with tender affections and commitment.

Behavior-Based Theories

The duality between empiricism and rationalism has a long history in philosophy and psychology. Empiricism is most often identified with the English philosophers John Locke and David Hume. Locke emphasized the role of direct experience in knowledge, believing that knowledge must be built up from collections of sensations. Locke's position became known as associationism. Here, learning is seen as occurring through a small collection of processes which associate one sensation with another. Empiricism found a counterpoint in the rationalism of continental philosophers, notably the Dutch philosopher Spinoza, the French philosopher Descartes, and the German philosopher Leibniz. In contrast, the empiricists held that innate ideas could not exist. Locke, for example, maintained that the mind was a *tabula rasa,* or blank slate, on which experience writes. Eventually, however, the elements of learning were recast in the language of stimulus and response. The foundations of behaviorism are perhaps more associated with J. B. Watson than with any other psychologist, though Watson was preceded by other important figures in the history of learning theory, notably Thorndike and Pavlov. Although a variety of learning theories eventually developed, behaviorism as a formal dogma is most associated with the views of B. F. Skinner. According to Skinner's strict behaviorism, it is unnecessary to posit the existence of unobservable emotional states or cognitive expectancies to account for behavior and its pathologies. Hypothetical inner states are discarded and explanations are formulated solely in terms of external sources of stimulation and reinforcement. Thus, all disorders become the simple product of environmentally based reinforcing experiences. These shape the behavioral repertoire of the individual, and differences between adaptive and maladaptive behaviors can be traced entirely to differences in the reinforcement patterns to which individuals are exposed.

By the mid-1980s a number of crucial reinterpretations of traditional assessment had been made which allowed clinically applied behavioral approaches to become successively broader and more moderate. Most notably, the diagnoses of Axis I, regarded in psychiatry as substantive disease entities, were reinterepreted with the behavioral paradigm as inductive summaries, labels which bind together a body of observations for the purpose of clinical communication. For example, while depression refers to a genuine pathology in the person for a traditional clinician, a behavioral clinician sees only its operational criteria and their label, not a disease. As a result, behavioral assessment and traditional assessment could thus speak the same tongue while retaining their respective identities and distinctions. This allowed behavioral therapists to rationalize their use of diagnostic concepts without being untrue to their behavioral core. Likewise, as the cognitive revolution got under way in earnest in the late 1960s and early 1970s, behavioral psychologists began seeking ways to generalize their own perspective in order to bring cognition under the behavioral umbrella. In time, cognitive activity was reinterpreted as covert behavior. Finally, the organism itself began to be seen a source of reinforcement and punishment, with affective mechanisms being viewed as the means through which reinforcement occurs. Contemporary behavioral assessment, then, is no longer focused merely on surface behavior. Instead, behavioral assessment is now seen as involving three "response systems," namely the verbal–cognitive mode, the affective–physiological mode, and the overt–motor response system, a scheme originated by Lang (1968).

Interpersonally Based Theories

In the previous section, personality was discussed from the behavioral perspective as a patterning of behavioral acts. Although there is no one behaviorism, several core features can nevertheless be summarized. First, behaviorism is contextual. The emphasis is on situations and the stimulus properties of situations which control behavior. No inferences are made about internal dispositions or personality traits. Second, behaviorism is positivistic in the sense that it is focused on events or responses which are circumscribed in time. Third, behaviorism is idiographic. The unique sequence of situations to which any individual is exposed creates unique patterns of behavior, both normal and pathological.

In contrast, the interpersonal domain argues that personality is best conceptualized as the social product of interactions with significant others. For behavioral psychologists, psychology is the study of behavior. For interpersonalists, behavior is simply one level of information, the raw data from which more complex inferences should be made. Although behavior is certainly constrained by the properties of situations, these properties cannot be objectively specified apart from their interpersonal significance. All situations possess a distinctly human import and, so, are best conceptualized through principles of human interaction. Few of our needs can be satisfied, our goals reached, or our potentials fulfilled in a nonsocial world. Even when we are alone, interpersonal theorists argue, the internal representations of significant others continue to populate our mental landscape and guide our actions. We are always, then, transacting either with real others or with our expectations about them. Frances (quoted in Benjamin, 1993) states that "the essence of being a mammal . . . is the need for, and to ability to participate in, interpersonal relationships. The interpersonal dance begins at least as early as birth and ends only with death. Virtually all of the most important events in life are interpersonal in nature and most of what we call personality is interpersonal in expression" (p. v). Work in the interpersonal domain has developed in two distinct but interdependent directions (Pincus, 1994), interpersonal theory and the interpersonal circumplex.

The circumplex first debuted in an article by Freedman, Leary, Ossorio, and Coffey (1951) and was then further developed by Timothy Leary (1957). These theorists crossed two orthogonal dimensions, dominance–submission and hostility–affection (also called love–hate and communion), creating an interpersonal circle further divided into eight segments or themes, each representing a different mix of the two fundamental variables. The dependent, for example, was represented as consisting of approximately equal levels of affection and submission, while the compulsive, which Leary called the responsible–hypernormal, consisted of approximately equal levels of affection and dominance. The four quadrants of the circumplex, Leary suggested, parallel the temperaments or humors of Hippocrates, while the axes of the circle parallel Freud's two basic drives. Each segment of the circle was further differentiated into a relatively normal region, closer to the center, and a relatively pathological region, closer to the edge. Thus, the circumplex may be used not only to generate a taxonomy of personality traits but also to represent continuity between normality and pathology. The most radical development of interpersonal theory is Benjamin's (1974, 1993) Structural Analysis of Social Behavior (SASB), which integrates interpersonal conduct, object relations, and self psychology in a single geometric model. Benjamin's point of departure lies in the synthesis of Leary's classic interpersonal circle with Earl Schaefer's (1965) circumplex of parental behavior. As every parent knows, there is a fundamental tension between controlling and guiding children and allowing them to gradually become masters of their own destiny. Parents must either let their children grow up to become genuinely mature beings who realize their own intrinsic potentials along a unique developmental path or else demand submission and deny autonomy, effectively making the child an extension of the parent. Schaefer's model thus places autonomy giving at the opposite of control, not submission, as with the Leary circle. The horizontal axis, however, remains the same.

Cognitively Based Theories

The cognitive view is extremely popular. Almost all clinical syndromes possess cognitive elements, and surveys show that cognitive therapy is widely practiced among clinicians. When viewed more broadly, the cognitive focus may be seen as being essentially identical with the information-processing perspective, so that cognitive models may be highly operationalized and flowcharted. Verbal sources of data feature prominently in cognitive therapies, but only as the final common pathway of beliefs and assumptions, perceptual distortions, heuristic biases, and automatic thoughts that occur across all levels of awareness. The beginning of the DSM-IV definition of personality traits as "enduring patterns of perceiving, relating to, and thinking about the environment and oneself" (p. 630) acknowledges the central role of cognition in these constructs. The cognitive perspective follows the general plan of science, seeking to explain a diversity of instances through the application of a small number of simple rules. Trait theorists, for example, explain individuality in terms of a few personality dimensions, the five-factor model being only one example. Chemists explain the behavior of molecules as combinations of a few chemical elements. Similarly, cognitive therapists hold internal cognitive structures and processes that mediate and explain behavior. Among these structures, the schema holds a particularly prominent place. Given its focus on processes, personality is naturally understood as a tenacious collection of interrelated schemas. Schematic change thus promises potentially sweeping change in a great many problematic behaviors. This provides a point of contrast between the behavioral and cognitive perspectives: For behavioral therapists, assessment and therapy operate at the same level of information. The behaviors assessed are the very behaviors eventually treated. In contrast, cognitive assessment and therapy occur at two different levels. Assessment is conducted at the level of behavior, but the nature of the inquiry is guided by cognitive theory, which seeks to uncover the maladaptive beliefs, attributions, and other appraisal processes that cause maladaptive behavior. Therapeutic change occurs not at the level of individual behaviors but at the level of core cognitive structures. Cognitive therapy seeks to preserve the rigor of behaviorism but nevertheless maintains that the raw flux of behavior must be ordered in some logical fashion if its significance for personality therapy and change is to be understood.

Although cognitive psychology would seem to be the natural foundation for theory and research on the role of cognitive constructs in the personality disorders, this has not been the case. Instead, theoretical speculation and research has come mostly from those involved in cognitive therapy. In turn, cognitive therapy, like the rest of psychotherapy, has developed almost independently semiautonomously from its natural pure science foundation, here cognitive psychology. Ideally, cognitive therapy would thus grow naturally from a pure science foundation, much as engineering grows naturally from its foundation in physics. The still expanding number of psychotherapies provides ample proof that the applied branches of our discipline need not be strongly coupled to a pure science foundation to become progressively more variegated. For example, Aaron Beck is without a doubt a seminal figure in the history of psychotherapy. Almost every book about cognitive therapy written by Beck or his associates includes a paragraph that states that cognitive therapy began in the mid-1950s when Beck was searching for empirical support for the psychodynamic theory of depression. Beck believed the theory was correct but found that depressed subjects, far from having a masochistic need to suffer, actually embraced experiences of success (Alford & Beck, 1997). No mention is made of the cognitive revolution that was occurring simultaneously, or that it influenced Beck's thinking in the least.

Nevertheless, Beck and his associates have been particularly successful in developing cognitive therapies for a wide range of Axis I disorders (Beck, 1976; Beck, Rush, Shaw, & Emery, 1979). More recently, Beck, Freeman, and Associates (1990) developed a cognitive theory of personality pathology, describing cognitive schemas that shape the experiences and behaviors of individuals with these disorders. Dysfunctional and distorting schemas give rise to maladaptive interaction strategies which, in turn, trigger automatic thoughts which make the individual susceptible to repetitive and pervasive life difficulties (Pretzer & Beck, 1996). Also included are affect and interpersonal behavior, integrated through the central component of cognition, which lead to pathological and self-perpetuating cognitive–interpersonal transaction cycles (Pretzer & Beck, 1996). The model of Beck et al. (1990) is anchored to evolution, and it speculates how personality pathology might relate to strategies that have facilitated survival and reproduction through natural selection. Derivatives of these evolutionary strategies may be identified, according to Beck, in exaggerated form among the Axis I clinical syndromes, and in less dramatic expression among the personality disorders. Further, Beck et al. (1990) state that these schemas may be either overdeveloped or underdeveloped, inhibiting or even displacing other schemas that may be more adaptive or more appropriate for a given situation. As a result, they introduce a persistent and systematic bias into the individual's processing machinery. For example, the dependent personality is hypersensitive to the possibility of a loss of love and help and quickly interprets signs of such loss as signifying its reality. Conversely, antisocials are likely to have an underdeveloped schema to be responsi-

ble or to feel guilt for their behavioral transgressions. In contrast, obsessive–compulsives are disposed to judge themselves responsible and guilt-ridden but are underdeveloped in the inclination to interpret events spontaneously, creatively, and playfully. Beck (1992) presented a list of "primeval" strategies for some personality disorders, elaborated as a "cognitive taxonomy" anchored across view of self, view of others, main beliefs, and strategy (reported in Pretzer & Beck, 1996). By 1997, Alford and Beck, striving to increase the integrative scope of cognitive therapy, noted numerous parallels between the theory of cognitive therapy, as derived from clinical observation, and academic cognitive psychology, including the concept of the cognitive unconscious. Later they state that "cognitive theory is a theory about the role . . . of cognition in the interrelationships among such variables as emotion, behavior, and interpersonal relationships. 'Cognition' includes the entire range of variables implicated in information processing, as well as consciousness of the cognitive products" (p. 106). Modern cognitive therapy, then, which began as a kind of refabricated introspectionism interested only in conscious contents, is now in the process of transition to a fully cognitive therapy with a solid foundation in cognitive psychology. Thus, the applied and pure science branches are closing together, and cognitive therapy has at last escaped the orbit of behaviorism.

Neurobiologically Based Theories

Temperament is often referred to as the soil, the biological foundation, of personality. The ontogenetic priority of temperament, the fact that it is the first domain of personality to come into existence in the development of the organism, perhaps gives it a taxonomic priority that other domains lack. The argument is that the contents of all aspects of personality are forever constrained by the first domain to develop. Accordingly, once temperament is determined by the individual's biological constitution, some developmental pathways in other domains are forever excluded whereas others are reinforced. Thus, although it is not impossible that an irritable and demanding infant will become a diplomat famous for calmly taking the perspectives of others to thereby negotiate resolutions satisfactory to all parties, the odds against it are greater than they would otherwise have been. Similarly, we might expect that children whose personal tempo is somewhat slower than average are unlikely to develop a histrionic personality disorder, and that those who are especially agreeable are unlikely to develop a negativistic personality disorder.

Probably the first explanatory system to specify pseudo–neurobiological dimensions was the doctrine of body humors posited by early Greeks some 25 centuries ago. Hippocrates concluded in the 4th century B.C. that all diseases stem from an excess of or imbalance of yellow bile, black bile, blood, and phlegm, the embodiment of earth, water, fire, and air, the declared basic components of the universe according to the philosopher Empedocles. Excesses of these humors led respectively to the choleric, melancholic, sanguine, and phlegmatic temperaments. Modified by Galen centuries later, the choleric temperament was associated with a tendency toward irascibility, the sanguine temperament with optimism, the melancholic temperament with sadness, and the phlegmatic temperament with apathy. The doctrine of humors is today preserved through studies on such topics as neurohormonal chemistry and neurotransmitter systems as its more modern parallels. In the 1920s, Kretschmer (1922) developed a classification system based on thin, muscular, and obese types of physiques. Kretschmer was interested mainly in the relation of physique to psychopathology, and he viewed these physiques as discrete types. For his student, Sheldon (Sheldon & Stevens, 1942), the three types became the dimensions of ectomorphy, mesomorphy, and endomorphy, as applicable to normal persons in clinical samples. According to Sheldon, each body type corresponded to a particular temperament, viscerotonia, somatotonia, and cerebrotonia.

Temperament, however, is only one aspect of human biology. Not only are we biological beings, we are also material and chemical beings. Although our experience of our own moment-to-moment existence is one of a continuous and unified consciousness, an anatomical examination of the structure of the nervous system shows that it is composed of many discrete units, called neurons, each of which communicates with many thousands of others through chemical messengers called neurotransmitters, which bridge the gaps between neurons and thus allow the system to work as whole. Because some neurotransmitters seem to be specialized for certain functions rather than others, it makes sense that a taxonomy based on neuro-

transmitter types might have particular relevance to personality. Ideally, such a model would be put forward so that each neurotransmitter type would relate to some content dimension of personality in a one-to-one fashion. Personality would thus reduce to a profile of neurotransmitter dimensions, and by changing the level of a particular neurotransmitter through a pill or procedure, personality change could be easily affected.

Cloninger (1986, 1987) proposed an elegant theory based on the interrelationship of three genetic-neurobiological trait dispositions, each of which is associated with a particular neurotransmitter system. Specifically, novelty seeking is associated with low basal activity in the dopaminergic system, harm avoidance with high activity in the serotonergic system, and reward dependence with low basal noradrenergic system activity. Novelty seeking is hypothesized to dispose the individual to exhilaration or excitement in response to novel stimuli, which leads to the pursuit of potential rewards as well as an active avoidance of both monotony and punishment. Harm avoidance reflects a disposition to respond strongly to aversive stimuli, leading the individual to inhibit behaviors to avoid punishment, novelty, and frustrations. Reward dependence is seen as a tendency to respond to signals of reward, verbal signals of social approval, for example, and to resist extinction of behaviors previously associated with rewards or relief from punishment. These three dimensions form the axes of a cube whose corners represent various personality constructs. Thus, antisocial personalities, who are often seen as fearless and sensation seeking, are seen as low in harm avoidance and high in novelty seeking, while the imperturbable schizoid is seen as low across all dimensions of the model. Interestingly, the personality disorders generated by Cloninger's model correspond only loosely to those in DSM-IV. A number of DSM-IV personality disorders are not represented at all. However, because DSM is itself atheoretical, it cannot be used as a criterion against which any strong structural model can be evaluated. From the standpoint of a theoretical model, it is the disorder categories of DSM that are spurious and not vice versa.

Evolution-Based Theories

In contrast to the perspectives outlined previously, which appeal to organizing principles that derive from a single domain of personality, we might ask whether any theory honors the nature of personality as the patterning of variables across the entire matrix of the person. Such a theory is necessary for a number of reasons. First, the natural direction of science is toward theories of greater and greater scope. In theoretical physics, for example, quantum gravity is an attempt to unify quantum mechanics with the theory of relativity. Second, the theoretical perspectives presented earlier do not treat personality in a manner congruent with the formal synthetic properties of the construct itself. Personality is not exclusively behavioral, exclusively cognitive, or exclusively interpersonal but, instead, an integration of all these. Advancement in the hard sciences often occurs through the construction of falsifying experiments. An experimental situation is conceived, the results of which are intended to support one theory but reject another. In contrast, the social sciences are intrinsically less boundaried, with advancement more often occurring when a heretofore neglected, but nevertheless highly relevant, set of variables surges to the center of scientific interest. Far from overturning established paradigms, the new perspective simply allows a given phenomena to be studied from an additional angle, becoming a new "research program" in Lakatosian sense (Lakatos, 1978). Agnostic scholars with no strong allegiance may thus avail themselves of a kaleidoscope of different views. By turning the kaleidoscope, by shifting paradigmatic sets, the same phenomenon can be viewed from any of a variety of internally consistent perspectives. Eclecticism thus becomes the scientific norm. But no theory which represents a partial perspective on the total phenomenon of personality can be complete. As we have seen, constructs which are considered taxonomically fundamental in one perspective may not emerge as such within another perspective. The interpersonal model of Lorna Benjamin (1993) and the neurobiological model of Robert Cloninger (1987) are both structurally strong approaches to personality. Yet their fundamental constructs are different. Rather than inherit the construct dimensions of a particular perspective, then, a theory of personality as a total phenomenon should seek some set of principles which can be addressed to the whole person, thereby capitalizing on the synthetic properties of personality as the total matrix of the person. The alternative is an uncomfortable eclecticism of unassimilated partial views.

But how are we to create a theory which breaks free of the "grand theories of human nature" that are all part of the history of psychology? The key lies in finding theoretical principles for personality which fall outside the field of personality proper. Otherwise, we could only repeat the errors of the past by asserting the importance of some new set of variables heretofore unemphasized, building another perspective inside personality as a total phenomenon but thereby missing a scientific understanding of the total phenomenon itself. Herein lies the distinction between the terms "personality" and "personology." Strictly speaking, a science of personality is limited to partial views of the person. These may in fact be highly internally consistent, but they cannot be total. In contrast, personology is from the beginning a science of the total person. In the absence of falsifying experiments, various perspectives on personality tend to develop to high states of internal coherence, becoming "schools" which intrinsically resist integration and contribute to the fragmentation of psychology as a unified discipline. In so doing, they also create conceptions of personality that intrinsically conflict with the nature of the construct itself. A science of personology ends this long tradition of fractiousness and creates a theoretical basis for a completely unified science of personality and psychopathology. As we see later, there can be only one science of personology. However, there is probably no limit to the number of variable domains that might call themselves personality.

Evolution is the logical choice as a scaffold from which to develop a science of personality (Millon, 1990). Just as personality is concerned with the total patterning of variables across the entire matrix of the person, it is the total organism that survives and reproduces, carrying forth both its adaptive and maladaptive potentials into subsequent generations. Although lethal mutations sometimes occur, the evolutionary success of organisms with "average expectable genetic material" is dependent on the entire configuration of the organism's characteristics and potentials. Similarly, psychological fitness derives from the relation of the entire configuration of personality characteristics to the environments in which the person functions. Beyond these analogies, the principles of evolution also serve as principles that lie outside personality proper and thus form a foundation for the integration of the various historical schools which escapes the part–whole fallacy of the dogmatic past. In creating a taxonomy of personality styles and disorders based on evolutionary principles, there is one central question: How can these processes can best be segmented so that their relevance to the individual person is drawn into the foreground?

The first task of any organism is its immediate survival. Organisms which fail to survive have been selected out, so to speak, and fail to contribute their genes and characteristics to subsequent generations. Whether a virus or a human being, every living thing must protect itself each against simple entropic decompensation, predatory threat, and homeostatic misadventure. There are literally millions of ways to die. Evolutionary mechanisms related to survival tasks are oriented toward life enhancement and life preservation. The former are concerned with improvement in the quality of life and gear organisms toward behaviors which improve survival chances and, ideally, lead them to thrive and multiply. The latter are geared toward orienting organisms away from actions or environments that threaten to jeopardize survival. Phenomenologically speaking, such mechanisms form a polarity of pleasure and pain. Behaviors experienced as pleasurable are generally repeated and generally promote survival, whereas those experienced as painful generally have the potential to endanger life and thus are not repeated. Organisms which repeat painful experiences or fail to repeat pleasurable ones are strongly selected against. Among the various personalities deduced from the theory, we find that some individuals are conflicted in regard to these existential aims. The sadistic personality, for example, finds pleasure in actively establishing conditions that will be experienced as painful. Other personalities possess deficits in these crucial substrates. The schizoid personality, for example, has little capacity to experience pleasurable affects.

The second universal evolutionary task faced by every organism relates to homeostatic processes employed to sustain survival in open ecosystems. To exist is to exist within an environment, and once an organism exists, it must either adapt to its surroundings or adapt its surroundings to conform to and support its own style of functioning. Every organism must satisfy lower-order needs related, for example, to nutrition, thirst, and sleep. Mammals and human beings must also satisfy other needs, for example, those related to safety and attachment. Whether the environment is intrinsically bountiful or hostile, the choice is essentially between a passive versus an active orientation, that is, a tendency to accommodate to a given ecological niche and accept what the environment offers, versus a tendency to modify or intervene in the environment, thereby adapting it to oneself. Organisms which fail to adapt to their environment or to restructure their environment to meet their own needs are strongly selected against. These modes of adaptation differ from the first phase of evolution, "being," in that they regard how that which is endures. Among the various personalities deduced from the theory, we find antisocials, who impulsively affect their environment, often with complete disregard for consequences.

The third universal evolutionary task faced by every organism pertains to reproductive styles that maximize the diversification and selection of ecologically effective attributes. All organisms must ultimately reproduce to evolve. To keep the chain of the generations going, organisms have developed strategies by which to maximize the survivability of the species. At one extreme is what biologists have referred to as the r-strategy. Here, an organism seeks to reproduce a great number of offspring, which are then left to fend for themselves against the adversities of chance or destiny. At the other extreme is the K-strategy, in which relatively few offspring are produced and are given extensive care by parents. Although individual exceptions always exist, these parallel the more male "self-oriented" versus the more female "other-nurturing" strategies of sociobiology. Psychologically, the former strategy is often judged to be egotistic, insensitive, inconsiderate, and uncaring, whereas the latter is judged to be affiliative, intimate, protective, and solicitous (Gilligan, 1981; Rushton, 1985; Wilson, 1978). Organisms which make reproductive investments in many offspring, so that their resources are spread too thin, or who make a long gestational investment but then fail to nurture their offspring, are strongly selected against. Among the various personalities deduced from the theory, we find a strong self-orientation among narcissists and a strong other-orientation among dependents.

In addition to the three content polarities, Millon's (1990) evolutionary theory also posits a content-free dimension which specifies a major pathway along which various personality styles develop and change. Such transformational principles are often important in revealing relationships between diverse personality styles and also suggest pathways along which personality might be changed in therapy. The evolutionary theory incorporates the interpersonal domain through the self and other polarities. In addition, however, it also includes the idea of conflictedness or ambivalence between polarities, a fundamentally psychodynamic construct. By representing self–other and active–passive as orthogonal in a two-dimensional plane, and depicting conflict as a third, vertical dimension, a number of personality disorder constructs can be interrelated and differentiated. The compulsive and negativistic (passive–aggressive) personalities, for example, share an ambivalence concerning whether to put their own priorities and expectations first or to defer to others. The negativistic acts out this ambivalence, repressed in the compulsive. The two personalities are thus theoretically linked, and the theory predicts that if the submerged anger of the compulsive can confronted consciously, the subject may tend to act out in a passive–aggressive manner until this conflict can be constructively refocused or resolved. Once the role of chance and necessity in the evolution of human psychology is understood, several conclusions readily follow. While the polarities and their derived constructs are necessary and universal, it is highly unlikely that the various content domains of personality will ever be put on a similar footing, one from which a domain of unconscious defenses, a domain of cognitive styles, a domain of interpersonal conduct, and so on, can be derived as an inevitable result. Domains of personality just exist, and the taxonomic principles of these domains are, at least in part, the particular product of our own evolutionary adaptations. As such, they contain specificities which render them unassimilable to any other perspective, including the evolutionary theory, and justify their very existence as domains.

Three important facts of the history of psychology are thus brought together. First, as history has shown, each perspective, once exposed to scientific enthusiasm, perpetuates itself ad nauseam, never becoming truly susceptible to falsification. Instead, it waxes and wanes in accord with the fashion of the times, eventually developing to a highly dogmatic state of internal consistency. Second, once drawn into a particular perspective, clinicians and researchers seem to spend their lives involved in "horizontal refinements," working out the particular

problems of their area even while the generality or clinical importance of their findings to the clinical treatment of the total organism remains unclear. And, finally, it explains why the contention between various perspectives never really fades but never really produces much of anything either. The "research programs" of Lakatos (1978), then, should not be viewed simply as an inductive fact wrought from an inspection of the history of the social sciences. At least in psychology, Lakatos's conception of "research programs" would seem to have a solid footing in the interplay between chance and necessity in human evolution. We can also conclude that neither the evolutionary theory nor any other theory will tell us that defense mechanisms, or any other personality domain, must exist as an inevitable part of the human psyche. Psychology is thus fundamentally different from sciences such as physics. Although physics contains numerous universal constants, such as the weight of a proton, the speed of light, Planck's constant, and so on, theoretical physics also explains why these particular values exist as they do and not otherwise. To be complete, a unified theory of the fundamental forces of nature must be able to account for these observed quantities. In contrast, it is doubtful that any "unified field theory" of personality will account for the existence of the various personality domains.

Nevertheless, although specific personality domains "just exist," the evolution of the structure and contents of each has not proceeded with total autonomy but is instead constrained by the evolutionary imperatives of survival, adaptation, and reproductive success, for it is always the whole organism that is selected and evolves. Accordingly, we should be able to discover the "footprints" of the evolutionary polarities within the history of the major psychological schools (Millon, 1990), a psychoarchaeological record of their role in mental life. This provides some empirical corroboration for the theory, although, as was argued at the beginning of this chapter, the progress of history is both contingent and meandering.

REFERENCES

Abraham, K. (1927a). The influence of oral eroticism on character formation. In *Selected papers on psychoanalysis* (pp. 393–406). London: Hogarth Press. (Original work published 1924)

Abraham, K. (1927). Contributions to the theory of the anal character. In *Selected papers on psychoanalysis* (pp. 370–392). London: Hogarth Press. (Original work published 1921)

Abraham, K. (1927b). A short study of the development of the libido. In *Selected papers on psychoanalysis*. London: Hogarth Press. (Original work published 1924)

Alford, B. A., & Beck, A. T. (1997). *The integrative power of cognitive therapy.* New York: Guilford Press.

Beck, A. T. (1976). *Cognitive therapy and the emotional disorders.* New York: International Universities Press.

Beck, A. T. (1992). Personality disorders (and their relationship to syndromal disorders). *Across-Species Comparisions and Psychiatry Newsletter, 5,* 3–13.

Beck, A. T., Freeman, A., & Associates. (1990). *Cognitive therapy of personality disorders.* New York: Guilford Press.

Beck, A. T., Rush, A. J., Shaw, B. F., & Emery, G. (1979). *Cognitive therapy of depression.* New York: Guilford Press.

Benjamin, L. S. (1974). Structured analysis of social behavior. *Psychological Review, 81,* 392–425.

Benjamin, L. S (1993). *Interpersonal diagnosis and treatment of personality disorders.* New York: Guilford Press.

Block, J. (1995). A contrarian view of the five-factor approach to personality description. *Psychological Bulletin, 117,* 187–215.

Bridgeman, P. W. (1927). *The logic of modern physics.* New York: Macmillian.

Cloninger, R. C. (1986). A unified biosocial theory of personality and its role in the development of anxiety states. *Psychiatric Developments, 3,* 167–226.

Cloninger, R. C. (1987). A systematic method for clinical description and classification of personality variants. *Archives of General Psychiatry, 44,* 573–588.

Costa, P. T., Jr., & McCrae, R. R. (1992). *Revised NEO Personality Inventory (NEO-PI-R) and NEO Five-Factor Inventory (NEO-FFI) professional manual.* Odessa, FL: Psychological Assessment Resources.

Digman, J. M. (1990). Personality structure: Emergence of the five-factor model. *Annual Review of Psychology, 41,* 417–440.

Fenichel, O. (1945). *The psychoanalytic theory of the neurosis.* New York: Norton.

Fiester, S., & Gay, M. (1991). Sadistic personality disorder: A review of data and recommendations for DSM-IV. *Journal of Personality Disorders, 5,* 376–385.

Freedman, M. B., Leary, T., Ossorio, A. G., & Coffey, H. S. (1951). The interpersonal dimension of personality. *Journal of Personality, 20,* 143–161.

Freud, S. (1915). The instincts and their vicissitudes. In *Collected papers* (Vol. 4). London: Hogarth Press.

Freud, S. (1931). Libidinal types. In *Collected papers* (Vol. 5). London: Hogarth Press.

Gilligan. C. (1981). *In a different voice.* Cambridge. MA: Harvard University Press.

Goldberg, L. R. (1993). The structure of phenotypic personality traits. *American Psychologist, 48,* 26–34.

Hempel, C. G. (1965). *Aspects of scientific explanation.* New York: Free Press.

John, O. P. (1990). The "Big Five" factor taxonomy: Dimensions of personality in the natural language and in questionnaires. In L. A. Pervin (Ed.), *Handbook of personality: Theory and research* (pp. 66–100). New York: Guilford Press.

John, O. P., Angleitner, A., & Ostendorf, F. (1988). The lexical approach to personality: A historical review of trait taxonomic research. *European Journal of Personality, 2,* 171–205.

Kernberg, O. F. (1984). *Severe personality disorders.* New Haven, CT: Yale University Press.

Kernberg, O. F. (1996). A psychoanalytic theory of personality disorders. In J. F. Clarkin & M. F. Lenzenweger (Eds.), *Major theories of personality disorder* (pp. 106–140). New York: Guilford Press.

Kohut, H. (1971). *The analysis of self.* New York: International Universities Press.

Kretschmer, E. (1922). *Korperbau und Charakter* (3rd ed.). Berlin: J. Springer.

Kukla, A. (1989). Non-empirical issues in psychology. *American Psychologist, 44,* 785–794.

Lakatos, I. (1978). *Philosophical papers: Vol. 2. Mathematics, science and epistemology.* (J. Worrall & G. Currie, Eds.). Cambridge, UK: Cambridge University Press.

Lang, P. J. (1968). Fear reduction and fear behavior: Problems in treating a construct. In J. M. Schlien (Ed.), *Research in psychotherapy* (Vol. III, pp. 90–102). Washington, DC: American Psychological Association.

Leary, T. (1957). *Interpersonal diagnosis of personality: A functional theory and methodology for personality evaluation.* New York: Ronald Press.

Meehl, P. E. (1962). Schizotaxia, schizotypy, schizophrenia. *American Psychologist, 17,* 827–838.

Meehl, P. E. (1978). Theoretical risks and tabular asterisks: Sir Karl, Sir Ronald, and the slow progress of soft psychology. *Journal of Consulting and Clinical Psychology, 46,* 806–834.

Meehl, P. E. (1995). Bootstraps taxometrics: Solving the classification problem in psychopathology. *American Psychologist, 50,* 266–275.

Meehl, P. E., & Golden, R. R. (1982). Taxometric methods. In P. Kendall & J. Butcher (Eds.), *Handbook of research methods in clinical psychology* (pp. 127–181). New York: Wiley.

Millon, T. (1981). *Disorders of personality: DSM-III, Axis II.* New York: Wiley-Interscience.

Millon, T. (1987). On the nature of taxonomy in psychopathology. In C. G. Last & M. Hersen (Eds.), *Issues in diagnostic research* (pp. 3–85). New York: Plenum.

Millon, T. (1990). *Toward a new personology.* New York: Wiley.

Millon, T., & Davis R. D. (1996). *Disorders of personality: DSM-IV and beyond* (2nd ed.). New York: Wiley-Interscience.

Pap, A. (1953). Reduction-sentences and open concepts. *Methods, 5,* 3–30.

Pepper, S. C. (1942). *World hypotheses: A study in evidence.* Berkeley: University of California Press.

Pincus, A. L. (1994). The interpersonal circumplex and the interpersonal theory: Perspectives on personality and its pathology. In S. Strack & M. Lorr (Eds.), *Dif-*

ferentiating normal and abnormal personality (pp. 114–136). New York: Springer.

Pretzer, J. L., & Beck, A. T. (1996). A cognitive theory of personality disorders. In J. F. Clarkin & M. F. Lenzenweger (Eds.), *Major theories of personality disorder* (pp. 36–105). New York: Guilford Press.

Quine, W. V. O. (1977). Natural kinds. In S. P. Schwartz (Ed.), *Naming, necessity, and natural groups.* Ithaca: Cornell University Press.

Reich, W. (1933). *Characteranalyse.* Leipzig: Serpol Verlag.

Rushton, J. P. (1985). Differential K theory: The socio-biology of individual and group differences. *Personality and Individual Differences, 6,* 441–452.

Schaefer, E. (1965). Configurational analysis of children's report of parent behavior. *Journal of Consulting Psychology, 29,* 552–557.

Sheldon, W. H., & Stevens, S. S. (1942). *The varieties of temperament.* New York: Harper & Row.

Widiger, T. A. (1993). The DSM-III-R categorical personality disorder diagnoses: A critique and an alternative. *Psychological Inquiry, 4,* 75–90.

Wilson, E. O. (1978). *On human nature.* Cambridge, MA: Harvard University Press.

CHAPTER 3

————◆————

Official Classification Systems

THOMAS A. WIDIGER

Disorders of personality are of concern to many different professions and agencies, whose participants hold an equally diverse array of beliefs regarding etiology, pathology, and treatment. It is imperative for these persons to be able to communicate meaningfully with one another. The primary purpose of an official classification system is to provide this common language of communication (Kendell, 1975; Sartorius et al., 1993).

Characterizing an official nomenclature as being simply a language does not imply that it is not important or powerful. On the contrary, clinicians think with their language, or, at least, it can be difficult to think otherwise. The current languages of modern psychiatry are the fourth edition of the American Psychiatric Association's (APA) *Diagnostic and Statistical Manual of Mental Disorders* (DSM-IV; APA, 1994) and the tenth edition of the World Health Organization's (WHO) *International Classification of Diseases* (ICD-10; WHO, 1992). As such, these nomenclatures have a substantial impact on how clinicians conceptualize personality disorders.

These two languages of psychopathology, however, are not the final word. DSM-IV and ICD-10 aspire to be but are not nearly as conclusive as chemistry's periodic table of elements. Interpreting DSM-IV or ICD-10 as conclusively validated nomenclatures is an idealized reification of working documents

(Frances, Pincus, Widiger, Davis, & First, 1990). On the other hand, they are not simply solipsistic whims. DSM-IV and ICD-10 are well-reasoned and scientifically researched nomenclatures that describe what is currently understood by most scientists, theorists, researchers, and clinicians to be the disorders of personality (Widiger & Trull, 1993).

This chapter describes and discusses DSM-IV and ICD-10 official classifications of personality disorder. The chapter begins with an historical overview, followed by a discussion of the major issues facing their future development and revision.

HISTORICAL OVERVIEW

Personality disorder classifications have been evident throughout the history of psychology, psychiatry, and medicine (Millon et al., 1996). The impetus for the development of official classifications has been the crippling confusion generated by their absence. "For a long time confusion reigned. Every self-respecting alienist [the 19th-century term for a psychiatrist], and certainly every professor, had his [sic] own classification" (Kendell, 1975, p. 87). The production of a new system for classifying psychopathology became a rite of passage for the young, aspiring professor.

To produce a well-ordered classification almost seems to have become the unspoken ambition of every psychiatrist of industry and promise, as it is the ambition of a good tenor to strike a high C. This classificatory ambition was so conspicuous that the composer Berlioz was prompted to remark that after their studies have been completed a rhetorician writes a tragedy and a psychiatrist a classification. (Zilboorg, 1941, p. 450)

Initial efforts to develop a uniform language did not meet with much success. The Statistical Committee of the British Royal Medico-Psychological Association produced a classification in 1892 and conducted formal revisions in 1904, 1905, and 1906. However, "the Association finally accepted the unpalatable fact that most of its members were not prepared to restrict themselves to diagnoses listed in any official nomenclature" (Kendell, 1975, p. 88). The Association of Medical Superintendents of American Institutions for the Insane (a forerunner to the American Psychiatric Association) adopted a slightly modified version of the British nomenclature in 1886 but was not any more successful in getting its membership to use it.

The American Bureau of the Census struggled to obtain national statistics in the absence of an officially recognized nomenclature (Grob, 1991). In 1908 the Bureau asked the American Medico-Psychological Association (which "rediagnosed" itself as the American Psychiatric Association in 1921) to appoint a Committee on Nomenclature of Diseases to develop a standard nosology. In 1917 this committee affirmed the need for a uniform system.

The importance and need of some system whereby uniformity in reports would be secured have been repeatedly emphasized by officers and members of this Association, by statisticians of the United States Census Bureau, by editors of psychiatric journals. . . . The present condition with respect to the classification of mental diseases is chaotic. Some states use no well-defined classification. In others the classifications used are similar in many respects but differ enough to prevent accurate comparisons. Some states have adopted a uniform system, while others leave the matter entirely to the individual hospitals. This condition of affairs discredits the science of psychiatry. (Salmon, Copp, May, Abot, & Cotton, 1917, pp. 255–256)

The American Medico-Psychological Association, in collaboration with the National Committee for Mental Hygiene, issued a nosology in 1918, titled *Statistical Manual for the Use of Institutions for the Insane* (Grob, 1991; Menninger, 1963). The National Committee for Mental Hygiene published and distributed the nosology. This nomenclature was of use to the census, but many hospitals failed to adopt the system for clinical practice, in part because of its narrow representation. There were only 22 diagnostic categories, which were confined largely to psychoses with a presumably neurochemical pathology (the closest to personality disorders were conditions within the category of "not insane," which included drug addiction without psychosis and constitutional psychopathic inferiority without psychosis; Salmon et al., 1917). Confusion continued to be the norm. "In the late twenties, each large teaching center employed a system of its own origination, no one of which met more than the immediate needs of the local institution. . . . There resulted a polyglot of diagnostic labels and systems, effectively blocking communication" (APA, 1952, p. v).

A conference was held at the New York Academy of Medicine in 1928 with representatives from various governmental agencies and professional associations. A trial edition of a proposed nomenclature (modeled after the *Statistical Manual*) was distributed to hospitals in 1932 within the American Medical Association's *Standard Classified Nomenclature of Disease*. Most hospitals and teaching centers used this system, or at least a modified version that was more compatible with the perspectives of the clinicians at that particular center. However, the *Standard Nomenclature* proved to be grossly inadequate when the attention of mental health clinicians expanded beyond the severe "organic" psychopathologies that had been the predominant concern of inpatient hospitals.

ICD-6 and DSM-I

Two medical statisticians, William Farr in London and Jacques Bertillon in Paris, had convinced the International Statistical Congress in 1853 of the value of producing a uniform classification of causes of death. Eventually Farr, Bertillon, and Marc d'Espine (of Geneva) developed a classification system. The *Bertillon Classification of Causes of Death* was substantially beneficial and informative to many governmental and public health agencies. In 1889 the International Statistical Institute urged that a more official governing body accept the task of sponsoring and revising the nomenclature. The French government therefore convened a series of international conferences in Paris in 1900, 1920, 1929, and 1938, producing successive revisions of the *International List of Causes of Death.*

The WHO accepted the authority to produce the sixth edition of the *International List,* renamed, in 1948, the *International Statistical Classification of Diseases, Injuries, and Causes of Death* (Kendell, 1975). It is sometimes said that this sixth edition was the first to include mental disorders. However, mental disorders were included within the 1938 fifth edition in the section on diseases of the nervous system and sense organs (Kramer, Sartorius, Jablensky, & Gulbinat, 1979). This section included the four subcategories of mental deficiency, dementia praecox, manic–depressive psychosis, and other mental disorders. Several other mental disorders (e.g., alcoholism) were included in other sections of the manual. ICD-6 was the first edition to include a specific (and greatly expanded) section devoted to the diagnosis of mental disorders (Kendell, 1975; Kramer et al., 1979). However, the "mental disorders section [of ICD-6] failed to gain acceptance and eleven years later was found to be in official use only in Finland, New Zealand, Peru, Thailand, and the United Kingdom" (Kendell, 1975, p. 91).

"In the United States, [the mental disorders section] of the ICD was ignored completely, in spite of the fact that American psychiatrists had taken a prominent part in drafting it" (Kendell, 1975, p. 92). American psychiatrists, however, were not any happier with the *Standard Nomenclature* because its neurochemical emphasis was not helpful to the many casualties of the war who dominated the attention and concern of mental health practitioners in the 1940s (Grob, 1991). "Military psychiatrists, induction station psychiatrists, and Veterans Administration psychiatrists, found themselves operating within the limits of a nomenclature specifically not designed for 90% of the cases handled" (APA, 1952, p. vi). Of particular importance was the inadequate coverage of somatoform, stress reaction, and personality disorders. As a result, the Navy, the Army, the Veterans Administration, and the Armed Forces each developed their own nomenclatures during World War II.

It should be noted, however, that ICD-6 had attempted to be responsive to the needs of the war veterans. As acknowledged by the APA (1952), ICD-6 "categorized mental disorders in rubrics similar to those of the Armed Forces nomenclature" (p. vii). The *Standard Manual,* the *Bureau of the Census Statistics,* and ICD were largely compatible (Menninger, 1963) and had expanded by the early 1940s to include psychoneurotic and behavior disorders, although not in the manner or extent desired by many of the mental health clinicians of the second world war (Grob, 1991). One specific absence from ICD-6, for example, was a diagnosis for passive–aggressive personality disorder, which was the most frequently diagnosed personality disorder by American psychiatrists during the war, accounting for 6% of all admissions to Army hospitals (Malinow, 1981).

The U.S. Public Health Service commissioned a committee, chaired by George Raines with representation from a variety of professional and public health associations, to develop a variant of ICD-6 for use within the United States. This nomenclature was coordinated with ICD-6, but it more closely resembled the Veterans Administration system developed by William Menninger. Responsibility for publishing and distributing the nosology was provided to the APA (1952) under the title *Diagnostic and Statistical Manual. Mental Disorders.*

DSM-I was more successful in obtaining acceptance across a wide variety of clinical settings than was the previously published *Standard Nomenclature.* This was due in large part to its inclusion of the many diagnoses of considerable interest to practicing clinicians. In addition, DSM-I, unlike ICD-6, included brief narrative descriptions of each condition which facilitated an understanding of the meaning, intention, and application of the diagnoses.

DSM-I, however, was not without significant opposition. The New York State Department of Mental Hygiene, which had been influential in the development of the original *Standard Nomenclature,* continued for some time to use its own classification. Fundamental objections and criticisms regarding the reliability and validity of psychiatric diagnoses were also being raised (e.g., Zigler & Phillips, 1961). For example, a widely cited reliability study by Ward, Beck, Mendelson, Mock, and Erbaugh (1962) concluded that most of the poor agreement among psychiatrists' diagnoses was due largely to inadequacies of DSM-I rather than to idiosyncrasies of the clinical interview or inconsistent patient reporting. "Two thirds of the disagreements were charged to inadequacies of the nosological system itself" (Ward et al., 1962, p. 205). The largest single disagreement was determining "whether the neurotic symptomatology or the characterological pathology is more extensive or 'basic'" (Ward et al., 1962, p. 202). Ward et al. criticized the DSM-I requirement that the clinician choose between a neurotic condition versus a personality disorder when both appeared to be present. The second most frequent cause of disagreement was said to be unclear diagnostic criteria.

The WHO was also concerned with the failure of its member countries to adopt ICD-6 and therefore commissioned a review by the English psychiatrist, Erwin Stengel. Stengel (1959) reiterated the importance of establishing an official diagnostic nomenclature.

> A . . . serious obstacle to progress in psychiatry is difficulty of communication. Everybody who has followed the literature and listened to discussions concerning mental illness soon discovers that psychiatrists, even those apparently sharing the same basic orientation, often do not speak the same language. They either use different terms for the same concepts, or the same term for different concepts, usually without being aware of it. It is sometimes argued that this is inevitable in the present state of psychiatric knowledge, but it is doubtful whether this is a valid excuse. (p. 601)

Stengel (1959) attributed the failure of clinicians to accept ICD-6 to the presence of theoretical biases within the nomenclature that were problematic to the diverse array of perspectives within the profession, cynicism regarding psychiatric diagnoses (with some theoretical perspectives opposing the use of any diagnostic terms), and the absence of specific, explicit diagnostic criteria (complicating the obtainment of agreement among clinicians who were in fact attempting to use the manual). Stengel recommended that future nomenclatures be shorn of their theoretical and etiological assumptions and provide instead behaviorally specific descriptions.

ICD-8 and DSM-II

Work began on ICD-8 soon after Stengel's (1959) report (ICD-6 had been revised to ICD-7 in 1955, but there were no revisions to the mental disorders). The first meeting of the Subcommittee on Classification of Diseases of the WHO Expert Committee on Health Statistics was held in Geneva in 1961. It was evident to all participants that there would be closer adherence by the member countries of the WHO to ICD-8 than had been the case for ICD-6. Considerable effort was extended in developing a system that would be usable by all countries. The United States collaborated with the United Kingdom in developing a common, unified proposal; additional proposals were submitted by Australia, Czechoslovakia, the Federal Republic of Germany, France, Norway, Poland, and the Soviet Union. These alternative proposals were considered within a joint meeting in 1963. The most controversial points of disagreement concerned mental retardation with psychosocial deprivation, reactive psychoses, and antisocial personality disorder (Kendell, 1975). The final edition of ICD-8 was approved by the WHO in 1966 and became effective in 1968. A companion glossary, in the spirit of Stengel's (1959) recommendations, was to be published conjointly, but work did not begin on the glossary until 1967 and was not completed until 1972. "This delay greatly reduced [its] usefulness, and also [its] authority" (Kendell, 1975, p. 95).

In 1965, the APA appointed the Committee on Nomenclature and Statistics, chaired by Ernest M. Gruenberg, to revise DSM-I to be compatible with ICD-8 and yet also to be suitable for use within the United States (a technical consultant to DSM-II was the young psychiatrist, Robert Spitzer). A draft was circulated in 1967 to 120 psychiatrists with a special interest in diagnosis, and the final version was approved in 1967, with publication in 1968 (APA, 1968).

Spitzer and Wilson (1968) summarized the changes to DSM-I. For example, deleted from the section for personality disorders were substance dependencies and sexual deviations that were closely associated with maladaptive personality traits but were not themselves necessarily disorders of personality. Deleted as well was the passive–dependent variant of the passive–aggressive personality trait disturbance. New additions were the explosive, hysterical, and asthenic personality disorders. Spitzer and Wilson (1975) subsequently criticized the absence of a diagnosis for depressive personality disorder, noting the inclusion of a cyclothymic personality disorder within DSM-II and an affective personality disorder within ICD-8. "No adequate classification is furnished for the much larger number of characterologically depressed patients" (Spitzer & Wilson,

1975, p. 842). Spitzer and Wilson (1975), however, also objected to other diagnoses. "In the absence of clear criteria and follow-up studies, the wisdom of including such categories as explosive personality, asthenic personality, and inadequate personality may be questioned" (p. 842).

The period in which DSM-II and ICD-8 were published was also highly controversial for mental disorder diagnoses (e.g., Rosenhan, 1973; Szasz, 1961). A fundamental problem continued to be the absence of empirical support for the reliability, let alone the validity, of these diagnoses (e.g., Blashfield & Draguns, 1976). Spitzer and Fleiss (1974) reviewed nine major studies of interrater diagnostic reliability. Kappa values for the diagnosis of a personality disorder ranged from a low of .11 to .56, with a mean of only .29. DSM-II was blamed for much of this poor reliability, although a proportion was also attributed to idiosyncratic clinical interviewing (Spitzer, Endicott, & Robins, 1975).

Many researchers had by now taken to heart the recommendations of Stengel (1959), developing more specific and explicit diagnostic criteria to increase the likelihood that they would be able to conduct replicable research (Blashfield, 1984). The most influential of these efforts was provided by Feighner et al. (1972). They developed criteria for 15 conditions, one of which was antisocial personality disorder. The inclusion of antisocial personality disorder within this influential project was due in large part to the interest and foresight of Robins (1966). Her criteria set was based in large part on the clinical research of Cleckley (1941), but she modified Cleckley's criteria for psychopathy to increase the likelihood of obtaining more reliable diagnoses. Many other researchers followed the lead of Feighner et al., and, together, they indicated empirically that mental disorders can be diagnosed reliably and can provide valid information regarding etiology, pathology, course, and treatment (Blashfield, 1984; Klerman, 1986; Nathan & Langenbucher, 1999).

ICD-9 and DSM-III

By the time Feighner et al. (1972) published, work was nearing completion on the ninth edition of ICD. Representatives from the APA were again involved, particularly Henry Brill, chairman of the Task Force on Nomenclature, and Jack Ewalt, past president of the APA (Kramer et al., 1979). A series of international meetings were held, each of which focused on a specific problem area (the 1971 meeting in Tokyo focused on personality disorders and drug addictions). It was decided that ICD-9 would include a narrative glossary describing each of the conditions, but it was apparent that ICD-9 would not include the more specific and explicit criteria sets being developed by many research programs (Kendell, 1975).

In 1974, the APA appointed a Task Force on Nomenclature and Statistics to revise DSM-II in a manner that would be compatible with ICD-9 but would also incorporate many of the innovations that were currently being developed. By the time this Task Force was appointed, ICD-9 was largely completed (the initial draft of ICD-9 was published in 1973). Spitzer and Williams (1985) described the mission of the DSM-III Task Force more with respect to developing an alternative to ICD-9 than with developing a manual that was well coordinated with ICD-9.

> As the mental disorders chapter of the ninth revision of the International Classification of Diseases (ICD-9) was being developed, the American Psychiatric Association's Committee on Nomenclature and Statistics reviewed it to assess its adequacy for use in the United States. . . . There was some concern that it had not made sufficient use of recent methodological developments, such as specified diagnostic criteria and multiaxial diagnosis, and that, in many specific areas of the classification, there was insufficient subtyping for clinical and research use. . . . For those reasons, the American Psychiatric Association in June 1974 appointed Robert L. Spitzer to chair a Task Force on Nomenclature and Statistics to develop a new diagnostic manual. . . . The mandate given to the task force was to develop a classification that would, as much as possible, reflect the current state of knowledge regarding mental disorders and maximize its usefulness for both clinical practice and research studies. Secondarily, the classification was to be, as much as possible, compatible with ICD-9. (Spitzer & Williams, 1985, p. 604)

DSM-III was published by the APA in 1980 and did indeed include many innovations (Spitzer, Williams, & Skodol, 1980). Four of the personality disorders that had been included in DSM-II were deleted (i.e., aesthenic, cyclothymic, inadequate, and explosive) and four new diagnoses were added (i.e., avoidant, dependent, borderline, and narcissistic) (Frances, 1980; Spitzer et al., 1980). Equally important, each of the personality disorders was now provided with more specific and explicit diagnostic criteria, with the hope that they would then be diagnosed reliably in general clinical practice.

Field trials indicated that the diagnostic criteria sets of DSM-III were indeed helpful in improving reliability (e.g., Spitzer, Forman, & Nee, 1979; Williams & Spitzer, 1980). "In the DSM-III field trials over 450 clinicians participated in the largest reliability study ever done, involving independent evaluations of nearly 800 patients. . . . For most of the diagnostic classes the reliability was quite good, and in general it was much higher than that previously achieved with DSM-I and DSM-II" (Spitzer et al., 1980, p. 154). However, there was less success with the personality disorders. For example, Spitzer et al. (1979) reported a kappa of only .61 for the agreement regarding the presence of any personality disorder for jointly conducted interviews. "Although Personality Disorder as a class is evaluated more reliably than previously, with the exception of Antisocial Personality Disorder . . . the kappas for the specific Personality Disorders are quite low and range from .26 to .75" (Williams & Spitzer, 1980, p. 468).

The inadequate reliability was attributed largely to the difficulty in developing behavioral indicators. "For some disorders, . . . particularly the Personality Disorders, a much higher order of inference is necessary" (APA, 1980, p. 7). Mellsop, Varghese, Joshua, and Hicks (1982) reported the agreement for individual DSM-III personality disorders in general clinical practice, with kappa ranging in value from a low of .01 (schizoid) to a high of .49 (antisocial). The relative "success" obtained for the antisocial diagnosis was attributed to the greater specificity of its diagnostic criteria, a finding that has been replicated many times since (Widiger & Sanderson, 1995a; Zimmerman, 1994). However, the overall lack of reliability was attributed by Mellsop et al. (1982) primarily to idiosyncratic biases among the clinicians rather than to inadequate criteria sets. They noted how one clinician diagnosed 59% of patients as borderline, whereas another diagnosed 50% as antisocial. Mellsop et al. (1982) concluded that "Axis II of DSM-III represents a significant step forward in increasing the reliability of the diagnosis of personality disorders in everyday clinical practice" (p. 1361). They acknowledged that further specification of the

diagnostic criteria might be helpful in increasing reliability, but they emphasized instead the development of more standardized and structured interviewing techniques to address idiosyncratic clinical interviewing.

Another innovation of DSM-III was the placement of the personality and specific developmental disorders on a separate "axis" to ensure that they would not be overlooked by clinicians whose attention might be drawn to a more florid and immediate condition and to emphasize that a diagnosis of a personality disorder was not mutually exclusive with the diagnosis of an anxiety, mood, or other mental disorder (Frances, 1980; Spitzer et al., 1980). The effect of this placement was indeed a boon to the diagnosis of personality disorders, dramatically increasing the frequency of their diagnosis (Loranger, 1990). The substantial growth in interest in the diagnosis of personality disorders over the past 15+ years (e.g., development of societies and journals devoted to their study) might be due in part to this special attention given to personality disorders in DSM-III (Blashfield & McElroy, 1987).

DSM-III-R

A disadvantage of the DSM-III explicit criteria was that systematic errors were as reliable as the diagnoses themselves, and a number of such errors were soon identified. "Criteria were not entirely clear, were inconsistent across categories, or were even contradictory" (APA, 1987, p. xvii). The APA therefore authorized the development of a revision to DSM-III to correct these errors, as well as to provide a few additional refinements and clarifications. A more fundamental revision to the manual was to be tabled until work began on ICD-10. The criteria were only to be "reviewed for consistency, clarity, and conceptual accuracy, and revised when necessary" (APA, 1987, p. xvii). However, it was perhaps unrealistic to expect the authors of DSM-III-R to confine their efforts to simply refinement and clarification, given the impact, success, and importance of DSM-III.

The impact of DSM-III has been remarkable. Soon after its publication, it became widely accepted in the United States as the common language of mental health clinicians and researchers for communicating about the disorders for which they have professional responsibility. Recent major textbooks of psychiatry and other textbooks that discuss psychopathology have either made extensive reference to DSM-III or largely adopted its terminology and concepts. In the seven years since the publication of DSM-III, over two thousand articles that directly address some aspect of it have appeared in the scientific literature. (APA, 1987, p. xviii)

It was not difficult to find persons who wanted to be involved in the development of DSM-III-R, and most persons who were (or were not) involved wanted to have a significant impact on the final decisions. There were more persons involved in making corrections to DSM-III than had been involved in its original construction (the DSM-III Personality Disorders Advisory Commitee consisted of only 10 persons, whereas the DSM-III-R Advisory Committee had 38) and, not surprisingly, there were many proposals for significant additions, revisions, and deletions. Work began on DSM-III-R in 1983, with an anticipated date of publication in 1985 (Spitzer & Williams, 1987), but DSM-III-R was not published until 1987, and the final edition included major revisions to the personality disorders section (Widiger, Frances, Spitzer, & Williams, 1988).

Two new diagnoses, sadistic and self-defeating, were included within an appendix for proposed categories needing further study (Widiger et al., 1988). These diagnoses had been approved by the Personality Disorders Advisory Committee, but this decision was overturned by the American Psychiatric Association Board of Trustees due to their controversial nature and questionable empirical support (Widiger, 1995). Most of the criteria sets were also revised substantially (e.g., the addition of frantic efforts to avoid abandonment to the borderline criteria set, the addition of lack of remorse to the antisocial, and the deletion of overlapping items from many of the criteria sets). One general revision was the conversion of the schizoid, avoidant, dependent, and compulsive monothetic criteria sets (all the criteria are required) to polythetic criteria sets (only a specified subset of optional criteria are required).

ICD-10 AND DSM-IV

By the time work was completed on DSM-III-R, work had already begun on ICD-10. The decision of the authors of DSM-III to develop an alternative to ICD-9 was instrumental in developing a highly innovative manual (Kendell, 1991; Spitzer & Williams, 1985; Spitzer et al., 1980). However, this was also at the cost of decreasing compatibility with the nomenclature being used throughout the rest of the world, which is problematic to the stated purpose of providing a common language of communication. International compatibility would only be achieved by a more cooperative, joint construction of DSM and ICD.

The American Psychiatric Association Committee on Psychiatric Diagnosis and Assessment recommended in 1987 that work begin on the development of DSM-IV in collaboration with the development of ICD-10, and in May 1988 the American Psychiatric Association Board of Trustees appointed a DSM-IV Task Force, chaired by Allen Frances (Frances, Widiger, & Pincus, 1989). Mandates for this Task Force were to revise DSM-III-R in a manner that would be more compatible with ICD-10, would be more user friendly to the practicing clinician, and would be more explicitly empirically based (Frances et al., 1990).

ICD-10 and DSM-IV Compatibility

Members of the ICD-10 and DSM-IV committees began meeting soon after the DSM-IV Task Force was formed (the personality disorder representatives from ICD-10 were Alv Dahl, Armand Loranger, and Charles Pull). These joint meetings were successful in increasing the congruency of the two nomenclatures. Table 3.1 provides the personality disorder diagnoses of ICD-10 (WHO, 1992) and DSM-IV (APA, 1994). For example, a borderline subtype was added to the ICD-10 emotionally unstable personality disorder that was closely compatible with DSM-IV borderline personality disorder. The DSM-IV Personality Disorders Work Group recommended that a diagnosis for the ICD-10 personality change after catastrophic experience be included in DSM-IV (Shea, 1996), but this recommendation was not approved by the Task Force (Gunderson, 1998). Many revisions to DSM-III-R criteria sets were also implemented to increase the congruency of respective diagnoses (Widiger, Mangine, Corbitt, Ellis, & Thomas, 1995). For example, the DSM-IV obsessive–compulsive criterion of rigidity and stubbornness and many of the DSM-IV criteria for schizoid personality disor-

TABLE 3.1. Personality Disorders of ICD-10 and DSM-IV

ICD-10	DSM-IV[a]
Paranoid	Paranoid
Schizoid	Schizoid
Schizotypal[b]	Schizotypal
Dissocial	Antisocial
Emotionally unstable, borderline type	Borderline
Emotionally unstable, impulsive type	
Histrionic	Histrionic
	Narcissistic
Anxious	Avoidant
Dependent	Dependent
Anankastic	Obsessive–compulsive
Enduring personality change after catastrophic experience	
Enduring personality change after psychiatric illness	
Organic personality disorder[c]	Personality change due to general medical condition[d]
Other specific personality disorders and mixed and other personality disorders	Personality disorder not otherwise specified

[a]Included within an appendix to DSM-IV are proposed criteria sets for passive–aggressive (negativistic) personality disorder and depressive personality disorder.
[b]ICD-10 schizotypal disorder is consistent with DSM-IV schizotypal personality disorder but included within the section for schizophrenia, schizotypal, and delusional disorders.
[c]Included within section for organic mental disorders.
[d]Included within section for mental disorders due to a general medical condition not elsewhere classified.

der were obtained from the ICD-10 research criteria.

Some of the effort to be congruent, however, was at times ironic. The 1994 DSM-IV histrionic criterion of self-dramatization, theatricality, and exaggerated expression of emotions was obtained from the 1992 ICD-10 research criteria, but this ICD-10 criterion had itself been obtained from the 1980 DSM-III criteria set (Widiger et al., 1995). An initial draft of ICD-10 included passive–aggressive personality disorder, largely in the spirit of compatibility with DSM-IV, but the authors of DSM-IV were recommending at the same time that this diagnosis be considered for removal, due in part to its failure to obtain recognition within the international nomenclature.

Clinical Utility

One difficulty shared by the authors of DSM-IV and ICD-10 was the development of criteria sets that would maximize reliability without being overly cumbersome for clinical practice. Maximizing the utility of the diagnostic criteria for the practicing clinician had been an important concern for the authors of DSM-III and DSM-III-R, but it did appear that more emphasis was at times given to the needs of the researcher (Frances et al., 1990). This was particularly evident in the lengthy, complex, and detailed criteria sets (e.g., DSM-III-R somatization, conduct, and antisocial personality disorders). Researchers are able to devote more than 2 hours to assess the personality disorder diagnostic criteria, but this is unrealistic for general practitioners. The WHO, therefore, provided separate versions of ICD-10 for the researcher and the clinician (Sartorius, 1988; Sartorius et al., 1993). The researcher's version includes relatively specific and explicit criteria sets, whereas the clinician's version includes only narrative descriptions. The DSM-IV Task Force considered this option but decided that it would complicate the generalization of research findings to clinical practice and vice versa (Frances et al., 1990). One might also question the implications of providing more detailed, reliable criteria sets for the researcher, and simpler, less reliable criteria sets for clinical decisions. The DSM-IV Task Force decided instead to try to simplify the most cumbersome and lengthy DSM-III-R criteria sets. The best example of their work for the personality disorders was the criteria set for antisocial personality disorder (Widiger et al., 1996; Widiger & Corbitt, 1995).

Empirical Support

One of the more common concerns regarding DSM-III and DSM-III-R was the extent of its empirical support. Persons reviewing the decisions that were made often suggested that these decisions were more consistent with the theoretical perspectives of the members of the Work Group or Advisory Committee than with the published research. "For most of the personality disorder categories there was either no empirical base (e.g., avoidant, dependent, passive–aggressive, narcissistic) or no clinical tradition (e.g., avoidant, dependent, schizotypal); thus their disposition was much more subject to the convictions of individual Advisory Committee members" (Gunderson, 1983, p. 30). Millon (1981) criticized the DSM-III criteria for antisocial personality disorder for being too heavily influenced by Robins (1966), a member of the DSM-III Personality Disorders Advisory Commitee. Gunderson (1983) and Kernberg (1984), on the other hand, criticized the inclusion of avoidant personality disorder as being too heavily influenced by Millon (1981), another member of the same committee.

The development of DSM-IV proceeded through three stages of review of empirical data, including systematic and comprehensive reviews of the research literature, reanalyses of multiple data sets, and field trials, all of which would be published in a series of archival texts (Frances et al., 1990; Nathan, 1994; Widiger, Frances, Pincus, Davis, & First, 1991). For example, systematic, comprehensive, and ostensibly neutral summaries of the clinical and empirical literature were provided with respect to all the major proposals for the DSM-IV personality disorders. Most of these reviews also contained the results of a series of internal consistency analyses of the DSM-III-R criteria sets using multiple data sets (Widiger & Trull, 1998). A field trial of the proposed revisions to the antisocial personality disorder was also conducted that included approximately 500 subjects from diverse, relevant sites (Widiger et al., 1996). Frances et al. (1989) concluded their initial presentation of the rationale and process for DSM-IV by stating that "it is in fact possible that the major innovation of DSM-IV will not be in its having surprising new content but rather will reside in the systematic and explicit method by which DSM-IV will be constructed and documented" (p. 375).

DSM-IV, however, did include many substantive revisions. Only 10 of the 93 DSM-III-R personality disorder diagnostic criteria were left unchanged, 21 received minor revisions, 10 were deleted, 9 were added, and 52 received a significant revision (Widiger et al., 1995). The personality disorder that was the most frequently diagnosed by clinicians during World War II (passive–aggressive) was downgraded to an appendix (Wetzler & Morey, 1999). A new diagnosis, depressive, was also added to this appendix (Ryder & Bagby, 1999).

The self-defeating and sadistic personality disorders, approved for inclusion by the DSM-III-R Advisory Committee, were deleted entirely from the manual (Widiger, 1995). A detailed summary of these revisions is beyond the scope of this chapter, but this information is available elsewhere (Gunderson, 1998; Livesley, 1995; Widiger et al., 1995).

ICD-11 AND DSM-V

The APA (2000) has already published revisions to the text of DSM-IV. No revisions were made to the criteria sets, and no diagnoses were deleted or added to the manual. The DSM-IV-Text Revision (DSM-IV-TR; APA, 2000) was confined solely to the description of the personality disorders' associated features, prevalence, course, familial pattern, differential diagnosis, and culture, age, or gender features.

A more fundamental revision may await the development of ICD-11. DSM-I, DSM-II, DSM-III, and DSM-IV were coordinated, at least in timing, with an edition of the ICD (ICD-6, ICD-8, ICD-9, and ICD-10, respectively). DSM-V would then be coordinated with ICD-11. However, the WHO experienced substantial difficulty completing all the sections of ICD in a timely fashion (Kendell, 1991). The mental disorders section of ICD-10 was published in 1992 but would not go into effect for sometime thereafter, awaiting the completion of other sections of the manual. Prior revisions of ICD have occurred approximately every 10 years, but the latest revision itself required more than 10 years to complete. It is possible that future revisions of ICD will be confined to individual sections of the manual, each being revised on its own schedule. Blashfield and Fuller (1996), using an empirically derived linear regression analysis, predicted that DSM-V will be published in 2007 (1998 with a logarithmic analysis), will include 390 diagnoses and 11 appendices; will be chaired by Gary Tucker; and will be published with a brown cover.

There are advantages to an earlier rather than a later revision. Substantial clinical, social, empirical, and theoretical attention is now being given to the diagnosis of mental disorders. The progress is perhaps so rapid that many sections of DSM-IV are quickly becoming antiquated. On the other hand, revisions are disruptive to clinical practice and research (Zimmerman, 1988), and most revisions generate significant disagreement and even controversy (Frances et al., 1990). Maser, Kaelber, and Wise (1991) surveyed clinicians from 42 countries with respect to DSM-III-R: "The personality disorders led the list of diagnostic categories with which respondents were dissatisfied" (p. 275). This could be an argument for substantial revision (i.e., address all their major concerns) or it could be an argument for minimal revision (i.e., wait until the solutions are clear to everyone before any more mistakes are made). In any case, initial planning meetings are now in progress for the development of DSM-V (McQueen, 2000). The authors of the personality disorders section of DSM-V will need to address a number of fundamental and difficult issues, including (1) criteria for revision, (2) number, specificity, and format of diagnostic criteria, (3) threshold for diagnosis, (4) dimensional versus categorical classification, (5) distinction between Axis I and Axis II, and (6) gender, ethnic, and cultural differences. Each of these issues is discussed briefly in turn.

Criteria for Revision

One of the more difficult issues for the authors of an official diagnostic system are the criteria for revision. The authors of DSM-III (APA, 1980) were intentionally liberal. Antisocial and borderline were the only two disorders for which specific diagnostic criteria had already been researched. The DSM-III Personality Disorders Advisory Committee based their construction of the other criteria sets on previously published descriptions, but there was otherwise little that would constrain the committee. The inclusion of new diagnoses was equally liberal.

> Because the DSM-III classification is intended for the entire profession, and because our current knowledge about mental disorder is so limited, the Task Force has chosen to be inclusive rather than exclusive. In practice, this means that whenever a clinical condition can be described with clarity and relative distinctness, it is considered for inclusion. If there is general agreement among clinicians, who would be expected to encounter the condition, that there are a significant number of patients who have it and that its identification is important in their clinical work, it is included in the classification. (Spitzer, Sheehy, & Endicott, 1977, p. 3)

This liberal policy, however, eventually led to the inclusion of diagnoses that were met with considerable opposition (e.g., Caplan, 1991). Blashfield, Sprock, and Fuller (1990) proposed substantially more conservative criteria for future editions, with particular emphasis on the presence of published empirical support: "there should be at least 50 journal articles published on the proposed diagnostic category in the last 10 years. Moreover, at least 25 of them should be empirical" (p. 17). Clark, Watson, and Reynolds (1995), however, have argued that a conservative approach to revision results in a continually outmoded, antiquated nomenclature that constrains rather than facilitates progress.

The authors of DSM-IV emphasized the obtainment of adequate empirical support for new diagnoses and for item revision (Frances et al., 1990; Nathan, 1994; Nathan & Langenbucher, 1999). As a result, diagnoses that were included in the appendix to DSM-III-R primarily "to facilitate further systematic clinical study and research" (APA, 1987, p. 367) were excluded from DSM-IV. The inclusion of new diagnoses is useful in generating highly informative research, but it was argued that "research should drive DSM and not the other way around" (Pincus, Frances, Davis, First, & Widiger, 1992, p. 114). DSM-IV is the primary source for officially recognized diagnoses. "Including an unproven experimental diagnostic category in DSM-IV may confer upon that category an approval which it does not yet merit" (Pincus et al., 1992, p. 367). Pincus et al. were clear in their rejection of the DSM-III-R Personality Disorder Advisory Committee decision to include the sadistic personality disorder: "the lack of any empirical support and historical tradition for this category as well as any compatibility with ICD-10 makes it impossible to recommend it for inclusion in DSM-IV" (p. 116).

A specific suggestion for DSM-V is to conduct field trials of all proposed revisions prior to the final decisions. The absence of systematic pilot testing of proposed revisions is perhaps remarkable given the substantial importance of the manual and the considerable impact that seemingly minor revisions can have (Blashfield, Blum, & Pfohl, 1992; Morey, 1988; Regier et al., 1998). Pilot data were obtained prior to the final decisions for the DSM-III borderline and schizotypal criteria sets (Spitzer, Endicott, & Gibbon, 1979), and for proposed revisions to the DSM-IV antisocial, schizotypal, and borderline criteria sets (Silverman, Siever, Zanarini, Coccaro, & Mitropoulou, 1998; Sternbach, Judd, Sabo, McGlashan, & Gunderson, 1992;

Widiger et al., 1996). However, there has never been a systematic effort to pilot a draft of all the proposed revisions to assess their likely effects prior to final approval (a field trial of the ICD-10 personality disorder criteria sets was conducted after the final decisions had been made; Loranger et al., 1994). A comprehensive and systematic field trial would be costly, but the expense of this project would be considerably less than the income that will ultimately be generated by the sales of the book.

Complicating the demand for adequate empirical support are the equally strong demands for a greater impact of theory and clinical experience (e.g., Cooper, 1987, 1993; Follette & Houts, 1996; Frances, 1980; Frances & Cooper, 1981; Gunderson, 1983; Kernberg, 1984; Livesley, 1985, 1998; Millon, 1981; Perry, 1990; Sarbin, 1997; Tyrer, 1988; Westen, 1997; Westen & Shedler, 1999) . It is not the case that relevant theoretical perspectives have failed to have an impact on the development of the diagnostic criteria. The influence of theory has often been substantial; for example, the impact of attachment theory on the revisions to the dependent criteria set (Hirschfeld, Shea, & Weise, 1991), the inclusion of the new histrionic criterion of excessive perception of intimacy (Pfohl, 1991), the inclusion of the passive–aggressive criterion of alternating between hostile defense and contrition (Millon, 1993), and the elevation of frantic efforts to avoid abandonment to the status of being the first diagnostic criterion (Gunderson, 1996; Gunderson, Zanarini, & Koesel, 1991).

Nevertheless, a related criticism has been the absence of a single, predominant, or unifying theoretical perspective (e.g., Davis & Millon, 1995; Frances & Widiger, 1986; Millon, 1981). Livesley (1998) characterized the DSM-IV personality disorders as "an arbitrary list drawn from diverse theoretical positions, including classical phenomenology, classical psychoanalytic theory, self-psychology, object-relations theory, and social learning concepts" (p. 138). Many theorists, clinicians, and researchers have therefore offered unifying theoretical models that would bring coherence to the nomenclature (e.g., Benjamin, 1993; Cloninger & Svrakic, 1994; Kiesler, 1996; Koerner, Kohlenberg, & Parker, 1996; Livesley, 1998; Millon et al., 1996; Pretzer & Beck, 1996; Sarbin, 1997; Siever & Davis, 1991; Westen & Shedler, 1999; Widiger & Costa, 1994). The obvious difficulty is that all (but one) of these authors would like-

ly be very critical of DSM-V if it adopted just one of the foregoing perspectives, although perhaps no less critical for trying to represent all of them. Livesley and Jackson (1992) suggested that "the classification be evaluated and revised using criteria derived from the theoretical and measurement models associated with each diagnosis" (p. 609). As noted previously, this has in fact been largely the intention of the authors of each edition of DSM (Frances, 1980; Livesley, 1995; Widiger et al., 1988). Nevertheless, it is also important to appreciate that there will be as much disagreement regarding which theoretical and measurement models should take priority for any particular diagnosis as there will be disagreement regarding which theoretical models should govern the entire class of disorders (Gunderson, 1992, 1998; Widiger & Trull, 1993).

The appropriate impact of clinical experience and tradition complicates the effort even further. Many systematic studies of the opinions, preferences, and practices of clinicians have been conducted (e.g., Adler, Drake, & Teague, 1990; Blashfield & Breen, 1989; Blashfield & Haymaker, 1988; Ford & Widiger, 1989; Gunderson et al., 1991; Kass, Skodol, Charles, Spitzer, & Williams, 1985; Kass, Spitzer, & Williams, 1983; Maser et al., 1991; Mellsop et al., 1982; Morey, 1988; Morey & Ochoa, 1989; Pfohl & Blum, 1991; Spitzer, Forman, & Nee, 1979; Spitzer, Fiester, Gay, & Pfohl, 1991; Sternbach et al., 1992) and this research influenced decisions regarding DSM-III-R and DSM-IV. However, many of these studies indicated that clinicians fail routinely to use the criteria sets in the manner that was intended, fail to assess the criteria in a comprehensive or systematic manner, and are even unable to identify the diagnoses in which the criteria are included (e.g., Blashfield & Breen, 1989; Morey, 1988; Westen, 1997; Zimmerman & Mattia, 1999). One interpretation of these findings is that the DSM lacks adequate face validity and should therefore be modeled more closely on how clinicians conceptualize and diagnose personality disorders within general clinical practice (Westen, 1997; Westen & Shedler, 1999). Another interpretation is that clinicians fail to appreciate the value and importance of learning, understanding, and using DSM in a reliable manner. There is much to be obtained from studying general clinical practice and surveying practitioners, but optimal clinical diagnosis of personality disorders is not necessarily that which is occurring in general clinical practice (e.g., Dawes, 1994).

If clinical experience does have an impact on decisions, it should not represent simply the experience of the members of the Work Group or their impressions of the experience of practicing clinicians. "Expert opinion [should] be sampled systematically . . . quantitative methods be used, and . . . sufficient experts be polled to ensure the representativeness and reliability of their pooled judgments" (Livesley & Jackson, 1992, p. 613). Proponents and opponents of proposed revisions will at times fail to appreciate how inadequately they understand or represent the perspectives of practicing clinicians. There might in fact be more diversity and disagreement concerning the diagnosis of personality disorders within 100 randomly selected clinicians than within 100 randomly selected researchers. For example, the authors of DSM-III-R recommended the inclusion of sadistic personality disorder in part because "many clinicians who evaluate individuals . . . who abuse spouses or children believe there is a need for identifying this particular pattern of personality disorder" (Work Group to Revise DSM-III, 1986, p. IX:43). However, a more systematic survey of forensic psychiatrists indicated that 66% believed that the diagnosis had considerable potential for misuse, only 11% believed that it would be "very useful and should be included," 29% felt that it was of "no or limited value and likely to be abused," and 16% felt that it was "perhaps useful, but inadequate data to justify its inclusion" (Spitzer et al., 1991, p. 877).

In sum, it is apparent from a review of the recent history that theorists, researchers, and clinicians are unlikely to agree as to the theory, research, and clinical experience that is adequate or necessary for a revision. In addition, theory, research, and clinical experience are often inconsistent, particularly in the context of competing theoretical models. Researchers and clinicians from one theoretical perspective do appear to be more favorable in their interpretation of findings consistent with their perspective and less favorable to the findings from an alternative perspective, at least in comparison to the researchers and clinicians with the alternative perspective. Spitzer et al. (1991) would likely disagree with the conclusion of Pincus et al. (1992) that there was no empirical support for the sadistic diagnosis. Caplan (1991) characterized the development of the recent editions

of DSM as being riddled with "pseudoscience and sloppy science" (p. 162), criticizing in particular the recognition of diagnoses that had inadequate empirical support. At the same time, Pantony and Caplan (1991) developed their own diagnosis of delusional dominating personality disorder and criticized the authors of DSM-IV for failing to give it adequate recognition.

Whatever criteria for revision are used for DSM-V, the authors should be as explicit as possible regarding the manner and extent to which their decisions were guided by theoretical, empirical, and clinical input (Livesley & Jackson, 1992; Nathan, 1994). This documentation is especially useful in facilitating informative critiques of the decisions (Widiger & Trull, 1993), as well as facilitating an accurate understanding and representation of the bases for the decisions. This was indeed the intention of the authors of DSM-IV (Frances et al., 1990; Nathan & Langenbucher, 1999). There is perhaps as much criticism regarding the decisions that were made for DSM-IV as there were for DSM-III (e.g., Bornstein, 1997; Livesley, 1995; Westen, 1997), but considerable effort was given to presenting the rationale for each of the decisions for each of the personality disorders. These presentations included the publication of the *DSM-IV Options Book* (Task Force on DSM-IV, 1991) and *DSM-IV Draft Criteria* (Task Force on DSM-IV, 1993), presentations at conferences, special sections within the *Journal of Personality Disorders* for each of the proposed diagnoses (Gunderson & Shea, 1991; Shea, 1993; Widiger, 1991), presentation within an edited volume accompanied by critiques of these decisions (i.e., Livesley, 1995), and publications of the literature reviews, data analyses, and field trials within the *DSM-IV Sourcebook* (Widiger et al., 1991).

Number, Specificity, and Format of Diagnostic Criteria

The authors of all prior editions of DSM and the ICD have struggled over the optimal number, specificity, and format of the diagnostic criteria. An innovation of DSM-III was the development of behaviorally specific criteria that could be diagnosed reliably in general clinical practice (Spitzer et al., 1980). As noted earlier, this effort was only partially successful for the personality disorders (APA, 1980). The criteria vary substantially within and across the personality disorders in their behavioral specificity (Clark, 1992; Shea, 1992). The DSM-III criteria for antisocial personality disorder are the most uniformally specific, providing the major reason this disorder is the most reliably diagnosed within clinical practice (Mellsop et al., 1982) and clinical research (Widiger & Sanderson, 1995a; Zimmerman, 1994). However, the antisocial criteria have been criticized precisely for being too behaviorally specific (Hare, Hart, & Harpur, 1991; Perry, 1992), and they have since been revised to include more general traits of psychopathy (Widiger et al., 1996; Widiger & Corbitt, 1995).

Inadequate reliability of personality disorder diagnoses is not necessarily due to the absence of sufficiently precise diagnostic criteria (Blashfield, 1984). All the personality disorders might be diagnosed reliably if clinicians used semistructured interviews (Rogers, 1995; Segal, 1997; Widiger & Sanderson, 1995a). Hare et al. (1991) have indicated that the more inferential constructs of psychopathy can be diagnosed as reliably as the more behaviorally specific antisocial criteria when psychopathy is assessed with a semistructured interview. A major source for the weak reliability and questionable validity of personality disorder diagnoses within general clinical practice does appear to be due in part to the failure of clinicians to assess systematically each of the diagnostic criteria (Adler et al., 1990; Morey & Ochoa, 1989). The solution to inadequate reliability may then be better training of clinicians as well as better diagnostic criteria.

Semistructured interviews, however, might be too cumbersome and impractical for routine clinical use. In addition, the interrater reliability reported by researchers might be somewhat overstated (Widiger & Sanderson, 1995a). The reliability that has been reported has been confined largely to the agreement in the rating of responses. This reliability is important, but it is unclear whether there is in fact much agreement in the administration of the same interview by different researchers at different sites. The reliability that has been obtained by researchers might be due in part to the development of a local consensus in how to interpret or code responses that goes well beyond the instructions provided within any particular interview manual.

A related goal for DSM-IV was to reduce and simplify the more lengthy and complex criteria sets to make them more suitable for routine clinical use (Frances et al., 1990). However, a complex constellation of personality traits may not be reducible to a small set of behaviorally specific indicators (Clark, 1992). It is difficult to have both simplicity and accuracy when diagnosing a personality disorder. For example, it might not be realistic to assess the identity disturbance of borderline psychopathology, the lack of empathy of narcissism, or the irresponsibility of psychopathy with just one or two behaviorally specific acts, even if these acts are prototypical (Widiger et al., 1988). One of the revisions for DSM-IV was to move some of the behaviorally specific indicators from the criteria sets into the text discussion (Gunderson, 1998; Widiger et al., 1995). For example, many researchers were confining their assessment of antisocial recklessness to simply the presence of the two behavioral indicators provided within the criteria set (i.e., driving under the influence and recurrent speeding), even though antisocial recklessness is much more than simply this particular reckless use of a car (Widiger & Corbitt, 1995). Placing the behavioral indicators within the text allows for the inclusion of more illustrations and clarifications of what is (and is not) meant by each particular feature of the disorder (Widiger et al., 1995).

A variety of alternative formats for the criteria sets have been proposed and piloted (Clark, 1992; Livesley, 1985, 1986; Perry, 1990; Schwartz, Wiggins, & Norko, 1995; Shea, 1992; Spitzer & Williams, 1987; Widiger & Frances, 1985). The current polythetic format avoids the unrealistically narrow requirement that all persons with the disorder share all the features. However, the polythetic format contributes to substantial heterogeneity among persons sharing the same diagnosis that is problematic to research and communication. Increasing the threshold for diagnosis would provide more homogeneity but at the expense of failing to diagnose persons who probably have enough of the features to warrant a diagnosis (Kass et al., 1985; Westen, 1997; Widiger & Corbitt, 1994). A compromise considered for DSM-IV was to require one essential or fundamental feature as a central anchor, but there was substantial disagreement regarding the criterion that would be emphasized and the basis for this selection (e.g., the feature that is theoretically central to the disorder or the feature that is empirically most diagnostic of the disorder; Gunderson, 1992). The final compromise was to provide the criteria sets in a descending order of diagnostic importance without indicating explicitly how much weight (if any) should be given to each criterion (Gunderson, 1998; Widiger et al., 1995).

Threshold for Diagnosis

DSM-III through DSM-IV provide specific rules for when there are enough features of the disorder for it to be diagnosed. For example, at least five of the eight features must be present in order to diagnose dependent personality disorder (APA, 1994). The provision of a specific rule is tremendously helpful in decreasing interrater unreliability, as clinicians will disagree substantially in their thresholds for a personality disorder diagnosis (Adler et al., 1990; Mellsop et al., 1982; Morey, 1988). However, current thresholds for diagnosis are largely unexplained and are perhaps weakly justified (Clark, 1992; Kass et al., 1985; Tyrer & Johnson, 1996; Widiger & Corbitt, 1994).

The DSM-III schizotypal and borderline diagnoses were the only two for which a published rationale has been provided, and the bases for their diagnostic thresholds may not even be sufficiently compelling to use as a model for other disorders. The DSM-III requirement that the patient have four of eight features for the schizotypal diagnosis and five of eight for the borderline (APA, 1980) was determined on the basis of maximizing agreement with diagnoses provided by clinicians (Spitzer, Endicott, & Gibbon, 1979). Setting the threshold to match clinically diagnosed cases is consistent with the spirit of modeling routine clinical diagnosis (Westen, 1997). The resulting thresholds might then be that point at which practicing clinicians would agree a sufficient number of features are present. However, there was no indication whether the clinicians' "borderline schizophrenia" or "borderline personality organization" cases had been reliably or validly diagnosed. There was no indication whether the cases were even typical, prototypical, or representative of persons with these disorders.

In any case, the borderline and schizotypal criteria sets have been revised substantially since DSM-III. No cross-validation of the diagnostic thresholds has been conducted, despite the substantial effects the subsequent revisions have had on clinical diagnosis. Blashfield et al. (1992) reported a kappa of only −.025 for the DSM-III and DSM-III-R schizotypal personality disorders, with a reduction in prevalence from 11% to 1% (Morey, 1988, reported a comparable decrease in prevalence from 17% to 9%).

There has been no comparable effort to develop a rationale for the establishment of the thresholds for any of the other personality disorders. In the absence of any data or rationale to guide the decision of where to set the thresholds, it is not surprising to find substantial variation across each edition (Frances, 1998). For example, Morey (1988) reported an 800% increase in the number of persons beyond the threshold for a schizoid diagnosis in DSM-III-R as compared to DSM-III, and a 350% increase for the narcissistic diagnosis. Some of this shift in prevalence might have been intentional (Widiger et al., 1988), but much of it was probably unanticipated (Blashfield et al., 1992).

It is stated in DSM-IV that it is "only when personality traits are inflexible and maladaptive and cause significant functional impairment or subjective distress do they constitute Personality Disorders" (APA, 1994, p. 630). A proposal for DSM-V would be to set the diagnostic thresholds for each personality disorder at that point at which the constellation of personality traits described therein would result in a clinically significant impairment to social or occupational functioning or personal distress. This would be consistent with the definition of a personality disorder, would result in a threshold for diagnosis that is more uniform across disorders, and would at least appear to be less arbitrary (Widiger & Corbitt, 1994). It would be difficult to reach a consensus of what is meant by clinically significant impairment (Frances, 1998; Spitzer & Williams, 1982; Strack & Lorr, 1997; Widiger & Corbitt, 1994), but this would only make explicit what is currently being decided implicitly without any guidelines.

Dimensional versus Categorical Classification

Establishing diagnostic thresholds would be easier if the disorders involved qualitatively distinct pathologies. Once a reasonably valid assessment of this pathology was obtained, the thresholds could be set at that point at which the diagnosis maximizes the likelihood of identifying the presence of this pathology. "The diagnostic approach used [in DSM-IV and ICD-10] represents the categorical perspective that Personality Disorders represent qualitatively distinct clinical syndromes" (APA, 1994, p. 633).

The empirical support for this perspective, however, does appear to be minimal relative to the alternative perspective that personality disorders are on a continuum with one another, with other mental disorders, and with normal personality functioning (Livesley, Schroeder, Jackson, & Jang, 1994; Widiger & Sanderson, 1995b). Personality and personality disorders appear to be the result of a complex interaction of biogenetic predispositions and environmental experiences that result in an array of possible constellations of adaptive and maladaptive personality traits (Clark, Livesley, & Morey, 1997; Paris, 1993). "There is an implicit and reasonable assumption that traits and their disordered counterparts exist on a continua, which means that the distinction is inherently arbitrary. Recognition of the universality of character types and the importance of documenting them is, I think, the single most important accomplishment of DSM-III" (Gunderson, 1983, pp. 20–21). Providing a diagnosis that refers to a particular constellation of traits is useful in highlighting certain features (e.g., the prototypical psychopathic profile; Widiger & Lynam, 1998), but a categorical diagnosis also suggests the presence of features that are not in fact present and fails to describe important features that are present. Many of the problems that bedevil the diagnosis of personality disorders are due in part to the imposition of arbitrary categorical distinctions upon underlying dimensions of personality functioning (Livesley et al., 1994; Widiger & Sanderson, 1995b).

A useful model for the diagnosis of personality disorders is perhaps provided by the diagnosis of mental retardation (Widiger, 1997). Personality and intelligence are both complex but relatively stable domains of functioning. The disorder of mental retardation is that point at which one's level of intelligence results in a clinically significant impairment to social and/or occupational functioning, currently diagnosed largely by an intelligence quotient score of 70 (APA, 1994). This point of demarcation is not unreasonable, random, or meaningless, but it is arbitrary and does not carve nature at a discrete joint. It is simply that point at which clinicians and researchers have determined is a meaningful and useful point at

which to characterize the limitations to intelligence as a disorder. Persons with a level of intelligence of approximately 79 (i.e., a DSM-IV diagnosis of borderline intellectual functioning) will also experience significant impairments to social and occupational functioning, but these impairments will not be as severe as those with levels of intelligence of 69. The distinction between normal and abnormal levels of intelligence is more quantitative than qualitative.

There are persons below an IQ of 70 for whom a qualitatively distinct disorder is evident. However, the disorder in these cases is not mental retardation. It is a physical disorder (e.g., Down syndrome) that can be traced to a specific biological event (e.g., trisomy 21). Intelligence, on the other hand, is a normally distributed, continuous dimension, as the level of intelligence in most persons (including most of the mentally retarded) is the result of a complex array of multiple genetic, fetal and infant development, and environmental influences. Down syndrome is a qualitatively distinct disorder, but the mental retardation that is associated with this medical disorder is not.

Personality disorders might also be conceptualized and diagnosed along an analogous continuum of personality functioning, with the disorder of personality being that point that results in a clinically significant level of impairment to social or occupational functioning (Livesley, 1998; Tyrer & Johnson, 1996; Widiger & Corbitt, 1994). There may indeed be specific etiologies for particular personality dispositions (e.g., Benjamin et al., 1996), but the phenotypical array of personality traits that constitute a disorder of personality will most likely have complex polygenetic and diversely interactive environmental etiologies (Clark et al., 1997; Paris, 1993). One is unlikely to find a discrete point of demarcation along this array of phenotypical characteristics. The diagnosis of a personality disorder may in fact also require a consideration of the maladaptivity of the personality dispositions relative to an equally diverse array of social and occupational contexts (Widiger & Costa, 1994).

Axis I versus Axis II

An additional issue for the authors of DSM-V is the distinction between personality disorders that are diagnosed on Axis II (along with mental retardation) and the disorders that are diagnosed on Axis I. Their separate axis placement has encouraged clinicians to diagnose both conditions "rather than being forced to arbitrarily and unreliably make a choice between them" (Frances, 1980, p. 1050). Ironically, however, the provision of a separate axis may have also increased interest in distinguishing between them, as the presence of a separate axis might imply the presence of some special, unique distinction (Gunderson & Pollack, 1985; Livesley, 1998).

Liebowitz (1992), the chair of the DSM-IV Anxiety Disorders Work Group, argued that most of the persons diagnosed with an avoidant personality disorder should be diagnosed instead with a generalized social phobia, due in large part to the apparent responsivity of these persons to the pharmacological treatment commonly used for social phobia. "One may have to rethink what the personality disorder concept means in an instance where 6 weeks of phenelzine therapy begins to reverse longstanding interpersonal hypersensitivity as well as discomfort in socializing" (Liebowitz, 1992, p. 251). Liebowitz (1992) suggested that misdiagnosing these persons with an avoidant personality disorder was even harmful, as many would then be treated with psychotherapy rather than pharmacotherapy. "The danger . . . is that, in my experience, practitioners tend to regard Axis II conditions as amenable to psychoanalytic psychotherapy rather than pharmacotherapy" (p. 251).

There are many rejoinders to the arguments of Liebowitz (1992). Personality disorders can be responsive to pharmacological interventions (Siever & Davis, 1991); pharmacotherapy is not necessarily better treatment than psychotherapy (Sanislow & McGlashan, 1998); shifting avoidant personality disorder to Axis I would only reify the misconception that personality disorders are unresponsive to pharmacotherapy; if responsivity to phenelzine is in fact a diagnostic indicator, then perhaps social phobia should itself be shifted to the mood disorders section of the manual (Widiger et al., 1995). Nevertheless, the diagnosis of generalized social phobia was expanded in DSM-IV to include "an onset in the mid-teens, sometimes emerging out of a childhood history of social inhibition or shyness" (APA, 1994, p. 414).

One proposal to address the problematic Axis I versus Axis II distinction is to revise substantially what is meant by a personality disorder. A proposal considered by the DSM-IV Personality Disorders Work Group was to shift to respective sections of Axis I all the personality disorders that were thought to be on a continuum with Axis I disorders (e.g., borderline, avoidant, schizotypal, schizoid, paranoid, and obsessive–compulsive; Siever & Davis, 1991), retaining on Axis II only those few remaining personality disorders that were considered to be on a continuum with normal personality functioning (e.g., dependent; Gunderson, 1992). This would be consistent with the ICD-10 placement of DSM-IV schizotypal personality disorder as a form of schizophrenia (WHO, 1992), and it might address the excessive effort that is at times given to defining what is perhaps an illusory boundary between Axis I and II (Livesley, 1998). The National Institute of Mental Health (NIMH) has recommended an even stronger variant of this proposal for DSM-V (American Psychiatric Association and National Institute of Mental Health, 1999). NIMH has proposed replacing Axis II with a measure of severity or disability, converting most of the existing personality disorders into early onset and chronic variants of Axis I disorders (the term "personality" might be included but only as an historical reference; the official classification and title of the disorder would be as an anxiety, mood, impulse dyscontrol, or other Axis I disorder), and relegating any remaining personality disorders to an appendix for other conditions that might be the focus of clinical attention (comparable to the current classification of sibling and other relational problems).

The majority of the DSM-IV Personality Disorders Work Group, however, did not support shifting any of the personality disorders to Axis I, in part because it was unclear which should move and which should stay (Gunderson, 1998). In addition, all the personality disorders might in fact be on a continuum with normal personality functioning as well as with Axis I mental disorders (Clark et al., 1995; Livesley et al., 1994; Widiger & Costa, 1994). The boundaries between the disorders within and across the respective sections of Axis I are also no less problematic than the boundaries between Axis I and Axis II (Clark et al., 1995; Widiger, 1997). Shifting individual personality disorders to respective sections of Axis I (e.g., avoidant personality disorder to the anxiety disorders section) would probably also have the effect of decreasing the consideration given to personality disorders and losing the construct itself (e.g., Akiskal & Akiskal, 1992; Keller, 1989; Liebowitz, 1992).

Differences across Gender and Culture

"Those diagnostic issues that have some relationship to gender . . . have been the focus of considerable and heated professional and public debate" (Ross, Frances, & Widiger, 1995, p. 205). The proposal to include masochistic personality disorder in DSM-III-R generated substantial controversy for DSM-III-R and DSM-IV (Caplan, 1991; Widiger, 1995), as have related concerns regarding the inclusion of and the diagnostic criteria for the histrionic and dependent personality disorders (Hirschfeld et al., 1991; Kaplan, 1983; Pfohl, 1991).

Kaplan (1983) and Frances, First, and Pincus (1995) argued that personality disorder diagnostic criteria should either be gender neutral or gender balanced. They suggested that the inclusion of (stereotypically feminine) gender-related behaviors within diagnostic criteria reflects a biased attitude toward and a misdiagnosis of normal women. They recommended that the criteria sets be revised so that no gender-related behaviors are included, or that a sufficient number of masculine-related behaviors be included to offset feminine-related behaviors. The criteria sets for the dependent and histrionic personality disorders were revised in part with this intention (Pfohl, 1991; Hirschfeld et al., 1991), although not to the extent recommended by Kaplan (1983) and Frances et al. (1995).

An alternative perspective is that some personality disorders represent, at least in part, maladaptive variants of gender-related traits (Widiger & Spitzer, 1991). The occurrence of differential sex prevalence rates is consistent with some theoretical models for these disorders. It is not particularly surprising to find that males and females differ on average with respect to some personality traits (Feingold, 1994); personality disorders that involve at least in part maladaptive variants of these gender-related traits should themselves obtain a differential sex prevalence rate (Corbitt & Widiger, 1995). Females tend to be higher, on average, than males in levels of anxiousness, trust, warmth, gregariousness, emotionality, tender-mindedness, compliance, modesty, and altruism (Corbitt & Widiger, 1995; Feingold, 1994), the maladaptive variants of which are evident in the dependent and histrionic personality disorders.

However, it is precisely because these disorders involve gender-related traits that there is the problem of gender-biased diagnoses. Clinicians do tend to overdiagnose histrionic personality disorder in females (Garb, 1997). Much of this overdiagnosis is attributable to a failure to adhere to the diagnostic criteria sets, but the direction of the error is the result of the close relationship of histrionic symptomatology to stereotypically feminine behaviors (Widiger, 1998). Antisocial personality disorder is comparably associated with stereotypically masculine behaviors, but there is less overdiagnosis of antisocial personality disorder in males (Garb, 1997) because its diagnostic criteria are more behaviorally specific and less prone to misapplication. The solution to the overdiagnosis of histrionic personality disorder in females might not be to revise histrionic personality disorder so that it is more masculine (Frances et al., 1995), no more than it would be to revise the antisocial personality disorder to be more feminine. Making the histrionic personality disorder more masculine would decrease the differential sex prevalence rates primarily by increasing the misdiagnoses of one sex relative to the other (overdiagnosing histrionic personality disorder in males). The preferable (but more difficult) solution for histrionic personality disorder is to decrease the likelihood of the misdiagnosis of normal women, perhaps by increasing the behavioral specificity of the diagnostic criteria.

Comparable issues have faced the authors of ICD-10 and DSM-IV with respect to cross-cultural issues (Alarcon, 1996; Rogler, 1996). Substantial inconsistencies still remain between DSM-IV and ICD-10. For example, DSM-IV narcissistic personality disorder does not have official recognition within ICD-10 (WHO, 1992), and ICD-10 personality change following a catastrophic experience is not recognized within DSM-IV (Gunderson, 1998; Shea, 1996). A more specific issue is whether the DSM-IV and ICD-10 criteria sets are equally applicable across all cultures (Alarcon, 1996; Rogler, 1999). Loranger et al. (1994) addressed this issue empirically and concluded that there were few difficulties. The only problematic criteria they identified were the DSM-III-R antisocial criterion pertaining to monogamous relationships and the DSM-III-R sadistic criterion pertaining to harsh treatment of spouses and children (both of which have since been deleted; Widiger, 1995; Widiger & Corbitt, 1995). "Otherwise, the clinicians viewed the two classification systems as applicable to their particular cultures" (Loranger et al., 1994, p. 223). Loranger et al. (1994) reported substantial agreement between the DSM-III-R and ICD-10 criteria sets for the diagnoses shared by the two nomenclatures. The agreement for DSM-III-R borderline and ICD-10 unstable personality disorder was 92% (kappa = .66) and for DSM-III-R avoidant and ICD-10 anxious it was 89% (kappa = .52). They also reported that all the DSM-III-R personality disorders can be diagnosed reliably within most countries. For example, they indicated that when a semistructured interview for DSM-III-R was administered, passive–aggressive personality disorder was diagnosed in 5% of patients assessed at 14 centers in 11 countries in North America, Europe, Africa, and Asia.

However, this success might have been to some extent illusory. Whenever a semistructured interview is administered that includes diagnostic criteria, at least some persons will meet the criteria for the proposed disorder. One can develop diagnostic criteria for an entirely illusory mental disorder and find that a proportion of the population are beyond the threshold for its diagnosis. Persons can meet the diagnostic criteria for a disorder that lacks meaning or validity within the culture in which the criteria set was applied (Rogler, 1999). In addition, the agreement that was obtained between DSM-III-R and ICD-10 was inflated by the absence of independent assessments of most of the diagnostic criteria from the two nomenclatures (i.e., the semistructured interview used the same questions to assess most of the alternative diagnostic criteria).

The general criteria for a personality disorder provided in DSM-IV require that the behavior pattern "deviates markedly from the expectations of the individual's culture" (APA, 1994, p. 633). The intention of this requirement is to decrease the likelihood that clinicians will impose the expectations of their culture onto a patient (Mezzich, Kleinman, Fabrega, & Parron, 1996; Rogler, 1993). "What is considered to be excessively inhibited in one culture may be courteously dignified within another" (Widiger et al., 1995, p. 212). However, requiring that a personality disorder be deviant from the expectations of a culture might also suggest that a disorder of personality, by definition, is deviancy from cultural expectations. Optimal, healthy functioning does not necessarily involve adaptation to cultural expectations, and adaptation to cultural expectations does not necessarily ensure the absence of maladaptive personality traits (Wakefield, 1992). In fact, many of the personality disorders may represent, at least in part, excessive or exaggerated expressions of traits that a culture values or encourages, at least within some members of that culture (Alarcon, 1996; Kaplan, 1983; Rogler, 1993; Widiger & Spitzer, 1991). The ICD-10 version of this requirement is perhaps preferable to its revision for DSM-IV. ICD-10 states that "for different cultures it may be necessary to develop specific sets of criteria with regard to social norms, rules, and obligations" (WHO, 1992, p. 202). It will be as difficult to develop culture-neutral diagnostic criteria as it is to develop gender-neutral diagnostic criteria, and it may be as problematic to develop culture-specific criteria as it is to develop gender-specific criteria, but it is perhaps better to acknowledge this complexity than to presume that there are no problems.

CONCLUSIONS

Nobody is fully satisfied with, or lacks valid criticisms of, the DSM-IV and ICD-10 classification of personality disorders. Zilboorg's (1941) suggestion that budding theorists and researchers must cut their first teeth by providing a new classification of mental disorders still applies, although the rite of passage for any leading investigator today is also to provide a critique of ICD and/or DSM.

However, few persons appear to suggest that all official diagnostic nomenclatures be abandoned. The benefits of such nomenclatures do appear to outweigh the costs (Salmon et al., 1917; Stengel, 1959; Regier et al., 1998). Everybody finds fault with this language, but at least everyone has the ability to communicate this disagreement. Communication among researchers, theorists, and clinicians would be much worse in the absence of the common language.

Official diagnostic systems are to some extent constraining. Clinicians, theorists, and researchers will at times experience the frustration of having to communicate in terms of DSM or ICD. For example, it can be difficult obtain a grant, publish a study, or receive insurance reimbursement without reference to a DSM or ICD diagnosis. However, these diagnostic systems also provide useful points of comparison that ultimately facilitate the presentation or understanding of a new way of conceptualizing personality disorders. The absence of an official diagnostic system would complicate the ability of persons with divergent theoretical perspectives to communicate with one another and to document the validity or utility of their new ideas. The DSM-IV and ICD-10 do have substantial authority and power, but their existence does not appear to have squelched the development, recognition, or appreciation of alternative diagnostic nomenclatures. There are today many viable alternatives to DSM-IV and ICD-10 whose recognition is due in part to the presence of, comparison to, and dissatisfaction with the official nomenclature.

DSM-IV and ICD-10 are the official diagnostic systems because of their substantial empirical support, theoretical cogency, and clinical utility. Everybody is critical of them, but people would be even more critical if the authors of DSM-V abandoned DSM-IV in favor of one of the current alternatives. No diagnostic system, including the alternatives, is without substantial, fundamental problems. The authors of the alternative nomenclatures have as much difficulty with establishing the number, specificity, and format of diagnostic criteria; with thresholds for diagnosis; and with gender and cultural differences as did the authors of DSM-IV. DSM-IV and ICD-10 are highly problematic, but most texts, including this one, will be more understandable, will have more utility, and will experience more success when the official diagnostic system is used.

REFERENCES

Adler, D., Drake, R., & Teague, G. (1990). Clinicians' practices in personality assessment: Does gender influence the use of DSM-III Axis II? *Comprehensive Psychiatry, 31,* 125–133.

Akiskal, H. S., & Akiskal, K. (1992). Cyclothymic, hyperthymic, and depressive temperaments as subaffective variants of mood disorders. In A. Tasman & M. B. Riba (Eds.), *Review of psychiatry* (Vol. 11, pp. 43–62). Washington, DC: American Psychiatric Press.

Alarcon, R. D. (1996). Personality disorders and culture in DSM-IV: A critique. *Journal of Personality Disorders, 10,* 260–270.

American Psychiatric Association. (1952). *Diagnostic and statistical manual. Mental disorders.* Washington, DC: Author.

American Psychiatric Association. (1968). *Diagnostic and statistical manual of mental disorders* (2nd ed.). Washington, DC: Author.

American Psychiatric Association. (1980). *Diagnostic and statistical manual of mental disorders* (3rd ed.). Washington, DC: Author.

American Psychiatric Association. (1987). *Diagnostic and statistical manual of mental disorders* (3rd ed., rev.). Washington, DC: Author.

American Psychiatric Association. (1994). *Diagnostic and statistical manual of mental disorders* (4th ed.). Washington, DC: Author.

American Psychiatric Association. (2000). *Diagnostic and statistical manual of mental disorders* (4th ed., rev.). Washington, DC: Author.

American Psychiatric Association and National Institute of Mental Health. (1999, September). *Research planning conference: Meeting summary.* Washington, DC: Author.

Benjamin, J., Lin, L., Patterson, C., Greenberg, B. D., Murphy, D. L., & Hamer, D. H. (1996). Population and familial association between the D4 dopamine receptor gene and measures of Novelty Seeking. *Nature Genetics, 12,* 81–84.

Benjamin, L. S. (1993). *Interpersonal diagnosis and treatment of personality disorders.* New York: Guilford Press.

Blashfield, R. K. (1984). *The classification of psychopathology. Neo-Kraepelinian and quantitative approaches.* New York: Plenum.

Blashfield, R. K., Blum, N., & Pfohl, B. (1992). The effects of changing Axis II diagnostic criteria. *Comprehensive Psychiatry, 33,* 245–252.

Blashfield, R. K., & Breen, M. (1989). Face validity of the DSM-III-R personality disorders. *American Journal of Psychiatry, 146,* 1575–1579.

Blashfield, R. K., & Draguns, J. G. (1976). Evaluative criteria for psychiatric classification. *Journal of Abnormal Psychology, 85,* 140–150.

Blashfield, R. K., & Fuller, A. K. (1996). Predicting the DSM-V. *Journal of Nervous and Mental Disease,184,* 4–7.

Blashfield, R. K., & Haymaker, D. (1988). A prototype analysis of the diagnostic criteria for DSM-III-R personality disorders. *Journal of Personality Disorders, 2,* 272–280.

Blashfield, R. K., & McElroy, R. A. (1987). The 1985 journal literature on the personality disorders. *Comprehensive Psychiatry, 28,* 536–546.

Blashfield, R. K., Sprock, J., & Fuller, A. (1990). Suggested guidelines for including/excluding categories in the DSM-IV. *Comprehensive Psychiatry, 31,* 15–19.

Bornstein, R. F. (1997). Dependent personality disorder in the DSM-IV and beyond. *Clinical Psychology: Science and Practice, 4,* 175–187.

Caplan, P. J. (1991). How do they decide who is normal?: The bizarre, but true, tale of the DSM process. *Canadian Psychology, 32,* 162–170.

Clark, L. A. (1992). Resolving taxonomic issues in personality disorders. *Journal of Personality Disorders, 6,* 360–378.

Clark, L. A., Livesley, W. J., & Morey, L. (1997). Personality disorder assessment: The challenge of construct validity. *Journal of Personality Disorders, 11,* 205–231.

Clark, L. A., Watson, D., & Reynolds, S. (1995). Diagnosis and classification of psychopathology: Challenges to the current system and future directions. *Annual Review of Psychology, 46,* 121–153.

Cleckley, H. (1941). *The mask of sanity.* St. Louis, MO: Mosby.

Cloninger, C. R., & Svrakic, D. M. (1994). Differentiating normal and deviant personality by the seven-factor personality model. In S. Strack & M. Lorr (Eds.), *Differentiating normal and abnormal personality* (pp. 40–64). New York: Springer.

Cooper, A. M. (1987). Histrionic, narcissistic, and compulsive personality disorders. In G. L. Tischler (Ed.), *Diagnosis and classification in psychiatry. A critical appraisal of DSM-III* (pp. 290–299). New York: Cambridge University Press.

Cooper, A. M. (1993). Psychotherapeutic approaches to masochism. *Journal of Psychotherapy Practice and Research, 2,* 1–13.

Corbitt, E. M., & Widiger, T. A. (1995). Sex differences among the personality disorders: An exploration of the data. *Clinical Psychology: Science and Practice, 2,* 225–238.

Davis, R., & Millon, T. (1995). On the importance of theory to a taxonomy of personality disorders. In W. J. Livesley (Ed.), *The DSM-IV personality disorders* (pp. 377–396). New York: Guilford Press.

Dawes, R. M. (1994). *House of cards. Psychology and psychotherapy built on myth.* New York: Free Press.

Feighner, J. P., Robins, E., Guze, S. B., Woodruff, R. A., Winokur, G., & Munoz, R. (1972). Diagnostic criteria for use in psychiatric research. *Archives of General Psychiatry, 26,* 57–63.

Feingold, A. (1994). Gender differences in personality: A meta-analysis. *Psychological Bulletin, 116,* 429–456.

Follette, W. C., & Houts, A. C. (1996). Models of scientific progress and the role of theory in taxonomy development: A case study of the DSM. *Journal of Consulting and Clinical Psychology, 64,* 1120–1132.

Ford, M. R., & Widiger, T. A. (1989). Sex bias in the diagnosis of histrionic and antisocial personality disorders. *Journal of Consulting and Clinical Psychology, 57,* 301–305.

Frances, A. J. (1980). The DSM-III personality disorders section: A commentary. *American Journal of Psychiatry, 137,* 1050–1054.

Frances, A. J. (1998). Problems in defining clinical significance in epidemiological studies. *Archives of General Psychiatry, 55,* 119.

Frances, A. J., & Cooper, A. M. (1981). Descriptive and dynamic psychiatry: A perspective on DSM-III. *American Journal of Psychiatry, 138,* 1198–1202.

Frances, A. J., First, M. B., & Pincus, H. A. (1995). *DSM-IV guidebook.* Washington, DC: American Psychiatric Press.

Frances, A. J., Pincus, H. A., Widiger, T. A., Davis, W. W., & First, M. B. (1990). DSM-IV: Work in progress. *American Journal of Psychiatry, 147,* 1439–1448.

Frances, A. J., & Widiger, T. A. (1986). The classification of personality disorders: an overview of problems and solutions. In A. Frances & R. Hales (Eds.), *Psychiatry update* (Vol. 5. pp. 240–257). Washington, DC: American Psychiatric Press.

Frances, A. J., Widiger, T. A., & Pincus, H. A. (1989). The development of DSM-IV. *Archives of General Psychiatry, 46,* 373–375.

Garb, H. N. (1997). Race bias, social class bias, and gender bias in clinical judgment. *Clinical Psychology: Science and Practice, 4,* 99–120.

Grob, G. N. (1991). Origins of DSM-I: A study in appearance and reality. *American Journal of Psychiatry, 148,* 421–431.

Gunderson, J. G. (1983). DSM-III diagnoses of personality disorders. In J. Frosch (Ed.), *Current perspectives on personality disorders* (pp. 20–39). Washington, DC: American Psychiatric Press.

Gunderson, J. G. (1992). Diagnostic controversies. In A. Tasman & M. B. Riba (Eds.), *Review of psychiatry* (Vol. 11, pp. 9–24). Washington, DC: American Psychiatric Press.

Gunderson, J. G. (1996). The borderline patient's intolerance of aloneness: Insecure attachments and therapist availability. *American Journal of Psychiatry, 153,* 752–758.

Gunderson, J. G. (1998). DSM-IV personality disorders: Final overview. In T. A. Widiger, A. J. Frances, H. A. Pincus, R. Ross, M. B. First, W. Davis, & M. Kline (Eds.), *DSM-IV Sourcebook* (Vol. 4, pp. 1123–1140). Washington, DC: American Psychiatric Association.

Gunderson, J. G., & Pollack, W. S. (1985). Conceptual risks of the Axis I-II division. In H. Klar & L. J. Siever (Eds.), *Biologic response styles: Clinical implications* (pp. 81–95). Washington, DC: American Psychiatric Press.

Gunderson, J. G., & Shea, M. T. (1991). DSM-IV reviews of the personality disorders: introduction to the second part of the special series. *Journal of Personality Disorders, 5,* 337–339.

Gunderson, J. G., Zanarini, M. C., & Kisiel, C. L. (1991). Borderline personality disorder: A review of data on DSM-III-R descriptions. *Journal of Personality Disorders, 5,* 340–352.

Hare, R. D., Hart, S. D., & Harpur, T. J. (1991). Psychopathy and the DSM-IV criteria for antisocial personality disorder. *Journal of Abnormal Psychology, 100,* 391–398.

Hirschfeld, R. M. A., Shea, M. T., & Weise, R. (1991). Dependent personality disorder: perspectives for DSM-IV. *Journal of Personality Disorders, 5,* 135–149.

Kaplan, M. (1983). A woman's view of DSM-III. *American Psychologist, 38,* 786–792.

Kass, F., Skodol, A. E., Charles, E., Spitzer, R. L., & Williams, J. B. W. (1985). Scaled ratings of DSM-III personality disorders. *American Journal of Psychiatry, 142,* 627–630.

Kass, F., Spitzer, R. L., & Williams, J. B. W. (1983). An empirical study of the issue of sex bias in the diagnostic criteria of DSM-III Axis II personality disorders. *American Psychologist, 38,* 799–801.

Keller, M. (1989). Current concepts in affective disorders. *Journal of Clinical Psychiatry, 50,* 157–162.

Kendell, R. E. (1975). *The role of diagnosis in psychiatry.* London, UK: Blackwell Scientific Publications.

Kendell, R. E. (1991). Relationship between the DSM-

IV and the ICD–10. *Journal of Abnormal Psychology,* *100,* 297–301.

Kernberg, O. F. (1984). Problems in the classification of personality disorders. *Severe personality disorders* (pp. 77–94). New Haven, CT: Yale University Press.

Kiesler, D. J. (1996). *Contemporary interpersonal theory & research. Personality, psychopathology, and psychotherapy.* New York: Wiley.

Klerman, G. L. (1986). Historical perspectives on contemporary schools of psychopathology. In T. Millon & G. L. Klerman (Eds.), *Contemporary directions in psychopathology* (pp. 3–28). New York: Guilford Press.

Koerner, K., Kohenlberg, R. J., & Parker, C. R. (1996). Diagnosis of personality disorder: A radical behavioral alternative. *Journal of Consulting and Clinical Psychology, 64,* 1169–1176.

Kramer, M., Sartorius, N., Jablensky, A., & Gulbinat, W. (1979). The ICD–9 classification of mental disorders. A review of its development and contents. *Acta Psychiatrica Scandinavika, 59,* 241–262.

Liebowitz, M. R. (1992). Diagnostic issues in anxiety disorders. In A. Tasman & M. B. Riba (Eds.), *Review of psychiatry* (Vol. 11, pp. 247–259). Washington, DC: American Psychiatric Press.

Livesley, W. J. (1985). The classification of personality disorder: I. The choice of category concept. *Canadian Journal of Psychiatry, 30,* 353–358.

Livesley, W. J. (1986). Trait and behavioral prototypes of personality disorder. *American Journal of Psychiatry, 143,* 728–732.

Livesley, W. J. (Ed.). (1995). *The DSM-IV personality disorders.* New York: Guilford Press.

Livesley, W. J. (1998). Suggestions for a framework for an empirically based classification of personality disorder. *Canadian Journal of Psychiatry, 43,* 137–147.

Livesley, W. J., & Jackson, D. N. (1992). Guidelines for developing, evaluating, and revising the classification of personality disorders. *Journal of Nervous and Mental Disease, 180,* 609–694.

Livesley, W. J., Schroeder, M. L., Jackson, D. N., & Jang, K. L. (1994). Categorical distinctions in the study of personality disorder: Implications for classification. *Journal of Abnormal Psychology, 103,* 6–17.

Loranger, A. W. (1990). The impact of DSM-III on diagnostic practice in a university hospital. *Archives of General Psychiatry, 47,* 672–675.

Loranger, A. W., Sartorius, N., Andreoli, A., Berger, P., Buchheim, P., Channabasavanna, S. M., Coid, B., Dahl, A., Diekstra, R. F. W., Ferguson, B., Jacobsberg, L. B., Mombour, W., Pull, C., Ono, Y., & Regier, D. A. (1994). The International Personality Disorder Examination. The World Health Organization/Alcohol, Drug Abuse, and Mental Health Administration international pilot study of personality disorders. *Archives of General Psychiatry, 51,* 215–224.

Malinow, K. (1981). Passive–aggressive personality. In J. Lion (Ed.), *Personality disorders* (2nd ed., pp. 121–132). Baltimore: Williams & Wilkins.

Maser, J. D., Kaelber, C., & Weise, R. F. (1991). International use and attitudes toward DSM-III and DSM-III-R: Growing consensus in psychiatric classification. *Journal of Abnormal Psychology, 100,* 271–279.

McQueen, L. (2000). Committee on psychiatric diagnosis and assessment update on publications and activities. *Psychiatric Research Report, 16*(2), 3.

Mellsop, G., Varghese, F., Joshua, S., & Hicks, A. (1982). Reliability of Axis II of DSM-III. *American Journal of Psychiatry, 139,* 1360–1361.

Menninger, K. (1963). *The vital balance.* New York: Viking Press.

Mezzich, J. E., Kleinman, A., Fabrega, H., & Parron, D. L. (Eds.). (1996). *Culture and psychiatric diagnosis: A DSM-IV perspective.* Washington, DC: American Psychiatric Press.

Millon, T. (1981). *Disorders of personality. DSM-III: Axis II.* New York: Wiley.

Millon, T. (1993). Negativistic (passive–aggressive) personality disorder. *Journal of Personality Disorders, 7,* 78–85.

Millon, T., Davis, R. D., Millon, C. M., Wenger, A., Van Zullen, M. H., Fuchs, M., & Millon, R. B. (1996). *Disorders of personality: DSM-IV and beyond* (2nd. ed.). New York: Wiley.

Morey, L. C. (1988). Personality disorders under DSM-III and DSM-III-R: an examination of convergence, coverage, and internal consistency. *American Journal of Psychiatry, 145,* 573–577.

Morey, L., & Ochoa, E. (1989). An investigation of adherence to diagnostic criteria: Clinical diagnosis of the DSM-III personality disorders. *Journal of Personality Disorders, 3,* 180–192.

Nathan, P. E. (1994). DSM-IV: Empirical, accessible, not yet ideal. *Journal of Clinical Psychology, 50,* 103–110.

Nathan, P. E., & Langenbucher, J. W. (1999). Psychopathology: Description and classification. *Annual Review of Psychology, 50,* 79–107.

Pantony, K-L., & Caplan, P. J. (1991). Delusional dominating personality disorder: A modest proposal for identifying some consequences of rigid masculine socialization. *Canadian Psychology, 32,* 120–133.

Paris, J. (1993). Personality disorders: A biopsychosocial model. *Journal of Personality Disorders, 7,* 255–264.

Perry, J. C. (1990). Challenges in validating personality disorders: Beyond description. *Journal of Personality Disorders, 4,* 273–289.

Perry, J. C. (1992). Problems and considerations in the valid assessment of personality disorders. *American Journal of Psychiatry, 149,* 1645–1653.

Pfohl, B. (1991). Histrionic personality disorder: a review of available data and recommendations for DSM-IV. *Journal of Personality Disorders, 5,* 150–166.

Pfohl, B., & Blum, N. (1991). Obsessive–compulsive personality disorder: A review of available data and recommendations for DSM-IV. *Journal of Personality Disorders, 5,* 363–375.

Pincus, H. A., Frances, A. J., Davis, W. W., First, M. B., & Widiger, T. A. (1992). DSM-IV and new diagnostic categories: Holding the line on proliferation. *American Journal of Psychiatry, 149,* 112–117.

Pretzer, J. L., & Beck, A. T. (1996). A cognitive theory of personality disorders. In J. F. Clarkin & M. F. Lenzenweger (Eds.), *Major theories of personality disorder* (pp. 36–105). New York: Guilford Press.

Regier, D. A., Kaelber, C. T., Rae, D. S., Farmer, M. E.,

Knauper, B., Kessler, R. C., & Norquist, G. S. (1998). Limitations of diagnostic criteria and assessment instruments for mental disorders. Implications for research and policy. *Archives of General Psychiatry, 55,* 109–115.

Robins, L. N. (1966). *Deviant children grown up.* Baltimore: Williams & Wilkins.

Rogers, R. (1995). *Diagnostic and structured interviewing. A handbook for psychologists.* Odessa, FL: Psychological Assessment Resources.

Rogler, L. H. (1993). Culturally sensitizing psychiatric diagnosis: A framework for research. *Journal of Nervous and Mental Disease, 181,* 401–408.

Rogler, L. H. (1996). Framing research on culture in psychiatric diagnosis: The case of the DSM-IV. *Psychiatry, 59,* 145–155.

Rogler, L. H. (1999). Methodological sources of cultural insensitivity in mental health research. *American Psychologist, 54,* 424–433.

Rosenhan, D. L. (1973). On being sane in insane places. *Science, 179,* 250–258.

Ross, R., Frances, A. J., & Widiger, T. A. (1995). Gender issues in DSM-IV. In J. M. Oldham & M. B. Riba (Eds.), *Review of psychiatry* (vol. 14, pp. 205–226). Washington, DC: American Psychiatric Press.

Ryder, A. G., & Bagby, R. M. (1999). Diagnostic viability of depressive personality disorder: theoretical and conceptual issues. *Journal of Personality Disorders, 13,* 99–117.

Salmon, T. W., Copp, O., May, J. V., Abbot, E. S., & Cotton, H. A. (1917). Report of the committee on statistics of the American Medico-Psychological Association. *American Journal of Insanity, 74,* 255–260.

Sanislow, C. A., & McGlashan, T. H. (1998). Treatment outcome of personality disorders. *Canadian Journal of Psychiatry, 43,* 237–250.

Sarbin, T. R. (1997). On the futility of psychiatric diagnostic manuals (DSMs) and the return of personal agency. *Applied and Preventive Psychology, 6,* 233–243.

Sartorius, N. (1988). International perspectives of psychiatric classification. *British Journal of Psychiatry, 152* (Suppl.), 9–14.

Sartorius, N., Kaelber, C. T., Cooper, J. E., Roper, M., Rae, D. S., Gulbinat, W., Ustun, T. B., & Regier, D. A. (1993). Progress toward achieving a common language in psychiatry. *Archives of General Psychiatry, 50,* 115–124.

Schwartz, M. A., Wiggins, O. P., & Norko, M. A. (1995). Prototypes, ideal types, and personality disorders: The return to classical phenomenology. In W. J. Livesley (Ed.), *The DSM-IV personality disorders* (pp. 417–432). New York: Guilford Press.

Segal, D. L. (1997). Structured interviewing and DSM classification. In S. M. Turner & M. Hersen (Eds.), *Adult psychopathology and diagnosis* (pp. 24–57). New York: Wiley.

Shea, M. T. (1992). Some characteristics of the Axis II criteria sets and their implications for assessment of personality disorders. *Journal of Personality Disorders, 6,* 377–381.

Shea, M. T. (1993). DSM-IV reviews of the personality disorders: introduction to the third part of the special series. *Journal of Personality Disorders, 7,* 28–29.

Shea, M. T. (1996). Enduring personality change after catastrophic experience. In T. A. Widiger, A. J. Frances, H. A. Pincus, R. Ross, M. B., First, & W. W. Davis (Eds.), *DSM-IV sourcebook* (Vol. 2, pp. 849–860). Washington, DC: American Psychiatric Association.

Siever, L. J., & Davis, K. L. (1991). A psychobiological perspective on the personality disorders. *American Journal of Psychiatry, 148,* 1647–1658.

Silverman, J. M., Siever, L. J., Zanarini, M. C., Coccaro, E. F., & Mitropoulou, V. (1998). Report on the proposed criteria for schizotypal personality disorder. In T. A. Widiger, A. J. Frances, H. A. Pincus, R. Ross, M. B. First, W. Davis, & M. Kline (Eds.), *DSM-IV sourcebook* (Vol. 4, pp. 343–356). Washington, DC: American Psychiatric Association.

Spitzer, R. L., Endicott, J., & Gibbon, M. (1979). Crossing the border into borderline personality and borderline schizophrenia. *Archives of General Psychiatry, 36,* 17–24.

Spitzer, R. L., Endicott, J., & Robins E. (1975). Clinical criteria for psychiatric diagnosis and DSM-III. *American Journal of Psychiatry, 132,* 1187–1192.

Spitzer, R. L., Fiester, S. J., Gay, M., & Pfohl, B. (1991). Results of a survey of forensic psychiatrists on the validity of the sadistic personality disorder diagnosis. *American Journal of Psychiatry, 148,* 875–879.

Spitzer, R. L., & Fleiss, J. L. (1974). A re-analysis of the reliability of psychiatric diagnosis. *British Journal of Psychiatry, 125,* 341–347.

Spitzer, R. L., Forman, J. B. W., & Nee, J. (1979). DSM-III field trials: I. Initial diagnostic reliability. *American Journal of Psychiatry, 136,* 815–817.

Spitzer, R. L., Sheehy, M., & Endicott, J. (1977). DSM-III: Guiding principles. In V. Rakoff, H. Stancer, & H. Kedward (Eds.), *Psychiatric diagnosis* (pp. 1–24). New York: Brunner/Mazel.

Spitzer, R. L., & Williams, J. B. W. (1982). The definition and diagnosis of mental disorder. In W. Gove (Ed.), *Deviance and mental illness* (pp. 15–31). Beverly Hills, CA: Sage.

Spitzer, R. L., & Williams, J. B. W. (1985). Classification of mental disorders. In H. Kaplan & B. Sadock (Eds.), *Comprehensive textbook of psychiatry* (4th ed., Vol. 1, pp. 591–613). Baltimore: Williams & Wilkins.

Spitzer, R. L., & Williams, J. B. W. (1987). Revising DSM-III: The process and major issues. In G. Tischler (Ed.), *Diagnosis and classification in psychiatry* (pp. 425–434). New York: Cambridge University Press.

Spitzer, R. L., Williams, J. B. W., & Skodol, A. E. (1980). DSM-III: The major achievements and an overview. *American Journal of Psychiatry, 137,* 151–164.

Spitzer, R. L., & Wilson, P. T. (1968). A guide to the American Psychiatric Association's new diagnostic nomenclature. *American Journal of Psychiatry, 124,* 1619–1629.

Spitzer, R. L., & Wilson, P. T. (1975). Nosology and the official psychiatric nomenclature. In A. M. Freedman, H. I. Kaplan, & B. J. Sadock (Eds.), *Comprehensive textbook of psychiatry* (2nd ed., vol. 1, pp. 826–845). Baltimore: Williams & Wilkins.

Stengel, E. (1959). Classification of mental disorders.

Bulletin of the World Health Organization, 21, 601–663.

Sternbach, S., Judd, A., Sabo, A., McGlashan, T., & Gunderson, J. (1992). Cognitive and perceptual distortions in borderline personality disorder and schizotypal personality disorder in a vignette sample. *Comprehensive Psychiatry, 33,* 186–189.

Strack, S., & Lorr, M. (1997). Invited essay: The challenge of differentiating normal and disordered personality. *Journal of Personality Disorders, 11,* 105–122.

Szasz, T. S. (1961). *The myth of mental illness.* New York: Hoeber-Harper.

Task Force on DSM-IV. (1991, September). *DSM-IV options book: work in progress.* Washington, DC: American Psychiatric Association.

Task Force on DSM-IV. (1993, March). *DSM-IV draft criteria.* Washington, DC: American Psychiatric Association.

Tyrer, P. (1988). What's wrong with DSM-III personality disorders? *Journal of Personality Disorders, 2,* 281–291.

Tyrer, P., & Johnson, T. (1996). Establishing the severity of personality disorder. *American Journal of Psychiatry, 153,* 1593–1597.

Wakefield, J. C. (1992). Disorder as harmful dysfunction: A conceptual critique of DSM-III-R's definition of mental disorder. *Psychological Review, 99,* 232–247.

Ward, C. H., Beck, A. T., Mendelson, M., Mock, J. E., & Erbaugh, J. K. (1962). The psychiatric nomenclature. Reasons for diagnostic disagreement. *Archives of General Psychiatry, 7,* 198–205.

Westen, D. (1997). Divergences between clinical and research methods for assessing personality disorders: Implications for research and the evolution of Axis II. *American Journal of Psychiatry, 154,* 895–903.

Westen, D., & Shedler, J. (1999). Revising and assessing Axis II: Part I: developing a clinically and empirically valid assessment method. *American Journal of Psychiatry, 156,* 258–272.

Wetzler, S., & Morey, L. C. (1999). Passive–aggressive personality disorder: The demise of a syndrome. *Psychiatry, 62,* 49–59.

Widiger, T. A. (1991). DSM-IV reviews of the personality disorders: introduction to special series. *Journal of Personality Disorders, 5,* 122–134.

Widiger, T. A. (1995). Deletion of self-defeating and sadistic personality disorders. In W. J. Livesley (Ed.), *The DSM-IV personality disorders* (pp. 359–373). New York: Guilford Press.

Widiger, T. A. (1997). Mental disorders as discrete clinical conditions: Dimensional versus categorical classification. In S. M. Turner & M. Hersen (Eds.), *Adult psychopathology and diagnosis* (3rd ed., pp. 3–23). New York: Wiley.

Widiger, T. A. (1998). Sex biases in the diagnosis of personality disorders. *Journal of Personality Disorders, 12,* 95–118.

Widiger, T. A., Cadoret, R., Hare, R., Robins, L., Rutherford, M., Zanarini, M., Alterman, A., Apple, M., Corbitt, E., Forth, A., Hart, S., Kultermann, J., Woody, G., & Frances, A. (1996). DSM-IV antisocial personality disorder field trial. *Journal of Abnormal Psychology, 105,* 3–16.

Widiger, T. A., & Corbitt, E. (1994). Normal versus abnormal personality from the perspective of the DSM. In S. Strack & M. Lorr (Eds.), *Differentiating normal and abnormal personality* (pp. 158–175). New York: Springer.

Widiger, T. A., & Corbitt, E. M. (1995). Antisocial personality disorder. In W. J. Livesley (Ed.), *The DSM-IV personality disorders* (pp. 103–126). New York: Guilford Press.

Widiger, T. A., & Costa, P. T. (1994). Personality and personality disorders. *Journal of Abnormal Psychology, 103,* 78–91.

Widiger, T., & Frances, A. (1985). The DSM-III personality disorders: Perspectives from psychology. *Archives of General Psychiatry, 42,* 615–623.

Widiger, T., Frances, A., Pincus, H., Davis, W., & First, M. (1991). Toward an empirical classification for DSM-IV. *Journal of Abnormal Psychology, 100,* 280–288.

Widiger, T., Frances, A., Spitzer, R., & Williams, J. (1988). The DSM-III-R personality disorders: An overview. *American Journal of Psychiatry, 145,* 786–795.

Widiger, T. A., & Lynam, D. R. (1998). Psychopathy and the five-factor model of personality. In T. Millon, E. Simonsen, M. Birket-Smith, & R. D. Davis (Eds.), *Psychopathy: Antisocial, criminal, and violent behavior* (pp. 171–187). New York: Guilford Press.

Widiger, T. A., Mangine, S., Corbitt, E. M., Ellis, C. G., & Thomas, G. V. (1995). *Personality Disorder Interview—IV. A semistructured interview for the assessment of personality disorders.* Odessa, FL: Psychological Assessment Resources.

Widiger, T. A., & Sanderson, C. J. (1995a). Assessing personality disorders. In J. N. Butcher (Ed.), *Clinical personality assessment. Practical approaches* (pp. 380–394). New York: Oxford University Press.

Widiger, T. A., & Sanderson, C. J. (1995b). Towards a dimensional model of personality disorders. In W. J. Livesley (Ed.), *The DSM-IV personality disorders* (pp. 433–458). New York: Guilford Press.

Widiger, T. A., & Spitzer, R. L. (1991). Sex bias in the diagnosis of personality disorders: Conceptual and methodological issues. *Clinical Psychology Review, 11,* 1–22.

Widiger, T. A., & Trull, T. J. (1993). The scholarly development of DSM-IV. In J. A. Costa e Silva & C. C. Nadelson (Eds.), *International review of psychiatry* (Vol. 1, pp. 59–78). Washington, DC: American Psychiatric Press.

Widiger, T. A., & Trull, T. J. (1998). Performance characteristics of the DSM-III-R personality disorder criteria sets. In T. A. Widiger, A. J. Frances, H. A. Pincus, R. Ross, M. B. First, W. W. Davis, & M. Kline (Eds.), *DSM-IV sourcebook* (Vol. 4, pp. 357–373). Washington, DC: American Psychiatric Association.

Williams, J. B. W., & Spitzer, R. L. (1980). DSM-III field trials: Interrater reliability and list of project staff and participants. *Diagnostic and statistical manual of mental disorders* (3rd ed., pp. 467–

469). Washington, DC: American Psychiatric Association.

Work Group to Revise DSM-III. (1986). *DSM-III-R in development, second draft.* Washington, DC: American Psychiatric Association.

World Health Organization. (1992). *The ICD–10 classification of mental and behavioural disorders. Clinical descriptions and diagnostic guidelines.* Geneva, Switzerland: Author.

Zigler, E., & Phillips, L. (1961). Psychiatric diagnosis: A critique. *Journal of Abnormal and Social Psychology, 63,* 607–618.

Zilboorg, G. (1941). *A history of medical ps*ᵧ New York: Norton.

Zimmerman, M. (1988). Why are we rushing to ɪ DSM-IV? *Archives of General Psychiatry*ᵧ 1135–1138.

Zimmerman, M. (1994). Diagnosing personᵼ disorders. A review of issues and research methoᵼ *Archives of General Psychiatry, 51,* 225–245.

Zimmerman, M., & Mattia, J. I. (1999). Psychiatriᵼ diagnosis in clinical practice: is comorbidity being missed? *Comprehensive Psychiatry, 40,* 182– 191.

———◆———

CHAPTER 4

Co-Occurrence with Syndrome Disorders

REGINA T. DOLAN-SEWELL
ROBERT F. KRUEGER
M. TRACIE SHEA

Following the introduction of DSM-III (American Psychiatric Association, 1980) and its innovative multiaxial format (which allowed for the diagnosis of both syndrome and personality disorders), the mid-1980s witnessed the first wave of empirical data documenting high levels of co-occurrence among Axis I and Axis II disorders (Dahl, 1986; Koenigsberg, Kaplan, Gilmore, & Cooper, 1985). This line of research demonstrates a striking tendency for Axis I and Axis II disorders to co-occur, with personality-disordered subjects tending to carry Axis I diagnoses at greater rates than vice versa. It is now clear that the modal treatment-seeking personality-disordered patient meets criteria for at least one Axis I disorder (e.g., Fabrega, Ulrich, Pilkonis, & Mezzich, 1992; Oldham et al., 1995). A review of this literature indicates that the percentage of personality-disordered subjects who also meet criteria for an Axis I disorder ranges from 66 (Dahl, 1986) to 97 (Alnaes & Torgersen, 1988). Examined from the reverse perspective, the number of subjects with Axis I disorders who also have a personality disorder ranges from approximately 13% (Fabrega, Pilkonis, Mezzich, Ahn, & Shea, 1990) to 81% (Alnaes & Torgersen, 1988).

When examining data on the rates of co-occurrence of personality and syndrome disorders, numerous questions arise. Are the co-occurring disorders truly distinct? Could there be an artifactual relationship between the disorders (e.g., due to overlapping diagnostic criteria)? Might the two apparently distinct conditions share the same etiology? Are specific Axis I and Axis II disorders more likely to occur with one another than with other disorders? Are there implications in terms of causality, course, or outcome of either of the disorders? What is the temporal relationship between the disorders? For example, does one disorder cause the second disorder or place a patient at risk for another disorder?

With these issues in mind, the purpose of this chapter is to examine the relationship between personality disorders (i.e., DSM system Axis II disorders) and syndrome disorders (i.e., DSM system Axis I disorders; American Psychiatric Association, 1980, 1987, 1994). Our emphasis is on the current (vs. lifetime) co-occurrence ("comorbidity") of these disorders. In the remainder of the chapter, we focus on the following issues: (1) conceptual problems associated with the term "comorbidity," (2) conceptual models for understanding relationships between Axis I and Axis II disorders, (3) specific relationships between Axis I and Axis II disorders that have received notable theoretical or empirical attention in the literature, and (4) our conclusions and suggested directions for future research.

THE PROBLEM OF COMORBIDITY

Recent discussions in psychiatric nosology have framed the observed high rates of covariation among multiple disorders in terms of "comorbidity" and have emphasized the conceptually problematic nature of these covariations (e.g., Clark, Watson, & Reynolds, 1995; Kendall & Clarkin, 1992; Lyons, Tyrer, Gunderson, & Tohen, 1997). Feinstein (1970) coined the term "comorbidity" to describe "any distinct additional clinical entity that has existed or that may occur during the clinical course of a patient who has the index disease under study" (pp. 456–457). Feinstein's definition presupposes that we understand enough about mental disorders that we would feel comfortable describing them as "distinct"—stating with confidence that a specific patient with a specific "index disease" has an "additional," co-occurring disorder. Although the use of the term "comorbidity" to refer to covariation among disorders is common, our understanding of mental disorders has not yet reached the level at which current nosological entities can be described as truly "distinct." We therefore agree with the assertion of Lilienfeld, Waldman, and Israel (1994) that the term "comorbidity" "implies a model of disease and a corresponding level of understanding that is absent for the vast majority of psychopathological entities" (p. 79). Thus, in this chapter, we refer to the co-occurrence of two or more disorders simply as co-occurrence to avoid the additional assumptions inherent in the term "comorbidity."

Although our understanding of mental disorders may not yet justify the use of the term "comorbidity, " it is readily apparent that "the comorbidity problem" has taken center stage in psychopathology research in recent years. A historical perspective may help us to understand the genesis of this problem.

How did the co-occurrence of mental disorders become a major topic of study in psychopathology research? This event may be traced to the neo-Kraepelinian revolution in psychiatric nosology, as codified in DSM-III (American Psychiatric Association, 1980). Among other things, the neo-Kraepelinian perspective is fundamentally concerned with the accurate splitting of diagnostic entities. In the neo-Kraepelinian tradition, "there is not one, but many mental illnesses" (Klerman, 1978, p. 104). Accordingly, DSM-III proposed the existence of various and separate psychopathological conditions. Hence, an accurate diagnosis of the patient's condition is made by applying extensive hierarchical exclusionary rules intended to enhance diagnostic precision.

These hierarchical exclusionary rules were reduced in the revision of DSM-III (DSM-III-R; American Psychiatric Association, 1987) due to objections to the assumptions of the hierarchies and because the rules were cumbersome and difficult to apply. These revisions allowed more possibilities for underlying "comorbidities" to reveal themselves. Empirical documentation of high rates of co-occurrence in both epidemiological and clinical samples followed (for a comprehensive, recent review, see Clark et al., 1995). It now appears that complex, "impure" symptom profiles are more the rule than the exception (Clark et al., 1995).

The "comorbidity" problem takes on special significance with regard to the relationship between Axis I and Axis II disorders. DSM-IV indicates that "the listing of Personality Disorders . . . on a separate axis ensures that consideration will be given to the possible presence of Personality Disorders . . . that might otherwise be overlooked when attention is directed to the usually more florid Axis I disorders" (American Psychiatric Association, 1994, p. 26). The distinction between persistent patterns of emotional, cognitive, and interpersonal functioning (i.e., personality traits) and problematic functioning during more circumscribed periods of time (i.e., episodic, state, or syndrome disorders) is more blurry than implied by assigning these domains to separate axes. That is, although a reasonably sharp distinction between personality and syndrome disorder is codified in the DSM system (as the Axis I–II distinction), various lines of evidence question this distinction. For example, meeting criteria for an Axis I disorder is a good indicator of having a personality profile that differs from that of the average person in the population (e.g., Krueger, Caspi, Moffitt, Silva, & McGee, 1996; Trull & Sher, 1994). With regard to Axis II disorders, Fabrega et al. (1992) found that 79% of their 2,344 patients with Axis II diagnoses also met criteria for an Axis I disorder. In addition, substantial correlations have been observed between measures of "normal" personality traits (e.g., the "Big Five") and measures of Axis II disorders (Widiger & Costa, 1994). The constructs of syndrome disorder (Axis I), personality disorder (Axis II), and personality traits are thus highly overlapping, both empirically and conceptually.

Although the existence of the "comorbidity" phenomenon is well established, various factors will affect the precise rate of co-occurrence between specific disorders assessed in specific studies (cf. Clark et al., 1995). First, the time frame sampled when the diagnoses are made may influence the rate of co-occurrence. The meaning of two disorders co-occurring over the course of a lifetime may be quite different from the implications of two disorders occurring at the same point in time. Second, sampling strategies will influence comorbidity rates. For example, relative to population samples, co-occurring cases are overrepresented in clinical samples and underrepresented in student samples (Newman, Moffitt, Caspi, & Silva, 1998). Third, diagnostic methods will influence co-occurrence rates. For example, self-report instruments have been found to yield higher prevalence estimates for Axis II disorders when compared with interview methods (e.g., Hyler, Skodol, Kellman, Oldham, & Rosnick, 1990). Fourth, if diagnostic criteria overlap, co-occurrence rates will increase, as persons will have a greater chance of meeting the criteria for "different" diagnoses while presenting with similar symptoms. Finally, the cutoff used to establish "caseness" will also influence co-occurrence rates. As this threshold is shifted, the base rate of the disorder changes—a higher threshold leads to less diagnosed cases, and a lower threshold leads to more diagnosed cases—and opportunities for disorders to co-occur are affected accordingly.

These considerations should always be borne in mind when interpreting the results from specific studies of co-occurrence. Nevertheless, a vast empirical literature on "comorbidity" indicates that the problem is manifest in diverse samples assessed using diverse techniques (cf. Clark et al., 1995). Nonetheless, the observation that putatively distinct Axis I and II disorders tend to co-occur is compatible with a number of theories or models of the relationship between the disorders. We turn now to review specific models that provide a conceptual framework for understanding the relationship between Axis I and Axis II disorders.

MODELS OF RELATIONSHIPS BETWEEN AXIS I AND AXIS II DISORDERS

Independence Model

This model presumes that no causal or risk relationship exists between the co-occurring disorders in question. The two disorders are occurring at the same time randomly, or due to "chance" (Lyons et al., 1997), and do not share the same etiology, disease processes, or symptom presentation. This is also referred to as the "null hypothesis" model for covariation.

Common Cause Model

A shared etiology between co-occurring conditions is postulated by this model. The co-occurring conditions have different presentations and different disease processes but share the same essential cause. This is also known as the "overlapping" model, and its similarity to the concept of pleiotropy (different phenotypical attributes being influenced by the same gene) has been noted (Lyons et al., 1997). The common cause may be genetic, biological, environmental, psychological, temperamental, or a combination of these factors (Kessler, 1995; Klein, Wonderlich, & Shea, 1993).

Spectrum/Subclinical Model

The spectrum or subclinical model of co-occurrence assumes that the two disorders are related in terms of etiology and mechanisms of action. Although there is variability in the presentation of the disorders (e.g., clinical features, severity, and impairment), they are not considered distinct disorders. The model typically presumes that one of the two disorders is a milder, or attenuated, version of the other disorder. In the Axis I–Axis II realm, this model has been used to describe the nature of the relationships between the Cluster A (odd/eccentric) personality disorders and psychotic disorders (most typically schizophrenia) and the Cluster C (anxious/fearful) personality disorders and Axis I anxiety disorders (e.g., social phobia and avoidant personality disorder). Lyons et al. (1997) suggest that individuals who manifest the more severe variant of the disorder possess "greater amounts" of the causal and pathophysiological factors than do individuals who only develop the milder version of the disorder.

Predisposition/Vulnerability Models

The predisposition or vulnerability models assume that one disorder both precedes a second disorder and increases the risk of a second disorder. Although the onset of the first disorder is not considered necessary for the development of the second disorder, the occurrence of the first disorder may act as a vulnerability that increases the likelihood of the onset of the second disorder. For example, avoidant personality features may increase an individual's risk for major depression. However, the development of major depression does not depend on the previous onset of avoidant personality traits. Using the framework generated by Lyons et al. (1997), the etiologies, pathophysiologies, and symptoms of the two disorders may be distinct, but the onset of one of these disorders makes it more likely than chance that an individual will develop the second disorder.

Complication/Scar Models

On the flip side of the predisposition/vulnerability models we find the complication or scar models. Similar to the vulnerability models, the complication or scar models presume that the co-occurring disorders are distinct entities. As Klein et al. (1993) illustrate, typically a second condition develops in the context of (or, perhaps, because of) a first condition. The second condition then continues on after the first condition remits, thus acting as a "scar" or "complication" of the first condition. An example of this might be the onset of panic attacks in the context of an acute stress disorder which then continue (in unexpected circumstances and leading to avoidance behavior) after the acute stress disorder subsides.

Pathoplasty/Exacerbation Model

The central assumption of this model is that whereas the co-occurring disorders may have independent etiologies (thus, co-occurring randomly), one may influence the manifestation or the course of the other. This may be due to an additive effect (pathoplasty) or a synergistic effect (exacerbation). The additive or synergistic effects of the disorders' distinct features result in subsequent symptom expression. For example, this model would suggest that the co-occurrence of obsessive–compulsive disorder and schizotypal personality disorder would result in more problematic symptom expression than either one disorder would produce independently. One can imagine the potentially impairing consequences of the interaction of obsessive thoughts regarding cleanliness or germs (obsessive–compulsive disorder) and perceptual disturbance or ideas of reference (schizotypal personality disorder). A patient with schizotypal personality disorder experiencing obsessive–compulsive disorder might experience greater difficulty being with others than a schizotypal personality disorder patient without obsessive–compulsive disorder due to an intensification of ideas of reference specifically related to obsessive–compulsive disorder behaviors (e.g., washing or checking). Formerly indistinct perceptual disturbances (e.g., seeing shadows and feeling tingling sensations) may be attributed to feared obsessive–compulsive disorder stimuli (e.g., bugs and germs) and result in frank psychotic symptoms.

Psychobiological Models

One promising approach for describing the development (and co-occurrence) of syndrome and personality disorders can be described as psychobiological in scope and orientation (e.g., Cloninger, Svrakic, & Przybeck, 1993; Siever & Davis, 1991). From this perspective, phenotypical personality variation results, in part, from heritable variation in underlying biological systems that regulate functioning in domains such as cognition, impulse control, and affect. Axis I disorders, Axis II disorders, and personality functioning in a broader sense (e.g., characteristic coping strategies and personality traits) are thus united as manifestations of (or indicators of activity in) these underlying biological systems.

Although psychobiological models emphasize biology and genetics, these models are comprehensive in scope and allow a place for environment and other nonbiological determinants of psychopathology (for a comprehensive review of these models, see Millon & Davis, 1996). These integrative models may be seen as complementary to the previously described models. In other words, psychobiological models may be consistent with common cause, spectrum, and vulnerability models. We now turn to a description of one particular psychobiological model (Siever & Davis, 1991) which can be used as a framework for understanding the co-occurrence of syndrome and personality disorders. This model also illustrates how the previously described models are not entirely separable.

To specifically explain the development of psychopathology, Siever and Davis (1991) proposed a dimensional model grounded in the core domains of cognitive/perceptual organization, affect regulation, impulse control, and anxiety modulation. The authors also present literature suggesting biological associations with each dimension. Each dimension is a continuum ranging from healthy to pathological functioning. Extreme, acute abnormalities on one or more dimensions may combine and manifest as Axis I disorders, whereas dimensional combinations of milder, more persistent disturbances may lead to presentation of Axis II disorders.

Siever and Davis (1991) describe the cognitive/perceptual dimension in terms of the "capacity to perceive and attend to important incoming stimuli, process this information in relation to previous experience, and select appropriate response strategies" (p. 1649). Abnormalities along this dimension may be reflected in attentional difficulties, confusion about and/or misunderstanding of other's social behaviors, or perceptual disturbances. Siever and Davis cite studies that suggest that the following biological indices can be used to demonstrate deficits along the cognitive/perceptual organization dimension: eye movement dysfunction, information-processing deficits, and dopamine activity (as evidenced by dopamine metabolites such as plasma HVA). Individuals with acute abnormalities along this dimension may present with schizophrenia or other psychotic disorders, whereas individuals with less intense and more chronic disturbances may present with one of the "odd" cluster personality disorders (i.e., schizotypal, schizoid, and paranoid personality disorders).

The impulsivity/aggression dimension refers to the threshold for behaviorally responding to internal (e.g., thoughts, affect, and physiological events) and external (e.g., noise and behavior of others) stimuli. Individuals who are high on this dimension are (1) limited in their ability to delay or inhibit their behavior when stimulated, (2) have difficulty anticipating the consequences of their behavior, and (3) fail to learn from undesirable consequences of previous behavior. To support the theoretical biological underpinnings of this dimension, Siever and Davis (1991) cite studies demonstrating a rela-

tionship between deficits in serotonergic functioning (e.g., decreased levels of the serotonin metabolite 5-HIAA) and aggressive, impulsive, and suicidal behaviors. Acute abnormalities along this dimension may be manifested in explosive disorders, pathological gambling, or kleptomania. Chronic disturbances along this dimension may be seen in persistent impulsive and aggressive behaviors such as those seen in borderline and antisocial personality disorders.

The affect regulation dimension encompasses variations in the experiencing, control, and expression of affective states. Insufficient affect regulation can result in a heightened sensitivity to environmental events (e.g., separation and disappointment) and distinct shifts in affective state. Siever and Davis (1991) review literature suggesting that shortened rapid eye movement latency and increased noradrenergic responsivity (i.e., catecholamine release) are principal biological correlates of affect dysregulation. The authors suggest that the instability and "hyperresponsiveness" of the catecholamine function may influence the instability of affect seen in borderline patients.

The core features of the anxiety/inhibition dimension are the cognitive and physiological symptoms that accompany the anticipation of potential danger or the aversive consequences of one's behavior (Gray, 1982; Siever & Davis, 1991). Individuals with pathological levels of anxiety/inhibition are quick to interpret environmental events, as well as their own behaviors and thoughts, as potentially harmful to themselves or to someone else. Reactions to perceived harm include increased physiological arousal and behavioral inhibition or withdrawal from the environment (Siever & Davis, 1991). Siever and Davis (1991) suggest that cortical and sympathetic arousal and lower thresholds for sedation may be biological correlates of pathological levels of anxiety/inhibition. Behaviors displayed by individuals with one or more of the anxious/fearful personality disorders (i.e., avoidant, dependent, obsessive–compulsive) or the Axis I anxiety disorders are thought to be indicators of abnormalities along the anxiety/inhibition dimension.

The advantages of using dimensional, psychobiological models to describe psychopathology and explain the co-occurrence of disorders are numerous. First, the use of a multidimensional framework encompassing Axis I and Axis II disorders averts the false distinction implied by the two axes. Second, these models provide testable predictions regarding underlying biological mechanisms (e.g., subjects with affective instability may have increased noradrenergic system activity). Finally, psychobiological models provide links to the environment by specifying the range of environmental stimuli that are "risky" for persons at the ends of the dimensions. For example, situations demanding the delay of gratification may be risky for impulsive people (cf. Krueger, Caspi, Moffitt, White, & Stouthamer-Loeber, 1996).

Although the psychobiological perspective provides a useful overarching viewpoint on personality and psychopathology, progress in this area will likely involve explicitly acknowledging and examining the possibility that different specific models may fit for different specific classes of disorder. Thus, the most satisfying research on patterns of covariance will likely be conducted with an eye toward testing the specific models outlined earlier. Therefore, we now examine specific pairings of diagnostic entities that are likely to represent the compass points for the next generation of research on personality and psychopathology.

CLUSTER A: THE ODD PERSONALITY DISORDERS

When considering the co-occurrence of Cluster A personality disorders and syndrome disorders, the most frequent association discussed (conceptually and empirically) is that between Cluster A personality disorders and psychotic disorders (e.g., schizophrenia) or psychotic symptoms (e.g., hallucinations and delusions). The hypothesized relationship between Cluster A personality disorders and psychotic disorders has often been referred to under the general rubric of a *spectrum of disorder* (but see Meehl, 1989, for an elucidating discussion of the conceptual strengths and weaknesses of the spectrum notion as applied to these disorders). The basic idea is that disorders such as the Cluster A personality disorders represent clinical variants of severe psychotic disorders such as schizophrenia. Indeed, the diagnosis of schizotypal personality disorder was added to DSM-III (American Psychiatric Association, 1980, pp. 309–310) to reflect the observation of a familial relationship between "various eccentricities of communication or behavior" and schizophrenia. We examine this idea from three complementary perspectives. First, we review

the literature regarding the contemporaneous co-occurrence of Cluster A personality disorders and Axis I disorders. Second, we examine patterns of co-occurrence longitudinally: Are there predictive relations between Cluster A signs and symptoms and the psychotic disorders? Third, we review family studies suggesting links between Cluster A signs and symptoms and psychotic disorders.

Contemporaneous Co-Occurrence of Cluster A Personality Disorders and Axis I Disorders

If Cluster A personality disorders and Axis I psychotic disorders lie on a unitary spectrum, one might expect persons with Cluster A personality disorders (but not Cluster B and C personality disorders) to have elevated rates of psychotic disorders (but not other Axis I disorders). The key research design for addressing this issue involves the examination of a reasonably large sample of diverse patients to ascertain *multiple* Axis I *and* II disorders and their patterns of co-occurrence. The typical research design, in which participants are initially selected based on the presence of a specific disorder and then examined for the presence of other disorders, cannot fully address this issue. For example, a study of persons with Cluster A personality disorders might find elevated rates of psychosis but cannot rule out the possibility that rates of psychosis are elevated in *all* personality disorders. This point was illustrated empirically in a careful study of 200 psychiatric in- and outpatients ascertained using semistructured diagnostic interviews broadly covering Axis I and II disorders (Oldham et al., 1995). These authors found that persons with Cluster A personality disorders had increased odds (odds ratio of 7.3) of having a concurrent Axis I psychotic disorder but not increased odds of having a concurrent Axis I mood, anxiety, substance use, or eating disorder. This finding appears highly supportive of the spectrum concept, as discussed previously. However, Cluster B and C personality disorders were *also* associated with increased rates of Axis I psychotic disorders (i.e., patients were more likely to have a Cluster B (odds ratio of 2.3) or C (odds ratio of 5.7) personality disorder co-occurring with a psychotic disorder (and vice versa) than to have either a Cluster B or C personality disorder or psychotic disorder occurring separately). Nevertheless, unlike Cluster A personality disorders, Cluster B personality disorders were also associated with anxiety, substance and eating disorders, and Cluster C personality disorders were also associated with mood, anxiety, and eating disorders. Thus, the "spectra" of mental disorder may be more subtle than previously thought. Perhaps personality disorders in general are *sensitive* indicators of proneness to Axis I disorders (including psychosis), but Cluster A personality disorders reflect a more *specific* proneness to psychosis.

Longitudinal Studies Linking Cluster A Signs and Symptoms with Psychotic Disorders

Contemporaneous studies are valuable because they tell us how psychopathological signs and symptoms "go together," thereby providing guidance in conceptualizing the complex presentations of many psychiatric patients. Nevertheless, more definitive investigations of the origins of psychiatric disturbance require a longitudinal approach. The spectrum notion suggests that clinical psychotic decompensation may be preceded by the more subtle yet pervasive oddities that constitute the Cluster A personality disorder criteria in recent DSMs. Evidence supporting this basic proposition has accumulated from the meticulous work of the Chapmans and their colleagues (e.g., Chapman, Chapman, Kwapil, Eckblad, & Zinser, 1994; Kwapil, Miller, Zinser, Chapman, & Chapman, 1997). The Chapmans worked to develop questionnaire indicators of what they term "psychosis proneness." These questionnaires (measuring physical anhedonia, perceptual aberration, magical ideation, impulsive nonconformity, and social anhedonia) were then administered to repeated samples of college students. Participants who scored deviantly on these measures and a non–deviantly-scoring control group were followed up 10 years later (Chapman et al., 1994). Psychotic outcomes were especially likely among participants who reported high levels of magical ideation *and* social anhedonia. Interestingly, these outcomes were not confined to a specific DSM-defined psychotic disorder and encompassed mood psychoses as well as schizophrenia. The utility of magical ideation combined with social anhedonia as a predictor of psychosis has also been confirmed in a separate 10-year follow-up study (Kwapil et al., 1997).

Berenbaum and Fujita (1994) have reviewed other studies of prospective links between personality and schizophrenia and concluded that preschizophrenics could be distinguished by their "peculiarity," that is, "deviant beliefs and perceptions" (p. 148) and introversion. Although peculiarity clearly maps onto the Cluster A criteria, introversion corresponds less clearly, being a very broad factor associated with the "normal" range of personality functioning. That is, introverted people might not especially enjoy social interaction, yet it is not clear that they are wholly indifferent to social approbation (i.e., schizoid). This specific interpretive difficulty highlights the general conceptual difficulty inherent in distinguishing normal from abnormal personality.

Family Studies of Cluster A Signs and Symptoms and Psychotic Disorders

Another approach to investigating the psychotic spectrum involves examining relatives of individuals with specific disorders. If "full-blown" schizophrenia represents the highest intensity within the spectrum, perhaps we will find "paler shades" (i.e., Cluster A personality disorders) among the relatives of schizophrenics. The corollary concern is again with the specificity of these relations—where does one spectrum end and another begin? Kendler, McGuire, Gruenberg, and Walsh (1995) examined these issues in the Roscommon Family Study—an epidemiological–family study conducted in western Ireland. Probands in the study were assigned to five groups: schizophrenia, other nonaffective psychosis, psychotic affective illness, nonpsychotic affective illness, and controls. A structured interview inquiring about 25 signs and symptoms of schizotypy was given to 1,544 first-degree relatives of the probands; the "sign" data are particularly valuable as they extend the data base beyond self-report to subtle observations of the participants' behavior. Specifically, six of seven schizotypy dimensions distinguished the relatives of schizophrenic probands from those of controls, three distinguished relatives of probands with nonaffective psychoses from controls, two distinguished relatives of probands with psychotic affective illness from controls, and only one distinguished relatives of probands with nonpsychotic affective illness from controls. These authors' conclusion about familial vulnerability to schizophrenia is informative: "It is neither highly specific nor highly nonspecific" (p. 302). As noted, Berenbaum and Fujita (1994) also reviewed family studies of schizophrenic probands and concluded that like preschizophrenics, relatives of schizophrenics could be distinguished by their peculiarity and introversion. These authors also noted that "it is not yet clear whether these characteristics are associated with vulnerability that is specific to schizophrenia" (p. 151). It appears, then, that should a schizophrenia spectrum exist, it is complex, with the risk to relatives of psychiatrically ill patients declining as the psychiatric illness of the patient moves away from the classic symptoms of schizophrenia. Nonetheless, it appears that risk of psychotic illness in relatives of mentally ill subjects exceeds that of control, or non–mentally ill subjects.

CLUSTER B: THE DRAMATIC PERSONALITY DISORDERS

The co-occurrence of Axis I disorders with the Cluster B (dramatic) personality disorders (antisocial, borderline, histrionic, and narcissistic) has been well documented. A recent review of the literature suggests that the relationship between Cluster B personality disorders and alcohol abuse and dependence is particularly strong (the association being greater than five times that expected by chance; Tyrer, Gunderson, Lyons, & Tohen, 1997). For example, Skodol, Oldham, and Gallaher (1995) found that the presence of a Cluster B personality disorder resulted in increased odds of having a lifetime diagnosis of alcohol, cannabis, stimulants, or other substance use disorder (odds ratios ranged from 2.6 to 8.2) where the diagnosis of a Cluster A or Cluster C personality disorder was not related to the increased probability of having a lifetime diagnosis of a substance use disorder. A moderate relationship (two to five times that expected by chance) appears to exist between Cluster B personality disorders and mood, stress, and eating disorders (Tyrer et al., 1997).

In their study of 200 treatment-seeking patients, Oldham et al. (1995) found that the presence of any Cluster B personality disorder resulted in elevated odds for having a current anxiety disorder (odds ratio = 2.3), psychotic disorder (odds ratio = 5.3), or substance use disorder (odds ratio = 5.0). (Notably, although these authors did not find elevated odds for the co-occurrence of Cluster B and mood disorders, they did find that elevations in borderline traits were associated with the presence of a mood disorder.) In the Epidemiologic Catchment Area study (ECA; Robins, Tipp, & Przybeck, 1991) greater than 90% of the antisocial personality disorder cases had an additional Axis I diagnosis. Not surprisingly, antisocial personality disorder was associated with alcohol and substance abuse; the more provocative finding was that antisocial personality disorder was also associated with a host of other Axis I disorders (including psychotic, affective, and anxiety disorders).

Similar to the relationship of Cluster A personality disorders to Axis I disorders, the mapping of Cluster B personality disorders to Axis I, with the exception of substance use disorders, does not appear to be specific. Other studies have also found that Cluster A personality disorders and Cluster C personality disorders co-occur at significant rates with psychosis (e.g., Oldham et al., 1995). Elevated rates of Cluster C personality disorders have also been documented in patients with mood, anxiety, or eating disorders (or vice versa) (e.g., Alnaes & Torgersen, 1988; Oldham et al., 1995; Skodol et al., 1993; Skodol, Oldham, Hyler, et al., 1995). It appears, then, that Cluster B personality disorders, while closely linked to substance use/dependence, are also linked, albeit less closely, to other Axis I syndromes.

A few issues in the realm of Cluster B personality disorders and Axis I disorders have received striking theoretical (and empirical) attention in the literature. Thus, we now turn to an examination of these issues, most notably the association between borderline personality disorder and mood disorders and posttraumatic stress disorder and between antisocial personality disorder and substance use disorders.

The Co-Occurrence of Borderline Personality Disorder and Depression

The oft-presumed spectrum relationship of borderline personality and depressive disorders (i.e., the two disorders are variant expressions of a shared etiology), has been investigated from numerous perspectives. These perspectives include the co-occurrence of the disorders (e.g., Oldham et al., 1995; Shea, Glass, Pilkonis, Watkins, & Doherty, 1987; Zanarini, Gunderson, & Frankenburg, 1989), family histories of subjects with either of these disorders (e.g., Reich, 1995; Riso et al., 1996), and response to antidepressant medications (e.g., Cornelius, Soloff, Perel, & Ulrich, 1990; Links, Steiner, Boiagio, & Irwin, 1990).

There is a wide literature describing the rates of personality disorders in depressed patients (for reviews, see Corruble, Ginestet, & Guelfi, 1996; Gunderson & Phillips, 1991; Gunderson, Triebwasser, Phillips, & Sullivan, 1999). Estimates of the presence of borderline personality disorder in depressed outpatients range from approximately 10% to 40%. Cluster C personality disorders, however, appear at higher rates than borderline personality disorder (most estimates for dependent personality disorder and avoidant personality disorder range from 25% to 65%).

In the few studies reporting rates of major depression in subjects with personality disorders (most studies report rates of "mood disorders"), subjects with borderline personality disorder are likely to experience major depression. However, depression also occurs at significant rates in subjects with other personality disorders. In a study of lifetime Axis I comorbidity of borderline patients, 83% of borderlines had major depressive disorder, whereas 67% of subjects with other personality disorders had major depressive disorder (Zanarini et al., 1998). Using data from a study of 571 subjects with personality disorders, percent co-occurrence rates were calculated for current major depression and personality disorders (Skodol et al., 1999). (Percent co-occurrence is a single number simultaneously representing the proportion of subjects with a mood disorder who have a personality disorder and the proportion with the personality disorder who have the mood disorder.) As expected, significant co-occurrence rates were found for borderline personality disorder and major depressive disorder (31%). Co-occurrence rates were also significant, though, for avoidant personality disorder (35%). Interestingly, the co-occurrence rates for dysthymia were not significant for borderline personality disorder (16%) but were significant for avoidant (21%), dependent (11%), and schizoid (6.8%) personality disorders. Results from the studies cited previously point to a relationship between borderline personality disorder and major depressive disorder, albeit a nonspecific relationship.

With regard to family history, borderline subjects do not appear to have a higher incidence of relatives with depression than do subjects without borderline personality disorder (Reich, 1995; Riso et al., 1996). Finally, subjects with borderline personality disorder do not respond as well to antidepressant medications as do depressed subjects without a borderline diagnosis (Gunderson & Phillips, 1991; Tyrer et al., 1997). Results from this line of research, although suggesting that there may be a shared etiological component, do not support a spectrum relationship (cf. Gunderson & Phillips, 1991; Tyrer et al., 1997). Thus, we agree with Gunderson and Phillips's conclusion of nearly 10 years ago that "a surprisingly weak and nonspecific relationship exists between these disorders" (p. 967).

Borderline Personality Disorder and/or Bipolar Disorder?

Controversy regarding the theoretical and phenotypical overlap between borderline personality disorder and the bipolar I and II disorders has intensified since the introduction of borderline personality disorder into DSM-III (e.g., Akiskal, 1994; Akiskal et al., 1985; Bolton & Gunderson, 1996; Fyer, Frances, Sullivan, Hurt, & Clarkin, 1988; Gunderson et al., 1999). The debate has evolved, at least in part, from the inclusion in the borderline personality disorder criteria set of criteria considered to be hallmarks of bipolar disorder. The variables stirring the most controversy are affective dysregulation and impulsivity. An important distinction can be made, however, between the "overlapping" criteria as defined for borderline personality disorder and bipolar disorder. First, the affective dysregulation of the borderline is due to "a marked reactivity of mood" (American Psychiatric Association, 1994) versus the autonomous mood shift of the patient with bipolar disorder. In other words, the mood of a patient with borderline personality disorder changes in reaction to an external event (e.g., a conflict with a partner or the perception of having been insulted by someone). The mood change of the patient with bipolar disorder, on the other hand, is theoretically due to an internal biological shift, independent of immediate external events. Next, the impulsivity that occurs in patients with borderline personality disorder is not limited to elevated, positive mood states, as is the case with patients with bipolar disorder, but may occur during states of depression, anger, or anxiety.

Due to the apparent criteria overlap and the co-occurrence rates of mood and borderline personality disorders, Akiskal and colleagues (Akiskal, 1994; Akiskal et al., 1985) argue that borderline personality disorder is better conceptualized as a mood disorder. In terms of the observed co-occurrence of bipolar personality disorder and borderline personality disorder, the pattern is notably nonspecific to borderline personality disorder. Investigators selecting subjects for the presence of mood disorders report rates of personality disorders in patients with bipolar disorder to range from 1% to 53% (e.g., Alnaes & Torgerson, 1989; Pica et al., 1990; Turley, Bates, Edwards, & Jackson, 1992; Ucok, Karaveli, Kundakci, & Yazici, 1998). Interestingly, histrionic, narcissistic, and obsessive–compulsive personality disorders occur with frequency exceeding that of borderline personality disorder in most of these samples, with rates of borderline personality disorder ranging from 10% to 23% and rates of the aforementioned personality disorders ranging from 12% to 53%.

Using samples of personality-disordered subjects, recent studies examining the co-occurrence of bipolar disorders have varied from approximately 2% to 10% (Skodol et al., 1999; Zanarini et al., 1998). Zanarini and colleagues, using DSM-III-R criteria, found that 10% of subjects with borderline personality disorder met lifetime criteria for bipolar II disorder, in comparison to 2% of subjects with other personality disorders. In a study using DSM-IV criteria (and the percent co-occurrence calculation described previously), Skodol and colleagues found that subjects with borderline personality disorder were no more likely than subjects with other personality disorders to have current bipolar I or II disorders. Co-occurrence rates for borderline personality disorder and bipolar I and II disorders were 9% and 4%, respectively. In contrast, subjects who met criteria for antisocial personality disorder or histrionic personality disorder were more likely than subjects without those disorders to have bipolar I disorder (co-occurrence rates of 9% between antisocial and bipolar I [$p < .05$] and 7% between histrionic and bipolar I disorders [$p < .01$]). In addition, antisocial personality disorder and bipolar II disorders co-occurred more frequently than did any other personality disorder and bipolar II (10% co-occurrence, $p < .001$).

Given that the aforementioned studies do not appear to support the assertion that borderline personality disorder is best conceptualized on a spectrum with bipolar disorder, a dimensional model of temperament may help us better understand the complex relationship between border-line personality disorder and bipolar disorder. In a recent study using Cloninger's (Cloninger, 1986; Cloninger et al., 1993; Cloninger, Przybeck, Svrakic, & Wetzel, 1994) dimensional model of personality, Atre-Vaidya and Hussain (1999) tested a continuum hypothesis of the relationship between borderline personality disorder and bipolar disorder. Cloninger's model presumes that various dimensions of character and temperament (which are biologically based and independent) distinguish individuals without mental disorders from those with mental disorders and also distinguish between various disorders. Early research using this model confirms these assumptions. For example, Starkowski, Stroll, Tohen, Paedda, and Goodwin (1993) found that depressed subjects evidenced high harm avoidance scores in comparison to a normative sample, whereas subjects with bipolar disorder did not differ from normals on any of the dimensions.

Although the Atre-Vaidya and Hussain study was small (28 borderline personality disorder and 13 bipolar subjects), the preliminary findings are intriguing. Similar to the study of Starkowski et al. (1993), the present study found that bipolar subjects did not differ from the normative sample on any of the seven scales of Cloninger's (Cloninger et al., 1994) Temperament and Character Inventory. Subjects with borderline personality disorder, however, scored higher on harm avoidance and lower on self-directedness and cooperativeness than did the normative sample and the bipolar comparison group. Moreover, the subjects with borderline personality disorder differed from the subjects with bipolar disorder on a number of subtrait scales. Namely, subjects with borderline personality disorder had higher scores on impulsivity and disorderliness and lower scores on persistence than did the subjects with bipolar disorder. In conclusion, further examination of dimensional aspects of personality appear to hold great promise for improving our understanding of the structure of borderline personality disorder and the bipolar disorders.

Borderline Personality Disorder and Trauma: A Complex Relationship

Prior to examining the literature on borderline personality disorder and posttraumatic stress disorder, one must first survey the literature on the incidence of trauma in patients with personality disorders. Research on the co-occurrence of personality disorders and childhood trauma (separation/loss, physical abuse, and/or sexual abuse) has been based largely on samples defined by the presence of a personality disorder, most frequently borderline. A notable literature exists regarding the incidence of traumatic events in subjects with borderline personality disorder (for comprehensive reviews, see Gunderson & Sabo, 1993; Paris, 1994, 1996; and Sabo, 1997). Estimates of the incidence of trauma in this group typically exceed 70% and are significantly greater than the incidence of trauma in comparison groups of other mental disorders (e.g., Herman, Perry, & van der Kolk, 1989; Links, Steiner, Offord, & Eppel, 1988; Ogata et al., 1990; Paris, Zweig-Frank, & Guzder, 1994a, 1994b; Weaver & Clum, 1993; Zanarini, Gunderson, Marino, Schwartz, & Frankenburg, 1989).

In a recent study, Fossati, Madeddu, and Maffei (1999) performed a meta-analysis of 21 studies (2,479 subjects) to evaluate the specific association between childhood sexual abuse and borderline personality disorder (i.e., the authors did not include studies examining other forms of trauma such as separation, loss, or physical abuse/neglect). Moderator variables (including gender, age, diagnostic criteria, clinical vs. nonclinical samples) were also examined. Counter to the oft accepted assumption, only a moderate association between borderline personality disorder and childhood sexual abuse was found (pooled effect size =. 279, $z = 14.07$, $p < .001$). There were no significant effects for moderator variables. The findings suggest that although there is an association between childhood sexual abuse and borderline personality disorder, the association is not specific. Thus, there is no simple explanatory model for the role childhood sexual abuse plays in the etiology of borderline personality disorder.

Using samples consisting of subjects with a range of personality disorders, at least two teams of researchers have documented a notable incidence of trauma across personality disorders (Norden, Klein, Donaldson, Pepper, & Klein, 1995; Paris et al., 1994a, 1994b). Paris and colleagues compared 78 subjects with borderline personality disorder and 72 subjects with other personality disorders on a number of trauma variables. Rates of self-reported history of childhood sexual abuse were 70% in the borderline personality disorder sample and 46% in the other personality disorder sample. Rates of physical abuse were 73% in the borderline personality disorder sample and 53% in the other personality disorder sample. While the differences between the two groups on these variables are significant, the existence of abuse is not particularly specific to a diagnosis of borderline personality disorder.

In their study of 90 subjects, Norden and colleagues found that borderline and self-defeating features were most consistently associated with a history of adverse experiences (including childhood sexual abuse). Nevertheless, narcissistic, histrionic, sadistic, and schizotypal traits were also significantly correlated with a history of childhood sexual abuse. Finally, antisocial traits were associated with a history of physical but not sexual abuse. An association between physical abuse and antisocial behavior has also been reported in a sample of young men (Pollock et al., 1990). Again, these findings point to the lack of specificity of trauma history in predicting the presence of borderline personality disorder.

An examination of the relationship between personality disorders and posttraumatic stress disorder from the perspective of samples selected for personality disorders, also reveals limited specificity for the co-occurrence between borderline personality disorder and posttraumatic stress disorder. In one of the only studies of its kind, Zanarini et al. (1998) assessed the lifetime rates of co-occurrence of a full range of Axis I disorders with borderline personality disorder and a comparison group of subjects with other personality disorders.[1] Although subjects with borderline personality disorder had significantly higher rates of posttraumatic stress disorder than did subjects with other personality disorders (56% vs. 22%), it remains important to note that nearly half of the borderline subjects did not have posttraumatic stress disorder and nearly one quarter of subjects with other personality disorders did have posttraumatic stress disorder.

Another set of studies have addressed the posttraumatic stress disorder/trauma/personality disorders quagmire from the perspective of two types of trauma samples: combat trauma victims (primarily Vietnam veterans with posttraumatic stress disorder) and childhood trauma victims (primarily sexual abuse). When assessed with structured clinical interviews, combat veterans with posttraumatic stress disorder have been found to have particularly high rates of borderline, avoidant, paranoid, and obsessive–compulsive personality disorders (Southwick, Yehuda, & Giller, 1993). Results from self-report measures of personality disorders yield elevated rates of borderline, avoidant, passive–aggressive, and schizoid personality disorders (Hyer, Woods, Boudewynes, Harrison, & Tamkin, 1990; Robert, Ryan, McEntyre, McFarland, Lips, & Rosenberg, 1985; Sherwood, Funari, & Piekarski, 1990).

Some data suggest that psychiatric patients with severe trauma histories (combat or childhood sexual abuse) may have similar patterns of personality features, which is furthermore distinct from psychiatric patients without such histories (Shea, Zlotnick, & Weisberg, 1999). The profiles of trauma history patients were characterized by particularly strong elevations in borderline, self-defeating, paranoid, and schizotypal criteria. Data from another sample suggest that elevations in borderline and self-defeating features are associated with a diagnosis of posttraumatic stress disorder rather than a history of trauma per sc (Shea et al., 2000).

In cross-sectional studies such as those noted, causal explanations of the association between personality disorder and trauma cannot be determined. It is unclear whether certain personality features represent risk factors for trauma exposure, vulnerabilities to the development of personality disturbance given exposure, direct consequences of severe or repeated traumatic experiences, consequences of living with chronic posttraumatic stress disorder, or some combination of causal pathways. Thus, although trauma and posttraumatic stress disorder occur frequently in borderline patients, the nature of a causal relationship (if present) is ambiguous. Sabo (1997) aptly concludes that "a complex set of constitutional and environmental factors interact to produce borderline personality disorder" (p. 65). Clearly, much more work is needed to clarify the relationship between different forms of trauma, and well as duration and severity of trauma, with personality features and disorders, using a prospective, longitudinal approach.

Antisocial Personality Disorder and the Substance Use Disorders

Antisocial personality disorder is strongly associated with substance dependence. Evidence for this proposition has accumulated from both community (e.g., Kessler et al., 1997; Nestadt, Romanoski, Samuels, Folstein, & McHugh, 1992) and clinical (e.g., Morgenstern, Langen-

bucher, Labouvie, & Miller, 1997; Skodol, Oldham, & Gallaher, 1995) samples. Concerns have been raised about the possibility that this connection could result simply from antisocial behavior that is directly attributable to illicit drug use—which is, after all, a crime (cf. Widiger & Corbitt, 1995). However, even when extraordinary care was taken to exclude drug-related antisocial behavior from the antisocial personality disorder diagnosis, antisocial personality disorder remained the most common personality disorder in a large clinical sample of persons entering treatment for drug and alcohol problems (Rounsaville et al., 1998).

Longitudinal evidence is also supportive of the antisocial personality disorder–substance dependence connection, in that substance dependence is often preceded by antisocial behavior. In a cohort of 21-year-olds studied since birth, childhood conduct disorder—a required antecedent of antisocial personality disorder—was the most common antecedent of substance dependence (Newman et al., 1996). These phenotypical associations are taken one step further by behavioral genetic studies, which suggest etiological links between antisocial personality disorder and substance dependence. For example, in a study of monozygotic twins reared apart, Grove et al. (1990) found substantial genetic correlations between antisocial personality disorder and substance dependence criteria. Indeed, these disorders may be usefully conceived of as indicators of a latent "externalizing disorder" continuum—a broad dimension undergirded by themes of acting out against the world and being at odds with mainstream goals and values (Krueger, Caspi, Moffitt, & Silva, 1998). In the National Comorbidity Survey, for example, antisocial personality disorder, alcohol abuse/dependence, and drug abuse/dependence formed a latent externalizing factor within both the participants' diagnoses and within the participants' reports of these diagnoses in their parents (Kendler, Davis, & Kessler, 1997). These authors also reported a positive correlation between their participant and parental externalizing factors, suggesting that externalizing behavior is transmittable across generations.

CLUSTER C: ANXIOUS/FEARFUL PERSONALITY DISORDERS

Investigators have documented significant relationships between Cluster C personality disorders (i.e., avoidant, dependent, obsessive–compulsive, and passive–aggressive) and anxiety, mood, eating, and somatoform disorders. The concurrent relationship between Cluster C personality disorders and anxiety disorders appears to be strong (Tyrer et al., 1997). In a study of 200 inpatients and outpatients (consecutive admissions), for example, the odds of an Axis I anxiety disorder co-occurring with a Cluster C personality disorder was more than five times greater than chance (Oldham et al., 1995). One must note, however, that the odds of a mood, psychotic, or eating disorder co-occurring with a Cluster C personality disorder were also significantly elevated (odds ratios of 3.3, 4.3, and 2.8, respectively) and not significantly different from the Cluster C/anxiety disorders odds ratio (5.7). For the remainder of this section, we examine in more detail those areas of co-occurrence that have received the most notable empirical and theoretical attention in the literature. We pay special attention to the relationships between obsessive–compulsive syndrome and personality disorders, avoidant personality disorder and social phobia, Cluster C personality disorders and mood disorders, and Cluster C personality disorders and the somatoform disorders.

Obsessive–Compulsive Personality Disorder and Obsessive–Compulsive Disorder

Numerous studies have examined the specific relationships between anxiety disorders and personality disorders. The results have been inconsistent. Although the vast majority of studies examining the question have found significant relationships between social phobia and avoidant personality disorder (e.g. Herbert, Hope & Bellack, 1992; Skodol, Oldham, Hyler, et al., 1995), the relationship between obsessive–compulsive disorder and obsessive–compulsive personality disorder is not predictable. For example, a number of investigators have documented a significant relationship between obsessive–compulsive disorder and obsessive–compulsive personality disorder (e.g., AuBuchon & Malatesta, 1994; Baer & Jencke, 1992; Skodol, Oldham, Hyler, et al., 1995), whereas a number of investigators have failed to find such a relationship (e.g., Black, Noyes, Pfohl, Goldstein, & Blum, 1993; Joffee, Swinson, & Regan, 1988). With the exception of the study by Skodol, Oldham, Hyler, et al.

(1995), subjects have been selected for the presence of an Axis I anxiety disorder and co-occurrence has been estimated from the perspective of subjects with obsessive–compulsive disorder. The majority of patients with obsessive–compulsive disorder do not meet criteria for obsessive–compulsive personality disorder and for those obsessive–compulsive disorder subjects who have a personality disorder, obsessive–compulsive personality disorder is no more common than other personality disorders. There does not appear to be sufficient information, then, to support a relationship between obsessive–compulsive disorder and obsessive–compulsive personality disorder (Pfohl & Blum, 1991).

Avoidant Personality Disorder and Social Phobia

Conceptual and empirical overlap are consistently observed between avoidant personality disorder and social phobia and have led to confusion regarding the nature of the relationship between these disorders. We now turn to an examination of issues central to the confusion in this area.

DSM-III (American Psychiatric Association. 1980) first officially recognized social phobia as a disorder characterized by fear and avoidance of specific social situations (e.g., speaking in public). Avoidant personality disorder was considered to be a more pervasive, chronic, and debilitating condition than social phobia. A spectrum model explaining the relationship between avoidant personality disorder and social phobia was implied in the decision rules requiring a diagnosis of avoidant personality disorder to take precedence over a diagnosis of social phobia. Evidence for the presumed greater severity of avoidant personality disorder (vs. social phobia) was found in one of a few studies using DSM-III criteria to compare subjects with avoidant personality disorder and social phobia (Turner, Beidel, Dancu, & Keys, 1986). The investigators found that subjects with avoidant personality disorder presented with more severe anxiety, greater levels of depression, and higher levels of interpersonal sensitivity than did subjects with social phobia.

DSM-III-R (American Psychiatric Association, 1987) dropped the avoidant personality disorder/social phobia hierarchy, as well as the trait criteria central to the previous definition of avoidant personality disorder (i.e., those pertaining to a desire for self-acceptance and low self-esteem; Millon & Martinez. 1995). Also, criteria were added that created increased overlap with social phobia (e.g., fears being embarrassed by blushing). Finally, a social phobia subtype was added, which created a more chronic and pervasive social phobia. The generalized social phobia subtype refers to social anxiety and avoidance behavior that extend to most social situations. Social phobia otherwise refers to social anxiety and avoidance behavior that is limited to fewer, more specific, situations (e.g., public speaking or eating in front of others). Although DSM-IV sought to further differentiate generalized social phobia from avoidant personality disorder in the criteria sets of the two disorders, studies examining the relationship between these disorders that are available for review at this time use DSM-III-R criteria and thus need to be considered in the context of this "overlap by definition."

Using DSM-III-R criteria, co-occurrence rates of avoidant personality disorder in subjects with social phobia range from 37% (Sanderson, Wetzler, Beck, & Betz, 1994) to 89% (Schneir, Spitzer, Gibbon, Fyer, & Liebowitz, 1991). Of note, the studies finding higher co-occurrence rates (50% and above) have been based on samples selected for the presence of generalized social phobia.

Due to the fact that selection criteria have typically been based on the presence of social phobia or an Axis I anxiety disorder (vs. selecting subjects for personality disorders or avoidant personality disorder), descriptions of differences between subjects with generalized social phobia and avoidant personality disorder have been limited to comparisons of subjects with generalized social phobia alone and subjects with both generalized social phobia and avoidant personality disorder. These studies have found that in comparison to subjects with generalized social phobia only, subjects with both generalized social phobia and avoidant personality disorder have higher levels of anxiety, increased impairment, and greater comorbidity with other disorders (Herbert et al., 1992; Holt, Heimberg, & Hope, 1992). The authors assert that these findings support the conceptualization of avoidant personality disorder and social phobia as quantitatively different disorders falling along the same spectrum of disease, but the possibility that other models of co-occurrence explain the relationship between avoidant personality disorder and social phobia

has not been ruled out. Similarly, whereas DSM-III-R suggested that social phobia is a "potential complication" of avoidant personality disorder, it is also possible that social phobia is a manifestation or associated feature of avoidant personality disorder (or vice versa) (i.e., they are really part of the same disorder; Widiger & Shea, 1991).

Cluster C Personality Disorders and the Mood Disorders

A review of studies reporting co-occurrence rates of Cluster C personality disorders with mood disorders suggests notable relationships among these disorders. Reported estimates of the concurrent co-occurrence of Cluster C and mood disorders range from approximately 20% to 85%. Most studies report that at least 30% to 40% of subjects with a current mood disorder also present with a current anxious cluster personality disorder (e.g., Alnaes & Torgersen, 1990; Mauri et al., 1992; Oldham et al., 1995; Reich & Noyes, 1987; Shea et al., 1987; Ucok et al., 1998; Zimmerman, Coryell, Pfohl, Corenthal, & Stangl, 1986). In one of the few studies selecting subjects on the basis of likelihood for a personality disorder, Oldham et al. (1995) found that when examining the relationship between mood and personality disorders, odds ratios were elevated only between mood and Cluster C disorders. Subjects with mood disorders were over three times more likely to have an anxious/fearful personality disorder (and vice versa) than were those subjects without mood disorders. In a recent study focusing on the course of four specific personality disorders (though all personality disorders were assessed), borderline and antisocial personality disorders co-occurred at significant rates with any mood disorder (10% and 39%, respectively). Two of the four Cluster C personality disorders, avoidant and obsessive–compulsive, co-occurred at significant rates with any mood disorder (48% and 11%, respectively).

Examined from a different perspective (i.e., in outpatient samples selected for depression or bipolar disorder), anxious/fearful personality disorders appear to occur more frequently than the dramatic or odd/eccentric personality disorders (e.g., Pilkonis & Frank, 1988; Rees, Hardy, & Barkham, 1997; Shea et al., 1987, Ucok et al., 1998). That Cluster C personality disorders appear to co-occur with mood disorders at greater rates than do Cluster B personality disorders may be a startling observation to theorists who have long asserted a unique relationship between Cluster B personality disorders (namely, borderline) and the mood disorders.

Rates of the co-occurrence of depression and Cluster C disorders appear to be dependent, in part, on the extent to which other Axis I anxiety disorders are also present. Alnaes and Torgersen (1990) found that subjects who met criteria for major depression only were significantly less likely to have a Cluster C personality disorder then were subjects who met criteria for depression and an Axis I anxiety disorder. Notably, subjects were selected for pure major depression, pure anxiety, or mixed anxiety and depression. Substance abusers and psychotic patients were excluded. In a sample assessed for inclusion into a psychotherapy study, Rees et al. (1997) found that the presence of a Cluster C personality disorder in depressed subjects was highly related to the presence of other comorbid conditions. Whereas only 1 of 29 subjects with pure major depression met criteria for a Cluster C personality disorder, 36% of 132 subjects with major depression and generalized anxiety or panic disorder had a Cluster C personality disorder.

Cluster C Personality Disorders and Somatoform Disorders

Research in this area has typically been conducted from the perspective of patients selected for the presence of a somatoform disorder. In these studies, rates of the co-occurrence of a personality disorder range from 59% to 83% (e.g., Barsky, Wyshak, & Klerman, 1992; Fishbain, Goldberg, Labbe, Steele, & Rosomoff, 1988; Fishbain, Goldberg, Meagher, Steele, & Rosomoff, 1986; Stern, Murphy, & Bass, 1993). The rates appear to be somewhat lower (ranging from 30% to 44%) when examining patients with somatoform disorder who were recruited into general studies of Axis I and Axis II disorders (Koenigsberg et al., 1985; Okasha et al., 1996).

A number of authors have argued that somatoform disorders would be better classified as personality disorders due to their rates of co-occurrence with personality disorders and the criteria overlap among the disorders (e.g., for somatization disorder: early age of onset, persistent course, and duration into adulthood). However, one must consider the possibility that the co-occurrence of personality disorders and somatoform disorders is an artifact of the help-seeking behavior of somatizers who have limited coping skills and problematic reactions to stressors (i.e., those with personality disorders) versus those somatizers who do not have significant personality pathology and thus do not tend to seek help (Barsky, 1995; Kirmayer, Robbins, & Paris, 1994).

Nonetheless, somatoform disorders appear to have a particularly strong relationship to Cluster C personality disorders. The association between somatoform and Cluster C personality disorders (in samples typically selected for the presence of a somatoform disorder) appears to be more than five times higher than that expected by chance and greater than the association with other personality disorders (cf. Tyrer et al., 1997). Specifically, hypochondriasis appears to have a specific relationship to Cluster C personality disorders (e.g., Kellner, 1986; Starcevic, 1990). Somatization disorder, on the other hand, appears to be related to both Cluster B and C personality disorders (e.g., Rost, Akins, Brown & Smith, 1992; Stern et al., 1993).

RESEARCH DIAGNOSES: THE CONTROVERSIAL (AND ILLUSTRATIVE) CASE OF DEPRESSIVE PERSONALITY DISORDER

Depressive personality disorder was introduced to DSM-IV as a research diagnosis, a criteria set identified for further study. The concept of a depressive personality type has been described for nearly a century; however, an empirical literature has only begun to emerge in the past decade (for recent reviews, see Huprich, 1998; Phillips, Hirschfeld, Shea, & Gunderson, 1996; Ryder & Bagby, 1999). The discussion that has arisen around the nosological appropriateness of depressive personality disorder has tended to focus on issues specific to depressive personality disorder (e.g., the internal consistency of the criteria set, the distinction of depressive personality disorder from other disorders). Arguments against the inclusion of depressive personality disorder emphasize conceptual overlap and the co-occurrence of depressive personality disorder with mood disorders, namely, dysthymia (e.g., Ryder & Bagby, 1999). Arguments for the inclusion of depressive personality disorder emphasize the conceptual uniqueness of depressive personality disorder and the relative distinction of depressive personality disorder from other disorders (e.g., Klein, 1999; Phillips & Gunderson, 1999). Were DSM to be totally reorganized, similar arguments could be had for and against many disorders based on their conceptual and empirical overlap (as illustrated in the present review of the co-occurrence of personality and syndrome disorders).

Thus, the current discussion regarding depressive personality disorder can also be used to illustrate broader issues germane to the categorization or description of personality disorders (Livesley, 1999). In his introduction to a special journal section pertaining to depressive personality disorder, Livesley (1999) outlines a number of issues that need to be resolved. These issues include (1) the relationship between personality and syndrome disorders, (2) the relationship between normal and disordered personality, (3) the definition of constructs that should be used to delineate personality pathology; and (4) the modification of categorical classification systems for the accommodation of related disorders (e.g., disorders considered to have a spectrum relationship).

CONCLUSIONS

A review of studies examining the co-occurrence of Axis I and Axis II disorders leads to the conclusion that having an Axis II disorder appears to place a patient at risk for an Axis I disorder and vice versa. Nearly three-quarters of patients diagnosed with a personality disorder also present with a syndrome disorder. Examined from the reverse perspective, fewer subjects diagnosed with a syndrome disorder will also be diagnosed with a personality disorder.

Questions of specificity need to be answered from the perspective of comprehensive data (e.g., interviews) from large samples which are unselected for specific disorders and cover a broad range of disorders across both axes. To date, few studies meet these criteria. Nonetheless, the strongest relationships appear to be between the substance use disorders and the Cluster B personality disorders and between the somatoform and Cluster C personality disorders. Beyond these conclusions, however, there is little evidence for specific relationships between disorders. For example, anxiety disorders are noted to occur at significant rates not only with the Cluster C personality disorders but also with the Cluster B personality disorders. Also, whereas psychotic disorders co-occur significantly with the Cluster A personality disorders, they also co-occur at significant rates with the Cluster B and Cluster C personality disorders.

When examining the relationship between Axis I and Axis II disorder criteria (measured dimensionally), a consistent and intriguing finding emerges from the study by Oldham et al. (1995): All classes of Axis I mental disorders examined were associated with elevated numbers of personality disorder criteria across the three personality disorder clusters (except for substance disorders, which were only consistently associated with the Cluster B personality disorders). Such a finding suggests the possible presence of a broad severity dimension, embedded in personality functioning and undergirding both Axis I and Axis II disorders. A search for the etiology of "severity" may be as valuable as a search for the etiology of various symptom constellations.

So where does the evidence of high rates of covariation among Axis I and II disorders leave us? Earlier in the chapter we outlined a number of models for explaining the nature of co-occurring disorders. These models provide opportunities for increased understanding of the co-occurrences. Research thus far in the area, however, is limited and allows us to describe the rates of co-occurrence between Axis I and Axis II disorders but not to explain the nature of the associations. Research on the co-occurrence among Axis I disorders may provide examples as to how questions regarding the nature of the relationships between Axis I and Axis II disorders may be addressed. For example, Kendler and colleagues used twin studies to search for common genetic vulnerabilities among disorders (e.g., genetic commonalties between depression and generalized anxiety disorder [Kendler, Neale, Kessler, Heath, & Eaves, 1992] and between depression and alcoholism [Kendler, Heath, Neale, Kessler, & Eaves, 1993]).

Further research in this area, including the testing of the covariation models outlined earlier (i.e., common cause, spectrum/subclinical, predisposition/vulnerability, complication/scar, pathoplasty/exacerbation, and psychobiological), is fraught with complexity. Nonetheless, researchers in the field have outlined important factors for consideration when developing hypotheses and designing research on the co-occurrence of mental disorders (e.g., Clark & Watson, 1999; Clark et al., 1995; Klein et al., 1993; Kessler, 1995; Lyons et al., 1997; Widiger & Shea, 1991).

Factors for consideration include the following:

1. Prospective, longitudinal designs should be used whenever possible as cross-sectional data limit us to descriptions of the covariation without avenues for testing causal models. Exceptions to this occur in cases in which reliable information is available regarding possible causes of covariation. For example, in genetically informative samples (e.g., twin samples), cross-sectional data can be used to determine the extent to which covariation among putatively separate mental disorders is genetic or environmental in origin.

2. Samples should be carefully chosen based on the population to which generalization is desired. For example, community samples should be used when investigating co-occurrence patterns in the general population in order to avoid the potential bias toward co-occurrence that may be present when selecting identified patients.

3. Personality and syndrome disorders (and/or facets thereof) need to be defined as distinct in order to eliminate artifactual associations due to overlapping criteria.

4. When investigating potentially meaningful dimensions of personality and psychopathology, it is necessary to identify and specifically define these dimensions in terms of severity, biological markers, phenotypical symptoms or traits, and/or genetic vulnerability.

5. When using traditional psychopathology research designs, clearly defined control or comparison groups need to be used (e.g., groups with psychopathological conditions other than those being examined, groups with the "pure" disorder (i.e., no co-occurring disorders), and groups with other "core defects" or potential causal factors).

6. Clear definitions of primacy need to be provided when investigating primary versus secondary disorder (e.g., age of onset, degree of impairment).

7. Genetically informative designs (e.g., twin studies) should be used to provide information regarding the extent to which genes and the environment act as independent or interacting causal factors.

Given the current state of the science, there are many directions for future research on the covariation of personality and syndrome disorders. Numerous models to describe the nature of these co-occurrences have been outlined and need to be tested. Data suggest that examining personality and syndrome constructs dimensionally will likely provide a wealth of information to better understand the multifaceted nature of psychopathology and adjustment. The dimensional approach, for one, avoids the problem of artificial overlap resulting from similar or identical criteria, and it is likely to provide a more precise assessment of the symptom and trait patterns under study. The use of prospective, longitudinal designs with clearly defined (and distinct) dimensions of personality and psychopathology and hypotheses stating the nature of the relationship between these dimensions appears to be the next logical step in this exciting area of research.

ACKNOWLEDGMENTS

This chapter was written while Regina T. Dolan-Sewell was a faculty member at Brown University and does not represent the opinions of the National Institute of Mental Health, the National Institute of Health, the Department of Health and Human Services, or the U.S. government. Work on this chapter was supported in part by Grant No. MH50837-02 from the National Institute of Mental Health.

NOTE

1. While the data presented in this chapter reflect lifetime rates of posttraumatic stress disorder, current rates of posttraumatic stress disorder in the borderline personality disorder and other personality disorder groups are not significantly different from lifetime rates (M. C. Zanarini, personal communication, January 31, 2000).

REFERENCES

Akiskal, H. S. (1994). The temperamental borders of affective disorders. *Acta Psychiatrica Scandinavica, 89* (Suppl. 379), 32–37.

Akiskal, H. S., Chen, S. E., Davis, G. C., Puzantian, V. R., Kashgarian, M., & Bolinger, J. M. (1985). Borderline: An adjective in search of a noun. *Journal of Clinical Psychiatry, 46,* 41–48.

Alnaes, R., & Torgersen, S. (1988). The relationship between DSM-III symptom disorders (Axis I) and personality disorders (Axis II) in an outpatient population. *Acta Psychiatrica Scandinavica, 78,* 485–492.

Alnaes, R., & Torgersen, S. (1990). DSM-III personality disorders among patients with major depression, anxiety disorders, and mixed conditions. *Journal of Nervous and Mental Disease, 178*(11), 693–698.

American Psychiatric Association. (1980). *Diagnostic and statistical manual of mental disorders* (3rd ed.). Washington, DC: Author.

American Psychiatric Association. (1987). *Diagnostic and statistical manual of mental disorders* (3rd ed., rev.). Washington, DC: Author.

American Psychiatric Association. (1994). *Diagnostic and statistical manual of mental disorders* (4th ed.). Washington, DC: Author.

Atre-Vaidya, N., & Hussain, S. M. (1999). Borderline personality disorder and bipolar mood disorder: Two distinct disorders or a continuum? *Journal of Nervous and Mental Disease, 187*(5), 313–315.

AuBuchon, R. G., & Malatesta, V. J. (1994). Obsessive–compulsive patients with comorbid personality disorder: Associated problems and response to a comprehensive behavior therapy. *Journal of Clinical Psychiatry, 55,* 448–453.

Baer, L., & Jencke, M. (1992). Personality disorders in obsessive compulsive disorder. *Psychiatric Clinics of North America, 15*(4), 803–812.

Barsky, A. J. (1995) Somatoform disorders and personality traits. *Journal of Psychosomatic Research, 39,* 399–402.

Barsky, A. J., Wyshak, G., & Klerman, G. L. (1992). Psychiatric comorbidity in DSM-III-R hypochondriasis. *Archives of General Psychiatry, 49,* 101–108.

Berenbaum, H., & Fujita, F. (1994). Schizophrenia and personality: exploring the boundaries and connections between vulnerability and outcome. *Journal of Abnormal Psychology, 103*(1), 148–158.

Black, D. W., Noyes, R. J., Pfohl, B., Goldstein, R. B., & Blum, N. (1993). Personality disorder in obsessive–compulsive volunteers, well comparison subjects, and their first degree relatives. *American Journal of Psychiatry, 150,* 1226–1232.

Bolton, D., & Gunderson, J. G. (1996). Distinguishing borderline personality disorder from bipolar disorder: Differential diagnosis and implications. *American Journal of Psychiatry, 153*(9), 1202–1208.

Chapman, L. J., Chapman, J. P., Kwapil, T. R., Eckblad, M., & Zinser, M. C. (1994). Putatively psychosis-prone subjects 10 years later. *Journal of Abnormal Psychology, 103*(2), 171–183.

Clark, L. A., & Watson, D. (1999). Personality, disorder, and personality disorder: A more rational conceptualization. *Journal of Personality Disorders, 13*(2), 142–151.

Clark, L. A., Watson, D., & Reynolds, S. (1995). Diagnosis and classification of psychopathology: Challenges to the current system and future directions. *Annual Review of Psychology, 46,* 121–153.

Cloninger, C. R. (1986). A unified biosocial theory of personality and its role in the development of anxiety states. *Psychiatric Developments, 3,* 167–226.

Cloninger, C. R., Przybeck, T. R., Svrakic, D. M., & Wetzel, R. (1994). *TCI—The temperament and character inventory: A guide to its development and use.* St. Louis, MO: Center for Psychobiology of Personality, Washington University.

Cloninger, C. R., Svrakic, D. M., & Przybeck, T. R. (1993). A psychobiological model of temperament and character. *Archives of General Psychiatry, 50,* 975–990.

Cornelius, J. R., Soloff, P. H., Perel, J. M., & Ulrich, R. F. (1990). Fluoxetine trial in borderline personality disorder. *Psychopharmacology Bulletin, 26,* 151–154.

Corruble, E., Ginestet, D., & Guelfi, J. D. (1996). Comorbidity of personality disorders and unipolar major depression: A review. *Journal of Affective Disorders, 37,* 157–170.

Dahl, A. A. (1986). Some aspects of the DSM-III personality disorders illustrated by a consecutive sample of hospitalized patients. *Acta Psychiatrica Scandinavica Supplement, 328,* 61–67.

Fabrega, H., Pilkonis, P., Mezzich, J., Ahn, C. W., & Shea, S. (1990). Explaining diagnostic complexity in an intake setting. *Comprehensive Psychiatry, 31*(1), 5–14.

Fabrega, H., Ulrich, R., Pilkonis, P., & Mezzich, J. E. (1992). Pure personality disorders in an intake psychiatric setting. *Journal of Personality Disorders, 6,* 153–161.

Feinstein, A. R. (1970). The pre-therapeutic classification of comorbidity in chronic disease. *Journal of Chronic Diseases, 23,* 455–468.

Fishbain, D. A., Goldberg, M., Meagher, B. R., Steele, R. & Rosomoff, H. (1986). Male and female chronic pain patients categorised by DSM-III psychiatric diagnostic criteria. *Pain, 26,* 181–197.

Fossati, A., Madeddu, F., & Maffei, C. (1999). Borderline personality disorder and childhood sexual abuse: A meta-analytic study. *Journal of Personality Disorders, 13*(3), 268–280.

Fyer, M. R., Frances, A. J., Sullivan, T., Hurt, S. W., & Clarkin, J. (1988). Comorbidity of borderline personality disorder. *Archives of General Psychiatry, 45,* 348–352.

Gray, J. A. (1982). *The neuropsychology of anxiety.* Oxford: Oxford University Press.

Grove, W. M., Eckert, E. D., Heston, L., Bouchard, T. J. Jr., Segal, N. & Lykken, D. T. (1990). Heritability of substance abuse and antisocial behavior: A study of monozygotic twins reared apart. *Biological Psychiatry, 27,* 1293–1304.

Gunderson, J. G., & Phillips, K. A. (1991). A current view on the interface between borderline personality disorder and depression. *American Journal of Psychiatry, 148,* 967–975.

Gunderson, J. G., & Sabo, A. N. (1993). The phenomenological and conceptual interface between borderline personality disorder and PTSD. *American Journal of Psychiatry, 150,* 19–27.

Gunderson, J. G., Triebwasser, J., Phillips, K. A., & Sullivan, C. N. (1999). Personality and vulnerability to affective disorders. In C. R. Cloninger (Ed.), *Personality and psychopathology* (pp. 3–32). Washington, DC: American Psychiatric Association Press.

Herbert, J. D., Hope, D. A., & Bellack, A. S. (1992). Validity of the distinction between generalized social phobia and avoidant personality disorder. *Journal of Abnormal Psychology, 101*(2), 332–339.

Herman, J., Perry, J. C., & van der Kolk, B. A. (1989). Childhood trauma in borderline personality disorder. *American Journal of Psychiatry, 146,* 490–495.

Holt, C. S., Heimberg, R. G., & Hope, D. A. (1992). Avoidant personality disorder and the generalized subtype in social phobia. *Journal of Abnormal Psychology, 101,* 318–325.

Huprich, S. K. (1998). Depressive personality disorder: Theoretical issues, clinical findings, and future research questions. *Clinical Psychology Review, 18,* 477–500.

Hyer, L., Woods, M. G., Boudewyns, P. A., Harrison, W. R., & Tamkin, A. S. (1990). MCMI and 16-PF with Vietnam veterans: Profiles and concurrent validation of MCMI. *Journal of Personality Disorders, 4*(4), 391–401.

Hyler, S. E., Skodol, A. E., Kellman, H. D., Oldham, J. M., & Rosnick, L. (1990). Validity of the Personality Diagnostic Questionnaire—Revised: Comparison with two structured interviews. *American Journal of Psychiatry, 147,* 1043–1048.

Joffee, R. T., Swinson, R. P., Regan, J. J. (1998). Personality features of obsessive–compulsive disorder. *American Journal of Psychiatry, 145,* 1127–1129.

Kellner, R. (1986). *Somatization and hypochondriasis.* New York: Praeger.

Kendall, P. C., & Clarkin, J. F. (1992). Introduction to special section: Comorbidity and treatment implications. *Journal of Consulting and Clinical Psychology, 60,* 833–834.

Kendler, K. S., Davis, C. G., & Kessler, R. C. (1997). The familial aggregation of common psychiatric and substance use disorders in the National Comorbidity Survey: A family history study. *British Journal of Psychiatry, 170,* 541–548.

Kendler, K. S., Heath, A. C., Neale, M. C., Kessler, R. C., & Eaves, L. J. (1993). Alcoholism and major depression in women: A twin study of the causes of comorbidity. *Archives of General Psychiatry, 50,* 690–698.

Kendler, K. S., McGuire, M., Gruenberg, A. M., & Walsh, D. (1995). Schizotypal symptoms and signs in the Roscommon Family Study: Their factor structure and familial relationship with psychotic and affective disorders. *Archives of General Psychiatry, 52,* 296–303.

Kendler, K. S., Neale, N. C., Kessler, R. C., Heath, A. C., & Eaves, L. J. (1992). Major depression and generalized anxiety disorder: Same genes (partly) different environments? *Archives of General Psychiatry, 49,* 716–727.

Kessler, R. C. (1995). Epidemiology of psychiatric comorbidity. In M. Tsuang, M. Tohen, & G. Zahner (Eds.), *Textbook in psychiatric epidemiology* (pp. 179–197). New York: Wiley-Liss.

Kessler, R. C., Crum, R. M., Warner, L. A., Nelson, C. B., Schulenberg, J. & Anthony, J. C. (1997). Lifetime co-occurrence of DSM-III-R alcohol abuse and dependence with other psychiatric disorders in the National Comorbidity Survey. *Archives of General Psychiatry, 54,* 313–321.

Kirmayer, L. J., Robbins, J. M., & Paris, J. (1994). Somatoform disorders: Personality and the social matrix of somatic distress. *Journal of Abnormal Psychology, 103,* 125–136.

Klein, D. H. (1999). Commentary on Ryder and Bagby's "Diagnostic viability of depressive personality disorder: Theoretical and conceptual issues." *Journal of Personality Disorders, 13*(2), 118–127.

Klein, M. H., Wonderlich, S., & Shea, M. R. (1993). Models of relationships between personality and depression: Toward a framework for theory and research. In M. H. Klein, D. J. Kupfer, & M. T. Shea (Eds.), *Personality and depression: A current view* (pp. 1–54). New York: Guilford Press.

Klerman, G. L. (1978). The evolution of a scientific nosology. In J. C. Shershow (Ed.), *Schizophrenia: Science and practice* (pp. 99–121). Cambridge, MA: Harvard University Press.

Koenigsberg, H. W., Kaplan, R. D., Gilmore, M. M., & Cooper, A. M. (1985). The relationship between syndrome and personality disorder in DSM-III: Experience with 2,462 patients. *American Journal of Psychiatry, 142,* 207–212.

Krueger, R. F., Caspi, A., Moffitt, T. E., & Silva, P. A. (1998). The structure and stability of common mental disorders (DSM-III-R): A longitudinal–epidemiological study. *Journal of Abnormal Psychology, 106,* 216–227.

Krueger, R. F., Caspi, A., Moffitt, T. E., Silva, P. A., & McGee, R. (1996). Personality traits are differentially linked to mental disorders: A multitrait–multidiagnosis study of an adolescent birth cohort. *Journal of Abnormal Psychology, 105,* 299–312.

Krueger, R. F., Caspi, A., Moffitt, T. E., White, J., & Stouthamer-Loeber, M. (1996). Delay of gratification, psychopathology, and personality: Is low self-control specific to externalizing situations? *Journal of Personality, 64,* 107–129.

Kwapil, T. R., Miller, M. B., Zinser, M. C., Chapman, J., & Chapman, L. J. (1997). Magical ideation and social anhedonia as predictors of psychosis proneness: A partial replication. *Journal of Abnormal Psychology, 106*(3), 491–495.

Lilienfeld, S. O., Waldman, I. D., & Israel, A. C. (1994). A critical examination of the use of the term and concept of comorbidity in psychopathology research. *Clinical Psychology: Science and Practice, 1,* 71–83.

Links, P. S., Steiner, M., Boiago, I., & Irwin, D. (1990). Lithium therapy for borderline patients: Preliminary findings. *Journal of Personality Disorders, 4,* 173–181.

Links, P. S., Steiner, M., Offord, D. R., & Eppel, A. (1988). Characteristics of borderline personality disorder: A Canadian study. *Canadian Journal of Psychiatry, 33*(5), 336–340.

Livesley, J. (1999). Depressive personality disorder: An introduction. *Journal of Personality Disorders, 13*(2), 970–998.

Lyons, M. J., Tyrer, P., Gunderson, J., & Tohen, M. (1997). Special feature: Heuristic models of comorbidity of axis I and axis II disorders. *Journal of Personality Disorders, 11*(3), 260–269.

Mauri, M., Sarno, N., Rossi, V. M., Armani, A., Zambotto, S., Cassano, G. B., & Akiskal, H. S. (1992). Personality disorders associated with generalized anxiety, panic, and recurrent depressive disorders. *Journal of Personality Disorders, 62*(2), 162–167.

Meehl, P. E. (1989). Schizotaxia revisited. *Archives of General Psychiatry, 46*(10), 935–944.

Millon, T., & Davis, R. D. (1996). Personality theories: Historical, modern, and contemporary. In T. Millon & R. O. Davis, *Disorders of personality: DSM-IV and beyond* (2nd ed., pp. 55–72). New York: Wiley.

Millon, T., & Martinez, A. (1995). Avoidant personality disorder. In W. J. Livesley (Ed.), *The DSM-IV personality disorders* (pp. 218–233). New York: Guilford Press.

Morgenstern, J., Langenbucher, J., Labouvie, E., & Miller, K. J. (1997). The comorbidity of alcoholism and personality disorders in a clinical population: Prevalence rates and relation to alcohol typology variables. *Journal of Abnormal Psychology, 106,* 74–84.

Nestadt, G., Romanoski, A. J., Samuels, J. F., Folstein, M. F., & McHugh, P. R. (1992). The relationship between personality and DSM-III Axis I disorders in the population: Results from an epidemiological survey. *American Journal of Psychiatry, 149,* 1228–1233.

Newman, D. L., Moffitt. T. E., Caspi, A., Magdol, L., Silva, P. A., & Stanton, W. R. (1996). Psychiatric disorder in a birth cohort of young adults: Prevalence, co-morbidity, clinical significance, and new case incidence from age 11 to 21. *Journal of Consulting and Clinical Psychology, 64,* 552–562.

Newman, D. L., Moffitt, T. E., Caspi, A., & Silva, P. A. (1998). Comorbid mental disorders: Implications for treatment and sample selection. *Journal of Abnormal Psychology, 107*(2), 305–311.

Norden, K. A., Klein, D. N., Donaldson, S. K., Pepper, C. M., & Klein, L. M. (1995). Reports of the early home environment in DSM-III-R personality disorders. *Journal of Personality Disorders, 9,* 213–223.

Ogata, S., Silk, K. R., Goodrich, S., Lohr, N. E., Weston, D., & Hill, E. M. (1990). Childhood sexual and physical abuse in adult patients with borderline personality disorder. *American Journal of Psychiatry, 147,* 1008–1013.

Okasha, A., Omar, A. M., Lotaief, F., Ghanem, M., Seif El Dawla, A., & Okasha, T. (1996). Comorbidity of Axis I and Axis II diagnoses in a sample of Egyptian patients with neurotic disorders. *Comprehensive Psychiatry, 37,* 95–101.

Oldham, J. M., Skodol, A. E., Kellman, H. D., Hyler, S. E., Doidge, N., Rosnick, L., & Gallaher, P. E. (1995). Comorbidity of axis I and axis II disorders. *American Journal of Psychiatry, 152*(4), 571–578.

Paris, J. (1994). *Borderline personality disorder: A multidimensional approach.* Washington, DC: American Psychiatric Press.

Paris, J. (1996). *Social factors in the personality disorders: A biopsychosocial approach to etiology and treatment.* New York: Cambridge University Press.

Paris, J., Zweig-Frank, H., & Guzder, J. (1994a). Psychological risk factors for borderline personality disorder in female patients. *Comprehensive Psychiatry, 35*(94), 301–305.

Paris, J., Zweig-Frank, H., & Guzder, J. (1994b). Risk factors for borderline personality disorder in male outpatients. *Journal of Nervous and Mental Disease, 182,* 375–380.

Pfohl, B., & Blum, N. (1991). Obsessive–compulsive personality disorder: A review of available data and recommendations for DSM-IV. *Journal of Personality Disorders, 5,* 150–166.

Phillips, K. A., & Gunderson, J. G. (1999). Depressive personality disorder: Fact or fiction? *Journal of Personality Disorders, 13*(2), 128–134.

Phillips, K. A., Hirschfeld, R. M. A., Shea, M. T., & Gunderson, J. G. (1996). Depressive personality disorder. In *DSM-IV Sourcebook, Volume II.* Washington, DC: American Psychiatric Association Press.

Pica, S., Edwards, J., Jackson, H. J., Bell, R. C., Bates, G. W., & Rudd, R. P. (1990). Personality disorders in recent-onset bipolar disorder. *Comprehensive Psychiatry, 31*(6), 499–510.

Pilkonis, P. A., & Frank, E. (1988). Personality pathology in recurrent depression: Nature, prevalence, and relationship to treatment response. *American Journal of Psychiatry, 145*(4), 435–441.

Pollock, V. E., Briere, J., Schneider, L., Knop, J., Mednick, S. A., & Goodwin, D. W. (1991). Childhood antecedents of antisocial behavior: Parental alcoholism and physical abusiveness. *American Journal of Psychiatry, 147*(10), 1290–1293.

Rees, A., Hardy, G. E., & Barkham, M. (1997). Covariance in the measurement of depression/anxiety and three Cluster C personality disorders (avoidant, dependent, obsessive–compulsive). *Journal of Affective Disorders, 45,* 143–153.

Reich, J. (1995). Family history of DSM-III-R dramatic personality disorder cluster and functioning in patients with major depressive disorder. *Journal of Nervous and Mental Disease, 183*(9), 587–592.

Reich, J., & Noyes, R. (1987). A comparison of DSM-III personality disorders in acutely ill panic and depressed patients. *Journal of Anxiety Disorders, 1*(2), 123–131.

Riso, L. P., Klein, D. L., Ferro, T., Kasch, K. L., Pepper, C. M., Schwartz, J. E., & Aaronson, T. A. (1996). Understanding the comorbidity between early-onset dysthymia and Cluster B personality disorders: A family study. *American Journal of Psychiatry, 153,* 900–906.

Robert, J. A., Ryan, J. J., McEntyre, W. L., McFarland, R. S., Lips, O. J., & Rosenberg, S. J. (1985). MCMI Characteristics of DSM-III posttraumatic stress disorder in Vietnam veterans. *Journal of Personality Assessment, 49*(3), 226–230.

Robins, L. N., Tipp, J., & Przybeck, T. (1991). Antisocial personality. In L. N. Robins & D. J. Regier (Eds.), *Psychiatric disorders in America* (pp. 258–290). New York: Free Press.

Rost, K. M., Akins, R. N., Brown, F. W., & Smith, G. R. (1992). The comorbidity of DSM-III-R personality disorders in somatization disorder. *General Hospital Psychiatry, 14,* 322–326.

Rounsaville, B. J., Kranzler, H. R., Ball, S., Tennen, H., Poling, J., & Triffleman, E. (1998). Personality disorders in substance abusers: Relation to substance use. *Journal of Nervous and Mental Disease, 186,* 87–95.

Ryder, A. G., & Bagby, R. M. (1999). Diagnostic viability of depressive personality disorder: Theoretical and conceptual issues. *Journal of Personality Disorders, 13*(2), 99–117.

Sabo, A. N. (1997). Etiological significance of association between childhood trauma and borderline personality disorder: Conceptual and clinical implications. *Journal of Personality Disorders, 11*(1), 50–70.

Sanderson, W. C., Wetzler, S., Beck, A. T., & Betz, F. (1994). Prevalence of personality disorders among patients with anxiety disorders. *Psychiatry Research, 51,* 167–174.

Schneir, F. R., Spitzer, R. L., Gibbon, M., Fyer, A. J., & Liebowitz, M. R. (1991). The relationship of social phobia subtypes and avoidant personality disorder. *Comprehensive Psychiatry, 32,* 496–502.

Shea, M. T., Zlotnick, C., Dolan, R. T., Warshaw, M. G., Phillips, K. A., Brown, P., & Keller, M. B. (2000). Personality disorders, history of trauma, and PTSD in subjects with anxiety disorders. *Comprehensive Psychiatry, 41,* 315–325.

Shea, M. T., Zlotnick, C., & Weisberg, R. B. (1999). Commonality and specificity of personality disorder profiles in subjects with trauma histories. *Journal of Personality Disorders, 13,* 199–210.

Shea, M. T., Glass, D., Pilkonis, P. A., Watkins, J., & Doherty, J. P. (1987). Frequency and implications of personality disorders in a sample of depressed outpatients. *Journal of Personality Disorders, 1*(1), 27–42.

Sherwood, R. J., Funari, D. J., & Piekarski, A. M. (1990). Adapted character styles of Vietnam veterans with posttraumatic stress disorder. *Psychological Reports, 66,* 623–631.

Siever, L. J., & Davis, K. L. (1991). A psychobiological perspective on the personality disorders. *American Journal of Psychiatry, 148,* 1647–1658.

Skodol, A. E., Oldham, J. M., & Gallaher, P. E. (1995). *Comorbidity of substance use and personality disorders.* Paper presented at the 148th annual meeting of the American Psychiatric Association, Miami, FL.

Skodol, A. E., Oldham, J. M., Hyler, S. E., Kellman, H. D., Doidge, N., & Davies, M. (1993). Comorbidity of DSM-III-R eating disorders and personality disorders. *International Journal of Eating Disorders, 14*(4) 403–416.

Skodol, A. E., Oldham, J. M., Hyler, S. E., Stein, D. J., Hollander, E., Gallaher, P. E., & Lopez, A. E. (1995). Patterns of anxiety and personality disorder comorbidity. *Journal of Psychiatric Research, 29*(5), 361–374.

Skodol, A. E., Stout, R. L., McGlashan, T. H., Grilo, C. M., Gunderson, J. G., Shea, M. T., Morey, L. C., Zanarini, M. C., Dyck, I. R., & Oldham, J. M. (1999). Co-occurrence of mood and personality disorders: A report from the Collaborative Longitudinal Personality Disorders Study (CLPS). *Depression and Anxiety, 10,* 175–182.

Southwick, S. M., Yehuda, R., & Giller, E. L. (1993). Personality disorders in treatment-seeking combat veterans with post traumatic stress disorder. *American Journal of Psychiatry, 150,* 1020–1023.

Starcevic, V. (1990). Relationship between hypochondriasis and obsessive–compulsive disorder: Close relatives separated by nosological schemes? *American Journal of Psychotherapy, 44,* 340–347.

Starkowski, S. M., Stroll, A. L., Tohen, M., Paedda, G.

L., & Goodwin, D. C. (1993). The trideminsional questionnaire: A predictor of six-month outcome in first episode mania. *Psychiatry Research, 48,* 1–8.

Stern, J., Murphy, M., & Bass, C. (1993). Personality disorders in patients with somatisation disorder: A controlled study. *British Journal of Psychiatry, 163,* 785–789.

Trull, T. J., & Sher, K. J. (1994). Relationship between the five-factor model of personality and axis I disorders in a nonclinical sample. *Journal of Abnormal Psychology, 103,* 350–360.

Turley, B., Bates, G. W., Edwards, J., & Jackson, H. J. (1992). MCMI-II personality disorders in recent-onset bipolar disorders. *Journal of Clinical Psychology, 48*(3), 320–329.

Turner, S. M., Beidel, D. C., Dancu, C. V., & Keys, D. J. (1986). Psychopathology of social phobia and comparison to avoidant personality disorder. *Journal of Abnormal Psychology, 95,* 389–394.

Tyrer, P., Gunderson, J., Lyons, M., & Tohen, M. (1997). Special feature: Extent of comorbidity between mental state and personality disorders. *Journal of Personality Disorders, 11,* 242–259.

Ucok, A., Karaveli, D, Kundakci, T., & Yazici, O. (1998). Comorbidity of personality with bipolar mood disorders. *Comprehensive Psychiatry, 39*(2), 72–74.

Weaver, T. L., & Clum, G. A. (1993). Early family environments and traumatic experiences associated with borderline personality disorder. *Journal of Consulting and Clinical Psychology, 61,* 1068–1075.

Widiger, T. A., & Corbitt, E. M. (1995). Antisocial personality disorder. In W. J. Livesley, (Ed.), *The DSM-IV personality disorders.* (pp. 103–126). New York: Guilford Press.

Widiger, T. A., & Costa, P. T., Jr. (1994). Personality and personality disorders. *Journal of Abnormal Psychology, 103,* 78–91.

Widiger, T. A., & Shea, T. (1991). Differentiation of axis I and axis II disorders. *Journal of Abnormal Psychology, 100,* 399–406.

Zanarini, M. C., Frankenburg, F. R., Dubo, E. D., Sickel, A. E., Trikha, A., Levin, A., & Reynolds, V. (1998). Axis I comorbidity of borderline personality disorder. *American Journal of Psychiatry, 155*(12), 1733–1739.

Zanarini, M. C., Gunderson, J. G., & Frankenburg, F. R. (1989). Axis I phenomenology of borderline personality disorder. *Comprehensive Psychiatry, 30*(2), 149–156.

Zanarini, M. C., Gunderson, J. G., Marino, M. F., Schwartz, E. O., & Frankenburg, F. R. (1989). Childhood experiences of borderline patients. *Comprehensive Psychiatry, 30,* 18–25.

Zimmerman, M., Coryell, W., Pfohl, B., Corenthal, C., & Stangl, D. (1986). ECT response in depressed patients with and without a DSM-III personality disorder. *American Journal of Psychiatry, 143,* 1030–1032.

PART II

ETIOLOGY AND DEVELOPMENT

CHAPTER 5

Epidemiology

JILL I. MATTIA
MARK ZIMMERMAN

Specific constellations of traits, behavior, and self-perception represented as disordered have been defined, modified, included, or excluded across successive generations of the diagnostic nomenclature, but the epidemiology of personality disorders still remains somewhat elusive. Lyons (1995) noted that with the possible exception of antisocial personality disorder, DSM-III (American Psychiatric Association, 1980) essentially marked the beginning of the systematic study of personality disorders. Prior efforts to study personality disorder epidemiology were substantially hampered by a lack of explicit criteria sets and consequently standardized assessment tools. Twenty years after DSM-III, researchers still struggle with both the methodology and the cost of conducting broadband personality disorder investigations.

Although the current version of the nosology, DSM-IV (American Psychiatric Association, 1994), has been available for 5 years, data have yet to be reported in the literature regarding the prevalence and clinical/demographic correlates of DSM-IV personality disorders. Thus, this chapter discusses the prevalence and clinical correlates of personality disorders as defined in DSM-III and DSM-III-R (American Psychiatric Association, 1980, 1987). Merikangas and Weissman (1986) and Weissman (1993) have published excellent reviews including information regarding the epidemiology of personality disorders prior to the advent of DSM-III.

OVERVIEW OF STUDIES INCLUDED IN THE REVIEW

This first section describes the studies included in the review (see Table 5.1 for a summary). These studies are then referenced in the second and third sections when reporting personality disorder prevalences and clinical/demographic correlates, respectively. Of course, diagnosis in mental health is inextricably nested within assessment methodology. The most common instruments used for epidemiological investigations are structured interviews. Similarly, experimental investigations assessing personality disorders also used some sort of structured or semistructured measure, although some have used self-report questionnaires instead. These measures are described elsewhere in this book and are only mentioned briefly here.

No epidemiological survey of the full range of personality disorders has been conducted in the post DSM-III era. As described later, several epidemiological studies of Axis I syndromes included DSM-III antisocial personality disorder in their assessment batteries. A reanalysis of this data or reexamination of participating subjects has provided some information regarding the prevalence of other personality disorders. Because of the paucity of formal epidemiological data, quasi-epidemiological data based on studies of nonpatient samples are included in this review. Some of these were studies of

TABLE 5.1. Overview of Studies Included in the Review

Study	N	Sample type	Criteria used	Axis II measure	Disorders assessed
Baron et al. (1985)	374	Control-Exp	DSM-III	SIB-SADS	Par, Szoid, Stypl, Bord, Anti, Avoid, Dep
Black et al. (1993)	127	Control-Fam	DSM-III	SIDP	All
Blanchard et al. (1995)	93	Control-Exp	DSM-III-R	SCID-II	Par, Anti, Bord, Avoid, Dep, OC
Bland et al. (1988)*	3,258	Epidemiology	DSM-III	DIS	Anti
Coryell & Zimmerman (1989)	185	Control-Fam	DSM-III	SIDP	All
Drake & Vaillant (1985)	369	Control-Exp	DSM-III	Unspecified	Cluster A, Cluster B, Avoid Dep
Erlenmeyer-Kimling et al. (1995)	93	Control-Fam	DSM-III-R	PDE	Cluster A
Kendler et al. (1993)*	580	Control-Fam	DSM-III-R	SIS	Par, Szoid,[a] Stypl, Bord,[a] Avoid[a]
Lenzenweger et al. (1997)	810	Undergrads	DSM-III-R	IPDE	Presence of at least one personality disorder
Kessler et al. (1994)	8,098	Epidemiology	DSM-III-R	CIDI	Anti
Maier et al. (1992, 1995)*	320	Control-Fam	DSM-III-R	SCID-II	All
Nestadt et al. (1990, 1991, 1992)	810	Epidemiology	DSM-III	SPE	Hist, OC
Regier et al. (1988)	18,571	Epidemiology	DSM-III	DIS	Anti
Reich et al. (1989)	235	Community	DSM-III	PDQ	All
Swartz et al. (1990)	1,541	Epidemiology	DSM-III	DIB-DIS	Bord
Wells et al. (1989)*	1,498	Epidemiology	DSM-III	DIS	Anti

Note. Exp, experimental study with a control group; Fam, family study of control probands; CIDI, Composite International Diagnostic Interview (World Health Organization, 1990); DIS, Diagnostic Interview Schedule (Robins, Helzer, Croughan, & Ratcliff, 1981); IPDE, International Personality Disorders Examination (Loranger et al., 1994; Loranger, Sartorious, & Janca, 1996); PDQ, Personality Diagnostic Questionnaire (Hyler, Lyons, et al., 1990; Hyler, Rieder, & Spitzer, 1983; Hyler, Skodol, Kellman, Oldham, & Rosnick, 1990); PDE, Personality Disorder Examination (Loranger, Susman, Oldham, & Russakoff, 1987); SADS-L, Schedule for Affective Disorders and Schizophrenia Lifetime Version (Endicott & Spitzer, 1978); SPE, Standardized Psychiatric Examination (Nestadt et al., 1992); SCID-II, Structured Clinical Interview for DSM-III-R Personality Disorders (Spitzer, Williams, Gibbon, & First, 1990b); SIDP, Structured Interview for DSM-III Personality (Pfohl, Stangl, & Zimmerman 1982); SIS, Structured Interview for Schizotypy (Kendler, Lieberman, & Walsh, 1989); Par, paranoid personality disorder; Szoid, schizoid personality disorder; Stypl, schizotypal personality disorder; Hist, histrionic personality disorder; Anti, antisocial personality disorder; Bord, borderline personality disorder; Avoid, avoidant personality disorder; Dep, dependent personality disorder; OC, obsessive–compulsive personality disorder; All, all DSM-III personality disorders.
*non-U.S. sample.
[a]All criteria not assessed.

first-degree family members of healthy control probands, and some were studies of control samples that were not selected based on the sophisticated sampling methods of epidemiological investigations.

Epidemiological Studies

The two largest epidemiological efforts in the United States using DSM-III or DSM-III-R criteria are the National Institute of Mental Health's Epidemiologic Catchment Area study (ECA; Regier et al., 1988) and the National Co-

morbidity Survey (NCS; Kessler et al., 1994). The ECA is the largest effort in the United States to derive population estimates of DSM-III psychiatric disorders. More than 18,000 subjects were interviewed across five sites (New Haven, Baltimore, St. Louis, North Carolina, Los Angeles) with the Diagnostic Interview Schedule (DIS; Robins, Helzer, Croughan, & Ratcliff, 1981), a fully structured interview designed to be administered by lay interviewers. Results were weighted to account for nonresponse as well as to approximate national population distributions of age, gender, and ethnicity. DSM-III antisocial personality disorder was the only personality disorder included in the ECA assessment battery.

Swartz, Blazer, George, and Winfield (1990) reanalyzed data for the 1,541 subjects from the ECA-North Carolina site to estimate the prevalence of DSM-III borderline personality disorder. Borderline personality disorder was not included in the DIS; however, an algorithm was constructed to use information from the DIS interview to approximate prevalence of borderline personality disorder. At the Baltimore site, Nestadt et al. (1990, 1991, 1992) reported the results of a second-stage clinical reappraisal of subjects who participated in the ECA. All subjects considered to have filtered positive for a DSM-III psychiatric disorder and a 17% random subsample of filtered-negative subjects were reassessed as part of the clinical reappraisal. In all, 1,086 subjects were selected for reappraisal, and 810 subjects (or 759 subjects; the reported final sample varies across publications) completed this assessment. The reappraisal was completed by psychiatrists administering the Standardized Psychiatric Examination (Romanoski et al., 1988), and interview results were used to estimate the prevalence of histrionic and obsessive–compulsive personality disorders.

The second national effort toward establishing the epidemiology of psychiatric disorders, the NCS, assessed 8,098 individuals ages 15–54 across the United States. In contrast to the ECA, which drew subjects from five discrete catchment areas, the NCS selected subjects from the 48 contiguous states. Thus, the NCS was designed to estimate the prevalence, comorbidity, and risk factors of DSM-III-R psychiatric disorders in a representative national sample in the United States. Participants were interviewed with the Composite International Diagnostic Interview (CIDI; World Health Organization, 1990), a structured interview based on the DIS and administered by trained nonclinician interviewers. Like the ECA study, antisocial personality disorder was the only personality disorder included in the NCS assessment battery, and results were weighted to account for nonresponse as well as to approximate national population characteristics of gender, ethnicity, marital status, education, living arrangements, region, and urbanicity.

Two epidemiological studies conducted outside the United States also confined assessment of personality disorders to antisocial personality disorder. Bland, Orn, and Newman (1988) reported the results of an epidemiological investigation in Edmonton, Canada. Over 3,000 randomly selected residents were interviewed with the DIS. Wells, Bushnell, Hornblow, Joyce, and Oakley-Browne (1989) reported the results of an epidemiological study in Christchurch, New Zealand. A sample of 1,498 residents were randomly selected and interviewed with the DIS. Both investigations used DSM-III criteria, and both investigations weighted their results according to age and sex distributions of their respective populations.

Controlled Studies

Because epidemiological investigations have been narrowly focused in terms of personality disorder assessment, the vast majority of information regarding the prevalence and clinical/demographic correlates of personality disorders is obtained from experimental normal control or family study normal control groups. Results derived from experimental control groups have been included here provided that potential control subjects were not screened and excluded for psychopathology. Family-study control groups were similarly included, regardless of whether their corresponding control probands were screened to exclude individuals with psychopathology. Although these controlled studies can provide valuable information, they fall short of the selection rigor and sampling representation found in epidemiological investigations and should be interpreted in that light.

Experimental Studies with Control Groups

Baron et al. (1985) interviewed 374 normal controls with the Schedule for Affective Disorders and Schizophrenia Lifetime Version (SADS-L; Endicott & Spitzer, 1978) and the Schedule for Interviewing Borderlines (SIB; Baron & Gruen, 1980). Additional questions were included as a supplement to assess DSM-III criteria for paranoid, schizoid, schizotypal, borderline, antisocial, avoidant, and dependent personality disorders. The normal control sample was obtained by randomly selecting acquaintances of the non-ill relatives (although not confirmed with a diagnostic interview) of patients with schizophrenia. This normal control sample was part of a larger study examining the risk of Axis I and Axis II disorders in the relatives of individuals with schizophrenia.

Blanchard, Hickling, Taylor, and Loos (1995) recruited a sample of normal controls for comparison to a group of individuals with posttraumatic stress disorder secondary to a motor vehicle accident (MVA). Normal controls were obtained through advertisements, from staff at referral sources, and some were friends of the MVA subjects. Controls were screened only to be MVA free within the prior 12 months and were matched on age and gender distribution with the MVA group. The 93 individuals in the control group were interviewed with the Structured Clinical Interview for DSM-III-R (SCID; Spitzer, Williams, Gibbon, & First, 1990a) and the Structured Clinical Interview for DSM-III-R Personality Disorders (SCID-II; Spitzer, Williams, Gibbon, & First, 1990b) by trained doctoral level psychologists. Although the SCID-II assesses all DSM-III-R Axis II diagnoses, only the prevalences of paranoid, antisocial, borderline, avoidant, dependent, and obsessive–compulsive personality disorders were reported.

Drake and Vaillant (1985) longitudinally followed 369 (80%) of 456 men who were originally recruited as normal control probands in a study of juvenile delinquency (Glueck & Glueck, 1950). Subjects were interviewed with an unspecified 2-hour interview by experienced clinicians and included ratings of health, social competence, alcoholism, and criteria for all the DSM-III personality disorders. Clinicians who did the ratings and the interviews were blind to information gathered on subjects when they were adolescents.

Family Studies of Normal Control Probands

Coryell and Zimmerman (1989) interviewed 185 first-degree relatives of normal control probands with the DIS and the Structured Interview for DSM-III Personality (SIDP; Pfohl, Stangl, & Zimmerman, 1982). Probands were recruited with advertisements targeting hospital personnel, and only individuals who were interviewed with the SADS-L and the SIDP and not diagnosed with either an Axis I or Axis II disorder were included. The normal control group of family members was part of a larger study examining the relative risk of DSM-III psychiatric disorders in the family members of depressed or schizophrenic probands. There are several reports published on this data set (e.g.,

Coryell & Zimmerman, 1989; Zimmerman & Coryell, 1989). Other reviews of personality disorder epidemiology (e.g., Lyons, 1995; Weissman, 1993) report prevalences based on all family members in the larger investigation (i.e., first-degree relatives of normal control probands and first-degree relatives of psychiatric probands). Because including relatives of psychiatric probands might inflate prevalence estimates, only results derived from the assessment of normal probands' family members ($n = 185$; Coryell & Zimmerman, 1989) are reported in the personality disorder prevalence section of this review. It is possible, however, that results based on these family members may underestimate true population prevalences given that probands were screened to exclude individuals with any psychiatric difficulties. Data regarding the demographic/clinical correlates of personality disorder diagnoses in normal control family members were not reported. For the purposes of this review, these correlates based on *all* family members in the study (i.e., 185 first-degree relatives of control probands *and* the 612 first-degree relatives of psychiatric probands; Zimmerman & Coryell, 1989) are discussed.

Black, Noyes, Pfohl, Goldstein, and Blum (1993) used a methodology comparable to Coryell and Zimmerman's (1989) to ascertain a second normal control group at the same site. These normal controls served as a comparison group in a family study of individuals with obsessive–compulsive disorder. The resulting 127 family members of similarly screened hypernormal probands were interviewed with the DIS and the SIDP. Again, it is possible that results based on these family members may underestimate true population prevalences given that probands were screened to exclude individuals with psychiatric difficulties.

Erlenmeyer-Kimling et al. (1995) gathered a control group as a part of a larger study comparing the offspring of probands with schizophrenia or a mood disorder. Normal probands were parents identified through two large school districts in the New York City metropolitan area. These parents were screened to have had no psychiatric treatment history and to have at least one child age 7 to 12 years without current symptoms or a treatment history of psychiatric disturbance. Normal probands were also matched on demographic characteristics to psychiatric probands, and the offspring of both groups were followed and compared. Ninety-three of the original 100 children in the normal control group were contacted approximately two decades later (mean age 30.84 ± 1.83). This normal control group was interviewed with the SADS-L and the Personality Disorder Examination (PDE; Loranger, Susman, Oldham, & Russakoff, 1987).

Kendler et al. (1993) assessed 580 relatives of 150 unscreened control subjects selected from an electoral registry in a rural county in the west of Ireland. As part of a larger family study of probands with schizophrenia or a mood disorder, the 150 control probands were matched for age and sex to two other study groups comprised of schizophrenic or mood disorder individuals. One first-degree relative, the informant, of control probands was questioned regarding other first-degree relatives' possible symptoms of paranoid and schizotypal personality disorder. The informant was also interviewed with the SCID for Axis I disorders and the Structured Interview for Schizotypy (SIS; Kendler, Lieberman, & Walsh, 1989) for some Axis II disorders. The SIS assesses the schizotypal signs and symptoms relevant to the identification of nonpsychotic but symptomatic relatives of individuals with schizophrenia. The interview process and the 25 SIS content items reflect all the DSM-III-R criteria for schizotypal and paranoid personality disorders, five of the seven criteria for schizoid personality disorder, five of the seven criteria for avoidant personality disorder, and five of the eight criteria for borderline personality disorder. Psychiatric hospital records, if available, were also used.

Maier, Minges, Lichtermann, and Heun (1995) randomly recruited 109 control subjects from the community as part of a larger family study of DSM-III-R schizophrenia and mood disorders. Control probands were recruited from the Rhein–Main area by a marketing company and were not screened for psychiatric status. All available first-degree relatives of the 109 control probands were interviewed with the SADS-L and the SCID-II, yielding a sample of 320 family control subjects. Interviews were conducted by 10 physicians and research assistants trained on the measures, and DSM-III-R criteria for all the personality disorders were assessed. For the purposes of this review, only results derived from the assessment of normal probands' family members are reported in the personality disorder prevalence section. Data regarding the demographic/clinical correlates of personality disorder diagnoses in normal control family members were not reported. However, information regarding correlates of personality disorders was reported based on a mixed group of normal control probands, their spouses, and their first-degree relatives (Maier, Lichtermann, Klinger, & Heun, 1992).

Survey Studies

Two large-scale surveys included assessment of personality traits. The first study examined a fairly specialized population—university undergraduates. Lenzenweger, Loranger, Korfine, and Neff (1997) used a two-stage method to estimate the prevalence of at least one DSM-III-R personality disorder in nonclinical undergraduates. Subjects were recruited from approximately 2,000 incoming freshmen at Cornell University. Fifteen research assistants used a door-to-door epidemiological style survey distribution and collection method and recruited 1,684 subjects into the first stage of the study. Subjects were paid $5 for participation with the possibility of being invited for later interviews for a $50 payment. All subjects initially completed the IPDE-S, a self-report version of the International Personality Disorder Examination (IPDE; Loranger et al., 1994; Loranger, Sartorius, & Janca, 1996) that screens for the presence of personality disorders. Results from the screening questionnaire indicated that 43% screened positive for a probable personality disorder. A subset ($ns = 134$ and 124, respectively) of the screen-probable and screen-negative groups was randomly selected to be interviewed with the IPDE and the SCID. These sampling procedures resulted in a slight overrepresentation of screen probables in the final study sample.

The second survey study reported prevalences of DSM-III personality disorders in a community sample confined to a specific geographical area. Reich, Yates, and Nduaguba (1989) recruited a community sample in a midwestern university town by random questionnaire mailings to 401 of approximately 36,697 adults whose names and addresses were listed in the Iowa City directory. Selected subjects were mailed the Personality Diagnostic Questionnaire (PDQ; Hyler, Rieder, & Spitzer, 1983; Hyler, Lyons, et al., 1990; Hyler, Skodol, Kellman, Oldham, & Rosnick, 1990), a self-report measure that assesses criteria related to the 11 DSM-III personality disorders. The PDQ arrived with instructions that recipients were to randomly choose one individual within the household to complete the survey. Surveys not returned within 6 weeks were followed with a second mailing, and both mailings included a stamped self-addressed envelope to increase compliance. Approximately 62% ($n = 235$) of those selected returned the mailing with a completed PDQ.

PREVALENCE OF PERSONALITY DISORDERS

Cluster A Personality Disorders: Odd/Eccentric

Paranoid

The median prevalence of paranoid personality disorder across all studies was 1.1% (see Table 5.2). The prevalence rates of DSM-III-defined paranoid personality disorder ranged from 0.5% (Coryell & Zimmerman, 1989) to 2.7% (Baron et al., 1985) with a median of 1.6%. The range according to DSM-III-R criteria was narrower, 0.4% (Kendler et al., 1993) to 1.8% (Maier et al., 1995), and the median was lower—1.0%. The studies reporting both the highest (2.7%; Baron et al., 1985) and lowest (0.4%; Kendler et al., 1993) prevalences in their control groups were investigations of schizophrenia and in the latter case also mood disorders. There appeared to be no pattern in prevalences related to methodology or assessment instrument, and the two studies (Black et al., 1993; Coryell & Zimmerman, 1989) with the closest methods showed a threefold differ-

ence in rates (0.5% and 1.6%, respectively). This is a consistent pattern that tends to repeat itself for these two investigations with every personality disorder except narcissistic personality disorder.

Schizoid

The median prevalence of schizoid personality disorder was 0.6% (see Table 5.2). Methodology appeared to have no relationship with prevalence. The range of schizoid personality disorder according to DSM-III criteria was 0% (Baron et al., 1985; Black et al., 1993) to 5.7% (Drake & Vaillant, 1985) with a median of 0.9%. A narrower range appeared to be associated with DSM-III-R criteria—0.2% (Kendler et al., 1993) to 1.1% (Erlenmeyer-Kimling et al., 1995) and with a lower median of 0.3%. The Kendler et al. (1993) data might be a slight underestimate of schizoid personality disorder in their sample given that all criteria were not assessed.

Schizotypal

The median prevalence of schizotypal personality disorder was 1.8% (see Table 5.2). The rates of DSM-III-defined schizotypal personality disorder ranged from 0.3% (Drake & Vaillant, 1985) to 5.1% (Reich et al., 1989) with a median of 2.2%. DSM-III-R criteria schizotypal personality disorder ranged more narrowly— 0% (Erlenmeyer-Kimling et al., 1995) to 1.4% (Kendler et al., 1993) with a lower median of 0.3%.

TABLE 5.2. Prevalence (%) of Cluster A Personality Disorders

Study	Paranoid	Schizoid	Schizotypal	Any Cluster A
Baron et al. (1985)[3]	2.7	0	2.1	—
Black et al. (1993)[3]	1.6	0	3.9	5.5
Blanchard et al. (1995)[3-R]	1.1	—	—	—
Coryell & Zimmerman (1989)[3]	0.5	1.6	2.2	3.8
Drake & Vaillant (1985)[3]	1.6	5.7	0.3	—
Erlenmeyer-Kimling et al. (1995)[3-R]	1.1	1.1	0	2.2
Kendler et al. (1993)*[3-R]	0.4	0.2	1.4	—
Maier et al. (1995)*[3-R]	0.9	0.3	0.3	—
Reich et al. (1989)[3]	0.9	0.9	5.1	—
Median prevalence	1.1	0.6	1.8	—
Median prevalence DSM-III	1.6	0.9	2.2	—
Median prevalence DSM-III-R	1.0	0.3	0.3	—

Note. [3]DSM-III; [3-R]DSM-III-R; *non-U.S. sample.

Comment

Most Cluster A studies included in this review are part of larger family studies of psychotic probands. However, there was no evidence that the rates of these schizophrenic spectrum personality disorders were higher in the family studies than in the other studies. The most common Cluster A personality disorder was schizotypal personality disorder, although this was true only for the studies using DSM-III criteria. Across studies it seems that rates of personality disorders tended to be higher according to DSM-III versus DSM-III-R criteria, although no study directly compared prevalence rates derived from both sets. This would not have been predicted from changes in criteria from DSM-III to DSM-III-R. DSM-III schizoid personality disorder required the presence of three out of three criteria whereas DSM-III-R employed an easier subset strategy of four out of seven criteria. Likewise, criteria for paranoid personality disorder seems easier to meet in DSM-III-R than in DSM-III. The schizotypal criteria are essentially the same in both DSM-III and DSM-III-R. Consequently, it is more likely that the difference in median prevalence rates between DSM-III and DSM-III-R is due to methodological differences between studies than differences in the broadness of criteria sets.

Cluster B Personality Disorders: Dramatic

Histrionic

The median prevalence of histrionic personality disorder across all studies was 2.0% (see Table 5.3). The range of DSM-III histrionic personality disorder was 1.6% (Coryell & Zimmerman, 1989) to 3.9% (Black et al., 1993), with a median of 2.1%. The piece of data associated with an epidemiological investigation (Nestadt et al., 1990) reported a rate right at the median of 2.1%. Only Maier et al. (1995) reported a prevalence of DSM-III-R-defined histrionic personality disorder—1.3%.

Antisocial

Far and away antisocial personality disorder has been the most frequently studied personality disorder with 12 reports of its prevalence rate. The median prevalence of antisocial personality disorder was 1.2% (see Table 5.3). The range of antisocial personality disorder according to DSM-III criteria was 0% (Baron et al., 1985) to 3.7% (Bland et al., 1988) with a median of 1.9%. Unlike most other personality disorders, a similar range appeared to be associated with DSM-III-R criteria—0% (Blanchard et al., 1995) to 3.5% (Kessler et al., 1994) but with a lower median of 0.3%.

TABLE 5.3. Prevalence (%) of Cluster B Personality Disorders

Study	Histrionic	Antisocial	Borderline	Narcissistic	Any Cluster B
Baron et al. (1985)[3]	—	0	1.6	—	—
Black et al. (1993)[3]	3.9	0.8	5.5	0	7.9
Blanchard et al. (1995)[3-R]	—	0	1.1	—	—
Bland et al. (1988)*[3]	—	3.7	—	—	—
Coryell & Zimmerman (1989)[3]	1.6	1.6	1.1	0	4.3
Drake & Vaillant (1985)[3]	1.9	2.2	0.8	5.7	—
Kendler et al. (1993)*[3-R]	—	0.2	0	—	—
Kessler et al. (1994)[3-R]	—	3.5	—	—	—
Maier et al. (1995)*[3-R]	1.3	0.3	1.3	0	—
Nestadt et al. (1990)[3]	2.1	—	—	—	—
Reich et al. (1989)[3]	2.1	0.4	0.4	0.4	—
Regier et al. (1988)[3]	—	2.5	—	—	—
Swartz et al. (1990)[3]	—	—	1.8	—	—
Wells et al. (1989)*[3]	—	3.1	—	—	—
Median prevalence	2.0	1.2	1.1	0	—
Median prevalence DSM-III	2.1	1.9	1.4	0.2	—
Median prevalence DSM-III-R	1.3[a]	0.3	1.1	0[a]	—

Note. [3]DSM-III; [3-R]DSM-III-R; *non-U.S. sample.
[a] Only prevalence in category.

Regier et al. (1988) reported the lifetime prevalence of DSM-III antisocial personality disorder in the ECA study to be 2.5%; 1-month and 6-month prevalences of this disorder were 0.5% and 0.8%, respectively. The NCS reported a somewhat higher prevalence of 3.5% based on DSM-III-R criteria. The two epidemiological studies conducted outside the United States and using DSM-III criteria reported rates of antisocial personality disorder similar to that found in the NCS. Bland et al. (1988) found a rate of 3.7% in Edmonton, Canada. Wells et al. (1989) reported 3.1% of their New Zealand sample merited the diagnosis of antisocial personality disorder. The median epidemiological prevalence of antisocial personality disorder was 3.3%

Borderline

The median prevalence of borderline personality disorder across all studies was 1.1% (see Table 5.3). The range of DSM-III borderline personality disorder was 0.4% (Reich et al., 1989) to 5.5% (Black et al., 1993) with a median of 1.4%. DSM-III-R criteria was associated with a narrower range—0% (Kendler et al., 1993) to 1.3% (Maier et al., 1995) with a median of 1.1%. The rate of borderline personality disorder from the Kendler et al. (1993) study might be an underestimate of the disorder in their sample given that all criteria were not assessed.

Narcissistic

The median prevalence of narcissistic personality disorder is 0% (see Table 5.3). Black et al. (1993) and Coryell and Zimmerman (1989) reported that none of their subjects met criteria for narcissistic personality disorder. This is the only time these two investigations agree. The other two studies to use DSM-III criteria, Drake and Vaillant (1985) and Reich et al. (1989), were quite disparate, the former reporting a rate of 5.7% while the latter reported a rate of 0.4%. Only Maier et al. (1995) used DSM-III-R criteria, and they found that none of their subjects merited the diagnosis. Thus, narcissistic personality disorder seems to be the least prevalent personality disorder according to both criteria sets.

Comment

The most common Cluster B personality disorder was histrionic personality disorder, al-

though its prevalence declined like all Cluster B personality disorders when comparing studies using DSM-III-R to DSM-III criteria. Because antisocial personality disorder has been examined in the four formal epidemiological investigations included in this review, it is instructive to compare results from these studies with results obtained from experimental control groups to determine if methodology systematically biased prevalence estimates. Relative to experimental control research, epidemiological investigations as a group reported the highest prevalence of antisocial personality disorder. The median epidemiological prevalence of antisocial personality disorder was 3.3% compared to the median experimental control group prevalence of 0.4%. Looking at this another way, the prevalence of antisocial personality disorder was less than 1.0% in six of the eight non-epidemiological studies, and it was 2.5% or higher in all four of the epidemiological studies. Perhaps the difference between studies is due to the period of assessment. When confined to 1-month and 6-month time periods, prevalence of antisocial personality disorder based on epidemiological data begins to resemble rates from normal control research. However, when Zimmerman and Coryell (1989) suspended the 5-year rule of the SIDP and included any lifetime evidence of the disorder, the prevalence of antisocial personality disorder in their family study sample increased by a modest 15% (from 26 subjects to 30). Thus, although the period of assessment may be related to the differences between epidemiological and normal control research, there is sufficient variance for additional methodological factors.

Cluster C Personality Disorders: Anxious/Fearful

Avoidant

The median prevalence of avoidant personality disorder across all studies was 1.2% (see Table 5.4). The range of DSM-III avoidant personality disorder was 0% (Baron et al., 1985; Reich et al., 1989) to 4.6% (Drake & Vaillant, 1985) with a median of 1.6%. Using DSM-III-R criteria, Blanchard et al. (1995) and Maier et al. (1995) reported that 1.1% and 1.3% of their samples, respectively, met criteria for avoidant personality disorder. The third study to use DSM-III-R criteria, Kendler et al. (1993), found none of their subjects with the diagnosis, although not all criteria were assessed.

Dependent

The median prevalence of dependent personality disorder was 2.2% (see Table 5.4). Using DSM-III criteria, rates of dependent personality disorder vary widely. Baron et al. (1985) reported that no subjects in their sample received a diagnosis of dependent personality disorder. Drake and Vaillant (1985) found that 7.9% of their sample merited the diagnosis. The median prevalence of DSM-III dependent personality disorder was 2.4%. Only Blanchard et al. (1995) and Maier et al. (1995) reported prevalences of dependent personality disorder using DSM-III-R criteria—2.2% and 1.6%, respectively.

Passive–Aggressive

The median prevalence of passive–aggressive personality disorder was 2.1% (see Table 5.4). Black et al. (1993) reported that a high 12.6% of their sample met criteria for passive–aggressive personality disorder while the median prevalence was 2.2%. Maier et al. (1995), the only study using DSM-III-R criteria to report a rate of passive–aggressive personality disorder, found that 1.9% of their sample merited the diagnosis.

Obsessive Compulsive

The median prevalence of this personality disorder was 4.3% (see Table 5.4). Rates of obsessive–compulsive personality disorder varied almost as much as dependent personality disorder. Using DSM-III criteria, prevalences of obsessive–compulsive personality disorder ranged from 1.5% (Nestadt et al., 1991) to 7.9% (Black et al., 1993) with a median of 4.8%. The two studies to use DSM-III-R criteria found prevalence rates of 2.2% (Maier et al., 1995) and 5.4% (Blanchard et al., 1995) of obsessive–compulsive personality disorder.

Comment

The Cluster C personality disorders were the most common of the three clusters. The two studies estimating the presence of any Cluster C personality disorder found that these rates were higher than the rates of any Cluster A or B personality disorder. All four studies that examine the full range of personality disorders found that obsessive–compulsive personality disorder was the most common. Obsessive–compulsive personality disorder may differ from the other personality disorders in that some of the traits of this disorder (e.g., perfectionism and excessive responsibility) are associated with achievement. There is some evidence that prevalence rates are lower when based on DSM-III-R criteria. Again, this would not be predicted from the change in diagnostic algorithms from DSM-III to DSM-III-R. Because no study has directly compared prevalence rates based on the two nosological sets, it is not possible to determine the reason for this discrepancy.

TABLE 5.4. Prevalence (%) of Cluster C Personality Disorders

Study	Avoidant	Dependent	Passive–aggressive	Obsessive–compulsive	Any Cluster C
Baron et al. (1985)[3]	0	0	—	—	—
Black et al. (1993)[3]	3.2	2.4	12.6	7.9	18.1
Blanchard et al. (1995)[3-R]	1.1	2.2	—	5.4	—
Coryell & Zimmerman (1989)[3]	1.6	0.5	2.2	3.2	7.0
Drake & Vaillant (1985)[3]	4.6	7.9	—	—	—
Kendler et al. (1993)*[3-R]	0	—	—	—	—
Maier et al. (1995)*[3-R]	1.3	1.6	1.9	2.2	—
Nestadt et al. (1991)[3]	—	—	—	1.5	—
Reich et al. (1989)[3]	0	5.1	0	6.4	—
Median prevalence	1.2	2.2	2.1	4.3	—
Median prevalence DSM-III	1.6	2.4	2.2	4.8	—
Median prevalence DSM-III-R	1.1	1.9	1.9[a]	3.8	—

Note. [3]DSM-III; [3-R]DSM-III-R; *non-U.S. sample.
[a] Only prevalence in category.

Prevalence of Any One Personality Disorder

Six studies reported the prevalence of any personality disorder, and the rates varied nearly fivefold from a low of 6.7% to a high of 33.1% (see Table 5.5). Drake and Vaillant (1985), using an unstructured clinical interview, found the rate of at least one DSM-III personality disorder in their sample to be 23%. Two of the family studies, Coryell and Zimmerman (1989) and Maier et al. (1995), reported that 14.6% and 9.4%, respectively, of their samples met criteria for at least one personality disorder. The lower rate found in the Maier et al. (1995) study is consistent with the trend for prevalences based on DSM-III-R personality disorder criteria to be lower than prevalences found with DSM-III criteria. In another family study of health probands, Black et al. (1993) reported a 33.1% prevalence rate of at least one personality disorder in their sample, approximately two and a half times higher than the Coryell and Zimmerman (1989) study. This broad discrepancy is consistent with the pattern of disagreement between the two research groups out of the same site regarding prevalences of each specific personality disorder. Reich et al. (1989), also studying a sample obtained in Iowa, found a prevalence of 11.1% for at least one DSM-III personality disorder. In spite of slightly oversampling the screen-positive personality disorder group, only 6.7% of the college students in the Lenzenweger et al. (1997) study came up positive for any definite personality disorder (and 11.0% for any definite/probable personality disorder). Selection for high academic achievement (hence university admission) may have biased the sample toward less pathology. Also, as university freshmen,

the sample had not yet completed the risk age cohort for developing or manifesting a personality disorder.

DEMOGRAPHIC AND CLINICAL CORRELATES OF PERSONALITY DISORDERS

Clinical Correlates

Axis I Comorbidity

Personality disorders appear to be associated with substantial Axis I comorbidity. Maier et al. (1995) reported that of those individuals who merited a personality disorder diagnosis, 63.3% were also diagnosed with an Axis I disorder. Half or more of those subjects with paranoid, histrionic, borderline, avoidant, dependent, or obsessive–compulsive personality disorders also met criteria for an Axis I disorder. No subjects with schizoid or schizotypal personality disorder were diagnosed with an Axis I disorder.

Prevalence ratios from the Canadian epidemiological data (Swanson, Bland, & Newman, 1994) indicate that subjects with antisocial personality disorder were three times more likely to merit an Axis I diagnosis compared to subjects who did not receive a diagnosis of antisocial personality disorder. Overall, 90.4% of antisocial personality disorder subjects also were diagnosed with an Axis I disorder— 85.6% were diagnosed with alcohol abuse/dependence, 34.6% were diagnosed with drug abuse/dependence, and 25.0% were diagnosed with depression.

The most detailed examination of the comorbidity between Axis I and Axis II was reported by Zimmerman and Coryell (1989). They examined the demographic and clinical correlates of personality disorders in their cohort of first-degree relatives of control and psychiatric probands. All 12 Axis I disorders assessed (mania, major depression, dysthymia, alcohol abuse/dependence, drug abuse/dependence, schizophrenia, obsessive–compulsive disorder, phobic disorders, panic disorder, bulimia, tobacco use disorder, and psychosexual dysfunction) were significantly more common in subjects with versus without a personality disorder. Individuals with a personality disorder were also seven times more likely to have made a suicide attempt (14.0% vs. 2.0%).

When examining the individual personality

TABLE 5.5. Prevalence (%) of Any Personality Disorder

Study	Prevalence (%)
Black et al. (1993)[3]	33.1
Coryell & Zimmerman (1989)[3]	14.6
Drake & Vaillant (1985)[3]	23.0
Lenzenweger et al. (1997)[3-R]	6.7
Maier et al. (1995)*[3-R]	9.4
Reich et al. (1989)[3]	11.1
Median prevalence	12.9

Note. [3]DSM-III; [3-R]DSM-III-R; *non-U.S. sample.

disorders, Zimmerman and Coryell (1989) used two comparison strategies. First, subjects with each specific personality disorder were compared to the group of subjects who received no personality disorder diagnosis. Second, subjects with each specific personality disorder were compared to subjects who were diagnosed with at least one of the other 9 personality disorders (only 10 personality disorders were examined with this strategy because narcissistic personality disorder was not diagnosed in any subject). Thus, the comparison group using the first strategy was always the 654 subjects who received no personality disorder diagnosis of any kind whereas the comparison group in the latter strategy changed with each analysis (e.g., 7 subjects with paranoid personality disorder vs. 136 subjects with a nonparanoid personality disorder, 14 subjects with dependent personality disorder vs. 129 subjects with a nondependent personality disorder, etc.). Each set of analyses consisted of 120 comparisons (10 personality disorders x 12 Axis I disorders).

In all, 68 (56.7%) of the 120 comparisons between subjects with a specific personality disorder and subjects with no personality disorder were significant, and 16 (13.3%) of the comparisons between subjects with a specific personality disorder and subjects with any other personality disorder were significant. Individuals with paranoid personality disorder had increased rates of all 12 Axis I disorders compared to individuals without a personality disorder, although only six differences were significant (alcohol abuse/dependence, drug abuse/dependence, schizophrenia, obsessive–compulsive disorder, phobic disorder, and bulimia). There was only one significant difference between individuals with paranoid and nonparanoid personality disorders (higher rate of bulimia in the paranoid subjects), and this was thought to be due to the high comorbidity between paranoid personality disorder and the other personality disorders (six of the seven subjects with paranoid personality disorder had another Axis II disorder). Individuals with schizoid and dependent personality disorder had the lowest rates of Axis I diagnoses. Individuals with schizoid personality disorder had a significantly lower rate of major depressive disorder, and dependent subjects a significantly lower rate of alcohol abuse/dependence, compared to subjects with other personality disorders. Axis I disorder rates were most often elevated in subjects with schizotypal and bor-

derline personality disorder. Compared to subjects without a personality disorder, individuals with schizotypal personality disorder had significantly higher rates of all disorders except bulimia, and individuals with borderline personality disorder significantly higher rates of all Axis I disorders except psychosexual dysfunction. In addition, the schizotypal subjects had significantly higher rates of major depressive disorder and obsessive–compulsive disorder compared to subjects with other personality disorders, and borderline subjects had higher rates of alcohol abuse/dependence, schizophrenia, phobic disorder, and tobacco use disorder. The Axis I correlates of histrionic and passive–aggressive personality disorder were similar. Individuals with each of these personality disorders had significantly higher rates of eight Axis I disorders (mania, major depressive disorder, alcohol abuse/dependence, drug abuse/dependence, schizophrenia, obsessive–compulsive disorder, phobic disorder, and psychosexual dysfunction), and there were no significant differences between subjects with each of these personality disorders and subjects with other personality disorders. The only difference in the pattern of Axis I correlates between histrionic and passive–aggressive personality disorder was that only the former was associated with a significantly higher rate of tobacco use disorder. Obsessive–compulsive personality disorder had a similar pattern of Axis I correlates to histrionic and passive–aggressive personality disorder except that it was not associated with an increased rate of drug abuse/dependence or schizophrenia. Subjects with antisocial personality disorder had the highest rates of drug and alcohol abuse/dependence and tobacco use disorder, whereas subjects with avoidant personality disorder had the highest rate of major depressive disorder and dysthymia.

Axis II Comorbidity

Personality disorders tend to covary with each other. Whether that is an artifact of symptom overlap or the true co-occurrence of distinct underlying clinical syndromes is beyond the scope of this review. Drake and Vaillant (1985) reported that half of those subjects who received a personality disorder diagnosis in their sample met criteria for more than one personality disorder diagnosis. Maier et al. (1992) found that approximately one-quarter of subjects with at least one personality disorder met criteria for more than one personality disorder, similar to results of Zimmerman and Coryell (1989). Zimmerman and Coryell (1989) found that paranoid, avoidant, and borderline personality disorders were most commonly diagnosed with at least one other personality disorder. In contrast, schizoid and dependent personality disorders were most frequently diagnosed as the sole personality disorder. The greatest percentage overlap was between avoidant and schizotypal personality disorders—half of the individuals with avoidant personality disorder also met criteria for schizotypal personality disorder. Also, more than 40% of individuals with paranoid personality disorder received a diagnosis of histrionic personality disorder or borderline personality disorder.

Demographic Correlates

Gender

Receiving a diagnosis of at least one personality disorder does not appear to favor gender. Maier et al. (1992) found that approximately 9.6% of males and 10.3% of females were diagnosed with at least one personality disorder. Of those who met for criteria a personality disorder in the Reich et al. (1989) study, approximately half (46%) were male. Zimmerman and Coryell (1989) also reported that approximately half (52.4%) of their personality disorder subjects were male.

There is some evidence that specific personality disorders tend to occur differentially between the genders. Maier et al. (1992) reported that dependent, passive–aggressive, and histrionic personality disorders tended to be more frequently diagnosed in females, and obsessive–compulsive, schizotypal, and antisocial personality disorders tended to be more frequently diagnosed in male subjects. No statistical tests of these trends were reported. Swartz et al.'s (1990) reexamination of the ECA data from the North Carolina site indicated that approximately 73% of those categorized as borderline personality disorder were female. Zimmerman and Coryell (1989) statistically compared subjects with and without personality disorders. Compared to subjects without a personality disorder, subjects with antisocial and obsessive–compulsive personality disorders were significantly more likely to be male, and subjects with dependent personality disor-

der were significantly more likely to be female. There was a nonsignificant tendency for individuals diagnosed with schizoid personality disorder to be male and individuals diagnosed with avoidant personality disorder to be female. Of note, there was no association between gender and the diagnosis of histrionic and borderline personality disorders. All four epidemiological studies that included assessment of antisocial personality disorder found a male predominance among antisocial subjects.

Age

It appears that personality disorders tend to favor youth and rates of personality disorders may decline with age. Although neither means nor statistical tests were reported, subjects diagnosed with a personality disorder in the Maier et al. (1992) study tended to be younger than those without. Zimmerman and Coryell (1989) found that individuals in all but one personality disorder category (schizoid) tended to be younger than individuals without a personality disorder diagnosis. These differences were statistically significant for borderline, antisocial, passive–aggressive, and schizotypal personality disorders. Subjects with borderline personality disorder were the youngest ($M = 30.3$) of all subjects with a personality disorder followed closely by individuals with antisocial personality disorder ($M = 32.5$). Individuals with schizoid personality disorder were the oldest ($M = 43.3$). Reich, Nduaguba, and Yates (1988) found that personality disorder traits and age were significantly and negatively correlated with age across all three personality disorder clusters. In addition, the relationship between age and Cluster B and C traits in this sample appeared to follow a J distribution wherein the mean number of traits declined with advancing age followed by a slight upturn in number of traits for the oldest age group. Data from three of the epidemiological studies (Bland et al., 1988; Regier et al., 1988; Wells et al., 1989) indicated that the majority of subjects diagnosed with antisocial personality disorder were below the age of 45, and rates of antisocial personality disorder appeared to decline with increasing age.

Marital Status

Presence of a personality disorder may be associated with lower rates of marriage and higher marital discord. In the Zimmerman and Coryell (1989) study, of those who merited a personality disorder diagnosis, 55.9% were married, 3.5% were separated, 13.3% were divorced, 3.5% were widowed, and 23.8% were single. Compared to subjects without a personality disorder diagnosis, individuals with a personality disorder diagnosis were significantly more likely to be single or divorced. Among those who ever married, subjects who merited a personality disorder diagnosis were twice as likely (54.1%) as subjects without a personality disorder diagnosis (25.6%) to have had a lifetime history of separation or divorce. All married subjects with borderline personality disorder had a lifetime history of being separated or divorced, as did a substantial majority of subjects with dependent personality disorder (78.6%) or antisocial personality disorder (70.0%). In contrast, no married subject with schizoid personality disorder had a history of being separated or divorced.

Education

No study has compared subjects with and without a personality disorder on educational attainment. The mean number of years of education for individuals who met for a personality disorder in the Reich et al. (1989) study was 14.9 (*SD* = 3.0). Swartz et al. (1990) found that 75% of those categorized as borderline personality disorder had graduated from high school.

Occupation

There are some data suggesting that occupational difficulties may be associated with personality disorders, although there is no study comparing individuals with and without a personality disorder on occupational functioning. Twenty-three percent of subjects diagnosed with a personality disorder in the Reich et al. (1989) study were unemployed for longer than 6 months in the preceding 5 years. Drake and Vaillant (1985) reported more substantial impairment. Forty-two percent of those with an Axis II personality disorder were unemployed for more than 4 years.

ASSESSMENT

Who should be questioned when assessing personality disorders in epidemiological investiga-

tions: the target individual or someone who knows the target individual well? The evaluation of personality disorders presents special problems that may require the use of informants. In contrast to the symptoms of major Axis I disorders, the defining features of personality disorders are based on an extended longitudinal perspective of how individuals act in different situations, how they perceive and interact with a constantly changing environment, and the perceived reasonableness of their behaviors and cognitions. Only a minority of the personality disorder criteria are discrete, easily enumerated behaviors. For any individuals to describe their normal personality they must be somewhat introspective and aware of the effect that their attitudes and behaviors have on others. But insight is the very thing usually lacking in individuals with a personality disorder. DSM-IV notes that the characteristics defining a personality disorder may not be considered problematic by the affected individual (i.e., ego-syntonic) and suggests that supplemental assessment information be obtained from informants. Research comparing patient and informant report of personality pathology has found rather marked disagreement between the two sources of information (Dowson, 1992a, 1992b; Tyrer, Alexander, Cicchettic, Cohen, & Remington, 1979; Zimmerman, Pfohl, Coryell, Stangl, & Corenthal, 1988). It is probable that a similar discrepancy would be found between the individuals participating in an epidemiological investigation (i.e., a nonpatient sample) and the people who know them well.

So should informants be included in epidemiological assessment for personality disorders? Although it certainly makes empirical sense to obtain as much information as possible, an algorithm regarding how to use that information is needed first. Psychiatric assessment of patients with informants relies on "best clinical judgment" to combine discrepant information, a vague and unsatisfying procedure for an epidemiological approach which tends to use nonclinician interviewers. Even if clinicians were used, the increased personnel cost on top of the added costs of recruiting and interviewing informants makes the value of the extra information somewhat uncertain.

Personality disorder assessment in epidemiological investigations also cannot be as flexible as clinical evaluations. Clinicians not only assess for criteria per se but also generally judge the reliability of patients as historians. Depending on a patient's mental status and apparent forthrightness, a clinician can extend his or her assessment over subsequent appointments and continue to identify or accumulate evidence of personality disorder characteristics and criteria. Assessment for epidemiological investigations, indeed for most research efforts, usually is confined to one opportunity. Clear algorithms deciding "caseness" must be defined *and* implemented uniformly—similarity of methodology and instrument are not enough. For example, in spite of nearly identical methodologies, Black et al. (1993) found the prevalence of specific personality disorders to be two to five times higher than that found in the Coryell and Zimmerman (1989) study.

There are two possible explanations of the interstudy differences in prevalence rates—true sample differences or systematic diagnostic bias. Reich et al.'s (1989) community survey using the PDQ found that 11.1% of respondents had a personality disorder. Zimmerman and Coryell (1990) compared 697 subjects of their original sample who completed both the PDQ and SIDP. The rate of any personality disorder was 10.3% according to the PDQ, similar to the rate found by Reich and colleagues using the same measure. Black and colleagues also used the PDQ in their study. In an unpublished comparison of the two Iowa family study samples Zimmerman, Coryell, and Black found that there were no demographic differences between samples. PDQ scores in the Black et al. (1993) sample also were not different from those in the Coryell and Zimmerman (1989) sample. These data suggest that the discrepancy in prevalence rates between the Zimmerman–Coryell and Black studies was probably due to a systematic diagnostic bias. Diagnostic raters in the two research groups probably held different evidence thresholds to count a symptom as "present" and contributing to a personality disorder diagnosis.

If investigators from the same institution using similar methodologies can produce such disparate results, epidemiological investigations are at a rather substantial risk of producing inconsistent results across sites. The incurred risk for bias to operate, although not unique to Axis II disorders, is perhaps greater than that for Axis I disorders as personality disorder criteria rely more heavily on latent constructs rather than overt symptomatology. As such, fully structured interviews like the DIS may not completely address the problem.

CONCLUSION

Due to the relative paucity of national efforts, the epidemiology of personality disorders in the general population is a difficult issue about which to draw firm conclusions. The National Institute of Mental Health's ECA study, the largest program estimating the lifetime prevalences of mental disorders in the general population, excluded assessment of all personality disorders with the exception of antisocial personality disorder. This was no doubt due in part to a lack of structured instruments for the full range of Axis II personality disorders. The NCS, another large effort to derive prevalence estimates of psychiatric disorders in the community, followed a similar strategy. Thus, with the exception of antisocial personality disorder, the two largest epidemiological efforts in the United States can yield only a small amount of information about the prevalence of these disorders. Inquiry into the epidemiology of personality disorders must rely on evidence derived from an admixture of quasi-epidemiological investigations based on experimental, family, and survey designs.

Based on the accumulated data, the prevalence of at least one personality disorder appears to be approximately 10–15%, a significant number when taken in the context that personality disorders are a source of long-term impairment in both treated and untreated populations (Merikangas & Weissman, 1986). The prevalence of each specific personality disorder tends to vary between 1% and 3%. These rates may represent the lower prevalence boundary of personality disorders; a comparison of experimental and epidemiological research in antisocial personality disorder suggests that experimental research tended to be lower than rates found in epidemiological research. There appears to be significant comorbidity among the personality disorders themselves, and a substantial number of individuals with a personality disorder diagnosis also seem to have a comorbid Axis I disorder. Overall, males and females may be similar in terms of receiving a diagnosis of at least one personality disorder, although diagnosis of specific personality disorders may be more common in one gender versus the other. Personality disorders seem to favor youth and may be associated with disturbances in marital and occupational functioning.

Unfortunately, Axis II disorders are not nearly as well researched as Axis I disorders. While epidemiological data for this disorder class are scarce, demographic characteristics and clinical correlates, important descriptive information of individuals with personality disorders, are even rarer. Few controlled studies report such information on their personality disorder subjects as they are usually only a subgroup of a larger, well-described sample. Clearly more research is needed. Of course, the largest stumbling block for such a large-scale study has been cost. Because of the low base rates of personality disorders, it is extremely expensive to recruit and cull the massive sample sizes needed to examine the nature of personality disorders. Hand in glove with the fiscal difficulties of such research are nosological considerations; theoretical conceptualizations have changed, diagnostic specificity has increased in service to assessment reliability, and criteria sets for personality disorders have evolved. A continuing source of variability among prevalence estimates and the relationships among clinical correlates may come from different criteria sets. Another source of variability comes from differing assessment methodologies among studies, and it may be the latter that are the biggest stumbling blocks to further research in the area. Although the SIDP (Pfohl et al., 1982) is a comprehensive instrument, it was perhaps its semistructured nature (vs. a fully structured instrument) that allowed the widely discrepant findings from the two studies conducted at the same site and using similar recruitment strategies. If lay interviewers are to be used in a large-scale epidemiological study of Axis II (as they were in the ECA and NCS), then it is unlikely that semistructured interviews could be used because of potential for systematic diagnostic biases. The four investigations based on fully structured instruments like the DIS yielded somewhat similar rates of antisocial personality disorder. Perhaps these instruments can be expanded to include all personality disorders. Whether or not fully structured personality disorder interviews would be valid is an empirical question.

REFERENCES

American Psychiatric Association. (1980). *Diagnostic and statistical manual of mental disorders* (3rd ed.). Washington, DC: Author.

American Psychiatric Association. (1987). *Diagnostic and statistical manual of mental disorders* (3rd ed., rev.). Washington, DC: Author.

American Psychiatric Association. (1994). *Diagnostic and statistical manual of mental disorders* (4th ed.). Washington, DC: Author.

Baron, M., & Gruen, R. (1980). *The schedule for interviewing borderlines (SIB)*. New York: New York State Psychiatric Institute.

Baron, M., Gruen, R., Rainer, J. D., Kane, J., Asnis, L., & Lord, S. (1985). A family study of schizophrenic and normal control probands: Implications for the spectrum concept of schizophrenia. *American Journal of Psychiatry, 142,* 447–455.

Black, D. W., Noyes, R., Pfohl, B., Goldstein, R. B., & Blum, N. (1993). Personality disorder in obsessive–compulsive volunteers, well comparison subjects, and their first degree relatives. *American Journal of Psychiatry, 150,* 1226–1232.

Blanchard, E. B., Hickling, E. J., Taylor, A. E., & Loos, W. (1995). Psychiatric morbidity associated with motor vehicle accidents. *Journal of Nervous and Mental Disease, 183,* 495–504.

Bland, R. C., Orn, H., & Newman, S. C. (1988). Lifetime prevalence of psychiatric disorders in Edmonton. *Acta Psychiatrica Scandinavica, 77*(Suppl. 338), 24–32.

Coryell, W. H., & Zimmerman, M. (1989). Personality disorder in the families of depressed, schizophrenic, and never-ill probands. *American Journal of Psychiatry, 146,* 496–502.

Dowson, J. H. (1992a). Assessment of DSM-III-R personality disorders by self-report questionnaire: The role of informants and a screening test for comorbid personality disorders (STCPD). *British Journal of Psychiatry, 161,* 344–352.

Dowson, J. H. (1992b). DSM-III-R narcissistic personality disorder evaluated by patients' and informants' self-report questionnaires: Relationships with other personality disorders and a sense of entitlement as an indicator of narcissism. *Comprehensive Psychiatry, 33,* 397–406.

Drake, R. E., & Vaillant, G. E. (1985). A validity study of Axis II of DSM-III. *American Journal of Psychiatry, 142,* 553–558.

Endicott, J., & Spitzer, R. L. (1979). Use of the Research Diagnostic Criteria and the Schedule for Affective Disorders and Schizophrenia. *American Journal of Psychiatry, 136,* 52–59.

Erlenmeyer-Kimling, L., Squires-Wheeler, E., Hilldoff Adamo, U., Bassett, A. S., Cornblatt, B. A., Kestenbaum, C. J., Rock, D., Roberts, S. A., & Gottsman, I. I. (1995). The New York High-Risk Project: Psychoses and Cluster A personality disorders in offspring of schizophrenic parents at 23 years of follow-up. *Archives of General Psychiatry, 52,* 857–865.

Glueck, J., & Glueck, E. (1950). *Unravelling juvenile delinquency.* New York: Commonwealth Fund.

Hyler, S., Lyons, M., Rieder, R., Young, L., Williams, J., & Spitzer, R. (1990). The factor structure of self-report DSM-III Axis II symptoms and their relationship to clinician's ratings. *American Journal of Psychiatry, 147,* 751–757.

Hyler, S., Rieder, R., & Spitzer, R. (1983). *Personality Diagnostic Questionnaire (PDQ).* New York: New York State Psychiatric Institute.

Hyler, S., Skodol, A., Kellman, H., Oldham, J., & Rosnick, L. (1990). Validity of the Personality Diagnostic Questionnaire—Revised: Comparison with two structured interviews. *American Journal of Psychiatry, 147,* 1043–1048.

Kendler, K. S., Lieberman, J. A., & Walsh, D. (1989). The Structured Interview for Schizotypy (SIS); A preliminary report. *Schizophrenia Bulletin, 15,* 559–571.

Kendler, K. S., McGuire, M., Gruenberg, A. M., O'Hare, A., Spellman, M., & Walsh, D. (1993). The Roscommon family study: III. Schizophrenia-related personality disorders in relatives. *Archives of General Psychiatry, 50,* 781–788.

Kessler, R. C., McGonagle, K. A., Zhao, S., Nelson, C. B., Hughes, M., Eshleman, S., Wittchen, H-U, & Kendler, K. S. (1994). Lifetime and 12-month prevalence of DSM-III-R psychiatric disorders in the United States. *Archives of General Psychiatry, 51,* 8–19.

Lenzenweger, M. F., Loranger, A. W., Korfine, L., & Neff, C. (1997). Detecting personality disorders in a nonclinical population. *Archives of General Psychiatry, 54,* 345–351.

Loranger, A. W., Sartorius, N., Andreoli, A., Berger, P., Buchheim, P., Channabasavanna, S. M., Coid, B., Dahl, A., Diekstra, R. F. W., Ferguson, B., Jacobsberg, L. B., Mombour, W., Pull, C., Ono, Y., & Regier, D. (1994). The International Personality Disorder Examination (IPDE): The World Health Organization/Alcohol, Drug Abuse, and Mental Health Administration International Pilot Study of Personality Disorders. *Archives of General Psychiatry, 51,* 215–224.

Loranger, A. W., Sartorius, N., & Janca, A. (1996). *Assessment and diagnosis of personality disorders: The International Personality Disorder Examination (IPDE).* New York: Cambridge University Press.

Loranger, A. W., Susman, V. L., Oldham, J. M., & Russakoff, L. M. (1987). The Personality Disorder Examination: A preliminary report. *Journal of Personality Disorders, 1,* 1–13.

Lyons, M. J. (1995). *Epidemiology of personality disorders.* In M. T. Tsuang, M. Tohen, & G. E. P. Zahner, *Textbook in psychiatric epidemiology.* New York: Wiley-Liss.

Maier, W., Lichtermann, D., Klinger, T., & Heun, R. (1992). Prevalences of personality disorders (DSM-III-R) in the community. *Journal of Personality Disorders, 6,* 187–196.

Maier, W., Minges, J., Lichtermann, D., & Heun, R. (1995). Personality disorders and personality variations in relatives of patients with bipolar affective disorders. *Journal of Affective Disorders, 53,* 173–181.

Merikangas, K., & Weissman, M. (1986). Epidemiology of DSM-III Axis II personality disorders. In A. Frances & R. Hales (Eds.), *Psychiatry update: American Psychiatric Association annual review* (Vol. 5). Washington, DC: American Psychiatric Association.

Nestadt, G., Romanoski, A. J., Brown, C. H., Chahal, R., Merchant, A., Folstein, M. F., Gruenberg, E. M., & McHugh, P. R. (1991). DSM-III compulsive personality disorder: An epidemiologic survey. *Psychological Medicine, 21,* 461–471.

Nestadt, G., Romanoski, A. J., Chahal, R. Merchant, A., Folstein, M. F., Gruenberg, E. M., & McHugh, P. A.

(1990). An epidemiological study of histrionic personality disorder. *Psychological Medicine, 20,* 413–422.

Nestadt, G., Romanoski, A. J., Samuels, J. F., Folstein, M. F., Gruenberg, E. M., & McHugh, P. R. (1992). The relationship between personality and DSM-III Axis I disorders in the population: Results from an epidemiological survey. *Amercian Journal of Psychiatry, 149,* 1228–1233.

Pfohl, B., Stangl, D., & Zimmerman, M. (1982). *The Structured Interview for DSM-III Personality Disorders (SIDP).* Iowa City, Department of Psychiatry, University of Iowa.

Reich, J., Yates, W., & Nduaguba, M. (1988). Age and sex distribution of DSM-III personality cluster traits in a community population. *Comprehensive Psychiatry, 29,* 298–303.

Reich, J., Yates, W., & Nduaguba, M. (1989). Prevalence of DSM-III personality disorders in the community. *Social Psychiatry and Psychiatric Epidemiology, 24,* 12–16.

Regier, D. A., Boyd, J. H., Burke, J. D., Rae, D. S., Myers, J. K., Kramer, M., Robins, L. N., George, L. K., Karno, M., & Locke, B. Z. (1988). One-month prevalence of mental disorders in the United States. *Archives of General Psychiatry, 45,* 977–986.

Robins, L. N., Helzer, J. E., Croughan, J., & Ratcliff, K. S. (1981). National Institute of Mental Health Diagnostic Interview Schedule: Its history, characteristics, and validity. *Archives of General Psychiatry, 38,* 381–389.

Romanoski, A. J., Nestadt, F., Chahal, R., Merchant, A., Folstein, M. F., Gruenberg, E. M., & McHugh, P. R. (1988). Inter-observer reliability of a Standardized Psychiatric Examination (SPE) for case ascertainment (DSM-III). *Journal of Nervous and Mental Disease, 176,* 63–71.

Spitzer, R. L., Williams, J. B. W., Gibbon, M., & First, M. (1990a). *Structured Clinical Interview for DSM-III-R Non-Patient Edition (SCID-NP; Version 1. 0).* Washinton, DC: American Psychiatric Association.

Spitzer, R. L., Williams, J. B. W., Gibbon, M., & First, M. (1990b). *Structured Clinical Interview for DSM-III-R Personality Disorders (SCID-II; Version 1.0).* Washington, DC: American Psychiatric Association.

Swanson, M. C., Bland, R. C., & Newman, S. C. (1994). Antisocial personality disorder. *Acta Psychiatrica Scandinavica, 376*(Suppl.), 63–70.

Swartz, M., Blazer, D., George, L., & Winfield, I. (1990). Estimating the prevalence of borderline personality disorder in the community. *Journal of Personality Disorders, 4,* 257–272.

Tyrer, P., Alexander, M. S., Cicchettic, D., Cohen, M. S., & Remington, M. (1979). Reliability of a schedule for rating personality disorders. *British Journal of Psychiatry, 135,* 168–174.

Weissman, M. M. (1993, Spring). The epidemiology of personality disorders: A 1990 update. *Journal of Personality Disorders, 44–62.

Wells, J. E., Bushnell, J. A., Hornblow, A. R., Joyce, P. R., & Oakley-Browne, M. A. (1989). Christchurch psychiatric epidemiology study, part I: Methodology and lifetime prevalence for specific psychiatric disorders. *Australian and New Zealand Journal of Psychiatry, 23,* 315–326.

World Health Organization. (1990). *Composite International Diagnostic Interview (CIDI) version 1. 0.* Geneva, Switzerland: World Health Organization.

Zimmerman, M., & Coryell, W. (1989). DSM-III personality disorder diagnoses in a nonpatient sample: Demographic correlates and comorbidity. *Archives of General Psychiatry, 46,* 682–689.

Zimmerman, M., & Coryell, W. (1990). Diagnosing personality disorders in the community: A comparison of self-report and interview measures. *Archives of General Psychiatry, 47,* 527–531.

Zimmerman, M., Pfohl, B., Coryell, W., Stangl, D., & Corenthal, C. (1988). Diagnosing personality disorder in depressed patients: A comparison of patient and informant interviews. *Archives of General Psychiatry, 45,* 733–737.

CHAPTER 6

———◄═══►———

Biological and Treatment Correlates

EMIL F. COCCARO

The notion that disorders of personality are due purely to developmental or other environmental factors has been refuted over the past 15 to 20 years by accumulating data from psychobiological research studies. First, various dimensions of personality have been shown to be moderately heritable in twin studies (Plomin, Owen, & McGuffin, 1994). Accordingly, to a substantial degree, individual differences in personality must be influenced by genetic, and therefore biological, factors. Second, various dimensions of personality have been shown to correlate with various measures of biological and neurophysiological/psychological/structural function (Coccaro & Siever, 1995).

This chapter reviews the existing data specifically regarding the biological and neurophysiological/psychological/structural correlates of personality in personality-disordered subjects. This review is organized first by neurotransmitter, second by neurophysiological/psychological/structural function, and third by pharmacological treatment correlates.

NEUROTRANSMITTER FUNCTION

Serotonin

The most heavily researched neurotransmitter with regard to personality and personality disorder is serotonin (5-HT). Over the course of 20 years, research in this area has suggested a strong role for 5-HT in aggression and impulsiv-

ity whereby 5-HT is inversely related to aggression and/or impulsivity. Whereas some studies suggest that impulsivity may have primacy over aggression specifically, most studies, in fact, report a 5-HT relationship with both impulsivity and aggression (e.g., "impulsive aggression") rather than with one personality dimension or the other. One of the most remarkable aspects of this literature is the consistency of the findings across different study samples using various assessments of 5-HT function.

Evidence for a role of 5-HT in aggression was first reported in studies of nonprimate mammals such as mice and rats (Valzelli, 1980). In these studies, conditions that reduced or enhanced 5-HT were associated with an increase or decrease, respectively, in aggressive responding in rodents.

Neurochemical Studies

Later, studies of the concentration of 5-hydroxyindoleacetic acid (the main 5-HT metabolite in the cerebrospinal fluid; CSF 5-HIAA) were applied to the study of aggression in humans. CSF 5-HIAA is thought to represent turnover of 5-HT, a view supported by the observation that CSF 5-HIAA is highly correlated with brain concentrations of 5-HIAA (Stanley, Ttaksman-Bendz, & Dorovini-Zis, 1985). A more conservative interpretation, however, suggests that CSF 5-HIAA represents an index of the number of viable 5-HT neurons in the central nervous system (Murphy et al., 1990).

The first evidence of an inverse relationship between 5-HT and aggression was reported by Asberg, Traksman, and Thoren (1976). In their study of CSF 5-HIAA concentration in depressed patients as a function of history of suicide attempting behavior, a disproportionate number of patients with history of suicide attempt had categorically low CSF 5-HIAA concentrations. Those who had made violent suicide attempts exclusively fell into the group with categorically low CSF 5-HIAA concentrations, whereas patients who had made nonviolent suicide attempts were approximately split between categorically low and normal CSF 5-HIAA concentrations.

Brown, Goodwin, Ballenger, Goyer, and Major (1979) reported a specific inverse relationship between CSF 5-HIAA concentrations and life history of actual aggressive behavior ($r = -.78$, $p < .001$) in male personality-disordered subjects with a variety of DSM-II personality disorder diagnoses. In addition, CSF 5-HIAA was reduced among those subjects with a life history of suicide attempt. In 1982, Brown et al. reported a replication study and further noted a trivariate relationship between aggression history, suicide history, and reduced CSF 5-HIAA whereby history of aggression and suicide attempt were correlated directly, while each historical variable correlated inversely, with CSF 5-HIAA. Almost simultaneously, Linnoila et al. (1983) reported reduced CSF 5-HIAA in impulsive, but not nonimpulsive, violent offenders (i.e., individuals who had committed murder, attempted murder, or serious assault) with a variety of DSM-II personality disorder diagnoses. The observation that impulsive, rather than nonimpulsive, aggression was associated with reduced CSF 5-HIAA concentration suggested that "impulsiveness" might be the more specific phenomenological correlate to 5-HT function. Later work by the same group (Virkkunen, Nuutila, Goodwin, & Linnoila, 1987), studying impulsive arsonists with borderline personality disorder, noted that impulsive arsonists had significantly reduced CSF 5-HIAA concentrations compared with normal volunteers but similar CSF 5-HIAA concentrations compared with those of the impulsive violent offenders. These data suggest that reduced CSF 5-HIAA concentration is related specifically to impulsivity rather than violence. However, evidence from later studies (see below) suggests that the critical phenomenological factor in this regard may be impulsive aggression rather than simply impulsivity alone.

The finding of reduced CSF 5-HIAA concentration in aggressive personality-disordered subjects has generally been replicated when the subjects studied were criminal offenders. However, when personality-disordered subjects do not have a history of criminal activity, CSF 5-HIAA studies are equivocal in terms of a relationship with aggression. At least four studies (Coccaro et al., 1997a; Coccaro, Kavoussi, Cooper, & Haugher, 1997c; Gardner, Lucas, & Cowdry, 1990; Simeon et al., 1992) report no correlation between CSF 5-HIAA and aggression in personality-disordered patients without history of criminal activity. This may be due to differences in the severity of aggressive behavior between these two populations. It is likely that CSF 5-HIAA, being a relatively insensitive index of 5-HT activity, is most reduced in the most severely aggressive individuals and that it is difficult to detect this relationship in less severely aggressive individuals.

Pharmacological Challenge Studies

A variety of 5-HT pharmacological challenge studies have been performed in personality-disordered subjects in the context of aggression. In the first such study in personality-disordered subjects, prolactin (PRL) responses to the 5-HT releaser/uptake inhibitor d,l-fenfluramine (i.e., PRL[d,l-FEN]) were noted to correlate inversely with various measures of aggression and impulsivity (e.g., $r = -.77$, $p < .002$; Coccaro et al., 1989). An inverse relationship between the PRL[d,l-FEN] response and aggression has been replicated in several, though not all, studies of personality-disordered subjects (Coccaro et al., 1997a, 1997c; O'Keane et al., 1992; Siever & Trestman 1993).

Pharmacological challenge studies of personality disorder using 5-HT agents other than fenfluramine are limited but generally support the hypothesis of an inverse relationship between 5-HT and measures of aggression. 5-HT agents used in these studies include direct 5-HT agonists and 5-HT$_{1a}$ partial agonists. Moss, Yao, and Panzak (1990) reported reduced PRL responses to the postsynaptic 5-HT agonist meta-chlorophenylpiperazine (PRL[m-CPP]) in male antisocial personality-disordered patients with comorbid alcohol abuse compared with normal volunteers. An inverse correlation between PRL[m-CPP] responses and assaultiveness was also reported across all subjects. While Coccaro et al. (1997a) could not replicate this finding in 20 male and female personality-disordered subjects, PRL[m-CPP] responses demonstrated had similar inverse correlations to those seen with PRL[d,l-FEN] responses in the subgroup of 10 male subjects in whom both PRL[m-CPP] and PRL[d,l-FEN] response data were available. This was due to a strong intercorrelation between PRL[m-CPP] and PRL[d,l-FEN] responses in these subjects. With regard to specific 5-HT receptor subtypes, Coccaro, Gabriel, and Siever (1990) reported an inverse correlation between the prolactin response to the 5-HT$_{1a}$ partial agonist buspirone and self-reported "assaultiveness" and "irritability" in 10 personality-disordered subjects. A follow-up study using a more potent and selective 5-HT$_{1a}$ agonist, ipsapirone, also found an inverse correlation between measures of aggression and cortisol and thermal responses to ipsapirone in eight male personality-disordered subjects (Cocccaro, Kavoussi, & Hauger, 1995). PRL[d-FEN] responses were also found to correlate inversely with aggression in the same subjects.

Behavioral responses to 5-HT stimulation in personality-disordered subjects has not received as much attention as have neuroendocrine responses. However, a recent study reported a significant reduction in anger in 12 borderline personality disorder subjects after administration of m-CPP but not placebo (Hollander et al., 1994). In addition, a reduction in fear was observed in the male subjects with borderline personality disorder.

Most interesting have been the early results of brain imaging (i.e., FDG–PET) studies during pharmacological challenge. Siever et al. (1999) recently reported reduced glucose utilization in the orbital frontal and adjacent ventral medial and cingulate cortex of impulsive aggressive personality-disordered patients, compared with normal controls, during challenge with d,l-FEN. While not a pharmacological challenge study, Goyer et al. (1994) had previously found reductions in glucose utilization (i.e., basal FDG–PET study) in similar areas in the brains of six borderline personality-disordered subjects compared with controls. In addition, these authors reported an inverse correlation between glucose utilization in these areas and a life history of aggression in the larger sample ($N = 16$) of general personality-disordered patients studied. Taken together, these data suggest that orbital frontal and adjacent areas of the prefrontal cortex are critical in impulsive aggression and that altered function of these areas may also involve a reduction in brain 5-HT function.

Platelet Receptor Markers

Receptor markers on circulating blood platelets have long been used as a model of 5-HT receptors in the central nervous system. Despite considerable platelet receptor work in other psychiatric populations, relatively little research in this area has been published on personality-disordered subjects. Simeon et al. (1992) reported an inverse correlation between the number of platelet [^{3}H]impiramine (5-HT transporter) binding sites and self-mutilation and impulsivity in personality-disordered subjects with, but not without, a history of self-mutilation. Coccaro, Kavoussi, Sheline, Lish, and Csernansky (1996) reported that the number of platelet [^{3}H]paroxetine (5-HT transporter) binding sites was inversely correlated with life history of aggression in personality-disordered subjects. In a study of overlapping subjects, the same authors noted a positive relationship between platelet 5-HT$_{2a}$ receptors and aggression (Coccaro, Kavoussi, Sheline, Berman, & Csernansky, 1997b).

DNA Polymorphism Studies

Polymorphisms are different forms of DNA sequences which represent either "anonymous" DNA markers (for gene mapping purposes) or DNA markers of known genes coding for specific specific proteins. Work with specific polymorphic markers of candidate genes is now being applied to subjects with personality disorders.

Several studies have been published in this area. Nielsen et al. (1994) reported that impulsive violent offenders (nearly all were personality disordered) with at least one copy of the AL allele for the tryptophan hydroxylase (TPH) gene had significantly lower CSF 5-HIAA compared with impulsive violent offenders with the AUU genotype. Because TPH is the rate-limiting step in the synthesis of 5-HT, it suggests that the AL allele is associated with reduced function of TPH and, by logical extension, reduced synthesis of 5-HT. Curiously, this finding did not generalize to nonimpulsive violent offenders (many of whom were also personality disordered) or to normal controls. In the same study, the AL allele was also associated with history of suicidal behavior. This latter finding has been replicated by these authors (Nielsen et al., 1998). More recently, New et al. (1998) reported that the self-reported tendency toward aggression varied as a function of TPH genotype. In this study of 21 white personality-disordered males, subjects with the ALL genotype had higher aggression scores than did those with the AUU genotype. Although PRL[d,l-FEN] responses did not significantly differ as a function of genotype in the subgroup with these data, PRL[d,l-FEN] responses among those with the ALL geneotype were 30% lower than among those with the ALU and AUU genotype. Most recently, Lappalainen et al. (1998) reported an association between antisocial alcoholism (i.e., alcoholism with antisocial personality disorder or intermittent explosive disorder) and the AC allele for the 5-HT$_{1d}$ beta receptor polymorphism. As the 5-HT$_{1d}$ beta receptor is a critical receptor involved in the regulation of 5-HT release on neuronal impulse, this finding could be highly relevant to the understanding of antisocial personality disorder comorbid with alcoholism.

Catecholamines

The study of norepinephrine (NE) and dopamine (DA) in personality disorder has not received the attention that 5-HT has. Although indices of these three neurotransmitters are often investigated simultaneously, typically the findings of relevance have focused on 5-HT.

Behavioral Activation Studies

The first studies in this area examined the behavioral responses to agents that activate both DA and NE systems. Based on the hypothesis that borderline and schizotypal personality-disordered subjects might show different mood and cognitive/perceptual responses to DA/NE stimulants, Schulz et al. (1985) administered acute doses of amphetamine to a series of personality-disordered subjects and carefully assessed their responses over a period of hours in a controlled setting. Schulz et al. (1985) reported that eight borderline personality-disordered subjects had greater behavioral sensitivity to amphetamine challenge, demonstrating an increase in clinician-rated well-being and in global psychopathology. Notably, half these subjects, compared to none of the normal volunteers, were rated as transiently psychotic

during the session. In a replication study in 16 subjects, Schulz et al. (1988) reported that global deterioration after amphetamine was typical of subjects with both borderline and schizotypal personality disorder while global improvement was typical of borderline subjects without comorbid schizotypal personality disorder. These data suggest that there are important biological differences among borderline personality-disordered subjects as a function of comorbid schizotypy. Elevation of dopaminergic function in schizotypal personality-disordered subjects (Siever et al., 1991, 1993), as noted below, may contribute to this adverse behavioral response to amphetamine in subjects with comorbid schizotypy.

Dopamine

Studies involving assessments of dopamine function in personality disorder fall into two main areas: schizotypy and aggression. Two studies support the hypothesis that DA function is directly related to schizotypy. One study reports higher CSF homovanillic acid (HVA) concentrations in 11 subjects with schizotypal personality-disordered subjects compared with 6 healthy volunteer controls (Siever et al., 1993). In addition, the number of psychotic-like schizotypal symptoms correlated positively with CSF HVA concentration ($r = .61, p = .007$) in a combined group of 18 schizotypal and nonschizotypal personality-disordered subjects. There was no correlation between non-psychotic-like schizotypal symptoms and CSF HVA concentration. Another study examining plasma HVA concentrations in 10 schizotypal and 14 nonschizotypal subjects also found a significant elevation in plasma HVA in the schizotypal personality-disordered subjects (Siever et al., 1991). As with CSF HVA concentration, plasma HVA concentration was found to correlate positively with psychotic-like ($r = .59, p = .002$), but not non-psychotic-like ($r = .11, p = $ ns), schizotypal symptoms. These data provide preliminary evidence that DA function may be higher in schizotypal subjects and that it may covary with the psychotic-like symptoms (suspiciousness, ideas of reference, recurrent illusions, magical thinking) of schizotypal personality which may also respond to treatment with low-dose neuroleptics in selected subjects (Coccaro, 1998b). Studies of schizotypal relatives of schizophrenic patients reveal the same basic finding with regard to plasma

HVA. Here, however, schizotypal relatives have been reported to have lower mean plasma HVA compared with other relatives regardless of the presence or absence of personality disorder. When examined closely, these relatives were found to primarily have deficit-type symptoms (e.g., constricted affect and lack of close friends) and that plasma HVA correlated inversely with these symptoms (Amin, Siever, & Silverman, 1997). These data suggest, then, that dopamine function may correlate directly with positive-type symptoms while correlating inversely with deficit-type symptoms.

Evidence for the role of DA in human aggression is limited, with some studies demonstrating no relationship between CSF HVA concentration and aggression (Brown et al., 1979; Virkkunen et al., 1987) and other studies suggesting an inverse relationship between the variables. Among the positive studies, Linnoila et al. (1983) reported a reduction in CSF HVA in antisocial, though not explosive, impulsive violent offenders, and Virkkunen, DeJong, Bartko, Goodwin, and Linnoila (1989) reported that recidivist violent offenders had lower CSF HVA concentrations than did their nonrecidivist violent offender controls. It is of note that in each of these studies a strong inverse relationship between CSF 5-HIAA concentration and the aggression variable was reported. Given the widely acknowledged observation that CSF 5-HIAA and CSF HVA concentrations are strongly intercorrelated, it is possible that findings with CSF HVA may be related to similar findings with CSF 5-HIAA concentration. In fact, Agren, Mefford, Rudorfer, Linnoila, and Potter (1986) have argued that CSF 5-HIAA "drives" CSF HVA. If so, a specific assessment of CSF HVA may not be made unless the effect of CSF 5-HIAA concentration is accounted for. Although this statistical adjustment has not been made to date in published studies, we have found a significant inverse relationship between CSF HVA, adjusted for CSF 5-HIAA, and life history of aggression in male and female personality-disordered subjects. Given that animal studies suggest a direct relationship between DA function and aggression (Coccaro, 1998a), it is possible that an inverse relationship between CSF HVA and aggression indirectly reflects the positive relationship between postsynaptic DA receptor sensitivity and aggression or arousal, which, in turn, can increase the likelihood of aggression given the proper circumstances. In this regard, it is noteworthy that a strong positive relationship between positive emotionality and PRL response to DA receptor agents has been reported in nonpsychiatric subjects (DePue, Luciana, Arbisi, Collins, & Leon, 1994)

Norepinephrine

Studies involving assessments of NE function in personality disorder have largely been in the area of aggression. As with DA, animal studies suggest a direct relationship between NE function and aggression (Coccaro, 1998a). Brown et al. (1979) reported a positive correlation between CSF 3-methoxy-4-hydroxyphenylglycol (MHPG) concentrations and life history of aggression in 12 male personality-disordered subjects. Despite this correlation, however, multiple regression, including CSF 5-HIAA, revealed that CSF 5-HIAA accounted for 80% of the variance in aggression scores. Accordingly, the influence of NE on aggression appeared to be small. Supporting this modest finding, Siever and Trestman (1993) reported that plasma NE was modestly but positively correlated with self-reported impulsivity in male personality-disordered subjects. In contrast to these studies, however, Virkkunen et al. (1987) reported a significant reductions in CSF MHPG concentration in violent offenders. Recently, we found a significant reduction in plasma free MHPG in male personality-disordered subjects when compared with normal volunteers. Among the former group, borderline personality disorder subjects had lower plasma free MHPG compared with their nonborderline controls. In addition, there was a modest but significant inverse correlation between plasma free MHPG and life history of aggression across all personality-disordered subjects.

NE pharmacological challenge studies in personality-disordered subjects have been limited. Coccaro et al. (1991) reported a positive correlation between the growth hormone response to the alpha-2 NE agonist clonidine and self-reported "irritability" (a correlate of aggression) in a small sample of male personality-disordered and healthy volunteer subjects. Together with our findings of an inverse relationship between plasma free MHPG and aggression, it is possible that there may be variable dysregulation of presynaptic (i.e., reflected by plasma free MHPG) and postsynaptic (i.e., reflected by growth hormone [clonidine] responses) NE function in personality-disordered subjects with prominent histories of aggression.

Other Neurotransmitters

This category includes data relevant to acetylcholine and vasopressin function. Studies of acetylcholine function in personality disorder have been limited to one study. Because enhanced acetylcholine sensitivity has been implicated in affective disorders, it is possible that this neurotransmitter may contribute to the heightened affective sensitivity of selected personality-disordered subjects such as those with borderline personality disorder. Steinberg et al. (1997) examined the behavioral response to acute infusions of the acetylcholinesterase inhibitor physostigmine in 10 borderline personality-disordered subjects compared with 24 nonborderline personality-disordered and 10 healthy volunteer subjects. In this study, borderline personality disorder subjects report greater self-rated depression scores than did the nonborderline or healthy volunteer controls. Peak physostigmine-induced depression scores correlated positively with the number of affective instability ($r = .45$, $p < .01$), but not with the number of impulsive aggressive ($r = .08$, p = ns), borderline personality traits, suggesting that physostigmine-induced dysphoria was a specific correlate of affective instability and not other borderline personality disorder traits. Accordingly, these data suggest that the trait of affective lability in borderline personality-disordered subjects may be mediated, in part, by a heightened sensitivity to acetylcholine.

Only one study of central vasopressin activity has been performed in personality-disordered subjects. Animal studies in lower mammals suggest a positive relationship between central vasopressin and aggression (Ferris & Delville, 1994). In our laboratory we have found a significant positive correlation between CSF vasopressin concentrations and life history of aggression, and of aggression against persons in particular. Most important, this relationship was present even after accounting for a separate relationship with 5-HT (Coccaro, Kavoussi, Hauger, Cooper, & Ferris, 1998).

NEUROPHYSIOLOGICAL/ PSYCHOLOGICAL/ STRUCTURAL CORRELATES

Findings from studies in these areas have largely focused on patients with schizotypal personality disorder. These studies have involved work examining smooth pursuit eye movement (SPEM), facility in continuous performance tasks, performance in tasks of executive cognitive function, and structural neuroimaging.

Attentional Function/Information Processing

Schizotypal personality-disordered subjects, like schizophrenics, display impairment of eye-movement tracking a smoothly moving target. Moreover, abnormalities in SPEM appear to be specifically associated with the "deficit-like" traits of schizotypal personality disorder (Siever et al., 1994). Subjects with schizotypal personality disorder show abnormalities on other attentional tasks as well, including continuous performance tasks (CPT) and backward masking tasks (BMT). The CPT is a test of sustained attention. Poor performance on the CPT has been observed in studies of schizotypal volunteers, patients, and offspring of schizophrenic patients (Siever, Kalus, & Keefe, 1993) and has been correlated with social detachment in offspring of schizophrenic patients (Cornblatt, Lenzenweger, Dworkin, & Erlenmeyer-Kimling, 1992). The BMT is a visual information-processing task which has also been reported to be abnormal in both patients with schizotypal personality disorder and volunteers with schizotypal traits (Merritt & Balough 1989).

Schizotypal personality-disordered subjects (or patients), like subjects with schizophrenia, also demonstrate impaired performance on tests sensitive to prefrontal function, including the Wisconsin Card Sorting Test (Raine, Sheard, Reynolds, & Lencz, 1992; Siever et al., 1993). However, because performance on the verbal fluency test and Wechsler Adult Intelligence Scale vocabulary and block design is similar to that of normal controls, cortical impairment is apparently not global and, instead, may be more selective for brain circuits including frontal and perhaps temporal regions in schizotypal individuals.

Structural Imaging

Neuroimaging studies suggest that there may be increased ventricular size both in patients with schizotypal personality disorder (Cazzullo, Vita, Giobbio, Diecie, & Sacchetti, 1991) and in schizotypal relatives of schizophrenics (Silverman et al., 1998). In one report, increased ventricular size was associated with reduced concentrations of plasma HVA and deficit-like symptoms (Siever et al., 1993). If replicated, this finding raises the possibility that frontal cortical impairment may be associated with increased ventricular size and reduced DA function in this area. Other structural abnormalities reported in schizotypal patients include reduced volume in the temporal lobe and hippocampus (Downhill et al., 1997; McCarley et al., 1995). Magnetic resonance imaging studies of schizotypal subjects also note abnormalities of the cavum septum pellucidum. While reduced frontal lobe volume has not been reported (as in schizophrenics) in schizotypal individuals (Shihabuddin et al., 1999), frontal lobe volume has been reported to correlate inversely with performance on tests of executive function in schizotypal subjects (Raine et al., 1992) and in schizotypal patients (Siever et al., 1993). Notably, poor performance on the Wisconsin Card Sorting Test tends to be associated with reduced concentrations of plasma HVA (Siever et al., 1993). Furthermore, increased ventricular size also tends to be associated with reduced concentrations of plasma HVA which, in turn, appears to be negatively related to the deficit-like symptoms (i.e., increased social withdrawal and constricted affect). Accordingly, these findings suggest that schizotypal personality-disordered subjects, particularly those with deficit-like symptoms, are characterized by impairment on a variety of cortical processing tasks, increased ventricular size, and reduced indices of dopamine activity (probably in frontal cortex).

PHARMACOLOGICAL TREATMENT CORRELATES

The data reviewed previously suggest that aspects of personality disorder that correlate with specific biological/neurotransmitter factors should be amenable to treatment with agents that work through these systems. Given the data available, the aspects of personality disorder most studied in this regard are impulsive aggression and schizotypy.

Impulsive Aggression in Personality Disorder

The most logical approach to the treatment of impulsive aggression in personality disorder, given available data, is to use agents that increase central 5-HT function. To date, at least three placebo-controlled studies involving 5-HT uptake inhibitor agents have been published in the area of personality disorder. In the first study a significant reduction in anger in 13 volunteer subjects with borderline personality disorder or traits treated with fluoxetine was seen compared with 9 subjects treated with placebo (Salzman et al., 1995). Preliminary data from another placebo-controlled study of fluoxetine (Markovitz, 1995) conducted in 17 patients with highly (Axis I/II) comorbid borderline personality disorder report general efficacy for fluoxetine in a variety of areas, some relevant to anger and aggression. The most recent published study was designed specifically to examine the effect of treatment with a 5-HT-specific agent on impulsive aggression in 40 personality-disordered subjects (Coccaro & Kavoussi, 1997). Compared with placebo, fluoxetine was noted to reduce events of verbal aggression as well as aggression against objects after at least 9 to 10 weeks of treatment. Entry into this 12-week study was confined to nondepressed personality-disordered subjects with recurrent, problematic, impulsive aggressive behavior. Accordingly, these data indicate that treatment with a 5-HT agent is associated with an antiaggressive effect in the absence of any possible antidepressant effect. Curiously, examination of pretreatment 5-HT function revealed a positive, rather than an inverse, relationship with clinical response to fluoxetine (Coccaro, Kavoussi, & Hauger, 1997d). This suggests that the more dysfunctional the 5-HT system, the less efficacious 5-HT uptake inhibitors may be in these subjects. However, it also suggests that the more aggressive a subject (and the more dysfunctional the 5-HT system) the less efficacious these agents will be. A possible reason for this is that 5-HT uptake inhibitors increase 5-HT in the synapse but do not necessarily increase 5-HT neurotransmission, particularly when postsynaptic receptors are dysfunctional. If so, other neuropsychopharmacological strategies will be needed. One strategy involves the use of anticonvulsants which have already been shown to be have antiaggressive efficacy in personality-disordered patients (Cowdry & Gardner, 1988). In an open 8-week trial of subjects who had failed to respond to fluoxetine, Kavoussi and Coccaro (1998) found that divalproex sodium was effective in reducing aggressive events. Another study with the same agent (E. Hollander, personal communication, 1999) has observed a similar finding in patients with borderline personality disorder. Using a different anticonvulsant (diphenhydantoin), Barratt, Stanford, Felthous, and Kent (1997) reported that impulsive, but not nonimpulsive, antisocial offenders displayed an anti-aggressive response to anticonvulsants.

Other neurotransmitter targets might be investigated as well. These include agents that might affect catecholamine function. To date, most placebo-controlled controlled studies with neuroleptics (dopamine receptor antagonists) have found only modest therapeutic effects for neuroleptics in patients with borderline (Cowdry & Gardner, 1988), borderline and/or schizotypal (Soloff, Cornelius, et al., 1993, Soloff, George, et al., 1989), and schizotypal personality disorder (Goldberg et al., 1986). In contrast, agents that increase catecholamine function may be associated with a risk for an increase in agitation and hostility in some personality-disordered patients, often those with prominent histories of impulsive aggressive behavior (Soloff et al., 1986a). Increases in "episodic dyscontrol" in borderline personality-disordered patients have similarly been noted during treatment with alprazolam (Cowdry & Gardner, 1988). This raises the possibility that both antidepressants and anxiolytics should be avoided when treating personality-disordered patients with prominent histories of impulsive aggression.

On the other hand, lithium, which may dampen catecholamine function while increasing 5-HT function, has been shown to have efficacy in this regard. One double-blind placebo-controlled study examined the efficacy of lithium carbonate on impulsive aggression in prison inmates with a probable diagnosis of antisocial personality disorder (Sheard, Marini, Bridges, & Wapner, 1976). This study, yet to be replicated in this population, demonstrated an unequivocal effect of lithium carbonate treatment on actual frequency of impulsive aggressive behavior. Efficacy of lithium on these behaviors was manifest within 1 month of treatment and returned to pretreatment levels within the same time frame after withdrawal. While beta-blockers may reduce aggression in selected psychiatric populations (Yudofsky, Silver, & Schneider, 1987), these agents have yet to be formally studied in personality-disordered subjects.

Agents that act on nonmonoaminergic systems have not yet been studied in placebo-controlled trials in personality-disordered subjects. However, it is noteworthy that 5-HT uptake inhibitor agents also reduce CSF levels of vasopressin (Altemus et al., 1994; DeBellis, Gold, Geracioti, Listwak, & King, 1993) in human subjects. Finally, open-label studies involving opiate antagonists have been reported to reduce self-injurious behavior (Roth, Ostroff, & Hoffman, 1996) as well as dissociative symptoms in patients with borderline personality disorder (Bohus, Landwehrmeyer, Stiglmayr, Limberger, & Bohme, 1999).

Schizotypy in Personality Disorder

As reviewed earlier, available data suggest that psychotic-like symptoms of the schizotypal personality disorder are related to increased dopamine function in subcortical brain regions and deficit-like symptoms are related to reduced dopamine function in cortical brain regions. Accordingly, psychotic-like symptoms may be ameliorated by agents that reduce (i.e., neuroleptics), and deficit-like symptoms by agents that increase, dopamine activity.

Neuroleptic treatment has generally been associated with global improvement in patients with either borderline and/or schizotypal personality disorder (Coccaro, 1998b). In two relatively large placebo-controlled trials in patients with either borderline and/or schizotypal personality disorder, psychotic-like symptoms (as well as symptoms of anxiety) were reduced by treatment with a neuroleptic (thiothixene, in Goldberg et al., 1986, and haloperidol, in Soloff et al., 1986a). The generalizability of the data from one trial may be limited, however, to personality-disordered patients with histories of brief transient psychotic-like symptoms prior to the start of the trial (Goldberg et al., 1986). A smaller study involving females with severe borderline personality disorder found only modest efficacy for the neuroleptic (trifluroperizine) over placebo (Cowdry & Gardner, 1988). While these data are in general agreement with those of several other studies involving neuroleptic treatment in personality-disordered patients, the most recent study found no efficacy for the neuroleptic (haloperidol) on psychotic-like symptoms in borderline and/or schizotypal personality-disordered patients (Soloff et al., 1993). The authors noted, however, that the patients in their previous study, where haloperidol had been efficacious in treating psychotic-like symptoms, had significantly higher ratings of "psychoticism," "schizotypal symptom severity," and "global impairment" than those in the more recent study. In conjunction with the finding that "severity of schizotypal symptoms" was a favorable predictor of response to thiothixine (Goldberg et al., 1986), these results suggest that neuroleptic treatment may be best indicated for moderately to severely impaired patients with prominent histories of psychotic-like schizotypal symptoms.

If the theory discussed previously regarding deficit-like symptoms (and cognitive processing abnormalities) and dopaminergic function is correct, deficits in cortical function and their associated social deficits might be improved with administration of agents that enhance dopaminergic activity. Preliminary data from Siegel et al. (1996) suggest that amphetamine (which increases central dopamine activity) may improve cognitive performance in schizotypal subjects on tests sensitive to prefrontal function (e.g., Wisconsin Card Sorting Test). If so, therapeutic trials with dopamine reuptake inhibitors, psychostimulants, L-dopa, or monoamine oxidase B inhibitors might be warranted. Because D_1 receptors are located in frontal cortex, D_1 agonists might selectively enhance cognitive function in such patients. If social deficits are related to this underlying cognitive impairment, an improvement in the interpersonal functioning of schizotypal personality-disordered subjects may also be observed.

ACKNOWLEDGMENTS

Portions of this work have previously appeared in Coccaro (1998c). Copyright 1998 by APA Press. Adapted by permission.

REFERENCES

Agren, H., Mefford, I. N., Rudorfer, M.V., Linnoila, M., & Potter, W. Z. (1986). Interacting neurotransmitter systems: A non-experimental approach to the 5-HIAA-HVA correlation in human CSF. *Journal of Psychiatric Research, 20,* 175–193.

Altemus, M., Swedo, S. E., Leonard, H. L., Richter, D., Rubinow, D. R., Potter, W. Z., & Rapoport, J. L. (1994). Changes in cerebrospinal fluid neurochemistry during treatment of obsessive–compulsive disorder with clomipramine. *Archives of General Psychiatry, 51,* 794–803.

Amin F., Siever, L. J., Silverman, J. M. (1997). Plasma HVA in schizotypal personality disorder. In A. J. Friedhoff & F. Amin (Eds.), *Plasma homovanillic acid studies in schizophrenia: Implications for presynaptic dopamine dysfunction* (pp. 133–149). Washington, DC: APA Press.

Asberg, M., Traksman, L., & Thoren, P. (1976). 5-HIAA in the cerebrospinal fluid: A biochemical suicide predictor? *Archives of General Psychiatry, 33,* 1193–1197.

Barratt, E. S., Stanford, M. S., Felthous, A. R., & Kent, T.A. (1997). The effects of phenytoin on impulsive and premeditated aggression: A controlled study. *Journal of Clinical Psychopharmacology, 17,* 341–349.

Bohus, M., Landwehrmeyer, G. B., Stiglmayr, C., Limberger, M., & Bohme, R. (1999). Naltrexone in the treatment of dissociative symptoms in patients with borderline personality disorder: An open-label trial. *Journal of Clinical Psychiatry, 60,* 598–603.

Brown, G. L., Ebert, M. H., Goyer, P. F., Jimerson, D. C., Klein, W. J., Bunney, W. E., & Goodwin, F. K. (1982). Aggression, suicide, and serotonin: Relationships to CSF amine metabolites. *American Journal of Psychiatry, 139,* 741–746.

Brown, G. L., Goodwin F. K., Ballenger, J. C., Goyer, P. F., & Major, L. F. (1979). Aggression in humans correlates with cerebrospinal fluid amine metabolites. *Psychiatry Research, 1,* 131–139.

Cazzullo, C. L., Vita, A., Giobbio, G. M., Diecie, M., & Sacchetti, E. (1991). Cerebral structured abnormalities in schizophreniform disorder in schizophrenia spectrum personality disorders. In C. A. Tamminga & S. C. Schultz (Eds.), *Advances in neuropsychiatry and psychopharmacology: Vol. 1. Schizophrenia research* (pp. 209–217). New York: Raven Press.

Coccaro, E. F. (1998a). Central neurotransmitter function in human aggression and impulsivity. In M. Maes & E. F. Coccaro (Eds.), *Neurobiology and clinical views on aggression and impulsivity* (pp. 143–168). Chichester, UK: Wiley.

Coccaro, E. F. (1998b). Clinical outcome of psychopharmacologic treatment of borderline and schizotypal personality disordered subjects. *Journal of Clinical Psychiatry, 59*(Suppl. 1), 30–35.

Coccaro, E. F. (1998c). Neurotransmitter function in personality disorder. In J. M. Oldham & M. B. Riba (Series Eds.) & K. R. Silk (Vol. Ed.), *APA annual review of psychiatry: Biology of personality disorders* (Vol. 17, pp. 1–25). Washington, DC: APA Press.

Coccaro, E. F., Gabriel, S., & Siever, L. J. (1990). Buspirone challenge: Preliminary evidence for a role for 5-HT-1a receptors in impulsive aggressive behavior in humans. *Psychopharmacology Bulletin, 26,* 393–405.

Coccaro, E. F., & Kavoussi, R. J. (1997). Fluoxetine and impulsive aggressive behavior in personality disordered subjects. *Archives of General Psychiatry, 54,* 1081–1088.

Coccaro, E. F., Kavoussi, R. J., Cooper, T. B., & Hauger, R. L. (1997c). Central serotonin and aggression: Inverse relationship with prolactin response to d-fenfluramine, but not with CSF 5-HIAA concentration in human subjects. *American Journal of Psychiatry, 154,* 1430–1435.

Coccaro, E. F., Kavoussi, R. J., & Hauger, R. L. (1995). Physiologic responses to d-fenfluramine and ipsapirone challenge correlate with indices of aggression in males with personality disorder. *International Clinical Psychopharmacology, 10,* 177–180.

Coccaro, E. F., Kavoussi, R. J., & Hauger, R. L. (1997d). Serotonin function and antiaggressive responses to fluoxetine: A pilot study. *Biological Psychiatry, 42,* 546–552.

Coccaro, E. F., Kavoussi, R. J., Hauger, R. L., Cooper, T. B., & Ferris, C. F. (1998). Cerebrospinal fluid vasopressin: Correlates with aggression and serotonin function in personality disordered subjects. *Archives of General Psychiatry, 55,* 708–714.

Coccaro, E. F., Kavoussi, R. J., Sheline, Y. I., Berman, M., & Csernansky, J. (1997b). Impulsive aggression in personality disorder: Correlates with ^{125}I-LSD binding in the platelet. *Neuropsychopharmacology, 16,* 211–216.

Coccaro, E. F., Kavoussi, R. J., Sheline, Y. I., Lish, J., & Csernansky, J. (1996). Impulsive aggression in personality disorder: Correlates with ^{3}H-paroxetine binding in the platelet. *Archives of General Psychiatry, 53,* 531–536.

Coccaro, E. F., Kavoussi, R. J., Trestman, R. L., Gabriel, S. M., Cooper, T. B., & Siever, L. J. (1997a). Serotonin function in personality and mood disorder: Intercorrelations among central indices and aggressiveness. *Psychiatry Research, 73,* 1–14.

Coccaro, E. F., Lawrence, T., Trestman, R., Gabriel, S., Klar, H. M., & Siever, L. J. (1991). Growth hormone responses to intravenous clonidine challenge correlates with behavioral irritability in psychiatric patients and in healthy volunteers. *Psychiatry Research, 39,* 129–139.

Coccaro, E. F., & Siever, L. J. (1995). The neuropsychopharmacology of personality disorder. In F. Bloom & D. Kupfer (Eds.), *Psychopharmacology: The fourth generation of progress.* New York: Raven Press.

Coccaro, E. F., Siever, L. J., Klar, H. M., Maurer, G., Cochrane, K., Cooper, T. B., Mohs, R. C., & Davis, K. L. (1989). Serotonergic studies in affective and personality disorder: Correlates with suicidal and impulsive aggressive behavior. *Archives of General Psychiatry, 46,* 587–599.

Cornblatt, B. A., Lenzenweger, M. F., Dworkin, R. H., & Erlenmeyer-Kimling, L. (1992). Childhood attentional dysfunctions predict social deficits in unaffected adults at risk for schizophrenia. *British Journal of Psychiatry, 161*(Suppl. 18), 59–64.

Cowdry, R. W., & Gardner, D. L. (1988). Pharmacotherapy of borderline personality disorder, Alprazolam, carbamazepine, trofluroperazine, and tranylcypromine. *Archives of General Psychiatry, 45,* 111–119.

DeBellis, M. D., Gold, P. W., Geracioti, T. D., Listwak, S. J., & Kling, M. A. (1993). Association of fluoxetine treatment with reductions in CSF concentrations of corticotropin-releasing hormone and arginine vasopressin in patients with major depression. *American Journal of Psychiatry, 150,* 656–657.

Depue, R. A., Luciana, M., Arbisi, P., Collins, P., & Leon, A. (1994). Dopamine and the structure of personality: Relation of agonist-induced doapmine activity to positive emotionality. *Journal of Personality and Social Psychology, 67,* 485–498.

Downhill, J. E., Buchsbaum, M. S., Hazlett, E. A., et al. (1997). Temporal lobe volume in schizotypal personality disorder and schizophrenia. *APA New Research Abstracts* (#172).

Ferris, C. F., & Delville, Y. (1994). Vasopressin and serotonin interactions in the control of agonistic behavior. *Psychoneuroendocrinology, 19,* 593–601.

Gardner, D. L., Lucas, P. B., & Cowdry, R. W. (1990). CSF metabolites in borderline personality disorder compared with normal controls. *Biological Psychiatry, 28,* 247–254.

Goldberg, S. C., Schulz, S. C., Schulz, P. M., Resnick, R. J., Hamer, R. M., & Friedel, R. O. (1986). Borderline and schizotypal personality disorders treated with low-dose thiothixine versus placebo. *Archives of General Psychiatry, 43,* 680–686.

Goyer, P. F., Andreason, P. J., Semple, W. E., Clayton, A. H., King, A. C., Compton-Toth, B. A., Schulz, S. C., & Cohen, R. M. (1994). Positron-emission tomography and personality disorders. *Neuropsychopharmacology, 10,* 21–28.

Hollander, E., Stein D., DeCaria, C. M., Simeon, D., Ghen, I., Hwang, M., & Islam, M. (1994). Serotonergic sensitivity in borderline personality disorder: Preliminary findings. *American Journal of Psychiatry, 151,* 277–280.

Kavoussi, R. J., & Coccaro, E. F. (1998). Divalproex sodium for impulsive aggressive behavior in patients with personality disorder. *Journal of Clinical Psychiatry, 59,* 676–680.

Lappalainen, J., Long, J. C., Eggert, M., Ozaki, N., Robin, R. W., Brown, G. L., Naukkarinen, H., Virkkunen, M., Linnoila, M., & Goldman, D. (1998). Linkage of antisocial alcoholism to the serotonin 5-HT-1B receptor gene in two populations. *Archives of General Psychiatry, 55,* 989–994.

Linnoila, M., Virkkunen, M., Scheinin, M., Nuutila, A., Rimon, R. J., & Goodwin, F. K. (1983). Low cerebrospinal fluid 5-hydroxyindoleacetic acid concentration differentiates impulsive from nonimpulsive violent behavior. *Life Sciences, 33,* 2609–2614.

Markovitz, P. J. (1995). Pharmacotherapy of impulsivity, aggression and related disorders. In D. Stein & E. Hollander (Eds.), *Impulsive aggression and disorders of impulse control* (pp. 263–287). Sussex, UK: Wiley.

McCarley, R. W., Salisbury, D., Voglmaier, M. M., et al. (1995). Temporal lobe dysfunction and schizotypal personality disorder. *APA New Research Abstracts* (#34D).

Merritt, R. D., & Balough, D. W. (1989). Backward masking spatial frequency effects among hypothetically schizotypal individuals. *Schizophrenia Bulletin, 15*(4), 573–583.

Moss, H. B., Yao, J. K., & Panzak, G. L. (1990). Serotonergic responsivity and behavioral dimensions in antisocial personality disorder with substance abuse. *Biosocial Psychiatry, 28,* 325–338.

Murphy, D. L., Mellow, A. M., Sunderland, T., Aulakh, C., Lawlor, B. L., & Zohar, J. (1990). Strategies for the study of serotonin in humans. In E. F. Coccaro &

D. L. Murphy (Eds.), *Serotonin in major psychiatric disorders* (pp. 3–25). Washington, DC: American Psychiatric Press.

New, A. S., Gelernter, J., Yovell, Y., Trestman, R. L., Nielson, D. A., Silverman, J., Mitropoulou, V., Siever, L. J. (1998). Tryptophan hydroxylase genotype is associated with impulsive aggression measures. *American Journal of Medical Genetics, 81*, 13–17.

Nielsen, D. A., Goldman, D., Virkkunen, M., et al. (1994). Suicidality and 5-hydroxyindoleacetic acid concentration associated with a tryptophan hydroxylase polymorphism. *Archives of General Psychiatry, 51*, 34–38.

Nielsen, D. A., Virkkunen, M., Lappalainen, J., Eggert, M., Brown, G. L., Long, J. C., Goldman, D., & Linnoila, M. (1998). A tryptophan hydroxylase gene marker for suicidality and alcoholism. *Archives of General Psychiatry, 55*, 593–602.

O'Keane. V., Moloney, E., O'Neill, H., et al. (1992). Blunted prolactin responses to *d*-fenfluramine in sociopathy: Evidence for subsensitivity of central serotonergic function. *British Journal of Psychiatry, 160*, 643–646.

Plomin, R., Owen, M. J., & McGuffin, P. (1994). The genetic basis of complex human behaviors. *Science, 264*, 1733–1739.

Raine, A., Sheard, C., Reynolds, G. P., & Lencz, T. (1992). Pre-frontal structural and functional deficits associated with individual differences in schizotypal personality. *Schizophrenia Research, 7*, 237–247.

Roth, A., Ostroff, R., & Hoffman, R. (1996). Naltrexone as a treatment for repetitive self-injurious behavior. *Journal of Clinical Psychiatry, 57*, 233–237.

Salzman, C., Wolfson, A. N., Schatzberg, A., Looper, J., Henke, R., Albanese, M., Schwartz, J., & Miyawaki, E. (1995). Effect of fluoxetine on anger in symptomatic volunteers with borderline personality disorder. *Journal of Clinical Psychopharmacology, 15*, 23–29.

Schulz, S. C., Cornelius, J., Schulz, P. M., et al. (1988). The amphetamine challenge test in patients with borderline personality disorder. *American Journal of Psychiatry, 145*, 809–814.

Schulz, S. C., Schulz, P. M., Dommisse, C., et al. (1985). Amphetamine response in borderline patients. *Psychiatry Research, 15*, 97–108.

Sheard, M., Marini, J., Bridges, C., & Wapner, A. (1976). The effect of lithium on impulsive aggressive behavior in man. *American Journal of Psychiatry, 133*, 1409–1413.

Shihabuddin, L. S., Buchsbaum, M. S., Siever, L. J., et al. (1999). Striatal [18]fluorodeoxyglucose PET and MRI in schizotypal personality disorder. *APA New Research Abstracts* (718).

Siegel, B. V., Treatman, R. L., O'Flaithbheartaigh, S., et al. (1996). D-amphetamine challenge effects in Wisconsin Card Sort test: Performance in schizotypal personality disorder. *Schizophrenia Research, 20*, 29–32.

Siever, L. J., Amin, F., Coccaro, E. F., Bernstein, D., Kavoussi, R. J., Kalus, O., Horvath, T., Warne, P., Davidson, M., & Davis, K. C. (1991). Plasma homovanillic acid in schizotypal personality dis-

order. *American Journal of Psychiatry, 148*, 1246–1248.

Siever, L. J., Amin, F., Coccaro, E. F., Trestman, R., Silverman, T., Horath, T. B., Mahon, T. R., Knott, P., Alstiel, L., Davidson, M., & Davis, L. (1993). CSF homovanillic acid in schizotypal personality disorder. *American Journal of Psychiatry, 150*, 149–151.

Siever, L. J., Buchsbaum, M., New, A., Spiegel-Cohen, J., Wei, T., Hazlett, E., Sevin, E., Nunn, M., & Mitropoulou, V. (1999). *d,l*-fenfluramine response in impulsive personality disorder assessed with [18]Fluorodeoxyglucose positron emission tomography. *Neuropsychopharmacology, 20*, 413–423.

Siever, L. J., Freidman, L., Moskowitz, J., Mitropoulou, V., Keefe, R., Roitman, S. L., Merhie, D., Trestman, R., Silverman, J., & Mohs, R. (1994). Eye movement impairment and schizotypal pathology. *American Journal of Psychiatry, 151*, 1209–1215.

Siever, L. J., Kalus, O. F., & Keefe, R. S. (1993). The boundaries of schizophrenia. *Psychiatric Clinics of North America, 16*, 217–244.

Siever, L., & Trestman, R. L. (1993). The serotonin system and aggressive personality disorder. *International Clinical Psychopharmacology, 8*(Suppl. 2), 33–39.

Silverman, J. M., Smith, C. J., Guo, S. L., Mohs, R. C., Siever, L. J., & Davis, K. (1998). Ventricular volume and asymmetry in schizotypal personality disorder and schizophrenia assessed with magnetic resonance imaging. *Schizophrenia Research, 27*, 45–53.

Simeon, D., Stanley, B., Frances, A., Mann, J. J., Winchel, R., & Stanley, M. (1992). Self-mutilation in personality disorders: Psychological and biological correlates. *American Journal of Psychiatry, 149*, 221–226.

Soloff, P. H., Cornelius, J., George, A., Nathan, S., Perel, J. M., & Ulrich, R. F. (1993). Efficacy of phenelzine and haloperidol in borderline personality disorder. *Archives of General Psychiatry, 50*, 377–385.

Soloff, P. H., George, A., Nathan, R. S., Schulz, P. M., Cornelius, J. R., Herring, J., & Perel, J. M. (1989). Amitriptyline versus haloperidol in borderlines: Final outcomes and predictors of response. *Journal of Clinical Psychopharmacology, 9*, 238–246.

Soloff, P. H., George, A., Nathan, R. S., Schulz, P. M., & Perel, J. M. (1986b). Paradoxical effects of amitriptyline in borderline patients. *American Journal of Psychiatry, 143*, 1603–1605.

Soloff, P. H., George, A., Nathan, R. S., Schulz, P. M., Ulrich, R. F., & Perel, P. M. (1986a). Progress in the pharmacotherapy of borderline disorders: A double-blind study of amitriptyline, haloperidol, and placebo. *Archives of General Psychiatry, 43*, 691–697.

Stanley, M., Ttaksman-Bendz, L., & Dorovini-Zis, K. (1985). Correlations between aminergic metabolites simultaneously obtained from human CSF and brain. *Life Sciences, 37*, 1279–1286.

Steinberg, B. J., Trestman, R., Mitroupolou, V., Serby, M., Silverman, J., Coccaro, E. F., Weston, S., deVegvar, M., & Siever, L. J. (1997). Depressive response to physostigmine challenge in borderline personality disorder patients. *Neuropsychopharmacology, 17*, 264–273.

Valzelli, L. (1980). *Psychobiology of aggression and violence.* New York: Raven Press.

Virkkunen, M., DeJong, J., Bartko, J., Goodwin, F. K., & Linnoila, M. (1989). Relationship of psychobiological variables to recidivism in violent offenders and impulsive fire setters. *Archives of General Psychiatry, 46,* 600–603.

Virkkunen, M., Nuutila, A., Goodwin, F. K., & Linnoila, M. (1987). Cerebrospinal fluid monoamine metabolite levels in male arsonists. *Archives of General Psychiatry, 44,* 241–247.

Yudofsky, S. C., Silver, J. M., & Schneider, S. E. (1987). Pharmacologic treatment of aggression. *Psychiatric Annals, 17,* 397–406.

CHAPTER 7

A Neurobehavioral
Dimensional Model

RICHARD A. DEPUE
MARK F. LENZENWEGER

Since formal derivation of diathetic threshold models of psychiatric disorders (Heston, 1973; Meehl, 1973; Rosenthal & Kety, 1969), there has been increasing interest in the problem of integrating psychobiological dimensions with taxonomic entities. Nowhere has a focus on dimensionality been more prevalent than in modeling personality disorders (Clarkin & Lenzenweger, 1996; Cloninger, 1987; Cloninger, Svrakic, & Przybeck, 1993; Depue, 1996; Francis & Widiger, 1986; Livesley, 1987; Livesley, Jackson, & Schroeder, 1992; Millon, 1996; Rutter, 1987; Siever & Davis, 1991; Wiggins & Pincus, 1989) because (1) there is extensive phenotypical blending across prototypical Axis II entities, suggesting a continuous multidimensional phenotypical gradient rather than distinct disorders (Cloninger, 1987; Widiger, 1992, 1993); and (2) the behavioral features of personality disorders are suggested to reflect extreme variation of normal personality traits (Harkness, 1992; Widiger & Costa, 1994; Widiger, Trull, Clarkin, Sanderson, & Costa, 1994). In the case of personality disorders, viewing the disorder as lying at the extreme of normal personality dimensions is based solely on a phenotypical correlational level of analysis, but no assumption is made herein that phenotypical dimensions are biologically continuous. The phenotypical continuity could well represent

several underlying distinct genotypical distributions (Gottesman, 1997), as may be the case even within the normal range of variation of some personality traits (Benjamin, 1996; Ebstein, 1996).

As a means of providing a framework for all subsequent sections of our discussion, Figure 7.1 outlines several types of extant personality disorder models and the complex issues they embody. As illustrated in Figure 7.1, dimensional models have focused on three pathways (designated A, B, and C) along which sets of variables influence the delineation of personality disorders. Each pathway is associated with complex issues that involve basic assumptions and decisions on the part of the theorist (left column of figure). We discuss these complexities in detail within respective sections focusing on the different pathways. Pathway B has received the most attention to date and represents models of personality disorders that attempt to delineate personality disorder entities or continua through the extreme extension of multiple lower- and/or higher-order personality traits (e.g., Clark, Livesley, Schroeder, & Irish, 1996; Cloninger, 1987; Harkness, 1992; Livesley et al., 1992; Millon, 1996; Widiger & Costa, 1994; Wiggins & Pincus, 1989). Because most dimensional models of personality disorders, including those incorporating neurobiological Pathway C as a component, are completely dependent on the positions adopted in Pathway *B,* this step in modeling personality disorders may be viewed as one of the most critical for the validity of any model. There are great complexities involved at the level of Pathway *B* that are associated with assumptions about the very structure of personality, including (1) its multidimensional composition, (2) the heterogeneity and primary versus emergent status of higher-order traits, and (3) the manner in which multiple traits combine to elaborate personality disorder phenotypes. Therefore, we devote the next entire section of our discussion to this pathway.

Pathway *C* attempts to delineate the neurobiological foundation of the personality traits assumed to elaborate personality disorder phenotypes and, by extension, the neurobiology of personality disorders. Pathway *C* requires a conceptual strategy for selecting neurobiological systems, as well as for extending those systems, by analogy, to personality traits. Thus, by integrating Pathway *C* with Pathway *B,* the complexities of modeling are multiplied substantially. Often the end result of this process is essentially the insufficient one of naming, of stating that neurobiological variable *X* underlies trait *Y.* To provide a more comprehensive foundation for future research on the neurobiology of personality disorders, the functional principles of the neurobiological variables must be derived (i.e., the manner in which they influence behavior), as must the way in which the variables interact with salient environmental stimuli to produce behavior. In view of these complexities, it is not surprising that Cloninger's (1987; Cloninger et al., 1993) work on such a model currently stands alone [note: we concern ourselves only with the temperament dimensions of Cloninger's model, ignoring the character dimensions until sufficient research is available for meaningful analysis). We believe, however, that Cloninger's model suffers from significant limitations with respect to the structure of personality and its neurobiological foundation (Depue & Collins, 1999). Thus, in the spirit of providing an alternative model as a means of promoting comparative research, we outline a neurobehavioral foundation of personality (Pathway C) which we argue resolves a number of taxonomic, measurement, and theoretical issues that currently remain unclear in the extant literature. We then apply that foundation to our own neurobehavioral model of personality disorders.

Pathway *A* represents the model of Siever and Davis (1991) that suggests that Axis I and II disorders lie on a continuum defined by behavioral processes, namely, cognitive/perceptual, impulsivity/aggression, affective instability, and anxiety/inhibition. Thus, understanding the neurobiology of those behavioral processes may delineate the biological nature of disorders of both axes. This is a novel personality disorder model, and although we believe it has significant merit, we do not address it further for three major reasons. First, it lies outside, or at least has not been integrated with, Pathways *B* and C, which serve as the foundation of our proposed model. Second, the selection of behavioral processes that form the substance of the continua in the model seems to us limited. Processes were selected on the basis of the core behavioral features of the broad categories of Axis I disorders (Siever & Davis, 1991), as shown in the top right row of Figure 7.1. We suggest, as shown on the bottom right of Figure 7.1, that this approach to modeling personality disorders would be on firmer ground if a taxonomy of normal behavioral processes derived in the animal research literature (e.g., motivation, emotion, attention, arousal, and cognition) were used, because such behavioral processes would be independent of presumed entities and disturbances found in both Axis I and II disorders. By using such a taxonomy, a Pathway A model would become more broadly dimensional in nature, attempting to integrate behavioral processes from normal functioning through Axis II and I conditions. Third, by selecting behavioral processes associated with disorders, and by characterizing them in some cases in a disturbed form (e.g., affective instability), the focus on particular behavioral processes, per se, runs the risk of missing a more central modulator that influences all the behavioral processes in a uniform manner. For instance, altered values of a central neurobiological modulator (e.g., serotonin; Coccaro & Siever, 1991; Depue & Spoont, 1986; Spoont, 1992) could produce variations in regulation of all behavioral processes, leading to cognitive and behavioral impulsivity, increased aggression, affective instability, and enhanced autonomic arousal. Put differently, focusing on behavioral processes on the basis of their alteration in Axis I disorders rather than on their taxonomic classes is equivalent to predicting personality by sole use of lower-order traits. Higher-order traits provide additional

Dimensional Models of Personality Disorders

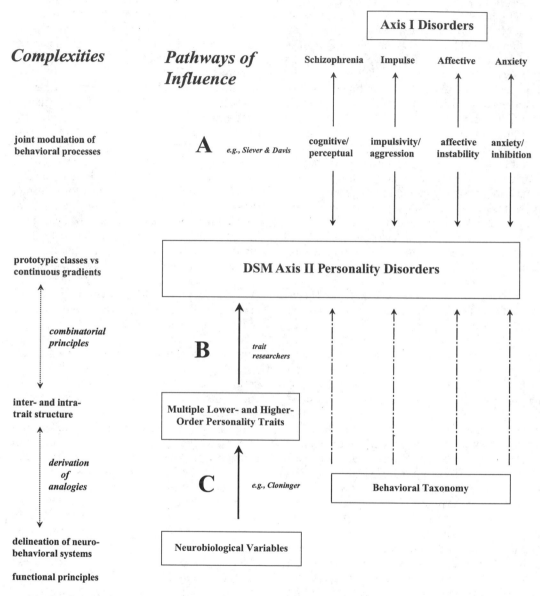

FIGURE 7.1. A framework for visualizing the contribution of several lines of empirical work to pathways of influence (designated *A, B, C*) on personality disorders and the complex issues involved in each pathway. See text for details.

meaning to the lower-order traits because they reflect central modulating factors that jointly influence the lower-order traits (Depue & Collins, 1999).

ISSUES RELATED TO THE STRUCTURE OF PERSONALITY

The higher-order structure of personality is converging on three to seven factors that account for the phenotypical variation in behavior (Digman, 1990; Eysenck & Eysenck, 1985; Tellegen & Waller, in press; Zuckerman, 1994). Although there is considerable agreement on the robustness of at least four higher-order traits, there is nevertheless substantial variation in the definition of these traits because researchers emphasize different characteristics depending on their trait concepts. Our model focuses on the following four higher-order traits that, although robustly identified in the psychometric literature, we uniquely delimit and define with reference to coherent neurobehavioral systems. Higher-order traits resembling *extraversion* and *neuroticism* (anxiety) are identified in virtually every taxonomy of personality (Buss & Plomin, 1984; Cattell, Eber, & Tatsuoka, 1980; Cloninger et al., 1993; Comrey, 1970; Costa & McCrae, 1985, 1992; Digman, 1990; Eysenck & Eysenck, 1985; Goldberg, 1981; Guilford & Zimmerman, 1949; Jackson, 1984; Tellegen & Waller, in press; Watson & Clark, 1996; Zuckerman, Kuhlam, Thornquist, & Kiers, 1991). Affiliation, termed "agreeableness" (Costa & McCrae, 1992; Goldberg & Rosolack, 1994) or "social closeness" (Tellegen & Waller, in press), has emerged more recently as a robust trait, and it comprises affiliative tendencies, cooperativeness, and feelings of warmth and affection. Finally, some form of impulsivity, more recently termed "constraint" (Tellegen & Waller, in press) or "conscientiousness" (due to an emphasis on the unreliability, unorderliness, and disorganization accompanying an impulsive disposition) (Costa & McCrae, 1992; Digman, 1990; Goldberg & Rosolack, 1994), typically emerges in factor studies. Significant complexities are associated with each of these traits which need to be addressed in any model of personality disorders, and we consider these in turn here.

The Agentic and Affiliative Components of Extraversion

Extraversion comprises behavioral and emotional characteristics including social dominance, positive emotional feelings, sociability, achievement, and motor activity. Trait psychologists have emphasized different subsets of these characteristics depending on their concept of extraversion (Watson & Clark, 1997). Despite terminological variation, a higher-order trait resembling extraversion is identified in virtually every taxonomy of personality (Buss & Plomin, 1984; Cattell et al., 1980; Cloninger et al., 1993; Comrey, 1970; Costa & McCrae, 1985, 1992; Digman, 1990; Eysenck & Eysenck, 1985; Goldberg, 1981; Guilford & Zimmerman, 1949; Jackson, 1984; Tellegen & Waller, in press; Zuckerman et al., 1991).

The interpersonal engagement aspect of extraversion is not a unitary characteristic but, rather, has two components. One component, sociability or affiliation, reflects enjoying and valuing close interpersonal bonds, and being warm and affectionate; the other component, agency, reflects social dominance, assertiveness, exhibitionism, and a subjective sense of potency in accomplishing goals. These two components are represented in lower-order traits of extraversion (Cattell et al., 1980; Costa & McCrae, 1992; Goldberg & Rosolack, 1994; Guilford & Zimmerman, 1949; Hogan, 1983; Tellegen & Waller, in press), and are also consistent with the two independent major traits identified in the theory of interpersonal behavior: warm–agreeable versus assured–dominant (Wiggins, 1991; Wiggins, Trapnell, & Phillips, 1988). Recent studies have consistently supported a two-component structure of extraversion in joint factor analyses of multidimensional personality questionnaires (Church, 1994; Church & Burke, 1994; Costa & McCrae, 1989; Morrone, Depue, Scherer & White 2000; Tellegen & Waller, in press), where two general traits were identified in each case as affiliation and agency (Depue & Collins, 1999). Lower-order traits of social dominance, achievement, endurance, persistence, efficacy, activity, and energy all loaded much more strongly on agency than on affiliation, whereas traits of sociability, warmth, and agreeableness showed a reverse pattern. Such findings have led trait psychologists to propose that affiliation and agency represent distinct dispositions (Hogan,

1983; Tellegen & Waller, in press). Whereas affiliation is clearly interpersonal in nature, agency represents a more general disposition that is manifest in a range of achievement-related, as well as interpersonal, contexts (Cattell et al., 1980; Costa & McCrae, 1992; Goldberg & Rosolack, 1994; Guilford & Zimmerman, 1949; Hogan, 1983; Tellegen & Waller, in press; Watson & Clark, 1996; Wiggins, 1991; Wiggins et al., 1988).

The lower-order traits associated with the agency factor represent different manifestations of a single underlying process that activates or motivates *both* social (e.g., social dominance) and work-related (e.g., achievement) goal acquisition (Depue & Collins, 1999). Tellegen has demonstrated that the type of activation linked with extraversion is positive affect, where *affect* means a joint experience of emotional feelings and motivation (Tellegen, 1985; Tellegen et al., 1988; Tellegen & Waller, in press). Accordingly, we (Depue & Collins, 1999) and others (Gray, 1973, 1992; Zuckerman, 1991) have suggested that the positive affect associated with extraversion reflects *positive incentive motivation,* a neurobehavioral system found in all mammals (Schnerla, 1959). Incentive motivational processes encode incentive stimuli for their intensity or salience, thereby attributing a motivational value to the stimuli (Robinson & Berridge, 1993). Subsequent exposure to the incentive stimuli (or activation of their central representation) elicits an incentive motivational state that facilitates and guides approach behavior to a goal. In humans, incentive motivational states are associated with strong positive affect characterized by feelings of desire, wanting, excitement, enthusiasm, energy, potency, and self-efficacy. These feelings are distinct from, but typically co-occur with, feelings of pleasure and liking (MacLean, 1986; Robinson & Berridge, 1993; Watson & Tellegen, 1985). We have proposed that variation in this process of encoding incentive salience is the basis of individual differences in the frequency and intensity of incentive motivation and, by extension, is the main source of individual differences in the agentic form of extraversion (Depue & Collins, 1999).

In contrast, when broadly conceived, affiliation is a neurobehavioral system observed in all mammals which promotes and maintains sexual and social contact and cohesion among members of kinship groups for varying temporal durations, depending on the species. As a neurobehavioral system, affiliation involves a number of components elicited by various specific types of nonaversive tactile, olfactory, visual, and vocal stimulation. These components include *facilitation* of (1) a positive reinforcement mechanism (social reward); (2) sensory processing pathways; (3) sexual, reproductive, and parenting functions; (4) formation of social memories; and (5) subjective feelings of warmth, affection, and caring in humans (Carter, Lederhendler, & Kirkpatrick, 1997; Dichiara, Acquas, & Carboni, 1992). Generally, the strong activational component of incentive motivation that characterizes the approach and initial interactive phases of sociosexual behavior gives way in later affiliative stages to a state of calm affection and pleasure that facilitates maintenance of interactions.

Independence of Neuroticism (Anxiety) and Harm Avoidance (Fear)

On the basis of neuroanatomical and behavioral studies, Davis, Walker, & Younglim, 1997) and others (LeDoux, 1996) proposed that fear evolved as a means of escaping unconditioned aversive stimuli that are inherently dangerous to survival, such as tactile pain, predator smells, injury contexts, snakes, spiders, heights, approaching strangers, and sudden sounds. These *discrete, explicit* stimuli elicit short-latency, high-magnitude phasic responses of autonomic arousal and behavioral escape, whereas conditioned fear stimuli elicit freezing, suppression of operant behavior, autonomic arousal, pain inhibition, and reflex potentiation. If present, safety cues (incentives) activate incentive motivation, which facilitates active avoidance behavior (Depue & Collins, 1999). In contrast, *nondiscrete, contextual* stimuli denoting potential danger (e.g., constant environmental bright light for nocturnal rats and darkness for humans), where no explicit aversive stimuli are present to inherently activate escape circuitries, are associated with autonomic arousal and *anxiety* that lasts as long as the contextual threat but not with behavioral inhibition (Davis et al., 1997). Because stimulus conditions for anxiety are associated with uncertainty, autonomic arousal reverberates until the uncertainty is resolved, which may be the functional goal of the heightened attentional scanning and cognitive worrying and rumination so typical of anxiety states. Thus, Davis et al. (1997) and Barlow (1988) suggest that the

TABLE 7.1. Correlation between Trait Measures of Fear and Anxiety

Fear	Anxiety		
	Tellegen NEM	Eysenck N	STAI
Tellegen Harm Avoidance	−.03	−.02	
Jackson Harm Avoidance			.05
Lykken Physical Activity		−.01	.05
Hodges Physical Danger			.02
Zuckerman SSS reversed	.08	.04	

stimulus conditions and behavioral characteristics of fear and anxiety are different, but that a similar state of intense autonomic arousal is associated with both emotional states, rendering them similar at the subjective level.

The trait literature demonstrates that anxiety (neuroticism) and fear (harm avoidance) are independent and subject to distinct sources of genetic variation (Tellegen et al., 1988). As the averaged correlations derived from numerous studies in Tables 7.1, 7.2 and 7.3 show, the relation between neuroticism and harm avoidance is essentially zero (White & Depue, 1999). As shown in Tables 7.2 and 7.3, the magnitude of emotional distress and autonomic arousal elicited by discrete stimuli associated with physical harm (Table 7.2) is significantly related to harm avoidance but not to neuroticism, whereas conditions of uncertainty associated with external evaluations of the self (Table 7.3) are significantly related to neuroticism but not to harm avoidance (White & Depue, 1999). Furthermore, Table 7.2 shows that, in contrast

to Gray's (1973, 1992) and Cloninger's (1987; Cloninger et al., 1993) theoretical position that anxiety is associated with behavioral inhibition, it is harm avoidance rather than neuroticism that correlates significantly with indices of behavioral inhibition in contexts of physical danger. This point is also supported by the fact that in most multidimensional personality questionnaires, neuroticism is orthogonal to higher-order traits of behavioral constraint (Costa & McCrae, 1992; Eysenck & Eysenck, 1985; Goldberg & Rosolack, 1994; Tellegen & Waller, 1998; Zuckerman et al., 1991), whereas harm avoidance loads preferentially on such a trait (Tellegen & Waller, in press). Indeed, one of the most reliable indices of conditioned fear in animals is behavioral inhibition (Davis et al., 1997; LeDoux, 1996a; Panksepp, 1998), which is not the case for stimulus-induced anxiety (Davis et al., 1997). Thus, from the standpoint of eliciting stimuli and behavioral inhibition, neuroticism and harm avoidance are distinctly different traits, and analysis of clinical anxiety disorders reached equivalent conclusions (Barlow, 1988).

Impulsivity as a Heterogeneous Construct

Impulsivity comprises a heterogeneous cluster of lower-order traits that includes sensation seeking, risk taking, novelty seeking, boldness, adventuresomeness, boredom susceptibility, unreliability, and unorderliness. This lack of specificity is reflected in the fact that the content of the measures of impulsivity is heterogeneous, and that not all these measures are highly interrelated (Depue & Collins, 1999). Despite this heterogeneity, Zuckerman (1991, 1999) argues that there is a specific sensation-seeking motive underlying this trait complex that activates interest in and exploration of nov-

TABLE 7.2. Correlation of Emotional Distress, Behavioral Inhibition, and Heart Rate (HR) and Electrodermal Responses to Aversive Stimuli with Trait Measures of Fear and Anxiety

Trait	Emotional distress					Behavioral inhibition				Threatened shock		
											Electrodermal	
	Dark	Heights	Rat	Snake	Shock	Heights	Rat	Snake	Cockroach	HR	Specific	Nonspecific
Fear	.40	.43	.54	.62	.64	.44	.35	.51	.46	.48	.43	.53
Anxiety	.17	.20		.14	.04	.15		.07		.09	.14	.17

TABLE 7.3. Correlation of Emotional Distress to Contexts Associated with Threats to the Self with Trait Measures of Fear and Anxiety

Trait	Exam	Intelligence test	Public speaking	Failure feedback
Fear	.11	.09	.05	.08
Anxiety	.48	.47	.57	.52

el and intense stimulation. We (Depue & Collins, 1999) demonstrated elsewhere, however, that at least five different neurobehavioral systems may underlie this trait complex:

1. *Positive incentive motivation,* associated with exploration of novel stimulus conditions (Bindra, 1978; Cloninger, 1987; Cloninger et al., 1993; Fink & Reis, 1980).
2. *Fear,* as indicated in risk taking, attraction to physically dangerous activities, and lack of fear of physical harm.
3. *Aggression,* which Zuckerman (1999) views as integral to sensation seeking and risk taking as a means of acquiring resources. This may involve two forms of aggression that may be neurobiologically different: (a) *affective aggression* that supports removal of obstacles to acquiring resources; and (b) *competitive or instrumental aggression* that is involved in striving for priority to resources, such as social dominance (Davis et al., 1997; Depue & Collins, 1999; LeDoux, 1996b; Panksepp, 1998);
4. *Low levels of a nonaffective form of impulsivity,* which results in disinhibition of the above neurobehavioral systems, as suggested by several researchers (Depue, 1995, 1996; Depue & Spoont, 1986; Panksepp, 1998; Spoont, 1992; Zuckerman, 1991, 1999).

Thus, impulsivity emerges from the interaction of at least four to five independent neurobehavioral systems. This complexity is increased when a postulated interaction of impulsivity with extraversion is considered, where positions vary from complete independence (Costa & McCrae, 1992; Eysenck & Eysenck, 1985; Goldberg & Rosolack, 1994; Guilford, 1975, 1977; Rocklin & Revelle, 1981; Tellegen & Waller, in press; Zuckerman, 1994) to interaction (Cloninger, 1987; Cloninger et al., 1993; Eysenck, 1981; Gray, 1973, 1992).

For instance, on the basis of Jung's concept of extraversion, Eysenck and Eysenck (1985) included impulsivity in their measure of extraversion, only to remove it later because evidence indicated that impulsivity and extraversion were independent traits (Guilford, 1975, 1977; Rocklin & Revelle, 1981). Nevertheless, Eysenck (Eysenck, 1981; Eysenck & Eysenck, 1985) continued to define nine lower-order traits of extraversion that include sensation seeking, venturesomeness, carefree, and lively, whereas impulsivity itself is included in the higher-order trait of psychoticism. Moreover, Gray (1973, 1992) proposed that impulsivity represents an interaction of the higher-order traits of extraversion, neuroticism, and psychoticism. Similarly, Cloninger's (1987) personality questionnaire replaces extraversion with a higher-order trait of novelty seeking which is aligned closely with impulsivity and sensation seeking ("disorderly and unpredictable," "seeks thrilling adventures," "spends on impulse"; p. 576). For instance, the Novelty Seeking scale correlated only moderately with Eysenck Personality Questionnaire (EPQ) Extraversion, fell on a different factor than Extraversion in two twin samples (Heath, Cloninger, & Martin, 1994; Stallings, Hewitt, Cloninger, Heath, & Eaves, 1996), and only partially accounted for genetic influences on Extraversion in a twin sample (Heath et al., 1994). On the other hand, the Novelty Seeking scale correlated .70 with the impulsivity-sensation seeking scale from the Zuckerman–Kuhlman Personality Questionnaire (Zuckerman et al., 1991; Zuckerman, personal communication, 1995), correlated positively with EPQ Psychoticism in males (Heath et al., 1994) and loaded on a factor along with EPQ Psychoticism (Stallings et al., 1996). Not surprisingly, then, four of the lower-order scales of Novelty Seeking emphasize a mixture of impulsivity, sensation seeking, agency, and activation (Cloninger, Przybeck, & Svrakic, 1991, Cloninger et al., 1993; Heath et al., 1994; Stallings et al., 1996), and correlate low with EPQ Extraversion (.45, .17, .20, .18; Stallings et al., 1996). Furthermore, a comparison of Cloninger's and Tellegen's multidimensional questionnaires also appeared to clarify the much stronger association of Novelty Seeking with impulsivity, as five of the six lower-order Novelty Seeking scales correlated from −.32 to −.64 with Tellegen's lower-order scale of Impulsivity, and the latter had the highest loading of all of both Tellegen's and

Cloninger's lower-order scales on the higher-order Novelty Seeking trait (Waller, Lilienfeld, Tellegen, & Lykken, 1991). Conversely, the remaining Novelty Seeking lower-order scale, Dramatic versus Laconic, produced the only correlation above .30 with any of Tellegen's lower-order extraversion scales (specifically, .49 with Social Potency, a primary marker of agentic extraversion).

As a means of disentangling and clarifying this complexity (see Figure 7.2), we plotted the trait loadings derived in 11 studies (Depue & Colins, 1999) in which two or more multidimensional personality questionnaires were jointly factor-analyzed to derive general, higher-order traits of personality. All studies identified a higher-order trait of impulsivity that *lacks affective content*, which in Figure 7.2 was labeled as "constraint" following Tellegen (1985; Tellegen & Waller, in press), who introduced the term to emphasize its independence from affective traits such as extraversion and neuroticism. All studies also found constraint to be orthogonal to a general, higher-order extraversion trait. Figure 7.2 shows a continuous distribution of traits within the two intersecting orthogonal dimensions of extraversion and constraint. Nevertheless, three relatively homogeneous clusterings of traits can be delineated on the basis of the position and content of traits, relative to extraversion and constraint. First, lower-order traits associated with agentic extraversion (sociability, dominance, achievement, positive emotions, activity, energy) cluster at the high end of the extraversion dimension without substantial association with constraint. A tight clustering of most traits to extraversion is evident. Second, various traits of impulsivity that *do not incorporate strong positive affect* (e.g., Conscientiousness) cluster tightly around the high end of the constraint dimension without substantial association with extraversion; Eysenck's Psychoticism trait and various aggression measures are located at the low end of constraint and show little association with extraversion. The anchoring of the two extreme ends of constraint by Conscientiousness and Psychoticism was also observed by Zuckerman (1991). Third, all but one trait measure of impulsivity *that incorporate positive affect* (sensation seeking, novelty seeking, risk-taking) are located within the dashed lines in Figure 7.2, and are moderately associated with both extraversion and constraint. Thus, currently most trait models of personality separate a nonaffec-

tive form of impulsivity and extraversion into distinct traits, although the terms used for the former vary from Conscientiousness (Costa & McCrae, 1985, 1992; Goldberg & Rosolack, 1994) to Constraint (Tellegen & Waller, in press) and Impulsivity–Unsocialized Sensation Seeking (Zuckerman, 1994; Zuckerman et al., 1991).

Conceptually, the complexity of impulsivity can be clarified by hypothesizing that *nonaffective* constraint lacks ties to a specific motivational system (Depue & Collins, 1999). As discussed in detail later, a vast body of animal and human literature demonstrates that constraint so conceived functions as a central nervous system variable that modulates the threshold of stimulus elicitation of motor behavior, both positive and negative affective systems, and cognition (Coccaro & Siever, 1991; Depue, 1995, 1996; Depue & Spoont, 1986; Mandel, 1984; Panksepp, 1998; Spoont, 1992; Zald & Depue in press; Zuckerman, 1991). This formulation is consistent with findings that low constraint is associated in both animals and humans with a generalized motor–cognitive–affective impulsivity but is not preferentially associated with any specific motivational system (Depue & Spoont, 1986; Spoont, 1992; Zald & Depue, in press). Alternatively, *affective* impulsivity emerges from the interaction of nonaffective constraint with other distinct affective–motivational systems, such as positive incentive motivation–agentic extraversion (as in Figure 7.2) or anxiety–neuroticism. Gray's (1973, 1992) theoretical treatment of neuroticism as a general amplifier of reactivity to both signals of reward and punishment, hence influencing the magnitude of both positive affective impulsivity and anxiety, is consistent with this concept of constraint. Similarly, Eysenck's psychoticism trait and Zuckerman et al.'s (1991) Impulsivity–Unsocialized Sensation Seeking trait partially overlap this conceptualization. Thus, two separate neurobehavioral systems, in interaction, create those traits/behaviors that other theorists have merged into a common dimension (Cloninger, 1986; Gray, 1973, 1992; Zuckerman et al., 1991).

Lines of Causal Neurobiological Influence in the Structure of Personality

Although much has been learned about the structure of personality, Gray's (1973, 1992)

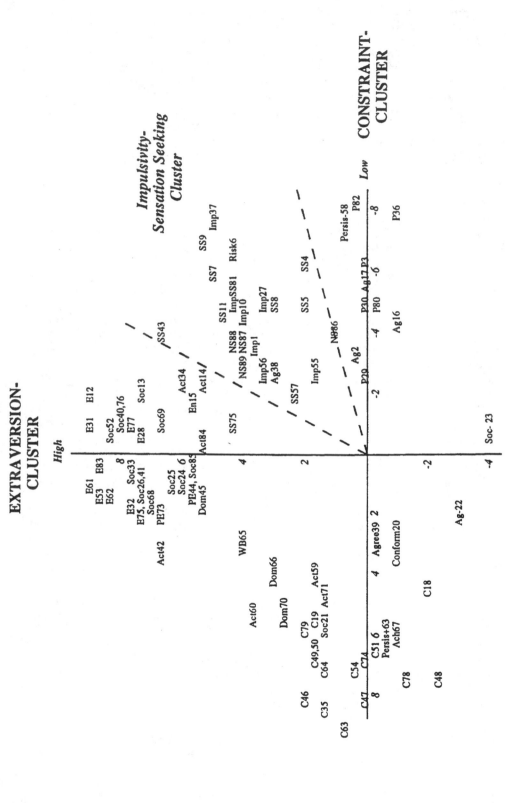

FIGURE 7.2 A plotting of loadings of personality traits derived in 11 studies in which more than one multidimensional personality questionnaire was jointly factor-analyzed as a means of deriving general traits of personality. All these studies defined a general nonaffective impulsivity trait, referred to as constraint (horizontal dimension in the figure), that was separate from the general extraversion trait (vertical dimension in the figure). The figure illustrates three clusterings of traits: an extraversion cluster at the high end of the extraversion dimension; conscientiousness and psychoticism–aggression clusters at the high and low end of the constraint dimension, respectively; and an impulsivity–sensation seeking cluster within the dashed lines. The figure also illustrates that extraversion and *nonaffective* constraint dimensions are generally identified and found to be orthogonal, and that impulsivity–sensation seeking traits *associated with strong positive affective* arise as a joint function of the interaction of extraversion and constraint. See Depue and Collins (1999) for the identity of the trait measure abbreviations with numbers, the questionnaires to which the abbreviations correspond, and the studies providing the trait loadings.

challenge concerning where the lines of causal influence lie within that structure remains cogent. The most critical issue here is that psychometrically derived higher-order traits often represent heterogeneous phenotypes, which may be reflected in a heterogeneous set of lower-order traits that have different sources of genetic variation (Livesley, Jang, & Vernon, 1998; Tellegen et al., 1988). Such heterogeneous higher-order traits as typically conceived are likely associated with two or more behavioral systems and neurobiological networks, rendering the search for neurobiological foundations of personality and personality disorders problematic. Perhaps the heterogeneous, emergent trait complex of impulsive sensation seeking will turn out to be a much richer way to index behavior than, for instance, using extraversion and nonaffective constraint in a combinatorial way (though from a measurement standpoint, such measures should be somewhat less reliable as they seek to capture an interactive product rather than a homogeneous latent dimension). But, when the research focus concerns the best way to discover the underlying neurobiological networks and neurotransmitters associated with phenotypical traits, we believe that less heterogeneous higher-order traits related to single evolutionarily preserved neurobehavioral systems provide the clearest path to causal neurobiological influences within personality structure. This position involves a psychometric strategy that purposefully attempts to remove covariation between traits that may exist naturally at the phenotypical level in order to derive trait measures that index neurobehavioral systems as purely as possible (Tellegen & Waller, in press). This is the reverse of the strategy espoused by others (Cloninger, 1987; Gray, 1973) of developing trait measures that attempt to assess that phenotypical heterogeneity.

Our (Depue & Collins, 1999) analysis of the trait literature suggests that neuroticism (anxiety), fear, agentic extraversion, and affiliation are relatively homogeneous traits based on coherent neurobehavioral systems. We hypothesize that these traits represent primary sources of causal neurobiological influence within the structure of personality. The vast majority of studies reviewed previously have also identified a higher-order trait of nonaffective constraint that is orthogonal to extraversion, neuroticism, and affiliation. Its scales, however (e.g., Conscientiousness, Costa & McCrae, 1992; Gold-

berg & Rosolack, 1994; Constraint, Tellegen, & Waller, in press), are composed of several behavioral domains, including nonaffective impulsivity, traditionalism, and fear. Phenotypically, all these domains modulate the level of expressed impulsivity, but they are not neurobiologically equivalent (Depue, 1995, 1996). It is specifically the nonaffective impulsivity component that best conforms to our concept of constraint as a central threshold variable. In this specific manner, we hypothesize that nonaffective constraint represents another primary line of causal neurobiological influence in personality.

It is positive affective impulsivity where the greatest disagreement lies concerning lines of causal influence. Gray (1973, 1992), Cloninger (1986, 1987; Cloninger et al., 1991), and Zuckerman (1991) have argued that a major line of *neurobiological* influence lies with the cluster of impulsivity and sensation seeking traits shown in Figure 7.2. Indeed, Cloninger (1986, 1987; Cloninger et al., 1991) has consistently argued that Novelty Seeking was designed to assess an underlying biogenetic dimension of personality and, therefore, reflects more directly the relevant causal neurobiological influences than does extraversion. We are in basic disagreement with the positions of Gray, Cloninger, and Zuckerman concerning the lines of causal *neurobiological* influence. On the basis of the foregoing discussion, we locate the causal lines of neurobiological influence along the two orthogonal dimensions of agentic extraversion and nonaffective constraint. Because agentic extraversion and constraint have genetically independent neurobiological influences (Tellegen et al., 1988), the emergent trait of positive affective impulsivity would necessarily have heterogeneous neurobiological sources of influence. For instance, in Gray's (1973, 1992) model, impulsivity emerges from two levels of complex interactions between the higher-order traits of extraversion and neuroticism. First, extraversion in Gray's model represents the interaction of the relative strength of sensitivities to two distinct classes of stimulus—signals of reward (more the extravert) and punishment (more the introvert). The model is affectively bipolar, with high and low extremes of extraversion being associated with different predominant affective states—positive versus negative. Sensitivities to these two stimulus classes undoubtedly have distinct neurobiological foundations. Second, Gray's intrinsically complex trait of extraversion interacts with neuroticism (defined as a modulator of the stimulus-elicited magnitude of all affective systems—similar to our concept of nonaffective constraint), entailing the further influence of at least one more neurobiological variable. The result is the emergent trait of impulsivity, and research attempting to detect a neurobiological variable strongly and specifically associated with that heterogeneous trait may likely produce weaker and more inconsistent results than with the more primary traits. Therefore, although neurobiological variables associated with those contributing sources will be correlated with the emergent trait, we believe that neurobehavioral systems underlying personality are more directly modeled when homogeneous traits are studied (Depue & Collins, 1999).

It is worth noting that bipolar construction of higher-order trait measures, where the phenotypical expression marking the opposite ends of the dimension is dissimilar, often signal heterogeneity of underlying neurobehavioral systems, as in Gray's conception of extraversion discussed earlier. Higher-order traits based on single affective neurobehavioral–motivational systems are naturally affectively unipolar. Positive incentive motivation, for instance, is associated with a unipolar dimension of positive affect, ranging from strong presence to complete absence at the extremes, rather than a bipolar dimension of positive versus negative affect (Tellegen & Waller, in press; Watson & Tellegen, 1985). Similarly, anxiety or a negative affective system is associated with a unipolar dimension of negative affect, ranging from strong presence of anxiety at one extreme of the dimension to an absence of negative affect (i.e., contentment and calmness) at the other extreme, rather than a bipolar dimension of negative versus positive affect, respectively (Tellegen & Waller, in press; Watson & Tellegen, 1985).

Argument far exceeds data in the debate over where to locate lines of causal influence within the structure of personality. However, data, such as they exist, do provide some measure of meaning and direction in this area. Nevertheless, a theoretical position is important because it ultimately directs the search in the animal literature for the neurobiological foundations of those traits. Moreover, it directs comparative analyses between personality disorder models, and in this sense our divergence from Cloninger's (1986, 1987) personality and Tridimensional Personality Questionnaire (TPQ)

model and the five-factor model of personality is important to summarize. Our model differs from the five-factor model (Costa & McCrae, 1992; Goldberg & Rosolack, 1994) in that, *to us,* the higher-order traits and their lower-order scales lack a clear theoretical basis in neurobehavioral systems that would help to delimit heterogeneity and to clarify a neurobiological foundation. With respect to Cloninger's model, the heterogeneity of both TPQ Novelty Seeking (predominantly impulsivity–sensation seeking with some agentic extraversion) and TPQ Harm Avoidance (multiply associated with low agentic extraversion and fear, but predominantly with anxiety), which may contribute to the relatively low internal reliabilities of lower-order TPQ traits, places those traits outside our approach to structuring personality (Heath et al., 1994; Stallings et al., 1996; Waller et al., 1991). The same is true of TPQ Reward Dependence, which required splitting the persistence scale off from that factor. Whether *persistence* is an independent trait needs investigation, as Waller et al. (1991) found it most closely associated with Tellegen's Multidimensional Personality Questionnaire (MPQ) Achievement, which is a component of agentic extraversion. Second, the lack of differentiation of fear and anxiety in Cloninger's conception of harm avoidance is not supported by data. Third, Cloninger's personality structure and TPQ does not define nor independently measure four traits that we believe are important in modeling personality disorders: (1) nonaffective constraint, (2) affiliation (although components of Reward Dependence may be related), (3) fear, and (4) aggression (e.g., Waller et al., 1991, found no correlate in the TPQ of MPQ Aggression).

A NEUROBEHAVIORAL FOUNDATION OF PERSONALITY TRAITS

Behavioral systems may be understood as behavior patterns that evolved to adapt to stimuli critical for survival and species preservation (Gray, 1973; MacLean, 1986; Panksepp, 1986; Schneirla, 1959). As opposed to specific behavioral systems that guide interaction with very specific stimulus contexts, *general* behavioral systems are more flexible and have less immediate objectives and more variable topographies (Blackburn, Phillips, Jakubovic, & Fibiger, 1989; MacLean, 1986). General systems are activated by broad *classes* of stimuli (Depue, in press; Gray, 1973; Rolls, 1986), and regulate general emotional–behavioral dispositions, such as desire–approach or fear–inhibition, that modulate goal-directed activity. It is the general systems that directly influence the structure of mammalian behavior at higher-order levels of organization, because, like higher-order personality traits, their modulatory effects on behavior derive from frequent activation by broad stimulus classes. Thus, the higher-order traits of personality, which are general and few, are most likely to reflect the activity of a few, general neurobehavioral systems.

In developing neurobehavioral models of personality traits below, we followed the strategy outlined in Figure 7.3. Personality psychology was used to define a trait's behavioral, emotional, and motivational characteristics. Next, we identified a mammalian behavior pattern with corresponding characteristics, as described in the psychological and ethological literatures. Once an analogous motivation was identified, animal neurobiological research provided empirical links to its neural organization and neurochemical modulation. These hypotheses were then extended to personality.

Agentic Extraversion

We (Depue & Collins, 1999) recently provided a comprehensive neurobehavioral framework of the incentive motivational foundation of agentic extraversion. Thus only an outline is presented here. Described in all animals across phylogeny (Bindra, 1978; Hebb, 1949; Schneir-

la, 1959), a behavioral approach system based on incentive motivation is activated by, and serves to bring an animal in contact with, unconditioned and conditioned positive incentive stimuli (Beninger, 1983; Depue, in press; Gray, 1973; Hebb, 1949; Koob, Robledo, Markou, & Caine, 1993; Panksepp, 1986; Schneirla, 1959; Stewart, de Wit, & Eikelboom, 1984). We reviewed (Depue & Collins, 1999) an immense body of literature which demonstrates that the ventral tegmental area (VTA) dopamine (DA) projections to the caudomedial shell region of the NAS (NAS$_{shell}$) play a critical role in the facilitation of incentive motivation, temporal maintenance of an incentive motivational state, and many goal-directed behaviors that are dependent on incentive motivation. Indeed, VTA DA neurons preferentially respond to stimuli that consistently predict reward, thereby facilitating early in a behavioral sequence the approach to rewards (Schultz et al., 1995; Schultz, Dayan, & Montague, 1997).

Animal research demonstrates that *individual differences in DA* functioning contribute significantly to variation in incentive-motivated behavior (Cabib & Puglisi-Allegra, 1996; Le Moal & Simon, 1991; Phillips, 1997; Piazza & Le Moal, 1996; Puglisi-Allegra & Cabib, 1997; Robinson, 1988). Inbred mouse and rat strains with variation in the number of neurons in the VTA DA cell group or several indicators of enhanced DA transmission show marked differences in behaviors dependent on DA transmission in the VTA–NAS pathway, including levels of spontaneous exploratory activity and DA agonist-induced locomotor activity, and increased

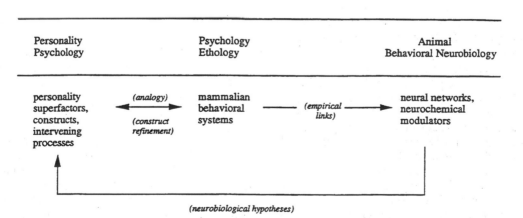

FIGURE 7.3. A modeling strategy for deriving neurobiological hypotheses about higher-order traits of personality. See text for details.

acquisition of self-administration of psycho-
stimulants (Cabib & Puglisi-Allegra, 1996;
Camp, Bowman, & Robinson, 1994; Fink &
Reis, 1981; George & Goldberg, 1988; George,
Porrino, Ritz, & Goldberg, 1991; Oades, 1985;
Phillips, 1997; Puglisi-Allegra & Cabib, 1997;
Ross, Judd, Pickel, Joh, & Reis, 1976; Segal &
Kuczenski, 1987; Shuster, Yu, & Bates, 1977;
Sved, Baker & Reis, 1984, 1985).

Models of individual differences in DA-in-
duced behavioral facilitation often employ a
minimum threshold that represents a central
nervous system weighting of the external and
internal factors that contribute to response facilitation (Stricker & Zigmond, 1986; White,
1986). The threshold is weighted most strongly
by the joint function of two main variables:
magnitude of incentive stimulation, and level of
DA postsynaptic receptor activation (Blackburn
et al., 1989; Cools, 1980; Mogenson, Grudzynski, Wu, Yang, & Yin, 1993; Oades, 1985; Scatton, D'Angio, Driscoll, & Serrano, 1988;
White, 1986). The relation between these two
variables is represented in Figure 7.4 as a trade-
off function (Grill & Coons, 1976; White,
1986), where pairs of values (of incentive magnitude and DA activation) specify a diagonal
representing the minimum threshold value for
response facilitation. Because the two input
variables are interactive, independent variation
in either one not only modifies the probability
of response facilitation but also simultaneously
modifies the value of the other variable that is
required to reach a minimum threshold for facilitation. The main determinant of facilitatory
efficacy of incentive stimuli is the magnitude of
reward because it is stongly related to the induced level of DA transmission and to the probability of response facilitation (Blackburn et
al., 1989; Koob, 1992; Koob et al., 1993;
Schultz, 1986; Schultz et al., 1995; White,
1986).

This facilitation model allows behavioral predictions that help to conceptualize the effects of
individual differences in DA functioning in extraversion. A trait dimension of VTA DA postsynaptic receptor activation is represented on the
horizontal axis of Figure 7.4, where two individuals with divergent trait levels are demarcated: A
(low trait level) and B (high trait level). First, for
any given incentive stimulus, the degree of state
DA response will, on average, be larger in individual B versus A. Because degree of state DA
activity affects the salience of incentive stimuli,
the subjective emotional and motivational expe-

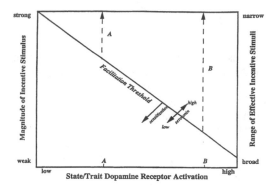

FIGURE 7.4. A minimum threshold for behavioral
facilitation is illustrated as a trade-off function between incentive stimulus magnitude (left vertical
axis) and dopamine postsynaptic receptor activation
(horizontal axis). Range of effective (facilitating) incentive stimuli is illustrated on the right vertical axis
as a function of level of dopamine activation. Two
hypothetical individuals with low and high *trait*
dopamine postsynaptic receptor activation (demarcated on the horizontal axis as A and B, respectively)
are shown to have narrow (A) and broad (B) ranges
of effective incentive stimuli, respectively. Threshold
effects due to serotonin modulation and sensitization
of dopamine transmission are illustrated as well.
Adapted from Depue and Collins (1999). Copyright
1999 by Cambridge University Press. Adapted by
permission.

riences that are naturally elicited by incentive
stimuli and that are part of extraversion—elation–euphoria, desire, incentive motivation,
sense of potency or self-efficacy—will also be
more enhanced in B versus A (Koob, 1992;
Koob et al., 1993; Stewart et al., 1984). Second,
the difference between individuals A and B in
magnitude of subjective experience may contribute to variation in the contemporaneous encoding of a stimulus's incentive intensity or
salience (a form of state-dependent learning)
and, hence, in the incentive salience encoded
during subsequent memory consolidation
(Robinson & Berridge, 1993). Accordingly, individuals A and B may develop differences in the
capacity of mental representations of incentive
contexts to activate incentive motivational
processes, which is significant due to the predominant motivation of behavior in humans by
symbolic representations of goals (Mishkin,
1982). Third, as shown on the right horizontal
axis of Figure 7.4, trait differences in DA transmission may have marked effects on the *range* of
effective (i.e., facilitating) incentive stimuli. The
broader range of effective incentives for individ-

ual *B* suggests that, on average, *B* will experience more frequent elicitation of approach behavior and more pervasive positive emotional and motivational feelings associated with extraversion. This may help to explain the *high stability* of extraversion over time (Costa & McCrae, 1992). Because VTA DA functioning plays an integral part in (1) determining the range of effective incentive stimuli that have access to an individual, and (2) the extent to which those stimuli are connected to and gain influence over VTA DA and NAS neurons, individual differences in VTA DA functioning will modulate both of these processes and, hence, the extent to which salient incentive contexts facilitate incentive motivational and behavioral processes over time. Finally, because variation in DA facilitation is associated with behavioral flexibility when changes in motor, affective, and cognitive response patterns are required by environmental circumstances (Oades, 1985), individual *B* versus *A* is predicted to manifest more flexible (or facilitated) adaptation to environmental contingencies as they fluctuate over time.

Dopamine's Facilitation of Connections between the Salient Incentive Context and Incentive Motivational Processes

The foregoing view of DA functioning in agentic extraversion does not address how salient environmental incentives actually become neurally connected to, and continue to elicit, incentive motivational processes such that individual differences develop in agentic extraversion. Recent work provides a framework for such considerations.

The salient context of incentive reward includes distinctive attributes of incentive stimuli (modality, size, color, scent, texture, etc.) as well as their immediate sensory surround (position, location of targets of action, etc.), both of which are integrated with respect to internal drive states, desirability of action, and intended actions in the near future. This context is transmitted to VTA DA and NAS neurons via glutamatergic excitatory afferents arising from several sources (Christie, Summers, Stephenson, Cook, & Beart, 1987; Fuller, Russchen, & Price, 1987; Gronewegen, Berendse, Wolters, & Lohman, 1990; Groves et al., 1995; Kapp, 1992; Meredith et al., 1993; Mishkin & Appenzeller, 1987; Sesack & Pickel, 1990, 1992; Takagishi & Chiba, 1991):

1. The basolateral complex of the amygdala, which associates *discrete, explicit* stimuli with reinforcement (Aggleton, 1992; Everitt & Robbins, 1992; Gaffan, 1992; Kalivas, Churchill, & Klitenick, 1993; Kalivas, Bush, & Hanson, 1995; Wright, Beijer, & Groenwegen, 1996).
2. Regions comprising the extended amygdala, which integrate information related to reinforcement, stimulus–reward associations, and motivation (Heimer, Alheid, & Zahm, 1993; Koob et al., 1993; Everitt & Robbins, 1992; Mogenson et al., 1993; Pert, Post, & Weiss, 1992). As shown in Figure 7.5, the extended amygdala stretches from the central and medial nuclei of the amygdala through the sublenticular area and bed nucleus of the stria terminalis (BNST) and merges specifically with the NAS_{shell}.
3. The hippocampus, which associates spatial and contextual interrelations of environmental stimuli with reinforcement (Annett, McGregor, & Robbins, 1989; Everitt & Robbins, 1992; Gaffan, 1992; Selden, Everitt, Jarrard, & Robbins, 1991; Sutherland & McDonald, 1990).
4. Posterior medial orbital prefrontal cortical area 13, which abstracts an integrated structure of appetitive and aversive behavioral contingencies from the environment, allowing a comparison of the valence and magnitude of outcome expectancies associated with several possible response strategies (Deutch, Bourdelais, & Zahm, 1993; Goldman-Rakic, 1995; Houk, Adams, & Barto, 1995; Kalivas et al., 1993; Rolls, 1986, 1999; Thorpe, Rolls, & Madisson, 1983; Watanabe, 1990).

Indeed, a recent human PET study showed that, after DA-agonist facilitated association of context with incentive motivation, subsequent presentation of that same context activates prefrontal and amygdala regions, as well as an increase in positive affect (Grant, London, & Newlin, 1996).

A glutamate–DA interaction is an important dynamic between the cortical and limbic contextual inputs and VTA DA and NAS neurons. As illustrated on the right of Figure 7.6, VTA DA efferents to medium spiny neurons in the NAS interdigitate on dendritic spines with the contextual corticolimbic glutamatergic inputs, reciprocally strengthening release of both transmitters (Kalivas, 1995; Lu, Chen, Xue, &

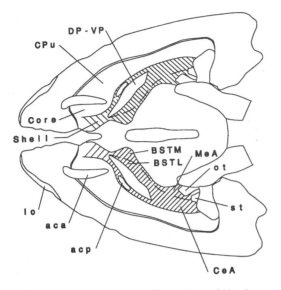

FIGURE 7.5. Schematic illustration of the large forebrain continuum referred to as the extended amygdala (hatched area). This drawing was composed with the aid of several angiotensin II–immunostained horizontal sections of the rat brain ventral to the crossing of the anterior commissure. Because the sublenticular part of the central extended amygdala is located lateral and slightly rostral and dorsal to the medial division of the extended amygdala, the structure appears broader in the diagram where the outline of these divisions are projected onto one horizontal plane than it would in a single histological section. Note the extension of the extended amygdala into the shell of the acuumbens. Abbreviations: aca, anterior commissure, anterior limb; acp, anterior commisusure, posterior limb; BSTL, lateral division of the bed nucleus of the stria terminalis; BSTM, medial division of the bed nucleus of the stria terminalis; CeA, central amygdaloid nucleus; MeA, medial amygdaloid nucleus; CPu, cuadate putamen; DP, dorsal pallidum; lo, lateral olfactory tract; ot, optic tract; st, stria terminalis; VP, vental pallidum. Adapted from Heimer, Alheid, and Zahm (1993).

Wolf, 1997; Nestler & Aghajanian, 1997; Pierce, Duffy, & Kalivas, 1995; Pierce, Born, Adams, & Kalivas, 1996; Shi, Hayashi, & Petalia, 1999; Zamanillo, Sprengel, & Hvalby, 1999; Zhang, Hu, White, & Wolf, 1997). As shown in Figure 7.7, this neuroanatomic association allows DA to facilitate the synaptic strength of the glutamatergic inputs to the NAS in a manner that increases the contrast gradient between weak and strong glutamatergic inputs in relation to the salient incentive context (Houk et al., 1995; Schultz et al., 1995, 1997;

Wickens & Kotter, 1995). With repeated strong glutamatergic and DA efferent input to NAS neurons, DA release increases this contrast gradient via induction of long-term potentiation (Begg, Wickens, & Arbuthnott, 1993; Wickens & Kotter, 1995). Because the learning capabilities of the isolated striatum are limited (Graybiel, Aosaki, Flaherty, & Kimura, 1994), in this way DA plays an important role in selective strengthening of the corticolimbic antecedents of previously successful responses, and hence in activating incentive motivation by, and approach behavior toward, the most salient context (Houk et al., 1995; Kalivas, 1995; Pierce et al., 1996; Schultz et al., 1995, 1997; Toshihiko, Graybiel, & Kimura, 1994; Wickens & Kotter, 1995).

As modeled on the left of Figure 7.6, stimulation by contextual inputs of glutamate receptors on VTA DA soma and/or dendrites increases *somatodendritic* DA release onto D1 receptors located on the terminals of the glutamatergic efferents (Kalivas, 1995; Nestler & Aghajanian, 1997; Pierce et al., 1996). *Repeated* context-activated VTA somatodendritic DA release reciprocally strengthens the heterosynaptic connections between glutamate efferents conveying contextual information and VTA DA neurons (Johnston, 1997; Kalivas, 1995; Murphy & Glanzman, 1997; Nestler & Aghajanian, 1997). Prefrontal glutamatergic efferents to VTA DA neurons may be particularly influential in this process because the primary pathway for prefrontal regulation of NAS DA release is via projections directly to the VTA (Taber, Das, & Fibiger, 1995): Prefrontal input strongly regulates burst firing of VTA DA cells, which is associated with a doubling of DA release per action potential in the NAS (Johnson, Sentin, & North, 1992; Suaud-Chagny, Dhergui, Chouvet, & Gonon, 1992).

When a salient context predicts an incentive goal, it is critical that that context gains access to, and subsequently influence over, the VTA and NAS circuitries that activate incentive motivational processes that support goal acquisition. DA facilitation of contextual glutamatergic connections in the VTA and NAS is critical for this process of heterosynaptic plasticity (Houk et al., 1995; Kalivas, 1995; Pierce et al., 1996; Schultz et al., 1995, 1997; Toshihiko et al., 1994; Wickens & Kotter, 1995). Nevertheless, the contextual input to both the VTA DA and NAS neurons acts as an *occasion-setter* for the elicitation of incentive motivation (Anag-

Salient Context of Incentive Reward

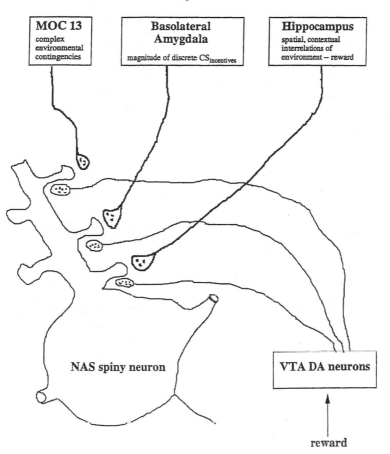

FIGURE 7.6. Interdigitation of cortical (medial orbital prefrontal) and limbic (basolateral amygdala, hippocampus) sources of the salient context of reward with VTA DA projections on the dendritic shafts of an NAS medium-spiny neuron. Synaptic contacts with NAS neurons of the more active cortical and limbic efferents are strengthened by dopamine, a process referred to as heterosynaptic plasticity. In this way, dopamine is thought to strengthen the connections between inputs of the salient incentive context and incentive processes integrated in the NAS_{shell}. Abbreviations: MOC 13, medial orbital prefrontal cortex, Brodmann's area 13; VTA, ventral tegmental area; DA, dopamine; NAS_{shell}, shell subterritory of the nucleus accumbens, a part of the ventral striatum. See text for details. Adapted from Depue and Collins (1999). Copyright 1999 by Cambridge University Press. Adapted by permission.

nostaras & Robinson, 1996; Bell & Kalivas, 1996; Stewart, 1992; Post, Weiss, Fontana, & Pert, 1992; Wolf, Dahling, Hu, & Xue, 1995). Indeed, lesions of the glutamatergic efferents representing contextual inputs to VTA DA or NAS regions prevent incentive-motivated responding, despite the fact that the intact VTA DA and NAS neurons are activated by a DA agonist (Dahlin et al., 1994; Kalivas, 1995; Kalivas & Stewart, 1991; Pert et al., 1992; Yoshikawa, Shibuya, Kaneno, & Toru, 1991). Thus, the expression of DA's facilitation of in-

centive motivational processes is *context-dependent.*

Our (Depue & Collins, 1999; Depue, Luciana, Arbisi, Collins, & Leon, 1994) conception is that variation in the expression of agentic affect and behavior is due in large part to the effects of stable individual differences in the extent to which VTA DA functioning facilitates the connections of salient contextual inputs to VTA DA and NAS neurons. Indeed, a positive correlation between (1) individual differences in DA functioning in the VTA and

No Dopamine Activity

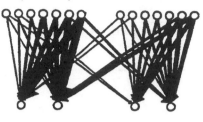

Dopamine-Facilitated Contrast of Afferent Input

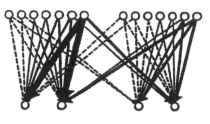

Dopamine-Facilitated Long-Term Potentiation

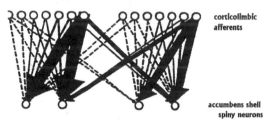

corticolimbic afferents

accumbens shell spiny neurons

FIGURE 7.7. Progressive, differential effects of dopamine release on weak (depressing) and strong (facilitating) cortical and limbic inputs to NAS spiny neurons. In the bottom of the figure, the salient inputs to the NAS have been enduringly strengthened by dopamine release via a process thought to be similar to long-term potentiation. Adapted from Schultz et al. (1995). Copyright 1995 by the MIT Press. Adapted by permission.

NAS and (2) the degree of subsequent expression of incentive-induced motor activity by an occasion-setting incentive context was observed in several studies, in some cases being substantial (.84; Hooks, Jones, Neill, & Justice, 1992). We argue that it is the effects of individual differences in VTA DA functioning on facilitation of context linking in the VTA and NAS, as well as variation in DA facilitation at the time of subsequent occurrence of that context, that together contribute to differences in agentic extraversion.

In conclusion, although we believe that agentic extraversion is the most homogeneous and direct reflection of the operation of posi-

tive incentive motivation and its DA facilitation, *this in no way implies that positive incentive motivation and its DA facilitation will show an association only to agentic extraversion.* Any trait with a heterogeneous phenotype that incorporates behavioral expression that is the result, in part, of elicitation by incentive stimuli will show some degree of association with positive incentive motivation and its DA facilitation. As shown in Figure 7.2, many traits labeled sensation seeking, novelty seeking, and risk taking are complex traits that incorporate positive incentive motivational processes, and therefore such traits would be expected to correlate with DA functioning as well. For instance, some but not all studies have found a relation between a genotypical variant of the D4 receptor and Cloninger's Novelty Seeking scale, which correlates highly with Zuckerman's Impulsivity Sensation Seeking scale ($r = .68$). However, the relation accounts for only 10% of trait variance, and the correlation was more robust with E, Positive Emotions, and Excitement Seeking than with the impulsivity subscale of Cloninger's Novelty Seeking scale (Benjamin, 1996), suggesting a possibly stronger relation with core extraversion than impulsivity. Concordantly, we (Depue, 1995, 1996) found that DA agonist-induced prolactin secretion, as an index of DA reactivity, was not related to Tellegen's MPQ Constraint (.09) or any of its primary scales, nor to Zuckerman's sensation seeking scales of Social Disinhibition (–.12) or Boredom Susceptibility (–.06), but was moderately related to Venturesomeness (.34) and Risk Taking (.34), which have a positive incentive component (Depue & Collins, 1999).

Affiliation

The need to preserve the species through reproduction and group cohesion has resulted in a number of mammalian neurobehavioral processes that support sexual mating, parturition, nursing, and parenting. Collectively, we refer to these as sociosexual processes, which vary in behavioral manifestation depending on the species and social and hormonal context. We divide them into four arbitrary functional groups: (1) sexual approach, where unconditioned and conditioned visual, gestural, vocal, and olfactory stimuli activate positive incentive motivation, desire, lust, and approach to mates; (2) sexual interaction, including courtship and copulation; (3) parturition, lactation, and parental behavior; and (4) longer-term affective bonding between parent–infant and adult pairs, whose processes may also extend to other forms of prosocial interactions and filial bonds within the same species (Insel, 1992, 1997). Because processes associated with (1), (2) and partially (3) operate in many mammalian species without the development of affective attachments that extend beyond short-term infant–parent bonding, we suggest that the personality construct of *affiliation* relates predominantly to neurobiological processes which promote longer-term affective bonds. We also take the position, with others (Insel, 1992, 1997), that such affiliative processes are not the same as those involved in social separation, because affiliation is not simply the absence of separation.

Gonadal Steroids

Recently, there has been intense focus on the role of gonadal steroids and the neuropeptides oxytocin (OT), vasopressin (VP), and opiates as modulators of all types of sociosexual interaction. In many mammalian species, acute or prolonged internally or sociosexually induced gonadal steroid (estrogen, progesterone, testosterone) secretion temporally sets the occasion for most types of sociosexual interaction and can play a permissive role in the action of the other neuropeptides in a regionally specific manner. For instance, peripheral and central OT synthesis rate, release, and receptor density (Carter, Devries, & Detz, 1995; Carter et al., 1997; Insel, 1992, 1997; Insel, Young, & Wang, 1997; McCarthy & Altemus, 1997; Witt, 1995, 1997); OT-induced sexual (Witt, 1995, 1997) and maternal behaviors (Insel, 1997) and reduction in autonomic arousal (Insel, 1997); mating- (Witt, 1995, 1997), grooming- (Argiolas & Gessa, 1991; Insel, 1997), and stress-induced OT release (Jezova, Juranlova, Mosnarova, Kriska, & Skultetyova, 1996); VP-induced aggression in male rodents (Carter et al., 1995); increased dendritic processes of OT and VP neurons (Carter et al., 1997); and opiate release (Keverne, 1996) can all be dependent, at least in initial phases of sociosexual interactions (Keverne, 1996), on gonadal steroid levels depending on the species. In primates and humans, sexual and parental functions are much more loosely linked to gonadal steroid levels (Keverne, 1996), indicating that neurobiological organization of sociosexual processes may vary in these species.

Oxytocin and Vasopressin

It has been well documented that OT and VP play a critical role in all the above sociosexual interactions. From a phylogenetic point of view, OT and VP, which are found only in mammals (Insel, 1997), are nevertheless two of the most highly conserved hormones (Argiolas & Gessa, 1991), and across mammalian phylogeny, the limbic structures that manifest OT and VP receptors are largely unchanged (LeDoux, 1987, 1996b), indicating that human sociosexual processes are likely influenced by these neuropeptides. Most neuroanatomical and behavioral data on OT and VP, however, relate to rodents, and significant differences occur across mammalian species (Carter et al., 1995, 1997; Richard, Mood, & Freund-Mercier, 1991). Therefore, extension to human behavior requires further empirical study.

In rodents and humans, a host of unconditioned and conditioned (Carter, 1992) sociosexual stimuli elicit OT neuron activity, including vaginocervical stimulation at birth (Insel, 1992, 1997; Keverne, 1996; Nissen, Gustavsson, Widstram, & Uvnas-Moberg, 1998; Richard et al., 1991), genital and breast stimulation and copulation (Argiolas & Gessa, 1991; Carter, 1992; Carter, Devries, & Detz, 1995; Insel, 1992, 1997; Insel & Shapiro, 1992; Keverne, 1996; McCarthy & Altemus, 1997; Richard et al., 1991; Witt, 1995, 1997), olfactory stimuli (Carter, 1992), and suckling (Richard et al., 1991). Nonsexual stimuli (Carter, 1992; Carter et al., 1995, 1997; Insel, 1992; Uvnas-Moberg, 1997b), such as grooming, nongenital touch, massage, hair stroking, pleasant vocalizations, warmth, and pup and lamb exposure (Carter, 1992; McCarthy & Altemus, 1997; Nissen et al., 1998) have also induced OT release and OT dendritic arborization (Carter, 1992). In turn, stimulus-induced OT activity facilitates numerous sociosexual functions in rodents, sheep, and humans (Altemus, Deuster, Gallivan, Carter, & Gold, 1995; Argiolas & Gessa, 1991; Carter, 1992; Carter et al., 1995, 1997; Engelmann, Ebner, Wotjak, & Landgraf, 1998; Insel, 1992, 1997; Insel et al., 1997; Insel & Shapiro, 1992; McCarthy & Altemus, 1997; Nissen et al., 1998; Richard et al., 1991; Williams, Insel, Harbugh, & Carter, 1994; Witt, 1995, 1997; Uvnas-Moberg, 1997b; Young, Wang, & Insel, 1998), including affiliation (mother-infant interaction, partner preference, and nonsexual social contact) (Carter et al., 1995; Insel, 1997; McCarthy & Altemus, 1997; Nissen et al.,

1998; Williams et al., 1994; Witt, 1995, 1997; Young et al., 1998). Less is known about VP, but in male rodents it can facilitate aggressive territorial mate protection, partner preference even without mating, paternal care, perhaps social recognition memory, and in human males, VP levels peak during sexual arousal (Carter et al., 1995, 1997; Insel, 1997; Young et al., 1998). Although OT (female) and VP (male) *functions* are gender dependent in some rodents, the fact that both neuropeptides are found in both sexes in rodents and humans indicates that their role in each gender requires further specification (Argiolas & Gessa, 1991; Strand, 1999).

Three points concerning the functional role of OT and VP are important. First, in view of the diverse physiological targets and sociosexual functions influenced, the role of these neuropeptides appears to be one of facilitative modulation rather than mediation (Carter et al., 1997). Second, some evidence suggests that their importance is predominant in the initiation rather than maintenance of certain sociosexual functions (Carter et al., 1997; Insel & Shapiro, 1992; Keverne, 1996). For instance, whereas acute sexual activity in rodents promotes OT and VP release, mating behaviors, and social memories; the decreased copulatory frequency, increased social contact, prolonged reduction in sympathetic autonomic and neuroendocrine activation, increased vagal tone, and calm sedation that are associated with *repeated* sexual activity over several days are blocked by opiate rather than OT antagonists (Carter et al., 1997).

Third, *peripheral* versus *central* OT and VP systems in rodents and humans can differ in their functional effects (Carter et al., 1997; Insel, 1992, 1997; Uvnas-Moberg, 1997a), receptor regulation and distribution (Insel, 1992, 1997; Strand, 1999), and stimulus elicitors (Carter et al., 1995; Keverne, 1996). They are therefore potentially dissociable (Insel, 1992). The peripheral system involves OT and VP *magnocellular* neurons in the paraventricular (PVN) and supraoptic nuclei of the hypothalamus that activate OT and VP secretion from the neurohypophysis. In turn, OT and VP traverse the blood stream locally to the anterior pituitary as well as more broadly to affect many peripheral functions, such as uterine contractions and milk ejection. In contrast, the central system involves OT and VP *parvocellular* neurons in the PVN that project to many coticolimbic regions,

such as the amygdala, BNST, NAS, and prelimbic cortex (Carter, 1992; Carter et al., 1995, 1997; Hulting, Genback, & Pineda, 1996; Insel, 1992, 1997; Insel et al., 1997; Insel & Shapiro, 1992; Ivell & Russell, 1996; McCarthy & Altemus, 1997; Richard et al., 1991; Strand, 1999; Witt, 1995, 1997; Uvnas-Moberg, Widstrom, Nissen, & Bjorvell, 1990). Thus, whereas the peripheral system seems well positioned to facilitate basic bodily processes related to sociosexual functions, the broad central corticolimbic distribution may correspond to an increased capacity to guide sociosexual interactions by more general motivational processes and by social memories. In this case, OT and VP may play a critical role in facilitating limbic-based memory and motivational processes that associate mate and offspring stimuli with primary positive reinforcement (Carter et al., 1997; Insel, 1992; Insel & Shapiro, 1992). For instance, OT activation facilitates association of the odor of a mate with copulation in male rodents, thereby motivating partner preference (Young et al., 1998). Such processes would be particularly important in humans, where sociosexual behavior is less tightly linked to gonadal steroids and neuropeptides, but is significantly influenced by social stimuli (Keverne, 1996).

Opiates

Effects of opioid drugs are mediated by at least three opiate receptor (OR) families having as many as nine subtypes (e.g., mu, delta, and kappa) (Mansour, Khachaturian, Lewis, Akil, & Watson, 1988; Olson, Olson, & Kastin, 1997; Schlaepfer, Strain, & Greenberg, 1998; Strand, 1999; Uhl, Sora, & Wang, 1999). In general, a critical role for opiates in sociosexual interactions is suggested because opiate release is increased in monkeys and humans in late pregnancy and by parturition, lactation and nursing, sexual activity, vaginocervical stimulation, maternal social interaction, and grooming and other nonsexual tactile stimulation (Insel, 1992; Keverne, 1996; Mansour et al., 1988; Nelson & Panksepp, 1998; Niesink, Vanderschuen, & van Ree, 1996; Nissen et al., 1998; Olson et al., 1997). The facilitatory effects of opiates on sociosexual behavior are thought to be exerted by fibers that terminate in corticolimbic brain regions that partially overlap OT and VP receptor distibution (Keverne, 1996; Mansour et al., 1988; Strand, 1999).

Perhaps most relevant to sociosexual interactions and a human trait of affiliation is the mu (μ) OR family, which is the main site of morphine action and whose μ_3 subtype may be the receptor for the newly discovered endogenous morphine (Olson et al., 1997; Schlaepfer et al., 1998; Stefano, Scharrer, & Smith, 1996; Stefano & Scharrer, 1996). μORs are not only the main site for the analgesic effects of β-endorphins, but also for the subjective feelings in humans of *increased* interpersonal warmth, euphoria, well-being, and peaceful calmness, as well as of *decreased* elation, energy, and incentive motivation (Cleeland, Nakamura, & Howland, 1996; Ferrante, 1996; Greenwald, June, Stitzer, & Marco, 1996; Olson et al., 1997; Schlaepfer et al., 1998). VTA-localized μORs are involved in increased sexual activity (Leyton & Stewart, 1996; van furth & van Ree, 1996) and maternal behaviors (Callahan, Baumann, & Rabii, 1996), and in the chronically increased play behavior, social grooming, and social approach of rats subjected to morphine *in utero* (Hol, Niesink, van Ree, & Spruijt, 1996). The μOR-agonist morphine versus naltrexone promotes or blocks, respectively, the ability of vaginocervical stimulation to induce maternal behavior and mother–infant bonds in sheep and humans (Keverne, 1996). Moreover, naltrexone leads to maternal neglect in monkeys that is similar to the neglect shown by mothers who abuse opiates (Keverne, 1996), and it blocks the sociosexual effects of increased social contact, reduced autonomic arousal, and calmness that is induced by repeated sexual activity in rodents (Carter et al., 1997; Porges, 1998).

μORs may mediate the positive reinforcement associated with the consummatory phase of many motivated behaviors (Bozarth, 1994; Keverne, 1996; Koob & Le Moal, 1997; Koob et al., 1993; Nelson & Panksepp, 1998; Niesink et al., 1996; Olson et al., 1997; Strand, 1999). Animals will work for the μ-agonists morphine and heroin, and morphine can serve as an unconditioned stimulus in conditioned place preference (Olson et al., 1997), whereas μ-antagonists block rewarding effects of sucrose and in neonatal rats persistently impair the response to the inherently rewarding properties of novel stimulation (Kehow & Tiano, 1996). These rewarding effects may involve two processes in that, during the anticipatory phase of goal acquisition, μOR activation in the VTA can increase DA release in the NAS and locomotor activity, as well as decrease the latency of maternal behavior (Bozarth, 1994; Callahan et al., 1996; Jaeger & van der Kooy, 1996; Kehow & Tiano, 1996; Marinelli et al., 1996: Olson et al., 1997; Shaham & Stewart, 1996). Subsequently, μOR (with dOR; Churchill, Roques, & Kalivas, 1995) activation in the NAS, perhaps stimulated by opiate release from the higher-threshold NAS terminals that colocalize DA and opiates (Le Moal & Simon, 1991), decreases NAS DA release (Stewart, Grabowski, Wang, & Meisch, 1996; Subrahmanyam, Paris, Chang, & Woodward, 1996). Thus, in contrast to the incentive motivational effects of DA during the anticipation of reward, opiates may subsequently induce calm pleasure and bring consummatory behavior to a gratifying conclusion (Bozarth, 1994).

μORs may play a critical role in two aspects of sociosexual processes. First, they may mediate the primary positive reinforcement necessary in limbic-based sociosexual associative processes whereby stimulus characteristics of others take on positive valence. For instance, the μOR-agonist morphine versus naltrexone promotes or blocks, respectively, the establishment of odor–mother and male–female recognition associations (Leyton & Stewart, 1996; Nelson & Panksepp, 1998; Panksepp, 1998), and naloxone blocks the sociosexual effects induced by *repeated* sexual activity in rodents (Carter et al., 1997). Second, μOR activation in the VTA appears to enhance DA facilitation of the heterosynaptic plasticity that connects salient context to VTA DA neurons described previously (Carlezon, Boundy, Kalb, Neve, & Nestler, 1996; Jaeger & van der Kooy, 1996; Kuribara, 1996; Leyton & Stewart, 1996; Miller, Livermore, & Nation, 1996; Sora, Takahashi, & Funada, 1997), thereby specifically facilitating the ability of sociosexual contextual stimuli to activate sociosexual behavior. Both of these μOR-dependent processes, then, may play a significant role in not only the *establishment* but also in the *maintenance* of long-term affiliative bonds.

In conclusion, whether central OT, VP, or opiate receptor (or other) variations are associated with differences in the affiliative trait dimension is an important area of investigation. Sources of individual differences in OT and VP neuropeptide systems have not been identified, although sociosexual differences between some species appear to be related to receptor brain distribution and density rather than to presynaptic features (Insel, 1997; Strand, 1999; Young et al., 1998). Individual differences in humans and rodents, however, have been demonstrated in levels of μOR expression, μ-dependent nociceptive thresholds, and preference for μ-agonists such as morphine (Belknap, Modil, & Helms, 1995; Berrettini, Alexander, Ferraro, & Vogel, 1994; Berrettini, Ferraro, Alexander, Buchberg, & Vogel, 1994; Sora et al., 1997; Uhl et al., 1999). These differences appear to be due in large part to variation at the μOR gene locus rather than to μOR affinities (Uhl et al., 1999). Moreover, in humans, individual differences in central nervous system μOR densities have shown a range of 75% between lower and upper thirds of the distribution (Frost, Mayberg, & Fisher, 1988; Frost, Douglas, & Mayberg, 1989; Pfeiffer, Pasi, Mehrain, & Herz, 1982; Uhl et al., 1999) differences that, when located in midbrain and limbic regions, may be related to variation in the rewarding effects of alcohol and in nociceptive thresholds (De Wacle, Kiianmaa, & Gianoulakis, 1996; Gianoulakis, 1996; Gianoulakis, De Wacle & Thavundayil, 1996; Gianoulakis, Krishnan & Thavundayil, 1996; Loiselle, Giannini, Martin, & Turner, 1996; Olson et al., 1997).

Neuroticism (Anxiety) and Harm Avoidance (Fear)

Roles of the Central Versus Extended Amygdala

The psychometric independence of neuroticism and harm avoidance noted previously is mirrored in a dissociable neuroanatomy of anxiety and fear. Species-specific unconditional stimuli that have an evolutionary history of danger elicit fear and defensive motor escape, facial and vocal signs, autonomic activation, and antinociception specifically from the lateral longitudinal cell column in the midbrain periaquiductal gray (PAG; see Figure 7.8) (Bandler & Keay, 1996). In turn, PAG efferents converge on the ventromedial and rostral ventrolateral regions of the medulla, where somatic and autonomic information, respectively, is integrated and transmitted to the spinal cord (Guyenet et al., 1996; Holstege, 1996). Whereas these processes can occur without cortex (Panksepp, 1998), association of *discrete, explicit* neutral stimuli (CS_{fear}) with the UCS and primary negative reinforcement occurs via cortical uni- and polymodal sensory efferents that converge on the basolateral complex of the amygdala, al-

though crude representations of external stimuli can rapidly reach the basolateral amygdala subcortically from the thalamus (Aggleton, 1992; Aggleton & Mishkin, 1986; Davis, 1992a, 1992b; Davis et al., 1997; LeDoux, 1987, 1996a, 1966b). CS_{fear} elicits a host of behavioral, neuropeptide, and autonomic responses via input to the central amygdala, which in turn sends *separable* efferents to many hypothalamic and brainstem targets (Aggleton, 1992; LeDoux, Cicchetti, Xagoraris, & Romanski, 1990). In the case of CS_{fear}, the motor response is not escape but rather freezing or *behavioral inhibition*, which involves activation of the caudal ventrolateral cell column of the PAG shown in Figure 7.8 (LeDoux et al., 1990); if safety cues are present, they act as incentive stimuli, engaging positive incentive motivational processes and forward locomotion, collectively known as active avoidance (Gray, 1973, 1992).

The neuroanatomic distinction between fear and anxiety has been further delineated in the fear-potentiated auditory-induced startle paradigm. In this paradigm, an explicit light CS_{fear} traverses a neural pathway from the basolateral to central amygdala, which in turn monosynaptically potentiates startle reflex circuitry in the reticular nucleus of the caudal pons. This potentiation is *phasic* in nature, occurring almost immediately after light onset but returning to baseline amplitude shortly after light offset (Davis, 1992a, 1992b; Davis et al., 1997). Lesions of the central amygdala reliably block CS_{fear}-potentiated startle and behavioral inhibition, whereas lesions of other extended amygdala structures, including the lateral BNST and sublenticular area, have no such effect. Thus, in line with other evidence, these findings suggest that *explicit* CS_{fear} is specifically associated with reinforcement in, and finds expression through, the basolateral and central amygdala, respectively.

In contrast, nondiscrete, contextually related aversive stimulation (e.g., prolonged bright light in an unfamiliar environment, which are aversive UCSs for nocturnal rats) elicits robust startle potentiation that endures tonically as long as the aversive conditions (Davis et al., 1997). As noted earlier, contextual stimuli are associated with reinforcement in the hippocampus rather than the amygdala, and this information is conveyed to the BNST via hippocampal glutamatergic efferents (Annett et al., 1989; Bechara et al., 1995; Everitt & Robbins, 1992;

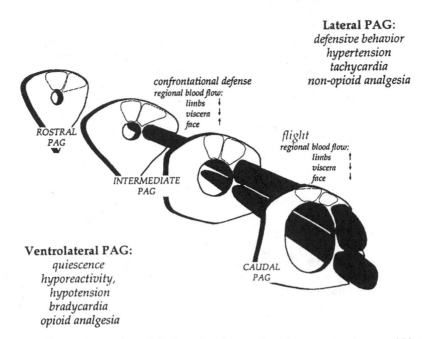

FIGURE 7.8. Schematic illustration of the lateral and ventrolateral neuronal columns within (from left to right) the rostral midbrain periacquiductal gray (PAG), the intermediate PAG (2 sections), and the caudal PAG. Injections of excitatory amino acids (EAA) within the lateral and ventrolateral PAG column evoke fundamentally opposite alterations in sensory responsiveness, and somatic and autonomic adjustments. EAA injections made within the intermediate, lateral PAG evoke a confrontational defensive reaction, tachycardia, and hypertension associated with decreased blood flow to limbs and viscera and increased blood flow to extracranial vascular beds. EAA injections made within the caudal, lateral PAG evoke flight, tachycardia, and hypertension associated with decreased blood flow to visceral and extracranial vascular beds and increased blood flow to limbs. In contrast, EAA injections made within the ventrolateral PAG evoke cessation of all spontaneous activity (i.e., quiescence), a decreased responsiveness to the environment, hypotension, and bradycardia. The lateral and ventrolateral PAG also mediate different types of analgesia. Adapted from Bandler and Keay (1996). Copyright 1996 by Elsevier Science. Adapted by permission.

Gaffan, 1992; Heimer et al., 1993; Phillips & LeDoux, 1992; Selden et al., 1991; Sutherland & McDonald, 1990). Other hippocampal efferents activated by stress release corticotophin-releasing hormone (CRH) into the BNST, which also potentiates startle in a prolonged, dose-dependent manner (Davis et al., 1997). It is not surprising then that lesions of the BNST, or injection of a CRH antagonist in the BNST, significantly attenuate both bright light- or CRH-enhanced startle without having any effect on discrete CS_{fear}- potentiated startle, whereas lesions of the central amygdala eliminate the latter without affecting the former. Prolonged bright light-induced startle potentiation is also blocked by lesions of the fornix, which carries hippocampal efferents conveying salient context to the BNST (Amaral & Witter, 1995; Canteras & Swanson, 1992; Cullinan, Herman,

& Watson, 1993), by glutamatergic antagonists injected into the BNST that block hippocampal efferent input, and by buspirone, a potent anxiolytic (Davis, Cassella, & Kehne, 1988; Davis et al., 1997). Conversely, lesions of, or glutamate antagonists injected in, the central amygdala blocked CS_{fear}-potentiated startle but had no effect on startle elicited by bright light conditions or on anxiolytic effects in the elevated plus maze, where benzodiazepines have a robust anxiolytic effect (Davis et al., 1997; Treit, Pesold, & Rotzinger, 1993). The basolateral amygdala is involved in both bright light- and CS_{fear}-potentiated startle due to processing of visual information but not in CRH-enhanced startle.

Thus, there is a multivariate double dissociation of the central amygdala and the BNST. As summarized in Figure 7.9, the nature of the different stimulus conditions that activate these two structures suggests that the amygdala connects explicit phasic stimuli that predict aversive UCSs with rapidly activated evasive responses and subjective fear. In contrast, prolonged contextual unfamiliar stimuli that connote uncertainty about expected outcome are associated with a neurobehavioral response system that coordinates activation of (1) the negative affective state of anxiety to inform the organism that the current context is uncertain and potentially dangerous, (2) autonomic arousal to mobilize energy for potential action, (3) selective attention in order to maximize sensory input, and (4) cognition in order to derive a response strategy.

Due to the prolonged nature of the stimulus conditions, this response system must be capable of iterative reverberation until the uncer-

tainty is resolved. Prolonged reverberatory activation of startle associated with the BNST may derive from three sources: (1) CRH release from hippocampal efferents to the BNST (Davis et al., 1997); (2) dense intrinsic connections among structures of the central division of the extended amygdala, including the central amygdala, sublenticular area, lateral BNST, and NAS$_{shell}$ (Heimer et al., 1993); and (3) activation of extended amygdala structures via these intrinsic connections by neurons in the sublenticular area that show maximal prolonged responsiveness to unfamiliar stimuli (Rolls, 1999; Wilson & Rolls, 1990). Viewing the sublenticular area and lateral BNST as a foundation for anxiety processes is also supported by the fact that, in contrast to the amygdala, electrical stimulation or lesions of the BNST did not initiate or block, respectively, the behavioral inhibition elicited by an explicit CS$_{fear}$ (LeDoux et al., 1990), which mirrors the lack of association of behavioral inhibition with trait neuroticism cited previously. Thus, anxiety and fear appear to differ in their stimulus elicitation and neuroanatomical base. Nevertheless, as shown in Figure 7.9, efferents from the BNST and sublenticular area innvervate many of the same hypothalamic and brainstem regions as the central amygdala (Heimer et al., 1993), suggesting that fear and anxiety derive their similar subjective nature from common neuroendocrine and autonomic response systems (Davis et al., 1997; LeDoux, 1996a, 1996b; Rolls, 1999).

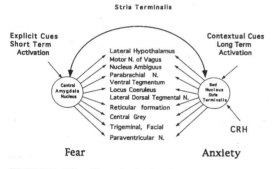

FIGURE 7.9. Hypothetical schematic suggesting that the central nucleus of the amygdala and the bed nucleus of the stria terminalis may be differentially involved in fear versus anxiety, repsectively. Both brain areas have highly similar hypothalamic and brainstem targets known to be involved in specific signs and symptoms of fear and anxiety. However, the stress peptide corticotropin releasing hormone (CRH) appears to act on receptors in the bed nucleus of the stria terminalis rather than the amygdala, at least in terms of an increase in the startle reflex. Futhermore, the bed nucleus of the stria terminalis seems to be involved in the anxiogenic effects of a very bright light presented for a long time but not when that very same light was previously paired with a shock. Just the opposite is the case for the central nucleus of the amygdala, which is critical for fear conditioning using explicit cues such as a light or tone paired with aversive stimulation (i.e., conditioned fear). Adapted from Davis, Walker, and Younglim (1997). Copyright 1997 by the New York Academy of Sciences. Adapted by permission.

Norepinephrine

Major outputs of both the central amygdala and the lateral BNST directly, or indirectly via PAG efferents, innervate the paragiganticocellularis (PGi) nucleus located in the ventral rostrolateral medulla (Aston-Jones, Rajkowski, Kubiak, Valentino, & Shipley, 1996; Heimer et al., 1993). As a major integrative region of extero- and interoceptive stimulation, the PGi coordinates and triggers reactivity to potentially urgent stimulus conditions by modulating two nonspecific emotional activation systems (Aston-Jones et al., 1996). One involves triggering *peripheral* activation via dense innervation of the rostral ventrolateral region of the medulla, which integrates arousal inputs from many brain regions and transmits that information to the intermediolateral cell column of the spinal cord to influence sympathetic preganglionic neurons. The other involves elicitation of *central* electroencephalogram (EEG) activation via the norepinephrine (NE) neurons of the locus coeruleus (LC), neurons long thought to be involved in the experience of both fear and anxiety (Charney, Grillon, & Bremner, 1998). Thus, emotional activation induced by PGi activity functions to interrupt ongoing behavior and reset cognitive activity, increase energy metabolism peripherally, increase sensory input to produce an "on line" stimulus–response mode of behavioral reactivity, and initiate selective central attentional and cognitive processes in order to determine adaptive emotional and behavioral responses to the urgent stimulus conditions (Aston-Jones et al., 1996).

The LC consists of only ~20,000 neurons, but their extensive collateralization results in innervation of all brain regions. They are the only source of NE in the cortex, hippocampus, cingulate gyrus, olfactory and cerebellar cortices, and many limbic areas, especially the central amygdala. Densest innervation is of the sensorimotor areas, prefrontal cortex, and parietal areas connected to the pulvinar nucleus of the thalamus and the superior colliculus. Descending efferents from a subgroup of LC neurons innervate the spinal cord and other brainstem regions as a means of modulating autonomic and visceral functions directly. All LC neurons respond with short latency (15–50 msec) in unity to tonic and phasic stimuli requiring orientation and vigilance, of all sensory modalities of both positive and negative valence (Aston-Jones et al., 1996; Cirelli, Pompeiano, & Tononi, 1996). Thus, the information relayed by LC activity is of a general nature that mainly creates EEG arousal. Via B_1-adrenergic receptors, stimulation- or stress-CRF-induced LC NE transmission increases signal-to-noise ratios in broad cortical regions, whereby target neurons respond with preference to the strongest inputs, a function referred to as tuning of information (Aston-Jones et al., 1996; Mason, 1981; Oades, 1985).

An NE tuning function has been found to increase the efficacy of sensory selection and attentional and cognitive processes by enhancing discrimination between relevant and irrelevant information (Oades, 1985). For instance, LC input to the thalamic reticular nucleus is critical in differentially activating the entire set of ascending thalamocortical sensory relay pathways. Second, the reticular nucleus of the thalamus is composed of gatelets, each of whose open-closed status is modulated by a number of inputs including the LC. When a gatelet is opened, it will pass information to other thalamic structures that process the information and relay it to the cortex. Only those gatelets are opened that carry information that is relevant to the current environmental conditions (Andersen, Snyder, Bradley, & Xing, 1997). For instance, imagine a tiger in a cage who is always fed through a door in a specific spatial location. As feeding time approaches, the tiger's brain directs attention to the relevant parts of extrapersonal space, which are determined, for instance, by their position in the visual field at any particular moment and their motivational significance. This means that the tiger's brain, in order to attend to what is relevant, needs to emphasize those visual parts of space that are currently relevant and guide the motor system accordingly. In this case, we wish to open the reticular gatelets that pass biasing information to the medial pulvinar of the thalamus, because the latter provides visual information that is weighted for salience to cortical regions concerned with mapping extrapersonal space (e.g., visual sensory receptive area, inferior parietal area, and dorsolateral prefrontal cortex) (Andersen et al., 1997).

An association of NE to *human* traits of harm avoidance and neuroticism has not been systematically investigated, although an association of LC activity to fear and anxiety has been noted in rodents (Blizzard, 1988) and monkeys (Redmond, 1987). The fact that the BNST is one of the most densely NE-innervated structures and is subject to stress-induced CRH facilitated activity is consistent with an NE-modulated stress-related role in the BNST. Chronic stress-induced NE is increased in inbred rat strains with high negative emotionality (Blizzard, 1988) and in posttraumatic stress disorder patients (Charney et al., 1998), and it creates in monkeys and humans distracted and scattered attentional and cognitive processes dependent on prefrontal working memory functions (Arnsten, 1998; Aston-Jones et al., 1996; Mason, 1981). Moreover, *stress reaction* (negative emotions, ruminative worrying, overreaction to minor stressors) is the predominant lower-order marker of Tellegen's neuroticism scale (Tellegen & Waller, in press). It may be that the convergence on stress reactivity and NE in neuroticism and anxiety is related to the fact that NE plays an important role in facilitating stress-induced behavioral sensitization that may provide the foundation of the persistent overreactivity that typifies trait neuroticism and anxiety disorders (Charney et al., 1998).

Because cortical and pupillary NE systems have a similar neurodevelopmental origin and are both responsive to emotionally arousing states (Aston-Jones et al., 1996), we (White & Depue, 1999) used pupillary dilation as a model system to study the relation of NE to harm avoidance and neuroticism. As a reverse analog to bright light in nocturnal rats, dark conditions in humans induce a significant increase in startle amplitude is correlated with self-ratings of childhood fear of the dark, and is enhanced in subjects who rate an experiment as more unpleasant in the dark than in the light (Davis et al., 1997). Concordantly, we found that neuroticism was significantly associated with the magnitude of pupil dilation induced by darkness (.66, $p < .01$), whereas relations with harm avoidance were nonsignificant (–.23). Because LC NE activity modulates central structures that *tonically* modulate pupil dilation (Christensen, Mutzig, & Koss, 1990; Gherezghiher & Koss, 1979; Heal, Prow, & Buckett, 1989; Loewenfeld, 1993), these findings encourage more direct assessment of a *tonic* NE influence on neuroticism. In addition, we found that the phasic response in pupil dilation to an alpha$_1$-adrenergic agonist, which is a reliable and genetically influenced indicator of alpha$_1$-receptor sensitivity (Loewenfeld, 1993; Mullen et al., 1981; Ziegler, Lake, Wood, & Ebert, 1976) and is significantly related to circulating plasma NE (Sitaram, Gillin, & Bunney, 1984), was significantly related to harm avoidance (.69, $p < .01$) but not at all to neuroticism ($r = .01$). Taken together, these findings support the possibility that anxiety (neuroticism) is associated with sensitivity to nondiscrete uncertain conditions that produces a relatively tonic NE-induced arousal, whereas fear (harm avoidance) is associated with a sensitivity to explicit stimuli that elicits strong phasic NE activation of specific response systems. Whether a putative NE involvement in fear and anxiety is primary or secondary to variation in BNST or amygdalar function needs to be addressed.

Nonaffective Constraint

Serotonin Modulation of a Response Threshold

Elicitation of behavior can be modeled neurobiologically by using a minimum threshold construct, which represents a central nervous system weighting of the external and internal factors that contribute to the probability of response expression (Depue & Collins, 1999; Stricker & Zigmond, 1986; White, 1986). External factors are characteristics of environmental stimulation, including magnitude, duration, and psychological salience. Internal factors consist of both state (e.g., stress-induced endocrine levels) and trait biological variation. We proposed earlier that nonaffective constraint is the personality trait analog of the neurobiological construct of a response threshold. As such, constraint embodies the influence of all modulators of threshold and exerts a general influence over behavior that is not preferentially associated with any specific neurobehavioral–motivational system. Other higher-order personality variables reflect the influence of trait neurobiological variables that strongly modulate the threshold for responding. We demonstrated this most explicitly through DA's role in a response facilitation model of agentic extraversion (Figure 7.4), but the neuropeptides related to affiliation and NE's role in the tuning of information may be conceived in the same modulatory manner (Depue & Collins, 1999; Oades, 1985).

Functional levels of neurotransmitters that provide a strong, relatively *tonic inhibitory* influence are particularly significant modulators of response threshold and, hence, likely account for a large proportion of the variance in the trait of nonaffective constraint. We and others previously (Coccaro & Siever, 1991; Depue, 1995, 1996; Depue & Spoont, 1986; Mandel, 1984; Panksepp, 1998; Spoont, 1992; Stein, Hollander, & Leibowitz, 1993; Zald & Depue, in press; Zuckerman, 1991) and most recently Lesch (1998) suggested that serotonin (5-HT), acting at multiple receptor sites in most brain regions, is such a modulator (Azmitia & Whitaker-Azmitia, 1997; Blakely, De Felice, & Hartzell, 1994; Tork, 1990). As reviewed many times in animal and human literatures (Coccaro et al., 1989; Coccaro & Siever, 1991; Depue, 1995, 1996; Depue & Spoont, 1986; Lesch, 1997, 1998; Mandel, 1984; Spoont, 1992; Stein et al., 1993; Zald & Depue in press; Zuckerman, 1991), 5-HT modulates a diverse set of functions—including emotion, motivation, motor, affiliation, cognition, food intake, sleep, sexual activity, and sensory reactivity such as nociception, sensitization to auditory and tactile startle stimuli, and escape latencies following PAG stimulation—and is associated with many clinical conditions, including violent suicide across several types of disorder, obsessive–compulsive disorder, disorders of impulse control, aggression, depression, anxiety, arson, and substance abuse (Coccaro & Siever, 1991; Depue & Spoont, 1986; Lesch, 1998; Spoont, 1992; Stein et al., 1993). Furthermore, *reduced* 5-HT functioning in animals (Depue & Spoont, 1986; Spoont, 1992) and humans (Coccaro et al., 1989) is also accompanied by *irritability* and *hypersensitivity* to stimulation in most sensory modalities (Spoont, 1992), which may be due to the important role played by 5-HT in the inhibitory modulation of sensory input at several levels of the brain (Azmitia & Whitaker-Azmitia, 1997; Tork, 1990), as well as to significant 5-HT modulation of the lateral hypothalamic region that activates autonomic reactivity under stressful conditions (Azmitia & Whitaker-Azmitia, 1997). Thus, 5-HT plays a substantial modulatory role in general neurobiological functioning that affects many forms of motivated behavior.

An important but difficult area of research is to determine which personality traits best assess the general modulatory role of 5-HT as opposed, for instance, to a single specific marker of that role. For instance, Tellegen's MPQ Constraint consists of three primary scales which assess generalized nonaffective Impulsivity, Harm Avoidance (fear), and Traditionalism. These scales apparently relate to different neurobiological systems, because we found that 5-HT agonist-induced increases in serum prolactin secretion were correlated significantly with only Impulsivity (−.44, $p < .01$) but not with Harm Avoidance (.01) or Traditionalism (.04) (Depue, 1995, 1996).

The Interactive Nature of Constraint and Behavioral Stability

A vast body of animal and human evidence consistently associates reduced functioning of 5-HT neurotransmission with *behavioral instability*. This instability is manifested as lability (i.e., a heightened probability of competing behavioral responses due to a reduced threshold of response elicitation) and hence an increased stimulus access to neural circuits, even when those circuits are currently engaged in processing other emotional responses (Mandel, 1984; Spoont, 1992). Therefore, instability or lability will increase as a function of increasing facili-

tatory influences on response elicitation (Depue & Spoont, 1986).

The effects of constraint depend on interactions with other personality traits. The *qualitative content* of unstable behavior will depend on which neurobehavioral–motivational system, or *affective* personality trait, is being elicited at any point in time (Zald & Depue, in press), although differential strength of various personality traits will obviously produce relative predominance of particular affective behaviors within individuals. For example, in considering a constraint × agentic extraversion interaction, 5-HT is an inhibitory modulator of a host of DA-facilitated behaviors, including the reinforcing properties of psychostimulants, novelty-induced locomotor activity, the acquisition of self-administration of cocaine, and DA utilization in the NAS_{shell} (Ashby, 1996; Depue & Spoont, 1986; Herve et al., 1981; Kelland & Chiodo, 1996; Loh & Roberts, 1990; Lucki, 1992; Piazza et al., 1991; Ritz, Lamb, Goldberg & Kuhar, 1987; Spoont, 1992). This modulatory influence arises in large part from the dense dorsal raphe efferents to the VTA and NAS_{shell}, connections that are known to modulate DA activity (Ashby, 1966; Azmitia & Whitaker-Azmitia, 1997; Deutch et al., 1993; Kalivas et al., 1993; Schultz, 1986). A 5-HT-related reduction in the threshold of DA facilitation of behavior results in an exaggerated response to incentive stimuli which is most apparent in reward–punishment conflict situations. In such situations, exaggerated responding to incentives results in (1) a greater weighting of immediate versus delayed future rewards, (2) increased reactivity to the reward of safety or relief associated with active avoidance (e.g., suicidal behavior), (3) impulsive behavior (i.e., a propensity to respond to reward when withholding or delaying a response may produce a more favorable long-term outcome), and (4) various attempts to experience the increased magnitude and frequency of incentive reward (e.g., self-administration of DA-active substances) (Babor, Hofmann, & Delboca, 1986; Coccaro & Siever, 1991; Depue & Iacono, 1989; Lesch, 1998). All these effects impair the ability to sustain long-term goal-directed behavior programs (e.g., obtaining a college degree) by mental representations of expected rewards that can be repeatedly accessed, be held on-line in prefrontal cortex, and thereby symbolically motivate behavior (Depue & Collins, 1999; Goldman-Rakic, 1995).

A 5-HT-DA interaction is more formally illustrated in the threshold model of behavioral facilitation in Figure 7.4, where 5-HT values modulate the probability of DA response facilitation across the entire range of incentive stimulus magnitude (Depue & Collins, 1999). This interaction is also modeled in Figure 7.10 within a personality framework, where the affectively unipolar dimension of agentic extraversion (DA facilitation) is seen in interaction with nonaffective constraint (5-HT inhibition) (Depue, 1996). The interaction of these two traits creates a diagonal dimension of *behavioral stability* that applies equally to affective,

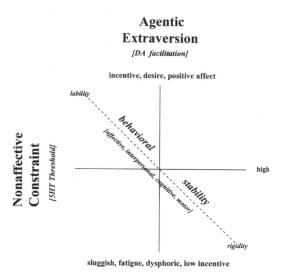

FIGURE 7.10. A hypothetical personality framework illustrating the interaction of the higher-order personality traits of agentic extraversion (vertical axis) and nonaffective constraint (horizontal axis). Agentic extraversion is hypothesized to be associated with dopamine (DA) functioning, whereas nonaffective constraint is proposed as being related to serotonin (5-HT) functioning. The interaction of the affectively unipolar dimension of agentic E (DA facilitation) and nonaffective constraint (5-HT inhibition) creates a diagonal dimension of *behavioral stability* that applies equally to affective, cognitive, interpersonal, motor, and incentive processes. The diagonal represents the line of greatest variance in stability, ranging from lability in the upper left quadrant (low 5-HT, high DA) to rigidity in the lower right (high 5-HT, low DA). The extent of lability is affected not only by a 5-HT influence but also by DA's more general facilitatory effects on the flow of neural information, where increased DA activity promotes *switching* between response alternatives (i.e., behavioral flexibility). See text for details.

cognitive, interpersonal, motor, and incentive processes. The diagonal represents the line of greatest variance in stability, ranging from lability in the upper left quadrant of the two-space (low 5-HT, high DA) to rigidity in the lower right (high 5-HT, low DA).

It is important to note that the extent of lability is affected not only by a 5-HT influence but also by DA's more general facilitatory effects on the flow of neural information, where increased DA activity promotes switching between response alternatives (i.e., behavioral flexibility) (Cools, 1980; Depue & Iacono, 1989; Le Moal & Simon, 1991; Louilot, Taghzouti, Deminiere, Simon, & Le Moal, 1987; Oades, 1985; Spoont, 1992). Indeed, when DA transmission is very low, a problem in exceeding the facilitation threshold of any response occurs, whereas at very high DA transmission levels, a high rate of switching between response alternatives is seen, which can evolve into a low variety of responses when abnormally high (e.g., stereotypy) (LeMoal & Simon, 1991; Oades, 1985; Oades & Halladay, 1987). Interpreting these notions within our neurobiological framework of DA, the establishment and selection of salient contexts in the NAS could be viewed as DA's contribution to switching from one response strategy to another (Depue & Collins, 1999). DA's role in switching may explain several of the *non*affective manifestations of extraverted behavior, such as rapidity of attentional shifts and cognitive switching between ideas (Eysenck, 1981).

This conceptualization of the interaction of 5-HT and DA may be relevant to interpersonal behavior. Brothers and Ring (1992) argued that humans have an innate cognitive alphabet of ethologically significant behavioral signs that signal the emotional intention of others. This alphabet is integrated into its highest representation in human social cognition as a person with propensities and dispositions that have valence for the observer, a social construct akin to personality. Personality research has demonstrated that the representation of others exists in two independent, contrasted forms as the familiar–good other and the unfamiliar–evil other, and the representation of the self is similarly represented in two independent positive and negative forms (Tellegen & Waller, in press). This is consistent with the fact that most percepts and concepts are represented in the brain as separate unified entities (Squire & Kosslyn, 1998). Interestingly, increased DA activation

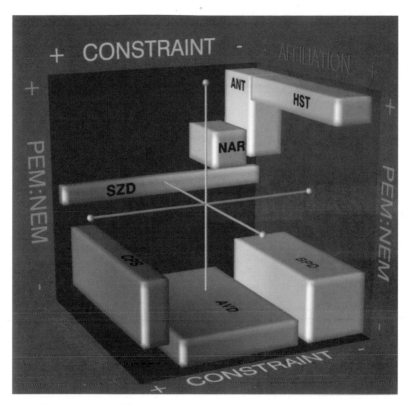

PLATE 7.1. A multidimensional model of personality disorders comprising Clusters B and C and schizoid personality disorder shown in a predominant agentic extraversion:neuroticism perspective on spatial relations between personality disorders. Positive Emotionality (PEM) and Negative Emotionality (NEM) are modeled as a ratio of their relative strength (PEM:NEM). Prototypical exemplars of personality disorder represent the convergence of the most extreme value ranges of multiple traits. (See Table 7.4 for the multitrait dimensional coordinates of each personality disorder.) Personality disorder phenotypical variation and merging are illustrated by the use of color coding of each trait dimension; hence, personality disorder categories show variation throughout their range in color saturation and hue as a function of the changing values of the traits contributing to the personality disorder category. See text for details.

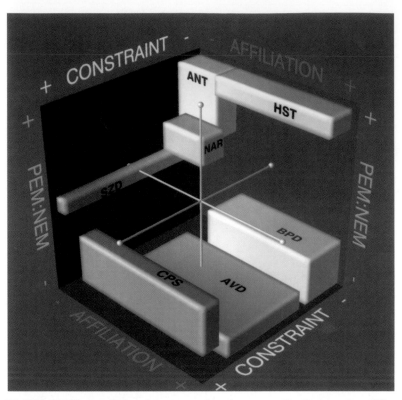

PLATE 7.2. Same as Plate 7.1, except this plate more clearly shows an affiliation perspective. See text for details.

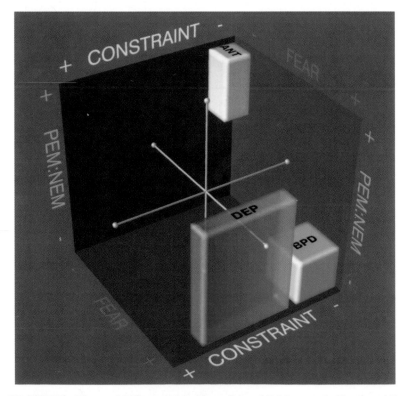

PLATE 7.3. The model illustrated in Plates 7.1 and 7.2 is extended by the addition of a dimension of fear, because this trait is necessary to account for the full range of phenotypical features of antisocial, dependent, and borderline personality disorders. See text for details.

results in a more rapid switching between contrasting percepts, such as two perceptual orientations of the Necker cube or of an ascending–descending staircase (Oades, 1985). Speculatively, we suggest that the frequent, sometimes rapid fluctuation in or switching between mental representations of others and/or the self that characterize several forms of personality disorders is related to an interactive condition of increased DA and reduced 5-HT functioning.

As illustrated in Figure 7.11, interaction between constraint–5-HT and neuroticism–NE dimensions may create a range of anxious phenotypes that vary in their stability, ranging from most highly labile and stress reactive in the up-

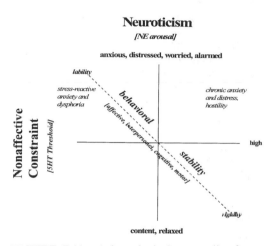

Neuroticism

[NE arousal]

anxious, distressed, worried, alarmed

lability

stress-reactive anxiety and dysphoria

behavioral

[affective, interpersonal, cognitive, motor]

chronic anxiety and distress, hostility

high

stability

highly

content, relaxed

Nonaffective Constraint

[5HT Threshold]

FIGURE 7.11. A hypothetical personality framework illustrating the interaction of the higher-order personality traits of neuroticism and nonaffective constraint. Neuroticism is hypothesized to be associated with norepinephrine (NE) functioning, whereas nonaffective constraint is proposed as being related to serotonin (5-HT) functioning. The interaction between constraint–5-HT and neuroticism–NE dimensions may create a range of anxious phenotypes that vary in stability, ranging from most highly labile and stress reactive in the upper left quadrant to chronically anxious with persistent reverberating negative affect and attitudinal hostility in the upper right quadrant. This framework would account for the weak, also unreplicable, relation (accounting for 3–4% of the variance in behavior) between neuroticism and a genotypical variant of the 5-HT uptake transporter, which may lead to reduced 5-HT functioning via negative feedback effects on 5-HT cells. In this case, reduced 5-HT functioning may disinhibit the locus coeruleus NE activity-induced autonomic arousal thought to underlie subjective anxiety. See text for details and evidence.

per left quadrant to chronically anxious with persistent reverberating negative affect and attitudinal hostility in the upper right quadrant (Zald & Depue, in press). In support of this interaction, Charney et al. (1998) recently demonstrated in normal subjects that, when combined with a 5-HT antagonist, activation of the LC NE system by an NE agonist resulted in significantly greater (1) NE release in the brain, and (2) subjective feelings of anxiety, nervousness, and restlessness than when the NE agonist was administered without a 5-HT antagonist. Moreover, together with these findings, our model would account for the weak relation (accounting for 3–4% of the variance in behavior) between neuroticism and a genotypical variant of the 5-HT uptake transporter, which may lead to reduced 5-HT functioning via negative feedback effects on 5-HT cells (Lesch, 1998; Lesch, Bengel, & Heils, 1996). In this case, reduced 5-HT functioning may disinhibit the LC NE activity-induced autonomic arousal thought to underlie subjective anxiety (Azmitia & Whitaker-Azmitia, 1997).

Based on animal work, interaction of constraint–5-HT with harm avoidance (fear) may result in variation in latencies to escape behavior mediated through PAG circuitries (Bandler & Keay, 1996; Spoont, 1992). However, this interaction is likely more complex in that behavioral expression of fear is relative to the strength of a separate but tightly linked neurobehavioral system of affective aggression (Gray, 1992; Panksepp, 1998). Affective aggression, which is strongly enhanced by DA agonists, is a goal-oriented pattern of attack behavior that is strongly modulated by incentive motivational processes and is disinhibited by conditions of reduced 5-HT functioning (Coccaro & Siever, 1991; Depue & Spoont, 1986; Lesch, 1998; Panksepp, 1998; Spoont, 1992; Stein et al., 1993; Valzelli, 1981). Joint consideration of fear and affective aggression is not inconsistent with our previous desire for homogeneity, because we view these two motivational systems as independent but as a special case in modeling due to their being neurobiologically tightly linked by *bistable* neural interconnections in both the PAG, somatic integrative zone in the ventromedial medulla, and spinal cord (Bandler & Keay, 1996; Cabot, 1996; Guyenet et al., 1996; Holstege, 1996). Thus, in Figure 7.12, the horizontal axis is represented as a ratio of the strength of fear to affective aggression, and this ratio is modulated by con-

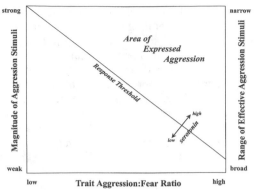

FIGURE 7.12. A minimum threshold for expression of affective aggression is illustrated as a trade-off function between the magnitude of aggression stimuli (left vertical axis) and the ratio of trait affective aggression to trait fear or harm avoidance (horizontal axis). The interaction of these two axes creates a diagonal line demarcating a response threshold, above which is the area of expressed affective aggression. Range of effective (aggression-inducing) aggression stimuli is illustrated on the right vertical axis as a function of level of the aggression:fear ratio. Threshold effects due to serotonin modulation associated with nonaffective constraint are illustrated as well.

straint–5-HT to produce an area of expressed aggression to the right of the diagonal. The common finding that reduced 5-HT functioning is associated with increased affective aggression is thus expressed in Figure 7.12 but is seen as a function of fear as well.

Finally, the effects of 5-HT variation on neurobiological variables associated with affiliation have not been well studied, although Higley, Mehlman, Taub, and Higley (1992) demonstrated that monkeys with low 5-HT functioning are overly aggressive and socially rejected by peers. Such monkeys manifest appropriate sociosexual behavior, but its expressive features, in terms of timing and magnitude, appear to be poorly modulated, thereby negatively arousing peers (Higley et al., 1992).

Conclusion

Models of personality traits based on only one neurotransmitter are clearly simplistic and require addition of other modifying factors (Ashby, 1996). In addition, individual differences of psychobiological origin in lower-order traits will represent error variance in predicting higher-order traits from any one variable alone

(Livesley et al., 1998). Using agentic E as an example, serotonin will certainly not be the only tonic inhibitory modulator of threshold for responding. For instance, functional levels of GABA tonic inhibitory activity may also influence the threshold of behavioral facilitation as an inhibitor of substance P, a neuromodulator having excitatory effects on VTA DA neurons (Kalivas et al., 1993; Le Moal & Simon, 1991). Moreover, receptors for GABA, opiates, substance P, and neurotensin are found in the VTA, and their activation can markedly affect DA activity (Deutch et al., 1993; Kalivas et al., 1993; LeMoal & Simon, 1991). Also, because MAO is responsible for presynaptic degradation of biogenic amines, it may be an important variable in interaction with DA functioning, particularly MAO-B that predominates in primates and has DA as a specific substrate (Mitra, Mohanakumar, & Ganguly, 1994).

Despite the complexity inherent in the interaction of neurotransmitters in emotional traits, there is good reason to start with one neurotransmitter, explore the details of its relation to a trait first, and then gradually build complexity by adding additional factors one at a time. This is particularly true of biogenic amines (DA, serotonin, norepinephrine) and neuropeptides, because they are phylogenetically old and modulate brain structures associated with behavioral processes relevant to personality, including emotions, motivation, motor propensity, and cognition (Depue & Collins, 1999; Lesch, 1998; Luciana & Collins, 1997; Luciana, Depue, Arbisi, & Leon, 1992; Luciana, Collins, & Depue, 1998; Oades, 1985). Furthermore, considering their nonspecific modulatory influence and broad distribution patterns in the brain (Ashby, 1996; Aston-Jones et al., 1996; Insel, 1997; Oades, 1985; Oades & Halliday, 1987; Tork, 1990), variation in a single neuromodulator can have widespread effects on behavior and on the functioning of multifocal neural networks (Mesulam, 1990), as animal research on the behavioral effects of DA, NE, OT, opiates, and 5-HT has clearly demonstrated. Therefore, variation in the biogenic amines and neuropeptides may provide a powerful predictor of human behavioral variation. Thus, single neuromodulators may serve as important building blocks for more complex models of personality traits.

The simplicity of our model, nevertheless, does not prevent comparison with Cloninger's (1986) biological model of personality, which equates novelty seeking with DA, harm avoidance with 5-HT, and reward dependence with NE. As we discussed previously, we would also expect DA to be associated with novelty seeking, although we predict that the relation of DA to personality will be stronger with a more direct measure of agentic extraversion uncontaminated by impulsivity. Our model differs from Cloninger's in most other respects, because his harm avoidance combines anxiety with fear, neither of which appears to be *primarily* related to 5-HT (Depue, 1995, 1996; Lesch, 1998). The relation of NE to reward dependence is not clear to us because the scale is not psychometrically homogeneous (Waller et al., 1991), and because, contrary to Cloninger's (1986) assertions, NE plays no mediating role in positive nor negative *reinforcement* in the animal literature (Depue & Collins, 1999; Mason, 1981). Finally, Cloninger's model provides no role for the neuropeptides OT, VP, and opiates.

A MODEL OF PERSONALITY DISORDERS

We conceive of personality disorders as emergent phenotypes arising from the interaction of the foregoing neurobehavioral systems underlying major personality traits. Plates 7.1, 7.2, and 7.3 illustrate our multidimensional model. In the plates, agentic extraversion (Positive Emotionality [PEM], to emphasize the emotional nature of the trait) and neuroticism (Negative Emotionality [NEM]) are modeled as a ratio of their relative strength, because the opposing nature of their eliciting stimuli affects behavior in a reciprocal manner, such that the expression of one trait is influenced by the strength of the other (Gray, 1973, 1992). This trait combination strongly influences the nature of emotional behavior, as does the affiliation dimension in the model, whereas the nonaffective constraint dimension modulates the expressive features of the other traits. Plate 7.1 provides a predominant PEM:NEM perspective on spatial relations between personality disorders, whereas Plate 7.2 more clearly shows an affiliation perspective. Plate 7.3 adds a dimension of fear to the model because we believe this trait is necessary to account for the full range of phenotypical features of antisocial, dependent, and borderline personality disorders. Taken together, then, the model proposes that the interaction of at least five dimensional personality traits is nec-

essary to account for the emergent phenotypes observed in personality disorders.

In the model, prototypical categories of personality disorder represent the convergence of the most extreme values of multiple traits. In large populations of personality disorders, however, phenotypes will both vary *within* a category and merge imperceptibly with other *related* categories as trait values vary continuously along the contributing multiple dimensions. This variation and merging are illustrated in the plates by the use of color coding of each trait dimension; hence, personality disorder categories show variation throughout their range in color saturation and hue as a function of the changing values of the traits contributing to the personality disorder category. For instance, in Plate 7.1, the changing color of schizoid personality disorder, which is modeled as extremely low on PEM, NEM, and affiliation, is a function of variation in yellow-coded nonaffective constraint.

Several aspects of the model are important. First, spatial placement of the personality disorders relative to the personality traits was based on the content of their DSM-IV criteria (with special attention to the ranked order of criteria), clinical literature, and personality questionnaire studies of personality disorders, although variation in questionnaires, study foci, and subject populations limits use of the latter. Table 7.4 gives the multidimensional coordinates of each personality disorder, but it must be emphasized that the volume of each personality disorder is not meant to mathematically estimate exact or relative personality disorder prevalence or the bounds of phenotypical extremity on any particular trait. Moreover, *generally* the broader the percent range, the less discriminatory power a trait has in delineating a personality disorder, although the unrepresented portion of the range can be important (e.g., histrionic behavior merges with antisocial features in the 0–25% range of affiliation and the 0–20% range of fear). Second, whereas the *emotional* nature of the personality disorder phenotype is strongly influenced by PEM:NEM, the model is relatively novel in proposing that *nonaffective* constraint and affiliation provide major sources of variation in other aspects of the phenotype, which is consistent with the clinical picture of personality disorders. For instance, behavioral instability (e.g., histrionic personality disorder) or rigidity (e.g., compulsive personality disorder) and interpersonal problems represent two

TABLE 7.4. Hypothetical Spatial Coordinates of Personality Disorders Represented in Figure 7.12 and Plates 1 and 2 as a Function of Percent Range on Five Personality Traits

Personality disorder	PEM:NEM	Constraint	Affiliation	Fear
Histrionic	85–100	0–20	25–100	20–100
Antisocial	60–100	0–20	0–25	0–20
Narcicistic	60–80	25–45	15–45	0–100
Borderline	0–30	0–30	30–100	70–100
Compulsive	10–40	85–100	15–100	0–100
Dependent	0–70	30–85	0–100	85–100
Avoidant	0–15	30–85	20–100	0–100
Schizoid	45–55	0–100	0–10	0–100

major criteria in almost every personality disorder category, and both these criteria likely reflect a combination of extreme values in nonaffective constraint and affiliation. Third, as discussed earlier and shown in Table 7.3, an important component of anxiety (NEM) but not fear (harm avoidance) is distress induced by social evaluation and potential disapproval and rejection. Therefore, NEM in the model also incorporates a social component, which we assume in part influences the fear of social evaluation and rejection so strongly evident in the higher-NEM avoidant and borderline personality disorders.

Fourth, the role of fear (or harm avoidance of physical and animal dangers and injury) in the model is novel and requires empirical confirmation. In particular, we propose that fear is a major source of influence on the phenotype of dependent personality disorder because extreme fear inhibits active coping, thereby requiring the protection and support of significant others. That is, developmentally, extreme fearfulness leads to the belief in one's inability to care for oneself and one's incompetence in coping with novel situations, thereby requiring others to provide. The fear of losing such support would be excessive and expressed as "fears of separation" (American Psychiatric Association, 1994, p. 665). In this sense, it may be that chronic forms of childhood separation anxiety disorder represent an early expression of trait fear and a precursor to dependent personality disorder. Concordant with these views is that separation disorder is more common in fearful, shy, inhibited children (Kagan, 1994), and that both clinical cases with separation disorder and fearful children are overrepresented in first-degree offspring of probands with panic disorder (American Psychiatric Association, 1994, p. 112; Kagan, 1994; Last, 1991), which itself

has been conceptualized as dysregulated fear rather than anxiety (Barlow, 1988; Charney et al., 1998; Davis et al., 1997; White & Depue, 1999). Moreover, we (Depue, 1995, 1996) found that fear (harm avoidance) is inversely related to agentic extraversion and to DA agonist-induced prolactin inhibition (-.47, $p < .05$), suggesting that fear inhibits incentive-motivated goal behavior.

Fifth, the model may help to understand sex differences in some personality disorders. The increased prevalence of males in antisocial personality disorder may reflect the lower mean of males in the population on both traits of fear and nonaffective C (including 5-HT), whereas the increased prevalence of females in borderline and dependent personality disorders may reflect a combination of (1) the higher mean of females in the population on neuroticism (borderline) and fear (dependent); (2) their higher mean on affiliation, thereby increasing the need for social relationships whose loss is feared (albeit, for different reasons); and (3) their lower mean on agentic extraversion, particularly social dominance, hence enhancing the effects of neuroticism and fear (Depue & Collins, 1999; Kohnstamm, 1989; Tellegen & Waller, in press). According to our model, histrionic and antisocial personality disorders share trait similarities, but the increased prevalence of females in histrionic personality disorder may reflect the higher female mean on affiliation and fear, whereas the lower male mean on both latter traits may contribute to an antisocial personality disorder phenotype.

Implications of the Model

Several implications of the model can be outlined. First, the model suggests that research on the lines of causal neurobiological influence within the structure of normal personality will need to be a primary focus if the neurobiological nature of personality disorders is to be fully understood. At present, there is a paucity of systematic research in this domain (Depue & Collins, 1999). Second, the multidimensional nature of the model indicates that univariate biological research in personality disorders will inadequately discriminate different phenotypic forms of personality disorders. Thus, not only is multivariate assessment suggested, but methods of combinatorial representation of those multiple variables—as in, for instance, profile, cluster, discriminant function, and multivariate taxonomic analyses—will need to be more fully integrated in personality disorder research. Third, in a similar fashion, research on classification and diagnosis of personality disorders using these same multivariate methods of analysis, but with personality trait values as dependent variables, may prove useful. But such effort will likely only be rewarded if psychometrically refined *and* biologically validated personality trait measures are established empirically rather than solely theoretically. Finally, the trend in development of neurotransmitter-specific drugs may not fully complement the pharmocotherapy requirements of personality disorders. If personality disorders represent emergent phenotypes of multiple neurobehavioral systems, then pharmacotherapy of personality disorders might be more effective when also designed to modulate multiple neurotransmitter–neuropeptide systems.

ACKNOWLEDGMENTS

This work was supported in part by NIH Research Grant No. 55347 and NIH Research Training Grant No. 17069 awarded to Richard A. Depue, and by NIMH Research Grant No. 45448 awarded to Mark F. Lenzenweger.

REFERENCES

Aggleton, J. (1992). *The amygdala: Neurobiological aspects of emotion, memory, and mental dysfunction* (pp. 124–141). New York: Wiley-Liss.

Aggleton. J., & Mishkin, M. (1986). Anatomy and functions of the amygdala. In R. Plutchik & H. Kellerman (Eds.), *Emotion: Theory, research and experience* pp. 52–83). New York: Academic Press.

Altemus, M., Deuster, P., Gallivan, E., Carter, C., & Gold, P. (1995). Suppression of hypothalamic–pituitary–adrenal axis to stress in lactating women. *Journal of Clinical Endocrinology and Metabolism, 80,* 2954–2959.

Amaral, D., & Witter, M. (1995). Hippocampal formation. In G. Paxinos (Ed.), *The rat nervous system* (pp. 443–494). New York: Academic Press.

American Psychiatric Association. (1994). *Diagnostic and statistical manual of mental disorders* (4th ed.). Washington, DC: Author.

Anagnostaras, S., & Robinson, T. (1996). Sensitization to the psychomotor stimulant effects of amphetamine: Modulation by associative learning. *Behavioral Neuroscience, 110,* 1397–1414.

Andersen, R., Snyder, L., Bradley, D., & Xing, J. (1997). Multimodal representation of space in the posterior parietal cortex and its use in planning movements. *Annual Review of Neuroscience, 20,* 303–330.

Annett, L., McGregor, A., & Robbins, T. (1989). The effects of ibotenic acid lesions of the nucleus accumbens on spatial learning and extinction in the rat. *Behavioral Brain Research, 31,* 231–242.

Argiolas, A., & Gessa, G. (1991). Central functions of oxytocin. *Neuroscience and Biobehavioral Reviews, 15,* 217–231.

Arnsten, A. (1998). The biology of being frazzled. *Science, 280,* 1711–1712.

Ashby, C. (1996). (1996). *The modulation of dopaminergic neurotransmission by other neurotransmitters.* Boca Raton, FL: CRC Press.

Aston-Jones, G., Rajkowski, J., Kubiak, P., Valentino, R., & Shipley, M. (1996). Role of the locus coeruleus in emotional activation. In G. Holstege, R. Bandler, & C. Saper (Eds.), *The emotional motor system.* New York: Elsevier.

Azmitia, E., & Whitaker-Azmitia, P. (1997). Development and adult plasticity of serotonergic neurons and their target cells. In H. Baumgarten & M. Gothert (Eds.), *Serotonergic neurons and 5-HT receptors in the CNS (vol. 129, pp. 1–39).* New York: Springer.

Babor, T., Hofmann, M., & Delboca, F. (1986). Types of alcoholics: 1. Evidence for an empirically derived typology based on indicators of vulnerability and severity. *Archives of General Psychiatry, 49,* 599–608.

Bandler, R., & Keay, K. (1996). Columnar organization in the midbrain periaqueductal gray and the integration of emotional expression. In G. Holstege, R. Bandler, & C. Saper (Eds.), *The emotional motor system.* New York: Elsevier.

Barlow, D. H. (1988). *Anxiety and its disorders: The nature and treatment of anxiety and panic.* New York: Guilford Press.

Bechara, A., Tranel, D., Damasio, H., Adolphs, R., Rockland, C., & Damasio, A. (1995). Double dissociation of conditioning and declarative knowledge relative to the amygdala and hippocampus in humans. *Science, 269,* 1115–1118.

Begg, A., Wickens, J., & Arbuthnott, G. (1993). A long-lasting effect of dopamine on synaptic transmission in the corticostriatal pathway, in vitro. *Proceedings of the 11th International Australasian Winter Conference on Brain Research, International Journal of Neuroscience.*

Belknap, J. K., Modil, J., & Helms, M. (1995). Localization to chromosome 10 of a locus influencing morphine analgesia in crosses derived from C57BL/6 and DBA/2 strains. *Life Sciences, 57,* PL117–PL128.

Bell, K., & Kalivas, P. (1996). Context-specific cross-sensitization between systemic cocaine and intra-accumbens AMPA infusion in the rat. *Psychopharmacology, 127,* 377–383.

Beninger, R. (1983). The role of dopamine in locomotor activity and learning. *Brain Research Review, 6,* 173–196.

Benjamin, E. (1996). Personality and the D4 receptor gene. *Nature Genetics, 12,* 81–84.

Berrettini, W. H., Alexander, R., Ferraro, T., & Vogel, W. (1994). A study of oral morphine preference in inbred mouse strains. *Psychiatric Genetics, 4,* 81–86.

Berrettini, W. H., Ferraro, T., Alexander, R., Buchberg, A., & Vogel, W. (1994). Quantitative trait loci mapping of three loci controlling morphine preference using inbred mouse strains. *Nature Genetics, 7,* 54–58.

Bindra, D. (1978). How adaptive behavior is produced: A perceptual-motivation alternative to response reinforcement. *Behavioral Brain Science, 1,* 41–91.

Blackburn, J. R., Phillips, A. G., Jakubovic, A., & Fibiger, H. C. (1989). Dopamine and preparatory behavior: II. A neurochemical analysis. *Behavioral Neuroscience, 103,* 15–23.

Blakely, R., De Felice, L., & Hartzell, H. (1994). Molecular physiology of norepinephrine and serotonin transporters. *Journal of Experimental Biology, 196,* 263–281.

Blizzard, D. A. (1988). The locus ceruleus: A possible neural focus for genetic differences in emotionality. *Experientia, 44,* 491–495.

Bozarth, M. (1994). Opiate reinforcement processes: Re-assembling multiple mechanisms. *Addiction, 89,* 1425–1434.

Brothers, L., & Ring, B. (1992). A neuroethological framework for the representation of minds. *Journal of Cognitive Neuroscience, 4,* 107–118.

Buss, A., & Plomin, R. (1984). *Temperament: Early developing personality traits.* Hillsdale, NJ: Erlbaum.

Cabib, S., & Puglisi-Allegra, S. (1996). Stress, depression and the mesolimbic dopamine system. *Psychopharmacology, 128,* 331–342.

Cabot, J. (1996). Some principles of the spinal organization of the sympathetic preganglionic outflow. In G. Holstege, R. Bandler, & C. Saper (Eds.), *The emotional motor system* (pp. 16–51). New York: Elsevier.

Callahan, P., Baumann, M., & Rabii, J. (1996). Inhibition of tuberoinfundibular dopaminergic neural activity during suckling: Involvement of *u* and *k* opiate receptor subtypes. *Journal of Neuroendocrinology, 8,* 771–776.

Camp, D., Browman, K., & Robinson, T. (1994). The effects of methamphetamine and cocaine on motor behavior and extracellular dopamine in the ventral striatum of Lewis versus Fischer 344 rats. *Brain Research, 668,* 180–193.

Canteras, N., & Swanson, L. (1992). Projections of the ventral subiculum to the amygdala, septum, and hypothalamus: A PHAL anterograde tract-tracing study in the rat. *Journal of Comparative Neurology, 324,* 180–194.

Carlezon, W., Boundy, V., Kalb, R., Neve, R., & Nestler, E. (1996). Increased sensitivity to the stimulant ac-

tions of morphine after infection of vTA with an HSV vector expressing GluR1. *Society for Neuroscience Abstracts, 22,* 171.

Carter, C. (1992). Oxytocin and sexual behavior. *Neuroscience and Biobehavioral Review,16,* 131–144.

Carter, C., Devries, A., & Detz, L. (1995). Physiological substrates of mammalian monogamy: The prairie vole model. *Neuroscience and Biobehavioral Review, 19,* 303–314.

Carter, C., Lederhendler, I., & Kirkpatrick, B. (1997). The integrative neurobiology of affiliation. *Annals of the New York Academy of Sciences, 807.*

Cattell, R., Eber, H., & Tatsuoka, M. (1980). *Handbook for the Sixteen Personality Questionnaire* (16PF). Champaign, IL: Institute for Personality and Ability Testing.

Charney, D. S., Grillon, C., & Bremner, D. (1998). The neurobiological basis of anxiety and fear: Circuits, mechanisms, and neurochemical interactions (Part I.). *Neuroscientist, 4,* 35–44.

Christensen, H. D., Mutzig, M., & Koss, M. C. (1990). CNS alpha2-adrenoceptor induced mydriasis in conscious rats. *Journal of Ocular Pharmacology, 6,* 123–129.

Christie, M., Summers, R., Stephenson, J., Cook, C., & Beart, P. (1987). Excitatory amino acid projections to the nucleus accumbens septi in the rat: A retrograde transport study utilizing D[^{3}H]aspartate and [^{3}H]GABA. *Neuroscience, 22,* 425–438.

Church, A T. (1994). Relating the Tellegen and five-factor models of personality structure. *Journal of Personality and Social Psychology, 67,* 898–909.

Church, T., & Burke, P. (1994). Exploratory and confirmatory tests of the big five and Tellegen's three- and four-dimensional models. *Journal of Personality and Social Psychology, 66,* 93–114.

Churchill, L., Roques, B., & Kalivas, P. (1995). Dopamine depletion augments endogenous opioid-induced locomotion in the nucleus accumbens using both μ1 and *d* opioid receptors. *Psychopharmacology, 120,* 347–355.

Cirelli, C., Pompeiano, M., & Tononi, G. (1996). Neuronal gene expression in the waking state: A role for the locus coeruleus. *Science, 274,* 1211–1215.

Clark, L., Livesley, W., Schroeder, M., & Irish, S. (1996). Convergence of two systems for assessing personality disorder. *Psychological Assessment, 8,* 294–303.

Clarkin, J., & Lenzenweger, M. (Eds.). (1996). *Major theories of personality disorders.* New York: Guilford Press.

Cleeland, C., Nakamura, Y., & Howland, E. (1996). Effects of oral morphine on cold pressor tolerance time and neuropsychological performance. *Neuropsychopharmacology, 15,* 252–262.

Cloninger, C. R. (1986). A unified biosocial theory of personality and its role in the development of anxiety states. *Psychiatric Development, 3,* 167–226.

Cloninger, C. R. (1987). Neurogenetic adaptive mechanisms in alcoholism. *Science, 236,* 410–416.

Cloninger, C. R., Przybeck, R., & Svrakic, D. (1991). The Tridimensional Personality Questionnaire: U.S. normative data. *Psychological Reports, 69,* 1047–1057.

Cloninger, C. R., Svrakic, D., & Przybeck, T. (1993). A psychobiological model of temperament and character. *Archives of General Psychiatry, 50,* 975–990.

Coccaro, E., & Siever, L. (1991). *Serotonin and psychiatric disorders.* Washington, DC: American Psychiatric Association Press.

Coccaro, E., Siever, L., Klar, H., Maurer, G., Cochrane, K., Cooper, T., Mohs, R., & Davis, K. (1989). Serotonergic studies in patients with affective and personality disorders. *Archives of General Psychiatry, 46,* 587–599.

Comrey, A. (1970). *Manual for the Comrey Personality Scales.* San Diego, CA: Educational and Industrial Testing Service.

Cools, A. R. (1980). The role of neostriatal dopaminergic activity in sequencing and selecting behavioral strategies: Facilitation of processes involved in selecting the best strategy in a stressful situation. *Behavioral Brain Research, 1,* 361–374.

Costa, P., & McCrae, R. (1985). *The NEO Personality Inventory manual.* Odessa, FL: Psychological Assessment Resources.

Costa, P., & McCrae, R. (1989). *The NEO-PI/NEO-FFI manual supplement.* Odessa, FL: Psychological Assessment Resources.

Costa, P., & McCrae, R. (1992). *Revised NEO Personality Inventory (NEO-PI-R) and NEO Five-Factor Inventory (NEO-FFI) professional manual.* Odessa, FL: Psychological Assessment Resourses.

Cullinan, W., Herman, J., & Watson, S. (1993). Ventral subicular interaction with the hypothalamic paraventricular nucleus: Evidence for a relay in the bed nucleus of the stria terminalis. *Journal of Comparative Neurology, 332,* 1–20.

Dahlin, S., Hu, X-T., Xue, C-J., & Wolf, M. (1994). Lesions of prefrontal cortex or amygdala, but not fimbria fornix, prevent sensitization of amphetamine-stimulated horizontal locomotor activity. *Society for Neuroscience Abstracts, 20,* 1621.

Davis, M. (1992a). The role of the amygdala in conditioned fear. In J. Aggleton (Ed.), *The amygdala: Neurobiological aspects of emotion, memory, and mental dysfunction (pp. 255–306).* New York: Wiley-Liss.

Davis, M. (1992b). The role of the amygdala in fear and anxiety. *Annual Review of Neuroscience, 15,* 353–375.

Davis, M., Cassella, J., & Kehne, J. (1988). Serotonin does not mediate anxiolytic effects of buspirone in the fear-potentiated startle paradigm: Comparison with 8-OH-DPAT and ipsapirone. *Psychopharmacology, 94,* 14–20.

Davis, M., Walker, D., & Younglim, L. (1997). Roles of the amygdala and bed nucleus of the stria terminalis in fear and anxiety measured with the acoustic startle reflex. *Annals of the New York Academy of Sciences, 821,* 305–331.

Depue, R. (1995). Neurobiological factors in personality and depression. *European Journal of Personality, 9,* 413–439.

Depue, R. (1996). Neurobiology and the structure of personality: Implications for the personality disorders. In J. Clarkin & M. Lenzenweger (Eds.), *Major theories of personality disorders* (pp. 149–163). New York: Guilford Press.

Depue, R. (in press). *A neurobehavioral model of temperament and personality.* New York: Springer-Verlag.

Depue, R., & Collins, F. (1999). Neurobiology of the structure of personality: Dopamine, facilitation of incentive motivation, and extraversion. *Behavioral Brain Science, 22,* 491–569.

Depue, R., & Iacono, W. (1989). Neurobehavioral aspects of affective disorders. *Annual Review of Psychology, 40,* 457–492.

Depue, R., Luciana, M., Arbisi, P., Collins, P., & Leon, A. (1994). Dopamine and the structure of personality: Relation of agonist-induced dopamine activity to positive emotionality. *Journal of Personality and Social Psychology, 67,* 485–498.

Depue, R., & Spoont, M. (1986). Conceptualizing a serotonin trait: A behavioral dimension of constraint. *Annals of the New York Academy of Sciences, 487,* 47–62.

Deutch, A., Bourdelais, A., & Zahm, D. (1993). The nucleus accumbens core and shell: Accumbal compartments and their functional attributes. In P. Kalivas & C. Barnes (Ed.), *Limbic motor circuits and neuropsychiatry* (pp. 239–257). New York: CRC Press.

De Wacle, J-P., Kiianmaa, K., & Gianoulakis, C. (1996). Distribution of the μ and d opiod binding sites in the brain of the alcohol-preferring AA and alcohol-avoiding ANA lines of rats. *Journal of Pharmacology and Experimental Therapeutics, 275,* 518–527.

Di Chiara, G., Acquas, E., & Carboni, E. (1992). Drug motivation and abuse: A neurobiological perspective. *Annals of the New York Academy of Sciences, 654,* 207–219.

Digman, J. (1990). Personality structure: Emergence of the five-factor model. *Annual Review of Psychology, 41,* 417–440.

Ebstein, A. (1996). The D4DR locus and personality. *Nature Genetics, 12,* 78–80.

Engelmann, M., Ebner, K., Wotjak, C., & Landgraf, R. (1998). Endogenous oxytocin is involved in short-term olfactory memory in female rats. *Behavioral Brain Research, 90,* 89–94.

Everitt, B., & Robbins, T. (1992). Amygdala-ventral striatal interactions and reward-related processes. In J. Aggleton (Ed.), *The amygdala: Neurobiological aspects of emotion, memory, and mental dysfunction* (pp. 312–329). New York: Wiley-Liss.

Eysenck, H. (1981). *A model for personality.* New York: Springer-Verlag.

Eysenck, H., & Eysenck, S. (1985). *Personality and individual differences: A natural science approach.* New York: Plenum.

Ferrante, F. (1996). Principles of opioid pharmacotherapy. *Journal of Pain Symptom Management, 11,* 265–273.

Fink, J. S., & Reis, D. J. (1981). Genetic variations in midbrain dopamine cell number: Parallel with differences in responses to dopaminergic agonists and in naturalistic behaviors mediated by dopaminergic systems. *Brain Research, 222,* 335–349.

Francis, A., & Widiger, R. (1986). The classification of personality disorders: An overview of problems and solutions. In A. Francis & R. Hales (Eds.), *Psychiatry update* (Vol. 5, pp. 240–278). Washington DC: American Psychiatric Press.

Frost, J. J., Douglass, K., & Mayberg, H. (1989). Multicompartmental analysis of [^{11}C]-carfentanil binding to opiate receptors in humans measured by positron emission tomography. *Cerebral Blood Flow and Metabolism, 9,* 398–409.

Frost, J. J., Mayberg, H., & Fisher, R. (1988). Mu-opiate receptors measured by positron emission tomography are increased in temporal lobe epilepsy. *Annals of Neurology, 23,* 231–237.

Fuller, T., Russchen, F., & Price, J. (1987). Sources of presumptive glutamatergic/aspartergic afferents to the rat ventral striatopallidal region. *Journal of Comparative Neurology, 258,* 317–339.

Gaffan, D. (1992). Amygdala and the memory of reward. In J. Aggleton (Ed.), *The amygdala: Neurobiological aspects of emotion, memory, and mental dysfunction* (pp. 95–121). New York: Wiley-Liss.

George, F., & Goldberg, S. (1988). Genetic differences in responses to cocaine. *NIDA Research Monograph, 88,* 239–249.

George, F., Porrino, L., Ritz, M., & Goldberg, S. (1991). Inbred rat strain comparisons indicate different sites of action for cocaine and amphetamine locomotor stimulant effects. *Psychopharmacology, 104,* 457–462.

Gherezghiher, T., & Koss, M. C. (1979). Clonidine mydriasis in the rat. *European Journal of Pharmacology, 57,* 263–266.

Gianoulakis, C. (1996). Implications of endogenous opioids and dopamine in alcoholism: Human and basic science studies. *Alcohol and Alcoholism, 31,* 33–42.

Gianoulakis, C., De Waele, J-P., & Thavundayil, J. (1996). Implication of the endogenous opioid system in excessive ethanol comsumption. *Alcohol, 13,* 19–23.

Gianoulakis, C., Krishnan, B., & Thavundayil, J. (1996). Enhanced sensitivity of pituitary B-endorphin to ethanol in subjects at high risk of alcoholism. *Archives of General Psychiatry, 53,* 250–257.

Goldberg, L. (1981). Language and individual differences: The search for universals in personality lexicons. In L. Wheeler (Ed.), *Review of personality and social psychology* (vol. 2, pp. 141–165). Beverly Hills, CA: Sage.

Goldberg, L., & Rosolack, T. (1994). The big five factor structure as an integrative framework. In C. Halverson, G. Kohnstamm, & R. Marten, *The developing structure of temperament and personality from infancy to adulthood* (pp. 25–50). Hillside, NJ: Erlbaum.

Goldman-Rakic, P. (1995). Toward a circuit model of working memory and the guidance of voluntary motor action. In J. Houk, J. Davis, & D. Beiser (Eds.), *Models of information processing in the basal ganglia* (pp. 317–329). Cambridge, MA: MIT Press.

Gottesman, I. I. (1997). Twins: En route to QTLs for cognition. *Science, 276,* 1522–1523.

Grant, S., London, E., & Newlin, D. (1996). Activation of memory circuits during cue-elicited cocaine craving. *Proceedings of the National Academy of Sciences, 93,* 12040–12045.

Gray, J. A. (1973). Causal theories of personality and how to test them. In J. R. Royce (Ed.), *Multivariate analysis and psychological theory* (pp. 192–248). New York: Academic Press.

Gray, J. (1992). Neural systems, emotion and personality. In J. Madden, S. Matthysee, & J. Barchas (Eds.), *Adaptation, learning and affect.* New York: Raven Press.

Graybiel, A., Aosaki, T., Flaherty, A., & Kimura, M. (1994). The basal ganglia and adaptive motor control. *Science, 265,* 1826–1831.

Greenwald, M., June, H., Stitzer, M., & Marco, A. (1996). Comparative clinical pharmacology of short-acting Mu opioids in drug abusers. *Journal of Pharmacology and Experimental Therapeutics, 277,* 1228–1236.

Grill, H., & Coons, E. (1976). The CNS weighting of external and internal factors in feeding behavior. *Behavioral Biology, 18,* 563–569.

Groenewegen, H., Berendse, H., Wolters, J., & Lohman, A. (1990). The anatomical relationship of the prefrontal cortex with the striatopallidal system, the thalamus and the amygdala: Evidence for a parallel organization. In H. Uylings, C. Van Eden, J. De Bruin, M. Corner, & M. Feenstra (Eds.), *The prefrontal cortex: Its structure, function, and pathology* (pp. 72–91). New York: Elsevier.

Groves, P., Garcia-Munoz, M., Linder, J., Manley, M., Martone, M., & Young, S. (1995). Elements of the intrinsic organization and information processing in the neostriatum. In J. Houk, J. Davis, & D. Beiser (Eds.), *Models of information processing in basal ganglia* (pp. 270–289). Cambridge, MA: MIT Press.

Guilford, J. P. (1975). Factors and factors of personality. *Psychological Bulletin, 82,* 802–814.

Guilford, J. P. (1977). Will the real factor of extraversion-introversion please stand up!: A reply to Eysenck. *Psychological Bulletin, 84,* 412–416.

Guilford, J. P., & Zimmerman, W. (1949). *The Guilford-Zimmerman Temperament Survey: Manual.* Beverly Hills, CA: Sheridan Supply.

Guyenet, P., Koshiqa, N., Huangfu, D., Baraban, S., Stornetta, R., & Li, Y-W. (1996). Role of medulla oblongata in generation of sympathetic and vagal outflows. In G. Holstege, R. Bandler, & C. Saper (Eds.), *The emotional motor system* (pp. 110–121). New York: Elsevier.

Harkness, A. (1992). Fundamental topics in the personality disorders: Candidate trait dimensions from lower regions of the hierarchy. *Psychological Assessment, 4,* 251–259.

Heal, D. J., Prow, M. R., & Buckett, W. R. (1989). Clonidine produces mydriasis in conscious mice by activating central (2-adrenoceptors. *European Journal of Pharmacology, 170,* 11–18.

Heath, A., Cloninger, C. R., & Martin, N. (1994). Testing a model for the genetic structure of personality: A comparison of the personality systems of Cloninger and Eysenck. *Journal of Personality and Social Psychology, 66,* 762–775.

Hebb, D. O. (1949). *The organization of behavior.* New York: Wiley.

Heimer, L., Alheid, G., & Zahm, D. (1993). Basal forebrain organization: An anatomical framework for motor aspects of drive and motivation In P. Kalivas & C.

Barnes (Eds.), *Limbic motor circuits and neuropsychiatry* (pp. 17–31). New York: CRC Press.

Herve, D., Simon, H., Blanc, G., Le Moal, M., Glowinski, J., & Tassin, J. (1981). Opposite changes in dopamine utilization in the nucleus accumbens and the frontal cortex after electrolytic lesion of the median raphe in the rat. *Brain Research, 216,* 422–428.

Heston, L. (1973). Genes and psychiatry. In J. Mendels (Ed.), *Biological psychiatry* (pp. 42–61). New York: Wiley Interscience.

Higley, J., Mehlman, P., Taub, D., & Higley, S. (1992). Cerebrospinal fluid monoamine and adrenal correlates of aggression in free-ranging rhesus monkeys. *Archives of General Psychiatry, 49,* 436–441.

Hogan, R. (1983). A socioanalytic theory of personality. In M. Page (Ed.), *1982 Nebraska symposium on motivation* (pp. 55–89). Lincoln: University of Nebraska Press.

Hol, R., Niesink, M., van Ree, J., & Spruijt, B. (1996). Prenatal exposure to morphine affects juvenile play behavior and adult social behavior in rats. *Pharmacological and Biochemical Behavior, 55,* 615–618.

Holstege, G. (1996). The somatic motor system. In G. Holstege, R. Bandler, & C. Saper (Eds.), *The emotional motor system* (pp. 392–408). New York: Elsevier.

Hooks, M., Jones, G., Neill, D., & Justice, J. (1992). Individual differences in amphetamine sensitization: Dose-dependent effects. *Pharmacological and Biochemical Behavior, 41,* 203–210.

Houk, J., Adams, J., & Barto, A. (1995). A model of how the basal gaglia generate and use neural signals that predict reinforcement. In J. Houk, J. Davis, & D. Beiser (Eds.), *Models of information processing in the basal ganglia* (pp. 215–237). Cambridge, MA: MIT Press.

Hulting, A., Genback, E., & Pineda, J. (1996). Effect of ocytocin on growth hormone release *in vitro. Regulatory Peptides, 67,* 69–73.

Insel, R., & Shapiro, L. (1992). Oxytocin receptor distribution reflects social organization in monogamous and polygamous voles. *Proceedings of the National Academy of Sciences, 89,* 5981–5985.

Insel, R., Young, L., & Wang, Z. (1997). Molecular aspects of monogamy. *Annals of the New York Academy of Sciences, 807,* 302–316.

Insel, T. (1992). Oxytocin—A neuropeptide for affiliation: Evidence from behavioral, receptor autoradiographic, and comparative studies. *Psychoneuroendocrinology, 17,* 3–35.

Insel, T. (1997). A neurobiological basis of social attachment. *American Journal of Psychiatry, 154,* 726–735.

Ivell, R., & Russell, J. (1996). Oxytocin: Cellular and molecular approaches in medicine and research. *Review of Reproduction, 1,* 13–18.

Jackson, D. (1984). *Personality Research Form manual* (3rd ed.). Port Huron, MI: Research Psychologists Press.

Jaeger, T., & van der Kooy, D. (1996). Separate neural substrates mediate the motivating and discriminative properties of morphine. *Behavioral Neuroscience, 110,* 181–201.

Jezova, D., Juranlova, E., Mosnarova, A., Kriska, M., &

Skultetyova, I. (1996). Neuroendocrine response during stress with relation to gender differences. *Acta Neurobiologiae Experimentalis, 56,* 779–785.

Johnson, S., Seutin, V., & North, R. (1992). Burst firing in dopamine neurons induced by N-methyl-D-aspartate: Roles of electrogenic sodium pump. *Science, 258,* 665–667.

Johnston, D. (1997). A missing link? LTP and learning. *Science, 278,* 401–402.

Kagan, J. (1994). *Galen's prophecy.* New York: Basic Books.

Kalivas, P. (1995). Interactions between dopamine and excitatory amino acids in behavioral sensitization to psychostimulants. *Drug and Alcohol Dependence, 37,* 95–100.

Kalivas, P., Bush, L., & Hanson, G. (1995). High and low behavioral response to novelty is associated with differences in neurotensin and substance P content. *Annals of the New York Academy of Sciences, 187,* 164–167.

Kalivas, P., Churchill, L., & Klitenick, M. (1993). The circuitry mediating the translation of motivational stimuli into adaptive motor responses. In P. Kalivas & C. Barnes (Eds.), *Limbic motor circuits and neuropsychiatry* (pp. 391–420). New York: CRC Press.

Kalivas, P., & Stewart, J. (1991). Dopamine transmission in the initiation and expression of drug- and stress-induced sensitization of motor activity. *Brain Research Review, 16,* 223–244.

Kapp, B. (1992). Amygdaloid contributions to conditioned arousal and sensory information processing. In J. Aggleton (Ed.), *The amygdala: Neurobiological aspects of emotion, memory, and mental dysfunction* (pp. 410–415). New York: Wiley-Liss.

Kehow, P., & Tiano, L. (1996). Chronic neonatal opioid blockade modulates behavior and brain dopamine response to stress in day 10 rats. *Society for Neuroscience Abstracts, 22,* 2059.

Kelland, M., & Chiodo, L. (1996). Serotonergic modulation of midbrain dopamine systems. In C. Ashby Jr. (Ed.), *The modulation of dopaminergic neurotransmission by other neurotransmitters.* Boca Raton, FL: CRC Press.

Keverne, E. (1996). Psychopharmacologyacology of maternal behaviour. *Journal of Psychopharmacology, 10,* 16–22.

Kohnstamm, G. (1989). Temperament in childhood: Cross-cultural and sex differences. In G. Kohnstamm, J. Bates, & M. Rothbart (Eds.), *Temperament in childhood* (pp. 89–101). New York: Wiley.

Koob, G. (1992). Drugs of abuse: Anatomy, pharmacology, and function of reward pathways. *Trends in Pharmacological Science, 13,* 177–198.

Koob, G., & Le Moal, M. (1997). Drug abuse: Hedonic homeostatic dysregulation. *Science, 278,* 52–58.

Koob, G., Robledo, P., Markou, A., & Caine, S. B. (1993). The mesocorticolimbic circuit in drug dependence and reward A role for the extended amygdala? In P. Kalivas & C. Barnes (Eds.), *Limbic motor circuits and neuropsychiatry* (pp. 217–245). New York: CRC Press.

Kuribara, H. (1996). Interval-dependent inhibition of morphine sensitization of ambulation in mice by post-morphine treatment with naloxone or restraint. *Psychopharmacology, 125,* 129–134.

Last, C. (1991). Anxiety disorders in children and their families. *Archives of General Psychiatry, 48,* 928–934.

LeDoux, J. (1987). Emotion. In V. Mountcastle (Ed.), *Handbook of physiology* (pp. 517–536). New York: American Physiological Society.

LeDoux, J. (1996a). *The emotional brain.* New York: Simon & Schuster.

LeDoux, J. (1996b). Emotional networks and motor control: A fearful view. In G. Holstege, R. Bandler, & C. Saper (Eds.), *The emotional motor system* (pp. 460–475). New York: Elsevier.

LeDoux, J., Cicchetti, P., Xagoraris, A., & Romanski, L. (1990). The lateral amygdaloid nucleus: Sensory interface of the amygdala in fear conditioning. *Journal of Neuroscience, 10,* 1062–1069.

Le Moal, M., & Simon, H. (1991). Mesocorticolimbic dopaminergic network: Functional and regulatory roles. *Physiological Reviews, 71,* 155–234.

Lesch, K. (1997). Molecular biology, pharmacology, and genetics of the serotonin transporter: Psychobiological and clinical implications. In H. Baumgarten & M. Gothert (Eds.), *Serotonergic neurons and 5-HT receptors in the CNS* (Vol. 129, pp. 671–705). New York: Springer.

Lesch, K-P. (1998). Serotonin transporter and psychiatric disorders. *The Neuroscientist, 4,* 25–34.

Lesch, K., Bengel, D., & Heils, A. (1996). Association of anxiety-related traits with a polymorphism in the serotonin transporter gene regulatory region. *Science, 274,* 1527–1531.

Leyton, M., & Stewart, J. (1996). Acute and repeated activation of male sexual behavior by tail pinch: Opioid and dopaminergic mechanisms. *Physiological Behavior, 60,* 77–85.

Livesley, J. (1987). A systematic approach to the delineation of personality disorer. *American Journal of Psychiatry, 144,* 772–777.

Livesley, J., Jackson, D., & Schroeder, M. (1992). Factorial structure of traits delineating personality disorders in clinical and general population samples. *Journal of Abnormal Psychology, 101,* 432–440.

Livesley, W., Jang, K., & Vernon, P. (1998). Phenotypic and genetic structure of traits delineating personality disorder. *Archives of General Psychiatry, 55,* 941–948.

Loewenfeld, I. E. (1993). *The pupil: Anatomy, physiology, and clinical applications* (Vol. 1.). Detroit, MI: Wayne State University Press.

Loh, E., & Roberts, D. (1990). Break-points on a progressive ratio schedule reinforced by intravenous cocaine increase following depletion of forebrain serotonin. *Psychopharmacology, 101,* 262–266.

Loiselle, R., Giannini, A., Martin, D., & Turner, C. (1966). Differential symptomatic presentation in premenstrual syndrome (PMS) as a function of beta-endorphin. *Society for Neuroscience Abstracts, 22,* 1314.

Louilot, A., Taghzouti, K., Deminiere, J., Simon, H., & Le Moal, M. (1987). Dopamine and behavior: Functional and theoretical considerations. In M. Sandler (Ed.), *Neurotransmitter interactions in the basal ganglia* (pp. 15–33). New York: Raven Press.

Lu, W., Chen, H., Xue, C., & Wolf, M. (1997). Repeated amphetamine administration alters the expression of mRNA for AMPA receptor subunits in rat nucleus accumbens and prefrontal cortex. *Synapse, 26,* 269–278.

Luciana, M., & Collins, P. (1997). Dopaminergic modulation of working memory for spatial but not object cues in normal humans. *Journal of Cognitive Neuroscience, 9,* 330–347.

Luciana, M., Collins, P., & Depue, R. (1998). Opposing roles for dopamine and serotonin in the modulation of human spatial working memory functions. *Cerebral Cortex, 8,* 218–226.

Luciana, M., Depue, R. A., Arbisi, P., & Leon, A. (1992). Facilitation of working memory in humans by a D2 dopamine receptor agonist. *Journal of Cognitive Neuroscience, 4,* 58–68.

Lucki, I. (1992). 5-HT1 receptors and behavior. *Neuroscience Biobehavioral Review, 16,* 83–93.

MacLean, P. (1986). Ictal symptoms relating to the nature of affects and their cerebral substrate. In E. Plutchik & H. Kellerman (Eds.), *Emotion: Theory, research, and experience. Vol. 3: Biological foundations of emotion* (pp. 45–63). New York: Academic Press.

Mandel, M. (1984). Constrained randomness. In R. M. Post & J. C. Ballenger (Eds.), *Neurobiology of mood disorders* (pp. 425–449). Baltimore, MD: Williams & Wilkins.

Mansour, A., Khachaturian, H., Lewis, M., Akil, H., & Watson, S. (1988). Anatomy of CNS opioid receptors. *TINS, 11,* 308–315.

Marinelli, M., Aouizerate, B., Barrot, M., Auriacombe, M., LeMoal, M., & Piazza, P. (1996). Blockade of type II glucocorticoid receptors reduces behavioral and dopaminergic responses to morphine. *Society for Neuroscience Abstracts, 22,* 171.

Mason, S. T. (1981). Noradrenaline in the brain: Progress in theories of Behavioural function. *Progress in Neurobiology, 16,* 263–303.

McCarthy, M., & Altemus, M. (1997). Central nervous system actions of oxytocin and modulation of behavior in humans. *Molecular Medicine Today, 1,* 269–275.

Meehl P. (1973). *Psychodiagnosis: Selected papers.* Minneapolis: University of Minnesota Press.

Meredith, G., Agolia, R., Arts, R., Groenewegen, H., & Zahm, D. (1993). Morphological diversity of projection neurons in the core and shell of the nucleus accumbens in the rat. *Neuroscience, 50,* 149–158.

Mesulam, M. (1990). Large-scale neurocognitive networks and distributed processing for attention, language, and memory. *Annals of Neurology, 28,* 597–613.

Miller, D., Livermore, C., & Nation, J. (1996). Cadmium exposure prevents sensitization to morphine. *Society for Neuroscience Abstracts, 22,* 172.

Millon T. (1996). *Disorder of personality: DSM-IV and beyond* (2nd ed.). New York: Wiley.

Mishkin, M. (1982). A memory system in the monkey. *Philosophical Transactions of the Royal Society, B298,* 85–95.

Mitra, N., Mohanakumar, K., & Ganguly, D. (1994). Resistance of golden hamster: Relationship to MAO-B. *Journal of Neurochemistry, 62,* 1906–1912.

Mogenson, G., Grudzynski, S., Wu, M., Yang, C., & Yim, C. (1993). From motivation to action. In P. Kalivas & C. Barnes (Eds.), *Limbic motor circuits and neuropsychiatry* (pp. 334–352). New York: CRC Press.

Morrone, J., Depue, R., Sherer, A., & White, T. (2000). Film-induced incentive motivation is associated with agentic extraversion but not affiliative extraversion. *Personality and Individual Differences, 29,* 199–216.

Mullen, P. E., Lightman, S., Linsell, C., McKeon, P., Sever, P. S., & Todd, K. (1981). Rhythms of plasma noradrenaline in man. *Psychoneuroendocrinology, 6,* 213–222.

Murphy, G., & Glanzman, D. (1997). Mediation of classical conditioning in *Aplysia californica* by long-term potentiation of sensorimotor synapses. *Science, 278,* 467–471.

Nelson, E., & Panksepp, J. (1998). Brain substrates of infant-mother attachment: Contributions of opioids, oxytocin, and norepinephrine. *Neuroscience and Biobehavioral Review, 22,* 437–452.

Nestler, E., & Aghajanian, G. (1997). Molecular and cellular basis of addiction. *Science, 278,* 58–63.

Niesink, R., Vanderschuen, L., & van Ree, J. (1996). Social play in juvenile rats in utero exposure to morphine. *Neurotoxicology, 17,* 905–912.

Nissen, E., Gustavsson, P., Widstrom, A-M., & Uvnas-Moberg, K. (1998). Oxytocin, prolactin, milk production and their relationship with personality traits in women after vaginal delivery or Cesarean section. *Journal of Psychosomatic Obstetrics and Gynecology, 19,* 49–58.

Oades, R. (1985). The role of noradrenaline in tuning and dopamine in switching between signals in the CNS. *Neuroscience Biobehavioral Review, 9,* 261–282.

Oades, R., & Halliday, G. (1987). Ventral tegmental (A10) system: Neurobiology. 1. Anatomy and connectivity. *Brain Research Review, 12,* 117–165.

Olson, G., Olson, R., & Kastin, A. (1997). Endogenous opiates: 1996. *Peptides, 18,* 1651–1688.

Panksepp, J. (1986). The anatomy of emotions. In E. Plutchik & H. Kellerman, *Emotion: Theory, research, and experience. Vol. 3: Biological foundations* (pp. 49–71). New York: Academic Press.

Panksepp, J. (1998). *Affective neuroscience.* New York: Oxford University Press.

Pert, A., Post, R., & Weiss, S. (1992). Conditioning as a critical determinant of sensitization induced by psychomotor stimulants. In L. Erinoff (Ed.), *Neurobiology of drug abuse: Learning and memory* (pp. 14–28). Washington, DC: NIDA.

Pfeiffer, A., Pasi, A., Mehraein, P., & Herz, A. (1982). Opiate receptor binding sites in human brain. *Brain Research, 248,* 87–96.

Phillips, R., & LeDoux, J. (1992). Differential contribution of amygdala and hippocampus to cued and contextual fear conditioning. *Behavioral Neuroscience, 106,* 274–285.

Phillips, T. (1997). Behavior genetics of drug sensitization. *Critical Review of Neurobiology, 11,* 21–33.

Piazza, P., & Le Moal, M. (1996). Pathophysiological basis of vulnerability to drug abuse: Role of an interaction between stress, glucocorticoids, and dopaminergic neurons. *Annual Review of Pharmacology and Toxicology, 36,* 359–378.

Piazza, P., Rouge-Pont, F., Deminiere, J., Kharoubi, M., Le Moal, M., & Simon, H. (1991). Dopamine activity is reduced in the prefrontal cortex and increased in the nucleus acumbens of rats predisposed to develop amphetamine self-administration. *Brain Research, 567,* 169–174.

Pierce, R., Born, B., Adams, M., & Kalivas, P. (1996). Repeated intra-ventral tegmental area administration of SKF-38393 induces behavioral and neurochemical sensitization to a subsequent cocaine challenge. *Journal of Pharmacology and Experimental Therapeutics, 278,* 384–392.

Pierce, R., Duffy, P., & Kalivas, P. (1995). Sensitization to cocaine and dopamine autoreceptor subsensitivity in the nucleus accumbens. *Synapse, 20,* 3–36.

Porges, S. (1998). Love: An emergent property of the mammalian autonomic nervous system. *Psychoneuroendocrinology, 23,* 837–861.

Post, R., Weiss, S., Fontana, D., & Pert, A. (1992). Conditioned sensitization to the psychomotor stimulant cocaine. *Annals of the New York Academy of Sciences,* 386–399.

Puglisi-Allegra, S., & Cabib, S. (1997). Psychopharmacologyacology of dopamine: The contribution of comparative studies in inbred strains of mice. *Progress in Neurobiology, 51,* 637–661.

Redmond, D. E. (1987). Studies of the nucleus locus coeruleus in monkeys and hypotheses for neuropsychopharmacology. In J. Y. Meltzer (Ed.), *Psychopharmacology: The third generation of progress* (pp. 967–975). New York: Raven Press.

Richard, P., Mood, R., & Freund-Mercier, M. (1991). Central effects of oxytocin. *Physiological Review, 71,* 331–370.

Ritz, M., Lamb, R., Goldberg, S., & Kuhar, M. (1987). Cocaine receptors on dopamine transporters are related to self-administration of cocaine. *Science, 237,* 1219–1223.

Robinson, T. (1988). Stimulant drugs and stress: Factors influencing individual differences in the susceptibility to sensitization. In P. Kalivas & C. Barnes (Eds.), *Sensitization in the nervous system* (pp. 145–173). Caldwell, NJ: Tetford Press.

Robinson, T., & Berridge, K. (1993). The neural basis of drug craving: An incentive sensitization theory of addiction. *Brain Research Review, 18,* 247–291.

Rocklin, T., & Revelle, W. (1981). The measurement of extraversion: A comparison of the Eysenck Personality Inventory and the Eysenck Personality Questionnaire. *British Journal of Social Psychology, 20,* 279–284.

Rolls, E. T. (1986). Neural systems involved in emotion in primates. In E. Plutchik & H. Kellerman (Eds.), *Emotion: Theory, research, and experience. Vol. 3: Biological foundations of emotion* (pp. 423–445). New York: Academic Press.

Rolls, E. T. (1999). *The brain and emotion.* New York: Oxford University Press.

Rosenthal, D., & Kety, S. (1968). *Transmission of schizophrenia.* New York: Pergamon Press.

Ross, R., Judd, A., Pickel, V., Joh, T., & Reis, D. (1976). Strain dependent variations in number of midbrain dopaminergic neurons. *Nature, 264,* 654–656.

Rutter, M. (1987). Temperament, personality, and personality disorder. *British Journal of Psychiatry, 150,* 443–458.

Scatton, B., D'Angio, M., Driscoll, P., & Serrano, A. (1988). An *in vivo* voltammetric study of the response of mesocortical and mesoaccumbens dopaminergic neurons to environmental stimuli in strains of rats with differing levels of emotionality. *Annals of the New York Academy of Sciences, 537,* 124–137.

Schlaepfer, T., Strain, E., & Greenberg, B. (1998). Site of opioid action in the human brain: Mu and kappa agonists' subjective and cerebral blood flow effects. *American Journal of Psychiatry, 155,* 470–473.

Schneirla, T. (1959). An evolutionary and developmental theory of biphasic processes underlying approach and withdrawal. In M. Jones (Ed.), *Nebraska symposium on motivation* (pp. 59–72). Lincoln: University of Nebraska Press.

Schultz, W. (1986). Responses of midbrain dopamine neurons to trigger stimuli in the monkey. *Journal of Neurophysiology, 56,* 1439–1461.

Schultz, W., Dayan, P., & Montague, P. (1997). A neural substrate of prediction and reward. *Science, 275,* 1593–1595.

Schultz, W., Romo, R., Ljungberg, T., Mirenowicz, J., Hollerman, J., & Dickinson, A. (1995). Reward-related signals carried by dopamine neurons. In J. Houk, J. J. Davis, & D. Beiser (Eds.), *Models of information processing in the basal ganglia* (pp. 301–349). Cambridge, MA: MIT Press.

Segal, D., & Kuczenski, R. (1987). Individual differences in responsiveness to single and repeated amphetamine administration: Behavioral characteristics and neurochemical correlates. *Journal of Pharmacology and Experimental Therapeutics, 242,* 917–926.

Selden, N., Everitt, B., Jarrard, L., & Robbins, T. (1991). Complementary roles of the amygdala and hippocampus in aversive conditioning to explicit and contextual cues. *Neuroscience, 42,* 335–350.

Sesack, S., & Pickel, V. (1990). Ultrastructural evidence for interactions between opiod and dopaminergic neurons in the rat mesolimbic system. In J. van Ree, A. Mulder, V. Wiegant, T. Van Wimersma Greidanus (Eds.), *New leads in opioid research* (pp. 241–264). Amsterdam, Holland: Excerpta Medica.

Sesack, S., & Pickel, V. (1992). Prefrontal cortical efferents in the rat synapse on unlabeled neuronal targets of catecholamine terminals in the nucleus accumbens septi and on dopamine neurons in the ventral tegmental area. *Journal of Comparative Neurology, 320,* 145–161.

Shaham, Y., & Stewart, J. (1996). Effects of opioid and dopamine receptor antagonists on relapse induced by stress and re-exposure to heroin in rats. *Psychopharmacology, 125,* 385–391.

Shi, S-H., Hayashi, Y., & Petalia R. (1999). Rapid spine delivery and redistribution of AMPA receptors after synaptic NMDA receptor activation. *Science, 284,* 1811–1816.

Shuster, L., Yu, G., & Bates, A. (1977). Sensitization to cocaine stimulation in mice. *Psychopharmacology, 52,* 185–190.

Siever, L., & Davis, K. (1991). A psychobiological perspective on personality disorders. *American Journal of Psychiatry, 148,* 1647–1658.

Sitaram, N., Gillin, J. C., & Bunney, W. E. (1984). Cholinergic and catecholaminergic receptor sensitivity in affective illness: Strategy and theory. In R. M. Post & J. C. Ballenger (Eds.), *Neurobiology of mood disorders* (pp. 629–651). Baltimore, MD: Williams & Wilkins.

Sora, I., Takahashi, N., & Funada, M. (1997). Opiate receptor knockout mice define mu receptor roles in endogenous nociceptive responses and morphine-induced analgesia. *Proceedings of the National Academy of Sciences, USA, 94,* 1544–1549.

Spoont, M. (1992). Modulatory role of serotonin in neural information processing: Implications for human psychopathology. *Psychological Bulletin, 112,* 330–350.

Squire, L., & Kosslyn, S. (1998). *Findings and current opinion in cognitive neuroscience.* Cambridge, MA: MIT Press.

Stallings, M., Hewitt, J., Cloninger, C. R., Heath, A., & Eaves, L. (1996). Genetic and environmental structure of the Tridimensional Personality Questionnaire: Three or four temperament dimensions. *Journal of Personality and Social Psychology, 70,* 127–140.

Stefano, G., & Scharrer, B. (1996). The presence of the µ3 opiate receptor in invertebrate neural tissue. *Comparative Biochemistry and Physiology, 113,* 369–373.

Stefano, G., Scharrer, B., & Smith, E. (1996). Opioid and opiate immunoregulatory processes. *Critical Reviews in Immunology, 16,* 109–144.

Stein, D., Hollander, E., & Liebowitz, M. (1993). Neurobiology of impulsivity and the impulse control disorders. *Journal of Neuropsychiatry, 5,* 9–17.

Stewart, J. (1992). Conditioned stimulus control of the expression of sensitization of the behavioral activating effects of opiate and stimulant drugs. In I. Gormezano & E. Wasserman (Eds.), *Learning and memory: The behavioral and biological substrates* (pp. 187–203). Hillsdale, NJ: Erlbaum.

Stewart, J., de Wit, H., & Eikelboom, R. (1984). Role of unconditioned and conditioned drug effects in the self-administration of opiates and stimulants. *Psychology Review, 91,* 51–268.

Stewart, R., Grabowski, J., Wang, N., & Meisch, R. (1996). Orally delivered methadone as a reinforcer in rhesus monkeys. *Psychopharmacology, 123,* 111–118.

Strand, F. (1999). *Neuropeptides.* Cambridge, MA: MIT Press.

Stricker, E., & Zigmond, M. (1986). Brain monoamines, homeostasis and adaptive behavior. In V. Mountcastle (Ed.), *Handbook of physiology. Section 1. The nervous system. Vol. IV. Intrinsic regulatory systems of the brain* (pp. 677–700). Bethesda, MD: American Physiological Society.

Suaud-Chagny, M., Dhergui, K., Chouvet, G., & Gonon F. (1992). Relationship between dopamine release in the rat nucleus accumbens and the discharge activity of dopaminergic neurons during local in vivo application of amino acid in the ventral tegmental area. *Neuroscience, 49,* 63–78.

Subrahmanyam, R., Paris, J., Chang, J., & Woodward, D. (1996). Ensemble neural activity in the nucleus accumbens (NAc) and prefrontal cortex (PFC) of the awake rat during food and water reinforcement and heroin self-administration. *Society for Neuroscience Abstracts, 22,* 174.

Sutherland, R., & McDonald, R. (1990). Hippocampus, amygdala and memory deficits in rats. *Behavioral Brain Research, 37,* 57–79.

Sved, A. F., Baker, H. A., & Reis, D. J. (1984). Dopamine synthesis in inbred mouse strains which differ in numbers of dopamine neurons. *Brain Research, 303,* 261–266.

Sved, A. F., Baker, H. A., & Reis, D. J. (1985). Number of dopamine neurons predicts prolactin levels in two inbred mouse strains. *Experientia, 41,* 644–646.

Taber, M., Das, S., & Fibiger, H. (1995). Cortical regulation of subcortical dopamine release: Mediation via the ventral tegmental area. *Journal of Neurochemistry, 65,* 1407–1410.

Takagishi, M., & Chiba, T. (1991). Efferent projections of the infralimbic (area 25) region of the medial prefrontal cortex in the rat. *Brain Research, 566,* 26–39.

Tellegen, A. (1985). Structures of mood and personality and their relevance to assessing anxiety, with an emphasis on self-report. In A. Tuma & J. Maser (Eds.), *Anxiety and the anxiety disorders.* Hillside, NJ: Erlbaum.

Tellegen, A., Lykken, D. T., Bouchard, T. J., Wilcox, K. J., Segal, N. L., & Rich, S. (1988). Personality similarity in twins reared apart and together. *Journal of Personality and Social Psychology, 54,* 1031–1039.

Tellegen, A., & Waller, N. G. (in press). Exploring personality through test construction: Development of the multidimensional personality questionnaire. In S. Briggs & J. Cheek (Eds.), *Personality measures: Development and evaluation* (Vol. 1, pp. 171–248). New York: JAI Press.

Thorpe, S., Rolls, E., & Maddison, S. (1983). The orbitofrontal cortex: Neuronal activity in the behaving monkey. *Experimental British Research, 49,* 93–113.

Tork, I. (1990). Anatomy of the serotonergic system. *Annals of the New York Academy of Sciences, 600,* 9–32.

Toshihiko, A., Graybiel, A., & Kimura, M. (1994). Effect of the nigrostriatal dopamine system on acquired neural responses in the striatuim of behaving monkeys. *Science, 265,* 412–415.

Treit, D., Pesold, C., & Rotzinger, S. (1993). Dissociating the anti-fear effects of septal and amygdaloid lesions using two pharmacologically validated models of rat anxiety. *Behavioral Neuroscience, 107,* 770–785.

Uhl, G., Sora, I., & Wang, Z. (1999). The *u* opiate receptor as a candidate gene for pain: Polymorphisms, variations, in expression, nociception, and opiate response. *Proceedings of the National Academy of Sciences, 96,* 7752–7755.

Uvnas-Moberg, K. (1997a). Oxytocin may mediate the benefits of positive social interaction and emotions.

Annals of the New York Academy of Sciences, 807, 222–239.

Uvnas-Moberg, K. (1997b). Physiological and endocrine effects of social contact. *Annals of the New York Academy of Sciences, 807,* 146–163.

Uvnas-Moberg, K., Widstrom, A-M., Nissen, E., & Bjorvell, H. (1990). Personality traits in women 4 days postpartum and their correlation with plasma levels of oxytocin and prolactin. *Journal of Psychosometric Obstetrics and Gynecology, 11,* 261–273.

Valzelli, L. (1981). *Psychobiology of aggression and violence.* New York: Raven Press.

van Furth, W., & van Ree, J. (1996). Sexual motivation: Involvement of endogenous opioids in the ventral tegmental area. *Brain Research, 729,* 20–28.

Waller, N., Lilienfeld, S., Tellegen, A., & Lykken, D. (1991). The Tridimensional Presonality Questionnaire: Structural validity and comparison with the Multidimensional Personality Questionnaire. *Multivariate Behavioral Research, 26,* 1–23.

Watanabe, M. (1990). Prefrontal unit activity during associative learning in the monkey. *Brain Research, 80,* 296–311.

Watson, C., & Clark, L. (1996). Extraversion and its positive emotional core. In S. Briggs, W. Jones, & R. Hogan (Eds.), *Handbook of personality psychology.* New York: Academic Press.

Watson, D., & Tellegen, A. (1985). Towards a consensual structure of mood. *Psychological Bulletin, 98,* 219–235.

White, N. (1986). Control of sensorimotor function by dopaminergic nigrostriatal neurons: Influence on eating and drinking. *Neuroscience and Biobehavioral Review, 10,* 15–36.

White, T., & Depue, R. (1999). Differential association of traits of fear and anxiety with norepinephrine- and dark-induced pupil reactivity. *Journal of Personality and Social Psychology, 77,* 863–877.

Wickens, J., & Kotter, R. (1995). Cellular models of reinforcement. In J. Houk, J. Davis, & D. Beiser (Eds.), *Models of information processing in the basal ganglia.* Cambridge, MA: MIT Press.

Widiger, T. (1992). Categorical versus dimensional classification: Implications from and for research. *Journal of Personality Disorders, 6,* 287–300.

Widiger, T. (1993). The DSM-III-R categorical personality disorder diagnoses: A critique and alternative. *Psychological Inquiry, 4,* 75–90.

Widiger, T., & Costa, P. (1994). Personality and personality disorders. *Journal of Abnormal Psychology, 103,* 78–91.

Widiger, T., Trull, T., Clarkin, J., Sanderson, C., & Costa, P. (1994). A description of the DSM-III-R and DSM-IV personality disorders with the five-factor model. In P. Costa & T. Widiger (Eds.), *Personality disorders and the five-factor model of personality* (pp. 41–56). Washington, DC: American Psychological Association.

Wiggins, J. (1991). Agency and communion as conceptual coordinates for the understanding and measurement of interpersonal behavior. In D. Cicchetti & W. Grove (Eds.), *Thinking clearly about psychology: Essays in honor of Paul Everett Meehl* (pp. 89–113). Minneapolis: University of Minnesota Press.

Wiggins, J., & Pincus, A. (1989). Conceptions of personality disorder and dimensions of personality. *Psychological Assessment, 1,* 305–316.

Wiggins, J., Trapnell, P., & Phillips, N. (1988). Psychometric and geometric characteristics of the revised Interpersonal Adjective Scales (IAS-R). *Multivariate Behavioral Research, 23,* 517–530.

Williams, J., Insel, R., Harbugh, C., & Carter, C. (1994). Oxytocin centrally administered facilitates formation of partner preference in female prairie voles. *Journal of Neuroendocrinology, 6,* 247–250.

Wilson, F., & Rolls, E. (1990). Neuronal responses related to the novelty and familiarity of visual stimuli in the substantia innominata, diagonal band of Broca, and perventricular region of the primate. *Experimental Brain Research, 80,* 104–120.

Witt, D. (1995). Oxytocin and rodent sociosexual responses: From behavior to gene expression. *Neuroscience and Biobehavioral Review, 19,* 315–324.

Witt, D. (1997). Regulatory mechanisms of oxytocin-mediated sociosexual behavior. *Annals of the New York Academy of Sciences, 807,* 287–301.

Wolf, M., Dahlin, S., Hu, X-T., & Xue, C-J. (1995). Effects of lesions of prefrontal cortex, amygdala, or fornix on behavioral sensitization to amphetamine: Comparison with N-methyl-D-aspartate antagonists. *Neuroscience, 69,* 417–439.

Wright, C., Beijer, A., & Groenewegen, H. (1996). Basal amygdaloid complex afferents to the rat nucleus accumbens are compartmentally organized. *Journal of Neuroscience, 16,* 1877–1893.

Yoshikawa, T., Shibuya, H., Kaneno, S., & Toru, M. (1991). Blockade of behavioral sensitization to methamphetamine by lesion of the hippocamp-accumbal pathway. *Life Sciences, 48,* 1325–1332

Young, L., Wang, Z., & Insel, T. (1998). Neuroendocrine bases of monogamy. *TINS, 21,* 71–75.

Zald, D., & Depue, R. (in press). Serotonergic modulation of both positive and negative affect. *Personality and Individual Differences.*

Zamanillo, D., Sprengel, R., & Hvalby, O. (1999). Importance of AMPA receptors for hippocampal synaptic plasticity but not for spatial learning. *Science, 284,* 1805–1810.

Zhang, X., Hu, X., White, F., & Wolf, M. (1997). Increased responsiveness of ventral tegmental area dopamine neurons to glutamate after repeated administration of cocaine or amphetamine is transient and selectively involves AMPA receptors. *Journal of Pharmacology and Experimental Therapeutics, 281,* 699–704.

Ziegler, M. G., Lake, C. R., Wood, J. H., & Ebert, M. H. (1976). Circadian rhythm in cerebrospinal fluid noradrenaline of man and monkey. *Nature, 264,* 656–657.

Zuckerman, M. (1991). *Psychobiology of personality.* New York: Cambridge University Press.

Zuckerman, M. (1994). An alternative five-factor model for personality. In C. Halverson, G. Kohnstamm, & R. Marten (Eds.), *The developing structure of temperament and personality from infancy to adulthood* (pp. 78–92). Hillside, NJ: Erlbaum.

Zuckerman, M. (1999). Incentive motivation: Just extraversion? *Behavioral Brain Science, 22,* 539–540.

Zuckerman, M., Kuhlman, D., Thornquist, M., & Kiers, H. (1991). Five (or three) robust questionnaire scale factors of personality without culture. *Personality and Individual Differences, 12,* 929–941.

CHAPTER 8

Genetics

KERRY L. JANG
PHILIP A. VERNON

Personality function has become the next great frontier for genetical research. Advances in mathematical modeling methodologies and the relative ease of obtaining genetically informative data (e.g., from identical and fraternal twins) have led to a virtual explosion of research in this area and produced one of the most replicable results ever found in the social sciences: About half the total variance in personality trait scores is directly attributable to genetic differences between individuals (see Bouchard, 1997, for a review). With the knowledge that personality is highly heritable, no matter how it is measured or from which model it is derived, researchers hoped that it would be relatively easy to localize the putative genes themselves. In stark contrast to the twin and adoption studies, however, efforts to localize these genes have met with little success. To date, no study or series of studies has unequivocally identified any loci for any personality trait or any of the personality disorder diagnoses. There have been several tantalizing reports of significant associations, but none of these has yet been consistently replicated on independent samples.

THE ELUSIVE PHENOTYPE

Genetic methodologies require a clear definition of the phenotype so that a proband or affected status can be assigned. The methods are predicated on the assumption that if a disorder has a genetic component, the responsible gene(s) would be passed from parents to offspring with certain probabilities in a predictable way. These probabilities and patterns will vary under different conditions (e.g., if the gene is autosomal dominant as opposed to recessive), as dictated by the laws of genetic transmission. However, any misdiagnosis due to unclear or overlapping diagnostic criteria will spuriously alter the observed pattern of inheritance and the results.

The definition of the phenotype remains the most important prerequisite for successful genetic studies. Despite years of effort, personality researchers have yet to provide such a definition and unresolved problems in the current psychiatric nosology are perhaps largely to blame for the slow progress in localizing putative genetic loci. For example, scanning the pages of any of the major psychological and psychiatric journals shows that competing models of personality and their measures—such as the Revised NEO Personality Inventory (NEO-PI-R; Costa & McCrae, 1992); the Multidimensional Personality Questionnaire (MPQ; Tellegen, 1982); the Revised Eysenck Personality Questionnaire (EPQ-R; Eysenck & Eysenck, 1992); or a host of weakly validated "home brew" measures—can be found prominently featured in any single issue. The existence of competing models would not be so much of a problem if the differences between them could be attributed to the fact that each is simply an imperfect measure of the same underlying trait. However, the differences that exist between some of the major models of personality are far more serious, revolving around whether or not some behaviors are actually part of the core definition of the trait in question. For example, NEO-PI-R Neuroticism contains items assessing impulsive behaviors, whereas these behaviors are lacking in the EPQ-R Neuroticism because the definition of trait neuroticism is fundamentally different in each model. How can one find the gene for personality when such fundamental differences exist?

The field of personality disorder research is no better, and likely in worse, shape as a result of the use of discrete categorical diagnostic systems such as the *Diagnostic and Statistical Manual of Mental Disorders* Axis II diagnoses (DSM-IV; American Psychiatric Association, 1994). It was thought that clear criteria would improve matters, but personality dysfunction in the real world continues to defy any orderly classification into distinct types. This is because the behaviors recognized as constituting personality are *pan diagnostic*. This is reflected by the large overlap in diagnostic criteria and by the fact that the present diagnostic system allows for a person to be simultaneously diagnosed with several personality disorders. This problem has not gone unnoticed. However, instead of directly addressing the problem, many psychiatric researchers have tried to circumvent it by discarding one method of genetic analysis for another. For example, consider the following quotation:

> A mathematical model will not produce meaningful results if the psychiatric diagnoses it analyzes do not correspond to genetically crisp categories. The dilemma we face is that the diagnoses were developed to serve many masters: clinicians, scientists, insurance companies, and more. There is no a priori reason why these categories would be ideal for genetic studies. Because of the difficulties facing mathematical modeling studies, psychiatric geneticists have turned to molecular genetic methods. Although these methods use mathematical procedures, they have one overriding advantage: their use of family members' actual genes make them powerful tools for discovering pathogenic genes. (Faraone, Tsuang, & Tsuang, 1999, p. 114)

The authors correctly suggest that genetic studies, and in particular, mathematical model-ing studies (e.g., the classic twin study), will be unsuccessful in finding the genes underlying psychiatric dysfunction because of the problems with psychiatric diagnoses. The solution they propose is that by working with people's actual DNA, the diagnostic problems would be mitigated. They are correct in some respects because mathematical genetic approaches typically identify broad "genetic factors" composed of several undefined genes. However, they are fundamentally incorrect because one would still have to link the DNA to behavior, and if the definition of behavior is ambiguous or changing, it would be difficult or impossible to obtain replicable results no matter what analytic technique is used.

THE STATE OF THE ART

This gloomy forecast does not suggest that genetic research must stop until the problems of personality measurement are resolved. Instead, the successes and failures in personality genetics are bringing about some fundamental changes in the way personality structure and organization are understood and the way in which personality is measured. With each change, the ability to localize and identify the putative genes is increased. This change is iterative in nature, where each finding informs the next phase of research. One purpose of this chapter is to examine some of the research that has brought about these changes. This research is best understood using the following general organizing principles or considerations:

1. The genetic methodology being used
2. The content of the personality measures
3. The specificity of the personality measures
4. The population under study

There is a specific genetic methodology to address different questions about the genetic basis of any phenotype:

1. Does it run in families - is personality function familial?
2. Is personality function heritable?
3. Is the phenotype caused by a particular allele?

In general, genetic studies tend to follow a progression of research beginning with the establishment of whether a genetic basis is present to the determination of its mode of inheritance to localization of the putative gene(s).

It might seem hardly necessary to mention scale content, but it is important because it determines the precise range of behavior under study. Do the scales, for example, focus on behavior within the normal range, the abnormal range, or the entire distribution? Until recently, the huge advances in personality measurement that occurred in psychology did little to influence the personality disorder classification so central to psychiatry, leading to a clear division between studies of personality and the personality disorders. This division is remediated in genetic studies by the *threshold liability model*. Figure 8.1 illustrates this model and it is instantly recognizable as the basis of the "dimensional model of personality disorder" that has received a great deal of support in the literature over the past decade. The distribution of personality function is seen to vary on a continu-um that ranges from a normal or not ill range of functioning (0 to T_1) to the spectrum conditions that refer to mild pathology—the interface between normal and disordered personality (T_1 to T_2)—to an extreme behavior or ill range of functioning (T_2 to ∞). As Figure 8.1 illustrates, most people have moderate levels of vulnerability, fewer have very high or very low levels. When a person's vulnerability exceeds the threshold denoted by T_2, that person will develop the full disorder; between T_1 and T_2, the person will develop a spectrum condition; below T_1, the individual will be unaffected and will not exhibit psychopathology.

The number of people in a population that will fall into each range is determined by the amount or dosage of genetic and environmental influence. The model is multifactorial in nature and assumes that several genes and environmental effects combine to create an individual's susceptibility; suggesting, then, that patients differ from nonpatients only in the number of pathogenic genetic and/or environmental events or experiences to which they have been exposed. The threshold liability model can be easily modified to explain disorders that exhibit clear discontinuities in the expression of pathology. These disorders are typically found by the appearance of a bimodal distribution (see Figure 8.2). Under this variant of the threshold liability model, the same multifactorial causes are still exerting an influence that creates much of the variability between people, with the addition of one or more significant genetic and/or environmental causes that create the patient group.

Genetic studies of personality function are designed to determine the extent to which the vulnerability or "dosage" is attributable to genetic causes. This task is made difficult given the varied content and response formats of different scales or personality measures. For example, some self-report scales such as the NEO-PI-R assess normal personality function, whereas the EPQ-R also assesses some pathological function. Still others, such as the Schedule of Nonadaptive and Adaptive Personality (SNAP; Clark, 1993), specialize in the assessment of personality dysfunction. It is interesting to note that some of these scales obtain their content from the diagnoses contained in DSM-IV; others use a traditional psychometric approach based on a rational assessment of the literature and expert judgments such as the Millon Clinical Multiaxial Inventory (MCMI-III; Millon, Davis, & Millon, 1994) or the Dimen-

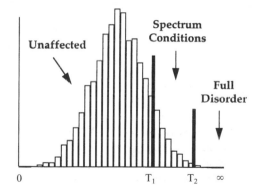

FIGURE 8.1. Threshold liability model. The distribution of personality function is seen to vary on a continuum that ranges from a normal or "not ill" range of functioning (0 to T_1) to the spectrum conditions that refer to mild pathology—the interface between normal and disordered personality T_1 to T_2) to an extreme behavior or ill range of functioning (T_2 to ∞). When a person's vulnerability exceeds the threshold denoted by T_2, he or she will develop the full disorder; if between T_1 and T_2, he or she will develop a spectrum condition, or if below T_1, he or she will be unaffected and will not exhibit psychopathology. The model assumes that multiple genetic and environmental effects combine to create an individual's susceptibility, suggesting, then, that patients differ from nonpatients only in the number of pathogenic genetic and/or environmental events or experiences to which they have been exposed. Adapted from Faraone, Tsuang, and Tsuang (1999). Copyright 1999 by The Guilford Press. Adapted by permission.

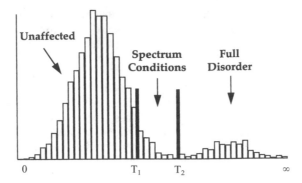

FIGURE 8.2. Modified threshold liability model that accounts for discontinuities in the expression of patholo-gy. Under this model, the same multifactorial causes are still exerting an influence that creates much of the vari-ability between people, 0 to T_1, T_1 to T_2, with the addition of one or more significant genetic and/or environ-mental causes that creates the patient group (T_2 to ∞). Adapted from Faraone, Tsuang, and Tsuang (1999). Copyright 1999 by The Guilford Press. Adapted by permission.

sional Assessment of Personality Pathology (DAPP; Livesley & Jackson, in press). Other scales, such as the Temperament and Character Inventory (TCI: Cloninger, Przybeck, Svrakic, & Wetzel, 1994) and the earlier Tridimensional Personality Inventory (TPQ: Cloninger, Przy-beck, & Svrakic, 1991) are wholly based on theories such as the hypothesized action of neu-rotransmitter systems on behavior. To add to the variety, there are also the clinical rating scales and structured interviews, epitomized by the Axis II DSM-IV diagnoses, which presently contain 10 overlapping diagnoses, down from 12 in the earlier DSM-III-R (American Psychi-atric Association, 1987).

Another complicating factor is the *specificity* of the scales. For example, although the NEO-PI-R measures five broad domains, each of these is composed of six specific facet traits. The question for genetic studies is: At what lev-el of analysis does one conduct a study? It may make sense to estimate the heritability of a broad trait such as "neuroticism," but does it make sense to try to find the specific genes for neu-roticism or for one of the specific subtraits com-prising this domain? Would we expect the genes influencing the broad trait to be the same ones influencing all the lower-level traits or only cer-tain ones? Hierarchical models of personality would predict that all the variation in lower-order traits could be accounted for by the super-ordinate traits, whereas critics might argue that only a portion of the total variance is shared. In the realm of personality function, the geneticist is faced with a wide variety of instruments and levels with which to begin the search for genes.

The great variety of content covered by dif-ferent personality measures is actually benefi-cial in some respects when the population char-acteristics have been taken into account. For example, with reference to Figure 8.1, the ge-netics of normal personality (the area bounded by 0 and T_1) would be addressed by genetic analyses of scales such as the NEO-PI-R ad-ministered to families or twins drawn from the general population. Spectrum disorders, bound-ed by T_1 and T_2 would be assessed by scales such as the DAPP or the SNAP. This same area could be assessed by the NEO-PI-R when ad-ministered to a sample drawn from an inpatient or outpatient personality disorder clinic, but the scores may be hampered by a ceiling effect. Re-gardless, to use measures that assess normal personality function with a clinical population (or vice versa), it must first be established that the scale psychometric properties (e.g., reliabil-ity and factorial structure) do not change from general population to clinical samples. Person-ality dysfunction, the area bounded by $T_2 - \infty$, would be assessed by dimensional measures such as the DAPP and MCMI-III as well as the DSM-IV system of diagnoses when applied to patients. However, the diagnostic overlap inher-ent in the DSM system is more likely to pro-duce erroneous results than is the case with the dimensional scales.

GENETIC METHODS

Several types of genetic analysis can be per-formed in each of the personality function areas delineated by the genetic liability model. Each method addresses a different question about the genetic basis of personality function, and each uses different types of data to answer these questions.

Family Studies

The first question usually addressed is whether or not behavior runs in families. A traditional family study uses a case-control methodology that determines whether a phenotype is familial by establishing that its frequency of diagnosis is greater among genetically related individuals than in a sample of matched controls. Note that familiality does not imply a genetic cause. The observed similarity of relatives is attributable not only to their genetic similarity but also to their common home environment, experiences, and culture. The family design is unable to separate the influence of common genes from common environment and the primary benefit of this type of study is to establish whether additional genetic analyses are warranted.

Family studies have typically been conducted using DSM-style categorical diagnoses because it is relatively simple to ascertain the affected status of different family members via standard clinical interviews. Second, the classification of study subjects amounts to no more than a frequency count of the disorder, and the statistical analyses amount to a simple test of whether the disorder appears in the proband families significantly more often than in the controls. Reich (1989) published a good example of this approach. He found that DSM-III (American Psychiatric Association, 1980) avoidant, dependent, and anxious clusters were familial, but he found only a trend in this direction for borderline personality disorder. The lack of significance for borderline personality disorder was contrary to what several other studies had found (see McGuffin & Thapar, 1993, for a review). It is interesting that Reich found a trend in the correct direction, and perhaps methodological problems (see Dahl, 1993, for a review), such as misdiagnosis due to the overlapping diagnostic criteria caused the discrepancy.

Family studies of dimensional or trait models of personality function are virtually nonexistent. To say that "anxiety" runs in families is meaningless because everybody displays anxiousness to some degree and because there is frequently no clear-cut threshold between "normal" and "abnormal" behavior for these types of scales. The usual approach to finding a threshold is to plot the distribution of scores and look for a discontinuity in the distribution, such as bimodality. However, several epidemiological studies suggest that for psychiatric dysfunction, there is no threshold for disorder in this traditional sense (e.g., Nesdadt, 1997; Nestadt, Romanoski, Brown, & Chahal, 1991). Several other genetic methods, such as linkage analysis (described later) require affected status to be clearly defined.

Segregation Analysis

Once the phenotype has been shown to run in families, the usual next step is to determine how the phenotype is transmitted from generation to generation. For example, is it transmitted in a dominant, recessive, x-linked, or multifactorial manner? How many genes are implicated—one, two, several, or many? The mode of transmission from generation to generation is typically studied using segregation analysis. Segregation analyses translate the laws of genetic transmission into a set of mathematical rules that express the probability that a gene (or gene variant) will be transmitted from parent to child. These probabilities differ for each of the modes of inheritance. These theoretical or "predicted" probabilities are compared against the actual probability that the disorder has been passed among members of a sample of families. Correspondence between the predicted and observed probabilities supports the presence of particular forms of genetic influence because the disorder is passed on in a manner consistent with genetic theory. This procedure is referred to as a "model-fitting" or "goodness-of-fit" approach. Like the family study, segregation analysis requires the assignment of affected status and any misdiagnoses can influence the results. This method is really not well equipped to handle quantitative data that characterize personality and, to an increasing extent, personality disorder assessment.

Twin Studies

A revised form of segregation analysis was developed to overcome this limitation: the twin study using path-analytic techniques (see Neale & Cardon, 1992). The comparison of identical to fraternal twin similarities on a variable of interest allows the separation of genetic from environmental influence, and the path-analytic statistical procedures used to compare twin similarities are designed to handle quantitative measures. These methods are extremely flexible, being able to analyze data from different populations and response formats, and have generated an explosion of studies over the past decade.

Most twin studies use data obtained from reared-together monozygotic (MZ) and dizygotic (DZ) twin pairs, although there are several other variations on the design, such as twins reared apart, and family-of-twin designs (see Plomin, DeFries, & McClearn, 1990). From twins reared together, the magnitude of genetic and environmental influences on a variable is estimated by comparing the relative similarity (e.g., measured by Pearson's r), of MZ pairs to DZ pairs on that variable. Greater MZ than DZ similarity suggests the presence of genetic influence: the greater MZ similarity being attributable to the twofold greater genetic similarity of MZ to DZ twins, assuming all other things being equal. For example, if $r_{MZ} = .42$ and $r_{DZ} = .25$,

$$\text{Heritability } (h^2) = 2(r_{MZ} - r_{DZ}) = 2(.42 - .25)$$
$$= .34 \ (100\%) = 34\%$$

The MZ correlation is due to the fact that these twins share 100% of their genetic material whereas DZ twins on average share only 50%. The difference between the MZ and DZ twin correlations estimates only half of their total genetic similarity so it is doubled to obtain the full complement. The heritability estimate yielded by this formula estimates the genetic influences from all sources, such as additive genetic influences (the extent to which genotypes "breed true" from parent to offspring) and genetic dominance (genetic effects attributable to the interaction of alleles at the same locus which results in a character that is not exactly intermediate in expression as would be expected between pure breeding [homozygous] individuals). Genetic dominance effects are suggested when the MZ correlation is more than twice the magnitude of the DZ correlation (see Plomin, Chipuer, & Loehlin, 1990).

Environmental factors are also estimable. The first is the "shared" environment. The shared component of the environment (e.g., socioeconomic status) distinguishes the general environment of one family from another, and influences all children within a family to the same degree. It is estimated as:

$$\text{Shared environment } (c^2) = r_{MZ} - h^2 = .42 - .34$$
$$= .08(100\%) = 8\%$$

The MZ twin correlation is due to the twin's genetic similarities and to the similarity of their environments. Subtraction of the heritable component yields an estimate of the variance in a variable shared by twins from the same family and differentiates between twins from different families.

The second class of environmental influence is "nonshared" environmental influence, which represents nongenetic factors unique to each person within a family. It is simply estimated with the following equation:

$$\text{Nonshared environment } (e^2) = 1.0 - h^2 - c^2$$
$$= 1.0 - .34 - .08 = .58(100\%) = 58\%$$

Nonshared environmental factors (Hetherington, Reiss, & Plomin, 1994; Rowe, 1994) include events that have differential effects on individual family members (e.g., illnesses, pre- and postnatal traumas, and differential parental treatment). These nonshared, within-family differences extend to the influence of extrafamilial networks, such as differences in peer groups, teachers, or relatives, which may cause siblings to differ. It should be noted that nonshared environmental influences are not estimated directly but represent the residual variance after the genetic and shared environmental influences have been removed. Thus, this component of variance also contains measurement error.

Although Falconer's estimates described above are easy to use, they are not versatile. For example, Falconer's method cannot estimate the magnitude of nonadditive genetic influences. Path-analytic approaches contained in statistical software packages such as LISREL (Jöreskog & Sörbom, 1999a, 1999b) can estimate this quantity as well as provide tests of statistical significance. Just as in classical segregation analysis, the hypothesized relationship between variables is expressed as a series of mathematical equations. This constitutes a "model." The actual correlations between the variables observed in a sample are then fed into the model. If the model is correct, the actual pattern of correlations observed will not differ from the pattern of correlations reproduced by the model. If the observed correlations differ significantly from those predicted by the model, the model does not "fit" the observed data and the hypothesized relationship between the variables is incorrect.

For example, the usual heritability model estimates the proportions of the variance attributable to additive genetic factors (a), nonadditive genetic variance due to genetic epistasis, primarily genetic dominance (d), shared environmental factors (c), and nonshared environmental factors (e). To illustrate the relationship between a hypothesized model and real data, if $r_{MZ} > 2(r_{DZ})$, the value of d is expected to be greater than zero and if the model allows for d to be estimated, the model would provide a good fit to the data. If the model did not include allowances for d, the fit of the model to the data would likely be poor.

The first model fit to the MZ and DZ correlations (or covariances) is the "full model," which specifies a, c, and e influences (or a, d, and e if appropriate). This model is modified to test the significance of a, d, c, and e by systematically removing the effects of (1) additive genetic variance (ce model); (2) shared environmental variance or nonadditive genetic effects (ae); and (3) both additive and nonadditive genetic and shared environmental variance (e only model). The fit of each of the modified models is assessed by testing the difference in χ^2 values between the full and reduced models. The critical value of χ^2 to test the χ^2 difference is determined by the difference in the number of degrees of freedom (df) between the full and reduced model under consideration. The reduced model is rejected whenever χ^2 difference exceeds the critical value of χ^2. The parameter estimates obtained from the best-fitting model are squared to yield the familiar proportions (%) of the variance attributable to each genetic and environmental influence: h^2, d^2 (where applicable), c^2, and e^2. A full treatment of the analytic procedures can be found in Neale and Cardon (1992).

The Assumption of Equal Environments

The results of any twin study are predicated on the assumption that the greater observed MZ than DZ twin similarity is not caused by nongenetic factors, such as MZ twins being treated more similarly than DZ twins. Asking MZ and DZ twins to rate the similarity of their environments usually tests this assumption. Twins are asked whether they were often dressed alike, went to the same schools, and so on. MZ and DZ agreement or concordance rates on these items are then compared.

If differences are found (suggesting that the environments of MZ and DZ twins are not the same), then the defaulting twin similarity variables are correlated with the study's dependent measures to determine whether they account for a significant proportion of the variance. The influence of these variables can be controlled for by computing the standardized residual from the regression of the twin similarity variable on the study variables prior to genetic analyses. To date, the assumption of "equal environments" has been shown to hold across different twin study designs (e.g., Rose, 1991) and for twin studies of psychiatric dysfunction, such as symptoms of depression and anxiety, major depression, phobia, generalized anxiety disorder, alcoholism, and traits delineating personality disorder (e.g., Andrews, Stewart, Morris-Yates, & Holt, 1990; Kendler, 1993; Jang, Livesley, Vernon, & Jackson, 1996). Other twin methodologies, such as studying MZ twins who were separated at birth and reared apart (e.g., Bouchard, Lykken, McGue, & Segal, 1990), dispense with this assumption altogether. Results from studies using twins reared apart yield results similar to those obtained from twins reared together (Bouchard et al., 1990), suggesting that the assumption of equal environments is valid.

The Problem of Sampling Adequacy

Twin studies require a relatively large number of twin pairs (Neale, Eaves, & Kendler, 1994) to have adequate power to detect genetic and environmental influences with any certainty. Unlike studies of normal personality function, it is difficult to recruit a large sample of twins who display personality dysfunction. If twins comprise approximately 2% of the general population and if the prevalence of personality dysfunction is itself no more than 2%, few pairs would be captured using conventional recruitment methods such as newspaper advertisements. This problem has been addressed in a number of ways. The simplest has been to develop a population-based twin registry that uses birth records to identify all twins born in a geographic area. Once the twins have been identified, each pair is systematically contacted and recruited into the study. From this huge sample, sufficient numbers of affected twin pairs may be found. Population-based studies are rare, given their expense, but are invaluable in the amount of information they can yield. Good examples of this type of study are the "Virginia 30,000" (e.g., Eaves et al., 1999) and the well-known Finnish and Swedish studies that find their twins through church birth registries (e.g., Pedersen, McClearn, Plomin, & Nesselroade, 1991). A listing of the world's major twin studies is described in the new journal *Twin Research* (e.g., Boomsma, 1998).

Volunteer twin studies of dysfunction have no option but to advertise for twins with a particular disorder, or to systematically screen for twins who come through a clinic specializing in the treatment of the dysfunction of interest. These strategies rarely find adequate numbers of affected twins and the sample is subject to more self-selection bias than any other recruitment method. It is possible to study dysfunction in general population samples by adopting a dimensional model of personality function and administering scales designed to measure abnormal personality function. This approach assumes that all the elements of personality dysfunction are present and measurable in the general population (albeit in subclinical form) and as such permit a study of the genetic basis of subclinical, or spectrum personality, dysfunction. This dimensional approach is justifiable because the pattern of responses of general population subjects to items assessing personality disorder and symptoms of psychopathology is similar to those of clinical samples (Jackson & Messnick, 1962; Livesley, Jackson, & Schroeder, 1992; Livesley, Jang, & Vernon, 1998).

Representitiveness of the sample can be assessed by comparing personality scores of twins who completed the study to those pairs that did not. In the usual twin design, both members of a twin pair will initially volunteer to participate in the study. If one member of the pair is dysfunctional, only the healthy (or healthier) member of the pair may complete the study. The data from twin pairs in which both members completed the study (concordant-participant) can be compared to the data obtained from pairs in which only one member completed the study (discordant-participant). Because they are twins, there is an expectation that data from the participant twin from a discordant-participant pair will be similar (especially among the MZ pairs) to the nonparticipant twins, and this could be used as a rough estimate of the level of psychopathology existing in the discordant-participant pair. Significant differences in test scores between concordant- and discordant-participant pairs would suggest that the concordant-participant pairs are not representative of the general population (i.e., they are *too* healthy).

Twin Studies of Personality Function

There are hundreds of twin studies of personality function. The results converge to two general findings. First, it is typically found that about 40 to 50% of the total phenotypical variance is due to additive genetic factors, that none or very little is due to shared environmental factors, and that the remainder of the variance is accounted for by nonshared environmental factors (e.g., see Bouchard, 1997, for a review). Second, of all the personality models extant, the results are most consistent when a variant of the five-factor model (FFM) (e.g., Costa & McCrae, 1992), consisting of the domains neuroticism, extraversion, openness to experience, agreeableness, and conscientiousness, is used as a measure of the phenotype.

One unresolved puzzle in this body of research is the fleeting influence of nonadditive genetic effects. The presence of genetic nonadditivity appears to vary by study methodology. For example, Bouchard (1997) notes that in his review of the Minnesota study of twins reared apart, nonadditive effects were not present, whereas in the Loehlin series of studies that used twins reared together (e.g., Loehlin, 1986, 1992, Loehlin, Horn, & Willerman, 1997; Loehlin & Nichols, 1976), they accounted for a sizable portion of the total genetic contribution. Nonadditive results also seem to appear as a function of the personality measure. In a number of studies, nonadditive genetic effects have been detected on the MPQ scales (e.g., Waller & Shaver, 1994) but not on scales such as the NEO-PI-R (e.g., Jang, Livesley, & Vernon, 1996; Jang, McCrae, Angleitner, Riemann, & Livesley, 1998; Riemann, Angleitner, & Strelau, 1997). The Reimann et al. (1997) study also showed that additive genetic influence actually increased when self-report measures of personality were replaced by observational ratings of personality.

Twin studies of personality dysfunction have been largely limited to the "spectrum" disorders in which scales assessing traits delineating personality disorder (e.g., DAPP and Minnesota Multiphasic Personality Inventory [MMPI]) have been administered to twin pairs recruited from the general population. DiLalla, Carey, Gottesman, and Bouchard (1996) estimated the heritability of the 10 standard MMPI clinical scales on a sample of 65 MZ and 54 DZ pairs reared apart. The twins-reared-apart design is the most powerful of twin designs because the usual assumption of equal environments does not apply. The heritability estimates reported were Hypochondriasis (35%), Depression (31%), Hysteria (26%), Psychopathic Deviate (61%), Masculinity–Femininity (36%), Paranoia (28%), Psychasthenia (60%), Schizophrenia (61%), Hypomania (55%), and Social Introversion (34%). They also estimated the heritability of the Wiggins's Content Scales (see Greene, 1991, and Wiggins, 1966, for description), which have demonstrated content validity and no item overlap and cover a wide range of thoughts, experiences, and behaviors associated with psychopathology. The heritability of these scales was estimated at Social Maladjustment (27%), Depression (44%), Feminine Interests (36%), Poor Morale (39%), Religious Fundamentalism (57%), Authority Conflict (42%), Psychoticism (62%), Organic Symptoms (42%), Family Problems (50%), Manifest Hostility (37%), Phobias (59%), Hypomania (45%), and Poor Health (56%). Over these two scales, the median heritability was 44%. Similarly, the heritability of the 18 DAPP dimensions on a large sample of general-population twins yielded similar results (Jang, Livesley, Vernon & Jackson, 1996). The estimates were Affective Lability (45%), Anxiousness (44%), Callousness (56%), Cognitive Distortion (49%), Compulsivity (37%), Conduct Problems (56%), Identity Problems (53%), Insecure Attachment (48%), Intimacy Problems (48%), Narcissism (53%), Oppositionality (46%), Rejection (35%), Restricted Expression (50%), Self-Harm (41%), Social Avoidance (53%), Stimulus Seeking (40%), Submissiveness (45%), and Suspiciousness (45%). The long version of the DAPP scale breaks these 18 basic dimensions into 69 defining facet scales, which were also found to be significantly heritable (0.0% to 58%, median = 45%). In short, the results from these studies are very much in line with those obtained with measures of normal personality function.

Superordinate traits were also found to be heritable to the same degree. For example, principal-components analysis of the 18 DAPP dimensions (e.g., Jang, Livesley, & Vernon, 1999;

Livesley et al., 1998; Schroeder, Wormworth, & Livesley, 1992) yields a four-factor structure that broadly resembles some of the DSM-IV diagnostic categories. The first factor, Emotional Dysregulation, represents unstable and reactive tendencies, dissatisfaction with the self and life experiences, and interpersonal problems. The factor subsumes the personality trait neuroticism as measured by Costa and McCrae's (1992) NEO-PI-R (Schroeder et al., 1992) or the EPQ (Jang et al., 1999). This factor broadly resembles the DSM-IV Cluster B diagnosis of borderline personality disorder. The second factor, Dissocial Behavior, describes antisocial personality characteristics and clearly resembles the DSM-IV Cluster B antisocial personality diagnosis. The third factor is Inhibition, defined by DAPP-DQ Intimacy Problems and Restricted Expression, which resemble the DSM-IV avoidant and schizotypal personality disorders. The fourth factor Compulsivity, clearly resembles DSM-IV Cluster C obsessive–compulsive personality disorder. Additive genetic influences accounted for 52%, 50%, 50% and 44% of the total variance in Emotional Dysregulation, Dissocial Behavior, Inhibition, and Compulsivity, respectively (Jang, Vernon, & Livesley, 2000).

Torgersen, Skre, Onstad, Evardsen, and Kringlen (1993) factor-analyzed DSM-III-R diagnostic criteria to create dimensional scales of personality disorder using data from a sample of healthy twin pairs and their relatives selected from a larger twin study of schizophrenia. Torgersen et al. (1993) interviewed 71 index twins, 106 co-twins, 190 siblings, and 77 parents using the Structured Clinical Interview for DSM-III-R personality disorders. Twelve factors resembling the DSM-III-R personality disorder diagnoses were obtained and, unlike other studies, several of these scales showed little genetic influence. They estimated the heritability for each scale at Self-effacive (63%), Affect-constricted (38%), Contrary (30%), Perfectionistic (30%), Suspicious (27%), Egocentric (24%), Appealing (12%), Disorganized (2%), Insecure (4%), Seclusive (0%), Unreliable (4%), and Submissive (0%). Unlike the other dimensional measures of personality dysfunction, Torgersen et al's (1993) factors are based on actual DSM criteria sets. The fact that they are not heritable suggests that true pathology is etiologically different from normal range function—thus supporting the categorical diagnostic model. However, contrary to expectations, their results suggest little genetic influence and that personality disorder is caused largely by environmental factors.

Results such as these clearly indicate the need for studies of personality dysfunction on clinical samples. Detailed reviews of the literature (e.g., Dahl, 1993; McGuffin & Thapar, 1993; Nigg & Goldsmith, 1994; Thapar & McGuffin, 1993) found few such studies. Most studies contained in these reviews drew their conclusions from the results of studies of normal personality function or from clinically based scales applied to healthy twins drawn from the general population. Of the studies that had been conducted on a clinical sample, these reviews concluded that the sample sizes were very small (e.g., less than 20 pairs) or that the study contained several methodological limitations that affect the accuracy of any heritability estimate. Furthermore, few of the studies used DSM criteria sets, and the abandonment of the DSM system in genetic studies is increasing. Instead, what has been appearing is a growing number of heritability studies on specific personality disorder traits measured using a variety of different scales, many of which were developed in the laboratory that conducted the study. Recent examples include twin studies of aggression (Seroczynski, Bergman, & Coccaro, 1999; Vernon, McCarthy, Johnson, Jang, & Harris, 1999), "pre-schizophrenic personality" (VanKampen, 1999), and juvenile antisocial traits (Lyons, True, Eisen, Goldberg, 1995). It appears as if the DSM diagnoses are now only mentioned to provide a reference point for those readers not familiar with their scales.

GENDER DIFFERENCES

Differences in the magnitude of genetic and environmental effects on a trait may vary by gender. In this form of gene expression, the same genes are assumed to affect both genders but differ only by some common multiple over all loci involved. The literature is full of examples of this research. Rose (1988), for example, reported greater heritability in females than males for the Psychoticism, Masculinity, Somatic Complaints, and Intellectual Differences scales from the MMPI. Zonderman (1982) estimated higher heritabilities in California Personality Inventory Scales (CPI) scales: Responsibility, Achievement via Independence, and Femininity in females. Finkel and McGue (1997) reported re-

sults of analyses using the MPQ that indicated lower female heritability for the Alienation and Control scales and higher female heritability for the Absorption scale. Eaves, Eysenck, and Martin (1989) reported that the heritability of EPQ Neuroticism and Extraversion scales was higher in females than males. However, Loehlin's (1992) combined analysis of the twin data obtained from major studies of personality suggested a different pattern; Neuroticism and Extraversion were more heritable in males. Macaskill, Hopper, White, and Hill (1994) failed to find significant sex differences in the heritability of Neuroticism but higher heritability in males for Extraversion. Loehlin (1982) suggested that these inconsistencies might be due to the use of broad personality trait measures that average out sex effects (Loehlin, 1982). Thus, consistent sex differences are more likely to be identified using measures of more specific personality traits.

Another form of sex-limited gene expression occurs when different genes control the expression of a trait that is measured exactly the same way in males and females. With this form of sex limitation, it is also possible that the same genes are present in both sexes but are only expressed in one sex. Neale and Cardon (1992) give the example of chest girth, in which some of the variation expressed in females may be due to loci that, although still present in males, are only expressed in females. Tests of sex limitation compare the similarities of opposite-sex twin pairs to that of same-sex DZ pairs. Sex-specific genetic influences are suggested when the similarity of opposite-sex pairs is significantly less than the similarities of male or female DZ pairs. The difference in the correlation is attributable to the gender composition of each zygosity group. When the same- and opposite-sex DZ correlations are similar, gender differences are not indicated.

Finkel and McGue (1997) reported the first major study of sex-limited gene expression in personality. This study simultaneously analyzed data from the usual twin groups and data from the twins' parents and siblings. It was concluded that the same genetic loci influence most (11 of 14) MPQ traits in males and females. The exceptions were the Alienation, Control, and Absorption scales. On these traits, genetic influences were sex-specific. It was also found that environmental influences were the same in both sexes. There are, however, several inconsistencies in the findings that may be the result of including data from families of twins in the analyses. For example, examination of the same and opposite-sex fraternal twin correlations suggests that other MPQ scales will show sex-limitation effects than those detected and reported. The $r_{DZ\ males}$, $r_{DZ\ females}$, and $r_{DZ\ opposite\ sex}$ correlations for the Social Potency scale are .33, .28, and .16, respectively. The smaller $r_{DZ\ opposite\ sex}$, which is about half the size of either same-sex correlation, suggests sex-specific effects as noted earlier. On the other hand, the authors report significant sex limitation for the Absorption scale, when the magnitude of $r_{DZ\ males}$, $r_{DZ\ females}$, and $r_{DZ\ opposite\ sex}$ are similar: .17, .13, and .16, respectively. These findings indicate the need for further studies to resolve the inconsistencies.

Jang, Livesley, and Vernon (1998) applied sex-limitation analyses to the DAPP to determine whether traits delineating personality disorders were influenced by gender-specific genetic and environmental influences. The sample consisted of 681 volunteer general-population twin pairs (128 MZ male, 208 MZ female, 75 DZ male, 174 DZ female, 96 DZ opposite-sex pairs). Heritability analyses showed that all dimensions except Submissiveness in males and Cognitive Dysfunction, Compulsivity, Conduct Problems, Suspiciousness, and Self-Harm in females were significantly heritable. Sex-by-genotype analyses suggested that the genetic influences underlying all but four DAPP dimensions (Stimulus Seeking, Callousness, Rejection, Insecure Attachment) were specific to each gender, whereas the influence of the environment was found to be the same in both genders across all dimensions. All four higher-order dimensions were also heritable across sex and in common to both genders except female Dissocial personality dimensions in females, for which no heritable basis was found.

These results are inconsistent with Finkel and McGue's (1997) study of normal personality traits and may be attributable to the insensitivity of the MPQ to detect sex differences. Examination of MPQ item content reveals that it is broad, assessing both positive and negative aspects of personality. The content of the DAPP is more specific, concentrating solely on pathological aspects of personality function and this specificity may permit detection of sex differences. Differences in scale content and specificity may also account for the lack of nonadditive genetic influences on the DAPP. As noted earlier, consistent nonadditive genetic effects have been detected with the MPQ but not with other measures of normal personality. These differences highlight the importance of studying the characteristics of each scale when interpreting the results of genetic studies. Heritability studies set the stage for genotype work by indicating on which traits genes would most likely be found, and, as shown here, this can vary considerably from measure to measure and even between measures of ostensibly the same trait.

MULTIVARIATE ANALYSES

Behavior does not occur in isolation, and the fact that we observe stable factor structures in personality clearly indicates that there are consistent and predictable relationships between behaviors. Genes can be pleiotropic, that is, they may influence one or more behaviors at the same time and may account for the consistent relationships observed between behaviors. Twin-study methodologies offer one avenue to explore these relationships, by estimating the genetic correlation (r_g), which estimates the extent to which two variables are influenced by the same genes. Variables may also covary because the same environmental factors influence their development. This is estimated by the environmental correlation (r_e). Genetic and environmental correlations yield an index that varies between +1.0 and −1.0, and which is interpretable in the same way as Pearson's r.

The method used to estimate the genetic correlation between two variables is similar to that used to estimate heritability. The heritability of a single variable is estimated by comparing the similarity of MZ to DZ twins. A higher within-pair correlation for the MZ twins than the DZ twins suggests that genetic influences are present, because the greater similarity is directly attributable to the twofold increase in genetic similarity in MZ as compared to DZ twins. In the multivariate case, common genetic influences are suggested when the MZ cross-correlation (i.e., the correlation between one twin's score on one of the variables and the other twin's score on the other variable) exceeds the DZ cross-correlation. Mathematically, the relationship between the observed correlation (r_p) between two variables (traits) x and y is explained by

$$r_p = (h_x \cdot h_y \cdot r_g) + (e_x \cdot e_y \cdot r_e)$$

where the observed correlation, r_p, is the sum of the extent to which the same genetic (r_g) and/or environmental factors (r_e) influence each variable, weighted by the overall influence of genetic and environmental causes on each symptom (h_x, h_y, e_x, e_y, respectively). The terms h and e are the square roots of the heritability estimates (h^2 and e^2), for variables x and y, respectively. Although genetic and environmental correlations can be estimated separately (Crawford & DeFries, 1978; Neale & Cardon, 1992), they can be incorporated into two general classes of multivariate genetic models that represent the different ways that genes and the environment can influence multiple symptoms (see McArdle & Goldsmith, 1990; Neale & Cardon, 1992, for detailed discussions).

A useful feature of genetic and environmental correlations is that they are amenable to factor analysis (Crawford & DeFries, 1978). Factor analysis of the matrices of genetic and environmental correlations permits the question of whether an observed (phenotypical) structure reflects a real underlying biological structure. If the factor analysis of the genetic correlations yields a solution similar to what is expected, this suggests that an observed structure reflects an underlying biological structure. This approach was used to study the higher-order structure of traits delineating personality disorder assessed by the DAPP. The DAPP was administered to three independent samples: 602 personality-disordered patients, 939 general-population subjects, and a volunteer sample of 686 twin pairs also recruited from the general population. The phenotypical, genetic, and environmental correlation matrices were computed in all three samples separately and subjected to separate principal-components analyses with rotation to oblimin criteria. In all three samples, four factors were extracted, as described earlier: Emotional Dysregulation, Dissocial, Callousness, and Conscientiousness. The loadings from the matrices of phenotypical correlation matrices were remarkably similar: congruence coefficients ranged from .94 to .99. The congruency coefficients between the genetic and phenotypical factors on Emotional Dysregulation, Dissocial, Inhibition, and Compulsivity were .97, .97, .98, and .95, respectively. The congruence between factors extracted from the phenotypical and nonshared environmental matrices is also very high at .99, .96, .99 and .96, respectively. These data clearly show that the phenotypical structure of personality and personality disorder traits closely reflects the underlying etiological architecture.

Of particular interest in these results is the great similarity of the genetic and phenotypical higher-ordered DAPP dimensions to the basic domains of the FFM (see Widiger, 1998). For example, DAPP Emotional Dysregulation resembles FFM Neuroticism; DAPP Inhibition is the opposite end of FFM Extraversion; DAPP Dissocial shares similar content, albeit in the opposite direction, as FFM Agreeableness; and DAPP Compulsivity resembles FFM Compulsivity. There is no DAPP equivalent to FFM Openness to Experience, which is not surprising given that these types of behaviors are not observed in personality-disordered populations. The similarity of the trait structures provides some strong circumstantial evidence that the same genetic factors underlie normal and abnormal personality, thus bolstering the cornerstone assumption of the dimensional model of personality disorder. A simple direct test would be to compute the genetic correlation between a measure of normal personality and personality dysfunction. Jang and Livesley (1999) computed the genetic correlations between the NEO-FFI scales (Costa & McCrae, 1992) and the DAPP scales on a sample of 545 volunteer general-population twin pairs (269 MZ and 276 DZ pairs). Note that because the data were collected on a general-population sample, the study examined the interface between normal personality and spectrum personality disorder. Between the 18 DAPP dimensions and NEO-FFI Neuroticism, genetic correlations ranged from .05 to .81 (median = .48); with Extraversion they ranged from −.65 to .33 (median = −.28); with Agreeableness they ranged from −.65 to .00 (median = −.38); and with Conscientiousness, the correlations ranged between −.76 and .52 (median = −.31). Not surprisingly, the smallest genetic correlations were found between the DAPP dimensions and NEO-FFI Openness (range = −.17 to .20; median = −.04). An interesting outcome from this study was the finding that the environmental correlations are lower in magnitude but show the same pattern of correlations between DAPP and NEO-FFI scales. In sum, these results indicate that these two scales, measuring normal and abnormal personality function, share to a significant degree a common genetic basis whereas the environmental influences show greater scale specificity.

These results have some implications for

clinical practice and research. First, the results support the use of normal personality inventories in assessing personality disorder, as proposed by Costa and Widiger (1994). Second, although the results show that NEO-FFI and DAPP scales share similar content and genetic basis, the two instruments are not equivalent forms. Unfortunately this study does not indicate the nature of these similarities and differences. This requires further research directed at the estimation of the r_g and r_e at the level of the scale items. Similarities and differences in item etiology between and within scales could then be used to evaluate the distinctiveness of related forms of behavior and to identify subsets of items that account for these similarities and differences. Such an approach has been used to identify distinct subsets of items from apparently homogeneous scales and to identify subtypes of personality function. For example, the EPQ consists of three broad scales composed of 21 to 25 items that assess Neuroticism, Extraversion, and Psychoticism. Heath, Eaves, and Martin (1989) extracted a common genetic and environmental factor for Neuroticism and Extraversion, indicating that these items are etiologically homogeneous. In contrast, little evidence was found for a common genetic basis among Psychoticism items. Subsequent analyses showed that the items formed into two distinct genetic factors: paranoid attitudes and hostile behavior. This analysis is a fine example of the iterative approach in which genetic research can be used to address some issues in personality that will eventually lead to a clear definition of the phenotype and clear the way for replicable genotyping studies.

MOLECULAR GENETIC METHODS

Unlike twin-study methods, linkage and association methods are designed to localize the actual alleles causing behavior as opposed to "genetic factors" or "genetic influences" in which nothing is known about the actual genes themselves. These two methods track the inheritance of DNA segments in families and populations to localize the location of the alleles to a relatively small part of the chromosome.

Linkage studies use the known locations of genes as road signs or "markers" for the disease gene to obtain an approximate idea of where the disease gene is located on a chromosome. For example, if it is thought that the disease gene is on a particular chromosome, a known gene on that chromosome (which may or may not be related to the disease gene) is selected as a marker. It may be, for example, a blood group gene. If the disease gene is physically close to the marker gene, the likelihood of the disease and the marker gene being transmitted together from parent to offspring will be high. The likelihood of them being separated during meiosis is much less than if the marker and the disease genes were far apart. The likelihood that the disease and marker genes will be transmitted together given the distance they are apart can be computed (referred to as a LOD, or "likelihood odds ratio" score) and tracked in families. Two genes are "linked" if they are transmitted together as expected. Linkage studies are popular but appear to work only if the disease gene has a defined mode of inheritance and is clearly defined. For example, several linkages for schizophrenia have been reported (see Faraone et al., 1999) with few replicated results. This is not unexpected given the multifactorial and polygenic basis of behavior, and it comes as no surprise that linkage studies of personality and their disorders are virtually nonexistent.

Personality researchers have tended to avoid linkage methods and have adopted association methodologies. Association study methods are more suited for psychiatric disorder because they require no information on the mode of inheritance, and variants of the method can handle quantitative or qualitative data with equal ease (i.e., quantitative trait loci, or QTL, methods; see Plomin & Caspi, 1998, for a detailed review). This method tests for whether or not the gene of interest is present in more affected individuals than nonaffected individuals: Is the disease form of the gene more common in patients with the disease than in nonpatient controls? The trade-off for not needing to know the mode of inheritance is having some clear idea of which gene is the actual disease gene. Unlike linkage studies, association studies do not pick road signs but require that the gene selected for analysis is actually involved with the disorder of interest. For example, if the neurotransmitter dopamine is found to be implicated in novelty-seeking behavior, it makes sense to choose one of the genes implicated in dopamine production as a "candidate" gene.

Recognizing the need to choose an appropriate candidate gene, Cloninger (1986) developed the Biosocial Model of Personality (see also Cloninger, 1994; Cloninger, Svrakic, & Przybeck, 1993) to provide some guidance in its selection. This model has become a significant model in psychiatry because it makes specific predictions about the neurochemical basis of both normal personality and its disorders and has guided the selection of candidate genes in just about all the association studies of personality. The Biosocial Model divides personality into two broad domains: temperament traits, which resemble stable inherited differences in emotional response, and character traits, which reflect learned, maturational variations in goals, values, and self-concepts. The initial version of the model was implemented through the TPQ, which focused on four temperament traits, each of which was postulated to be influenced by inherited variations in monoamine neurotransmitter systems: serotonin for harm avoidance, dopamine for novelty seeking, and norephinephrine for reward dependence and persistence. The current version of the model, assessed using the TCI, also includes three character traits: Self-Directedness, Cooperativeness, and Self-Transcendence (Cloninger et al., 1993; Cloninger et al., 1994).

Association studies based on predictions from this model have yielded mixed results. Cloninger, Adolfsson, and Svrakic (1996) reported an allelic association between the personality trait Novelty Seeking from Cloninger's TPQ and a gene for a dopamine receptor known as DRD4 or Dopamine D4. The DRD4 marker exists in two forms. The first is a short form in which the alleles that compose the gene are shorter in length and codes for a receptor that is more efficient in binding dopamine. The long form of the allele is less efficient, and it is predicted that individuals with the long DRD4 allele are dopamine deficient and seek novelty to increase dopamine release. As such, an allelic association would be found if the Novelty Seeking scores of individuals with the long form of the allele are significantly higher than those of individuals with the short form of the allele. Since the Cloninger et al. (1996) report of this association, there have been a number of notable replications (Benjamin, Greenberg, & Murphy, 1996; Ebstein, Novick, & Umansky, 1996; Ebstein, Segman, & Benjamin, 1997), but more important, there have been as many failures to replicate the results (e.g., Ebstein, Gritsenko, & Nemanov, 1997; Gebhardt et al., 1997; Malhotra, Goldman, Ozaki, & Breier, 1996; Ono et al., 1997; Pogue-Geile, Ferrell, Deka, Debski,

& Manuck, 1998; Vandenbergh, Zonderman, Wang, Uhl, & Costa, 1997).

Another line of genetic association studies involving trait neuroticism has produced similarly mixed results. Studies on humans and primates indicate that altered brain serotonin activity is related both to negative emotional states such as depression, anxiety, and hostility and to social behaviors such as dominance, aggression, and affiliation with peers. For example, Knutson et al. (1998) found that administration of paroxetine, a specific serotonin reuptake inhibitor that targets the serotonin transporter, both decreased negative affect and increased scores on a behavioral index of social affiliation in normal human subjects. Recently it was reported that expression of the human serotonin transporter gene 5-HTTLPR also exists in long and short forms. The short form of this allele is dominant to the long version of the allele, with the long version of 5-HTTLPR genotype producing more serotonin transporter mRNA and protein than the short form in cultured cells, platelets, and brain tissue. Results have shown that individuals possessing the short form of the allele have significantly increased NEO-PI-R scores (e.g., Lesch et al., 1996) and related traits, such as Harm Avoidance as measured by the TPQ (e.g., Katsuragi et al., 1999). However, at least two other recent studies have found no associations between Harm Avoidance (Hamer, Greenberg, Sabol, & Murphy, 1999) and NEO-PI-R Neuroticism (Gelernter, Kranzler, Coccaro, Seiver, & New, 1998) with the serotonin receptor genes.

Although no definitive allelic associations have been found for the personality traits studied to date, the mixed results are important in shaping how personality is understood. First, the fact that the results are mixed regarding allelic association between the temperament traits Harm Avoidance and 5-HTTLPR and between Novelty Seeking and DRD4 suggests that the neurochemical basis of the popular Biosocial Model is simplistic or incorrect. Second, Hamer et al. (1999) also found significant allelic associations with the "learned" TCI Cooperativeness and Self-directedness character traits and the 5-HTTLPR allele. This finding questions the adequacy of the biosocial model's commonly accepted division of personality into character and temperament. An overview of the molecular genetics of character and temperament traits can be found in Ono et al. (1999) and Herbst, Zonderman, McCrae, and Costa

(2000). In summary, these results suggest that it is unlikely that further studies using the Biosocial Model will be successful at finding the genes for personality. This model needs to be revised and more work needs to be conducted at the phenotypical level before jumping directly to genotyping studies based on theoretical as opposed to empirical grounds. For example, it is not entirely clear why some studies failed to replicate the initial reports of allelic association: Is it due to significant sample differences, or is the content or the psychometric properties of the scales to blame? These questions presently remain unresolved.

ENVIRONMENTAL INFLUENCES ON PERSONALITY FUNCTION

Within the social sciences, the term "environmental factors" has come to broadly include the social environment of the family (e.g., the degree of family conflict, achievement orientation, and moral–religious emphasis), extrafamilial factors such as the social environment of the classroom (e.g., peers and discipline), and factors unique to each person (e.g., traumatic events and differential parental favoritism) as they were growing up. Environmental influences usually refer to objectively measured circumstances, such as poverty or number of books in the home, and to physical factors, such as temperature and degree of sunlight exposure, important in the etiology of some forms of depression, for example. The environment also includes perceptions of the environment, which may be poor representations of reality but which are what people react and respond to. These and other environmental factors have long had central roles in psychiatric and psychological theories on the development of dysfunction and its treatment, epitomized by behavior modification approaches (e.g., cognitive-behavioral therapy). Despite knowing that the environment is important, years of research attempting to identify specifically what these environmental factors are have met with limited success. For example, research identifying family environmental variables that influence alcohol abuse (e.g., Tarter, Kabene, Escallier, Laird, & Jacob, 1990) has typically accounted for approximately 3% or less of the variance in alcohol misuse, leaving 97% accountable by as to yet to be identified factors. This research is characterized by the simple correlation of environmental measures with measures of psychopathology.

IDENTIFYING THE ENVIRONMENTAL INFLUENCES ON THE PERSONALITY TRAIT VARIANCE

Nonshared environmental influences are important because they have been shown to have as much influence on personality as do genes and far more than do shared environmental influences (Bouchard, 1994; Plomin, Chipuer, & Neiderhiser, 1994). In an attempt to identify what these nonshared environmental influences are, several studies have used twin-difference scores on measures of the environment and have then correlated these differences with sibling differences in personality (e.g., Vernon, Jang, Harris, & McCarthy, 1997). Another approach has been to create measures of differential sibling experience in which twins are asked to what degree they were treated differentially by parents, peers, and so on (e.g., Baker & Daniels, 1990; Hetherington et al., 1994). Although some of the findings have been suggestive, few if any nonshared influences on personality have yet been identified. Part of the reason may be the fact that most studies have remained at the level of the phenotype. Recent research has shown that measures of the environment also have a heritable component (e.g., Plomin, Lichtenstein, Pedersen, McClearn, & Nesselroade, 1990; Vernon et al., 1997).

A number of studies have computed genetic correlations between measures of the environment and personality. Several of these correlations were significant, suggesting that an individual's personality plays a significant role in the selection or creation of his or her environment. EPQ Neuroticism and Extraversion, for example, have been shown to be good predictors of life events (e.g., Magnus, Diener, Fujita, & Pavot, 1993; Poulton & Andrews, 1992). Saudino, Pedersen, McClearn, and Plomin (1997) showed that all genetic variance on controllable, desirable, and undesirable life events in women was common to the genetic influences underlying Neuroticism, Extraversion from the EPQ, and Openness to Experience measured by a short version of the NEO Personality Inventory (NEO-PI: Costa & McCrae, 1985). Genetic influences underlying personality scales had little influence on uncontrollable life events simply because this variable was not heritable. Kendler and Karkowski-Shuman (1997) showed that the genetic risk factors for major depression increased the probability of experiencing significant life events in the interpersonal and occupational/financial domains. This is possibly because individuals play an active role in creating their own environments. Heritable factors, such as personality and depression, influence the types of environments sought or encountered. Jang et al. (2000) report significant genetic correlations between FES Cohesiveness and DAPP-DQ Emotional Dysregulation (–.45) FES Cohesiveness and DAPP-DQ Inhibition (–.39); FES Achievement Orientation and DAPP-DQ Dissocial Behavior (.38) and DAPP-DQ Inhibition (–.58); and FES Intellectual Cultural Orientation and DAPP-DQ Emotional Dysregulation (–.34). All these results explain why so-called measures of the "environment" can have a heritable component: They are often a reflection of genetically influenced characteristics of the individual (Saudino, Pedersen, Lichtenstein, & McClearn, 1997).

CONCLUSIONS

Genetic research in personality is coming to a crossroads. Twin research has shown that genetic factors are implicated in personality function but that molecular genetic research has been inconsistent. The reason for this is clear—personality function as a phenotype remains ill defined. Normal personality function can be assessed by any one of a number of scales, each often being developed from quite different theoretical underpinnings or perhaps from no theoretical basis at all. With regard to personality dysfunction, the current DSM system of overlapping and arbitrary categorical diagnoses clearly produces an obscure phenotype. Furthermore, although there is agreement that such a categorical system is no longer tenable, none of the dimensional scales has been developed far enough to replace the current diagnostic system.

For the search for genes to be successful, a great deal of work remains on the definition of personality function. Genetic studies, particularly twin studies using path-analytic techniques, are well placed to bring about definitions of the phenotype that correspond to what Faraone et al. (1999) refer to as "genetically crisp categories" (p. 114). The development of

measures of personality that are only influenced by genetic factors will be the most useful in the search for the putative genes. The development of such measures requires an iterative approach in which genetic studies inform us about the nature of personality and bring about modified measures, which in turn generates genetic studies on these modifications, and so on until replicable results using several different methods are found. This iterative process has clearly begun. For example, Parker (1997) reviewed the genetic research (adoption, twin, molecular genetic, etc.) published to date and used these results to develop and propose a new tripartite model of personality. The viability of Parker's tripartite model is open to empirical test, but the debate it has sparked (e.g., Cloninger, 1997) demonstrates that genetic research of personality function does not end with the discovery of putative gene(s).

REFERENCES

American Psychiatric Association. (1980). *Diagnostic and statistical manual of mental disorders* (3rd ed.). Washington, DC: Author.

American Psychiatric Association. (1987). *Diagnostic and statistical manual of mental disorders* (3rd ed., rev.). Washington, DC: Author.

American Psychiatric Association. (1994). *Diagnostic and statistical manual of mental disorders* (4th ed.). Washington, DC: Author.

Andrews, G., Stewart, G., Morris-Yates, A., & Holt, P. (1990). Evidence for a general neurotic syndrome. *British Journal of Psychiatry, 157,* 6–12.

Baker, L. A., & Daniels, D. (1990). Nonshared environmental influences and personality differences in adult twins. *Journal of Personality and Social Psychology, 58,* 103–110.

Benjamin, J., Greenberg, B., & Murphy D. L. (1996). Mapping personality traits related to genes: Population and family association between the D4 dopamine receptor and measures of novelty seeking. *Nature Genetics, 12,* 81–84.

Boomsma, D. I. (1998). Twin registers in Europe: An overview. *Twin Research, 1,* 34–51.

Bouchard, T. J. (1994). Genes, environment, and personality. *Science, 264*(5166): 1700–1701.

Bouchard, T. J., Jr. (1997). The genetics of personality. In K. Blum & E. P. Noble (Eds.), *Handbook of psychiatric genetics* (pp. 273–296). Boca Raton, FL: CRC Press.

Bouchard, T. J., Lykken, D. T., McGue, M., & Segal, N. L. (1990). Sources of human psychological differences: The Minnesota Study of twins reared apart. *Science, 250*(4978), 223–228.

Clark, L. A. (1993). *Manual for the Schedule of Nonadaptive and Adaptive Personality.* Minneapolis: University of Minnesota Press.

Cloninger, C. R. (1986). A unified biosocial theory of personality and its role in the development of anxiety states. *Psychiatric Developments, 3,* 167–226.

Cloninger, C. R. (1994). Temperament and personality. *Current Opinion in Neurobiology, 4,* 266–273.

Cloninger, C. R. (1997). Etiology of personality disorders: A commentary on Dr. Parker's tripartite model. *Journal of Personality Disorders, 11,* 370–374.

Cloninger, C. R., Adolfsson, R., & Svrakic, N. M. (1996). Mapping genes for human personality. *Nature Genetics, 12,* 3–4.

Cloninger, C. R., Przybeck, T., & Svrakic, D. (1991). The Tridimensional Personality Questionnaire: US normative data. *Psychological Reports, 69,* 1047–1057.

Cloninger, C. R., Przybeck, T., Svrakic, D., & Wetzel, R. D. (1994). *The Temperament and Character Inventory (TCI): A guide to its development and use.* St. Louis, MO: Center for Psychobiology and Personality, Washington University.

Cloninger, C. R., Svrakic, D. M., & Przybeck, T. R. (1993). A psychobiological model of temperament and character. *Archives of General Psychiatry, 50,* 975–990.

Costa, P. T., & McCrae, R. R. (1985). *Manual for the NEO Personality Inventory.* Odessa, FL: Psychological Assessment Resources.

Costa, P. T., & McCrae, R. R. (1992). *Revised NEO Personality Inventory and NEO Five-Factor Inventory.* Odessa, FL: Psychological Assessment Resources.

Costa, P. T. Jr., & Widiger, T. A. (Eds.). (1994). *Personality disorders and the five-factor model of personality.* Washington, DC: American Psychological Association.

Crawford, C. B., & DeFries, J. C. (1978). Factor analysis of genetic and environmental correlation matrices. *Multivariate Behavioral Research, 13,* 297–318.

Dahl, A. A. (1993). The personality disorders: A critical review of family, twin, and adoption studies. *Journal of Personality Disorders, Suppl. 1,* 86–99.

DiLalla, D. L., Carey, G., Gottesman, I. I., & Bouchard, T. J. Jr. (1996). Heritability of MMPI personality indicators of psychopathology in twins reared apart. *Journal of Abnormal Psychology, 105,* 491–499.

Eaves, L. J., Eysenck, H. J., & Martin, N. G. (1989). *Genes, culture and personality.* Berkeley, CA: Academic Press.

Eaves, L., Heath, A., Martin, N., Maes, H., Neale, M., Kendler, K., Kirk, K., & Corey, L. (1999). Comparing the biological and cultural inheritance of personality and social attitudes in the Virginia 30,000 study of twins and their relatives. *Twin Research, 2,* 62–80.

Ebstein, R. P., Gritsenko, I. & Nemanov, L., (1997). No association between the serotonin transporter gene regulatory region polymorphism and the tridimensional personality questionnaire (TPQ) temperament of harm avoidance. *Molecular Psychiatry, 2,* 224–226.

Ebstein, R. P., Novick, O., & Umansky, R. (1996). D4DR exon III polymorphism associated with the personality trait of novelty seeking in normal human volunteers. *Nature Genetics, 12,* 78–80.

Ebstein, R. P., Segman, R., & Benjamin, J. (1997). 5-HT2C (HTR2C) serotonin receptor gene polymor-phism associated with the human personality trait of reward dependence: Interaction with dopamine D4 receptor (D4DR) and dopamine D3 (D3DR) polymorphisms. *American Journal of Medical Genetics, 74,* 65–72.

Eysenck, H. J., & Eysenck, S. B. G. (1992). *Manual for the Eysenck Personality Questionnaire—Revised.* San Diego, CA: Educational and Industrial Testing Service.

Faraone, S. V., Tsuang, M. T., & Tsuang, D. W. (1999). *Genetics of mental disorders: A guide for students, clinicians, and researchers.* New York: Guilford Press.

Finkel, D., & McGue, M. (1997). Sex differences and nonadditivity in heritability of the Multidimensional Personality Questionnaire Scales. *Journal of Personality and Social Psychology, 72,* 929–938.

Gebhardt, C., Fureder, T., Fuchs, K., Urmann, A., Gerhard, E., Heiden, A., Stompe, T., Fathi, N., Meszaros, K., Hornik, K., Sighart, W., Kasper, S., & Aschauer, H. N. (1997, October). *No evidence for normal personality traits related to dopamine 4 receptor gene polymorphism.* Paper presented at the 1997 World Congress on Psychiatric Genetics, Santa Fe, NM.

Gelernter, J., Kranzler, H., Coccaro, E. F., Siever, L. J., & New, A. S. (1998). Serotonin transporter protein gene polymorphism and personality measures in African American and European American subjects. *American Journal of Psychiatry, 155,* 1332–1338.

Greene, R. L. (1991). *The MMPI-2/MMPI: An interpretive manual.* Boston: Allyn & Bacon.

Hamer, D. H., Greenberg, B. D., Sabol, S. Z., & Murphy, D. L. (1999). Role of serotonin transporter gene in temperament and character. *Journal of Personality Disorders, 13,* 312–328.

Heath, A. C., Eaves, L. J., & Martin, N. G. (1989). The genetic structure of personality: III. Multivariate genetic item analysis of the EPQ scales. *Personality and Individual Differences, 10,* 877–888.

Herbst, J. H., Zonderman, A. B., McCrae, R. R., & Costa, P. T. (2000). Do the dimensions of the Temperament and Character Inventory map a simple genetic architecture?: Evidence from modelcular genetics and factor analysis. *American Journal of Psychiatry, 157,* 1285–1290.

Hetherington, E. M., Reiss, D., & Plomin, R. (Eds). (1994). *Separate social worlds of siblings: The impact of nonshared environment on development.* Hillsdale, NJ: Erlbaum.

Jackson, D. N., & Messnick, S. (1962). Response styles on the MMPI: Comparison of clinical and normal samples. *Journal of Abnormal and Social Psychology, 65,* 285–299.

Jang, K. L., & Livesley, W. J. (1999). Why do measures of normal and disordered personality correlate?: A study of genetic comorbitity. *Journal of Personality, 13,* 10–17.

Jang, K. L., Livesley, W. J., & Vernon, P. A. (1996). Heritability of the big five personality dimensions and their facets: A twin study. *Journal of Personality, 64,* 577–591.

Jang, K. L., Livesley, W. J., & Vernon, P. A. (1998). A twin study of genetic and environmental contributions to gender differences in traits delineating personality disorder. *European Journal of Personality,* *12,* 331–344.

Jang, K. L., Livesley, W. J., & Vernon, P. A. (1999). The relationship between Eysenck's P-E-N model of personality and traits delineating personality disorder. *Personality and Individual Differences, 26,* 121–128.

Jang, K. L., Livesley, W. J., Vernon, P. A., & Jackson, D. N. (1996). Heritability of personality disorder traits: A twin study. *Acta Psychiatrica Scandinavica, 94,* 438–444.

Jang, K. L., McCrae, R. R., Angleitner, A., Riemann, R., & Livesley, W. J. (1998). Heritability of facet-level traits in a cross-cultural twin sample: Support for a hierarchical model of personality. *Journal of Personality and Social Psychology, 74,* 1556–1565.

Jang, K. L., Vernon, P. A., & Livesley, W. J. (2000). Personality disorder traits, family environment, and alcohol misuse: A multivariate behavioural genetic analysis. *Addiction, 95,* 873–888.

Jöreskog, K. G., & Sörbom, D. (1999a). *PRELIS 8.2., A preprocessor for LISREL.* Chicago, IL: Scientific Software International.

Jöreskog, K. G., & Sörbom, D. (1999b). *LISREL 8.3.* Chicago, IL: Scientific Software International.

Katsuragi, S., Kunugi, A. S., Sano, A., Tsutsumi, T., Isogawa, K., Nanko, S., & Akiyoshi, J. (1999). Association between serotonin transporter gene polymorphism and anxiety-related traits. *Biological Psychiatry, 45,* 368–370.

Kendler, K. S. (1993). Twin studies of psychiatric illness: Current status and future directions. *Archives of General Psychiatry, 50,* 905–915.

Kendler, K. S., & Karkowski-Shuman, L. (1997). Stressful life events and genetic liability to major depression: Genetic control of exposure to the environment? *Psychological Medicine, 27,* 539–547.

Knutson, B., Wolkowitz, O. M., Cole, S. W., Chan, T., Moore, E. A., Johnson, R. C., Terpstra, J., Turner, R. A., & Reus, V. I. (1998). Selective alteration of personality and social behavior by serotonergic intervention. *American Journal of Psychiatry, 155,* 373–379.

Lesch, K. P., Bengel, D., Heils, A., Zhang Sabol, S., Greenberg, B. D., Petri, S., Benjamin, J., Muller, C. R., Hamer, D. H., & Murphy, D. L. (1996). Association of anxiety-related traits with a polymorphism in the serotonin transporter gene regulatory region. *Science, 274,* 1527–1530.

Livesley, W. J., & Jackson, D. N. (in press). *Manual for the Dimensional Assessment of Personality Problems—Basic Questionnaire (DAPP).* London, Ontario: Research Psychologists' Press.

Livesley, W. J., Jackson, D. N., & Schroeder, M. L. (1992). Factorial structure of traits delineating personality disorders in clinical and general population samples. *Journal of Abnormal Psychology, 101,* 432–440.

Livesley, W. J., Jang, K. L., & Vernon, P. A. (1998). Phenotypic and genetic structure of traits delineating personality disorder. *Archives of General Psychiatry, 55,* 941–948.

Loehlin, J. C. (1982). Are personality traits differentially heritable? *Behavior Genetics, 12,* 417–428.

Loehlin, J. C. (1986). Are California Psychological Inventory items differentially heritable? *Behavior Genetics, 16,* 599–603.

Loehlin, J. C. (1992). *Genes and environment in personality development.* Newbury Park, CA: Sage.

Loehlin, J. C., Horn, J. M., & Willerman, L. (1997). Heredity, environment, and IQ in the Texas adoption study. In R. J. Sternberg & E. L. Grigorenko (Eds.), *Heredity, environment, and intelligence* (pp. 105–125). New York: Cambridge University Press.

Loehlin, J. C., & Nichols, R. C. (1976). *Heredity, environment, & personality: A study of 850 sets of twins.* Austin: University of Texas Press.

Lyons, M. J., True, W. R., Eisen, S. A., & Goldberg, J. (1995). Differential heritability of adult and juvenile antisocial traits. *Archives of General Psychiatry, 52,* 906–915.

Macaskill, G. T., Hopper, J. L., White, V., & Hill, D. J. (1994). Genetic and environmental variation in Eysenck Personality scales measured on Australian adolescent twins. *Behavior Genetics, 24,* 481–491.

Magnus, K., Diener, E., Fujita, F., & Pavot, W. (1993). Extraversion and neuroticism as predictors of objective life events: A longitudinal analysis. *Journal of Personality and Social Psychology, 65,* 1046–1053.

Malhotra, A. K., Goldman, D., Ozaki, N., & Breier, A., (1996). Lack of association between polymorphisms in the 5-HT-sub(2A) receptor gene and the antipsychotic response to clozapine. *American Journal of Psychiatry, 153,* 1092–1094.

McArdle, J. J., & Goldsmith, H. H. (1990). Alternative common factor models for multivariate biometric analyses. *Behavior Genetics, 20,* 569–608.

McGuffin, P., & Thapar, A. (1993). The genetics of personality disorder. In P. Tyrer & G. Stein (Eds.), *Personality disorder reviewed* (pp. 42–63). London: Gaskell/Royal College of Psychiatrists.

Millon, T., Davis, R., & Millon, C. (1994). *Manual for the MCMI-III.* Minneapolis, MN: National Computer Systems.

Neale, M. C., & Cardon, L. R. (1992). *Methodology for genetic studies of twins and families.* London: Kluwer.

Neale, M. C., Eaves, L. J., & Kendler, K. S. (1994). The power of classical twin study to resolve variation in threshold traits. *Behavior Genetics, 24,* 239–258.

Nestadt, G. (1997). Response to Dr. Gordon Parker's paper: An epidemiological perspective. *Journal of Personality Disorders, 11,* 375–380.

Nestadt, G., Romanoski, A. J., Brown, C. H., & Chahal, R. (1991). DSM-III compulsive personality disorder: An epidemiological survey. *Psychological Medicine, 21,* 461–471.

Nigg, J. T., & Goldsmith, H. H. (1994). Genetics of personality disorders: Perspectives from personality and psychopathology research. *Psychological Bulletin, 115,* 346–380.

Ono, Y., Manki, H., Yomishura, K., Muramatsu, T., Higuchi, S., Yagi, G., Kanba, S., & Asai, M. (1997). Association between dopamine D4 receptor (D4DR) exon III polymorphism and novelty seeking in Japanese subjects. *American Journal of Genetics, 47,* 501–503.

Ono, Y., Yoshimura, K., Mizushima, H., Manki, H., Yagi, G., Kanba, S., Nathan, J., & Asai, M. (1999). Environmental and possible genetic contributions to character dimensions of personality. *Psychological Reports, 84,* 689–696.

Parker, G. (1997). The etiology of personality disorders: A review and consideration of research models. *Journal of Personality Disorders, 11,* 345–369.

Pedersen, N. L., McClearn, G. E., Plomin, R., & Nesselroade, J. R. (1991). The Swedish Adoption/Twin Study of Aging: An update. *Acta Geneticae Medicae et Gemellologiae, 40,* 7–20.

Plomin, R., & Caspi, A. (1998). DNA and personality. *European Journal of Personality, 12,* 387–407.

Plomin, R., Chipuer, H. M., & Loehlin, J. C. (1990). Behavioral genetics and personality. In L. A. Pervin (Ed.), *Handbook of personality: Theory and research* (pp. 225–243). New York: Guilford Press.

Plomin, R., Chipuer, H. M., & Neiderhiser, J. M. (1994). Behavioral genetic evidence for the importance of nonshared environment. In E. M. Hetherington & D. Reiss (Eds.), *Separate social worlds of siblings: The impact of nonshared environment on development* (pp. 1–31). Hillsdale, NJ: Erlbaum.

Plomin, R., DeFries, J. C., & McClearn, G. E. (1990). *Behavioral genetics: A primer* (2nd ed.). New York: Freeman.

Plomin, R., Lichtenstein, P., Pedersen, N. L., McClearn, G. E., & Nesselroade, J. R. (1990). Genetic influence on life events during the last half of the life span. *Psychology and Aging, 5,* 25–30.

Pogue-Geile, M., Ferrell, R., Deka, R., Debski, T., & Manuck, S. (1998). Human novelty seeking personality traits and dopamine D4 receptor polymorphisms: A twin and genetic association study. *American Journal of Medical Genetics, 81,* 44–48.

Poulton, R. G., & Andrews, G. (1992). Personality as a cause of adverse life events. *Acta Psychiatrica Scandinavica, 85,* 35–38.

Reich, J. H. (1989). Familiality of DSM III dramatic and anxious personality clusters. *Journal of Nervous and Mental Disease, 177,* 96–100.

Riemann, R., Angleitner, A., & Strelau, J. (1997). Genetic and environmental influences on personality: A study of twins reared together using the self- and peer-report NEO-FFI scales. *Journal of Personality, 65,* 449–475.

Rose, R. J. (1988). Genetic and environmental variance in content dimensions of the MMPI. *Journal of Personality and Social Psychology, 55,* 302–311.

Rose, R. J. (1991). Twin studies and psychosocial epidemiology. In M. T. Tsuang & K. S. Kendler (Eds.), *Genetic issues in psychosocial epidemiology: Series in psychosocial epidemiology* (Vol. 8, pp. 12–32). New Brunswick, NJ: Rutgers University Press.

Rowe, D. C. (1994). *The limits of family influence: Genes, experience, and behavior.* New York: Guilford Press.

Saudino, K. J., Pedersen, N. L., Lichtenstein, P., & McClearn, G. E. (1997). Can personality explain genetic influences on life events? *Journal of Personality and Social Psychology, 72,* 196–206.

Schroeder, M. L., Wormworth, J. A., & Livesley, W. J. (1992). Dimensions of personality disorder and their relationships to the Big Five dimensions of personality. *Psychological Assessment, 4,* 47–53.

Seroczynski, A. D., Bergeman, C. S., & Coccaro, E. F. (1999). Etiology of the impulsivity/aggression relationship: Genes or environment? *Psychiatry Research, 86,* 41–57.

Tarter, R. E., Kabene, M., Escallier, E. A., Laird, S. B., & Jacob, T. (1990). Temperament deviation and risk for alcoholism. *Alcoholism: Clinical and Experimental Research, 14,* 380–382.

Tellegen, A. (1982). *Brief manual for the Differential Personality Questionnaire.* Unpublished manuscript, University of Minnesota, Minneapolis, MN.

Thapar, A., & McGuffin, P. (1993). Is personality disorder inherited? An overview of the evidence. *Journal of Psychopathology and Behavioral Assessment, 15,* 325–345.

Torgersen, S., Skre, I., Onstad, S., Edvardsen, J., & Kringlen, E. (1993).The psychometric–genetic structure of DSM-III-R personality disorder criteria. *Journal of Personality Disorders, 7,* 196–213.

Vandenbergh, D. J., Zonderman, A. B., Wang, J., Uhl, G. R., & Costa, P. T. (1997). No association between novelty seeking and dopamine D4 receptor (DRD4) exon III seven repeat alleles in Baltimore Longitudinal Study of Aging participants. *Molecular Psychiatry, 2,* 417–419.

VanKampen, D. (1999). Genetic and environmental influences on pre-schizophrenic personality: MAXCOV-HITMAX and LISREL analyses. *European Journal of Personality, 13,* 63–80.

Vernon, P. A., Jang, K. L., Harris, J. A., & McCarthy, J. M. (1997). Environmental predictors of personality differences: A twin and sibling study. *Journal of Personality and Social Psychology, 72,* 177–183.

Vernon, P. A., McCarthy, J. M., Johnson, A. M., Jang, K. L., & Harris, J. A. (1999). Individual differences in multiple dimensions of aggression: A univariate and multivariate genetic analysis. *Twin Research, 2,* 16–21.

Waller, N. G., & Shaver, P. R. (1994). The importance of nongenetic influences on romantic love styles: A twin-family study. *Psychological Science, 5,* 268–274.

Widiger, T. A. (1998). Four out of five ain't bad. *Archives of General Psychiatry, 55,* 865–866.

Wiggins, J. S. (1966). Substantive dimensions of self-report in the MMPI item pool. *Psychological Monographs: General and Applied, 80,* 42.

Zonderman, A. B. (1982). Differential heritability and consistency: a reanalysis of the National Merit Scholarship Qualifying Test (NMSQT) California Psychological Inventory (CPI) data. *Behavior Genetics, 12,* 193–208.

CHAPTER 9

Attachment

KIM BARTHOLOMEW
MARILYN J. KWONG
STEPHEN D. HART

Attachment theory and research can help provide a much needed developmental perspective on personality pathology. In addition, attachment theory highlights the interpersonal dimensions of personality difficulties, both as an important aspect of personal adaptation and as a social context in which pathology may develop. Although attachment research has tended to focus on early childhood functioning and adult close relationships, the theory was developed to provide an understanding of personality development, emotional regulation, and psychopathology.

Attachment theory provides a useful framework for understanding personality pathology independent of any claims of continuity between childhood and adult attachment orientations. But the more exciting and controversial implication of the theory is that attachment patterns and associated patterns of adaptation established in the family of origin tend to be carried forward into adulthood. To quote Bowlby (1988b), a key hypothesis of the theory is that "variations in the way these [attachment] bonds develop and become organized during the infancy and childhood of different individuals are major determinants of whether a person grows up to be mentally healthy" (p. 2). Therefore, consideration of the various forms that insecure attachment can take may help clarify the paths leading to forms of personality pathology.

In this chapter, we first provide an overview of attachment theory and research, including a discussion of attachment and child psychopathology and the application of attachment theory to adult relationships. We describe one model of individual differences in attachment in some detail, the two-dimensional four-category model of adult attachment (Bartholomew & Horowitz, 1991). Next, we discuss continuity of attachment, with particular attention to the conceptualization of continuity in attachment orientation and the mechanisms that may mediate such continuity. We then apply this understanding of attachment to adult personality pathology, including links between attachment and dimensional models of personality disorder and between attachment and particular personality disorders. Finally, we discuss the potential implications of an attachment perspective on personality pathology for intervention.

ATTACHMENT THEORY

Attachment theory, to quote Bowlby (1977), is "a way of conceptualizing the propensity of human beings to make strong affectional bonds to particular others" (p. 201). The theory was originally developed by Bowlby to explain the extreme emotional distress that follows unwilling separation from, or loss of, particular others (Bowlby, 1973, 1980, 1982). Bowlby proposed that the *attachment behavioral system,* an innate motivational system, has evolved in order to maintain proximity between children and their caregivers. The attachment system is proposed to have "its own internal motivation distinct from feeding and sex, and of no less importance for survival" (Bowlby, 1988a, p. 27). The system is hypothesized to promote the survival of young children by ensuring that they maintain proximity to a caregiver (the *attachment figure*), especially under conditions of threat (Bowlby, 1973, 1980). The attachment system is organized homeostatically: It is especially prone to activation when children are afraid, hurt, ill, or tired. Under such conditions, children will emit attachment behaviors such as crying, clinging, and following to establish contact with the attachment figure. If caregivers are successful in providing a sense of security, children's anxiety will be relieved and their attachment behavior will be terminated. This is the *safe haven* function of attachment relationships.

Although the goal of the attachment system is maintenance of proximity with the attachment figure, from the perspective of the attached individual, the goal is the regulation of a sense of *felt security* (Sroufe & Waters, 1977). More recent formulations view the attachment system as functioning continuously to provide a so-called secure base, a sense of security which facilitates children venturing from the proximity of the caregiver to explore the environment. Perceptions that others are available and willing to provide support in the event that such help is needed enables individuals to attempt demanding or potentially stressful undertakings.

The quality of early attachment relationships is seen as rooted largely in the history of interactions between infants and their primary caregivers (or attachment figures). Especially crucial is the degree to which infants can rely on their attachment figures as sources of security and support. Based on a laboratory procedure (called the Strange Situation) designed to observe infant exploratory and proximity-seeking behavior under conditions of increasing stress, Ainsworth, Blehar, Waters, and Wall (1978) identified three distinct patterns of attachment organization—secure, ambivalent, and avoidant. *Secure* infants confidently explore their environments under nonthreatening conditions, and when distressed, they seek contact with their caregivers and are readily soothed and reassured by that contact. This pattern of interaction suggests that secure infants perceive their

caregivers to be reliable sources of protection and security. In contrast, infants showing *anxious–resistant* or *ambivalent* attachment patterns are less confident in their exploration, show a mix of contact seeking and angry resistance when distressed, and are not readily comforted. Finally, infants showing *avoidant* patterns of attachment actively avoid contact with their caregivers when distressed. Thus, neither ambivalent nor avoidant infants appear to successfully use their caretakers to gain security when distressed or to provide a secure base for exploration. Extensions of Ainsworth's model have involved the addition of attachment categories: Crittenden (1988) identified an *avoidant/ambivalent* pattern, for children who exhibit a combination of ambivalence and avoidance, and Main and Soloman (1990) identified a *disorganized–disoriented* pattern, for infants who show contradictory or disoriented behaviors, reflecting an inability to maintain a consistent strategy for handling stress in the Strange Situation.

Attachment theory proposes that the caregiver's sensitivity to the infant's signals is of fundamental importance in the development of a secure attachment. Ainsworth (1973) found that mothers of securely attached infants tended to be consistently responsive, mothers of ambivalent infants tended to be inconsistent and inept in dealing with their infants, and mothers of avoidant infants tended to be cold and rejecting toward their infants. Subsequent research suggests that maternal lack of responsivity is related to infant ambivalence, and maternal intrusiveness and overcontrol to infant avoidance (Belsky, 1999). However, recent meta-analytic reviews indicate that the associations between parental sensitivity and infant attachment are modest (DeWolff & van IJzendoorn, 1997; Goldsmith & Alansky, 1987), with maternal sensitivity showing stronger associations with security than paternal sensitivity shows (Belsky, 1999).

There has been much attention in the childhood attachment literature to the role temperament may play in influencing child attachment patterns. In a review of the theoretical and empirical literature on the relation between attachment and temperament, Vaughn and Bost (1999) concluded that the two domains should not be considered redundant but, rather, independent or interactive contributors to personality and interpersonal development. A review of 54 published papers indicated only modest and inconsistent associations between infant temperament and attachment security. When differences between secure and insecure infants (as assessed by the Strange Situation) are examined, parental reports of temperamental difficulty generally do not distinguish the two groups. However, neonatal irritability does appear to increase the risk for insecurity later in the first year. And because the temperament assessments often precede the establishment of attachment, this establishes a temporal, though not necessarily causal, association.

Three interpretations of this association are outlined and evaluated by Vaughn and Bost (1999). They argue that the extant data do not support the proposition that individual differences in attachment security can be explained by preexisting temperamental differences. The associations between temperament and attachment security are too modest and could be partially explained by common content across assessment instruments (Vaughn et al., 1992). A second, and less direct, interpretation is that difficult temperament may be either an additional stressor for a parent or an independent factor that leads to unfavorable interactions and thus insecurity. For example, a difficult child may elicit suboptimal caregiving in a parent who is under economic, social, and/or psychological stress, thereby increasing the risk of insecure attachment. Some support for this three-stage pathway has been found (Crockenberg, 1981; Susman-Stillman, Kalkoske, Egeland, & Waldman, 1996; van den Boom, 1994). A final interpretation is that individual differences in both temperament and attachment stem from the history of infant–caregiver interactions but are not causally related to each other. This interpretation is consistent with findings that show only modest concordance between temperament reports from different informants and between attachment patterns with mothers and fathers (e.g., Belsky, Fish, & Isabella, 1991; Seifer et al., 1998). In sum, the existing data do not justify any strong conclusions about the nature of the association between temperament and attachment quality. It does, however, seem clear that "temperament need not imply attachment destiny, even in at-risk groups" (Vaughn & Bost, 1999, p. 219).

Bowlby (1973, 1980, 1982) proposed that over time, children internalize repeated interactions with caregivers in *internal working models* or schemas about the self, close others, and the self in relation to others. Bowlby (1973) de-

scribes the basic process through which such internal representations come to be formed:

> Confidence that an attachment figure is, apart from being accessible, likely to be responsive can be seen to turn on at least two variables: (a) whether or not the attachment figure is judged to be the sort of person who in general responds to calls for support and protection; (b) whether or not the self is judged to be the sort of person towards whom anyone, and the attachment figure in particular, is likely to respond in a helpful way. . . . Once adopted, moreover, and woven into the fabric of the working models, [the model of the attachment figure and the self] are apt henceforward never to be seriously questioned. (p. 204)

Internal working models are a system of expectations and beliefs about the self and others that allow children to predict and interpret an attachment figure's behavior. These working models become integrated into the personality structure and thereby provide the prototype for later social relations. Throughout the lifespan, these models serve as templates that guide behavior in subsequent relationships and provide a basis for interpretation of later relationship experiences (Bowlby, 1973). If caregivers have been consistently responsive and supportive, children are hypothesized to develop positive expectations of close others and confidence in their own worthiness as someone deserving of support. Such secure models then facilitate the development of secure attachment relationships in adulthood, relationships that provide a safe haven and secure base. In contrast, a family history characterized by various forms of inconsistent and rejecting caregiving would be expected to give rise to schemas of others as unavailable and rejecting in times of need. Through an active process of construction, these insecure models would tend to lead individuals to recreate insecure patterns in their adult relationships.

Attachment and Child Psychopathology

Some attention has been given to problematic childhood attachments in current diagnostic systems. Childhood attachment disorders, as classified by DSM-IV and ICD-10, are comprised of two atypical attachment patterns—a withdrawn or unresponsive style and a disinhibited or indiscriminately social style (Zeanah, 1996). It is important to note that these disorders reflect extremely impaired attachment relations which should be distinguished from insecure but nonpathological attachments. As Zeanah (1996) emphasized, "disordered attachments are all insecure attachments, but most insecure attachments are not disordered" (p. 42). Though this distinction can be difficult, it is guided by the degree to which children's emotions and behaviors reflect profound disturbances in their feelings of safety and security, placing them at risk for persistent distress or disability.

The substantial body of child attachment research has not been used in the development of the criteria for the diagnostic categories of attachment disorders (Zeanah, 1996). Several problems have been identified in the current classification systems. First, although these disorders are labeled attachment disorders, the criteria focus on general socially aberrant behaviors rather than specific attachment behaviors. Second, an etiological presumption is made that these disorders are due to severe deprivation and maltreatment when it is possible for them to develop in stable but unhealthy relationships not characterized by maltreatment. Third, as attachment disorders are by nature relational, they do not fit well into a classification system that conceptualizes disorders as person-centered.

Lieberman and Zeanah (1995) have proposed an alternative conceptualization of attachment disorders that focuses specifically on the child's attachment behaviors and relationships. Three distinct attachment disorders are defined: nonattachment, disordered attachment, and disrupted attachment. Nonattachment describes infants who have attained a cognitive age of 10 to 12 months yet do not exhibit a preferred attachment to anyone. Two subcategories, emotionally withdrawn and indiscriminately social, are also specified to parallel the two subtypes in DSM-IV and ICD-10. Disordered attachment refers to children who are unable to successfully use their caregivers to provide a secure base and safe haven, with the diagnosis being applied only to those children who are so extremely insecure that they fall within the pathological range. There are three subcategories: with inhibition (children who are clingy and extremely reluctant to explore), with self-endangerment (children who fail to use their caregiver in times of risk), and with role reversal (children who are excessively worried about their caregiver). Although a couple of these subcategories seem to have commonalities with standard insecure categories (e.g., extreme inhibition could be a characteristic of an ambivalent style and self-endangerment of an avoidant style), they do not directly map onto the dominant attachment models. Finally, disrupted attachment describes the grief response of young children who lose their major attachment figure. This category was predicated on the belief that loss of a primary caregiver in infancy is inherently pathogenic (Greenberg, 1999), even if the attachment relationship prior to loss was healthy. Though this proposed system is based on attachment theory and research, empirical validation of the diagnostic categories is needed.

Researchers have typically hypothesized that avoidant attachment will be predictive of the development of externalizing disorders, and that ambivalent attachment will be predictive of the development of internalizing disorders (e.g., Rubin, Hymel, Mills, & Rose-Krasnor, 1991). Greenberg (1999) reviewed the empirical literature on the role of infant attachment in later maladaptation. Some research has confirmed links between avoidance and later conduct problems and between ambivalence and later anxiety disorders (e.g., Renken, Egeland, Marvinney, Mangelsdorf, & Sroufe, 1989; Warren, Huston, Egeland, & Sroufe, 1997). However, Greenberg (1999) concluded that there is not yet clear evidence of specific links between forms of insecurity and particular disorders. Rather, it may be that attachment insecurity is an important nonspecific risk factor for various childhood disorders.

Attachment in Adult Relationships

Bowlby strongly maintained that the attachment system continues to operate throughout the lifespan and that how "an individual's attachment behavior becomes organized within his [sic] personality . . . [determines] the pattern of affectional bonds he [sic] makes during his [sic] life" (Bowlby, 1980, p. 41). Hazan and Shaver (1987) observed that the same attachment dynamics observed between caregivers and young children also characterize adult intimate relationships. Individual differences in adult attachment are expected to be highlighted in romantic relationships, with research suggesting that long-term sexual or romantic partners typically serve as primary attachment figures for one another (Hazan & Zeifman, 1994; Trinke &

Bartholomew, 1997). However, any number of adult relationships could meet the criteria for an attachment bond to be present—a desire for proximity with the attachment figure, especially under stressful conditions; a sense of security derived from contact with the attachment figure; and distress or protest when threatened with loss or separation from the attachment figure (see Weiss, 1982). There are important differences between childhood and adult attachment relationships (see Bartholomew, 1990; Hazan & Zeifman, 1994). Notably, in adult relationships, unlike parent–child relationships, attachment is typically reciprocal; that is, partners function as attachment figures for one another. However, the underlying dynamics may be surprisingly similar (see also Shaver, Hazan, & Bradshaw, 1988).

Individual Differences in Attachment Strategies

Two major lines of research have investigated individual differences in attachment patterns in adulthood. First, Main and colleagues (George, Kaplan, & Main, 1985; Main, Kaplan, & Cassidy, 1985) were interested in how adults' representations of their childhood experiences, or "states of mind with respect to attachment," may affect their childrearing practices, which in turn affect the attachment patterns of their young children. Main initially described three primary adult attachment patterns—a secure *autonomous* category and two insecure categories, dismissing and preoccupied. These patterns were identified by analyzing how adults grouped by the attachment classifications of their infants in the Strange Situation talked about their childhood family relationships in a semistructured interview, the Adult Attachment Interview (AAI). Within this research tradition, trained coders assess individuals' attachment patterns from their transcribed responses on the AAI, with the focus on *how* individuals discuss their childhood rather than the content of their descriptions. Infants classified as secure in the Strange Situation had caregivers who were *free and autonomous* with respect to attachment, showing coherence and balance in their interview responses. Infants classified as avoidant had primary caregivers who were *dismissing* of attachment-related memories and feelings, and infants classified as anxious had primary caregivers who were anxiously *preoccupied* with attachment-related issues. Subse-

quent studies using the AAI have confirmed that parents' attachment classifications are associated with independent assessments of their infants' attachment classifications (see van IJzendoorn, 1995, for a review). Main's system has also been refined and expanded over time. The infant disorganized pattern was found to be associated with caregivers who were *unresolved* with respect to losses and traumas in their attachment history. Adults who are rated unresolved are also assigned one of the three primary attachment categories. Finally, a cannot-classify category has been added to account for those adults who show aspects of two incompatible attachment strategies, such as preoccupied and dismissing.

In an independent line of work, Hazan and Shaver (1987) extended the childhood attachment paradigm to adult love relationships, speculating that orientations to romantic relationships might be an outgrowth of previous attachment experiences. They developed a brief self-report measure to assess adult parallels of the three infant attachment patterns identified by Ainsworth et al. (1978). *Secure* adults were characterized by ease of trusting and getting close to others, *ambivalent* (or preoccupied) adults by anxiety and overdependency in close relationships, and *avoidant* adults by distrust of others and avoidance of closeness in relationships. Responses on this measure, as well as a number of subsequent variations of the measure, have been found to be predictive of a broad range of theoretically relevant measures of individual differences and experiences in close relationships (for reviews, see Shaver & Clark, 1994; Shaver & Hazan, 1993). Although adult attachment as assessed within this tradition is correlated with retrospective reports of childhood experiences with parents, the focus of research has remained on understanding adult intimate relationships from an attachment perspective.

In summary, there have been two distinct approaches to applying attachment theory to adults. These approaches differ in several important ways: in method of assessment (interview vs. self-report), focus on structure versus content, and content domain (family vs. love relationships). However, there is an emerging consensus that two latent dimensions may underlie individual differences in adult attachment, potentially providing a unifying framework within which the range of approaches taken to assessing adult attachment may be integrated (Brennan, Clark, & Shaver, 1998; Feeney & Noller, 1996; Griffin & Bartholomew, 1994b; Hazan & Shaver, 1994; Shaver & Clark, 1994). One dimension, *anxiety,* reflects the propensity to experience attachment-related anxiety (including anxiety stemming from fears of rejection, separation, and abandonment). The other dimension, *avoidance* or (conversely) *closeness,* reflects the individual's response to attachment anxiety— approach toward attachment figures to seek reassurance or defensive avoidance (which can encompass both emotional and behavioral avoidance). These same dimensions may underlie individual differences in infant attachment (Shaver & Clark, 1994). A secure attachment strategy stems from low anxiety and the willingness to seek closeness when under stress, with the various insecure patterns showing high anxiety and/or high avoidance.

The dimensions of anxiety and avoidance can also be conceptualized in terms of the content of working models, with the anxiety dimension corresponding to feelings about the self and the avoidance dimension corresponding to feelings about the other. These two conceptualizations are complementary, with each guiding a set of measures of adult attachment. Though Fraley and Shaver (2000) make a convincing argument for the greater utility and parsimony of the functional definition, both conceptualizations are used in the field and are drawn on here in discussing individual differences in adult attachment. Not only may the dimensions of anxiety and avoidance underlie various measures of adult attachment, but Fraley and Waller (1998) further suggest that these dimensions may be sufficient for describing individual differences in adult attachment. They have questioned the meaningfulness of the typological approach, showing that, at least for one self-report measure of attachment, variations in adult attachment can be accounted for by a latent dimensional model and there is no evidence of an underlying taxonomy. However, we have included descriptions of attachment types or patterns for ease of presentation and because previous literature has tended to be based on typological models of attachment. The next section describes the two-dimensional, four-category model of adult attachment (Bartholomew & Horowitz, 1991) in some detail. Though no claim is being made that this is the best approach to assessing adult attachment, this model has the advantage of being explicitly based on a two-dimensional structure. In addition, attachment patterns defined by this model overlap in largely predictable ways with other approaches to assessing attachment, facilitating the subsequent review of research linking attachment and personality pathology.

The Two-Dimensional, Four-Category Model of Attachment

The two-dimensional, four-category model of attachment (Bartholomew, 1990; Bartholomew & Horowitz, 1991) initially drew on Bowlby's conceptual analysis of internal working models of self and other to provide a framework for exploring the potential range of adult attachment patterns (see Figure 9.1). Four prototypical attachment patterns are defined in terms of the intersection of two underlying dimensions, the positivity of the self model and the positivity of the other model. Alternatively, the self-model dimension can be conceptualized in terms of attachment anxiety and the other-model dimension can be conceptualized in terms of avoidance of closeness. In the following description of the two-dimensional model, we incorporate both conceptualizations of the underlying dimensions.

The positivity of the self dimension (on the horizontal axis) indicates the degree to which individuals have an internalized sense of their own self-worth. Thus, a positive self model reflects an internalized sense of self-worth that is not dependent on ongoing external validation. In terms of the attachment behavioral system, a positive self-model facilitates individuals feeling self-confident, rather than anxious, in close relationships. In contrast, a negative other model indicates a dependency on others' ongoing approval to maintain feelings of self-worth, a dependency that fosters anxiety regarding acceptance and rejection in close relationships. The positivity of the other dimension (on the vertical axis) reflects expectations of others' availability and supportiveness. In terms of the attachment system, a positive other model facilitates the willingness to seek intimacy and support from close others. In contrast, a negative other model is associated with the tendency to withdraw and maintain a safe distance within close relationships, particularly when feeling threatened.

Each combination of self and other models defines a prototypical attachment pattern, or a particular strategy of regulating felt security

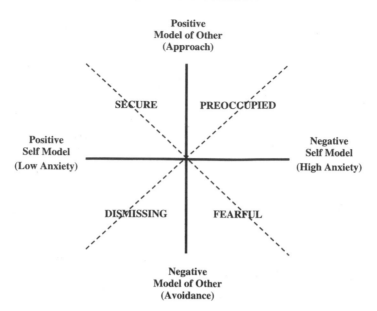

FIGURE 9.1. Two-dimensional, four-category model of adult attachment.

within close relationships (Bartholomew, Cobb, & Poole, 1997). A heuristic model of the dynamics of the attachment system (see Figure 9.2) will be used to characterize each of four attachment patterns defined by the two-dimensional model. Because of their relevance to personality pathology, particular attention is given to the insecure patterns. For each attachment pattern, we also present a circumplex analysis of the interpersonal difficulties associated with the pattern. From this perspective, interpersonal behaviors are seen as being jointly defined by two dimensions: a vertical dimension of control (dominance to submission) and a horizontal di-

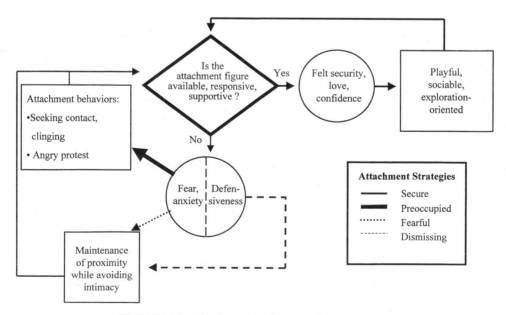

FIGURE 9.2. The dynamics of the attachment system.

mension of affiliation (warmth to coldness or distance) (e.g., Kiesler, 1983; Wiggins, 1982). Maladaptive interpersonal behavior is characterized by a lack of flexibility in moving around the circle in response to situational demands. Interpersonal problems were assessed with the Inventory of Interpersonal Problems (IIP; Horowitz, Rosenberg, Baer, Ureno, & Villasenor, 1988), a measure of a broad cross-section of interpersonal problems that arise in therapy. A circumplex scoring procedure for the IIP yields eight problem subscales, one for each octant of the Interpersonal Circle (Alden, Wiggins, & Pincus, 1990). The profiles presented have been observed in multiple studies, including both self-reports and reports of knowledgeable others (friends and romantic partners) (Bartholomew & Horowitz, 1991; Bartholomew & Scharfe, 1994).

Secure Attachment

Experiences of consistent responsive caretaking in childhood are hypothesized to facilitate the development of both an internalized sense of self-worth and a trust that others will generally be available and supportive. Secure individuals are characterized by high self-esteem and an ability to establish and maintain close intimate bonds with others without losing a sense of self. They are able to use others as sources of support when needed, and they are likely to form intimate relationships in which both partners act as safe havens and secure bases for one another. The secure pattern is represented by a solid dark line in Figure 9.2: Secure individuals expect their attachment figures to be supportive, facilitating inner security and behavioral competence. Secure attachment is associated with satisfying intimate relationships and high personal adjustment (for a review, see Shaver & Clark, 1994).

As expected, circumplex analysis confirms that secure individuals tend to be well adjusted in the interpersonal domain. They show relatively low levels of interpersonal difficulties, especially according to the reports of their intimates. Moreover, the secure group's profile of interpersonal problems, though somewhat elevated on the warm side of the interpersonal space, is not distinctive. That is, no subscale scores tend to be extreme, indicating flexibility in being able to respond appropriately to specific interpersonal situations.

Preoccupied Attachment

Preoccupied (or anxious–ambivalent) attachment is characterized by the combination of a negative self model and a positive model of others. Preoccupied individuals are preoccupied with their attachment needs and actively seek to have those needs fulfilled in their close relationships. Experiences of inconsistent and insensitive caretaking are thought to contribute to preoccupied attachment. This kind of parenting may lead children to conclude that they are to blame for lack of love from the caretaker. Because past attachment figures are likely to have responded inconsistently to their distress, the preoccupied have learned to express their needs actively and unrelentingly in order to maximize their chances of gaining support. The result is an overly dependent style in which personal validation is sought through gaining others' acceptance and approval.

Turning to Figure 9.2, preoccupied individuals are hypervigilant to potential sources of stress or threat. They show high general levels of distress and anxiety (Bartholomew & Horowitz, 1991; Kobak & Sceery, 1988; Mikulincer & Orbach, 1995) and intense negative reactions to external stress (Mikulincer, Florian, & Weller, 1993). They often question the availability of attachment figures, both because they do not expect consistent responsiveness and because their unrealistically high demands for supportiveness are unlikely to be met. When they feel that attachment figures are not responsive, they experience anxiety and respond with high levels of attachment behaviors in an attempt to get their needs for support met (see bold arrow in Figure 9.2). They often express their needs for support in a demanding, histrionic, and/or manipulative manner, overrely on potential supporters, and are indiscriminant in self-disclosure and help-seeking behaviors (Bartholomew & Horowitz, 1991; Mikulincer & Nachshon, 1991). These forms of support seeking only alienate potential support providers, leading to further anxiety and frustration and further demands.

Driven by their active attempts to get their attachment needs met, preoccupied individuals demonstrate an intrusive and demanding interpersonal style. In attachment terms, they show exaggerated attachment behaviors, including both emotional displays (especially anger and anxiety) and behavioral displays (at times even resorting to violence, see Bartholomew, Henderson, & Dutton, 2001). A typical quote of a preoccupied individual is, "I scare away partners. I want to be so close, all the time, and they get nervous." In terms of the Interpersonal Circle, preoccupied individuals tend to show elevations in the quadrant characterized by dominance and warmth, especially problems associated with being overly expressive. Typical items endorsed by this group are "It is hard for me to spend time alone," "I am overly disclosing," and "I want to be noticed too much." Such problems are consistent with the preoccupied person's dependency on others' acceptance and their active strategies to gain the acceptance and support of others. At the extreme, preoccupied individuals would be expected to exhibit histrionic and borderline tendencies.

In contrast, *avoidant attachment,* defined in terms of avoidance or negative models of others, is characterized by the inhibition of displays of distress and behavioral withdrawal from others, especially under conditions of stress. This strategy has presumably developed, at least in part, because of a history of attachment figures either not responding to or actively rejecting the child's displays of distress and attempts at comfort seeking. Thus avoidance is a defensive strategy in which the natural inclination to seek proximity to attachment figures when threatened is suppressed. This strategy is expected to be especially evident under high levels of anxiety or distress (e.g., Mikulincer et al., 1993; Simpson, Rholes, & Nelligan, 1992). The two avoidant patterns identified by the four-category model, fearful avoidance and dismissing avoidance, share the behavioral strategy of withdrawing when distressed. However, individuals with the two avoidant patterns differ in their proneness to experience attachment anxiety or distress, in their conscious reasons for avoidance, and in their investment in close relationships.

Fearful Attachment

This pattern is characterized by negative other models and negative self models. Fearful individuals have concluded both that others are uncaring and unavailable and that they themselves are unlovable. Although they desire acceptance by others—in fact, they are hypersensitive to social approval—they avoid intimacy due to a fear or expectation of rejection which further contributes to their difficulties in obtaining adequate support. Not surprisingly, fearful individuals report chronically high levels of subjective distress (Bartholomew & Horowitz, 1991) and poor-quality intimate relationships (e.g., Bartholomew & Horowitz, 1991; Carnelley, Pietromonaco, & Jaffe, 1994; Scharfe & Bartholomew, 1995).

Fearful individuals, similar to the preoccupied, do not expect others to be responsive, giving rise to fear and anxiety. However, opposite to the preoccupied pattern of actively seeking support, they inhibit expressing anxiety and asking for support. Instead, they deal with their anxiety by maintaining a comfortable distance within their close relationships (see dotted arrow in Figure 9.2). They can thereby avoid anticipated rejection of their attachment needs by the attachment figure while gaining some indirect support by not alienating the attachment figure. In extreme cases, fearful individuals may manage their fear of rejection by avoiding close relationships altogether.

Fearful individuals tend to be characterized by interpersonal passivity and difficulty in making their needs known within relationships. A typical quote of a fearful individual is, "I'm incapable of vocalizing my feelings because I'm afraid I'll say something that will ruin the relationship." A circumplex analysis reveals elevations in the lower quadrants of the Interpersonal Circle, especially on problems related to introversion and subassertiveness. Typical items assessing these forms of interpersonal problems are "I am too afraid of other people" and "It is hard for me to confront people with problems that come up." At an extreme, fearful attachment has much in common with the avoidant and dependent personality disorders.

Dismissing Attachment

This pattern is characterized by a positive self model and a negative model of others. Dismissing individuals have managed to maintain a positive self-image and to minimize anxiety by distancing themselves from attachment figures and by downplaying, devaluing, or denying the impact of negative attachment experiences. It is important to the dismissing to maintain a self-image as independent and not overly reliant on the support of others. Therefore, when these individuals do experience distress, they prefer to deal with that distress on their own rather than seeking support from others. With their characteristic compulsive self-reliance and emotional control, and a defensive downplaying of the importance of intimate relationships, they become relatively invulnerable to potential rejection by others. (For a discussion of the developmental pathways and psychological processes that may give rise to a dismissing orientation, see Fraley, Davis, & Shaver, 1998). Dismissing attachment appears to be a generally successful form of adaptation: Though it is related to low relationship satisfaction (Bartholomew, 1997; Scharfe & Bartholomew, 1995), it is also associated with high self-esteem and low levels of subjective distress and depression (Bartholomew & Horowitz, 1991).

As indicated by the broken line in Figure 9.2, dismissing individuals have learned to defensively deactivate the attachment system, reducing their tendency to experience the anxiety that typically follows from unmet attachment needs. Dismissing individuals downplay the importance of potential stressors, defensively avoiding acknowledgment of distress that could activate the attachment system (Bartholomew, 1990; Mikulincer & Orbach, 1995). This defensive emotional stance is complemented by an avoidant behavioral stance in which they maintain distance within close relationships. Interpersonal problems associated with dismissing attachment are centered on the cold side of the Interpersonal Circle. Typical items endorsed by the dismissing are "It is hard for me to feel close to others" and "A lot of people are not worth getting to know." Note that their problems tend to be associated with distance and alienation from others, not necessarily active hostility toward others.

Each of the four attachment patterns described in this model represents a theoretical ideal or prototype, with individuals varying in the degree to which they approximate each prototypical pattern. Thus, participants are rated on their correspondence with *each* of the attachment prototypes (secure, fearful, preoccupied, and dismissing), resulting in an *attachment profile* for each individual. In both the childhood and adult attachment fields it has been common to conceptualize individual differences in attachment in terms of three or more discrete categories. However, such approaches overlook meaningful variation *within* the attachment categories (Griffin & Bartholomew, 1994b). Most individuals show a complex profile across attachment patterns, with few showing prototypical patterns. Two individuals with the same primary attachment patterns will present very

differently if they have different secondary or even tertiary strategies. For example, a prototypically preoccupied individual will look quite different from an individual who shows a mix of preoccupied and fearful tendencies or even preoccupied and dismissing tendencies.

Within this model, there are three ways to treat attachment ratings: (1) an attachment *profile* gives participants' correspondence with each of the attachment prototypes, (2) the best fitting attachment *category* can be derived from the highest of the four prototype ratings, or (3) ratings of the underlying attachment *dimensions* of anxiety and avoidance can be derived from linear combinations of the four prototype ratings (e.g., Griffin & Bartholomew, 1994b; Scharfe & Bartholomew, 1994). Various methods of assessment have also been used, though we recommend the use of in-depth, semistructured attachment interviews. The Peer Attachment Interview (Bartholomew & Horowitz, 1991) explores individuals' experiences with friends and romantic partners, and the History of Attachments Interview (Henderson, 1998) asks participants for a chronological history of relationship experiences from childhood parent–child relationships to current peer and romantic relationships. In assessing attachment from such interviews, expert coders consider both the *content* of participants' relationship accounts and *how* participants discuss their experiences (including the coherence of their accounts, defensiveness in discussing difficult experiences, etc.).

Many of the approaches currently being taken to assess adult attachment can be organized within the framework of the four-category, two-dimensional model. Hazan and Shaver's (1987) original categorical measure of three styles of adult attachment yields ratings that correspond quite closely to three of the four attachment patterns defined in the four-category model: secure with secure, ambivalent with preoccupied, and avoidant with fearful (Bartholomew & Shaver, 1998; Brennan, Shaver, & Tobey, 1991). There is no equivalent of dismissing attachment in their original formulation. Within this research tradition, a number of multi-item self-report measures have been developed to assess dimensions underlying individual differences in adult attachment. Those that assess attachment anxiety and avoidance (or, conversely, closeness) in adult close relationships, such as those measures of Simpson et al. (1992) and Collins and Read (1990), closely correspond to the anxiety and avoidance dimensions (Griffin & Bartholomew, 1994a).

Connections between the two-dimensional model and the classifications derived from the AAI are somewhat more complex. In the one study that looked at these associations, high concordance was found on secure, preoccupied, and dismissing ratings from the two systems (Bartholomew & Shaver, 1998). Unfortunately, this study did not include unresolved or cannot-classify categorizations on the AAI. Conceptually, the fearful pattern has no clear equivalent in the AAI system and it was not associated with AAI classifications in the study by Bartholomew and Shaver (1998). But fearfulness is likely to overlap to some degree with a subcategory of preoccupied attachment that contains fearful elements (E3, fearfully preoccupied). Fearfulness may also be associated with a failure to resolve loss or trauma (as suggested, for instance, by Shaver & Clark, 1994). Although the criteria for coding fearfulness and lack of resolution have little overlap, there is evidence of associations between fearfulness and both retrospective reports of childhood abuse (Roche, Runtz, & Hunter, 1999; Shaver & Clark, 1994) and the experience of trauma symptoms that may be associated with childhood abuse (Alexander, 1993). The cannot-classify AAI categorization is reserved for cases that show evidence of two incompatible attachment strategies, such as preoccupied and dismissing. In the four-category scoring system, such individuals would be given relatively high ratings on the two strategies rather than being classified in a distinct category.

Kobak, Cole, Ferenz-Gillies, Fleming, and Gamble (1993) devised a two-dimensional measure of adult attachment security based on responses to the AAI. First, trained coders conduct a Q-sort on an individual's interview using items drawn from the AAI scoring system. Then the Q-sort results are used to derive ratings of two dimensions, a secure–insecure dimension and a deactivating–hyperactivating dimension. These dimensions are similar conceptually to the diagonals of Figure 9.1 (i.e., 45-degree rotations of the avoidance and anxiety dimensions). The secure–insecure dimension is parallel to the secure–fearful diagonal and the deactivating–hyperactivating dimension is parallel to the dismissing–preoccupied diagonal (see also Shaver & Hazan, 1993).

In general, different measures of adult attachment show moderate convergence when comparisons are made between measures assessing similar conceptual patterns or dimensions. However, these convergences are considerably attenuated when conceptually noncorresponding categorical systems are compared, when different methods of measurement are compared (such as interviews and self-reports), and when measures focusing on different content domains are compared (such as the parental and romantic relationship domains). (For discussions of the correspondence between different methods of assessing adult attachment, see Bartholomew & Shaver, 1998; Brennan et al., 1998.)

CONTINUITY OF ATTACHMENT ORIENTATIONS

It is not uncommon for those outside the field of attachment to believe that this theory assumes that adult attachment patterns, and even personality as a whole, are primarily determined by experiences with primary caregivers in early childhood, implying strong continuity in attachment organization from infancy to adulthood (e.g., Hendrick & Hendrick, 1994). This is not accurate. Attachment theory is neither a stage model nor a critical period theory. Rather attachment patterns are seen to reflect complex patterns of social interaction, emotional regulation, and cognitive processing that emerge over the course of development and tend to become self-perpetuating through adulthood.

Consistent with current conceptualizations of developmental psychopathology (e.g., Rutter, 1994), Bowlby (1988b) conceived of continuity in attachment patterns and associated personality functioning in terms of developmental pathways or trajectories: "my hypothesis is that the pathway followed by each developing individual and the extent to which he or she becomes resilient to stressful life events is determined to a very significant degree by the pattern of attachment he or she develops during the early years" (p. 7). Within such a model, early attachment experiences do not directly cause later personality organization and outcomes. Rather, they initiate the child along one of an array of potential developmental pathways. Some of these pathways reflect healthy development, and others deviate in various directions toward less healthy psychosocial outcomes. At each point, an individual's path is determined by an interaction between the individual (and his or her ability to flexibly respond to stress and challenges) and the environment. At any point in development, more or less favorable experiences will lead the path to deviate toward or away from healthy pathways. For example, the loss of a parent or an increase in marital conflict would tend to shift children toward less desirable paths, whereas an improvement in parenting, psychological intervention, or the support of a secondary caretaker might have the opposite effect.

Although change is possible at any point, the longer an individual follows a given path, the more difficult it will become to shift the direction of that path. Change will be constrained by prior functioning, as patterns of functioning associated with that pathway become increasingly habitual and entrenched with time. As children become older, they gain more influence over their environments (see section "Mechanisms of Continuity") and, therefore, they are more able to structure their social environments to reaffirm and perpetuate their patterns of adaptation. In Bowlby's (1988b) words, "during the earliest years, features of personality crucial to psychiatry remain relatively open to change because they are still responsive to the environment. As a child grows older, however, clinical evidence shows that both the pattern of attachment and the personality features that go with it become increasingly a property of the child himself or herself and also increasingly resistant to change" (p. 5).

Attachment insecurity (or, conversely, attachment security) can be conceptualized as a risk (or protective) factor. A risk factor is a particular experience or individual characteristic that increases the probability or risk of a future undesirable outcome (Kazdin, Kraemer, Kessler, Kupfer, & Offord, 1997). From a risk factor perspective, attachment insecurity would be seen as just one factor which, in concert with others, may contribute to negative outcomes. For instance, Greenberg (1999) proposes a model in which four risk domains are used to understand the development of childhood and adolescent disorders: difficult child temperament, insecure attachment, high family adversity, and ineffectual parenting practices. Attachment insecurity alone would be unlikely to be associated with any given disorder, but the more of these risk factors a given child has, the greater his or her likelihood of manifesting a psychosocial disorder. Extending the model to

adulthood, child or adult attachment insecurity could be a risk factor (in combination with other risk factors) for later marital conflict and disruption, for adult difficulties in regulating negative affect, or for a particular personality disorder. Conversely, attachment security can be considered a protective factor that helps buffer responses to stressful experiences that might otherwise have negative consequences for development. Attachment security could act as a protective factor in at least two ways. It could serve as a personal resource that facilitates the capacity of individuals to cope adaptively with adversity without compromising their feelings of self-worth and trust in others. Attachment security could also serve as an indicator of a relationship resource in that secure attachment is likely to be associated with supportive close relationships (with caregivers in childhood and later with peers) which may provide assistance in difficult times.

Evidence of Continuity

Several longitudinal studies have demonstrated temporal stability of attachment patterns during childhood (e.g., Main et al., 1985; Waters, 1978). As would be expected from a developmental pathways perspective, the stability of the caretaking environment appears to mediate the degree of stability of attachment patterns (e.g., Thompson, Lamb, & Estes, 1982; Vaughn, Egeland, Sroufe, & Waters, 1979). That is, continuity in attachment is stronger when childrearing environments are more stable. Also relevant to the question of continuity is a large body of research indicating that attachment patterns assessed in infancy predict various aspects of emotional functioning, self-concept, and social functioning in a range of settings in later childhood. For example, Waters, Wippman, and Sroufe (1979) found that attachment assessed at 15 months in the Strange Situation predicted Q-sort ratings of social competence and ego strength in preschool classrooms at 3½ years. Those few studies to look at the predictability of infant attachment classification over longer periods have also tended to show continuity in developmental adaptation. For example, Elicker, Englund, and Sroufe (1992) showed that infant attachment quality predicted a range of measures of emotional and social competence in summer camps at 10 to 11 years of age (including counselor, observational, and interview ratings). Although such findings are impressive, it is important to keep in mind that the obtained associations are generally moderate at best. (For reviews of this literature, see Rothbard & Shaver, 1994; Thompson, 1999; Weinfield, Sroufe, Egeland, & Carlson, 1999.)

To date, only a handful of studies have followed samples from infancy through young adulthood to investigate long-term continuity in attachment patterns, and the results have been somewhat inconsistent. Two studies have found relatively high continuity between security in infancy as assessed in the Strange Situation and security in late adolescence and young adulthood as assessed by the AAI (Hamilton, 1998; Waters, Merrick, Treboux, Crowell, & Albersheim, 2000; cited in Crowell, Fraley, & Shaver, 1999). In contrast, two studies have failed to show continuity using similar methods (see Weinfield, Sroufe, & Egeland, 2000, with a high-risk sample; Zimmermann, Fremmer-Bombik, Spangler, & Grossmann, 1997, with a German sample). Fraley (1998) reviewed the studies assessing continuity in attachment security from infancy to young adulthood and found that stability correlations over this period ranged from $r = -.10$ to $r = .50$. He constructed two mathematical models of continuity in attachment and tested which model provided the best fit for the data available. Fraley concluded that though working models of attachment are extremely plastic, these models continue to shape people's caregiving environments, contributing to an estimated stability correlation of .39 from age 1 to young adulthood. Moreover, he found that samples characterized by family instability, abuse, and other risk factors that might be expected to attenuate stability in the caretaking environment showed considerably less continuity than samples in more stable caregiving environments.

In contrast to the childhood literature, relatively little research has examined continuity in attachment orientations in adulthood. Bowlby (1973) saw the formative period for the development of attachment-related models as extending from childhood through adolescence, by which point attachment patterns would be expected to become relatively resistant to change. Therefore, relatively high stability of attachment orientation would be expected in adulthood. Consistent with this expectation, moderate to high stability has been demonstrated in adult attachment over periods of months to a few years (e.g., Kirkpatrick & Hazan,

1994; Scharfe & Bartholomew, 1994). One recent longitudinal study looking at attachment patterns of women avoidantly or securely attached at age 52 suggests reasonable stability in measures of intra- and interpersonal functioning over 31 years (Klohnen & Bera, 1998). Interestingly, using a new prototype measure of working models of attachment with this same sample, Klohnen and John (1998) documented that preoccupation declined over time and security increased.

Intergenerational Continuity

In contrast to research investigating continuity of attachment within the individual, a growing body of research focuses on intergenerational continuity by assessing the concordance of attachment patterns across generations. Although certainly not conclusive, evidence of intergenerational continuity suggests individual continuity over the lifespan. Most of this work has compared parental attachment representations as assessed by the AAI and infant attachment with the same parent as assessed in the Strange Situation. For example, Fonagy, Steele, and Steele (1991) assessed attachment in mothers expecting their first child and, in a follow-up, assessed attachment of their 12-month-old infants in the Strange Situation. There was 75% concordance between maternal attachment security and subsequent infant security, with infant security and anxious–avoidance (but not anxious–ambivalence) strongly predictable from maternal AAI ratings. In addition, paternal AAI ratings were predictive of infant security in the Strange Situation at 18 months (with the father) but less strongly and consistently so than maternal ratings (Steele & Steele, 1994).

van IJzendoorn (1995) conducted a meta-analysis of studies comparing adult attachment classifications based on the AAI and infant attachment classifications based on the Strange Situation. Strong associations were found between autonomous parents and secure infants ($r = .47$), dismissing parents and avoidant infants ($r = .45$), and preoccupied parents and ambivalent infants ($r = .42$). Parental responsiveness appears to play a mediating role in this transmission. A combined effect size of $r = .34$ was found for the association between security of attachment organization and sensitive responsiveness. However, the rest of the correspondence between parents' and children's attachment styles remains unexplained, and surprisingly little is known about the mechanisms underlying the intergenerational transmission of attachment.

Sources of Continuity

Attachment theory is consistent with a transactional model of development in which the social environment affects individual functioning and, conversely, individuals actively construct their social environments (Sameroff & Chandler, 1975). Within attachment theory, there has been a tendency to focus on internal working models as the key mediators linking experiences in the family and later functioning outside the family. These dynamic cognitive structures are hypothesized to operate largely automatically and outside of conscious awareness. To maintain stability and coherence of their perceptions of the self and of the world (cf. Epstein, 1987), individuals are expected to process social information and to behave so as to obtain feedback which confirms their preexisting models of themselves and others (see Caspi & Elder, 1988; Swann, 1983, 1987). It is precisely "because persons select and create later social environments that early relationships are viewed as having special importance" (Sroufe & Fleeson, 1986, p. 68).

Working models formed during childhood and adolescence are proposed to be self-perpetuating over time. But they are also expected to be open to change if people experience life events that are inconsistent with their existing models. Thus, although attachment patterns are expected to have some trait-like stability, they are also expected to be sensitive to changes in the social environment. In particular, experiences in emotionally significant relationships that contradict earlier relationship patterns may lead to the reorganization and revision of internal models (cf. Ricks, 1985).

The degree to which early experiences predict later social functioning *independently* of continuity in the social environment is still a controversial question. In the first few years, attachment quality is very much a property of the specific attachment relationship and, therefore, may readily shift if the nature of that relationship changes. Early attachment orientations may tend to be maintained, and be predictive of later outcomes, because the caretaking environment tends to be consistent in quality over time. Thus, early insecure attachment may persist when the conditions that contributed to the insecurity (insensitive parenting, family conflict, poverty, etc.) persist. Consistent with this perspective, a number of studies have documented lawful discontinuity in functioning over time in childhood when there have been intervening changes in the quality of the parent–child relationship. For example, a greater number of life stressors among low-income families was associated with infants shifting from secure to insecure attachments over a 6-month period (Vaughn et al., 1979). It seems likely, however, that over time attachment increasingly becomes a property of the child as he or she comes to impose established patterns on new relationship partners outside the family. Therefore, although early attachment orientation may not predict later functioning independently of the intervening environmental influences, neither is the current environment a sufficient explanation of current functioning. In one of the few studies that permit an examination of the roles of early experience and subsequent environmental conditions in predicting adaptation, Sroufe, Egeland, and Kreutzer (1990) followed a poverty sample from infancy through middle childhood. Children who differed in their early adaptation (as shown, in part, by security of attachment at 12 to 18 months), but who showed equally poor adaptation in the preschool period, differed in their later development. Specifically, those children with an early history of secure attachments showed greater rebound in the early elementary years, even controlling for intermediate and concurrent circumstances.

It is also likely that genetic factors associated with attachment orientations are an important source of continuity in development, though to date there is little evidence of the role of heritable factors in the attachment domain (Vaughn & Bost, 1999). Just one published study has looked at heritability of attachment patterns in infancy using a validated measure of attachment and a twin methodology (Finkel, Wille, & Matheny, 1998). Although the sample size was too small to permit the estimation of reliable heritability coefficients, findings suggested a moderate genetic basis for individual differences in infant attachment. One study has also examined the heritability of attachment in adulthood, using standard behavioral genetic methods and a self-report measure of the four-category model of attachment (Brussoni, Jang, Livesley, & MacBeth, 2000). Genetic effects, ranging from 25% to 43%, were found for three of the four attachment patterns; only the dismissing pattern showed no significant genetic variance. In addition, studies have indicated genetic influences on personality measures related to adult attachment. For example, Jang, Livesley, Vernon, and Jackson (1996) obtained a heritability estimate of 45% for a self-report measure of insecure attachment (a scale of the Dimensional Assessment of Personality Pathology), a measure that is likely to line up with the secure–fearful diagonal of Figure 9.1. Unfortunately, studies have not yet tested a plausible explanation for these findings: The genetic component of attachment may be accounted for by temperament or basic dimensions of personality that overlap, to some extent, with individual differences in attachment. Individuals may even vary in their susceptibility to environmental influences, including parenting practices, suggesting potential gene–environment interactions (cf. Belsky, 1999).

Mechanisms of Continuity

Attachment patterns are proposed to be externalized and maintained through a number of mechanisms, notably the choice of social environments and partners, habitual interaction patterns, and model-driven processing of socially relevant information. The system of expectations and associated behavioral strategies that define working models are assumed to be constructed as a reasonable adaptation to individuals' childrearing environments. But they may be more or less effective when applied within the social environments in which adults find themselves and create for themselves.

One potentially important mechanism through which patterns of adaptation may be maintained is selective affiliation, or the selection of social partners who are likely to confirm internal models (see Bartholomew, 1990). Selective affiliation is expected to play a more important role in adult than childhood attachment relationships because adults have greater control over the people with whom they become involved than do children. For example, dismissive individuals may show a preference for preoccupied partners to validate their need for psychological distance; preoccupied people tend to desire a pathological level of closeness in intimate relationships. One striking demonstration of selective affiliation was presented by Swann and Pelham (1999): College students with randomly assigned roommates showed a preference for keeping roommates (and maintaining a relationship with roommates) who held concordant views of their self-worth. Notably, students with well-defined negative self-images preferred roommates who also thought poorly of them.

To date, there is no evidence of selective affiliation in initial choice of relationship partners based on attachment orientations. But cross-sectional evidence does indicate nonrandom pairing of romantic partners based on attachment patterns. The most consistent finding has been moderately strong associations between romantic partners on scales related to security of attachment (e.g., Bartholomew, 1997; Collins & Read, 1990; Kirkpatrick & Davis, 1994; Senchak & Leonard, 1992). However, longitudinal work is needed to examine how adult attachment patterns may affect both the initial selection of relationship partners and the development of relationship dynamics over time.

Attachment orientations are associated with habitual patterns of affective and behavioral regulation that will be carried forward into new relationships. On the most general level, highly insecure individuals may simply lack the social skills to take advantage of more positive social opportunities (cf. Rutter, 1988). Specifically, differing interaction patterns may set in motion self-fulfilling interpersonal dynamics, independent of initial partner choice. For instance, when dismissing individuals actively maintain emotional distance in their close relationships, relationship partners tend to respond with greater insecurity and dependency, leading to greater distancing, further insecurity, and so on. Thereby, mutually frustrating positive feedback loops can become established. Complementing research documenting the interpersonal problems associated with various forms of insecure attachment (e.g., Bartholomew & Horowitz, 1991) and the interaction styles associated with adult attachment in daily social activities (e.g., Tidwell, Reis, & Shaver, 1996), a number of studies have observed social behavior in laboratory settings. For instance, Simpson et al. (1992) found that the avoidance dimension of attachment was associated with deficits in seeking and giving support between dating couples in an anxiety-provoking situation. Feeney (1994) found that the underlying dimensions of avoidance and anxiety were related to measures of couple communication and conflict strategies, and Kobak and Hazan (1991) documented associations between a Q-sort measure of security in the marital relationship and observed couple communication. The interpersonal patterns observed in such studies are expected to reflect the interaction of both partners' attachment orientations and the dynamics that have evolved within their relationships.

Less well documented is the potential impact of attachment patterns on interaction styles with strangers (or confederates) to examine whether attachment patterns are associated with interaction styles independent of partner choice and relationship histories. One such study assessed whether attachment patterns were predictive of forms of disclosure in initial encounters with social partners (Mikulincer & Nachshon, 1991). As expected, avoidant attachment was associated with low disclosure and negative responses to disclosure by partners and ambivalent attachment was associated with less flexibility of disclosure. This study also suggests that interaction styles associated with habitual interpersonal orientations may elicit feedback from social partners that reinforces existing mental models and interaction patterns (see Swann, 1983, 1987). Such dynamics have been illustrated in work by Downey, Freitas, Michaelis, and Khouri (1998), who have shown that women who anticipate rejection in their intimate relationships (i.e., are high on attachment anxiety) tend to behave in ways during conflict with partners that elicit the very rejecting partner behaviors they fear.

Working models of attachment are also proposed to guide the construal of social information, including directing attention to model-consistent information, organizing how new information is filtered and interpreted, and influencing the accessibility of past experiences in memory (Collins & Read, 1994). Through these and other information processing biases (see Swann, 1983), ambiguous social stimuli (arguably virtually all social stimuli) tend to be assimilated to existing working models. Collins and Read (1994) proposed a theory in which working models are conceived of as highly accessible schemas that will be automatically activated in response to attachment-relevant events. Once activated, these models have an impact on social information processing and emotional response patterns, in turn mediating behavioral strategies. Collins (1996) tested and confirmed aspects of this model by investigating how individuals' preexisting working models guide their interpretations of and explanations for hypothetical relationship events. For example, the anxiety dimension of attachment was predictive of a tendency to make negative interpretations of relationship events, including viewing partner behavior as rejecting and unresponsive, and with a tendency to experience emotional distress. In addition, attachment anxiety showed little association with the interpretation of attachment-irrelevant events, indicating that a general negative response bias or negative emotionality could not account for the findings.

IMPLICATIONS OF ATTACHMENT FOR ADULT PERSONALITY PATHOLOGY

Attachment theory, especially when viewed from a developmental psychopathology or pathways perspective, has the potential to offer a new framework through which to conceptualize personality pathology. From this perspective, personality disorder is viewed as a deviation from optimal development. Such deviation is presumed to have developed over an extended period and would be hypothesized to be associated with a number of interacting risk factors, which may differ across individuals and across disorders. Multiple pathways can lead to the same overt outcome—for instance, a particular form of personality disorder—and no specific risk factor would be expected to be necessary or sufficient for the development of a particular outcome. Attachment processes, in the past and present, may be one important factor affecting developmental pathways to personality disorder.

Approaching personality disorders from an attachment perspective focuses attention on the interpersonal contexts in which personality disorders develop and are maintained. As has often been discussed, a maladaptive interpersonal style is central to most personality disorders (e.g., West & Keller, 1994). However, the degree to which interpersonal difficulties, and difficulties with intimate relationships in particular, are key features of the disorders varies considerably. Extreme attachment insecurity may be associated with personality pathology (and associated interpersonal difficulties) in at least two ways. First, insecure attachment indicates a relatively fixed response to stress and interpersonal challenges, a response that is generally not helpful in moderating anxiety and contributing to well functioning relationships.

Such rigid response styles tend to be self-per-petuating, as discussed previously in the section "Mechanisms of Continuity." For example, the fearful attachment strategy of avoiding rejection by avoiding relationships, or not expressing attachment needs within relationships, precludes the possibility of establishing more secure relationships and thereby eventually developing greater trust in others and acceptance of the self. In contrast, secure attachment is associated with flexibility in responding to stress; secure individuals can both depend on close others for support and have the internal resources to effectively modulate negative affect (Bartholomew et al., 1997). In addition, inconsistency of insecure attachment strategies (indicating conflicting internal models and a lack of organization or even a break down in functioning) may be associated with especially problematic personality profiles.

It is important to remember that attachment theory is concerned with the psychological mechanisms underlying regulation of affect in close interpersonal relationships; it is not a theory of personality disorder. Personality disorder is, of course, usually associated with significant disruption of close personal relationships. However, many important aspects of personality disorder symptomatology (e.g., behavioral impulsivity, disturbances in cognition and perception, even disruption of relationships with strangers and acquaintances) fall outside this realm. Thus, attachment problems will be more relevant to some forms of personality disorder than to others or to some aspects of symptomatology more than others. In addition, based on a pathways perspective, we would not expect a high degree of specificity in the links between forms of insecure attachment and forms of personality pathology.

Just as insecure childhood attachment is not a disorder per se, adult attachment insecurity is not necessarily associated with adult personality difficulties. Between 25% and 50% of adults are typically categorized as insecure in community samples (Mickelson, Kessler, & Shaver, 1997; van IJzendoorn & Bakermans-Kranenburg, 1997). Although these individuals' insecurity would be expected to be reflected in some challenges in their intimate relationships, many, if not most, insecure adults are expected to be functioning quite adequately even in the interpersonal realm. In contrast, only about 10% to 15% of adults in community samples suffer from personality disorder (Weissman,

1993), as the diagnosis depends on symptoms that result in clinically significant distress or impairment. In short, although the large majority of individuals diagnosed with personality disorders may be insecurely attached (e.g., van IJzendoorn & Bakersmans-Kranenburg, 1996), many people with attachment problems will not be diagnosed with personality disorders.

Finally, the nature of the link between attachment problems and personality disorder is unclear. Any serious personality pathology is likely to undermine intimate relationships, potentially contributing to attachment insecurity. Moreover, attachment insecurity could be a nonspecific indicator of general malfunction. Thus, the co-occurrence of attachment insecurity with a personality disorder in no way indicates that the two are causally connected. However, forms of childhood and adulthood attachment insecurity may be risk factors that are probabilistically associated with specific personality difficulties, even though such insecurity is not inherently pathological.

Connections between Dimensions Underlying Attachment and Personality Disorders

As has been discussed already, it is common for people to discuss attachment patterns in terms of a number of distinct categories. The categorical model facilitates discussion and some forms of research. Capturing the complexity of attachment, however, requires dimensional measurement models. Dimensional models permit differentiation among people with the same attachment pattern on the basis of extremity or severity, recognize that many people do not have pure or simple attachment patterns, and acknowledge that the boundaries between attachment patterns are not always distinct and rigid. A focus in research on basic dimensions of attachment rather than descriptive categories—genotypes rather than phenotypes; symptoms rather than disorders—is also more likely to result in the identification of underlying causal mechanisms.

The same thing is true of personality disorder. Categorical models have been developed to facilitate communication and treatment decisions in clinical settings. For example, the fourth edition of the *Diagnostic and Statistical Manual of Mental Disorders* (DSM-IV; American Psychiatric Association, 1994) describes 10 specific categories of personality disorder, each defined by a set of symptoms/traits. However, substantial heterogeneity within categories and excessive comorbidity of personality disorders has led many to call for the replacement of categorical with dimensional models (Costa & Widiger, 1994; Stuart et al., 1998; Widiger & Frances, 1994; Widiger & Sanderson, 1995).

Dimensional models of personality disorder differ with respect to the nature of the symptomatology on which they focus (i.e., phenotypical or "surface" vs. genotypical or "source" traits), the generality of those traits (i.e., a relatively small number of general or "higher-order" vs. a relatively large number of more specific or "lower-order" dimensions); and the assumed relation among the traits (i.e., independent or "orthogonal" vs. correlated or "oblique" dimensions). Once a model is selected, a variety of statistical methods can be used to obtain a solution. Two models illustrate these differences. The first is the five-factor model (FFM), which originally was developed to describe normal personality but more recently has been applied to personality disorder (for excellent overviews, see Costa & Widiger, 1994; Wiggins, 1996). According to the FFM, five broad, bipolar, orthogonal dimensions are necessary and reasonably sufficient to account for the associations among phenotypical or manifest aspects of personality. One particular version of the FFM (Costa & McCrae, 1992) defines these factors as follows: neuroticism is a tendency to be emotionally unstable and experience negative affect, extraversion is a tendency

to be energetic and sociable, agreeableness is a tendency to be warm and nonconfrontational, conscientiousness is a tendency to be responsible and organized, and openness to experience is a tendency to value the exploration of new feelings and ideas over traditionalism. Each broad dimension comprises a number of specific lower-level facet traits (Table 9.1 summarizes this model). The dimensions and their facets have been explicated over the course of decades by numerous investigators via factor analysis of data from tests of normal personality.

The second model is the Dimensional Assessment of Personality Pathology (DAPP) developed by Livesley and colleagues (e.g., Livesley, Jackson, & Schroeder, 1989, 1992; Schroeder, Wormworth, & Livesley, 1994). They chose a "bottom-up" approach, which focuses primarily on lower-level traits and only secondarily on broad, general dimensions. In the DAPP model, 18 oblique dimensions are considered necessary and reasonably sufficient to describe the domain of personality pathology (see Table 9.2). The dimensions were identified through the factor analysis of data from comprehensive measures of personality disorder symptomatology. Subsequent analyses have examined the phenotypic and genotypic structure of the 18 dimensions (Livesley, Jang, & Vernon, 1998), identifying four broad, orthogonal factors.

The DAPP factors parallel those of the FFM in many respects. The DAPP neuroticism and compulsivity factors are isomorphic to the

---

TABLE 9.1. A Dimensional Model of Normal Personality: The Five-Factor Model as Measured by the Revised NEO Personality Inventory

NEO-PI-R factor and facet scales
Neuroticism
Anxiety, Hostility, Depression, Self-Consciousness, Impulsiveness, Vulnerability
Extraversion
Warmth, Gregariousness, Assertiveness, Activity, Excitement Seeking, Positive Emotions
Openness
Fantasy, Aesthetics, Feelings, Actions, Ideas, Values
Agreeableness
Trust, Straighforwardness, Altruism, Compliance, Modesty, Tendermindedness
Conscientiousness
Competence, Order, Dutifulness, Achievement Striving, Self-Discipline, Deliberation

Note. NEO-PI-R, Revised NEO Personality Inventory (Costa & McCrae, 1992).

TABLE 9.2. A Dimensional Model of Personality Disorder: Factors and Scales of the Dimensional Assessment of Personality Pathology—Basic Questionnaire

DAPP-BQ factors and scales

Neuroticism

    Insecure Attachment, Anxiousness, Diffidence, Affective Lability, Narcissism, Social Avoidance, Passive–Oppositionality

Disagreeableness

    Rejection, Interpersonal Disesteem, Conduct Problems, Stimulus Seeking, Suspiciousness

Introversion

    Intimacy Problems, Restricted Expression, Identity Problems

Compulsivity

    Compulsivity

Note. DAPP-BQ, Dimensional Assessment of Personality Pathology—Basic Questionnaire (Schroeder, Wormworth, & Livesley, 1994). Scales that were factorially complex appear under the factor on which they loaded highest. Two additional scales, Self-Harming Behaviors and Perceptual Cognitive Distortions, were not included in the factor analysis.

FFM neuroticism and conscientiousness factors, respectively. An important difference is that the DAPP neuroticism factor has a strong interpersonal component, whereas its FFM counterpart is more purely emotional in nature (i.e., "negative affectivity"). Similarly, the DAPP disagreeableness and introversion factors are reflections or polar reversals of the FFM agreeableness and extraversion factors, respectively. The two models do not correspond perfectly, however. Note that the FFM openness factor is not well represented in the DAPP. This is perhaps because traits related to openness are not salient aspects of personality disorder symptomatology, or because there are not enough of these traits assessed in the DAPP to form a coherent psychometric factor.

How do these dimensional models of personality disorder relate to the dimensional model of attachment discussed previously? First, attachment theory is concerned with people who are motivated to establish and maintain interpersonal relations. People with little social investment may be considered to suffer from disorders of nonattachment, appearing not to feel the typical human need for attachment relations. With respect to the FFM and DAPP models, such individuals would likely score low on the FFM factor of extraversion and high on the DAPP factor of introversion. In DSM-IV terms, they are most likely to be diagnosed as suffering from schizoid, schizotypal, paranoid, or antisocial personality disorder.

One of the two key dimensions underlying individual differences in attachment orientations is anxiety, the propensity to experience attachment-related anxiety. The neuroticism factors of the FFM and DAPP—and particularly that of the DAPP—have strong parallels to the dimension of attachment anxiety. Individuals high on neuroticism would, in general, be expected to be high on the attachment anxiety dimension and will be prone to symptoms such as sensitivity to criticism or disapproval by others, fears of abandonment and loss of intimates, and need for constant approval and reassurance (e.g., Griffin & Bartholomew, 1994b). In DSM-IV terms, such individuals would most likely be diagnosed with traits of borderline, histrionic, avoidant, or dependent personality disorder.

The second dimension underlying individual differences in attachment reflects the individual's response to attachment anxiety: approach versus defensive avoidance. Approach involves responding to attachment anxiety with active and often desperate attempts to gain support from others and forestall separation from others. In contrast, avoidance involves the suppression of attachment behaviors under anxiety. The FFM extraversion factor and the DAPP introversion factor show some parallels to the avoidance attachment dimension, though the FFM extraversion factor tends to focus on behavior in general social relations rather than in intimate relations (Griffin & Bartholomew, 1994b). In particular, the DAPP restricted expression scale, a facet of introversion, would likely to be a close marker of the avoidance dimension. Some of the scales of the FFM factor of agreeableness (notably, trust) and the DAPP factor of disagreeableness (notably, suspiciousness) may also show some correspondence with the avoidance dimension, though these FFM and DAPP factors also reflect general assertiveness in interpersonal relations. In DSM-IV terms, individuals who exhibit high levels of avoidance are most likely to be diagnosed as suffering from avoidant or dependent personality disorder, and those who exhibit high levels of closeness to be diagnosed as suffering from narcissistic, histrionic, and borderline personality disorder.

There have been surprisingly few attempts to examine empirically the general association between dimensions of attachment and personality disorder. One important exception is the study by Brennan and Shaver (1998). In a large college sample, they used self-report measures to assess both personality disorders (the PDQ-R) and adult attachment. Their analysis identified two attachment dimensions corresponding to the diagonals of Figure 9.1, Insecurity (secure vs. fearful) and Defensive Style (dismissing vs. preoccupied). These dimensions lined up with corresponding dimensions underlying personality disorders. Insecurity was strongly associated with generalized pathology, with avoidant, borderline, and schizotypal scales loading highly. Defensive Style was associated with dependency/counterdependency, defined by histrionic and dependent personality disorder at one pole and schizoid personality disorder at the other pole. A third personality disorder dimension, labeled *psychopathy,* was not associated with attachment. Unfortunately, the different sets of dimensions underlying personality disorders preclude a direct comparison with our conceptual analysis of the dimension linkages between attachment and personality disorder. However, the general conclusion that, at least in part, individual differences in adult attachment and personality disorders share a common underlying structure is consistent with our analysis.

RELEVANCE OF ATTACHMENT TO SPECIFIC PERSONALITY DISORDERS

As previously mentioned, from a developmental pathways perspective we would not necessarily expect simple links between forms of attachment insecurity and personality disorders. However, based on previous research and theoretical analysis, we can speculate about the attachment components of some personality disorders. In this section, we first discuss those disorders whose criteria overlap to a considerable degree with the criteria for forms of insecurity, specifically the histrionic, borderline, and avoidant. We then point out how attachment may be helpful in clarifying the covariation between some disorders, focusing on the covariation between the avoidant, dependent, and schizoid disorders. We then discuss the antisocial personality disorder, a disorder that shows considerable heterogeneity in terms of attachment orientation.

Histrionic Personality Disorder

The key features of the histrionic personality disorder overlap to a considerable extent with a preoccupied attachment orientation. The excessive emotionality and desperate need for attention and reassurance of the histrionic indicates high attachment anxiety, whereas the exaggerated display of emotion and active seeking and demanding of approval from others indicates an approach-oriented strategy of attempting to get attachment needs met. The impressionistic speech of the histrionic is consistent with the preoccupied tendency to idealize (and often derogate as well) relationship partners. However, though many histrionic features are classically preoccupied, other features are not. Notably, the impulsivity and sensation seeking often characteristic of the histrionic are not necessarily characteristic of even highly preoccupied individuals and are not necessarily even attachment related. Conversely, a histrionic pattern is just one form that extreme attachment preoccupation can take.

To illustrate, we provide an attachment analysis of a 32-year-old woman who meets all eight DSM-III-R (American Psychiatric Association, 1987) criteria for the histrionic personality disorder. This woman's presentation is classically histrionic: impressionistic speech, exaggerated emotionality, and extremely seductive behavior. Both of her parents were physically and psychologically unavailable, appearing to have no interest in parenting. As a child she was demanding and oppositional, in an attempt to gain attention and acceptance from her parents. Her efforts only occasionally met with success, resulting in hysterical outbursts from her mother and either affection or criticism from her father. She had an intense sexual relationship with a female babysitter (from the age of 10), as well as a number of early sexual experiences with peers, from which she was able to gain the attention that she could not gain from her parents. She felt positively about all these sexual experiences, describing them as "exciting" and as the best things to happen during her childhood. Thus, her basic needs for attachment security were not met by her parents, and she came to see sexual relations as the one arena in which she could gain acceptance and a sense of connection. She had little insight into her childhood experiences and their impact on her life, oscillating between blaming her unhappy experiences on food allergies and blaming her experiences on her parents (at which times she refused all contact with them for periods of a year or longer). As an adult, this individual sought acceptance through sexual relationships. When single, she was highly sexually active (describing getting men as "a hobby"), though these liaisons never satisfied her craving for love and attention. A series of serious relationships with men followed a typical pattern: idealization at the outset, difficulties arising when her partners were not sufficiently attentive and sexually interested in her, and a move to a new relationship. This woman's attachment orientation is predominantly preoccupied, with her obsessive need for attention and acceptance from others and her active strategies to meet this need. However, she also shows some secondary dismissing elements—a tendency to objectify others, and a tendency to cut off threatening feelings of vulnerability by derogating others and focusing on sexuality to the exclusion of intimacy within relationships. It is these dismissing elements, in combination with a preoccupied orientation, which are consistent with the shallow emotions and exaggerated emotionality of the histrionic personality.

Borderline Personality Disorder

Of the various personality disorders, the borderline has received the most attention from attachment theorists and researchers. This is not surprising given both the prevalence of this disorder and its defining features. Two key features of borderline personality organization are a pattern of unstable and intense interpersonal relationships and frantic efforts to avoid real or imagined abandonment. The affective instability characteristic of the borderline indicates a failure to regulate attachment anxiety effectively, with proneness to extreme anger and recurrent suicidal threats and gestures reflecting the desperation underlying the borderline's attempts to get attachment needs met. The borderline is further seen as having disturbances in the capacity to maintain a coherent representation of both childhood relationships and current intimate relationships, vacillating between idealization and devaluation. The strong approach orientation implicated in borderline criteria is suggestive of a preoccupied, hyperactivating strategy.

A number of studies have looked at attachment as assessed in the AAI and borderline personality disorder. Unfortunately, the classification systems used in these studies have varied, making comparisons across studies difficult. Patrick, Hobson, Castle, Howard, and Maughan (1994) looked at the attachment patterns of 12 women who met at least seven of the eight DSM-III-R criteria for borderline personality disorder. They found that all women in the group were preoccupied, with a preponderance classified into a preoccupied subcategory (E3) characterized by fearfulness and feelings of being overwhelmed in relation to past attachment figures—a combination of preoccupied and fearful tendencies in the four-category system. As well, the majority of borderlines were seen as unresolved regarding losses and/or traumas they had experienced. Similar associations were found by Fonagy et al. (1996) with a somewhat more diverse clinical sample and by Stalker and Davies (1995) in a sample of women with a history of childhood sexual abuse. Results were more mixed in Rosenstein and Horowitz's (1996) study of psychiatrically hospitalized adolescents. Preoccupied attachment was not associated with clinical elevations on borderline traits as assessed by the Millon Clinical Multiaxial Inventory (MCMI), but there was an overrepresentation of preoccupied attachment in borderlines as assessed by DSM-III-R criteria. However, contrary to expectations, 29% of those classified as borderline had a dismissing attachment organization. These authors did not include the AAI cannot-classify category, and they speculate that the heterogeneity within diagnostic groups may reflect the lack of specificity of attachment classifications. They suggest that some patients may show a multiplicity of working models or, in other words, elements of more than one insecure pattern, and that this variation is not captured by the AAI classification system.

Turning to research using non-AAI measures of attachment, Brennan and Shaver (1998) found that both preoccupied and fearful attachment (based on a self-report measure) were associated with borderline personality and overall, that the fearful showed the highest levels of personality pathology. In a sample of men in treatment for spousal assault, Dutton, Saunders, Starzomski, and Bartholomew (1994) showed strong associations between borderline personality organization (as assessed by the Self-Report Instrument for Borderline Personality Organization, Oldham et al., 1985) and both preoccupied and fearful attachment. Sack, Sperling, Fagen, and Foelsch (1996) assessed attachment in a sample of borderline patients (almost all of whom were women) using a number of self-report measures of attachment. They found that borderlines were characterized by elevations on three insecure attachment styles defined in terms of dependency and anger (avoidant, hostile, and ambivalent), on avoidant attachment (fearful) based on Hazan and Shaver's three-category measure, and on continuous measures of various aspects of insecure attachment, including fear of loss, compulsive careseeking, and angry withdrawal. These findings confirm that extreme attachment anxiety is a defining feature of the borderline disorder. They also suggest that borderlines may show both high approach behaviors (careseeking, clingyness) and avoidant behaviors (angry withdrawal, devaluation of relationship partners).

We have not looked systematically at the associations between attachment and borderline personality disorder in our work. But it is our impression, from both clinical and nonclinical samples and from previous literature, that the key defining feature of the borderline from an attachment perspective is a pathological level of attachment anxiety. The behavioral response to that anxiety may vary somewhat across those diagnosed as borderline, consistent with the heterogeneity in the borderline group. However, several borderline characteristics (intense anger, suicidal or self-mutilating behavior, frantic efforts to avoid abandonment) indicate a predominantly preoccupied, approach-oriented strategy. In some cases, this preoccupation is combined with avoidance when relationships become close, yielding a vacillation between strategies or a lack of organization of strategies. The specific mix of strategies, along with other risk factors, can give rise to different presentations. In addition, the instability of self-image, relationships, and affect of the borderline suggest a lack of coherence in internal models of the self and others. Such incoherence can be characteristic of extreme insecurity of any form (though, within the four-category model, most often the preoccupied), and it can also reflect a failure to show a consistent strategy to deal with negative affect. Consistent with this expectation, studies using continuous ratings of attachment have found that borderline personality disorder is associated with elevations in multiple forms of insecurity. Unfortunately, the studies assessing borderlines with the AAI have not included the cannot-classify category, which would be expected to be overrepresented if borderlines often show mixed attachment orientations (as suggested by Rosenstein & Horowitz, 1996). We would add that although the cannot-classify category does subsume mixed strategies (such as a preoccupied/dismissing strategies), it does not specify the specific mixture of strategies or the degree to which each is displayed.

From an attachment perspective, it is not surprising that the borderline and histrionic disorders often co-occur (Stuart et al., 1998). Both are characterized by attachment anxiety and an approach orientation. The major difference may be one of extremity. The borderline is expected to show the most extreme levels of attachment-related anxiety, and the approach strategies of the borderline tend to take on more destructive forms than those of the histrionic. In addition, the borderline would tend to show more extreme incoherence of internalized representations of the self and others and, in some cases, may also present an incoherent mix of approach and avoidance strategies.

To illustrate the attachment perspective on borderline personality disorder, we present a 30-year-old man who received the highest possible borderline rating (based on the Personality Disorder Examination; Loranger, 1988). On an attachment interview, he was assessed as showing high preoccupation, with some secondary dismissing characteristics and the lowest possible rating on attachment security. His mother was controlling, dominant, unpredictably abusive, both in private and in public, and, on very rare occasions, affectionate. As a child, he was terrified of his mother and yet desperate to gain her acceptance. The physical abuse ended when he became bigger than his mother as a teenager and was able to assume a dominant role in the relationship. But he continued to be caught in a typically preoccupied relationship with his mother, characterized by enmeshment and conflict and frustrating attempts to gain her acceptance. His feelings regarding his mother shifted between idealization and derogation, the one constant being a consuming anger for his mother's treatment of him as a child. His father was passive and uninvolved, spending much of his time "drunk and depressed." In contrast to his emotional engagement with his mother, he distanced himself from his father and expressed disdain for his father's weakness and passivity (showing dismissing tendencies). He felt humiliated by his mother's domination of the family and was determined not to feel controlled by another woman. Ironically, to deal with his humiliation he came to adopt the same interpersonal style as his mother, becoming dominant, controlling, and abusive in his relationships with peers and romantic partners. His intimate relationships, in particular, were marked by extreme attachment anxiety and frantic attempts to gain acceptance and validation. His preoccupation was evidenced in a history of quick involvements (moving in with partners almost immediately), an obsession with partners to the exclusion of other social relations, a vacillation between idealization and derogation of partners, and an inability to consider letting go of one relationship until another had taken its place. His feelings of well-being and self-worth were entirely dependent on the state of his close relationships, resulting in extreme fluctuations in mood. His attachment anxiety became overwhelming when he perceived any threat to a partner's accessibility and acceptance, such as a partner wanting to see independent friends or attending to children. In response to these perceived threats, he attempted to maintain contact with partners and ensure that their attention was focused on his needs by becoming controlling and abusive and engaging in threats of suicide. When this behavior led romantic partners to withdraw from him, he became even more insecure and jealous and increased his attempts to gain their attention and acceptance to increasingly dangerous levels. His strong approach orientation was also evident in a long history of seeking help from others, including individual and group therapy, self-help groups, and religious groups. The extremity of this individual's preoccupied orientation, as shown in a lack of internalized self-worth, an inability to regulate his negative affect, and obsessive and exaggerated attempts to get attachment needs met in relationships, is consistent with the borderline personality disorder.

Avoidant Personality Disorder

There is considerable overlap between fearful attachment and avoidant personality disorder: a desire for close relationships, a fear of disapproval or rejection, and a behavioral strategy of avoiding relationships. The characterizations differ, however, in their specificity: Fearfulness focuses on functioning in close attachment relationships, and the avoidant focuses on timidity across social contexts. Although temperament may play a significant role in social anxiety in general, difficult childhood experiences and associated fearful attachment would be expected to contribute to a pathway leading to the avoidant personality disorder (in interaction with other risk factors such as temperamental vulnerability). In particular, rejection by caretakers, unresolved losses, and childhood physical and sexual abuse have been associated with fearfulness (e.g., Roche et al., 1999; Shaver & Clark, 1994).

A 35-year-old male illustrates the attachment viewpoint on avoidant personality disorder. Based on an attachment interview, this man was assessed as having a fearful attachment pattern with some preoccupied features. He described himself as clumsy, awkward, shy, and consumed with loneliness. His family background was characterized by disengagement. When he was in kindergarten, his parents divorced, and to this day, he does not understand the reasons behind the divorce because his family refused to discuss it. After the divorce, he became increasingly introverted and started to have problems with severe acne and stammering. When he was upset, sick, or emotionally hurt, he would withdraw from people and try to deal with his problems on his own, a pattern that continued into adulthood. He never felt able to discuss problems with any of his caregivers, and he does not remember either parent expressing any physical or verbal affection to him. Currently, he claims to have one close friend; but he rarely sees this friend, he does not trust his friend enough to discuss personal issues with him, and there is evidence that this friend takes advantage of him in various ways. Despite his lack of satisfying friendships, he does not attempt to make new friends because he fears his overtures will not be reciprocated. Although he has never been involved in a romantic relationship, he is obsessed with meeting a romantic partner. In fact, his lack of a relationship is the major source of distress in his life. He has developed crushes on a number of women over time but is afraid to talk to them or initiate casual interactions, presumably because of his fear of being rejected. In some cases, he has written letters expressing his feelings, leading the women to become uncomfortable and distance themselves from him, further contributing to his fears of rejection. Furthermore, the solitary nature of his occupation hinders any opportunities to meet new people.

This case illustrates a prototypical avoidant pattern. But there is considerable heterogeneity of individuals qualifying as avoidant, perhaps indicating problems with the criteria for diagnosis. For example, a 29-year-old man diagnosed as avoidant and high on fearful attachment (based on independent interview measures) presents quite differently. This individual also reported a number of risk factors in his background: loss of his father at 5, loss of his mother at 7, subsequently being raised by strict and emotionally unavailable relatives, attention-deficit/hyperactivity disorder that led to school failure, and severe rejection by peers at school (tied to his school failures and his status as a visible minority). Although none of these factors on its own would necessarily have led to personality pathology, in combination and in interaction (e.g., he had no one he felt he could turn to when being harassed and assaulted at school), his entire history contributed to the development of a distrust of others and the adoption of a self-defensive stance in which he would not risk rejection. He had never established close friendships as a child or as an adult. In contrast to the first case described, this individual did occasionally socialize with acquaintances and he had become involved in two romantic relationships (initiated by his partners). However, in both of his intimate relationships his partners had been emotionally and physically abusive toward him, further contributing to his fearfulness.

This latter case highlights some of the potential weaknesses of the current criteria for avoidant personality disorder. As discussed by West and Keller (1994; see also Sheldon & West, 1990), from an attachment perspective, the shift in DSM-III-R to a focus on general social discomfort rather than a desire for, but fear of, dyadic intimacy is unfortunate. Though discomfort with both close and general social relations may tend to coexist (as in the first case), this is not necessarily the case. An individual may be extremely shy and timid in many social settings but have the capacity to form intimate and secure close relationships. Such a person may still qualify as avoidant but would not have the same level of impairment as an individual with deep fears of intimacy. Conversely, some individuals are relatively comfortable in superficial social situations but fearful of close relationships in which they are vulnerable to rejection. For example, the second avoidant man described was reasonably comfortable, and quite enjoyed, interacting with coworkers and acquaintances; but he was hesitant to let anyone come to know him better, for fear of further rejection. We would propose that the critical features of this disorder are a desire for close relationships, coupled with an extreme fear of disapproval and rejection, leading to avoidance of becoming intimately involved with others.

Covariation of Personality Disorders

The two-dimensional conception of adult attachment distinguishes between the tendency to experience attachment anxiety (an internal state) and the behavioral strategies triggered by that anxiety. This distinction may be helpful in clarifying the covariation among some of the personality disorders. In particular, attachment may be helpful in considering the covariation between the avoidant and both the schizoid and dependent personality disorders, an issue that has generated considerable attention (e.g., Trull, Widiger, & Frances, 1987).

From an attachment perspective, the avoidant and dependent would be expected to show high overlap, as they do in fact (e.g., Trull et al., 1987). Both are defined in terms of attachment anxiety, though the anxiety of the avoidant is shown more in fearfulness of becoming close to others (because of fear of rejection) and the anxiety of the dependent is shown more in fear of separation and rejection once in a relationship (cf. Trull et al., 1987). The prototypical avoidant would likely score more extremely on the avoidant attachment dimension than would the prototypical dependent, or, in terms of attachment patterns, the dependent would show some preoccupied/approach-oriented tendencies. However, individuals with both disorders take a basically avoidant and passive approach to dealing with their anxiety. Neither directly expresses their attachment needs: The avoidant actively avoids situations in which they are vulnerable to rejection, and the dependent acts in a passive and compliant manner within relationships to avoid rejection and abandonment. We have heard many stories (in conducting attachment interviews) of avoidant individuals who find their way into close relationships, usually with a friend or partner who has actively initiated the relationship, and then shift into a more dependent stance. Though their behavior will look different when in and out of close relationships, their basic personality dynamic remains unchanged. This would be true of the avoidant man described earlier.

In contrast, though the avoidant and schizoid share social withdrawal and behavioral avoidance of close relationships, they would be seen as fundamentally different from an attachment perspective. As previously discussed, the schizoid is uninterested in close relationships, showing a disorder of nonattachment, whereas the avoidant is intensely interested in close relationships but is incapable of initiating those relationships, showing a form of insecure attachment. Some researchers have drawn links between the schizoid and dismissing attachment (Brennan & Shaver, 1998). But we would not expect schizoid individuals to be characterized by dismissing attachment (or vice versa), just as nonattached children are not avoidantly attached. Although on some measures of attachment schizoid individuals may be classified as dismissing—because the two constructs do share some features—we feel that this would be a misleading classification. Dismissing individuals do form attachments; they just maintain a comfortable distance within those relationships, presumably in order to defensively avoid the activation of their attachment systems. Though dismissing individuals may be more or less extroverted, they are generally social integrated. Though they downplay the intimacy and support functions of relationships, they would not avoid sexual relations (in fact, they may even use casual sexual relations as a safe alternative to more intimate relationships; Brennan & Shaver, 1995). And though the dismissing orientation is associated with the tendency to defensively downplay negative emotions, and

with constricted expression of emotion, it is not associated with the same degree of emotional constriction of the schizoid. Of the many dismissing individuals we have assessed in studies over the years, we have not seen one individual whom we would consider schizoid.

Antisocial Personality Disorder

Antisocial personality disorder provides an example of how different developmental pathways (as reflected in different attachment orientations) may lead to phenotypically similar behavioral disturbances. There are a number of mechanisms through which a history of insecure attachment could increase the risk of antisocial behavior. Insecure models may predispose individuals to attribute hostile intent in ambiguous social situations, and they also may interfere with the ability to consider others' perspectives and feelings (whether through an egocentric focus or a disengagement and lack of psychological awareness). In addition, childhood insecurity may tend to make socialization practices less effective, putting the child at risk for being more susceptible to negative influences outside the family. In some cases, the parenting practices associated with insecure attachment, especially physical and emotional abuse, may actually be modeling antisocial behaviors for children.

Most commonly, researchers and theorists have proposed a link between dismissing attachment and externalizing disorders such as antisocial personality disorder. There is some evidence for such a link. Notably, Rosenstein and Horowitz (1996) studied a group of psychiatrically hospitalized adolescents and found a strong link between dismissing organization (as assessed by the AAI) and both conduct disorder (based on the Structured Clinical Interview for Diagnosis, SCID; Spitzer, Williams, & Gibbon, 1987) and antisocial disorder (based on the MCMI). However, the other studies to look at antisocial behavior from an attachment viewpoint have failed to confirm such a specific link. Allen, Hauser, and Borman-Spurrell (1996) looked at attachment organization (based on the AAI) and criminal behavior in a sample of young adults (some from a community sample and some who had been psychiatrically hospitalized in adolescence). Criminal behavior was associated with lack of resolution of trauma and dismissing attachment organization, though young adults in the AAI cannot classify category showed the highest rates of criminal behavior. In contrast, van IJzendoorn and Bakersmans-Kranenburg (1996) did not find any predictable associations between AAI classifications and personality disorders in a group of mentally disturbed criminal offenders. This group showed the full range of insecure attachment patterns (including the unresolved and cannot classify categories), with the dismissing individuals least likely to be diagnosed with a personality disorder. Finally, using a self-report measure of attachment in a nationally representative sample, Mickelson et al. (1997) found that anxious–ambivalence and avoidant attachment were both associated with antisocial disorder (as assessed by a structured interview). In sum, it appears that insecurity of attachment is related to antisocial tendencies, though perhaps extremity of insecurity (as shown in the unresolved category) is more predictive than a specific attachment orientation.

We looked at attachment orientations associated with antisocial personality disorder in a sample of men in treatment for assaulting their female partners and were struck by the heterogeneity in their attachment assessments. The majority of men who were diagnosed as antisocial also were diagnosed with one or more additional personality disorders (Hart, Dutton, & Newlove, 1993). Other than a lack of security, there was little consistency in the attachment patterns observed, suggesting that there are multiple pathways to antisocial personality disorder. Men were assessed with the full range of attachment insecurities, with some showing combinations of two insecure orientations (parallel to the cannot classify). Interestingly, the small subgroup of men whose personality problems appeared limited to antisocial (and perhaps sadistic) characteristics were most likely to be predominantly dismissing. In listening to these men's stories, we were impressed by how a dismissing strategy seemed to act as a risk factor for the development of antisocial tendencies. To varying degrees, these men lacked empathy with others and tended to objectify others, characteristics that would make it less unacceptable to be hurtful to others. They were also distrustful, tending to make negative attributions of others' intentions and behaviors, thereby fueling their own hostility. But, of course, the vast majority of dismissing individuals are not antisocial. Therefore, other factors, including genetic dispositions and socialization forces, appear to be necessary for

putting these men on a path toward antisocial behavior.

To illustrate, a 27-year-old man who was diagnosed with antisocial personality disorder showed a prototypical dismissing pattern. He had a superficial understanding of his childhood, downplayed or was unaware of any effects his upbringing had on him, and displayed an impoverished understanding of both his own feelings and the feelings of others. His family relationships were characterized by emotional disengagement. His mother, a single parent on social assistance, had a difficult time providing for the physical needs of her 8 children and had little energy left over for their emotional needs. She provided only minimal care and supervision of her children, and, though not actively rejecting, she was unresponsive to their attempts to gain attention and support. On multiple occasions his mother sent him away to live with relatives or put him in foster care. He dropped out of school at a young age, clearly alienated from the larger community. His childhood was also permeated with models of threats and violence as the means to assert authority and handle interpersonal conflict. His mother was unnecessarily harsh in her sporadic attempts at discipline, and one older brother was extremely violent toward him (until he was able to physically defend himself as a teenager). He found a sense of belonging and camaraderie in an antisocial peer group, beginning his criminal career in his early teens. He had a number of long-term male friends, who he clearly valued, though these friendships were based primarily on shared activities rather than emotional support. His long-term romantic relationship showed a classic pursuer–distancer pattern, with his partner actively seeking greater closeness (physically and emotionally) and he withdrawing from her demands and desiring greater autonomy. When he felt too overwhelmed by his partner's demands, he would attempt to escape from the conflict by either physically leaving or threatening his partner with violence. He did not understand or sympathize with his partner's desire for greater intimacy and support, feeling no such needs himself, yet he downplayed their problems, viewing them as typical of heterosexual relationships.

Consistent with prior research, we have also observed that many antisocial men show high attachment anxiety, anxiety that may actually drive their antisocial behavior. For example, a 43-year-old man in treatment for spousal assault was diagnosed as antisocial as well as borderline and histrionic. Based on an attachment interview, he was assessed as highly preoccupied (with some fearful and dismissing elements). He came from a background that had fostered a hypersensitivity to rejection and an active, aggressive style. His father was domineering and abusive to his children and wife and forcefully rejected any sign of vulnerability on his son's part. His mother was overwhelmed, prone to depression, and unpredictably moody. She sporadically (and ineffectually) tried to protect him from his father's violence, and she was occasionally warm and responsive if he actively sought out her attention. From a young age, this individual responded to any frustration or hurt with aggression and temper tantrums, which at least served to gain the attention of his parents. He had had a series of intense and volatile romantic relationships, all characterized by extremes of dependency, jealousy, conflict, and fears of abandonment. In these relationships, he became violent and controlling in a desperate attempt to hold on to his partners, especially when he felt that they were withdrawing from him (e.g., when they refused to engage him in conflict) or focusing attention on others (friends, family members, their children). However, his violent outbursts had the opposite effect—driving away his partners and thereby confirming his worst fears of being abandoned and being alone.

IMPLICATIONS FOR INTERVENTION

Though research on the therapeutic implications of attachment theory has been slow to develop, the availability of adult attachment measures has recently facilitated an increase in these investigations (Slade, 1999). This research has focused primarily on the relation between attachment theory and psychoanalysis, the treatment of infants and their parents, and the theory and practice of psychotherapy. Given its developmental perspective, attachment theory's most promising therapeutic implications are likely to reside in preventative efforts aimed at infants and their parents. As Bowlby (1977) stated, "My hope is that, in the long term, the greatest value of the theory proposed may prove to be the light it throws on the conditions most likely to promote healthy personality development" (p. 676). In fact, a meta-analysis of intervention studies found a substantial effect size ($d = .48$) for the effectiveness of short-term attachment interventions in enhancing maternal sensitivity and, subsequently, the likelihood that an infant will develop a secure attachment (van IJzendoorn, Juffer, & Duyvestyn, 1995). However, this discussion focuses on the implications of attachment for the theory and practice of adult psychotherapy.

Attachment theory can assist in the development and implementation of intervention plans for people with personality difficulties (e.g., Dozier & Tyrrell, 1998). However, it should not be considered an organizing framework for understanding problems of adjustment or personality or as a framework for therapy (Bartholomew & Thompson, 1995). Instead, it is most properly and usefully thought of as a way of informing, rather than defining or prescribing, intervention (Slade, 1999). Most generally, attachment theory should encourage therapists to conceptualize attachment styles and behaviors as *intervention targets* (i.e., problems that are a primary focus of therapy) and as *responsivity factors* (i.e., client characteristics that may mediate or moderate responses to interventions targeted at other problems). This is true regardless of the nature of the intervention. Attachment theory is clearly compatible with intervention models that are strongly focused on close interpersonal relations, such as family systems theory (e.g., Byng-Hall, 1999), but any intervention can benefit from explicit consideration of attachment feelings and behaviors— just as any intervention should consider people's cognitive and intellectual abilities.

The first step in intervention is assessment, and here attachment difficulties must be considered potential intervention targets. Therapists must have some understanding, however incomplete, of a person's problems and resources before they can determine what kinds of intervention are most appropriate for that person. Knowledge of attachment theory can help the therapist to conduct a more thorough and sophisticated assessment of the person's functioning in close personal relationships—in particular, relationships with family of origin, romantic partners, and friends. These relationships are, of course, of relevance and therefore routinely considered in virtually all forms of therapy. But attachment theory promotes the understanding of attachment as a process rather than a trait—the search for patterns in the person's attachment behaviors across relationships, consideration of the person's reactions to threats to relationships (real or imagined), and exploration of basic working models for self and others. Therapists should keep in mind one of the important points discussed earlier in this chapter: There is no simple correspondence between personality disorder and attachment pattern. Thus people suffering from the same personality disorder can differ with respect to attachment orientation. In addition, a person's attachment-related experiences and behaviors can differ across relationships and across time.

The second step in intervention is the establishment and maintenance of a stable, productive therapeutic relationship. Here, attachment patterns must be considered responsivity factors. Attachment theory encourages therapists to conceptualize at least part of their responsibility as providing a secure base that promotes safe exploration on the part of clients (Dozier & Tyrrell, 1998). At the very least, therapists should recognize that they must "work around" a client's attachment insecurities. For example, the client may have problems related to anxious attachment that are manifested in the therapeutic relationship, including behaviors that represent separation protest—feelings of anger or panic in response to the therapist's encouragement of independent action on the part of the client. Working around this, the therapist might attempt to find strategies for encouraging independent action that do not elicit feelings of abandonment and rejection in the client. Alternatively, the therapist might not change the primary interventions but, instead, might add strategies to help the client cope with the feelings of abandonment and rejection. A more sophisticated approach would be to "work with" the client's attachment style and behaviors rather than working around them. Continuing with the same example, the therapist might develop strategies that would use the client's anxious attachment to motivate or facilitate independent action. This could include encouraging the client to develop new close personal relationships in which the client is likely to be required to act independently. Perhaps the most sophisticated approach would be "working through" the client's attachment difficulties. Here, the therapist might directly explore with the client attachment behaviors in past close personal relationships and draw parallels with experiences in the therapeutic relationship, with the goal of removing actual or potential obstacles in the treatment of the primary intervention targets. (This process is similar to analysis of transference in psychodynamic psychotherapies, although here it is not necessarily expected that exploration of the therapeutic relationship would, in and of itself, have a direct impact on the primary intervention targets.) Note that these three applications of attachment theory in the establishment and maintenance of the therapeutic relationship—working around, working with, and working through attachment styles and behaviors—are possible regardless of the nature of the primary intervention target (e.g., spider phobia, dysthymia, parasuicidal behavior, marital distress, and antisocial behavior) and regardless of the nature of the intervention (e.g., cognitive-behavioral therapy, short-term psychodynamic psychotherapy, couple therapy, and group therapy).

The third step in intervention is action, that is, using therapeutic techniques to ameliorate target problems. When those target problems include difficulties in close personal relationships, attachment theory is directly relevant to the choice of therapeutic strategies. In such instances, the therapist's task is to help the client explore how feelings, thoughts, and behaviors in current interpersonal relationships are related to earlier experiences (Dozier & Tyrrell, 1998). The general aim is to revise the client's existing working models of self and others at both the psychological and behavioral levels. At the psychological level, Holmes (1998) suggested that the process of therapy involves helping the client to tell a coherent story and to reframe this story in a more positive and therapeutic way. Attachment patterns provide a type of story in which emotional regulation, experiences in primary relationships, and the interpretations of these experiences can be understood. In interpersonal terms, insight is gained when the individual is able to recognize, accept, and understand relationship patterns; in cognitive terms, changes in schemas and attitudes occur when the individual reinterprets the attachment behaviors of self and others in a more positive or realistic way. At the behavioral level, changing the ways in which one acts in close personal relationships can create more secure relationships, which should, in turn, lead to positive changes in internal working models.

Our discussion so far has been on individual treatment, but attachment theory is also relevant to dyadic, family, and group therapies. Importantly, attachment theory highlights the fact that in interactions, peoples' attachment problems and dynamics are mutually constructed. For example, one common pattern observed in couples seeking therapy is the pursuer–distancer dynamic, in which one partner constantly seeks reassurance from the other but is met with withdrawal. This leads to increased efforts of the shunned partner to seek comfort, which are again rejected. Byng-Hall (1999) interpreted this pattern as reflecting a preoccupied–dismissing pairing in which the pursuer, the preoccupied partner, is feeling deprived and abandoned while the withdrawer, the dismissing partner, is disdainful of his or her partner's dependency needs. The four-category model of attachment (Bartholomew & Horowitz, 1991) provides an additional interpretation of this pattern. Bartholomew et al. (2001) observed that a common pairing in abusive intimate relationships is a preoccupied female with a fearful male. In this context, the dynamic is a highly volatile one in which the female partner is extremely possessive, jealous, and demanding of her partner's time and attention. In turn, the male partner feels overwhelmed by her demands and unable to live up to his partner's expectations. His inclination to withdraw only leaves her feeling angrier and more desperate. This creates a high level of conflict that can escalate into violence and have disastrous consequences for both partners. From an attachment perspective, such relationship conflict results from perceptions that one's partner is inaccessible and emotionally unresponsive (Johnson, 1986). Attachment-based therapies can help relationship partners to better anticipate and communicate each other's underlying needs for security, protect against future misunderstandings, and develop appropriate ways of achieving these needs.

Empirical research on attachment and intervention has suggested that attachment organization may be predictive of seeking therapy, compliance, and therapeutic outcomes. Individuals with a dismissing attachment pattern discount the importance of relationships and deal with emotional distress through strategies of deactivation and minimization. These individuals would therefore be expected to find the treatment process emotionally challenging and difficult (Byng-Hall, 1999). Dozier (1990) found dismissing individuals to be resistant to treatment; they rarely asked for help and often rejected offers for help. Slade (1999) observed that it takes a substantial amount of time before dis-

missing individuals can acknowledge their feelings of loss, rejection, and need, and that these insights are frequently followed by periods of suppression and denial. Horowitz, Rosenberg, and Bartholomew (1993) pointed out that the dismissing tend to have interpersonal problems characterized by hostile dominance, and that people with these types of problems do not respond well to brief dynamic psychotherapy. Instead, long-term dynamic therapy, cognitive therapy, or pharmacotherapy may be more appropriate. Despite these negative outcomes for the dismissing, Fonagy et al. (1996) found that psychiatric patients assessed as dismissing on the AAI showed more clinical improvement after treatment than those who were assessed as preoccupied. They proposed that it may be easier to deal with avoidant strategies such as minimization than to attempt to reframe a protective and well-established set of perceptions about the past, as would be required with preoccupied clients. To the therapist, the preoccupied present as needy, dependent, and demanding, transforming the therapist–client relationship into one reminiscent of a parent–child relationship (Dozier, 1990).

A more sophisticated attachment analysis of the therapeutic relationship will take into consideration the interaction of the client's and therapist's attachment orientations and behaviors. Consistent with interpersonal theory, part of the therapist's task is to provide noncomplementary interpersonal responses which challenge clients' habitual interpersonal patterns and thereby challenge their internal working models (Dozier & Tyrrell, 1998). However, therapists with insecure attachment orientations may be less able than secure therapists to appropriately adjust their responses to clients. Consistent with this proposition, Dozier, Cue, and Barnett (1994) found that secure therapists were more apt to respond in noncomplementary ways—intervening in more depth with clients relying on deactivating strategies (i.e., those with dismissing tendencies) and in less depth with clients relying on hyperactivating strategies (i.e., those with preoccupied tendencies). Insecure therapists did just the opposite, intervening in ways consistent with their clients' characteristic strategies. In a subsequent study, Tyrrell, Dozier, Teague, and Fallot (1999) showed that clients appeared to form stronger therapeutic alliances and to gain more from therapy when they were paired with a therapist with noncorresponding attachment strategies.

CONCLUSIONS

Much work is needed in mapping out the associations between personality pathology and forms of attachment insecurity, both concurrently and longitudinally. The current body of research looking at these associations is plagued by inconsistencies in methods of assessing attachment (including different classification systems) and personality disorders and, for the most part, by reliance on small clinical samples with little range of disorders. It is not reasonable to expect future work in this area to adopt common methodologies, nor would it be desirable. However, as a larger body of research accumulates, ideally it will become possible to discern greater consistencies in patterns of findings.

In spite of these limitations in the literature, we hope we have demonstrated the usefulness of attachment theory in explicating the potential developmental and interpersonal components of personality disorder. The developmental pathways model conceptualizes personality pathology as being the outcome of a series of deviations which take the developing child (and later, adult) further and further from adaptive functioning. To fully understand personality disorders and the heterogeneity within disorders, it will be necessary to trace these pathways from a point before the presence of disorder. A case in point is Moffitt's (1993) distinction between "adolescent-limited" and "life-course persistent" (early emerging) antisocial behavior. These two groups are not on the same pathway as only the latter group has a higher likelihood of criminal behavior in adulthood. As argued by Sroufe (1997), more important than the mapping on of specific currently defined attachment and personality disorder categories would be work that follows individuals defined by early patterns of adaptation through to adulthood and observes what families of outcomes may be associated with different developmental pathways. This approach may "uncover new, coherent groupings of problems" (p. 264) as well as yield a rich picture of the antecedents of personality difficulties.

REFERENCES

Ainsworth, M. D. S. (1973). The development of infant–mother attachment. In B. Caldwell & H. Ricciuti (Eds.), *Review of child development Research* (Vol. 3, pp. 1–94). Chicago: University of Chicago Press.

Ainsworth, M. D. S., Blehar, M. C., Waters, E., & Wall, S. (1978). *Patterns of attachment: Psychological study of the Strange Situation*. Hillsdale, NJ: Erlbaum.

Alden, L. E., Wiggins, J. S., & Pincus, A. L. (1990). Construction of circumplex scales for the Inventory of Interpersonal Problems. *Journal of Personality Assessment, 55,* 521–536.

Alexander, P. C. (1993). The differential effects of abuse characteristics and attachment in the prediction of long-term effects of sexual abuse. *Journal of Interpersonal Violence, 8,* 346–362.

Allen, J. P., Hauser, S. T., & Borman-Spurrell, E. (1996). Attachment theory as a framework for understanding sequelae of severe adolescent psychopathology: An 11-year follow-up study. *Journal of Consulting and Clinical Psychology, 64,* 254–263.

American Psychiatric Association (1987). *Diagnostic and statistical manual of mental disorders* (3rd ed., rev.). Washington, DC: Author.

American Psychiatric Association. (1994). *Diagnostic and statistical manual of mental disorders* (4th ed.). Washington, DC: Author.

Bartholomew, K. (1990). Avoidance of intimacy: An attachment perspective. *Journal of Social and Personal Relationships, 7,* 147–178.

Bartholomew, K. (1997). Adult attachment processes: Individual and couple perspectives. *British Journal of Medical Psychology, 70,* 249–263.

Bartholomew, K., Cobb, R. J., & Poole, J. A. (1997). Adult attachment patterns and social support processes. In G. R. Pierce, B. Lakey, I. G. Sarason, & B. R. Sarason (Eds.), *Sourcebook of social support and personality* (pp. 359–378). New York: Plenum.

Bartholomew, K., Henderson, A. J. Z., & Dutton, D. G. (2001). Insecure attachment and abusive intimate relationships. In C. Clulow (Ed.), *Adult attachment and couple work: Applying the "secure base" concept in research and practise* (pp. 43–61). London: Routledge.

Bartholomew, K., & Horowitz, L. M. (1991). Attachment styles among young adults: A test of a model. *Journal of Personality and Social Psychology, 61,* 226–244.

Bartholomew, K., & Scharfe, E. (1994, August). *Adult attachment patterns and interpersonal problems in young adults.* Paper presented at the American Psychological Association Convention, Los Angeles.

Bartholomew, K., & Shaver, P. R. (1998). Methods of assessing adult attachment: Do they converge? In J. A. Simpson & W. S. Rholes (Eds.). *Attachment theory and close relationships* (pp. 25–45). New York: Guilford Press.

Bartholomew, K., & Thompson, J. M. (1995). An application of attachment theory to counseling psychology. *The Counseling Psychologist, 23,* 484–490.

Belsky, J. (1999). Interactional and contextual determinants of attachment security. In J. Cassidy & P. R. Shaver (Eds.), *Handbook of attachment: Theory, research, and clinical applications* (pp. 249–264). New York: Guilford Press.

Belsky, J., Fish, M., & Isabella, R. (1991). Continuity and discontinuity in infant negative and positive emotionality: Family antecedents and attachment consequences. *Developmental Psychology, 27,* 421–431.

Bowlby, J. (1973). *Attachment and loss: Vol. 2. Separation.* New York: Basic Books.

Bowlby, J. (1977). The making and breaking of affectional bonds. *British Journal of Psychiatry, 130,* 201–210.

Bowlby, J. (1980). *Attachment and loss: Vol. 3. Loss, sadness and depression.* New York: Basic Books.

Bowlby, J. (1982). *Attachment and loss: Vol. 1. Attachment* (2nd ed.). New York: Basic Books.

Bowlby, J. (1988a). *A secure base.* New York: Basic.

Bowlby, J. (1988b). Developmental psychiatry comes of age. *American Journal of Psychiatry, 145,* 1–10.

Brennan, K. A., Clark, C. L., & Shaver, P. R. (1998). Self-report measurement of adult attachment: An integrative overview. In J. A. Simpson & W. S. Rholes (Eds.), *Attachment theory and close relationships* (pp. 46–76). New York: Guilford Press.

Brennan, K. S., & Shaver, P. R. (1995). Dimensions of adult attachment, affect regulation, and romantic relationship functioning. *Personality and Social Psychology Bulletin, 21,* 267–283.

Brennan, K. A., & Shaver, P. R. (1998). Attachment styles and personality disorders: Their connections to each other and to parental divorce, parental death, and perceptions of parental caregiving. *Journal of Personality, 66,* 835–878.

Brennan, K. A., Shaver, P. R., & Tobey, A. E. (1991). Attachment styles, gender, and parental problem drinking. *Journal of Social and Personal Relationships, 8,* 451–466.

Brussoni, M. J., Jang, K. L., Livesley, W. J., & MacBeth, T. M. (2000). Genetic and environmental influences on adult attachment styles. *Personal Relationships, 7,* 283–289.

Byng-Hall, J. (1999). Family and couple therapy: Toward greater security. In J. Cassidy & P. R. Shaver (Eds.), *Handbook of attachment: Theory, research, and clinical applications* (pp. 625–645). New York: Guilford Press.

Carnelley, K. B., Pietromonaco, P. R., & Jaffe, K. (1994). Depression, working models of others, and relationship functioning. *Journal of Personality and Social Psychology, 66,* 127–140.

Caspi, A., & Elder, G. H. (1988). Emergent family patterns: The intergenerational construction of problem behavior and relationships. In R. A. Hinde & J. Stevenson-Hinde (Eds.), *Relationships within families* (pp. 218–240). Oxford, UK: Clarendon Press.

Collins, N. L. (1996). Working models of attachment: Implications for explanation, emotion, and behavior. *Journal of Personality and Social Psychology, 71,* 810–832.

Collins, N. L., & Read, S. J. (1990). Adult attachment, working models, and relationship quality in dating couples. *Journal of Personality and Social Psychology, 58,* 644–663.

Collins, N. L., & Read, S. J. (1994). Cognitive representations of adult attachment: The structure and function of working models. In D. Perlman & K. Bartholomew (Eds.), *Advances in personal relationships* (Vol 5, pp. 53–90). London: Jessica Kingsley.

Costa, P. T., Jr., & McCrae, R. R. (1992). *Revised NEO Personality Inventory (NEO-PI-R) and NEO Five-Factor Inventory (NEO-FFI): Professional manual.* Odessa, FL: Psychological Assessment Resources.

Costa, P. T., Jr., & Widiger, T. A. (1994). Introduction: Personality disorders and the five-factor model of personality. In P. T. Costa & T. A. Widiger (Eds.), *Personality disorders and the five-factor model of personality* (pp. 1–12). Washington, DC: American Psychological Association.

Crittenden, P. M. (1988). Relationships at risk. In J. Belsky & T. Nezworski (Eds.), *Clinical implications of attachment* (pp. 136–174). Hillsdale, NJ: Erlbaum.

Crockenberg, S. B. (1981). Infant irritability, mother responsiveness, and social support influences on the security of infant–mother attachment. *Child Development, 52,* 857–865.

Crowell, J. A., Fraley, R. C., & Shaver, P. R. (1999). Measurement of individual differences in adolescent and adult attachment. In J. Cassidy & P. R. Shaver (Eds.), *Handbook of attachment: Theory, research, and clinical applications* (pp. 434–465). New York: Guilford Press.

DeWolff, M., & van IJzendoorn, M. (1997). Sensitivity and attachment: A meta-analysis on parental antecedents of infant attachment. *Child Development, 68,* 571–591.

Downey, G., Freitas, A., Michaelis, B., & Khouri, H. (1998). The self-fulfilling prophecy in close relationships: Rejection sensitivity and rejection by romantic partners. *Journal of Personality and Social Psychology, 75*(2), 545–560.

Dozier, M. (1990). Attachment organization and treatment use for adults with serious psychopathological disorders. *Development and Psychopathology, 2,* 47-60.

Dozier, M., Cue, K., & Barnett, L. (1994). Clinicians as caregivers: Role of attachment organization in treatment. *Journal of Counseling and Clinical Psychology, 62,* 793–800.

Dozier, M., & Tyrrell, C. (1998). The role of attachment in therapeutic relationships. In J. A. Simpson & W. S. Rholes (Eds.), *Attachment theory and close relationships* (pp. 221–248). New York: Guilford Press.

Dutton, D. G., Saunders, K., Starzomski, A., & Bartholomew, K. (1994). Intimacy–anger and insecure attachment as precursors of abuse in intimate relationships. *Journal of Applied Social Psychology, 24,* 1367–1386.

Elicker, J., Englund, M., & Sroufe, L. A. (1992). Predicting peer competence and peer relationships in childhood from early parent–child relationships. In R. Parke & G. Ladd (Eds.), *Family–peer relations: Modes on linkage* (pp. 77–106). HIllsdale, NJ: Erlbaum.

Epstein, S. (1987). Impliations of cognitive self-theory for psychopathology and psychotherapy. In N. Cheshire & H. Thomas (Eds.), *Self, symptoms, and psychotherapy* (pp. 43–58). New York: Wiley.

Feeney, J. A. (1994). Attachment style, communication patterns, and satisfaction across the life cycle of marriage. *Personal Relationships, 4,* 333–348.

Feeney, J. A., & Noller, P. (1996). *Adult attachment.* Beverly Hills, CA: Sage.

Finkel, D., Wille, D. E., & Matheny, A. P. Jr. (1998).

Preliminary results from a twin study of infant-caregiver attachment. *Behavior Genetics, 28,* 1–8.

Fonagy, P., Leigh, T., Steele, M., Steele, H., Kennedy, R., Mattoon, G., Target, M., & Gerber, A. (1996). The relation of attachment status, psychiatric classification, and response to psychotherapy. *Journal of Consulting and Clinical Psychology, 64,* 22—31.

Fonagy, P., Steele, H., & Steele, M. (1991). Maternal representations of attachment during pregnancy predict the organization of infant–mother attachment at one year of age. *Child Development, 62,* 891–905.

Fraley, R. C. (1998). *Attachment continuity from infancy to adulthood: Meta-analysis and dynamic modeling of developmental mechanisms.* Manuscript submitted for publication.

Fraley, R. C., Davis, K. E., & Shaver, P. R. (1998). Dismissing–avoidance and the defensive organization of emotion, cognition, and behavior. In J. A. Simpson & W. S. Rholes (Eds.), *Attachment theory and close relationships* (pp. 249–279). New York: Guilford Press.

Fraley, R. C., & Shaver, P. R. (2000). Adult romantic attachment: Theoretical developments, emerging controversies, and unanswered questions. *Review of General Psychology, 4,* 132–154.

Fraley, R. C., & Waller, N. G. (1998). Adult attachment patterns: A test of the typological model. In J. A. Simpson & W. S. Rholes (Eds.), *Attachment theory and close relationships* (pp. 77–114). New York: Guilford Press.

George, C., Kaplan, N., & Main, M. (1985). *The adult attachment interview.* Unpublished manuscript, University of California at Berkeley, Department of Psychology.

Goldsmith, H. H., & Alansky, J. A. (1987). Maternal and infant temperamental predictors of attachment: A meta-analytic review. *Journal of Consulting and Clinical Psychology, 55,* 805 816.

Greenberg, M. T. (1999). Attachment and psychopathology in childhood. In J. Cassidy & P. R. Shaver (Eds.), *Handbook of attachment: Theory, research, and clinical applications* (pp. 469–496). New York: Guilford Press.

Griffin, D. W., & Bartholomew, K. (1994a). Models of the self and other: Fundamental dimensions underlying measures of adult attachment. *Journal of Personality and Social Psychology, 67,* 430–445.

Griffin, D. W., & Bartholomew, K. (1994b). The metaphysics of measurement: The case of adult attachment. In K. Bartholomew & D. Perlman (Eds.), *Advances in personal relationships: Vol. 5. Attachment processes in adulthood* (pp. 17–52). London: Jessica Kingsley.

Hart, S. D., Dutton, D. G., & Newlove, T. (1993). The prevalance of personality disorder among wife assaulters. *Journal of Personality Disorders, 7*(4), 329–341.

Hazan, C., & Shaver, P. R. (1987). Romantic love conceptualized as an attachment process. *Journal of Personality and Social Psychology, 52,* 511–524.

Hazan, C., & Shaver, P. R. (1994). Attachment as an organizational framework for research on close relationships. *Psychological Inquiry, 5,* 1–22.

Hazan, C., & Zeifman, D. (1994). Sex and the psycho-logical tether. In K. Bartholomew & D. Perlman (Eds.), *Advances in personal relationships: Vol. 5. Attachment processes in adulthood* (pp. 151–177). London: Jessica Kingsley.

Henderson, A. J. Z. (1998). *It takes two to tango: An attachment perspective exploring women's and men's relationship aggression.* Unpublished doctoral dissertation. Simon Fraser University, Burnaby, B.C., Canada.

Hendrick, C., & Hendrick, S. S. (1994). Attachment theory and close relationships. *Psychological Inquiry, 5,* 38–41.

Holmes, J. (1998). Defensive and creative uses of narrative in psychotherapy: An attachment perspective. In G. Roberts & J. Holmes (Eds.), *Narrative in psychotherapy and psychiatry* (pp. 49–68). Oxford, UK: Oxford University Press.

Horowitz, L. M., Rosenberg, S. E., Baer, B. A., Ureno, G., & Villasenor, V. S. (1988). Inventory of interpersonal problems: Psychometric properties and clinical applications. *Journal of Consulting and Clinical Psychology, 56,* 885–892.

Horowitz, L., Rosenberg, S., & Bartholomew, K. (1993). Interpersonal problems, attachment styles, and outcome in brief dynamic psychotherapy. *Journal of Consulting and Clinical Psychology, 61,* 549–560.

Jang, K. L., Livesley, W. J., Vernon, P. A., & Jackson, D. N. (1996). Heritability of personality disorder traits: A twin study. *Acta Psychiatra Scandinavica, 94,* 438–444.

Johnson, S. (1986). Bonds or bargains: Relationship paradigms and their significance for marital therapy. *Journal of Marital and Family Therapy, 12,* 259–267.

Kazdin, A. E., Kraemer, H. C., Kessler, R. C., Kupfer, D. J., & Offord, D. R. (1997). Contributions of risk-factor research to developmental psychopathology. *Clinical Psychology Review, 17,* 375–406.

Kiesler, D. J. (1983). The interpersonal circle: A taxonomy for complementarity in human transactions. *Psychological Review, 90,* 185–214.

Kirkpatrick, L. A., & Davis, K. E. (1994). Attachment style, gender, and relationship stability: A longitudinal analysis. *Journal of Personality and Social Psychology, 66,* 502–512.

Kirkpatrick, L. A., & Hazan, D. (1994). Attachment styles and close relationships: A four-year prospective study. *Personal Relationships, 1,* 123–142.

Klohnen, E. C., & Bera, S. (1998) Behavioral and experiential patterns of avoidantly and securely attached women across adulthood: A 31-year longitudinal perspective. *Journal of Personality and Social Psychology, 74,* 211–223.

Klohnen, E. C., & John, O. P. (1998). Working models of attachment: A theory-based prototype aproach. In J. A. Simpson & W. S. Rholes (Eds.), *Attachment theory and close relationships* (pp. 115–140). New York: Guilford Press.

Kobak, R. R., Cole, H., Ferenz-Gillies, R., Fleming, W., & Gamble, W. (1993). Attachment and emotional regulation during mother-teen problem solving: A control theory analysis. *Child Development, 64,* 231–245.

Kobak, R. R., & Hazan, C. (1991). Attachment in marriage: Effects of security and accuracy of working models. *Journal of Personality and Social Psychology, 60,* 861–869.

Kobak, R. R., & Sceery, A. (1988). Attachment in late adolescence: Working models, affect regulation, and representations of self and others. *Child Development, 59,* 135–146.

Lieberman, A. F., & Zeanah, C. H. (1995). Disorders of attachment in infancy. *Child and Adolescent Psychiatric Clinics of North America, 4,* 571–687.

Livesley, W. J., Jackson, D., & Schroeder, M. L. (1989). A study of the factorial structure of personality pathology. *Journal of Personality Disorders, 3,* 292–306.

Livesley, W. J., Jackson, D., & Schroeder, M. L. (1992). Factorial structure of traits delineating personality disorders in clinical and general population samples. *Journal of Abnormal Psychology, 101,* 432–440.

Livesley, J., Jang, K., & Vernon, P. (1998). Phenotypic and genotypic structure of traits delineating personality disorder. *Archives of General Psychiatry, 55,* 941–948.

Loranger, A.W. (1988). *Personality Disorder Examination (PDE) manual.* Yonkers, NY: DV Communications.

Main, M., Kaplan, N., & Cassidy, J. (1985). Security in infancy, childhood, and adulthood: A move to the level of representation. In I. Bretherton & E. Waters (Eds.), Growing points in attachment theory and research. *Monographs of the Society for Research in Child Development, 50,* 66–106.

Main, M., & Solomon, J. (1990). Procedures for identifying insecure–disorganized/disoriented infants: Procedures, findings, and implications for the classification of behavior. In M. Greenberg, D. Cicchetti, & M. Cummings (Eds.), *Attachment in the preschool years: Theory, research, and intervention* (pp. 121–160). Chicago: University of Chicago Press.

Mickelson, K. D., Kessler, R. C., & Shaver, P. R. (1997). Adult attachment in a nationally representative sample. *Journal of Personality and Social Psychology, 73,* 1092–1106.

Mikulincer, M., Florian, V., & Weller, A. (1993). Attachment styles, coping strategies, and post-traumatic psychological distress: The impact of the Gulf War in Israel. *Journal of Personality and Social Psychology, 64,* 817–826.

Mikulincer, M., & Nachshon, O. (1991). Attachment styles and patterns of self-disclosure. *Journal of Personality and Social Psychology, 61,* 321–331.

Mikulincer, M., & Orbach, I. (1995). Attachment styles and repressive defensiveness: The accessibility and architecture of affective memories. *Journal of Personality and Social Psychology, 68,* 917–925.

Moffitt, T. (1993). Adolescent-limited and life-course persistent antisocial behavior: A developmental taxonomy. *Psychological Review, 100,* 674–701.

Oldham, J., Clarkin, J., Appelbaum, A., Carr, A., Kernberg, P., Lotterman, A., & Haas, G. (1985). A self-report instrument for borderline personality organization. In T. H. McGlashan (Ed.), *The borderline: Current empirical research. The progress in psychiatry series* (pp. 1–18). Washington, DC: American Psychiatric Press.

Patrick, M., Hobson, R. P., Castle, D., Howard, R., &

Maughan, B. (1994). Personality disorder and the mental representation of early social experience. *Development and Psychopathology, 6,* 375–388.

Renken, B., Egeland, B., Marvinney, D., Mangelsdorf, S., & Sroufe, L. A. (1989). Early childhood antecedents of aggression and passive withdrawal in early elementary school. *Journal of Personality, 57,* 257–281.

Ricks, M. (1985). The social transmission of parental behavior: Attachment across generations. In I. Bretherton & E. Waters (Eds.), Growing points in attachment theory and research. *Monographs of the Society for Research in Child Development, 50,* 211–230.

Roche, D. N., Runtz, M. G., & Hunter, M. A. (1999). Adult attachment: A mediator between child sexual abuse and later psychological adjustment. *Journal of Interpersonal Violence, 14,* 184–207.

Rosenstein, D. S., & Horowitz, H. A. (1996). Adolescent attachment and psychopathology. *Journal of Consulting and Clinical Psychology, 64,* 244–253.

Rothbard, J. C., & Shaver, P. R. (1994). Continuity of attachment across the life span. In M. B. Sperling & W. H. Berman (Eds.), *Attachment in adults: Clinical and developmental perspectives* (pp. 31–71). New York: Guilford Press.

Rubin, K. H., Hymel, S., Mills, S. L., & Rose-Krasnor, L. (1991). Conceptualizing different developmental pathways to and from social isolation in childhood. In D. Cicchetti & S. L. Toth (Eds.), *Rochester symposium on developmental psychopathology: Vol. 2. Internalizing and externalizing expressions of dysfunction* (pp. 91–122). Hillsdale, NJ: Erlbaum.

Rutter, M. (1988). Functions and consequences of relationships: Some psychopathological considerations. In R. A. Hinde & J. Stevenson-Hinde (Eds.), *Relationships within families* (pp. 332–353) Oxford, UK: Clarendon Press.

Rutter, M. (1994). Continuities, transitions and turning points in development. In M. Rutter and D. F. Hay (Eds.), *Development through life: A handbook for clinicians* (pp. 1–25). Oxford, UK: Blackwell Scientific.

Sack, A., Sperling, M. B., Fagen, G., & Foelsch, P. (1996). Attachment style, history, and behavioral contrasts for a borderline and normal sample. *Journal of Personality Disorders, 10,* 88–102.

Sameroff A. J., & Chandler, M. J. (1975). Reproductive risk and the continuum of caretaking causality. In F. D. Horowitz (Ed.), *Review of child development research* (Vol. 4, pp. 187–244). Chicago: University of Chicago Press.

Scharfe, E., & Bartholomew, K. (1994). Reliability and stability of adult attachment patterns. *Personal Relationships, 1,* 23–43.

Scharfe, E., & Bartholomew, K. (1995). Accommodation and attachment representations in young couples. *Journal of Social and Personal Relationships, 12,* 389–401.

Schroeder, M. L., Wormworth, J. A., & Livesley, W. J. (1994). Dimensions of personality disorder and the five-factor model of personality. In P. T. Costa & T. A. Widiger (Eds.), *Personality disorders and the five-factor model of personality* (pp. 1–12). Washington, DC: American Psychological Association.

Seifer, R., Schiller, M., Sameroff, A., Hayden, L., Dickstein, S., Wheeler, E., Hermann, M., & St. Martin, A. (1998). *Individual patterns of change and longitudinal characteristics of infant temperament: Description and association with relationship development.* Unpublished manuscript.

Senchak, M., & Leonard, K. E. (1992). Attachment styles and marital adjustment among newlywed couples. *Journal of Social and Personal Relationships, 9,* 51–64.

Shaver, P. R., & Clark, C. L. (1994). The psychodynamics of adult romantic attachment. In J. M. Masling & R. F. Bornstein (Eds.), *Empirical perspectives on object relations theory* (Vol. 5, pp. 105–156). Washington, DC: American Psychological Association.

Shaver, P. R., & Hazan, C. (1993). Adult romantic attachment: Theory and evidence. In D. Perlman & W. Jones (Eds.), *Advances in personal relationships* (Vol. 4, pp. 29–70). London: Jessica Kingsley.

Shaver, P. R., Hazan, C., & Bradshaw, D. (1988). Love as attachment: The integration of three behavioral systems. In R. J. Sternberg & M. L. Barnes (Eds.), *The psychology of love* (pp. 68–99). New Haven, CT: Yale University Press.

Sheldon, A. E. R., & West, M. L. (1990). Attachment pathology versus low social skills in avoidant personality disorder: An exploratory study. *Canadian Journal of Psychiatry, 35,* 596–599.

Simpson, J. A., Rholes, W. S., & Nelligan, J. S. (1992). Support seeking and support giving within couples in an anxiety-provoking situation: The role of attachment styles. *Journal of Personality and Social Psychology, 62,* 434–446.

Slade, A. (1999). Attachment theory and research: Implications for the theory and practice of individual psychotherapy with adults. In J. Cassidy & P. R. Shaver (Eds.), *Handbook of attachment: Theory, research, and clinical applications* (pp. 575–594). New York: Guilford Press.

Spitzer, R. L., Williams, J. B. W., & Gibbon, M. (1987). *Structured Clinical Interview for DSM-III-R.* New York: New York State Psychiatric Institute, Biometric Research Unit.

Sroufe, L. A. (1997). Psychopathology as an outcome of development. *Development and Psychopathology, 9,* 251–268.

Sroufe, L. A., Egeland, B., & Kreutzer, T. (1990). The fate of early experience following developmental change: Longitudinal approaches to individual adaptation in childhood. *Child Development, 61,* 1363–1373.

Sroufe, L. A., & Fleeson, J. (1986). Attachment and the construction of relationships. In W. Hartrup & Z. Rubin (Eds.), *Relationships and development* (pp. 239–252). Hillsdale, NJ: Erlbaum.

Sroufe, L. A., & Waters, E. (1977). Attachment as an organizational construct. *Child Development, 48,* 1184–1199.

Stalker, C., & Davies, F. (1995). Attachment organization and adaptation in sexually abused women. *Canadian Journal of Psychiatry, 40,* 234–240.

Steele, H., & Steele, M. (1994). Intergenerational patterns of attachment. In K. Bartholomew & D. Perlman (Eds.), *Advances in personal relationships: Vol.*

5. *Attachment processes in adulthood* (pp. 93–120). London: Jessica Kingsley.

Stuart, S., Pfhol, B., Battaglia, M., Bellodi, L., Grove, W., & Cadoret, R. (1998). The co-occurrence of DSM-III-R personality disorders. *Journal of Personality Disorders, 12,* 302–315.

Susman-Stillman, A., Kalkoske, M., Egeland, B., & Waldman, I. (1996). Infant temperament and maternal sensitivity as predictors of attachment security. *Infant Behavior and Development, 19,* 33–47.

Swann, W. B. (1983). Self-verification: Bringing social reality into harmony with the self. In J. Suls & A. G. Greenwald (Eds.), *Psychological perspectives on the self* (Vol. 2, pp. 33–66). Hillsdale, NJ: Erlbaum.

Swann, W. B. (1987). Identity negotiation: Where two roads meet. *Journal of Personality and Social Psychology, 53,* 1038–1051.

Swann, W. B., & Pelham, B. W. (1999). *Who wants out when the going gets good? Psychological investment and preference for self-verifying college roommates.* Unpublished manuscript.

Thompson, R. A. (1999). Early attachment and later development. In J. Cassidy & P. R. Shaver (Eds.), *Handbook of attachment: Theory, research, and clinical applications* (pp. 265–286). New York: Guilford Press.

Thompson, R. A., Lamb, M. E., & Estes, D. (1982). Stability of infant–mother attachment and its relationship to changing life circumstances in an unselected middle-class sample. *Child Development, 53,* 144–148.

Tidwell, M. O., Reis, H. T., & Shaver, P. R. (1996). Attachment, attractiveness, and social interaction: A diary study. *Journal of Personality and Social Psychology, 71,* 729–745.

Trinke, S., & Bartholomew, K. (1997). Attachment hierarchies in young adults. *Journal of Social and Personal Relationships, 14,* 603–625.

Trull, T. J., Widiger, T. A., & Frances, A. (1987). Covariation of criteria sets for avoidant, schizoid, and dependent personality disorders. *American Journal of Psychiatry, 144,* 767–771.

Tyrrell, C., & Dozier, M., Teague, G. B., & Fallot, R. D. (1999). Effective treatment relationships for persons with serious disorders: The importance of attachment states of mind. *Journal of Consulting and Clinical Psychology, 67,* 725–733.

van den Boom, D. (1994). The influence of temperament and mothering on attachment and exploration: An experimental manipulation of sensitive responsiveness among lower-class mothers with irritable infants. *Child Development, 65,* 1457–1477.

van IJzendoorn, M. H. (1995). Adult attachment representations, parental responsiveness, and infant attachment: A meta-analysis on the predictive validity of the Adult Attachment Interview. *Psychological Bulletin, 117,* 387–403.

van IJzendoorn, M. H., & Bakermans-Kranenburg, M. J. (1996). Attachment representations in mothers, fathers, adolescents, and clinical groups: A meta-analytic search for normative data. *Journal of Consulting and Clinical Psychology, 64,* 8–21.

van IJzendoorn, M. H., & Bakermans-Kranenburg, M. J. (1997). Intergenerational transmission of attachment: A move to the contextual level. In L. Atkinson & K. J. Zucker (Eds.), *Attachment and psychopathology* (pp. 135–170). New York: Guilford Press.

van IJzendoorn M. H., Juffer, F., & Duyvesteyn, M. G. C. (1995). Breaking the intergenerational cycle of insecure attachment: A review of the effects of attachment-based interventions on maternal sensitivity and infant security from a contextual perspective. *Journal of Child Psychology and Psychiatry, 36,* 225–248.

Vaughn, B. E., & Bost, K. K. (1999). Attachment and temperament: Redundant, independent, or interacting influences on interpersonal adaptation and personality development? In J. Cassidy & P. R. Shaver (Eds.), *Handbook of attachment: Theory, research, and clinical applications* (pp. 198–225). New York: Guilford Press.

Vaughn, B. E., Egeland, B. R., Sroufe, L. A., & Waters, E. (1979). Individual differences in infant-mother attachment at 12 and 18 months: Stability and change in families under stress. *Child Development, 50,* 971–975.

Vaughn, B. E., Stevenson-Hinde, J., Waters, E., Kotsaftis, A., Lefever, G. B., Shouldice, A., Trudel, M., & Belsky, J. (1992). Attachment security and temperament in infancy and early childhood: Some conceptual clarifications. *Developmental Psychology, 28,* 463–473.

Warren, S. L., Huston, L., Egelend, B., & Sroufe, L. A. (1997). Child and adolescent anxiety disorders and early attachment. *Journal of the American Academy of Child and Adolescent Psychiatry, 36,* 637–644.

Waters, E. (1978). The reliability and stability of individual differences in infant–mother attachment. *Child Development, 49,* 483–494.

Waters, E., Merrick, S., Treboux, D., Crowell, J., & Albersheim, L. (2000). Attachment security in infancy and early adulthood: A twenty-year longitudinal study. *Child Development, 71,* 684–689.

Waters, E., Wippman, J., & Sroufe, L. A. (1979). Attachment, positive affect, and competence in the peer group: Two studies in construct validation. *Child Development, 50,* 821–829.

Weinfield, N., Sroufe, L. A., & Egeland, B. (2000). Attachment from infancy to early adulthood in a high risk sample: Continuity, discontinuity, and their correlates. *Child Development, 71,* 695–702

Weinfield, N. S., Sroufe, L. A., Egeland, B., & Carlson, E. A. (1999). The nature of individual differences in infant–caregiver attachment. In J. Cassidy & P. R. Shaver (Eds.), *Handbook of attachment: Theory, research, and clinical applications* (pp. 68–88). New York: Guilford Press.

Weiss, R. S. (1982). Attachment in adult life. In C. M. Parkes & J. Stevenson-Hinde (Eds.), *The place of attachment in human behavior* (pp. 171–184). New York: Basic Books.

Weissman, M. M. (1993, Spring). The epidemiology of personality disorders: A 1990 update. *Journal of Personality Disorders, 44–62.*

West, M., & Keller, A. (1994). Psychotherapy strategies for insecure attachment in personality disorders. In M. B. Sperling & W. H. Berman (Eds.), *Attachment in adults: Clinical and developmental perspectives* (pp. 313–330). New York: Guilford Press.

Widiger, T. A., & Frances, A. J. (1994). Toward a dimensional model for the personality disorders. In P. T. Costa & T. A. Widiger (Eds.), *Personality disorders and the five-factor model of personality* (pp. 19–39). Washington, DC: American Psychological Association.

Widiger, T. A., & Sanderson, C. J. (1995). Toward a dimensional model of personality disorders. In W. J. Livesley (Ed.), *The DSM-IV personality disorders* (pp. 433–458). New York: Guilford Press.

Wiggins, J. S. (1982). Circumplex models of interpersonal behavior in clinical psychology. In P. D. Kendall & J. N. Butcher (Eds.), *Handbook of research methods in clinical psychology* (pp. 183–221). New York: Wiley.

Wiggins, J. S. (Ed.). (1996). *The five-factor model of personality: Theoretical perspectives.* New York: Guilford Press.

Zeanah, C. H. (1996). Beyond insecurity: A reconceptualization of attachment disorders of infancy. *Journal of Consulting and Clinical Psychology, 64,* 42–52.

Zimmermann, P., Fremmer-Bombik, E., Spangler, G., & Grossmann, K. E. (1997). Attachment in adolescence: A longitudinal perspective. In W. Koops, J. B. Hoeksma, & D. C. van den Boom (Eds.), *Development of interaction and attachment: Traditional and non-traditional approaches* (pp. 281–292). Amsterdam: North-Holland.

CHAPTER 10

⤙❖⤚

Psychosocial Adversity

JOEL PARIS

ADVERSITIES ASSOCIATED WITH MENTAL DISORDERS

Mental health clinicians and researchers have long been interested in the impact on adults of adverse events during childhood. On theoretical grounds, it has often been assumed that psychosocial stressors occurring early in life must produce more sequelae than stressors occurring later in life. This theoretical principle can be termed "the primacy of early experience" (Paris, 1999).

Primacy has long been the conventional wisdom for clinicians. A large body of books on personality disorders, using either psychodynamic frameworks (e.g., Adler, 1985; Kohut, 1977) or empirical approaches (Benjamin, 1993; Millon & Davis, 1996) have all assumed that personality disorders are shaped by experiences during childhood.

Yet in spite of its ubiquity, primacy has a shaky evidence base. A large body of research (Garmezy & Masten, 1994; Rutter, 1989) shows that negative childhood experiences need not necessarily lead to psychopathological outcomes in adult life. Rather, adversities increase the eventual *risk* for mental disorders. In other words, risk factors are not causes but increase the likelihood of negative sequelae. Most people exposed to a particular risk do not develop any disorder, whereas people developing disorders may well have been exposed to different risks.

One useful way to frame these conclusions is to note that data from clinical and community populations can lead to very different conclusions. In clinical populations, patients with a variety of mental disorders report more psychosocial adversities during childhood than do nonpatients (Rutter & Maughan, 1997). Yet, in community populations, the same adversities lead to clinically significant pathology in only a minority of those exposed (Garmezy & Masten, 1994). In other words, whereas most individuals are resilient to adversity, people who develop clinical symptoms have an underlying vulnerability to the same risk factors.

These observations may come as a surprise to clinicians who routinely search for historical events to account for present distress. However, there is no contradiction between the fact that psychiatric patients suffer from adversities and the fact that most people manage to overcome them. Therapists need to take the meaning of individual differences in sensitivity to stress into account.

The failure to distinguish between risks and causes has also led to the misinterpretation of research findings linking adversities to mental disorders (Paris, 2000). If one reads, for example, that a large number of patients with a personality disorder report a history of child abuse, it is tempting to assume that these experiences must account for its etiology. However, correlations between risk factors and disorders do not, by themselves, prove causal relationships. In fact, simple associations can often be explained by *third variable* effects. Many examples demonstrate the importance of these latent variables. Thus, children exposed to any particular risk factor are often exposed to other risks at the same time (Rutter, 1987a). Long-term sequelae can be due to these coexisting adversities or to the cumulative effects of many risks.

Moreover, children with temperamental vulnerabilities are much more likely to experience adverse events. To consider an example that clinicians frequently see, children with difficult temperaments come into conflict with peers and parents, increasing the likelihood of either social rejection or physical abuse (Rutter & Quinton, 1984).

Even when the long-term effects of adversity are statistically significant, they tend to be more subtle than dramatic. Family breakdown provides an instructive example of this complexity. Children of divorce and children from intact families show few large-scale differences in their long-term risk for developing mental disorders, and a vulnerable minority accounts for the statistically higher prevalence of sequelae from family breakdown (Tennant, 1988). Moreover, many of the sequelae of divorce for children are due to third variables, involving additional adversities such as poverty, change of neighborhood, or depression in a custodial parent. The increase risk for psychopathology in children from broken families depends on "cascades" of adversity, which all too often follow family breakdown.

Of course, parental divorce is not the worst thing that can happen to children. Most clinicians assume that overtly traumatic events are particularly likely to lead to sequelae. Yet, when we review the empirical literature on adversities such as childhood sexual abuse (Browne & Finkelhor, 1986; Finkelhor, Hotaling, Lewis, & Smith, 1990) or childhood physical abuse (Malinovsky-Rummell & Hansen, 1993), the same pattern emerges. Research demonstrates statistical relationships between exposure to trauma and pathological sequelae, but negative outcomes occur only in a minority of cases, most often in about a quarter of those exposed.

The concept that most children are *resilient* to adversity is crucial for understanding the impact of negative events in childhood. The ubiquity of this protective mechanism is both fortunate and logical. Given the relatively greater adverse nature of life in the environment of evolutionary adaptiveness (Beck, Freeman, & Associates, 1990, Bowlby, 1969), resilience must have been favored by natural selection.

A large literature has developed to elucidate the precise mechanisms underlying resilience (see reviews in Garmezy & Masten, 1994; Rutter, 1987, 1989). Studies of children at risk (e.g., Werner & Smith, 1992) have documented both biological and psychosocial aspects involved in developing some degree of "immunity" to adverse experiences.

Some aspects of resilience are biological. Children with positive personality traits and higher levels of intelligence are more resourceful and therefore better at finding ways to cope with adversity. There is even some evidence that adversity can cause "steeling" (i.e., increased resilience to future adverse events) (Rutter, 1989). In contrast, children with negative personality traits and lower levels of intelligence tend to experience adversities as more stressful than do those with a stronger constitution.

Other aspects of resilience are psychosocial. The most important principle is that positive relationships buffer negative experiences. Thus, problems with nuclear family members can be compensated for by attachments to members of the extended family, or to nonfamily members in the community. For example, it is known that children whose parents have psychosis, substance abuse, or personality disorders carry an increased risk for pathology (Garmezy & Masten, 1994). Yet, the less time such children spend with their immediate family and the more time they spend outside the home with alternate attachment figures, the less likely they are to develop mental disorders (Anthony & Cohler, 1987; Kaufman, Grunebaum, Cohler, & Gamer, 1979).

A third problem in interpreting associations between early negative events and psychopathology is that most studies describing childhood adversities in clinical populations have used retrospective methodologies. It is difficult to know how much we can rely on information drawn from asking patients with serious current pathology to provide accurate reports of their childhood after the passage of several decades. Being ill creates a recall bias, and memories of the past can be negatively colored by present suffering (Paris, 1995, 1997).

The validity of retrospective studies must therefore be regarded with caution. Memories of childhood adversities can sometimes be confirmed through sibling concordance or through objective records (Brewin, Andrews, & Gotlib, 1993; Maughan & Rutter, 1997). However, patient reports should never be automatically assumed to be accurate without independent confirmation. Unfortunately, hardly any of the studies on adult patients who recollect adversities have collected corroborating data.

Only prospective research can overcome this problem. Thus, studies following large cohorts of normal children, or children with identified risks for psychopathology, are needed to determine the precise conditions under which adversities cause disorders. Unfortunately, this kind of research is expensive, and the number of existing studies necessarily limited (see reviews in Rutter, 1987a, 1989; Rutter & Maughan, 1997). At this point, four preliminary conclusions can be drawn from the existing literature on adversity and resilience:

1. A large number of children exposed to any specific adversity, usually constituting a majority, do not develop any mental disorder.
2. Multiple adversities have *cumulative* effects. The greater the number of negative events during childhood, the more likely are pathological sequelae in adolescence and adulthood (Rutter, 1989). Thus, resilience mechanisms usually buffer single adversities, and even when traumas are severe, positive experiences can prevent long-term sequelae. However, if, as so often happens, adversities follow each other in a cascade, resilience mechanisms can be overwhelmed.
3. Adversities rarely have any specific relationship to mental disorders. On the contrary, the psychosocial risk factors for many types of mental disorder are similar (Paris, 1999; Rutter, 1989).
4. There is little evidence that *timing* plays a crucial role in the effects of childhood adversities. Many models have assumed that the more severe the form of pathology, the earlier in childhood must be its origin (Paris, 1983, 1999). It seems intuitive that younger children could be more vulnerable to adversity because of a diminished ability for cognitive processing (Rutter, 1989). Yet, findings of longitudinal studies have not supported this hypothesis. The problem is that the effects of timing are confounded with those of cumulative dosing. In other words, when problems start early, they are much more likely to be chronic, making it difficult to separate these factors (Rutter & Rutter, 1993). For example, family breakdown can sometimes have more sequelae when it occurs in adolescence (Hethering-

ton, Cox, & Cox, 1985; Wallerstein, 1989, and these effects usually depend on prior levels of marital conflict (Amato, Loomis, & Booth, 1995).

In conclusion, although childhood adversities increase the risk for mental disorders, they need not be their primary causes. This principle is highly consistent with a *stress–diathesis* model of mental disorders (Cloninger, Martin, Guze, & Clayton, 1990; Monroe & Simmons, 1991). In this theoretical framework, psychopathology emerges when stressors uncover specific underlying vulnerabilities. These diatheses determine the type of pathology that any individual develops and account for the fact that there are similar risk factors for a wide range of different mental disorders.

Adversities Associated with Personality Disorders

Over the last two decades, a series of systematic investigations have provided empirical documentation for clinical observations of associations between adversities and personality disorders (Paris, 1997). The main risk factors that have been identified are (1) dysfunctional families (the effects of parental psychopathology, family breakdown, or pathogenic parenting practices, (2) traumatic experiences (e.g., childhood sexual abuse or physical abuse), and (3) social stressors.

Dysfunctional Families

Parental Psychopathology

As is the case for most psychiatric diagnoses, patients with personality disorders tend to have parents or other close relatives who also have significant psychopathology (Siever & Davis, 1991). The disorders tend to fall in the same "spectrum" (impulsive, affective, or cognitive), but given the low level of precision in the present diagnostic classification, it should not be surprising that probands and first-degree relatives do not always share the same diagnosis.

These relationships have been most thoroughly investigated in impulsive personality disorders. In a classical study, Robins (1966) examined the predictors of whether children with conduct disorder develop psychopathy (or antisocial personality disorder) as adults. By far, the most important risk factor consisted of having a psychopathic parent (usually the father). Even more strikingly, antisocial behavior in a parent predicted antisocial personality in the child independent of other co-occurring psychosocial risks.

The findings on borderline personality disorder have been similar. First-degree relatives of these patients tend to have either "impulsive spectrum" disorders (antisocial personality, substance abuse, borderline personality), or mood disorders (Links, Steiner, & Huxley, 1988; Silverman et al., 1991; Zanarini, 1993). Parallel findings also emerge concerning substance abuse (Schuckit & Smith, 1996), a condition in which fathers and sons frequently share a genetic risk. Zanarini (1993) has argued that because antisocial personality, borderline personality, and substance abuse segregate together in family studies, they form a group of "impulsive spectrum disorders," all associated with a common temperament. Similarly, patients with schizoid, paranoid, and schizotypal personality disorders tend to have relatives with schizophrenia or schizophrenia-spectrum disorders, whereas patients with avoidant, dependent, and compulsive personality disorders tend to have relatives with anxiety disorders (Paris, 1996).

Although these relationships undoubtedly reflect the genetic factors in personality disorders, environmental mechanisms are involved as well. Parental psychopathology is associated with a variety of psychosocial adversities, such as trauma, family dysfunction, and family breakdown. For example, being raised by a psychopathic father is a stressor, even if, as so often happens, the father eventually becomes absent. As shown by Cloninger, Sigvardsson, and Bohman (1982), adopted children with an antisocial parent are most likely to develop pathology when they also experience significant adversities in their family environment.

Family Breakdown

The long-term effects of family breakdown can be palpable but subtle. For example, experiencing parental divorce as a child may affect the quality of intimacy in early adulthood (Wallerstein, 1989) and clearly reduces the stability of marriage in the next generation (Riley, 1991). As discussed previously, most children of divorce are psychopathology-free. However, as these observations are drawn from community populations, they may not reflect the impact of separation or loss on highly vulnerable children: those who are temperamentally sensitive, and those who have been exposed to multiple adversities.

The rate of family breakdown in patients with personality disorders is greater than that seen in community populations. Paris, Zweig-Frank, and Guzder (1994a, 1994b) found that 50% of a large cohort of patients with a variety of Axis II diagnoses had experienced parental separation. (This is indeed a high rate, as most of the cohort had been raised in the 1960s, prior to the recent "epidemic" of divorce.)

A specific relationship between parental loss and borderline personality disorder has been reported in some studies (Bradley, 1979; Links, Steiner, Offord, & Eppel, 1988; Paris, Nowlis, & Brown, 1988; Soloff & Millward, 1983) but not in others (Ogata, Silk, & Goodrich, 1990; Paris et al., 1994a; Zanarini, Gunderson, & Marino, 1989). Most likely, these discrepancies depend on differences between samples, as well as on different control groups used for comparison. Moreover, patients with personality disorders who experience family breakdown also have histories of multiple adversities (Zanarini et al., 1997).

Parenting Practices

Theorists of the nature of parenting describe two basic components in the task of raising children: providing love and support and allowing them to become independent (Rowe, 1981). These two dimensions (affection vs. neglect and autonomy vs. overprotection) emerge consistently from empirical research on effective parenting practices (Parker, 1983).

The idea that children who develop serious personality pathology experience early emotional neglect derives from psychodynamic models such as Bowlby's (1969) attachment theory and Kohut's (1977) theory of self-pathology. Both these models assume that emotional security in adults is grounded in internalizations of consistent empathic and supportive responses from parents during childhood. Bowlby's concept of "secure attachment" and Kohut's concept of a "cohesive self" both assume that abnormal personality structures result from negative relationships with parents.

Levy (1943) was the first to propose that overprotective behavior by parents toward children may also increase the risk for psychopathology. Masterson and Rinsley (1975) applied this idea to personality disorders, suggesting that parents who prevent their children from developing autonomy produce an increased risk for borderline pathology.

Empirical studies of these dimensions of parenting have made use of self-report instruments such as the Parental Bonding Instrument (PBI; Parker, 1983), a measure that has been standardized in community samples. However, the validity of these scales are limited by their retrospective nature, with scores ultimately reflecting perceptions about childhood environment. In fact, the PBI, as well as all other self-report measures of childhood experience, has been shown to have a heritable component (Plomin & Bergeman, 1991), reflecting the effect of personality traits on perceptions of the past. Most probably, individuals with a greater temperamental need for affirmation and reassurance are more likely to perceive their parenting as inadequate.

There has been a large body of research on recollections of parenting among patients with borderline personality disorder. Adler (1985) hypothesized that this form of pathology, in which intimate attachments are problematical and difficult, results from problems in bonding and attachment during childhood. Empirical studies using Parker's instrument (Frank & Paris, 1981; Paris & Frank, 1989, Zweig-Frank & Paris, 1991; Torgersen & Alnaes, 1992) confirm that borderline patients describe both neglect and overprotection, and that they describe both parents in similar ways. The question remains, What do these reports mean? Do they reflect historical reality of biparental failure, a discrepancy between greater needs and what "good enough" parents can offer, or the tendency of borderline patients to perceive all forms of nurturance as inadequate?

However, one recent prospective community study (Johnson, Cohen, Brown, Smailes, & Bernstein, 1999) has at least shown that the symptoms of personality disorders (but not necessarily the full clinical picture) are more likely to develop in children who have been grossly neglected or abused (physically or sexually). This report was not dependent on recall alone but used court records to document these events. However, the children in the cohort who were most affected suffered from multiple, and not single, adversities. This study also confirms the principle that patients with a wide range of personality disorders tend to experience similar risk factors in their upbringing. It therefore

seems likely that temperament determines the category into which patients eventually fall (Paris, 1996).

In clinical samples, relationships between parental neglect have been most studied in impulsive disorders, whereas little empirical research exists on the relationship between parenting practices and personality disorders in the anxious cluster. Overprotection might be of particular relevance for patients with disorders in the avoidant and dependent categories. From a theoretical point of view, one of the main childhood precursors of avoidant personality could be extreme shyness. In a retrospective study of patients with dependent personality (Head, Baker, & Williamson, 1991), scores on the Family Experiences Questionnaire suggested that patients remembered their families as significantly interfering with their autonomy during childhood. A study by Kagan (1994) following a cohort of children with unusual levels of "behavioral inhibition" is particularly relevant here. Overprotective responses by parents may have interfered with the deconditioning of anxiety in this population. Follow-up of these children into adulthood will determine whether they are also at risk for anxious cluster personality disorders.

Traumatic Experiences

Childhood Sexual Abuse

Most of the work on sexual abuse as a risk factor has examined patients with borderline personality disorder. A large series of studies (Byrne, Cernovsky, Velamoor, Coretese, & Losztyn, 1990; Herman, Perry, & van der Kolk, 1989; Links, Steiner, Offord, & Eppel, 1988; Ludolph, Westen, & Misle, 1990; Ogata, Silk, Goodrich, Lohr, Westen, & Hill, 1990; Paris et al., 1994a, 1994b; Westen, Ludolph, Misle, Ruffins, & Block, 1990; Zanarini et al., 1989) has reported a high frequency, ranging as high as 50–70%, of childhood sexual abuse in this population. Some theorists (Herman & van der Kolk, 1987) have interpreted these findings as showing that traumatic experiences are the main etiological factor in borderline pathology, and they have reformulated this diagnosis as a chronic and complex form of posttraumatic stress disorder.

However, these conclusions are not warranted by the existing evidence. First, the relationship between trauma and borderline pathology is far from specific, with similar experiences being reported by patients with a wide range of diagnoses, including a wide range of other personality disorders (Paris, 1994). Moreover, most people who experience childhood trauma never develop personality disorders, or, for that matter, any form of mental disorder. Finally, research on posttraumatic stress disorder itself (Yehuda & McFarlane, 1995) shows that pathology is not the simple result of exposure to trauma but also depends on constitutional vulnerabilities.

There are also serious methodological problems with the data on trauma and borderline personality. In particular, most of the research in this area has failed to take into account the severity of the experiences under study (Paris & Zweig-Frank, 1996). Simple reports of a frequency of sexual abuse in a given population, with a variety of experiences lumped together, can be misleading. Research in community populations (Browne & Finkelhor, 1986; Finkelhor et al., 1990) consistently shows that the impact of sexual trauma depends on the identity of the perpetrator, the nature of the act, and the duration of the experience. In fact, most abuse reports in personality-disordered patients do not involve the type of experiences that most frequently produce pathological sequelae in community samples. In studies that have specifically examined the parameters of abuse (Ogata, Silk, Goodrich, et al., 1990; Paris et al., 1994a, 1994b), the range of reported trauma was not different from observations in community studies drawn from the general population. Thus, most of the cases, accounting for the high rates in borderline patients quoted earlier, do not involve repeated episodes, sexual intercourse, or incest but single events involving molestation by a nonrelative or stranger.

About one-third of patients with borderline personality do report severe abuse experiences, such as an incestuous perpetrator, severity of sexual act, or high frequency and duration. It seems reasonable to conclude that traumatic events play an important etiological role in this subpopulation (Paris, 1994). In a second third of patients who report milder forms of trauma, childhood experiences of this type are unlikely, by themselves, to be important etiological factors for developing a personality disorder. Finally, another third of borderline patients report no traumatic events at all during childhood.

There is an even more important problem. Much of the literature on trauma and personality disorders has failed to address the role of third variable effects derived from family dysfunction, parenting practices, or parental psychopathology (Paris, 1997). Thus, it is difficult to determine whether sequelae are attributable to trauma alone or to the cumulative effects of many adversities. Community studies show that child abuse does not usually occur in isolation, and that its negative effects can often be accounted for by coexisting family dysfunction (Nash, Hulsely, Sexton, Harralson, & Lambert, 1993). Because borderline patients describe a wide range of adversities from childhood, it is difficult to determine which are most pathogenic (Zanarini et al., 1997). One way to approach the problem is to conduct regression analyses of all risk factors. Two studies (Links & van Reekum, 1993; Paris et al., 1994a, 1994b) did find an independent association between childhood sexual abuse and borderline personality, but these results reflect the high rates of reported abuse in the samples, and neither found any relationship between outcome and parameters of abuse severity.

Finally, some studies (e.g., Herman et al., 1989) have been conducted on patient populations undergoing therapies designed to "recover" repressed memories of trauma and may therefore involve a certain percentage of false memories. In general, one should only accept memories that had never been forgotten, and which were not elicited for the first time by experiences in psychotherapy (Paris, 1995). Prospective research, such as the Johnson et al. (1999) study described previously, has addressed these issues to some extent and suggests that childhood sexual abuse does increase the risk for personality disorder symptoms. However, community studies, even in large populations, rarely find enough adults with any specific personality disorder to reach firm conclusions about these relationships.

Herman and van der Kolk (1987) have hypothesized that specific symptoms, such as dissociation and self-mutilation, commonly seen in patients with borderline personality, are "markers" for traumatic experiences. Relationships between scores on the Dissociative Experience Scale (Bernstein & Putnam, 1986) as well as wrist cutting and histories of child abuse have been reported in univariate studies (Chu & Dill, 1990; van der Kolk, Perry, & Herman, 1991). However, in multivariate studies (Zweig-Frank, Paris, & Guzder, 1994a, 1994b), these symptoms turn out to be largely a function of diagnosis and are equally common in nontraumatized as in traumatized borderline patients. In fact, the capacity to dissociate has a strong heritable component (Jang, Paris, Zweig-Frank, & Livesley, 1998). Other features of borderline personality disorder, such as defense styles and impulsive aggression, are also more strongly related to diagnosis than to psychological risk factors (Paris, Zweig-Frank, Bond, & Guzder, 1996).

In summary, research on the relationship between childhood sexual abuse and personality disorders supports the following conclusions:

1. Sexual abuse during childhood is one of several relevant psychosocial risk factors for personality disorders as a group.
2. Childhood sexual abuse may have a particular relationship to borderline pathology.
3. Sexual abuse seems to play a major etiological role only in a subgroup of borderline patients.

Childhood Physical Abuse and Verbal Abuse

Again, most of the research on the relationship between physical abuse during childhood and the development of personality disorders has been conducted on patients with borderline personality. However, the results are less consistent than for sexual abuse, with only four of the studies listed previously (Herman et al., 1989; Ludolph et al., 1990; Paris et al., 1994a; Westen et al., 1990) reporting higher frequencies in borderline patients than in near-neighbor disorders. Physical abuse has also been reported to predict the development of antisocial personality disorder (Pollock et al., 1990), but these associations may not be independently significant when parental psychopathy is taken into account (Robins, 1966). Finally, the Johnson et al. (1999) study suggests that physical abuse increases the risk for a variety of personality disorder symptoms.

Zanarini et al. (1989) reported that patients with borderline personality also describe severe verbal abuse. However, it is not clear whether these reports shed much light on etiological mechanisms. There is no clear boundary between parental criticism and "abuse," and be-

cause there are no community studies delineating the impact of such experiences, the meaning of this term remains subjective.

Social Stressors

The role of social stressors in psychopathology has not been well researched. Yet, indirect evidence suggests that they play an important role. In particular, social changes are necessary to explain time cohort effects on the prevalence of personality disorders. These findings include a well-established increase in the rate of antisocial personality (Robins & Regier, 1991) in North America, as well as probable increases in the prevalence of borderline personality (Millon, 1993).

Moreover, during the same postwar period during which these changes have been observed, there has also been a parallel increase in related phenomena, including those associated with emotional dysregulation (depression, parasuicide, and completed suicide) and those associated with impulsivity (substance abuse and criminality). Several hypotheses have been proposed to account for these changes. The breakdown of traditional social structures could be one important factor (Millon, 1993; Paris, 1992, 1996). Another mechanism may be related to a relative absence of secure attachments in contemporary society, resulting in increased affective instability (Linehan, 1993).

These hypotheses also help to account for striking cross-cultural differences in the prevalence of personality disorders. The best documented finding is the rarity of the antisocial diagnosis in Taiwan (Hwu, Yeh, & Change, 1989), a society whose traditional and more integrated structure provides buffering against impulsive behavior and also has protective effects against psychosocial adversities.

Social disintegration is an organizing principle that helps explain some of the effects of social factors on personality disorders. If these conditions are increasing in prevalence, it may not be because families themselves are any more dysfunctional than in the past but because of a breakdown of protective social factors: extrafamilial influences needed to buffer trait vulnerabilities and intrafamilial stressors. Although these social forces affect everyone, they have a greater effect on those who are vulnerable because of biological and psychological risk factors.

Moreover, in the modern world, these stresses are being amplified by *rapid social change*. Young people are now expected to find an "identity" in the absence of traditional guidance and support from the community. Those who have problematical personality traits and negative family experiences are less likely to find buffering and protection from the social environment, and are therefore more likely to develop personality pathology (Paris, 1996).

Summary

Three general conclusions about the relationship between psychosocial adversities and personality disorders seem justified by the evidence.

1. Parental psychopathology, family breakdown, and traumatic events are all risk factors. The evidence most clearly supports their role in impulsive personality disorders, and they may also play a role in anxious cluster disorders.
2. These risk factors show great heterogeneity within the categories of disorder, as well as large overlaps between categories.
3. Histories of adversity during childhood, by themselves, do not fully account for the development of personality disorders.

The lack of etiological specificity in these relationships points to the need to develop more comprehensive etiological models. To explain why personality disorders develop, we need to take individual differences into account. In other words, responses to adversity are linked to constitutional vulnerabilities rooted in temperamental variations.

ADVERSITY IN THE CONTEXT OF GENE–ENVIRONMENT INTERACTIONS

Gene–environment interactions are a key component of diathesis–stress models of psychopathology. These theories hypothesize that childhood adversities are more likely to be pathogenic when they interact with underlying genetic vulnerabilities. Thus, personality disorders are most likely to arise when temperamental and trait variants that predispose to behavioral and affective disturbances interact with psychosocial adversities (Rutter, 1987b). In other words, personality disorders can be conceptualized as the outcome of interactions between diatheses (trait profiles) and stressors (psychosocial adversities). Models of this type have been suggested by several authors (e.g., Beck et al., 1990; Linehan, 1993; Paris, 1994, 1996; Stone, 1993).

Empirical findings support a continuous relationship between traits and disorders (Livesley, Schroeder, Jackson, & Jang, 1994). A wide range of trait variability is entirely compatible with normality. Yet even though trait variations are insufficient by themselves to account for personality pathology, they are probably the main determinant of which type of personality disorder can develop in any individual. Thus, disorders characterized by extraversion, such as those in the impulsive or dramatic cluster on Axis II of DSM, should not appear in introverts. Conversely, disorders characterized by introversion, such as those in the odd and anxious clusters of Axis II, should not appear in extraverts. Moreover, trait profiles influence whether the individual is vulnerable to develop any disorder. The fact that siblings have surprisingly few personality traits in common (Dunn & Plomin, 1990) helps to explain why in most cases, even when exposed to the same family environment, only one child in a family develops a personality disorder.

Whereas traits reflect underlying vulnerabilities, psychological and social factors can be crucial determinants of whether underlying traits are *amplified,* thereby leading to overt disorders (Paris, 1994, 1996). However, individuals differ in their *exposure* to and *susceptibility* to environmental factors (Kendler & Eaves, 1986). Thus, impulsive traits can make exposure to adversity more likely (Rutter & Rutter, 1993). Traits for affective lability can make individuals more susceptible to adverse events (Linehan, 1993). An anxious temperament leads to a high level of environmental sensitivity, associated with social anxiety and avoidance (Kagan, 1994). These interactions lead to negative feedback loops, interfering with both peer relationships and parental attachments, followed by amplification of underlying temperamental characteristics.

RESEARCH IMPLICATIONS

The precise relationship between psychosocial adversities and the development of personality disorders remains uncertain. The most useful future directions to shed light on the many unanswered question in the field might include the following:

1. Long-term prospective studies of normal children, children at risk, or children in treatment, to document the effects of childhood adversity in adult life.
2. Multivariate studies examining both biological factors (as measured by temperamental observations, biological markers, and genotyping) and psychosocial adversities in the same patients.
3. Studies of twin populations, allowing researchers to control for genetic influences on personality development.
4. Epidemiological studies examining risk factors for personality traits and dimensions in the community.
5. Studies of clinical populations examining a wider range of categories of disorder, as well as of the trait dimensions underlying personality disorders.

CLINICAL IMPLICATIONS

Personality disorders are complex, multidimensional forms of psychopathology. The role of childhood adversities must therefore be seen within a broad etiological model that is multidimensional and takes into account interactions between multiple stressors and multiple diatheses.

These conclusions have implications for the treatment of patients with personality disorders. If childhood adversities increase the risk for personality pathology, but are not necessarily their primary cause, then clinicians should not assume that effective psychotherapy need always depend on the uncovering and working through of childhood traumas. At present, the most effective therapies for personality disorders tend to focus less on the past and more on methods of improving present levels of functioning by teaching patients to make more adaptive use of their personality traits (Kroll, 1988; Linehan, 1993, Paris, 1998; Stone, 1993).

REFERENCES

Adler, G. (1985). *Borderline psychopathology and its treatment.* New York: Jason Aronson..

Amato, P. R., Loomis, L. S., & Booth, A. (1995). Parental divorce, marital conflict, and offspring well-being during early adulthood. *Social Forces, 73,* 895–915.

Anthony, E. J., & Cohler, B. J. (Eds.). (1987). *The invulnerable child.* New York: Guilford Press.

Beck, A. T., Freeman, A., & Associates. (1990). *Cognitive therapy of personality disorders.* New York: Guilford Press.

Benjamin, L. S. (1993). *Interpersonal diagnosis and treatment of personality disorders: A structural approach.* New York: Guilford Press.

Bernstein, E. M., & Putnam, F. W. (1986). Development, reliability, and validity of a dissociation scale. *Journal of Nervous and Mental Disease, 174,* 727–734.

Bowlby J. (1969). *Attachment.* London: Hogarth Press.

Bradley S. J. (1979). The relationship of early maternal separation to borderline personality disorder in children and adolescents. *American Journal of Psychiatry, 136,* 424–426.

Brewin, C. R., Andrews, B., & Gotlib, I. H. (1993). Psychopathology and early experience: a reappraisal of retrospective reports. *Psychological Bulletin, 113,* 82–98.

Browne, A., & Finkelhor, D. (1986). Impact of child sexual abuse: A review of the literature. *Psychological Bulletin, 99,* 66–77.

Byrne C. P., Cernovsky A., Velamoor, V. R., Coretese L., & Losztyn S. (1990). A comparison of borderline and schizophrenic patients for childhood life events and parent–child relationships. *Canadian Journal of Psychiatry, 35,* 590–595.

Chu, J. A., & Dill, D. L. (1990). Dissociative symptoms in relation to childhood physical and sexual abuse. *American Journal of Psychiatry, 147,* 887–892.

Cloninger, C. R., Martin R. L., Guze S. B., & Clayton P. J. (1990). The empirical structure of psychiatric comorbidity and its theoretical significance. In J. D. Maser & C. R. Cloninger (Eds.), *Comorbidity of anxiety and depression* (pp. 439–462). Washington, DC: American Psychiatric Press.

Cloninger, C. R., Sigvardsson, S., & Bohman, M. (1982). Predisposition to petty criminality in Swedish adoptees II: cross-fostering analysis of gene-environment interaction. *Archives of General Psychiatry, 39,* 1242–1253.

Dunn, J., & Plomin, R. (1990). *Separate lives: Why siblings are so different.* New York: Basic Books.

Finkelhor D., Hotaling G., Lewis I. A., & Smith C. (1990). Sexual abuse in a national survey of adult men and women: Prevalence characteristics and risk factors. *Child Abuse Neglect, 14,* 19–28.

Frank, H., & Paris J. (1981). Family experience in borderline patients. *Archives of General Psychiatry, 38,* 1031–1034.

Garmezy, N., & Masten, A. S. (1994). Chronic adversities. In M. Rutter & L. Hersov (Eds.), *Child and adolescent psychiatry: Modern approaches* (3rd ed., pp. 191–208). London: Blackwell.

Head, S. B., Baker, J. D., & Williamson, D. A. (1991). Family environment characteristics and dependent personality disorder. *Journal of Personality Disorders, 5,* 256–263.

Herman, J. L., Perry, J. C., & van der Kolk, B. A. (1989). Childhood trauma in borderline personality disorder, *American Journal of Psychiatry, 146,* 490–495.

Herman, J. L., & van der Kolk, B. A. (1987). Traumatic antecedents of borderline personality disorder, In B. A. van der Kolk (Eds.), *Psychological trauma* (pp. 111–126). Washington, DC: American Psychiatric Press.

Hetherington, E. M., Cox, M., & Cox R. (1985). Long-term effects of divorce and remarriage on the adjustment of children. *Journal of the American Academy of Child Psychiatry, 24,* 518–530.

Hwu H. G., Yeh, E. K., & Change, L. Y. (1989). Prevalence of psychiatric disorders in Taiwan defined by the Chinese Diagnostic Interview Schedule. *Acta Psychiatrica Scandinavica, 79,* 136–147.

Jang, K., Paris, J., Zweig-Frank, H., & Livesley, W. J. (1998). A twin study of dissociative experience. *Journal of Nervouse and Mental Disease, 186,* 345–351.

Johnson, J. J., Cohen, P., Brown, J., Smailes, E M., Bernstein, D. P. (1999). Childhood maltreatment increases risk for personality disorders during early adulthood. *Archives of General Psychiatry, 56,* 600–606.

Kagan, J. (1994). *Galen's prophecy.* New York: Basic Books.

Kaufman C., Grunebaum H., Cohler B., & Gamer E. (1979). Superkids: Competent children of schizophrenic mothers. *American Journal of Psychiatry, 136,* 1398–1402.

Kendler, K. S., & Eaves, L. J. (1986). Models for the joint effect of genotype and environment on liability to psychiatric illness. *American Journal of Psychiatry, 143,* 279–289.

Kohut, H. (1977). *The restoration of the self.* New York: International Universities Press.

Kroll, J. (1988). *The challenge of the borderline patient.* New York: Norton.

Levy, D. (1943). *Maternal overprotection.* New York: Columbia University Press.

Linehan, M. M. (1993). *Cognitive-behavioral treatment of borderline personality disorder.* New York: Guilford Press.

Links, P. S., Steiner, B., & Huxley, G. (1988). The occurrence of borderline personality disorder in the families of borderline patients. *Journal of Personality Disorders, 2,* 14–20.

Links, P. S, Steiner, M., Offord, D. R., & Eppel, A. (1988). Characteristics of borderline personality disorder: A Canadian study. *Canadian Journal of Psychiatry, 33,* 336–340.

Links, P. S., & van Reekum, R (1993) Childhood sexual abuse, parental impairment, and the development of borderline personality disorder. *Canadian Journal of Psychiatry, 38,* 472–474.

Livesley, W. J., Schroeder, M. L., Jackson, D. N., & Jang, K (1994). Categorical distinctions in the study of personality disorder: implications for classification. *Journal of Abnormal Psycholology, 103,* 6–17.

Ludolph, P. S., Westen, D., & Misle, B. (1990). The borderline diagnosis in adolescents: Symptoms and developmental history. *American Journal of Psychiatry, 147,* 470–476.

Malinovsky-Rummell, R., & Hansen, D. J. (1993). Long-term consequences of physical abuse. *Psychological Bulletin, 114,* 68–79.

Masterson, J., & Rinsley, D. (1975). The borderline syndrome: role of the mother in the genesis and psychic structure of the borderline personality. *International Journal of Psychoanalysis, 56,* 163–177.

Maughan, B., & Rutter, M. (1997). Retrospective reporting of childhood adversity. *Journal of Personality Disorders, 11,* 19–33.

Millon, T. (1993). Borderline personality disorder: A psychosocial epidemic. In J. Paris (Ed.), *Borderline personality disorder: Etiology and treatment* (pp. 197–210). Washington, DC: American Psychiatric Press.

Millon, T., & Davis, R. (1996). *Personality disorders: DSM-IV and beyond.* New York: Wiley.

Monroe, S. M., & Simons, A. D. (1991). Diathesis–stress theories in the context of life stress research. *Psychological Bulletin, 110,* 406–425.

Nash, M. R., Hulsely, T. L., Sexton, M. C., Harralson, T. L., & Lambert, W. (1993). Long-term effects of childhood sexual abuse: Perceived family environment, psychopathology, and dissociation. *Journal of Consulting Clinical Psychology, 61,* 276–283.

Ogata, S. N., Silk, K. R., & Goodrich, S. (1990). The childhood experience of the borderline patient. In P. S. Links (Ed.), *Family environment and borderline personality disorder* (pp. 87–103). Washington, DC: American Psychiatric Press.

Ogata S. N., Silk K. R., Goodrich S., Lohr N. E., Westen D., & Hill E. M. (1990). Childhood sexual and physical abuse in adult patients with borderline personality disorder. *American Journal of Psychiatry, 147,* 1008–1013.

Paris, J. (1983). Family theory and character pathology. *International Journal of Family Psychiatry, 3,* 475–485.

Paris, J. (1992). Social risk factors in borderline personality disorder: A review and a hypothesis. *Canadian Journal of Psychiatry, 37,* 510–515.

Paris, J. (1994). *Borderline personality disorder: A multidimensional approach.* Washington, DC: American Psychiatric Press.

Paris, J. (1995). Memories of abuse in BPD: True or false? *Harvard Review of Psychiatry, 3,* 10–17.

Paris, J. (1996). *Social factors in the personality disorders.* New York: Cambridge University Press.

Paris, J. (1997). Childhood trauma as an etiological factor in the personality disorders. *Journal of Personality Disorders, 11,* 34–49.

Paris, J. (1999). *Nature and nurture in psychiatry: A predisposition–stress model of mental disorders.* Washington, DC: American Psychiatric Press.

Paris, J. (1998). *Working with traits: Psychotherapy of personality disorders.* Northvale, NJ: Jason Aronson.

Paris, J. (2000). *Myths of childhood.* Philadelphia: Brunner/Mazel.

Paris, J., & Frank, H. (1989). Perceptions of parental bonding in borderline patients. *American Journal of Psychiatry, 146,* 1498–1499.

Paris, J., Nowlis, D., & Brown, R. (1988). Developmental factors in the outcome of borderline personality disorder. *Comprehensive Psychiatry, 29,* 147–150.

Paris, J., & Zweig-Frank, H. (1996). The parameters of childhood sexual abuse in female patients with borderline personality disorder and Axis II controls. In M. C. Zanarini (Ed.), *The relationship between childhood sexual abuse and borderline personality disorder* (pp. 15–28). Washington, DC: American Psychiatric Press.

Paris, J., Zweig-Frank, H., Bond, M., & Guzder, J (1996). Defense styles, hostility, and psychological risk factors in male patients with personality disorders. *Journal of Nervous and Mental Disease, 184,* 155–160.

Paris, J., Zweig-Frank, H., & Guzder, J. (1994a). Psychological risk factors for borderline personality disorder in female patients. *Comprehensive Psychiatry, 35,* 301–305.

Paris, J., Zweig-Frank, H., & Guzder, J. (1994b). Risk factors for borderline personality in male outpatients. *Journal of Nervous Mental Disease, 182,* 375–380.

Parker, G. (1983). *Parental overprotection: A risk factor in psychosocial development.* New York: Grune & Stratton.

Plomin, R., & Bergeman, C. S. (1991). The nature of nurture: Genetic influence on "environmental" measures. *Behavioral and Brain Sciences, 14,* 373–427.

Pollock, V. E., Briere, J., Schneider, L., Knop, J., Mednick, S. A., & Goodwin, D. W. (1990). Childhood antecedents of antisocial behavior: parental alcoholism and physical abusiveness. *American Journal of Psychiatry, 147,* 1290–1293.

Riley, G. (1991). *Divorce: An american tradition.* New York: Oxford University Press.

Robins, L. N. (1966). *Deviant children grown up.* Baltimore: Williams & Wilkins.

Robins, L. N., & Regier, D. A. (Eds.). (1991). *Psychiatric disorders in America.* New York: Free Press.

Rowe, D. C. (1981). Environmental and genetic influences on dimensions of perceived parenting. A twin study. *Developmental Psychology, 17,* 203–208.

Rutter M. (1987a). Psychosocial resilience and protective mechanisms. *American Journal of Orthopsychiatry, 57,* 316–331.

Rutter, M. (1987b). Temperament, personality, and personality development. *British Journal of Psychiatry, 150,* 443–448.

Rutter, M. (1989). Pathways from childhood to adult life. *Journal of Child Psychology and Psychiatry, 30,* 23–51.

Rutter, M., & Maughan, B. (1997). Psychosocial adversities in psychopathology. *Journal of Personality Disorders, 11,* 4–18.

Rutter, M., & Quinton, D. (1984). Long-term follow-up of women institutionalized in childhood. *British Journal of Developmental Psychology, 18,* 225–234.

Rutter, M., & Rutter, M. (1993). *Developing minds: Challenge and continuity across the life span.* New York: Basic Books.

Schuckit, M. A., & Smith, T. L. (1996). An 8 year follow-up of 450 sons of alcoholic and control subjects. *Archives of General Psychiatry, 53,* 202–210.

Siever, L. J., & Davis, K. L. (1991). A psychobiological perspective on the personality disorders. *American Journal of Psychiatry, 148,* 1647–1658.

Silverman, J. M., Pinkham, L., Horvath, T. B., Coccaro, E. R., Klar, H., Schear, S., Apter, S., Davidson, M., Mohs, R. C., & Siever, L. J. (1991). Affective and impulsive personality disorder traits in the relatives of patients with borderline personality disorder. *American Journal of Psychiatry, 148,* 1378–1385.

Soloff, P. H., & Millward, J. W. (1983). Psychiatric disorders in the families of borderline patients. *Archives of General Psychiatry, 40,* 37–44.

Stone, M. H. (1993). *Abnormalities of personality.* New York: Norton.

Tennant, C. (1988). Parental loss in childhood to adult life. *Archives of General Psychiatry, 45,* 1045–1050.

Torgersen, S., & Alnaes, R. (1992). Differential perception of parental bonding in schizotypal and borderline personality disorder. *Comprehensive Psychiatry, 33,* 34–38.

van der Kolk, B. A., Perry, J. C., & Herman, J. L. (1991). Childhood origins of self-destructive behavior. *American Journal of Psychiatry, 148,* 1665–1671.

Wallerstein, J. (1989). *Second chances: men, women, and children a decade after divorce.* New York: Ticknor and Fields.

Werner, E. E., & Smith, R. S. (1992). *Overcoming the odds: High risk children from birth to adulthood.* New York: Cornell University Press.

Westen, D., Ludolph, P., Misle, B., Ruffins, S., & Block, J. (1990). Physical and sexual abuse in adolescent girls with borderline personality disorder. *American Journal of Orthopsychiatry, 60,* 55–66.

Yehuda, R., & McFarlane, A. C. (1995). Conflict between current knowledge about posttraumatic stress disorder and its original conceptual basis. *American Journal of Psychiatry, 152,* 1705–1713.

Zanarini, M. C. (1993). Borderline personality as an impulse spectrum disorder. In J. Paris (Ed.), *Borderline personality disorder: Etiology and treatment* (pp. 67–86). Washington, DC: American Psychiatric Press.

Zanarini, M. C., Gunderson, J. G., & Marino, M. F. (1989). Childhood experiences of borderline patients. *Comprehensive Psychiatry, 30,* 18–25.

Zanarini, M. C., Williams, A. A., Lewis, R. E., Reich, R. B., Vera, S. C., Marino, M. F., Levin, A., Yong, L., & Frankenburg, F. R. (1997). Reported pathological childhood experiences associated with the development of borderline personality disorder. *American Journal of Psychiatry, 154,* 1101–1106.

Zweig-Frank, H., & Paris, J. (1991). Recollections of emotional neglect and overprotection in borderline patients. *American Journal of Psychiatry, 148,* 648–651.

Zweig-Frank, H., Paris, J., & Guzder, J. (1994a). Psychological risk factors for dissociation in female patients with borderline and non-borderline personality disorders. *Journal of Personality Disorders, 8,* 203–209.

Zweig-Frank, H., Paris, J., & Guzder, J. (1994b). Psychological risk factors for disssociation and self-mutilation in female patients with personality disorders. *Canadian Journal of Psychiatry, 39,* 259–265.

CHAPTER 11

Can Personality Change?

JENNIFER J. TICKLE
TODD F. HEATHERTON
LAUREN G. WITTENBERG

Can personality change? Arguably, this is the most important and controversial issue facing contemporary personality psychology (Heatherton & Weinberger, 1994). William James claimed in 1890 that "for most of us, by age 30, the character has set like plaster and will never soften again" (p. 124). This grand pronouncement implies that personality changes little after early adulthood. Is personality really so stable?

From a functional perspective, it makes sense that personality should remain stable over time. It is a basic human desire to understand others and to be able to predict their behavior, especially the behavior of those people we care about or rely on. When people choose others to spend the rest of their lives with, they do so with the hope that the person will still be recognizable to them after they have been together many years. This understanding and predictability depends upon stability in people's underlying dispositions. When people choose partners and friends, they do so with the general expectation that their interactions with these people will be somewhat stable (or at least predictable) across time and situation. Similarly, having a stable sense of self helps people to cope with the vagaries of a changing world and assists them in setting goals, making plans, and regulating their behavior. Thus, a stable sense of self helps foster a coherent sense of identity.

At a more theoretical level, most models of personality include notions of enduring characteristics and temperamental styles as part of the basic definition of personality. Tremendous advances in the genetic, temperamental, and biological aspects of personality imply that personality characteristics should be relatively stable over time (assuming that the underlying neurobiological basis of personality does not change, as might occur from major brain injury). In addition, characteristics or adaptations that have an evolutionary basis would be expected to remain remarkably consistent. Thus, there are reasons to believe that some stability in personality is not only likely but quite desirable.

On the other hand, many theoretical perspectives on personality have emphasized its dynamic nature. Allport's (1937) classic definition of personality embodied this idea: "the dynamic organization within the individual of those psychophysical systems that determine his unique adjustments to his environment" (p. 48). Indeed, the malleability of personality is at the heart of psychological treatment. People often enter therapy because they are unhappy with basic personality dispositions, such as chronic anxiety, shyness, or long-term depressed affect. Moreover, people are strongly motivated to achieve personal growth and positive changes in their lives, and the legions of popular books that provide advice on how to change are testimony to the widespread belief that change is both desirable and possible.

Even at the societal level we expect people to be able to change. For instance, someone who takes back an unfaithful spouse hopes that the spouse will have changed his or her wandering ways. The penal system releases prisoners with the expectation that they will give up their criminal lifestyle and adopt less deviant roles in society. For many people the question is not whether personality *can* change but, rather, how one goes about making lasting change.

At the empirical level, there is evidence for both stability of personality (Caspi & Herbener, 1990; Costa & McCrae, 1980) and maturational changes and adaptations in personality (Helson & Moane, 1987; Ozer & Gjerde, 1989). This chapter reviews the basic arguments on both sides of the personality change question. Of course, the question of whether personality *can* change differs from the question of whether personality *does* change or whether an individual can *intentionally* change his or her personality. These questions presuppose answers to even more basic questions, such as "What is personality?" and "What is change?" In the past century, personality researchers have sought answers to all these questions in an attempt to better understand the important topic of personality. As we hope to show, whether personality can change really depends on how the constituent parts of the question are defined.

WHAT IS PERSONALITY?

How one defines the essential features of personality has tremendous implications for whether it is fixed or changeable. Although there is some agreement within the field regarding what is meant by the term "personality," there is sufficient diversity in how personality is viewed to preclude any rigid or clear-cut definitions. For instance, many contemporary researchers restrict the term "personality" to refer to objective and observable traits (such as the five-factor model), whereas more holistic definitions extend beyond traits to include roles, attitudes, goals, and behavioral tendencies. At the extreme, some social psychologists view personality as embedded and inseparable from social context. Each of these perspectives is explored in general terms and also examined in terms of their predictions about personality change.

Basic Trait Adjectives as Personality

When asked to describe someone's personality, laypeople tend to use trait adjectives (e.g., friendly, independent, conscientious, caring, arrogant). Similarly, trait psychologists believe that personality consists of a small group of basic, latent traits around which all dimensions of personality can be categorized. The list of which traits are considered essential has varied from Cattell's (1947) original 16 personality trait factors to today's five-factor theory (Digman, 1990; John, 1990; McCrae & Costa, 1990), or even three-factor models (Eysenck, 1952). Although there is debate over the correct number of basic factors, trait theories share the belief that personality can be characterized adequately by a relatively small number of basic trait dimensions. Even personality psychologists who believe that factor models of personality are overly simplistic agree that traits play an important role in depictions of personality.

Traits have been defined as "dimensions of individual differences in tendencies to show consistent patterns of thoughts, feelings and actions" (McCrae & Costa, 1990, p. 23). Continuity over time and across situation is inherent in this definition of "trait" and accordingly such stability is implied (Caspi & Bem, 1990). Given this definition, it should not be surprising that most research finds that personality traits are remarkably stable over the adult lifespan (McCrae & Costa, 1990).

The most influential recent trait model of personality, the five-factor model, consists of the following basic dimensions: agreeableness, conscientiousness, openness to experience, extraversion, and neuroticism (Costa & McCrae, 1985). Although there is not complete agreement as to what the names of these five factors should be (especially for the openness to experience factor), there is a growing consensus in the field of personality research that some variation of these basic five personality factors is core to the assessment of personality (Digman, 1990; Goldberg, 1981; John, 1990; McCrae & John, 1992; Wiggins & Pincus, 1992; Wiggins & Trapnell, 1997).

Empirical evidence supports the notion of stability in these basic trait factors over time. For instance, Costa and McCrae (1988), using their NEO—Personality Inventory (NEO-PI) to assess personality, examined both nomothetic and ideographic change in personality over the lifespan. They found that group means on the five factors did not change significantly over the assessment period, and that the personalities of individual adults also remain stable over this period (see also Conley, 1984; Costa & McCrae, 1977, 1988, 1994, for summary; Costa, McCrae, & Arenberg, 1980; Siegler, George, & Okun, 1979). An examination of these basic traits as personality, then, seems to suggest that personality does not change much over time, especially in adults.

The Whole Person

For many researchers, the question "What is personality?" is not fully satisfied by reference to basic traits (independent of the number of traits). For instance, in an attempt to construct a more complete representation of personality, McAdams (1994) presents a model that consists of three parallel levels: dispositional traits, personal concerns (which includes roles, motivations, coping strategies, and goals), and the life narrative (which brings together the past, present, and future into a meaningful, coherent narrative). This model dictates that malleability of personality may depend on the particular level under consideration. Although the dispositional trait level will likely remain stable over time, as Costa and McCrae have shown, other aspects of this model may be more likely to show variability over the life course.

Similarly, Helson and Stewart (1994) argue against using the five trait factors as a sum measure of personality, because they view trait approaches as reductionistic and biased against change. Their conception of personality encompasses all domains that personality psychologists study, including not only traits but motives, personal styles, roles, schemas, attitudes, the self-concept, coping strategies, and so forth. Like the varying extents of change expected in the levels of McAdam's model, some of the dimensions of personality in this framework are prone to stability whereas others are prone to change.

When personality is defined in terms broader than the basic five factors, greater evidence of change obtains. For example, over a 10-year span in middle age, researchers found that women increased in self-confidence and outgoingness and decreased in assertiveness, whereas both men and women increased in warmth (Haan, Millsap, & Hartka, 1986). In another study, women showed curvilinear change in masculinity/femininity (including measures of compassion, vulnerability, lack of confidence, and self-criticism) over a 30-year period (Helson, 1993). Evidence of change has also been obtained for men: In a sample of managerial candidates, men declined in ambition and increased in autonomy from their 20s to their 40s (Howard & Bray, 1988).

Roles may change in conjunction with normative roles associated with age (e.g., becoming a parent), and the traits affiliated with these roles may also shift. For instance, women who became mothers increase self-ratings of responsibility, self-control, tolerance, and femininity and decrease ratings of self-acceptance and sociability compared to women who do not become mothers (Helson, Mitchell, & Moane, 1984). Wink and Helson (1993) found that women increase in competence, independence and self-confidence and men increase in affiliativeness between early parental and postparental periods in their lives. Roberts (1997) examined personality change in women from age 27 to age 43 and the association of change with work experiences. Although there was some evidence for consistency in personality over time, specific work roles were associated with personality change after age 30, especially in the domains of norm adherence (including traits such as dependable, responsible, achievement oriented, and perseverant) and agency (assertive, ambitious, gregarious, and sociable). Roberts concluded that this is evidence for the plasticity of personality.

These more holistic approaches contradict the stability of personality inherent in trait-based theories (although even holistic research finds stability in a number of traits examined). According to this framework, personality needs to be moved beyond simple trait dimensions if we are to understand genuine change in personality. From this perspective, reliance on trait models may obscure any changes in personality that do occur. Researchers such as Helson, Stewart, Roberts, and McAdams maintain that there are hierarchies of personality and they argue that these multiple levels must be considered in order to derive a meaningful assessment of personality and its stability.

The Situationist Perspective

For some researchers, stable personality does not exist. Proponents of this situationist perspective believe that situations, not traits, largely determine behavior. In a seminal and controversial paper, Mischel (1968) stated that consistency in personality is an illusion and that any apparent consistency in personality is due entirely to the effects of a consistent environment. Evidence for this claim can be found in contexts that are conducive or nonconducive to eliciting specific behavior, such as honesty in children or strategies for coping with stress among spies (Hartshorne & May, 1928; OSS Assessment Staff, 1948). Because so many behaviors vary across situation, Mischel (1968) questions whether the traits that may underlie these behaviors are useful for predicting future behavior. Although there is not much current support for the hard-line version of the situationist perspective, most researchers acknowledge that personality interacts with the situation to produce behavior (Endler & Magnusson, 1976). Without stepping into this debate, we simply note that evidence for the relative stability of personality can be observed in our everyday interactions with people in their usual situations.

Reconciling Personality Theories

Costa and McCrae (1994) propose a meta-theoretical model of the person (*not the personality*) that incorporates each of the three perspectives on personality just described, although their model still relies on basic traits as central to personality. Their model contains six levels: basic tendencies, external influences, characteristic adaptations, objective biography, the self-concept, and dynamic processes. *Basic tendencies* refer to traits, dispositions and abilities and, as such, are representative of personality. *External influences* are the environment or the broader context of human experience (cultural, social, or historical). According to Costa and McCrae, basic tendencies interact with external influences to develop *characteristic adaptations,* which exist at the third level of their model. These adaptations consist of skills, beliefs, interests, roles, relationships and habits. A person's *objective biography* refers to one's life story including events, behaviors, thoughts, and feelings during the life course. One's thoughts and feelings about oneself make up the *self-concept.* Finally, *dynamic processes* are the mechanisms that connect each of the other five components of the model.

On the surface, the Costa and McCrae model of the person shares a number of features with McAdam's model (which we described earlier).

McAdam's dispositional traits, personal concerns, and life narrative appear quite similar to Costa and McCrae's basic tendencies, characteristic adaptations, and objective biography, respectively. Both models make consistent predictions regarding which of the levels are stable and which are more variable. In addition, both conceptions agree that the trait-based levels will remain stable in the adult life course and the other levels are likely to change.

The key difference between these two models, however, relates to how the respective theories represent personality. McAdams contends that all three levels are integral aspects of personality. For Costa and McCrae, the multiple levels reflect the *person,* not *personality.* Although this may seem like a semantic quibble, the distinction is important when one considers the issues of stability or change in personality. The level that represents personality in the Costa and McCrae model is the basic tendencies (or trait) level. The other levels (aside from external influences) may be affected by the basic tendencies via dynamic processes, but the basic tendencies are not affected in a bidirectional manner. For instance, though roles do change across the lifespan, roles (in this conception) are not part of personality and do not influence personality, even though personality may affect which roles people choose or how people interpret their roles and relationships. This relationship suggests that the basic tendencies are a framework for the structure of the person and are the core of personality. Evidence presented later in the chapter supports the idea that the basic tendencies (defined to include traits, dispositions and temperament) may be a useful framework for understanding personality throughout the life course.

To this point, we have established that traits are relatively stable whereas other aspects of self may exhibit change. The fact remains, however, that inclusion of these other aspects of self as part of basic personality is open to debate, and how the definitional issues are resolved will determine whether personality is malleable or stable. Our review of this literature leads us to believe that the question of whether personality can change is really a question of whether basic human dispositions and traits change. The fact that roles and situational contexts change and that these changed contexts have an influence on people's reactions, accommodations, or motivational pursuits is clear; the inability to adapt to new situations or respond to new challenges would have wiped out the homo sapiens early in our evolutionary history. But, does the essential core of personality change? Do extroverts become introverts? This is not asking whether extroverts occasionally feel shy, almost everyone feels shy at one time or another. But some people are seldom shy and some people are always shy. When the extroverted person feels temporarily shy or shows some sort of behavioral manifestation of feeling shy, does this represent a change in personality or a change in behavior?

Although behaviors may express or reflect aspects of personality, it is important to note that behavior is not the same as personality. The correlation between the stability of traits and the stability of related behavior is not particularly high (which is at the core of the situationist argument), but there is no reason to believe that examining behavior is a more accurate way to assess personality than using personality inventories. Simply because changes occur in behavior does not mean that personality has changed (Pervin, 1984). For instance, a woman high in extraversion may behave differently when she is a young adult (e.g., partying, thrill seeking, and having multiple sexual partners) than when she is close to 90 years old (when the parties are probably tamer and promiscuous sex is uncommon, but she may still have many friends and like to travel). Her behaviors at both times, however, will reflect the underlying trait of extraversion. In this way, the underlying disposition remains stable across situations and roles even though the expression of that trait may change over time (Costa & McCrae, 1994).

The possession of a certain trait does not dictate that the expression of that trait will always be the same, but the long-term stability of traits should constrain behavior in predictable ways (Pervin, 1985). Traits may be expressed as consistent patterns in action, motivation, and style over time and situation, but this does not imply that traits *determine* specific action, motivation, or style. Behavior may be enacted or traits suppressed depending on situational demands. In addition, a behavior may vary from situation to situation depending on the number of traits that are influencing that behavior in a particular situation. Multiple traits may interact to produce behavior that is not representative of any of the single traits when considered in isolation (Allport, 1961). This is a key point that is often neglected in personality research. There are few situations, roles, or circumstances in which one personality trait will entirely determine behavior. How extroverts react in a given situation will depend in part on whether they are also high or low in agreeableness, conscientiousness, and neuroticism.

The role of individual differences in personality stability is yet another aspect of personality that needs to be considered. Some people's personalities may be more consistent than others', whereas others may be highly consistent on a few central traits and variable on other traits (Bem & Allen, 1974; Kenrick & Stringfield, 1980). When asked to rate their own personality on a scale, some people claim it is difficult, because their level of the trait depends on the situation. For instance, when asked to rate one's own sociability, some people may respond that it depends on the context, whether they are at a party with friends or in a strange place. This conditional responding is a characteristic of some people who may be more likely to vacillate in the short term on personality measures (Thorne, 1989). Other research has directly examined personality "changers" and personality "nonchangers" (Block, 1971). This research finds that people who are more likely to change have different life outcomes than those whose personalities do not change.

WHAT IS STABILITY?

Whether one considers personality to be subject to change depends not only on how one defines personality but also on how one defines stability. Stability of a trait (or any aspect of the person, for that matter) does not imply that the trait cannot change. Fluctuation in the expression of traits is expected: personality traits seem to be stable over time, but they do undergo slight state fluctuations in the short term. In other words, traits provide a basic personality framework which remains stable in the long term and allows patterns of responses to be established. There exists, however, a range of behaviors and other trait expressions that occur within this framework of stability.

There is evidence that both long-term stability and short-term change in personality may occur during the life course. Helson and Stewart (1994), proponents of the idea that personality changes over the life course, find that many traits remain stable longitudinally, including stability within the context of job and role changes. This coincidental stability and change is not unusual in research on aspects of self. Constancy can be thought of in two ways: (1) as a stable characteristic or (2) as an attribute that is predictable overall, but that may vary considerably around this predictable level (see Nesselroade & Boker, 1994). Examples of self-aspects that are considered stable over the long term are work values, creativity, and the self-concept. Each of these characteristics is relatively stable over time but may have considerable variability in the short term. This distinction is often referred to as the state–trait distinction and this distinction has been useful in a number of domains. For instance, Heatherton and Polivy (1991) found that self-esteem has both trait and state aspects in that over time, self-esteem remains fairly stable, but in the short term it may fluctuate. The literature on anxiety distinguishes between persons high in anxiety over time (trait anxiety) and those who experience anxiety in the short term (state anxiety), often in relation to a situational factor. Following this logic, personality "traits" are so named because they remain consistent over the long term. However, day-to-day expression of traits may not be, and should not be expected to be, perfectly stable. There is evidence that trait expression may follow recurring systematic patterns, possibly in response to regular changes in social roles and context (Moskowitz, Brown, & Cote, 1997). Personality, then, is often variable over the short term, but stable over long periods.

HOW ARE STABILITY AND CHANGE MEASURED?

Findings of stability or change in personality also depend on a number of methodological factors. For instance, one important issue is the age of those under consideration. In general, personality stability increases as the age of the participants increases (Clark & Clark, 1984; Finn, 1986; Moss & Susman, 1980; Olweus, 1979). For instance, studies of people over 30 years of age are much more likely to find stability of personality than are studies are using younger participants. Before age 30, personality may not be fully established.

How often personality is assessed is also an important factor to consider, as there is evidence that stability decreases as the time between measurement intervals increases. However, this may be a measurement artifact. The similarity of the environment or situation at the two measurement times may have a stronger effect on personality stability than the intervals between measurements. This situational similarity may simply make it seem as if personality consistency increases as the measurement intervals decrease (see Caspi & Bem, 1990, for a discussion). Longitudinal studies that collect data at irregular intervals over long periods may be the way to approach the measurement of personality and personality change (see Nesselroade & Boker, 1994).

Another measurement issue that is important to address is how personality itself is measured. Some methods of assessing personality seem predisposed to find continuity (Heatherton & Nichols, 1994b). For instance, self-report methodologies that require people to rate themselves on a scale from 1 to 5 on global traits may not find much change over time. Individuals who choose 4 or 5 at one measurement period are unlikely to choose 1 or 2 at a follow-up session, even if they believe that they have changed. They may select a 3 because they have not changed "that much." It is also possible that the meaning of a "4" may change from the first assessment to the second. For instance, a person's report of extraversion in the liberal 1960s may differ from their report of extraversion in the 1980s. In a related vein, people may use the same reference group in the 1960s and 1980s and discover that although they may have changed in extraversion, relative to their peers they are still a 4 on the scale. Aside from using rating scales to measure personality, others have used life narratives or interviews to assess changes in a person's life. These methods allow for a greater richness in the data and typically evidence greater change. However, these methods are more likely to confuse personality changes with other types of life change.

Finally, even if group means suggest stability in personality, it is possible that a minority of people undergo major change in personality. Idiographic rather than nomothetic approaches may be valuable for understanding personality change that does occur. For individuals, the ability of the group to change is irrelevant; it is the personal perception of the ability to change that may motivate efforts to do so. It is the individual experience of being a different person now than in the past that provides personal evidence of change. For instance, consider the analogous case of weight loss. Evidence indicates that fewer than 5% of people manage to maintain weight loss over a 1-year period, and fewer than 2% can do so over 5 years. Yet, if we assume that even as few as 10 million Americans lose weight in a year (given that approximately half of adults will go on a diet), this means that hundreds of thousands do manage to maintain weight loss. We propose that it is important to identify people who have experienced genuine change in personality to establish what sorts of people are most likely to change.

WHY IS PERSONALITY STABLE?

Although there is evidence that some personal aspects change over time, there is general support for the stability of trait factors over the life course. The next portion of the chapter examines several theoretical perspectives that help explain the tendency for personality to be stable.

The Role of Genetic Influence

There is ample evidence that personality is determined in part by genetic mechanisms. Most research that examines the role of genetics in personality compares similarities between monozygotic twins (who share the same genes) and dizygotic twins (who only share as many genes as typical siblings). Genetic influence can also be assessed using adoption studies that examine the similarities of children's personalities with their biological versus adoptive parents, or by examining the similarities that exist between twins who are reared apart. Adoption studies allow researchers the possibility of distinguishing the role of genetics from the influence of the environment. Some caution needs to be taken in assuming, for instance, that twins raised apart do not share a common environment. Adoption agencies often try to place children in homes in which the adoptive parents are similar to the biological parents. Moreover, children evoke idiosyncratic reactions from others and also help shape their personal environments (genetic influence may predispose identical twins to choose similar recreational activities, relationship partners, or career paths). Thus, the environment cannot be artificially separated from the person. This built-in correlation between person and environment explains in part why identical twins

may be just as similar when raised apart as when raised together. Note, however, that this implies a high level of genetic determination of personality.

Genetics of Traits

Multiple studies show that genetic factors have a substantial influence on personality traits (e.g., Henderson, 1982; Loehlin, Willerman, & Horn, 1988; Tellegen et al., 1988). Correlations among personality traits are typically higher for monozygotic twins than for dizygotic twins (.5 vs. .3, respectively) (Loehlin & Nichols, 1976). These correlations are particularly strong for major personality traits, such as neuroticism, extraversion, and conscientiousness (Floderus-Myhred, Pedersen, & Rasmuson, 1980; Loehlin, 1982; Tellegen et al., 1988; see Loehlin, 1989, for a review).

It might be predicted that personality traits that are under the greatest genetic influence would show the best evidence of stability of personality, and some evidence supports this idea. For instance, some researchers have examined personality stability using the Multidimensional Personality Questionnaire (MPQ). The MPQ measures three trait categories: constraint (traditionalism, harm avoidance, control), negative emotionality (aggression, alienation, stress reaction), and positive emotionality (achievement, social potency, well-being, social closeness). Research has generally found these MPQ traits to be heritable, predictable from childhood, and stable from adolescence to adulthood (Caspi & Silva, 1995; McGue, Bacon, & Lykken, 1993; Tellegen et al., 1988).

Genetics of Dispositions

As mentioned previously, traits can be thought of as predispositions for behavior. From this perspective, traits represent a tendency toward expression of that particular trait that relies on, or is constrained by, the situation. Dispositions have been shown to play a larger role in behavior when the setting is unstructured than when structured, which makes sense because in the absence of structure, internal traits are relied on to "guide" behavior (Monson, Hesley, & Chernick, 1982; Snyder & Ickes, 1985). Indeed, monozygotic twins behave more similarly than do dizygotic twins in novel situations (Matheny

& Dolan, 1975). For instance, monozygotic and dizygotic pairs behave quite similarly with their mothers, but differences emerge when these pairs interact with strangers (Plomin & Rowe, 1979).

It follows that if dispositions emerge most strongly in unstructured settings, at points of life change (transitions and major life events that might require adjustment to new circumstance or novel people) dispositions would be most pronounced (as discussed in Caspi & Bem, 1990). Research supports this idea that personality continuity may become more clear if assessed at discontinuities in the life course. For instance, research assessing personality change in individuals who were affected by the Nazi revolution found that even this major life incident did not coincide with personality alteration. Any changes that did occur during the measured time span were mere strengthening of the personality that existed precrisis (Allport, Bruner, & Jandorf, 1941).

Genetics of Temperament

Another term often associated with the genetics of personality development is "temperament." Temperament is the term used to describe initial expressions of personality in infants and children and is generally believed to be biologically based and heritable (Kagan, 1992). Several different models of temperament have been proposed in the psychology literature. For instance, Buss and Plomin (1975, 1984) established three definitional conditions for temperament: heritability, stability, and evolutionary significance. Based on these criteria, Buss and Plomin identified three temperaments: activity level, emotionality, and sociability. These temperaments have shown stability over the lifespan, such that early temperament tends to persist from childhood to adulthood and is especially stable later in life.

In an alternative model, Thomas and Chess (1984) in their New York Longitudinal Study (NYLS) described nine basic temperaments (i.e., activity level, rhythmicity, approach/withdrawal, adaptability, intensity of reaction, attention span and persistence, distractibility, quality of mood, and responsiveness threshold) that they grouped into three general patterns: difficult temperament, easy temperament, and slow-to-warm-up temperament. When measured in the first 5 years of life, some of these nine temperaments do show stability from childhood to adulthood, but these relationships are often difficult to examine since the behavior associated with a particular temperament may change over time (even if the temperament itself stays the same). According to Chess and Thomas (1984) people make adaptations that "hide" temperaments until they are confronted with a novel situation, when basic temperaments are likely to emerge.

A number of questions have been raised in the literature about how temperament and personality are related. It seems that what many researchers have termed "temperament" may be the same thing as more widely used terms referring to personality traits. For instance, the emotionality temperament is similar to the trait factor of neuroticism. The temperament of sociability relates to aspects of agreeableness and extraversion. The trait factor of conscientiousness has many traits that relate to impulsivity, which is arguably one of the temperaments (discussed in Carver & Scheier, 1992). Although these relationships are not perfect, the similarities are striking.

A central question remains, however: Is temperament the foundation—or precursor—for personality or is temperament equivalent to personality? One answer to this question is that temperament can be thought of as the entirety of infant personality and as a precursor to adult personality (Goldsmith et al., 1987). Thus, it makes sense that temperament, on the whole, seems to be more heritable than individual personality traits, and that the traits that are most heritable seem to be those linked most closely to the temperaments. It is also possible that temperament is essentially equivalent to personality. The genetic mechanisms underlying childhood temperament may be the same that underlie adult personality. However, little research directly examines the relationship between temperament in childhood and personality dimensions in adults.

The Contribution of Biology to Stability

Many personality psychologists have turned their attention to the biological basis of human personality. Of course, it has long been known that the brain is related to personality. The earliest theories of personality were based on bodily fluids (humors) and the classic lesson learned from the case of Phineas Gage was that trauma to specific brain regions was associated with major change in personality. Theories such as Eysenck's (1967) classic theory of extraversion proposed that personality was, at the core, a matter of biological functioning. Kagan (1992) states that "concepts of temperament include, as part of their theoretical definition, an inherited neurochemical and physiological profile that is linked to emotion and behavior" (p. 33).

We do not have sufficient space in this chapter to provide a reasonable overview of research on the biological underpinnings of personality. Suffice it to say that recent research has focused on functional neuroanatomy, neurochemistry, the endocrine (hormonal) system, and psychophysiological responding. The recent excitement over fluoxetine (Prozac) occurred in part because of the anecdotal claims that administration of Prozac—above and beyond its effects on depression—led to dramatic (and positive) changes in personality (Kramer, 1993).

For the purposes of this chapter it is simply important to point out that if personality is rooted in biology, it will change only to the extent that the underlying biology changes. Thus, personality change may be expected to occur following brain injury or neurochemical alteration, during brain maturation, or during circadian or other hormonal cycles. The evidence is overwhelming that brain injury (as occurs following trauma or results from diseases such as Parkinson's, for example) is associated with fundamental changes in personality (see Santoro & Spiers, 1994). Moreover, personality change can be temporarily induced through changes in hormonal or neurotransmitter action, as might occur if a person self-administers anabolic steroids or drugs. Thus, it does appear that some aspects of personality are rooted in biological processes, which explains in part why personality is generally stable. In the absence of fundamental changes to brain neurochemistry or structure, personality would tend to be set following brain maturation (during which personality might be expected to be malleable). This notion suggests that personality can change, but it most often does not without some major biological event.

The Contribution of Evolutionary Processes to Personality Continuity

Evolutionary theory predicts that certain personality traits are (or were) adaptive for survival and reproductive success (Buss, 1994). Possession of personality traits that were useful for obtaining resources and for securing potential mates would mean the holder would be more likely to survive and pass along his or her genes to future generations. For instance, males who were aggressive might have been threatening to competitors, thereby increasing their social status and, in turn, making them more likely to attract the opposite sex, win mates, and subsequently pass along their genes (Buss, 1988; Daly & Wilson, 1988; Trivers, 1972). In the search for mates and sexual opportunities, traits such as kindness, dependableness, emotional stability, dominance, and intellect are highly favored. These traits are attractive to males and females in search of partners and would have been selected for during evolution.

Moreover, adaptations to recurrent situational dilemmas may lead to stable individual differences in personality (Buss, 1997). For instance, one long-standing dilemma is who to choose for a relationship partner. Personality trait expressions can be used to determine others' status, resources, and intentions, or their suitability as a friend, mate, or good community member. The fact that many of these traits are central to conceptions of personality is strong support for their adaptive role throughout evolution. The importance of particular traits (as represented by a five-factor model, for instance) may be a reflection of which traits have been evolutionarily adaptive and necessary for survival and continuance of the species (Buss, 1997).

There is also some evidence, in line with sociobiology, that assortative mating occurs for some personality traits (Klohnen & Mendelsohn, 1997). Assortative mating for personality involves choosing a partner with a similar personality so that certain traits will be likely in their offspring (Theissen & Gregg, 1980). People tend to choose mates who exhibit similar physical characteristics, values, and cognitive abilities in addition to personality (Epstein & Guttman, 1984; Jensen, 1978; Vandenberg, 1972). Having parents with similar traits may also create an environment that encourages the expression of that trait in their children (Buss, 1984).

The Contribution of Person–Environment Interactions to Stability

As was discussed previously, situationists proposed that stable situations give the illusion of stability in personality. Although it may be true that environments tend to be relatively stable, it may be that people immerse themselves in environments that promote stability (Buss, 1987; Plomin, DeFries, & Loehlin, 1977; Scarr & McCartney, 1983).

Caspi and Bem (1990) discuss three types of interaction of person with environment. *Reactive interactions* occur when a person reacts differently from others to a particular environment. For instance, an introvert will react differently from an extravert in many social situations. *Evocative interactions* occur when individuals induce responses from others to create a certain environment. For instance, an introvert will evoke different responses from others in an interaction than will an extravert. *Proactive interactions* occur when a person selects or creates the environment around him or her. For example, an introvert may choose to be a librarian rather than a salesperson because the role better suits his personality. Although the specific effects of these types of interactions are not discussed separately, it is important to realize that individuals interact with their environment in such a way that their personalities affect their environments and the environments simultaneously affect personality.

Environments support continuity by reinforcing tendencies and sustaining dispositions (Emmons, Deiner, & Larsen, 1986; Snyder & Ickes, 1985; see also Caspi & Herbener, 1990). A stable environment is predictive of less change than an unstable environment. The people in one's life are important aspects of the environment that influence personality consistency. Assortative mating involves choosing a partner who is similar to the self, which in turn promotes personality continuity (Buss, 1984; Caspi & Bem, 1990). Because those who are similar to us like to do similar things, relationship partners help to maintain a stable environment.

People also want their partners to remain consistent over time. People like to believe that they are able to make reasonable predictions about their partner's behavior. People typically do not choose mates expecting them to change, and indeed may actively try to discourage attempts at change (Heatherton & Nichols, 1994a). People also choose friends who have similar values and characteristics to themselves (Kandel, 1978; Newcomb, 1961). Friends, like partners, can encourage continuity in this respect. Family and friends often want to maintain homeostasis in their relationships, and this homeostasis promotes personality continuity.

Given a choice of environments, people are likely to choose those that are consistent with their personalities. People tend to choose occupations and interests that reflect significant aspects of their personalities (Scarr & McCartney, 1983). Even when a job is not perfectly suited to a person's personality, the personality may still be expressed in the manner in which the person performs the job.

Thus, there is a built-in correlation between personality and the environment. People actively select environments that suit their personalities and that support their basic behavioral tendencies. This includes choosing others who are compatible with their traits. Stability in environment discourages change in personality.

PREDICTIONS OF LONG-TERM OUTCOMES BASED ON EARLY PERSONALITY

The interaction of personality and environment also influences the trajectory of the life course (Caspi, Bem, & Elder, 1989). One way to examine this is to look at the predictions that can be made regarding adult traits and behavior based on childhood personality.

For example, people who score high on neuroticism tend to be maladjusted at all ages, have ineffective coping strategies, and have career and family difficulties including a higher likelihood of divorce and downward occupational change (Costa & McCrae, 1980; McCrae & Costa, 1986; Vaillant, 1977). Midlife crises have been linked to high neuroticism, although some research indicates that a combination of environment and neuroticism may be the significant precursor to midlife crises (Costa & McCrae, 1980, 1984). In general, psychological maladjustment appears to be relatively stable over time.

Various temperaments and dispositions also appear to have predictive utility. Children who had difficult temperaments at age 3 and 4 tend to have more coping difficulties as adults than do children who had easy temperaments (Thomas & Chess, 1984). Childhood temperament has also been shown to predict occupational status and stability after 20 years (Caspi, Elder, & Bem, 1987). Age 3 temperament as well as age 18 personality have been found to predict health-related risk behavior at age 21

(Caspi et al., 1997). In the latter study, under-controlled temperament (involving irritability, impulsivity, and emotion lability) predicted health risk behavior, including alcohol dependence, violent crime, sexual behavior, and driving habits. This relationship was mediated by age 18 personality profiles that indicated low ratings on traditionalism, harm avoidance, control, and social closeness and high ratings on aggression. In another study, personality measures at 3 and 4 years of age also predict drug use by age 14 (Block, Block, & Keyes, 1988).

Related to the life-course predictions for temperament, Caspi, Bem, and Elder (1989) discuss three interactional styles of childhood that shape the life course: ill temperedness, shyness, and dependency. Each of these three interactional styles has predictive utility over the lifespan, but the predictions differ for males and females. Ill-tempered children tend to have difficulties later in life, including relationship instability, divorce, and lower overall achievement. Ill-tempered male children become men who find their job statuses particularly unstable. Ill-tempered female children become women who are ill-tempered mothers (Caspi et al., 1987).

Shyness is evidenced throughout the life course in tendencies to delay or avoid action, hesitancies to enter novel situations, and slow adjustment to change. Men who were shy as children tended to be behind their peers in making role changes in life such as marriage or parenting. Females who were shy as children tended to be less likely than their peers to have held a job for a significant period and more likely to have undertaken domestic responsibilities (Caspi, Elder, & Bem, 1988). Shyness seems to be particularly stable from childhood to adulthood (Kagan & Moss, 1962).

People with dependent interaction styles tend to self-perpetuate their interaction style more than do shy or ill-tempered persons. Dependent male children tend to become adults who are quite well adjusted and who have stable relationships with satisfied wives. Dependent female children tend to become adults who are unassertive, moody, and anxious and who both marry and have children early (Caspi et al., 1989). Over all three interaction styles, the actual behavior of persons with those styles will not be immutable but is nevertheless predictable from the childhood interactional style.

The childhood disposition for aggression remains stable and predicts later antisocial personality (e.g., Huesmann, Eron, Lefkowitz, & Walder, 1984; Olweus, 1979). Longitudinal studies have shown that high aggression predicts low intelligence, poor scholastic achievement, and psychiatric problems for both men and women and additional health problems for women (Moskowitz & Schwartzman, 1989). Conversely, inhibited 21-month-olds were less likely to show delinquent or aggressive behavior as 13-year-olds (Schwartz, Snidman, & Kagan, 1996).

Another disposition with long-term predictive utility is the ability to delay gratification (Mischel, Shoda, & Rodriguez, 1989). Funder and Block (1989) define delay of gratification (as it relates to ego control) as "the individual's generalized disposition or capacity to modulate and contain impulses, feelings and desires; to inhibit action; and to be isolated from environmental distractors" (p. 1041). Funder and Block find that adolescents who delay gratification tend to be well-adjusted, reliable, productive, ethical, consistent, insightful, likable, and warm. Mischel, Shoda, and Peake (1988), in an attempt to examine predictive facets of delay behavior, used preschool measures of delay of gratification to predict adolescent competencies. They find that ability to delay gratification in children is positively related to adolescent verbal fluency, use of reason, concentration and attentiveness, confidence, and coping with stress. Preschoolers who were extreme in impulsivity were more likely to become delinquent adolescents (Kagan & Zentner, 1996).

CHANGES IN PERSONAL BELIEFS ABOUT PERSONALITY

The research discussed thus far in the chapter has been primarily concerned with finding objective evidence for personality stability or change. This objective examination of personality ignores personal beliefs and accounts of change processes that might add depth to the literature. This last section discusses some research that examines the equally important issue of people's subjective experiences of change.

In line with research that states that personality remains relatively stable over time, most people report that they have not changed very much in the past 10 years (see McCrae & Costa, 1990, for a discussion). Approximately 51% of respondents say they have remained the same, 35% claim to have changed a little, and 14% claim to have changed substantially. However, there does not appear to be any evidence in actual personality measures that supports these reported changes (Costa & McCrae, 1989). Woodruff and Birren (1972) reported similar findings over a 10-year span after asking people to complete personality forms as they had 10 years earlier. Many people perceived that they had changed, but in reality, trait ratings completed over that time period, both by the person and by other people assessing that person, did not tend to corroborate the perceived change.

But there are people who change, aren't there? As we mentioned earlier, even if as few as 10% of people change (and thereby group means would indicate little change), this means that millions of people do manage to make changes in their lives, and do experience change in their personality. Moreover, the evidence from trauma, disease, and brain injury suggests that some people have change thrust upon them.

If asked, some people report sudden, dramatic changes in personality that are confirmed by others, much akin to the transformation of Ebenezer Scrooge in Charles Dickens's *A Christmas Carol* or the shifts in self that ex-alcoholics report in Alcoholics Anonymous (Miller & C'deBaca, 1994). These quantum changes may be very different from the gradual change that most psychologists have studied. Using retrospective accounts of quantum change, Miller and C'deBaca (1994) have found that there are similarities between these accounts. The majority of people recalled such things as the specific day and time of the experience, that the change came suddenly and surprised them, and that the change seemed to be initiated by an external source. The year before the change occurred was often filled with distress and negative life events. After the change, most people reported an increased sense of life meaning and happiness, an increased closeness to God, and increased satisfaction. Ninety-six percent of respondents claimed that the change made their lives much better and 93% of respondents were confident that the change would endure. The aspects of the person that seemed to change in these accounts were tem-

perament, life goals, values, and perceptual style. Although temperament has clear ties to personality, there is no direct evidence that personality traits change after quantum change. Further examination of traits before and after quantum change would be necessary in order to draw firm conclusions regarding personality change.

Even if one accepts that some people might experience dramatic changes in core aspects of self, do people choose to change, or does change spontaneously occur? The types of change that were considered in the first part of the chapter related to changes involving roles, circumstance, and life story. These aspects of self are under some volitional control, but it is possible that they occur without a conscious decision to change. Are volitional attempts at personality change different from changes, such as quantum change, that are perceived to happen more spontaneously?

Heatherton and Nichols (1994a) examined this question by comparing narrative accounts of people who had made attempts at major life change and had succeeded versus accounts from people who had tried to make major life changes and had failed. Although some people did report attempts to change personality, other examples of attempted change were quitting habits or changing relationships. Despite the fact that the study did not focus exclusively on personality change, information about perceptions and attributions about change processes may be as applicable to personality change as to the other types of change examined. The successful change stories differed in substantial and predictable ways compared to the unsuccessful change stories. Individuals who reported making changes described extreme negative affect, and often suffering, before the change was made. One common theme in the successful change stories was the occurrence of a focal event that triggered the change attempt. An important part of this focal event may have been the prior crystallization of discontent that led to a sudden reevaluation of circumstance.

Baumeister (1991, 1994) has described the role of crystallization of discontent in the processes of major life change. Crystallization of discontent involves changes in attention to and attributions about negative life events that lead to life change in such domains as politics, religion, romance, marriage, or identity and personality. People make attributions that positive events are interrelated, typical, and permanent while negative events are isolated, atypical, and temporary. This allows people to exaggerate the positive aspects and dismiss the negative aspects of their lives. A focal incident may call attention to an overabundance of negative aspects or may allow a person to see an overarching pattern that has previously been dismissed or ignored. The focal incident reverses the typical attributions such that positive events are suddenly seen as external and unstable, while negative events are interpreted as typical and stable. This reinterpretation of life events leads to a sudden insight and subsequent sudden change in values, and even memory of associated events (Baumeister, 1991; Vaughan, 1986).

In Heatherton and Nichols's (1994a) examination of successful versus unsuccessful attempts at major life change, crystallization of discontent was observed much more often in successful change stories than in unsuccessful ones. Successful changers compared to unsuccessful changers were more likely to report that another person requested the change, helped with the change, supported the change, or commented on the process of change, thus eliminating one possible source of pressure for continuity that was still present in unsuccessful changers. There is evidence that social support is an important component of life change (Clifford, Tan, & Gorsuch, 1991; Marlatt, 1985). Successful changers were more likely than nonchangers to eliminate another pressure for stability by altering their environment. People who were unsuccessful at changing were less committed to making the change, more uncertain about the desirability of change, and more likely to be unwilling to change their current role or identity to accommodate the change. They were also more likely to report that they experienced external barriers to change. This could be a realistic difference, or it may be a difference in how the unsuccessful versus successful changers chose to focus their attributions and interpret their efforts at change.

Of course, there is no evidence that the change stories were true, and it is possible that people were misremembering their prior circumstances in order to create the perception that they had changed. However, the story that people tell themselves is important for predicting future behavior. The belief that one has changed in some fundamental way may provide the motivation necessary to engage in certain behaviors or act in specific ways. Whether this represents a genuine change in the core of personality is unclear at the present time.

CONCLUSIONS

So, can personality change? As we have described, the answer to this question depends on how one defines the basic features of the question, such as the basic definitions of personality and stability, and the methods used to assess personality and stability. If personality is restricted to traitlike behavioral tendencies, the evidence suggests that most people's personalities remain stable over time. Various theoretical perspectives provide functional accounts of why personality "should" be stable. The genetic, biological, and evolutionary theories suggest that personality, as it is grounded in genes, biological processes, and species adaptations, should not change a great deal across the lifespan (or even across close relatives in the case of genes or generations in the case of evolution). In addition to these scientific approaches to the issue of stability, social forces are also at work to promote stability in personality. Interactions with people and environments promote stability over the life course, and some child and adolescent personality characteristics have predictive utility for adult personality and behavior. Nonetheless, many people believe that personality changes, and for some people it may actually do so. We encourage idiographic research that examines all aspects of people's lives in order to clarify which aspects of personality change and which do not. Finally, there is considerable evidence that change is sometimes thrust on people, as when they develop certain disease states or have brain injury. In these cases it is clear that personality *does* change, but it remains to be seen whether personality *can* be changed through volitional effort. For the vast majority of people, personality remains stable after early adulthood.

REFERENCES

Allport, G. W. (1937). *Personality: A psychological interpretation.* New York: Holt, Rinehart & Winston.

Allport, G. W. (1961). *Pattern and growth in personality.* New York: Holt, Rinehart & Winston.

Allport, G. W., Bruner, J. S., & Jandorf, E. M. (1941). Personality under social catastrophe: Ninety life histories of the Nazi revolution. *Character and Personality, 10,* 1–22.

Baumeister, R. F. (1991). *Meanings of life.* New York: Guilford Press.

Baumeister, R. F. (1994). The crystallization of discontent in the process of major life change. In T. F. Heatherton & J. L. Weinberger (Eds.), *Can personality change?* (pp. 281–298). Washington, DC: American Psychological Association.

Bem, D. J., & Allen, A. (1974). On predicting some of the people some of the time: The search for cross-situational consistencies in behavior. *Psychological Review, 81*(6), 506–520.

Block, J. (1971). *Lives through time.* Berkeley, CA: Bancroft.

Block, J., Block, J. H., & Keyes, S. (1988). Longitudinally foretelling drug usage in adolescence: Early childhood personality and environmental precursors. *Child Development, 59*(2), 336–355.

Buss, D. M. (1984). Toward a psychology of person–environment (PE) correlation: The role of spouse selection. *Journal of Personality and Social Psychology, 47*(2), 361–377.

Buss, D. M. (1987). Selection, evocation, and manipulation. *Journal of Personality and Social Psychology, 53*, 1214–1221.

Buss, D. M. (1988). The evolution of human intrasexual competition: Tactics of mate attraction. *Journal of Personality and Social Psychology, 54*(4), 616–628.

Buss, D. M. (1994). Personality evoked: The evolutionary psychology of stability and change. In T. F. Heatherton & J. L. Weinberger (Eds.), *Can personality change?* (pp. 41–57). Washington, DC: American Psychological Association.

Buss, D. M. (1997). Evolutionary foundations of personality. In R. Hogan, J. Johnson, & S. Briggs (Eds.), *Handbook of personality psychology* (pp. 317–344). San Diego, CA: Academic Press.

Buss, A. H., & Plomin, R. (1975). *A temperament theory of personality development.* New York: Wiley-Interscience.

Buss, A. H., & Plomin, R. (1984). *Temperament: Early developing personality traits.* Hillsdale, NJ: Erlbaum.

Carver, C. S., & Scheier, M. F. (1992). *Perspectives on personality* (2nd ed.). Boston: Allyn & Bacon.

Caspi A., & Bem, D. J. (1990). Personality continuity and change across the life course. In L. A. Pervin (Ed.), *Handbook of personality: Theory and research* (pp. 549–575). New York: Guilford Press.

Caspi, A., Bem, D. J., & Elder, G. H., Jr. (1989). Continuities and consequences of interactional styles across the life course. Special issue: Long-term stability and change in personality. *Journal of Personality, 57* (2), 375–406.

Caspi, A., Elder, G. H., & Bem, D. J. (1987). Moving against the world: Life-course patterns of explosive children. *Developmental Psychology, 23*(2), 308–313.

Caspi, A., Elder, G. H., & Bem, D. J. (1988). Moving away from the world: Life-course patterns of shy children. *Developmental Psychology, 24*(6), 824–831.

Caspi, A., Harrington, H., Moffitt, T. E., Begg, D., Dickson, N., Langley, J., & Silva, P. A. (1997). Personality differences predict health-risk behaviors in adulthood: Evidence from a longitudinal study. *Journal of Personality and Social Psychology, 73*(5), 1052–1063.

Caspi, A., & Herbener, E. S. (1990). Continuity and change: Assortative mating and consistency of personality in adulthood. *Journal of Personality and Social Psychology, 58*(2), 250–258.

Caspi, A., & Silva, P. A. (1995). Temperamental qualities at age three predict personality traits in young adulthood: Longitudinal evidence from a birth cohort. *Child Development, 66*(2), 486–498.

Cattell, R. B. (1947). Confirmation and clarification of primary personality factors. *Psychometrika, 12,* 197–220.

Chess, S., & Thomas, A. (1984). *Origins and evolution of behavior disorders: From infancy to early adult life.* Cambridge, MA: Harvard University Press.

Clark, A. D. B., & Clark, A. M. (1984). Constancy and change in the growth of human characteristics. *Journal of Child Psychology and Psychiatry, 25,* 191–210.

Clifford, P. A., Tan, S. Y., & Gorsuch, R. L. (1991). Efficacy of a self-directed behavioral health change program: Weight, body composition, cardiovascular fitness, blood pressure, health risk, and psychosocial mediating variables. *Journal of Behavioral Medicine, 14,* 303–323.

Conley, J. J. (1984). The hierarchy of consistency: A review and model of longitudinal findings on adult individual differences in intelligence, personality, and self-opinion. *Personality and Individual Differences, 5,* 11–26.

Costa, P. T., Jr., & McCrae, R. R. (1977). Age differences in personality structure revisited: Studies in validity, stability and change. *Aging and Human Development, 8,* 261–275.

Costa, P. T., & McCrae, R. R. (1980). Influence of extraversion and neuroticism on subjective well-being: Happy and unhappy people. *Journal of Personality and Social Psychology, 38*(4), 668–678.

Costa, P. T., Jr., & McCrae, R. R. (1984). Personality as a lifelong determinant of well-being. In G. Malatesta & C. Izard (Eds.), *Affective processes in adult development and aging* (pp. 141–157). Beverly Hills, CA: Sage.

Costa, P. T., & McCrae, R. R. (1985). Concurrent validation after 20 years: Implications of personality stability for its assessment. In J. N. Butcher & C. D. Spielberger (Eds.), *Advances in personality assessment* (Vol. 4, pp. 31–54). Hillsdale, NJ: Erlbaum.

Costa, P. T., Jr., & McCrae, R. R. (1988). Personality in adulthood: A six-year longitudinal study of self-reports and spouse ratings on the NEO Personality Inventory. *Journal of Personality and Social Psychology, 54,* 853–863.

Costa, P. T., Jr., & McCrae, R. R. (1989). Personality continuity and the changes of adult life. In M. Storandt & G. R. VandenBos (Eds.), *The adult years: Continuity and change* (Vol. 8., pp. 41–77). Washington, DC: American Psychological Association.

Costa, P. T., Jr., & McCrae, R. R. (1994). Set like plaster? Evidence for the stability of adult personality. In T. F. Heatherton & J. L. Weinberger (Eds.), *Can personality change?* (pp. 21–40). Washington, DC: American Psychological Association.

Costa, P. T., Jr., McCrae, R. R., & Arenberg, D. (1980). Enduring dispositions in adult males. *Journal of Personality and Social Psychology, 38,* 793–800.

Daly, M., & Wilson, M. (1988). Evolutionary social psychology and family homicide. *Science, 242*(4878), 519–524.

Digman, J. M. (1990). Personality structure: Emergence of the five-factor model. *Annual Review of Psychology, 41,* 417–440.

Emmons, R. A., Diener, E., & Larsen, R. J. (1986). Choice and avoidance of everyday situations and affect congruence: Two models of reciprocal interactionism. *Journal of Personality and Social Psychology, 51*(4), 815–826.

Endler, N. S., & Magnusson, D. (1976). Toward an interactional psychology of personality. *Psychological Bulletin, 83*(5), 956–974.

Epstein, E., & Guttman, R. (1984). Mate selection in man: Evidence, theory, and outcome. *Social Biology, 31,* 243–278.

Eysenck, H. J. (1952). *The scientific study of personality.* London: Routledge & Kegan Paul.

Eysenck, H. J. (1967). *The biological basis of personality.* Springfield, IL: Thomas.

Finn, S. E. (1986). Stability of personality self-ratings over 30 years: Evidence for an age/cohort interaction. *Journal of Personality and Social Psychology, 50,* 813–818.

Floderus-Myrhed, B., Pedersen, N., & Rasmuson, I. (1980). Assessment of heritability for personality, based on a short form of the Eysenck Personality Inventory: A study of 12,898 twin pairs. *Behavior Genetics, 10,* 153–162.

Funder, D. C., & Block, J. (1989). The role of ego-control, ego-resiliency, and IQ in delay of gratification in adolescence. *Journal of Personality and Social Psychology, 57,* 1041–1050.

Goldberg, L. R. (1981). Language and individual differences: The search for universals in personality lexicons. In L. Wheeler (Ed.), *Review of personality and social psychology* (Vol. 2, pp. 141–165). Beverly Hills, CA: Sage.

Goldsmith, H. H., Buss, A. H., Plomin, R., Rothbart, M. K, Thomas, A., Chess, S., Hinde, R. A., & McCall, R. B. (1987). What is temperament? Four approaches. *Child Development, 58*(2) 505–529.

Haan, N., Millsap, R., & Hartka, E. (1986). As time goes by: Change and stability in personality over fifty years. *Psychology and Aging, 1,* 220–232.

Hartshorne, H., & May, M. A. (1928). *Studies in the nature of character: Studies in deceit.* New York: Macmillan.

Heatherton, T. F., & Nichols, P. A. (1994a). Personal accounts of successful versus failed attempts at life change. *Personality and Social Psychology Bulletin, 20*(6), 664–675.

Heatherton, T. F., & Nichols, P. A. (1994b). Conceptual issues in assessing whether personality can change. In T. F. Heatherton & J. L. Weinberger (Eds.), *Can personality change?* (pp. 3–18). Washington, DC: American Psychological Association.

Heatherton, T. F., & Polivy, J. (1991). Development and validation of a scale for measuring state self-esteem. *Journal of Personality and Social Psychology, 60,* 895–910.

Heatherton , T. F., & Weinberger, J. L. (1994). *Can personality change?* Washington, DC: American Psychological Association.

Helson, R. (1993). Comparing longitudinal studies of adult development: Toward a paradigm of tension between stability and change. In D. C. Funder, R. D. Parke, C. Tomlinson-Keasey, & K. Widaman (Eds.), *Studying lives through time: Personality and development* (pp. 93–120). Washington, DC: American Psychological Association.

Helson, R., Mitchell, V., & Moane, G. (1984). Personality and patterns of adherence and non-adherence to the social clock. *Journal of Personality and Social Psychology, 46,* 1079–1096.

Helson, R., & Moane, G. (1987). Personality change in women from college to midlife. *Journal of Personality and Social Psychology, 53,* 176–186.

Helson, R., & Stewart, A. (1994). Personality change in adulthood. In T. F. Heatherton & J. L. Weinberger (Eds.), *Can personality change?* (pp. 210–226). Washington, DC: American Psychological Association.

Henderson, N. D. (1982). Human behavior genetics. *Annual Review of Psychology, 33,* 403–440.

Howard, A., & Bray, D. (1988). *Managerial lives in transition: Advancing age and changing times.* New York: Guilford Press.

Huesmann, L. R., Eron, L. D., Lefkowitz, M. M., & Walder, L. O. (1984). Stability of aggression over time and generations. *Developmental Psychology, 20*(6), 1120–1134.

James, W. (1890). *Principles of psychology.* New York: Holt.

Jensen, A. R. (1978). Genetic and behavioral effects of non-random mating. In C. E. Noble, R. T. Osborne, N. Weyle (Eds.), *Human variation: Biogenetics of age, race, and sex* (pp. 51–105). New York: Academic Press.

John, O. P. (1990). The "big five" factor taxonomy: Dimensions of personality in the natural language and in questionnaires. In L. A. Pervin (Ed.), *Handbook of personality: Theory and research* (pp. 66–100). New York: Guilford Press.

Kagan, J. (1992). *Unstable ideas: Temperament, cognition, and self.* Cambridge, MA: Harvard University Press.

Kagan, J., & Moss, H. A. (1962). *From birth to maturity.* New York: Wiley.

Kagan, J., & Zentzer, M. (1996). Early childhood predictors of adult psychopathology. *Harvard Review of Psychiatry, 3*(6), 341–350.

Kandel, D. B. (1978). Similarity in real-life adolescent friendship pairs. *Journal of Personality and Social Psychology, 36*(3), 306–312.

Kenrick, D. T., & Stringfield, D. O. (1980). Personality traits and the eye of the beholder: Crossing some traditional philosophical boundaries in the search for consistency in all of the people. *Psychological Review, 87*(1), 88–104.

Klohnen, E.C., & Mendelsohn, G. A. (1997). Partner selection for personality characteristics: A couple-centered approach. *Personality and Social Psychology Bulletin, 24*(2), 268–278.

Kramer, P. D. (1993). *Listening to Prozac.* New York: Viking.

Loehlin, J. C. (1982). Are personality traits differentially heritable? *Behavior Genetics, 12*(4), 417–428.

Loehlin, J. C. (1989). Partitioning environmental and genetic contributions to behavioral development. *American Psychologist, 44,* 1285–1292.

Loehlin, J. C., & Nichols, R. C. (1976). *Heredity, environment, and personality.* Austin: University of Texas Press.

Loehlin, J. C., Willerman, L., & Horn, J. M. (1988). Human behavior genetics. In M. R. Rosenzweig & L. W. Porter (Eds.), *Annual review of psychology* (Vol. 39, pp. 101–133). Palo Alto, CA: Annual Reviews.

Marlatt, G. A. (1985). Cognitive factors in the relapse process. In G. A. Marlatt & J. R. Gordon (Eds.), *Relapse prevention: Maintenance strategies in the treatment of addictive behaviors* (pp. 128–200). New York: Guilford Press.

Matheny, A. P., Jr., & Dolan, A. B. (1975). Persons, situations, and time: A genetic view of behavioral change in children. *Journal of Personality and Social Psychology, 32,* 1106–1110.

McAdams, D. P. (1994). Can personality change? Levels of stability and growth in personality across the life span. In T. F. Heatherton & J. L. Weinberger (Eds.), *Can personality change?* (pp. 299–314). Washington, DC: American Psychological Association.

McCrae, R. R., & Costa, P. T. (1986). Personality, coping, and coping effectiveness in an adult sample. *Journal of Personality, 54*(2), 385–405.

McCrae, R. R., & Costa, P. T., Jr. (1990). *Personality in adulthood.* New York: Guilford Press.

McCrae, R. R., & John, O. P. (1992). An introduction to the five-factor model and its applications. Special Issue: The five-factor model: Issues and applications. *Journal of Personality, 60*(2), 175–215.

McGue, M., Bacon, S., & Lykken, D. T. (1993). Personality stability and change in early adulthood: A behavioral genetic analysis. *Developmental Psychology, 29*(1), 96–109.

Miller, W. R., & C'deBaca, J. (1994). Quantum change: Toward a psychology of transformation. In T. F. Heatherton & J. L. Weinberger (Eds.), *Can personality change?* (pp. 253–280). Washington, DC: American Psychological Association.

Mischel, W. (1968). *Personality and assessment.* New York: Wiley.

Mischel, W., Shoda, Y., & Peake, P. K. (1988). The nature of adolescent competencies predicted by preschool delay of gratification. *Journal of Personality and Social Psychology, 54*(4), 687–696.

Mischel, W., Shoda, Y., & Rodriguez, M. L. (1989). Delay of gratification in children. *Science, 244,* 933–938.

Monson, T. C., Hesley, J. W., & Chernick, L. (1982). Specifying when personality traits can and cannot predict behavior: An alternative to abandoning the attempt to predict single-act criteria. *Journal of Personality and Social Psychology, 43*(2), 385–399.

Moskowitz, D. S., Brown, K. W., & Cote, S. (1997). Reconceptualizing stability: Using time as a psychological dimension. *Current Directions in Psychological Science, 6*(5), 127–132.

Moskowitz, D. S., & Schwartzman, A. E. (1989). Painting group portraits: Studying life outcomes for aggressive and withdrawn children. *Journal of Personality, 57*(4), 723–746.

Moss, H. A., & Susman, E. J. (1980). Longitudinal study of personality development. In O. G. Brim, Jr. & J. Kagan (Eds.), *Constancy and change in human development* (pp. 530–595). Cambridge, MA: Harvard University Press.

Nesselroade, J. R., & Boker, S. M. (1994). Assessing constancy and change. In T. F. Heatherton & J. L. Weinberger (Eds.), *Can personality change?* (pp. 121–148). Washington, DC: American Psychological Association.

Newcomb, T. M. (1961). *The acquaintance process.* New York: Wiley.

Olweus, D. (1979). Stability of aggressive reaction patterns in males: A review. *Psychological Bulletin, 86,* 852–875.

OSS Assessment Staff. (1948). *Assessment of men.* New York: Rinehart.

Ozer, D. J., & Gjerde, P. F. (1989). Patterns of personality consistency and change from childhood through adolescence. *Journal of Personality, 57,* 483–507.

Pervin, L. A. (1984). *Current controversies and issues in personality.* New York: Wiley.

Pervin, L. A. (1985). Personality: Current controversies, issues, and directions. *Annual Review of Psychology, 36,* 83–114.

Plomin, R., DeFries, J. C., & Loehlin, J. C. (1977). Genotype–environment interaction and correlation in the analysis of human behavior. *Psychological Bulletin, 84,* 309–322.

Plomin, R., & Rowe, D. C. (1979). Genetic and environmental etiology of social behavior in infancy. *Developmental Psychology, 15*(2), 62–72.

Roberts, B. W. (1997). Plaster or plasticity: Are adult work experiences associated with personality change in women? *Journal of Personality, 65*(2), 205–232.

Santoro, J., & Spiers, M . (1994). Social cognitive factors in brain injury-associated personality change. *Brain Injury, 8*(3), 265–276.

Scarr, S., & McCartney, K. (1983). How people make their own environments: A theory of genotype-environment correlations. *Child Development, 54,* 424–435.

Schwartz, C. E., Snidman, N., & Kagan, J. (1996). Early childhood temperament as a determinant of externalizing behavior in adolescence. *Development and Psychopathology, 8*(3), 527–537.

Siegler, I. C., George, L. K., & Okun, M. A. (1979). Cross-sequential analysis of adult personality. *Developmental Psychology, 15*(3), 350–351.

Snyder, M., & Ickes, W. (1985). Personality and social behavior. In G. Lindzey & E. Aronson (Eds.), *Handbook of social psychology (3rd ed.). Vol. II: Special fields and applications* (pp. 883–947). New York: Random House.

Tellegen, A., Lykken, D. J., Bouchard, T. J., Jr., Wilcox, K. J., Segal, N. L., & Rich, S. (1988). Personality similarity in twins reared apart and together. *Journal of Personality and Social Psychology, 54,* 1031–1039.

Theissen, D., & Gregg, B. (1980). Human assortative mating and genetic equilibrium: An evolutionary perspective. *Ethology and Sociobiology, 1,* 111–140.

Thomas, A. T., & Chess, S. (1984). Genesis and evolution of behavioral disorders: From infancy to early adult life. *American Journal of Psychiatry, 141*(1), 1–9.

Thorne, A. (1989). Conditional patterns, transference, and the coherence of personality across time. In D. M. Buss & N. Cantor (Eds.), *Personality psychology: Recent trends and emerging directions* (pp. 149–159). New York: Springer-Verlag.

Trivers, R. L. (1972). Parental investment and sexual selection. In B. Campbell (Ed.), *Sexual selection and the descent of man: 1871–1971* (pp. 136–179). Chicago: Aldine.

Vaillant, G. E. (1977). *Adaptation to life.* Boston: Little, Brown.

Vandenberg, S. G. (1972). Assortative mating, or who marries whom? *Genetics, 2*(2–3), 127–157.

Vaughan, D. (1986). *Uncoupling.* New York: Basic Books.

Wiggins, J. S., & Pincus, A. L. (1992). Personality: Structure and assessment. *Annual Review of Psychology, 43,* 473–504.

Wiggins, J. S., & Trapnell, P. D. (1997). Personality structure: The return of the big five. In R. Hogan, J. A. Johnson, & S. R. Briggs (Eds.), *Handbook of personality psychology* (pp. 737–765). San Diego, CA: Academic Press.

Wink, P., & Helson, R. (1993). Personality change in women and their partners. *Journal of Personality and Social Psychology, 65,* 597–605.

Woodruff, D. S., & Birren, J. E. (1972). Age changes and cohort difference in personality. *Developmental Psychology, 6*(2), 252–259.

CHAPTER 12

Natural History and Long-Term Outcome

MICHAEL H. STONE

Personality disorders have been with us since earliest times. Yet, in the annals of psychiatry, they have become a "hot topic" only in the past generation. Interest in personality disorders was spurred greatly by their inclusion in a special section (Axis II) in the third edition of the American Psychiatric Association's (1980) *Diagnostic and Statistical Manual of Mental Disorders* (DSM-III), published in 1980. Also important were the personality types outlined in the ninth edition of the *International Classification of Diseases* (ICD-9; World Health Organization, 1977). Before DSM-III there was little unity in the realm of personality taxonomy. What we would now call the milder disorders of personality were often treated by psychoanalysts—who referred to these conditions as "character disorders." The psychoanalytic nomenclature derived from the pioneering works of Freud, Abraham and Wilhelm Reich. Among the various types described by Reich in the late 1920s (published along with several unrelated works in 1949) were the passive–feminine, the aristocratic, the hysterical, the compulsive, the phallic–narcissistic, and the masochistic. The passive–feminine type corresponds roughly to contemporary descriptions of the *avoidant* and *dependent* personality disorders. The aristocratic and phallic–narcissistic overlap with DSM's narcissistic personality disorder. The hysterical character disorder as formulated in the psychoanalytic community over-

laps with DSM's *histrionic* personality disorder, in that both refer to highly expressive and dramatic modes of self-presentation. But histrionic personality disorder describes a more serious disorder, akin to what Easser and Lesser (1965) called "hysteroid" and Kernberg (1967) called "infantile," or "hysteric personality functioning at the borderline level of personality organization." In histrionic personality disorder one encounters more impulsivity and hostility than would be typical of the hysteric, and a less secure sense of identity. The descriptions of compulsive character or personality do not differ greatly, although the compulsive patients of the earlier generation of psychoanalysts tended to be inhibited persons—not as routinely controlling and mean-spirited as those who conform to DSM's obsessive–compulsive personality disorder. Similarly, the "sadistic" characters of the older literature were more apt to speak of sadistic fantasies on the couch (Reich 1949, p. 199), whereas the sadistic persons of DSM-III were, by definition, outwardly cruel toward others (whether intimates or strangers).

In hospital-based psychiatry (in contrast to the ambulatory nature of the analyst's caseload) the term "personality disorder" (or the equivalent) was already in use at the turn of the century. Kraepelin (1905), and later, Kurt Schneider (1959), spoke of "*psychopathische Persoenlichkeiten*." Here, the term "psychopathic" had only the connotation of its Greek roots: *mental-*

ly ill. Although both Kraepelin and Schneider described antisocial and callous types among their many varieties, it is only in recent years, owing in large part to the influential works of Cleckley (1972) and Robert Hare (1993), that "psychopathic" has taken on the serious overtones of remorselessness, emotional coldness, and lack of conscience that give the term its special applicability in forensic psychiatric work.

Many of the personality types in Schneider's taxonomy resemble those of DSM and ICD in their recent editions. Corresponding to Schneider's fanatic type is our paranoid type; to his *attention seeking,* our *histrionic;* to his *affectionless,* our *antisocial* and *psychopathic types;* and so on. Elsewhere, I have shown the similarities between the 10 Schneider categories and those of DSM (Stone, 1993a).

As for the natural history and outcome of personality disorders, it quickly becomes apparent that these divide into two broad groups: one that relates primarily to fairly well-functioning persons who, if they seek psychiatric help at all, do so within the confines of private offices or outpatient clinics, and a sicker group of persons who sometimes require institutional (including forensic-hospital) care. The former group answers mainly to *inhibited* persons of the sort who were—and continue to be—treated by psychoanalysts and by other practitioners of verbal psychotherapy. This group includes the majority of avoidant, compulsive, dependent, hysteric, and masochistic persons, belonging at least in spirit to DSM's "anxious" cluster (Cluster C currently includes only the first three), and manifesting the characteristics of Cloninger's (1986) "harm-avoidant" temperament. The more dysfunctional personality-disordered patients often exhibit either *uninhibited* personality styles (e.g., antisocial, psychopathic, and sadistic) or else the socially awkward styles of DSM's "eccentric" Cluster (Cluster A: paranoid, schizoid, and schizotypal disorders).

Straddling these larger groups is the numerically smaller but psychiatrically important group of *narcissistic* and *borderline* disorders. Depending on the definitions used and on the severity of the disorder in any given patient, some will be amenable to the various forms of ambulatory care; others may require hospital or other forms of institutional treatment. Both narcissistic and borderline personality disorder's have been placed in DSM's "dramatic" Cluster (Cluster B)—which is appropriate enough for borderline personality disorder but less so for narcissistic personality disorder. Many narcissistic patients, as it turns out, are not at all "dramatic" and may even be shy and self-effacing. These are the "aristocratic" (fussy, compulsive, and un-self-confident) persons whom Reich described. In contrast, antisocial and psychopathic persons, all of whom by definition have narcissistic traits (they are all intensely egocentric) can be placed in the dramatic cluster with greater confidence.

From the standpoint of natural history, we can conjecture—before we even look at the follow-up data—that the inhibited, ambulatory persons start out at a generally higher level on measures of life function, whether their ultimate trajectory is flat (there is no significant improvement) or ascending (significant improvement occurs with treatment or with time). The impulsive, uninhibited (and especially the antisocial/psychopathic/sadistic) group generally start out at a lower level of overall function. Narcissistic persons can be found at all levels of function initially, whereas borderline patients, occupy at the outset of their life course—an intermediate level of function: They usually are more capable of social (and even intimate) relationships than are Cluster A persons, though they are often less successful initially in the interpersonal sphere than are the harm-avoidant types.

FOLLOW-UP STUDIES OF PATIENTS WITH PERSONALITY DISORDERS

Thus far in the literature there is a certain unrepresentative quality to follow-up studies in this area. To begin with, research has focused more on the most difficult of personality disorders. These are the disorders that, because they are so challenging from a therapeutic standpoint, stimulate the most interest within the psychiatric community. Much more has been written about outcome in borderline patients, for this reason, than about avoidant or dependent patients. Antisociality serves as another "attractor" because of the profound and adverse effects antisocial persons exert on society. When we turn our attention to antisocial, let alone psychopathic and sadistic persons, we are actually dealing with "patients" only occasionally—because most such persons do not come voluntarily for our help: They thus have personality disorders but generally not "patienthood." If they are seen by psychiatrists at all, it will customarily be in some forensic setting. As for the healthier and socially more appropriately functioning persons—with the milder personality disorders—who seek the help of psychotherapists in ambulatory settings, they have "patienthood" but are rarely the subjects of follow-up studies. Therapists in clinics and private offices almost never contact their former patients from many years past because of concerns about intrusiveness. Concerns about confidentiality militate against the use of objective raters in evaluating former private patients years later, but this means that methodical studies of former analytic and other psychotherapy patients are almost never attempted. An ironical result of this situation is that we know a fair amount about the fate of the most severe personality disorders, who constitute a numerically small group, and little about the long-term outcome of the vastly larger group of persons who exhibit the milder personality disorders.

THE NATURAL HISTORY OF PERSONALITY DISORDERS IN THE ANTISOCIAL REALM

I am choosing here for didactic purposes to speak of an "antisocial realm" embracing antisocial personality disorder as defined in DSM; psychopathy, as defined by Hare et al. (1990); and sadistic personality disorder, as defined in the Appendix of DSM-III. There is often considerable overlap among these distinctions, as all but a few persons scoring high on the Psychopathy Checklist also behave in antisocial ways, and all sadistic psychopaths (including recidivist rapists and serial killers, for example) are by definition antisocial. Because the definition of antisocial personality disorder in DSM-III-R (American Psychiatric Association, 1987) and DSM-IV (American Psychiatric Association, 1994) rely heavily on certain behaviors (e.g., performing acts that are grounds for arrest) and, in the earlier versions especially, less so on extreme narcissistic traits, it is possible to have antisocial personality disorder without being psychopathic. This means that antisocial personality disorder constitutes a large and heterogeneous group, as Hare (1996) has pointed out: the natural history of persons with antisocial personality disorder is correspondingly diverse.

In the studies of a generation ago, there were several comparatively brief follow-up reports (1½ to 6 years) of antisocial persons. This was before the era of the Hare Psychopathy Checklist—Revised (PCL-R; Hare et al., 1990), so rigorous distinctions had not been made between (1) psychopaths and (2) persons who were antisocial without scoring high on the PCL-R. Maddocks (1970) noted that in a 5-year follow-up, impulsivity had not changed appreciably but there was less recidivism (with regard to unlawful behavior). Martin, Cloninger, and Guze (1979) looked at a group of female antisocial persons, and found that about three-fourths (19 of 26) could still be considered antisocial 6 years later. Most of the antisocial patients followed briefly (average = 1½ years) by Robins, Gentry, Muñoz, and Marten (1977) were still "antisocial" (54 of 57) at trace time.

Perry (1988) noted stability of the *impulsivity* trait in antisocial persons, diagnosed by DSM-III criteria, though the follow-up time-interval was brief: 1 to 3 years. Black, Baumgard, and Bell (1995), in their 16- to 45-year follow-up of antisocial men (also using DSM-III criteria), reported little change in life course or diagnosis. High psychiatric comorbidity and persistent legal difficulties were common in their group. A similar pessimism was registered by Gabbard and Coyne (1987) in their study of 33 antisocial patients (DSM-III criteria) formerly admitted to the Menninger Clinic: At follow-up, 19 had been "completely unresponsive to treatment" (p. 1183), 21 had left hospital prematurely and against advice, and only 5 had met initial treatment goals. A history of previous felony arrest or a history of "conning" (manipulative deceitfulness) augured for a poor prognosis. Another predictor of poor outcome was early onset of dyssocial behavior during childhood (age 8 being a typical onset of severe conduct disorder in those who manifest this difficulty) (Offord & Reitsma-Street, 1983). In a study of incarcerated rapists, Rice, Harris, and Quinsey (1990), from the forensic hospital in Penatenguishene, Ontario, noted that the men who did not fulfill DSM-III criteria for antisocial personality disorder showed less recidivism on release than did those who met these criteria. In a recent study Dinwiddie and Daw (1998) assessed the temporal stability of antisocial personality disorder (as diagnosed by DSM-III-R; American Psychiatric Association, 1987). Narrow and broad definitions of antisocial personality disorder were made at initial evaluation and at 8-year follow-up. Their kappa values ranged from .31 to .68 (the more restrictive criteria yielding the lower kappas and "less" stability). The authors concluded that antisocial personality disorder showed considerable stability over time, when the attempt was not made to attribute the cause of individual symptoms to alcohol abuse.

More optimistically, Arboleda-Florez and Holley (1991) noted a tendency for criminality to decrease ("antisocial burnout") in their long-term (25- to 51-year) follow-up of patients diagnosed according to DSM-III-R criteria. Robins, Tipp, and Przybeck (1991) reported comparable findings in their epidemiological/follow-up study of (DSM-III) antisocial adolescents: Years later, only 47% had arrest records; only 37% still met antisocial personality disorder criteria.

In my long-term follow-up study of patients hospitalized with borderline and other personality disorders, or else with various psychoses (the "PI-500" study: Stone, 1990), there were some 13 patients with borderline personality disorder (by DSM-III) who were comorbid for antisocial personality disorder. There were another 7 who were borderline only by Kernberg criteria ("borderline personality organization"; Kernberg, 1967), who met criteria for antisocial personality disorder—but for borderline personality disorder. Not surprisingly, the borderline × antisocial personality disorder group had poorer outcomes (borderline personality disorder emphasizes self-destructive acts, inordinate anger, etc., and constitutes a more disturbed condition than borderline personality organization): Three committed suicide and only one reached a trace-time Global Assesment Scale (GAS) score (Endicott, Spitzer, Fleiss, & Cohen, 1967) above 60. One of the suicides concerned a former adolescent adoptee raised in a non-abusive home—who committed arson on several occasions. He was imprisoned briefly for one such offense, and when he was about to be apprehended for another arson, he jumped out his apartment window. The "best" borderline × antisocial personality disorder patient was one who had been alcoholic as an adolescent, and in continual trouble with the law for driving while intoxicated and petty larceny. He joined Alcoholics Anonymous in his 30s, became abstemious, worked his way up to a managerial post in a business, married, and is currently (30 years later) doing very well. One of the borderline personality organization × anti-

social personality disorder patients, also in trouble since adolescence, had run away from home after his mother died, and his father remarried to an abusive stepmother. This man became a heroin addict—and had a near-death experience after an overdose. He joined Narcotics Anonymous, became a lecturer to youth groups, warning youths against the dangers of drugs, and is currently married with two children. We did not appreciate it at the time (either when these last two men had been hospitalized, nor when traced years later), but neither would have scored in the "psychopathic" range on the Hare PCL-R. Both, as I had mentioned elsewhere (Stone, 1993b), were "of decent character, forced by parental rejection to take to the streets and survive by their wits" (p. 306). Altogether, six of the antisocial patients (one with borderline personality disorder; five with borderline personality organization) are now clinically well. They partook of the kind of spontaneous remission—once they passed age 40—Robins et al. (1991) had noted in their series. These favorable outcomes also reflect another factor discussed in the forensic literature: Among youthful delinquents, some are "continuous antisocials" with a higher loading of negative genetic and environmental influences who persist over the years in antisocial (including criminal) activity (Dilalla & Gottesman, 1990). There are also transitorily antisocial delinquents who do not go on to have criminal careers as adults. As Myner, Santman, Cappelletty, and Perlmutter (1998) mention, an *early age at first conviction* and a *history of (early) alcohol abuse* arc strong indicators of recidivism in juvenile offenders.

To get a better picture of the impact of psychopathy, in contrast to "antisociality" as diagnosed by DSM, it is necessary to tease apart the cases meeting Hare's criteria from the larger field of antisocial personality disorder cases, with which psychopathy is (especially in the pre-1980 literature) often conflated. Depending on the site and sample, PCL-R scores of 25 or more, or 30, or more are used to define *psychopathy*. The presence of this factor appears now to be the strongest predictor of continuing criminal violence (after release) in persons incarcerated for violent offenses (Quinsey, 1995). Other important factors included elementary school maladjustment (bully boys at 8 often became criminals at 28), age (early) at index offense, and a history of having been separated from parent(s) before age 16 (Villeneuve &

Quinsey, 1995). Lykken (1995) emphasizes fatherlessness as a key factor, inasmuch as boys reared without a father (or with very little contact with a law-abiding father) are much more at risk for committing offenses and for developing at least "secondary" (i.e., predominantly environment-driven) psychopathy. Many recent studies attest to the power of the PCL-R to predict (e.g., in the high-scoring psychopathic offenders) future recidivism and, particularly, future violence in those with an earlier record of violent crimes (Hart, 1998). Hart also outlined various factors that contributed to the decision to act violently. These include biological factors such as high testosterone, low central nervous system serotonin, and head injury; psychological factors such as psychosis, personality disorder, and cognitive impairment; and social factors such as exposure to violent role models and "machismo" (p. 357). The heightened risk for violent recidivism, given a high PCL-R score, was underlined by Hemphill, Templeman, Wong, and Hare (1998), who noted that whereas about half the released offenders with low PCL-R scores reoffended within 10 years of release, 80% of those with scores 30 (out of a possible 40) and over had reoffended—mostly within the first 3 years. The follow-up data of Serin and Amos (1995) also support the position that high PCL-R scores predict violent recidivism in psychopaths: In an average follow-up period of 5½ years, 35% of those with scores > 30 reoffended, in contrast to 5% for those with scores < 10, and 15% for those with intermediate (21–30) scores.

An interesting sidelight on the psychopathy factor concerns alcoholism: Though alcohol abuse is a common accompaniment of psychopathy, treatment for alcohol abuse in institutional settings seemed not to reduce the likelihood of violent recidivism in psychopathic detainees (Rice & Harris, 1995, p. 339).

In general, follow-up reports concerning antisocial and, particularly, psychopathic offenders need to be read with the caveat that persons convicted repeatedly of the most serious violent felonies tend not to be released once apprehended. There could be no ethical justification for releasing, for example, serial killers such as Ted Bundy, Jerry Brudos, or Ian Brady (Stone, 1993a), simply to put Hare's checklist to the test. By the same token, recidivism figures tend, if anything, to be conservative, because some released offenders, especially the more organized and cautious psychopaths, reoffend without being recaptured or commit many more crimes than are known to the authorities (Yochelson & Samenow, 1976).

Some recent work in the child psychiatric literature suggests that a subgroup of latency-age and early-adolescent children exists in whom "callous and unemotional" traits are prominent. These callous, unemotional children exhibited a greater number of conduct disturbances, a stronger history of parental antisociality, and a stronger history of police contacts than did other groups of conduct-disordered children who did not show the extreme callous unemotionality (Christian, Frick, Hill, Tyler, & Frazer, 1997). These callous, unemotional children not only showed a pattern of severe antisocial behavior but also resembled closely the kinds of persons designated "psychopaths" in the adult forensic literature. Long-term studies as to the fate of these young persons over time are not yet available.

In sum, contemporary research on the extreme narcissistic traits now subsumed under Hare's "Factor-I" (a subset of the descriptors in the 20-item PCL-R) is proving useful in distinguishing persons within the broad antisocial realm whose prognosis is somewhat encouraging (at least in their later years)—from others (psychopaths high on Factor-1 traits) whose prognosis is bleak. Ascertaining whether this proves true even of the callous, unemotional children with conduct disorder studied by Christian and her coworkers will (because of its forensic implications) be an important task for future follow-up investigation.

As for sadistic personality, one can only speak about *natural history,* as the effects of therapy can scarcely be measured in a condition that is largely untreatable, because it is found in persons who (for all intents and purposes) never come for help. Sadistic personality, as defined in DSM-III, is common among the murderers whose cases became the subject of a full-length biography in my series—which now includes 312 examples. The men in this series are twice as likely as the women to meet sadistic personality disorder criteria (84% as against 42%). Men committing serial sexual homicide ("serial killers") are almost all sadistic and psychopathic. Sadistic personality, in the typical case, germinates in adolescence in the form of sadistic sexual/paraphilic fantasies, which get acted out at first on animals (cats being the favorite target) and later on women (or in the rarer cases of homosexual serial homicide, men).

Given that the sadistic violation of their victims goes on unabated until capture (which sometimes does not occur before several years have gone by), there is little reason to assume that sadistic personality disorder "burns out" with the passage of time. None of the 80 serial killers in my series had ever sought treatment. The same could be said for the many men in my biography series who sadistically controlled, subjugated, and eventually killed their wives. The case of Fred and Sara Tokars (McDonald, 1998) is exemplary: Throughout the 7 years of their marriage, the prominent (but corrupt) attorney controlled every movement of his wife and every penny he doled out to her, progressed from verbal to physical abuse, and finally hired a "hitman" to kill her when she sued for divorce. His sadistic traits showed "stability"— even augmentation—over time, and he would have scoffed at the idea of "getting help."

FOLLOW-UP STUDIES IN THE BORDERLINE DOMAIN

Rivaling, if not equaling, in size—the literature on antisocial personality is the literature on borderline personality. Much of the latter has been reviewed in my book on the long-term follow-up of borderline patients (Stone, 1990). Briefly, the pre-DSM-III studies (Grinker, Werble, & Drye, 1968) used less methodical diagnostic criteria and tended to rely on comparatively small samples, in which the patients were traced after intervals of generally 2 to 5 years at most, and in which the trace rates seldom reached the 80% levels required if meaningful results are to be extracted.

The best study of this pre-1980 period was that of Gunderson, Carpenter, and Strauss (1975); a 2-year follow-up of 24 inpatients diagnosed borderline by the criteria of Gunderson and Singer (1975), who were compared with 29 schizophrenic patients. When only 2 years had gone by after discharge, the two groups of patients both functioned poorly, about equally so, in the areas of social adjustment, work history, and sexual relations. By 5 years, however, some divergence was apparent: The patients who were borderline showed better social adjustment and a trend toward better function and stability in the workplace, compared with the patients with schizophrenia (Carpenter, Gunderson, & Strauss, 1977). Improvement at work, with continuing social impairment had

been noted in an earlier study (a 3- to 5-year follow-up), using less rigorous diagnostic criteria, by Werble (1970).

The appearance in DSM-III (American Psychiatric Association, 1980) of *borderline personality disorder*—whose criteria, albeit polythetic, were more standardized and objectifiable than most preexisting criteria (apart from those of Gunderson & Singer, 1975, some of whose items, along with others of Kernberg, 1967, were amalgamated into the DSM criteria)—stimulated the follow-up work of the late 1980s. The largest of these studies were those of McGlashan (1985, 1986a, 1986b), with 81 traced patients with borderline personality disorder; Plakun, Burckhardt, and Muller (1985), with 63 patients with borderline personality disorder; Paris, Brown, and Nowlis (1987), with 100 cases, and my "PI-500" series (Stone, Hurt, & Stone, 1987; Stone, 1990), based on 299 inpatients meeting Kernberg's (1967) criteria for borderline personality organization. Of the latter, 206 also met DSM-III criteria for borderline personality disorder. The highest trace rates were achieved in McGlashan's (1986a) Chestnut Lodge study (86%) and in the PI-500 study (95%). The follow-up intervals in all these studies converged around the 15-year mark, with some patients having been located after 25 or even 30 years. All had originally been hospitalized patients. Convergence was also noted in the major studies as to global outcome (as estimated, for example, by the GAS of Endicott et al., 1967). About two-thirds of the former patients with borderline personality disorder were functioning at trace time in the GAS range of 61–70 or better. This meant they were only minimally symptomatic, in need of little therapy, able to work fairly well, though with some restrictions in their interpersonal life (GAS 61–70), or else "clinically recovered" (GAS > 70)—functioning at levels scarcely distinguishable from the general population. Among the third with poorer outcomes, some had already died from suicide. The rate was 3% in McGlashan's series and 9% in Paris's series and the PI-500. An important factor accounting for the difference was the age when first admitted: The Chestnut Lodge patients had been 26 on average when admitted; those of the PI-500 and of Paris's Montreal studies had been younger (about 22). Because, as it turned out, the late 20s was a high-risk age for suicide, the younger patients had more high-risk years to get through than was the case for the somewhat older Chestnut Lodge patients. At all events, the suicide risk in borderline personality disorder was comparable to that of schizophrenia and affective disorders (Stone et al., 1987), even though the majority of the patients with borderline personality disorder did much better than the patients with schizophrenia at trace times of 10 years or longer.

The life trajectory typical of the patients with borderline personality disorder in both the Chestnut Lodge and the PI-500 studies was that of a "ladle-shaped" curve, with a "dip" throughout the 20s, followed by a steady and stable improvement in function throughout the 30s and beyond. The patients with borderline personality disorder who remained chronically angry, however, tended to alienate those on whom they depended for emotional support. Such persons often experienced a downturn once again in their mid-40s, generally in connection with having finally worn out the patience of a spouse or other sexual partner.

Female patients with borderline personality disorder tended also to have been significantly depressed when first hospitalized; the males were more apt to show a mixture of antisocial features alongside the borderline attributes. Not surprisingly, the females tended to outperform their male counterparts at trace time. Also, the females were much more likely to have married and to have had children (though still only to rates half that of the general population) than were the males. The patients of the Chestnut Lodge and PI studies came from middle-class to upper-class backgrounds; many at trace time had become doctors, lawyers, social workers, psychologists, artists, musicians, accountants, and religious leaders, and there were even a few cheif executive officers. A few, however, had become drifters, or persons working at menial jobs; four males in the PI series had become murderers.

The large number of patients in the PI series could be subdivided into four main groups: those with borderline personality disorder × major affective disorder (the largest group); those with borderline personality disorder but no major affective disorder; those with borderline personality organization × major affective disorder (who would be called *dysthymic* in contemporary nosology); and those with borderline personality organization but no major affective disorder (most of whom were comorbid for other personality disorders, including schizotypal, antisocial, and histrionic). The

"dysthymic" group (similar to the Type-IV "anaclitic-depressed" group in Grinker's [1968] study) outperformed all the others: 75% were functioning at GAS > 60; none of the 34 traced (of an original 36) had committed suicide. This result is not surprising when we consider that patients who meet borderline personality organization criteria but fail to meet borderline personality disorder criteria generally lack the *self-destructive, inordinately angry* and *stormy relationship* items of the DSM definition.

In the series with the high trace rates, it was possible to tease out certain patient variables that either augured for a poor or a better than average prognosis and life course. I set forth these variables *in extenso* elsewhere (Stone, 1990, p. 207). Although the verbal IQs of the patients in both the Chestnut Lodge and PI series were high (average = 118), those with IQs > 130 did better than the group as a whole. Some of these former patients were still socially awkward or abrasive but able to hold down positions in mathematics, computing, or other high-tech areas that assured them a livelihood, even if their interpersonal lives were somewhat meager or ungratifying. The same was true for patients with borderline personality disorder who had notable artistic abilities (in music, art, dance, or writing). There were many patients with borderline personality disorder who abused alcohol, but those who joined, and who remained with, Alcoholics Anonymous all made excellent adjustments. Two other factors were also highly "protective" and were correlated with better than average outcomes: strong self-discipline and (in the female patients) physical beauty.

A number of other factors were associated with a poor outcome years later. Female patients with borderline personality disorder who had been victims of incest by a relative of the older generation (uncle, father, stepfather, etc.) had a heightened risk for suicide and tended to function only in the "marginal to fair" range (GAS = 41–60) when traced 10 to 25 years later. Subsequently, Paris (1994) noted in his study that incest when it involved penile penetration was associated with a poorer prognosis than when less severe forms of incest had taken place. van der Kolk (1996) has shown that the impact of incest is greater when the child victim is 10 years old or younger, compared with children who were first abused in adolescence. The association between sexual abuse in childhood and adult borderline personality disorder is stronger than for other personality disorders (Zanarini, Gunderson, Marino, Schwartz, & Frankenburg, 1989).

Other negative factors include parental brutality, antisocial traits, and chaotic impulsivity. Patients who met all eight items of the DSM-III borderline personality disorder definition tended to be extremely impulsive and reckless (e.g., allowing themselves to be picked up by strangers, and then being raped). These were often the same patients who had been incest victims in their early years—who were now unwittingly living out the victim role again (in what van der Kolk, 1989, refers to as "revictimization").

The majority of patients with borderline personality disorder, as mentioned, ended up a decade or more later with good outcomes and often outgrew their borderline personality disorder diagnosis. That is, having established more harmonious (rather than "stormy") relationships, becoming less angry, and no longer making suicidal acts, they no longer met five or more borderline personality disorder criteria. Similarly, many of the patients with borderline personality organization began to solidify in their sense of identity so that they in time "graduated" to the higher ("neurotic") level of personality organization and thus were not "borderline" by Kernberg's criteria either (Stone, 1990). borderline personality disorder has been noted by others as well not to manifest the stability over time that one assumes is characteristic of personality disorders (Grilo, McGlashan, & Oldham, 1998). The explanation for this counterintuitive result lies in the heavy reliance of the DSM definition of borderline personality disorder on symptoms (e.g., self-damaging acts and mood lability) rather than on pure personality traits (e.g., tactfulness or stinginess, which seldom change much over the life cycle).

Despite the agreement among the borderline personality disorder follow-up studies of the 1980s, one must keep in mind that these were not representative of the entire population of patients with borderline personality disorder (to say nothing of those from distinctly different cultures). There are many persons in the community who manifest all the signs of borderline personality disorder but who never present themselves to the mental health profession. There are others treated by private practitioners, who rarely report on the long-term follow-up of their former patients. Finally, there are patients with borderline personality disorder who live in reduced circumstances and struggle with many more disadvantages than the traced, relatively high-socioeconomic status borderlines of the studies cited previously. I have elsewhere reported on the outcomes of my own borderline patients seen in private practice since 1966 (Stone, 1995, 1997), 75% of whom (45 of 60) were traced at intervals ranging from 5 to 25 years. As with the inpatient series of the 1980s, two-thirds are now functioning at the level of GAS 61 or better. Among those with unfavorable outcomes were seven patients with borderline personality disorder seen only in consultation: Two were provocative women who were murdered by their husbands; two committed suicide some years later; one died while driving under the influence of alcohol.

Patients with borderline personality disorder who had been raised with the multiple disadvantages of poverty, abuse, neglect, meager education, and poor work skills have thus far not been the subjects of methodical, long-term outcome study. Unfortunately, there are many such patients, treated generally in low-cost or free clinics by overworked staff members who have little to provide for their patients beyond sympathy and pills. Having worked for 2 years in such a clinic (at Middletown Psychiatric Center in New York State), I can testify that fully 64% of the female patients with borderline personality disorder had been incest victims—and that few, even in their 30s, 40s, or 50s, ever escaped the misery of their earlier years. These were not the patients about whom Allen Frances was able to write (in the foreword of my 1990 book), "Dr. Stone has discovered that borderline patients tend to get better if only they live long enough" (p. vii). Nor was I aware of their typical life course when I wrote the book. Thus I would have to amend my original remarks to the effect that an optimistic outcome is indeed the lot of many borderline patients—as there also exists a large group, reared without love or money, crushed by maltreatment at the hands of their "caretakers," who can never look forward to the mellowing and the surcease of symptoms enjoyed by their better-off counterparts.

FOLLOW-UP AND NATURAL HISTORY OF OTHER PERSONALITY DISORDERS

Schizotypal Personality Disorder

There appears to be a closer relationship between schizophrenia and schizotypal personality disorder than is the case with other putative "spectrum" personality disorders: paranoid or schizoid (Siever, Bernstein, & Silverman, 1989; Stone, 1985). Schizotypal persons are, in general, more anxious than are paranoid and schizoid patients (granted that admixtures of the traits belonging to these disorders are more common than "prototypical" cases). As such, they are more apt to seek help, and as a result, therapists have more experience with schizotypal than with the other two "eccentric cluster" (DSM) disorders; there is, correspondingly, a larger literature devoted to the life course of schizotypal persons.

In my long-term follow-up series there were 16 schizotypal patients, of whom I could locate 14. Six of the 14 were comorbid for borderline personality disorder. Thus there is some arbitrariness in placing them here. This is a reflection of a common problem in writing about personality disorders: Mixtures are more the rule than the exception, so that classification depends on the preponderance, not on the uniformity, of one's traits. These more-schizotypal-than-borderline patients, at all events, fell more into the marginal-to-fair outcome levels (four of the six) than into the GAS > 60 level—but the numbers are too small to permit generalization. As for the whole group of 14 traced schizotypal patients, they were less likely to have good outcomes than were patients with borderline personality disorder. Less flamboyant than the borderlines, the schizotypals tended to lead constricted lives, with few friends but with fewer of the "crises" so routine among the patients with borderline personality disorder. In the Chestnut Lodge study, McGlashan (1986a) found that the "pure" schizotypal patients (not comorbid for borderline personality disorder) functioned only slightly better than those with schizophrenia: Their social and occupational success was considerably below what one would expect from their non-personality-disordered age mates.

Schizotypal personality disorder seems more common in Scandinavian countries than in the United States. The majority of the 50 patients with "borderline" disorder whose long-term (20-year) follow-up was reported by Tove Aarkrog (1981, 1993) in Copenhagen would be considered schizotypal by DSM criteria (though also borderline by Kernberg's borderline personality organization criteria). The typical life course in her series (with 95% trace rate) was one of marginal adaptation, social dysfunction, and poor work history. A similarly gloomy picture emerged from the follow-up study of Alv Dahl (1993) in Oslo. Thorkil Vanggaard (1979) a psychoanalyst in Copenhagen, has written extensively on "schizophrenic borderline states" (comparable to our schizotypal personality), drawing attention to the general need of patients in this category for long-term psychotherapy. Because of the cognitive difficulties schizotypal patients exhibit (though these are not as severe as those encountered in frank schizophrenia), therapists may need to serve as "auxiliary egos" for many years. As Fenton and McGlashan (1989) mention, schizotypal patients tend not to shed their magical thinking and suspiciousness no matter how long they remain in therapy. Schizotypal patients are also prone to concreteness of thought, such that suggestions made in one context are not easily generalized to similar contexts (Stone, 1989b). This makes each life situation "new" and keeps alive and active the need for ongoing supportive therapy.

Schizoid Personality Disorder

Persons who are predominantly or purely schizoid (by DSM standards) are rarities in psychiatric treatment facilities: Their aloofness is such that they seldom seek help. Those who do seek therapy usually have admixtures of other disorders, including schizotypal personality disorder (Widiger & Rogers, 1989). In a follow-up study by Wolff and Chick (1981), one of the few devoted to schizoid personality disorder, 18 of 22 boys with this disorder still met the requisite diagnostic criteria 10 years later, attesting to the stability of the diagnosis over this time span.

Narcissistic Personality Disorder

The literature on outcome in narcissistic personality disorder is sparse. Some studies have focused on patients with narcissistic personality disorder who were originally hospitalized. As with many personality disorders, "pure" types are less common than those with comorbidity. Antisocial, and particularly psychopathic, persons are narcissistic by definition. There is less, though still significant, overlap of narcissistic personality disorder with borderline personality disorder and with hysteric/histrionic persons. Here I limit myself to patients with narcissistic personality disorder without any prominent antisociality. Plakun (1989) noted in his long-term (approximately 14-year) follow-up study that patients with narcissistic personality disorder were more often readmitted to hospital than were patients with borderline personality disorder. The outcome, as to global function, in patients with narcissistic personality disorder and borderline personality disorder was about the same, both in the Chestnut Lodge (McGlashan & Heinssen, 1989) and the PI-500 studies (Stone, 1989a)—provided there was no antisocial personality disorder comorbidity. Strong narcissistic traits might predispose to suicide in certain persons who lose some narcissistic "supply" they consider vital (wealth, physical prowess, beauty, social position, etc.), but the follow-up studies have not shed light on this possibility: The numbers of patients with narcissistic personality disorder have been small and those who have committed suicide are rarer still. There are many highly narcissistic persons who never become "cases" (i.e., are never in treatment) about whose fate we read in newspapers and books. Brenda Frazier (DiLiberto, 1987), Archibald Douglas (Douglas, 1992), and Rebecca Harkness (Unger, 1988) are examples of narcissistic persons either ruined by power-hungry, narcissistic parents (Brenda Frazier), almost ruined by such parents (Geoffrey Douglas, whose father Archibald drove his wife to suicide and made life a horror for his children), or who ruined their families with their self-centeredness and disdain (Rebecca Harkness). The father of the actress Edie Sedgwick is another example—a man who sponged off his heiress wife, never worked, paraded around the family mansion in a bikini, molested his daughters sexually, and humiliated his sons (three of the eight children committed suicide) (Stein, with Plimpton, 1982). The protagonists of these books remained intensely narcissistic throughout their lives—so at least in their case there would have been "stability" to their diagnosis had they ever submitted to an evaluation. In contrast, the patients with "a pathological narcissism" evaluated by Ronningstam, Gunderson, and Lyons (1995), when rediagnosed 3 years later, often showed improvement, such that only 40% of the 20 traced patients still carried the narcissistic personality disorder diagnosis. This led the authors to comment that "the instability of narcissistic psychopathology found in [our] study raises questions about the construct validity of narcissistic personality disorder as a diagnostic category. . . ." (p. 253). It may well be the case,

however, that the degree to which persons originally diagnosed with narcissistic personality disorder remain so over time is highly sample dependent. The mere fact that theirs was a group willing to be in treatment (ideally conducing to some change for the better) marked their patients as quite different from the self-contented, eternally narcissistic persons of the aforementioned biographies.

Inhibited Personality Types

The personality disorders of DSM's "anxious" cluster—the obsessive-compulsive, dependent, and avoidant, along with the no-longer-included passive–aggressive—are all characterized by an inhibited, as opposed to impulsive, personality style. The same is true for *hysteric personality*, as this psychoanalytic literature about it. The latter represents a healthier version of what is now confusingly referred to in DSM as histrionic personality disorder—which is actually an amalgam of some hysteric traits and some borderline features (Kernberg, 1992). Still another personality configuration that belongs to the inhibited category is the *depressive–masochistic*—not found in DSM but in common psychoanalytic parlance.

These personality disorders are generally less severe or dysfunctional as the disorders of the preceding sections. In the forensic literature there are occasional instances in which obsessive–compulsive personality disorder is admixed with antisociality—as in the case of John List (Sharkey, 1990) who killed his entire family and then hid from the authorities for 18 years, or Len Fagot (Donahue & Hall, 1991), who killed two sons-in-law for insurance money. But these are the exception. The inhibited personality types much outnumber the impulse-ridden and violent types in the population as a whole, but they have seldom been the subject of methodical, long-term follow-up. The main reason, I believe, is that persons with these milder disorders are usually treated by private practitioners or in clinics. In these settings, various factors militate against the accumulation of the relevant data: concern about confidentiality, limited access to government funding, difficulties building up sufficiently large samples to permit valid statistical analysis, and a paucity of data (e.g., names and phone numbers of relatives) that are needed to trace people after many years since last contact.

I recently traced the neurotic-level (Kernberg, 1967) patients I had seen in private practice since 1966. In the 35 patients I was able to trace, the intervals ranged from 10 to 30 years (average = 17 years). These former patients—all treated with psychoanalysis or psychoanalytically oriented therapy—could be compartmentalized, according to their main personality type, as follows: hysteric, 4; obsessive–compulsive, 9; avoidant, 1; depressive–masochistic, 7; dependent, 1; narcissistic, 4; paranoid, 1; passive–aggressive, 1; antisocial, 1; schizoid, 3; mixed, 4. With the exception of the antisocial, the passive–aggressive, and one of the schizoid patients, all were functioning well when traced—even the three who had been briefly hospitalized (for affective illness) before I began working with them. None had ever been rehospitalized; there were no suicides. The (mildly) paranoid man, who was also avoidant and rather inhibited, made an excellent adjustment, and is now the head of his own thriving engineering company. This is not a methodical study, and I dwell on it only because psychoanalysts seldom do follow-ups on their patients at such long intervals, so these impressions may have some value. The main point here is that better-functioning patients, with the mostly inhibited-type personality disorders, ordinarily are resilient and have a favorable life course. In some cases, of course, recovery takes a long time. One of the schizoid women, for example, remained ensconced in a self-defeating relationship with a man who mistreated her and sponged off her all the years (4) she was in analysis with me. But when I located her 20 years later, she had finally left him, completed her doctorate after a long struggle, and recently remarried—to a much more suitable man. I attribute this outcome more to her perseverance than to my treatment—but, as Cloninger emphasizes (Cloninger, Svrakic, & Svrakic, 1997), *perseverance* is the personality trait that seems to divide the severely disordered (no matter what Axis II personality diagnosis) from the ordinary person.

There have, to be sure, been a few follow-up studies carried out within the context of psychoanalytic clinics in connection with "neurotic" patients exemplifying one or another of the inhibited-type personalities. One such study was that carried out at the Columbia Psychoanalytic Center (Weber, Bachrach, & Solomon, 1985; Bachrach, Weber, & Solomon, 1985). Unfortunately, this study did not use the more common outcome scales and did not analyze results in relation to standardized personality diagnosis at the outset. In an earlier study by Knapp, Levin, & McCarter, (1960), the patients with mainly obsessive characteristics did better (eight of nine cases) than did those with mainly hysteric features (whose outcomes varied over a wider range).

COMMENT

As I mentioned earlier (Stone, 1993a), follow-up studies and impressions about the natural history (the "life trajectory") of personality disorders have concentrated on the severe end of the personality spectrum. Many of the people in this range have been institutionalized, whether in psychiatric hospitals, forensic centers, or prisons. The social consequences of these severe disorders stimulate interest in investigators, government authorities, and the public. The most is known about the worst conditions. I have scarcely mentioned several of the more severe disorders—paranoid, hypomanic, and intermittent–explosive—but this is a reflection of the near-total absence of follow-up work on these disorders, all of which are difficult to treat in their more fully developed form and mostly consistent with a dysfunctional life course. Generalizations must always be tempered with the realization that mild forms of almost all the personality disorders exist, and the evidence suggests strongly that it is better to have a mild form of a "severe" disorder (even antisocial) than a severe form of an inhibited-type personality, such as obsessive–compulsive personality disorder. Kernberg's distinction among personality–*organizational levels* (neurotic, borderline, psychotic), though not accepted by DSM, is useful and deserves wider recognition in the field of personality diagnosis and treatment inasmuch as these distinctions point the way to important boundary markers with respect to prognosis. Suicide and other calamities, for example, are rare among neurotic-level persons; all too common among those at the borderline level (which would include borderline personality disorder, many persons with narcissistic personality disorder, most with antisocial personality disorder and psychopathic personality and most paranoid, hypomanic, explosive, schizotypal, histrionic (as opposed to hysteric), and schizoid persons).

The current definitions in DSM-IV of borderline personality disorder, antisocial personality disorder, and schizotypal personality disorder contain items more properly understood as symptoms rather than personality traits. Symptoms are often easier to control and minimize with treatment such that certain defining "items" disappear over time and the disorder is no longer diagnosable years later. The more rigorously defined disorders (which base definitions only on true traits) would appear to show more stability over long periods. *Stability* in this context means resistance to change. This in turn means that the severe personality disorders (e.g., those existing within the borderline organizational level) are difficult to treat and require years or even decades for substantial change for the better to occur. The higher-level disorders, along with the milder conditions not even meeting full DSM criteria—of the sort treated for the most part in clinics and private offices—also do not change radically in coloration over the years, but the life course is usually more favorable. This was the case in most of my former private patients, some of whom were probably nudged toward better function via their therapy, many of whom got better mainly through "true grit." The hysteric patients were still hysteric, only less so; the obsessives were still obsessive, only less so; and so on, throughout the wide spectrum of personality variation they demonstrated at the outset. As for the borderline patients (whether borderline personality disorder or just borderline personality organization), they had much more room to go "up" in life function (compared with their neurotic counterparts, whose GAS initially was already in the 65–70 range). And many of the borderline patients did ascend into the 60s or 70s on the Global Function scale, to the point of no longer manifesting borderline personality disorder. Instead, they would now be diagnosed via their (originally) second most prominent "comorbid" personality disorder (i.e., hysteric, dependent, or depressive–masochistic).

I have purposely not touched on the issue of treatment methods. Because of the long time usually required to bring about favorable change in personality disorders, especially in the more severe ones (e.g., the borderline and schizotypal), and because of the near impossibility of ameliorating psychopathic personality—the *controlled randomized treatment studies* that, at the end of chapters such as this, everyone says "ought to be done"—are extraordinarily difficult (and extraordinarily expensive) to mount. Absent scientifically ideal studies, we are left with what fuzzy-set mathematicians call "expert opinion" (Rocha, Theoto, Oliveira, & Gomide, 1992). At this time, experts are converging toward a consensus that it is no longer meaningful in the borderline domain, for example, to contend that method X is "superior" (globally) to method Y. Thus the debate concerning the merits of Kernberg's transference-focused psychotherapy (TFP; Kernberg, Selzer, Koenigsberg, Carr, & Appelbaum, 1989) versus those of Linehan's (1993) dialectical behavioral therapy (DBT) largely evaporates when one realizes that the more legitimate question is: For whom is TFP apt to be more successful? And, For whom is DBT apt to be more successful? For it is likely that a theoretically sensible, well-structured therapy in the hands of a competent, empathic therapist will surely be helpful for a good many, but never for all, personality-disordered patients. Certain methods will be especially well suited to a particular subset of patients; some patients will turn out to be equally amenable to several accepted therapies. For the foreseeable future the selection process—which method, for which personality-disordered patient—will depend more on intuition than on "exact science."

REFERENCES

Aarkrog, T. (1981). The borderline concept in childhood, adolescence and adulthood. *Acta Psychiatrica Scandinavica, 64*(Suppl. 243).

Aarkrog, T. (1993). *Borderline personality disorder adolescents 20 years later.* Paper presented at the third international conference of the International Society for the Study of Personality Disorders, Cambridge, MA. (Expanded version published 1994 by PJ Schmidt, Vojens, Denmark)

American Pyschiatric Association. (1980). *Diagnostic and statistical manual of mental disorders* (3rd ed.). Washington, DC: Author.

American Pyschiatric Association. (1987). *Diagnostic and statistical manual of mental disorders* (3rd ed., rev.). Washington, DC: Author.

American Pyschiatric Association. (1994). *Diagnostic and statistical manual of mental disorders* (4th ed.). Washington, DC: Author.

Arboleda-Florez, J., & Holley, H. L. (1991). Antisocial burnout: An exploratory study. *Bulletin of the American Academy of Psychiatry and the Law, 19*, 173–183.

Bachrach, H. M., Weber, J. J., & Solomon, S. (1985). Factors associated with the outcome of psychoanalysis (clinical and methodilogical considerations): Report of the Columbia Psychoanalytic Research Project: IV. *International Review of Psycho-analysis, 12*, 379–389.

Black, D. W., Baumgard, C. H., & Bell, S. E. (1995). A

16- to 45 year follow-up of 71 men with antisocial personality disorder. *Comprehensive Psychiatry, 36,* 130–140.

Carpenter, W. T., Jr., Gunderson, J. G., & Strauss, J. S. (1977). Considerations of the borderline syndrome: Longitudinal and comparative study of borderline and schizophrenic patients. In P. Hartocollis (Ed.), *Borderline personality disorders.* (pp. 231–253). New York: International Universities Press.

Christian, R. E., Frick, P. J., Hill, N. L., Tyler, L., & Frazer, D. R. (1997). Psychopathy and conduct problems in children: II. Implications for subtyping children with conduct problems. *Journal of the American Academy of Child and Adolescent Psychiatry, 36,* 233–241.

Cleckley, H. (1972). *The mask of sanity* (5th ed.). St. Louis: Mosby.

Cloninger, C. R. (1986). A unified biosocial theory of personality and its role in the development of anxiety states. *Psychiatric Developments, 3,* 167–226.

Cloninger, C. R., Svrakic, N. M., & Svrakic, D. M. (1997). Role of personality self-organization in development of mental order and disorder. *Developmental Psychopathology, 9,* 881–906.

Dahl, A. (1993). *Schizotypal personality disorder compared to chronic schizophrenia.* Paper presented at the Third International Conference of the International Society for the Study of Personality Disorders, Cambridge, MA.

Dilalla, L. F., & Gottesman, I. I. (1990). Heterogeneity of causes of delinquency and criminality: Lifespan perspectives. *Development and Psychopathology, 1,* 339–349.

DiLiberto, G. (1987). *Debutante: The story of Brenda Frazier.* New York: Knopf.

Dinwiddie, S. H., & Daw, E. W. (1998). Temporal stability of antisocial personality disorder: Blind follow-up study at 8-years. *Comprehensive Psychiatry, 39,* 28–34.

Donahue, C., & Hall, S. (1991). *Deadly relations: A true story of murder in a suburban family.* New York: Bantam.

Douglas, G. (1992). *Class: The wreckage of an American family.* New York: Holt.

Easser, R.-R., & Lesser, S. (1965). Hysterical personality: A reevaluation. *Psychoanalytic Quarterly, 34,* 390–402.

Endicott, J., Spitzer, R. L., Fleiss, J. L., & Cohen, J. (1967). The Global Assessment Scale. *Archives of General Psychiatry, 33,* 766–771.

Fenton, W. S., & McGlashan, T. H. (1989). Risk of schizophrenia in character-disordered patients. *American Journal of Psychiatry, 146,* 1280–1284.

Gabbard, G. O., & Coyne, L. (1987). Predictors of response of antisocial patients to hospital treatment. *Hospital and Community Psychiatry, 38,* 1181–1185.

Grilo, C. M., McGlashan, T. H., & Oldham, J. M. (1998). Course and stability of personality disorders. *Journal of Practical Psychiatry and Behavioral Health, 4,* 61–75.

Grinker, R. R., Sr., Werble, B., & Drye, R. C. (1968). *The borderline syndrome.* New York: Basic Books.

Gunderson, J. G., Carpenter, W. T., Jr., & Strauss, J. S. (1975). Borderline and schizophrenic patients: A comparative study. *American Journal of Psychiatry, 132,* 1257–1264.

Gunderson, J. G., & Singer, M. T. (1975). Defining border-line patients: An overview. *American Journal of Psychiatry, 132,* 1–10.

Hare, R. D. (1993). *Without conscience: The disturbing world of the psychopaths among us.* New York: Pocket Books

Hare, R. D. (1996). Psychopathy: A clinical construct whose time has come. *Crimianl Justice and Behavior, 23,* 25–54.

Hare, R. D., Harpur, T. J., Hakstian, A. R., Forth, A. E., Hart, S. D., & Newman, J. P. (1990). The revised Psychopathy Checklist: Reliability and factor structure. *Psychological Assessment, 2,* 338–341.

Hart, S. D. (1998). Psychopathy and risk for violence. In D. J. Cooke, A. E. Forth, & R. D. Hare (Eds.); *Psychopathy: Theory, research and implications for society* (pp. 355–373). Boston: Kluwer.

Hemphill, J. F., Templeman, R., Wong, S., & Hare, R. D. (1998). Psychopathy and crime: Recidivism and criminal careers. In D. J. Cooke, A. E. Forth, & R. D. Hare (Eds.), *Psychopathy: Theory, research and implications for society* (pp. 375–399). Boston: Kluwer.

Kernberg, O. F. (1967). Borderline personality organization. *Journal of the American Psychoanalytic Association, 15,* 641–685.

Kernberg, O. F. (1992). *Aggression in personality disorders and perversions.* New Haven: Yale University Press.

Kernberg, O. F., Selzer, M. A., Koenigsberg, H. W., Carr, A. C., & Appelbaum, A. II. (1989). *Psychodynamic psychotherapy of borderline patients.* New York: Basic Books.

Knapp, P., Levin, S., & McCarter, R. H. (1960). Suitability for psychoanalysis: A review of 100 supervised cases. *Psychoanalytic Quarterly, 29,* 459–477.

Kraepelin, E. (1905). *Einfuehrung in die Psychiatrische Klinik* (2nd ed.). Leipzig: Barth.

Linehan, M. M. (1993). *Cognitive-behavioral treatment of borderline personality disorder.* New York: Guilford Press.

Lykken, D. T. (1995). *The antisocial personalities.* Hillsdale, NJ: Erlbaum.

Maddocks, P. D. (1970). A five year follow-up of untreated psychopaths. *British Journal of Psychiatry, 116,* 511–515.

Martin, R. L., Cloninger, C. R., & Guze, S. B. (1979). The evaluation of diagnostic concordance in follow-up studies, II: A blind prospective follow-up of female criminals. *Journal of Psychiatric Research, 15,* 107–125.

McDonald, R. R. (1998). *Secrets never lie: The death of Sara Tokars—A southern tragedy of money, murder and innocence betrayed.* New York: Avon Books.

McGlashan, T. H. (1985). The prediction of outcome in borderline personality disorder: Part V of the Chestnut Lodge follow-up study. In T. H. McGlashan (Ed.). *The borderline: Current empirical research* (pp. 63–98). Washington, DC: American Psychiatric Press.

McGlashan, T. H. (1986a). The Chestnut Lodge follow-up study: III. Long-term outcome of borderline personalities. *Archives of General Psychiatry, 43,* 20–30.

McGlashan, T. H. (1986b). Chestnut Lodge follow-up study: VI. Long term follow-up perspectives. *Archives of General Psychiatry, 43,* 329–334.

McGlashan, T. H., & Heinssen, R. K. (1989). Narcissistic, antisocial and non-comorbid subgroups of borderline disorder: Are they distinct entities by long-term clinical profile? *Psychiatric Clinics of North America, 12,* 653–670.

Myner, J., Santman, J., Cappelletty, G. G., & Perlmutter, B. (1998). Variables related to recidivism among juvenile offenders. *International Journal of Offender Therapy and Comparative Criminology, 42,* 65–80.

Offord, D. R., & Reitsma-Street, M. (1983). Problems of studying antisocial behavior. *Psychiatric Developments, 1,* 207–224.

Paris, J. (1994, June 8). *Effects of incest in borderline patients.* Lecture presented at a symposium in honor of Otto Kernberg, New York Hospital/Westchester Division.

Paris, J., Brown, R., & Nowlis, D. (1987). Long-term follow-up of borderline patients in a general hospital. *Comprehensive Psychiatry, 28,* 530–535.

Perry, J. C. (1988). A prospective study of life stress, defenses, psychotic symptoms, and depression in borderline and antisocial personality disorders and bipoplar type II affective disorder. *Journal of Personality Disorders, 4,* 273–289.

Plakun, E. M. (1989). Narcissistic personality disorder. A validity study and comparison to borderline personality disorder. *Psychiatric Clinics of North America, 12,* 603–620.

Plakun, E. M., Burckhardt, P. E., & Muller, J. P. (1985). 14-year follow-up of borderline and schizotypal personality disorders. *Comprehensive Psychiatry, 26,* 448–455.

Quinsey, V. L. (1995). The prediction and explanation of criminal violence. *International Journal of Law and Psychiatry, 18,* 117–127.

Reich, W. (1949). *Character analysis.* New York: Farrar, Strauss & Giroux.

Rice, M. E., & Harris, G. T. (1995). Psychopathy, schizophrenia, alcohol abuse, and violent recidivism. *International Journal of Law and Psychiatry, 18,* 333–342.

Rice, M. E., Harris, G. T., & Quinsey, V. L. (1990). A follow-up of rapists assessed in a maximum security psychiatric facility. *Journal of Interpersonal Violence, 5,* 435–448.

Robins, E., Gentry, K. A., Munoz, R. A., & Marten, S. A. (1977). A contrast of the three more common illnesses with the ten less common in a study and 18-month follow up of 314 psychiatric emergency room patients, III: Findings at follow-up. *Archives of General Psychiatry, 34,* 285–291.

Robins, L. N., Tipp, J., & Przybeck, T. (1991). Antisocial personality. In L. N. Robins & D. Regier (Eds.). *Psychiatric disorders in America* (pp. 258–290). New York: Macmillan.

Rocha, A. F., Theoto, M., Oliveira, C. A. C., & Gomide, F. (1992). Approximate reasoning in diagnosis, therapy, and prognosis. In L. Sadeh & J. Kacprzyk (Eds.), *Fuzzy logic for the management of uncertainty* (pp. 437–446). New York: John Wiley.

Ronningstam, E., Gunderson, J. G., & Lyons, M. (1995). Changes in pathological narcissism. *American Journal of Psychiatry, 152,* 253–257.

Schneider, K. (1959). *Clinical psychopathology* (M. W. Hamilton, Trans.). New York: Grune & Stratton.

Serin, R. C., & Amos, N. L. (1995). The role of psychopathy in the assessment of dangerousness. *International Journal of Law and Psychiatry, 18,* 231–238.

Sharkey, J. (1990). *Death sentence: The inside story of the John List murders.* New York: Prentice Hall.

Siever, L. J., Bernstein, D. P., & Silverman, J. M. (1989). *Schizotypal, paranoid and schizoid personality disorders: A review of their current status.* Unpublished manuscript.

Stein, J., with Plimpton, G. (Ed.). (1982). *Edie: An American biography.* New York: Knopf.

Stone, M. H. (1985). Genetische Faktoren in schizotypen Patienten. In G. Huber (Ed.), *Basisstudien endogener Psychosen und das Borderline Problem* (pp. 225–237). Stuttgart: Schattauer.

Stone, M. H. (1989a). Long-term follow-up of narcissis-tic/borderline patients. *Psychiatric Clinics of North America, 12,* 621–641.

Stone, M. H. (1989b). Psychotherapy of the schizotypal patient. In T. Karasu (Ed.), *Treatment of psychiatric disorders* (pp. 2718–2727). Washington, DC: American Psychiatric Press.

Stone, M. H. (1990). *The fate of borderline patients: Successful outcome and psychiatric practice.* New York: Guilford Press.

Stone, M. H. (1993a). *Abnormalities of personality.* New York: Norton.

Stone, M. H. (1993b) Long-term outcome in personality disorders. *British Journal of Psychiatry, 162,* 299–313.

Stone, M. H. (1995). Follow-up a lungo termine di pazienti borderline: Risultati del campione P.I.-500 e della pratica privata. *Noos, 1,* 95–109.

Stone, M. H. (1997). Langzeit-Katamnesen von leichten und schweren Persoenlichkeitsstoerungen: Therapeutische Implikationen. *Psychotherapie, 2,* 29–36.

Stone, M. H., Hurt, S. W., & Stone, D. K. (1987). The P.I.-500: Long-term follow-up of borderline inpatients meeting DSM-III criteria. I: Global outcome. *Journal of Personality Disorders, 1,* 291–298.

Unger, C. (1988). *Blue blood: The Story of Rebecca Harkness and how one of the richest families in the world descended into drugs, madness, suicide and violence.* New York: Morrow.

van der Kolk, B. (1989). The compulsion to repeat the trauma. *Psychiatric Clinics of North America, 12,* 389–411.

van der Kolk, B. A. (1996). The complexity of adaptation to trauma: Self-regulation, stimulus discrimination, and characterological development. In B. A. van der Kolk, A. C. McFarlane, & L. Weisaeth (Eds.), *Traumatic stress: The effects of overwhelming experience on mind, body, and society* (pp. 182–213). New York: Guilford Press.

Vanggaard, T. (1979). *Borderlands of sanity.* Copenhagen: Munksgaard.

Villeneuve, D. B., & Quinsey, V. L. (1995). Predictors of general and violent recidivism among mentally disordered inmates. *Criminal Justice and Behavior, 22,* 397–410.

Weber, J. J., Bachrach, H. M., & Solomon, M. (1985). Factors associated with the outcome of psychoanalysis: Report of the Columbia Psychoanalytic Research Project: II, III. *International Review of Psycho-analysis, 12,* 13–26.

Werble, B. (1970). Second follow-up study of borderline patients. *Archives of General Psychiatry, 23,* 307.

Widiger, T. A., & Rogers, J. H. (1989). Prevalence and comorbidity of personality disorders. *Psychiatric Annals, 19,* 132–136.

Wolff, S., & Chick, J. (1981). Schizoid personality in childhood: A controlled follow-up study. *Annual Progress in Child Psychiatry and Child Development,* 550–580.

World Health Organization. (1977). *International classification of diseases* (9th ed.). Geneva, Switzerland: Author.

Yochelson, S., & Samenow, S. E. (1976). *The criminal personality: Vol. I. A profile for change.* (Reprinted 1993). Northvale, NJ: Aronson.

Zanarini, M. C., Gunderson, J. G., Marino, M. F., Schwartz, E. O., & Frankenburg, F. R. (1989). Childhood experience of borderline patients. *Comprehensive Psychiatry, 30,* 18–25.

PART III

DIAGNOSIS
AND ASSESSMENT

CHAPTER 13

━━◆◆◆◆━━

Assessment Instruments

LEE ANNA CLARK
JULIE A. HARRISON

Over the past two decades, instruments designed to assess personality disorder, maladaptive personality traits, or personality dimensions that are relevant to personality-based pathology have proliferated. Several forces have driven this proliferation. First, in 1980, the American Psychiatric Association (APA) officially recognized personality disorder as a distinct and important realm of psychopathology by according it a separate "Axis II" in the *Diagnostic and Statistical Manual of Mental Disorders* (DSM; APA, 1980). Both clinical and research interest in personality disorder—and, consequently, the need for assessment instruments—increased as a result. Second, in the discipline of psychology, the fields of personality and psychopathology developed along separate paths for decades, but in recent years their close interdependence has become the focus of much research (see Watson & Clark, 1994). Investigators of both personality and psychopathology began to recognize that the extensive knowledge accumulated about normal-range personality structure and the accompanying broad array of personality measures could be applied fruitfully in the domain of psychopathology. This recognition has led to expanded research in two directions. On the one hand, the clinical utility of measures originally developed for normal-range personality is being evaluated; on the other hand, measures designed to assess psychopathology are being studied in nonclinical samples to evaluate relations between normal and abnormal personality.

The purpose of this chapter is to familiarize readers with the wide range of instruments now available for investigating personality disorder. Both well-known and some less widely used instruments are included. The focus is on more comprehensive instruments, but selected measures of single constructs are discussed as well. Both (semi-)structured interviews and self-report instruments are covered, as well as measures designed originally to assess both normal and pathological personality.

For the most part, we provide references to primary sources rather than reiterate basic information (e.g., about instrument development and psychometric properties); on the other hand, in-depth reviews of the validity studies for each instrument would be prohibitively long. We try, therefore, to steer a middle course, highlighting measures' specific strengths and weaknesses and comparing similar instruments, as appropriate. We discuss certain key assessment issues as they are relevant to instrument selection, including the relative (dis)advantages of interviews and self-reports, categorical versus dimensional approaches to personality disorder assessment, the generally poor convergent and discriminant validity of measures, and the use (or not) of informants. However, we resist extended discussion of these issues because they are discussed by MacKenzie in Chapter 14 (this volume) and/or elsewhere (e.g., Clark, Livesley, & Morey, 1997; Kaye & Shea, 2000; Livesley, Schroeder, Jackson, & Jang, 1994; Perry, 1992; Zimmerman, 1994).

For the most part, it is possible to organize instruments assessing normal and abnormal personality into a two-by-two grid: trait-based versus diagnostically based instruments and self-report forms versus interviews (see Table 13.1). Instruments falling in the trait-based quadrants can be arranged further along a continuum ranging from the normal to pathological, depending on the primary target of assessment. Also, for self-report trait scales, both multitrait and single-trait measures are common; only multitrait measures are included in Table 13.1.

An instrument that derives from Benjamin's (1996a) Structural Analysis of Social Behavior (SASB) model resists simple categorization in this two-by-two grid because the SASB model addresses interpersonal behavior rather than either traits or diagnoses per se. However, we have included it in the trait-based section because of its conceptual links with trait measures based on the interpersonal circumplex (IPC) and because it can be used to describe traits (Benjamin, 1996b). The Schedule for Nonadaptive and Adaptive Personality (SNAP; Clark, 1993a) can be scored for both traits and diagnoses so it is included in two quadrants.[1]

When the range of available instruments is organized in this way, it is clear (and not surprising) that there are fewer interviews than self-report instruments. The most empty cells are trait-based and diagnostically based interviews ($N = 5$ each). Of the five trait-based interviews, two are multitrait interviews, designed to assess the broad domain of personality or personality disorder, whereas the other three focus on a single diagnostic category, providing more differentiated within-category assessment. All five of the diagnostically based interviews assess a full complement of diagnoses.

The fullest cell is trait-based self-report forms: There are at least seven multitrait instruments that are relatively well-known and used frequently in personality disorder research, an uncountable number of specific trait measures, a few of which we discuss, plus many classic instruments such as the California Psychological Inventory (CPI; Gough, 1987) that have not been widely used in personality disorder re-

search, even though they assess essentially the same domain as some of the more widely used instruments (Fleenor & Eastman, 1997). We do not report on this last set. Diagnostically based self-reports also are relatively common, with at least seven measures available.

For diagnostically based measures—both interviews and self-reports—our discussion is focused on important parameters of the set of measures as a whole, whereas for trait-based measures, our discussion is focused more on the individual interviews or inventories. The reason for this decision is that diagnostically based measures—whether interview or self-report—all address the same (or highly similar) content (i.e., the DSM Axis II personality disorders), so the primary features that distinguish them are such things as format and scoring procedures. By contrast, trait-based instruments tap different traits or set of traits, so the target of assessment is the key distinguishing feature between measures.

DIAGNOSTICALLY BASED INTERVIEWS

As mentioned, there are five well-known omnibus semistructured interviews for assessing the DSM personality disorders. An overview of these instruments is available in the "Personality Disorder" section (Kaye & Shea, 2000) of APA's *Handbook of Psychiatric Measures* (Rush, Pincus, & First, 2000); the reader is referred to that volume for additional information. Table 13.2 summarizes key features of these interviews.

As can be seen from the table, the interviews have several common features but also differ along a number of important parameters. All the omnibus instruments are now available in a DSM-IV version. Most of them include the appendixed diagnoses—negativistic (formerly passive–aggressive) and depressive personality disorder—while two also permit assessment of ICD-10 diagnoses. It is important to note that there are virtually no psychometric data on any of these DSM-IV-based revisions. For some parameters (e.g., interrater reliability) it is reasonable to hypothesize that the basic psychometric properties of the DSM-III-R version (summarized in the next section) will apply also to the DSM-IV version. However, Blashfield, Blum, and Pfohl (1992) demonstrated that even "apparently minor changes in the wording of crite-

TABLE 13.1. Multiscale Instruments Assessing Personality and Personality Pathology

Interviews	Self-reports
	Diagnostically based measures
Diagnostic Interview for DSM-IV Personality Disorders (DIPD-IV; Zanarini et al., 1996)	*Coolidge Axis II Inventory* (CATI; Coolidge & Merwin, 1992)
International Personality Disorder Examination (PDE; Loranger, 1995, 1999)	*Millon Clinical Multiaxial Inventory—III* (MCMI-III; Millon et al., 1994)
Personality Disorder Interview—IV (PDI-IV; Widiger et al., 1995)	*Minnesota Multiphasic Personality Inventory Personality Disorder Scales* (MMPI-PD; Morey et al., 1985)
Structured Clinical Interview for DSM-IV Axis II Personality Disorder (SCID-II; First et al., 1997)	*Personality Disorder Questionnaire—IV* (PDQ-IV; Hyler (1994)
Structured Interview for DSM Personality—IV (SIDP-IV; Pfohl et al., 1997)	*Schedule for Nonadaptive and Adaptive Personality* (SNAP; Clark, 1993)
	Wisconsin Personality Inventory (WISPI; Klein et al., 1993)
	Personality Assessment Inventory (PAI; Morey, 1991)[a]
	Trait-based measures
Diagnostic Interview for Borderline Patients (DIB; Gunderson et al., 1981)	*Dimensional Assessment of Personality Pathology— Basic Questionnaire* (DAPP-BQ; Livesley & Jackson, in press)
Diagnostic Interview for Borderline Patients— Revised (DIB-R; Zanarini et al., 1989)	*Schedule for Nonadaptive and Adaptive Personality,* (SNAP; Clark, 1993)
Diagnostic Interview for Narcissism (DIN; Gunderson et al., 1990)	*Inventory of Interpersonal Problems*—Personality Disorder scales (IIP-PD; Pilkonis et al., 1996)
Psychopathy Checklist—Revised (PCL-R; Hare, 1991)	*NEO-Personality Inventory—Revised* (NEO-PI-R; Costa & McCrae, 1992)
Personality Assessment Schedule (PAS; Tyrer, 1988)	*Extended Interpersonal Adjective Scales* (IASR-B5; Trapnell & Wiggins, 1990)
Structured Interview for the Five-Factor Model (SIFFM; Trull & Widiger, 1994)	*Personality Adjective Check List* (PACL; Strack, 1987)
	Tridimensional Personality Questionnaire (TPQ; Cloninger et al., 1991, 1993); *Temperament–Character Inventory* (TCI; Cloninger et al., 1994)
	Structural Analysis of Social Behavior Intrex Questionnaire (SASB-IQ; Benjamin, 1996a)[b]

Note. Only the last of multiple versions of an instrument is included, unless there was a substantive change between versions.
[a] Assesses "major clinical constructs" rather than diagnoses per se. See text for explanation.
[b] Assesses interpersonal dimensions rather than traits per se. See text for explanation.

ria can have major effects on which patients receive a diagnosis of personality disorder" (p. 245). Thus, it would be risky to hypothesize generalizability from the DSM-III-R to DSM-IV version of an instrument for other parameters (e.g., diagnostic frequencies or temporal stability).

Reliability

Reliability is a more complex concept, and empirically is more variable across studies, for interviews (particularly semistructured interviews, as the personality disorder interviews are) compared to questionnaires, because reliability is a function of not only the content of the interview questions but also the research design (e.g., joint vs. separate interviews) and, perhaps most important, interviewer quality. Specifically, interrater reliabilities are higher for joint compared to separate interviews (Zimmerman, 1994), and the interrater reliability of highly skilled versus newly trained interviewers likely would differ considerably. Thus, for interview-based measures it is important to establish reliability estimates for each new set of interviewers, and it is inappropriate to speak of the interrater reliability of the *measure* as if it were independent of the interviewers. With that caveat in mind, we offer a summary of the reliability data for the interviews listed in Table 13.2 based on Zimmerman's (1994) review, which provides details from individual studies. Interestingly, internal consistency reliabilities are rarely reported for interview-based measures, so our focus is on interrater reliability and temporal stability.

Most of the studies Zimmerman (1994) reviewed used small samples—only 5 of the 23 studies had *N*'s greater than 100. Because kappa (Cohen, 1968) is unstable with small *N*'s, results often were available for only a subset of personality disorder diagnoses, and the aggre-

gate statistics we present are more reliable than individual study results. Following Zimmerman, we distinguish between studies that used joint versus separate interviews and, for the latter, those with short versus longer retest intervals. Even when the retest interval is short, reliability is lower when separate (vs. joint) interviews are conducted, and longer retest intervals also are associated with lower reliability, because the greater possibility of change with the passage of time introduces an additional source of "error."

For the 15 joint-interview studies, the average ranges and overall reliabilities for individual personality disorder diagnoses were as follows: Structured Clinical Interview for DSM-III-R Personality Disorders (SCID-II) (5 studies), range = .57 to 86, mean = .71; Structured Interview for DSM-IV Personality (SIDP) (4 stud-

TABLE 13.2. Summary of Key Features of Diagnostically Based Personality Disorder Interviews

Interview (alphabetic order)	Primary author(s)	No. of items (sets)	Format	App. Dxes	Scoring (threshold)		Admin. (min.)	Screen	©	Availability
					Criteria	Dxes				
Diagnostic Interview for DSM-IV Personality Disorders (DIPD-IV)	Zanarini	108	Dx	Yes	0–2 (2)	0–2 (2)	90	No	Yes	Author
Comments: Psychometric data forthcoming; currently available for previous version (DSM-III-R). Training video and workshops available.										
International Personality Disorder Examination (PDE)	Loranger	67	T	—	0–2 (2)	No. of criteria	90	Yes	Yes	Author; WHO
Comments: Assesses ICD-10 diagnoses; DSM-IV version (99 questions) available from American Psychiatric Press. Well-constructed manual, training courses available.										
Personality Disorder Interview—IV (PDI-IV)	Widiger	93	Both	Yes	0–2 (1)	0–6 (4)	90–120	No	Yes	Psychological Assessment Resources
Comments: Extensive manual with thorough discussion of criteria and diagnoses; few psychometric data currently available.										
Structured Clinical Interview for DSM-IV Axis II Personality Disorders (SCID-II)	First/ Spitzer	119	Dx	Yes	1–3 (3)	No. of criteria	<60	Yes	Yes	American Psychiatric Press
Comments: Computer administered version available (Multi-Health Systems); training video/workshops available (authors). Psychometric data forthcoming; currently available for previous version (DSM-III-R).										
Structured Interview for DSM Personality—IV (SIDP-IV)	Pfohl	101	Both	Yes	0–3 (2)	No. of criteria	90	Yes	Yes	American Psychiatric Press
Comments: "Super SIDP" version assesses ICD-10, DSM-III-R and -IV; only DSM-IV version available in diagnostic format; computer scoring, computer administered, training video and courses available. Psychometric data forthcoming; currently available for previous versions (III and III-R). SIDP on the internet: http://home.att.net/~SIDP/										

Note. Format: Questions arranged by diagnosis (Dx), topic (T), or both (two versions available). App. Dxes, DSM Appendix diagnoses; depressive and negativistic (passive–aggressive). Scoring (threshold), rating scale for criteria and diagnoses (Dxes); rating corresponding to threshold is in parentheses. Admin. (min.), administration time in minutes indicated by the author.

ies), range = .46 to 99, mean = .70; Personality Disorders Examination (PDE) (3 studies), range = .60 to .84, mean = .71; PIQ (2 studies), range = .49 to .88, mean = .71; Diagnostic Interview for DSM-IV Personality Disorders (DIPD) disorder (1 study), range = .52 to 1.0, mean = .89. The average joint-interview interrater reliability of these five interviews is thus remarkably consistent—.70 to .71—with the single exception of the DIP data, which come from a single small N (43) study conducted by the interview author (Zanarini, Frankenburg, Chauncey, & Gunderson, 1987). For "any personality disorder," mean kappas were .75 (SCID-II, N = 32; Renneberg, Chambless, Dowdall, Fauerbach, & Gracely, 1992), .82 (SIDP, two studies, N's = 43 and 104; Stangl, Pfohl, Zimmerman, Bowers, & Corenthal, 1985; Zimmerman & Coryell, 1989), .61 (PDE, two studies, N's = 60 and 20; Loranger, Susman, Oldham, & Russakoff, 1987; Standage & Ladha, 1988), and .89 (DIDP, N = 43, Zanarini et al., 1987). Although somewhat more variation is seen across these studies, interrater reliability for "any personality disorder" is above the standard cutoff of .70 for good agreement in all but one case.

Fewer test-retest studies have been conducted. Zimmerman (1994) reviewed four short-term (< 1 week) and five longer-term interval studies (average = 132 days). Kappa reliabilities for any personality disorder in the short-interval studies were .50 (SCID-II), .58 (DIPD), and .66 (SIDP), whereas mean kappas for individual diagnoses were .49 (SCID-II), .68 (DIPD), and .66 (SIDP). The SIDP (Pfohl, Black, Noyes, Coryell, & Barrash, 1990) and DIPD (Zanarini et al., 1987) data are each based on a single small sample (N's = 20 and 54, respectively), whereas those for the SCID-II were on two samples of reasonable size (103 patients and 181 nonpatients; First et al., 1995b). As noted previously, these values are expectably lower than those from joint-interview studies. Although the range of reliabilities across instruments is greater than that for the joint interviews, given these limited data it would be unwise to draw any firm conclusions regarding differential reliability of these interviews.

Zimmerman (1994) reported longer term test–retest reliability data for only three interviews—the SCID-II, PDE (or IPDE), and SIDP. Kappa for any personality disorder in 17 depressed inpatients assessed with the SCID-II an average of 2 months apart was .68; mean kappa

for individual diagnoses was .36 (range = −.08 to .77) (O'Boyle & Self, 1990). For the PDE, average kappa for any personality disorder in three studies was .46 (total N = 131); mean kappa for individual diagnoses in these and an additional larger (N = 243) study was .37 (range = −.04 to .70). Finally, for the SIDP, mean kappa for individual diagnoses in 36 depressed inpatients interviewed 6–12 months apart was .48 (range = .16 to .84; Pfohl et al., 1990). These data indicate that individual personality disorder diagnoses—and even a diagnosis of any personality disorder—is quite unstable beyond a few weeks, regardless of the instrument used to assess the disorders.

It is important to consider the source of this unreliability, whether it reflects true change (which would belie the concept of personality disorder as stable), *state* influences on measurement, or error variance. Critical evidence in this regard is that when dimensional scores, rather than diagnoses, are used to calculate reliability, test–retest reliabilities are considerably higher. For example, Loranger et al. (1991) reported temporal stabilities of diagnostic dimensional scores ranging from .60 to .76, with a median value of .72 in a sample of 84 patients interviewed from 1 week to 6 months apart, whereas the kappa values in this same sample range from .26 to .57, with a median of .55. The observed unreliability of diagnoses, therefore, cannot be attributed either to true change or only to state influences on measurement, because the underlying personality *traits* are relatively stable. Thus, the observed unreliability over longer periods is most likely due to measurement error, for example, the use of arbitrary cutoffs to define categorical diagnoses (Clark, 1999; Heumann & Morey, 1990).

Although dimensional assessments of personality pathology show greater stability than categorical assessments, they are still less stable than normal personality. One reason for this is inherent in the distinction between normal and pathological personality. That is, at least some personality pathology involves dysregulation—and accordingly, instability—of affective states (Cowdry & Gardner, 1991; Jones & Morey, 1995). To the extent that this variation in state affect influences trait assessment, lower test–retest stability of personality pathology compared to normal range personality is theoretically predicted, because of the inherent affective instability of the former.

Thus, ironically, the somewhat lower test–retest stabilities may themselves be evidence of measurement validity of personality pathology.

Interview Format

A major consideration in selecting an interview for clinical or research use is format or organization (First, Spitzer, Gibbon, & Williams, 1995a). Questions are grouped diagnostically in two interviews (DIPD-IV and SCID-II) and arranged by topic (e.g., Work, Interpersonal Relations, Impulse Control) in one (PDE), whereas two interviews offer a version with each format (PDI-IV and SIDP-IV). The primary argument for a diagnostic arrangement is that because the personality disorder criteria are intended to be manifestations of a given personality disorder, when the questions relevant to that disorder are grouped together, it facilitates judgment of whether a particular behavior exemplifies a core characteristic of the target disorder. The weakness of this approach is the potential for biased judgment: If a patient appears to be above (or below) threshold for the first two or three criteria for a diagnosis, the clinician may develop a positive (or negative) set and not rate subsequent criteria with appropriate objectivity, perhaps over- (or under-) probing in a conscious or unconscious attempt to confirm the initial diagnostic impression.

Of even greater concern is that patients will be affected by the grouping of questions. It has been shown for self-report questionnaires, for example, that when items tapping a single construct are administered without buffer items, the internal consistency of the scale increases through the course of administration (Knowles, 1988). This appears to occur because responding to a set of questions all on the same topic activates respondents' "self-schema" so that later responses increasingly reflect internalized and perhaps somewhat stereotypical self-constructs rather than independent judgments about the veridicality of each item (Hamilton & Shuminsky, 1990). Thus, when questions are grouped so as to facilitate recognition of a given diagnosis, even if the clinician is able to avoid biased judgment, patients' responses may be affected by whether they do or do not "identify with" that particular disorder. It must be noted, however, that it is not clear whether these processes (in either clinicians or patients) necessarily lead to decreased accuracy (see Clark, 1989, for a discussion of this issue with regard

to ratings of anxiety and depression). That is, Hamilton and Shuminsky (1990) have argued that activating self-schemas *increases* the reliability and criterion-related validity of measurement, perhaps by facilitating access to schema-relevant memories.

A second potential advantage of the diagnostically arranged format is that the user can easily select a subset of diagnoses for assessment for a particular clinical or research use. However, given the high degree of comorbidity among personality disorders, selective assessments can give a misleading impression about the sample or individual. For example, if only the sections for borderline and schizotypal personality disorder are used, the fact that many of those scoring positive for one or both of these diagnoses may meet criteria also for avoidant, dependent, antisocial or other personality disorder is obscured.

Proponents of the topically arranged format, on the other hand, argue that topical organization creates a more natural interview, in part because it facilitates patients' reflection on the various domains of their lives much as they would in ordinary discourse. That is, people think about their lives in terms of their work, their relationships, their moods and emotions, and so forth, so interviews organized around these topics flow easily because they parallel the way that patients parse their daily behavior. A concern with topical organization is that specific behaviors are multidetermined and may reflect different underlying traits. Thus, even if a given maladaptive behavior is present, it may not be clear which diagnostic criteria the behavior represents. For example, indecisiveness may stem from either the low self-confidence of dependent personality disorder or the anxious, overconcern with perfection of obsessive–compulsive personality disorder. Therefore, determining that a patient is pathologically indecisive is not sufficient for rating the relevant diagnostic criteria. However, topical-arrangement proponents respond to this critique by noting that this is not a problem in practice, because the interview format makes it readily apparent for which criteria the questions are intended to provide information. Indeed, they argue that it is more efficient to ask a single initial question about indecisiveness, for example, and then probe for the underlying construct or motivation if warranted, rather than having to ask about indecisiveness twice in two different contexts.

Skodol, Oldham, Rosnick, Kellman, and Hyler (1991) compared these two approaches to each other as well as to clinical assessment, using Spitzer's (1983) LEAD (longitudinal expert evaluation using all available data) standard. They found only modest agreement (median kappa = .50) between the diagnostically organized SCID-II and the topically arranged PDE. Moreover, neither approach was clearly more valid than the other in terms of its relation to the clinical method (median kappa = .25 in both cases). The diagnostic approach had a slight edge (i.e., ignoring statistical significance, kappas were higher for more diagnoses), but this may have simply reflected method variance, that is, its greater similarity to the clinical method. In sum, absent strong empirical data supporting the validity of one format over the other, the choice would appear to be largely a matter of preference or theoretical predilection. Users may wish to consider other features (e.g., availability of a screener, options for training, or quality of the manual) more heavily in their decision of which instrument to use.

Scoring

The most common scoring scale for criteria is 0–2, with 0 representing (near-)absence of the criteria; 1, a subclinical manifestation; and 2, at or above threshold. On the Personality Disorder Interview—IV (PDI-IV; Widiger, Mangine, Corbitt, Ellis, & Thomas, 1995), subclinical manifestations are grouped with absence and rated 0, a score of 1 indicates an at-or-above threshold level of the criteria, whereas 2 marks a prominent characteristic. The SIDP-IV (Pfohl, Blum, & Zimmerman, 1997) combines these two systems and provides a 4-point rating scale.

Scoring of diagnoses also varies by interview. The number of criteria or a total score for each diagnosis can be computed in all cases, as can a dichotomous judgment of presence or absence of personality disorder. The fact that interrater reliability for these instruments is typically reported as a kappa statistic indicates that—despite the greater reliability of the former scoring methods—the latter is favored. Most likely this reflects the theoretical adherence of most interview authors to the DSM categorical system.

Two interviews also provide for alternative scoring schemes. On the DIPD-IV (Zanarini, Frankenburg, Sickel, & Yong, 1996), disorders may be scored on the same 0–2 scale as criteria, with a score of 1 indicating that the person meets one fewer criteria than needed for a DSM diagnosis. The PDI-IV provides a unique scoring method: Each diagnosis is scored 0–6, with a score of 4 corresponding to the DSM threshold. The rationale for this method is that it provides a scoring system that is calibrated consistently across diagnoses regardless of the number of criteria required for the DSM threshold. Thus, a patient who meets only three antisocial personality disorder criteria is at the DSM threshold, whereas one must meet five dependent personality disorder criteria to be at the DSM threshold. Using the PDI-IV scoring method, these cases would receive the same rating of 4, reflecting the underlying assumption (which, it must be noted, has not been established empirically) that the DSM thresholds have a constant meaning across diagnoses.

Screeners

Three of the interviews have a screening instrument. The International Personality Disorder Examination (IPDE; Loranger, 1995) and the SCID-II (First, Gibbon, Spitzer, Williams, & Benjamin, 1997) both have a self-administered true–false format questionnaire, whereas the SIDP-IV screener is a brief clinician-administered interview. In the case of the SCID-II screener, the initial questions are designed to have high sensitivity at the cost of specificity. Thus, interviewers are to assume that "no" answers are veridical (but to use clinical judgment if they have reason to suspect that this is not so) and to follow up "yes" answers by interview to ascertain whether the characteristic is truly at or above threshold. In the case of both the IPDE and SIDP-IV screener, the instrument provides a global assessment of the likelihood of a personality disorder diagnosis. If the respondent is below threshold on the screener, a presumption of "no personality disorder diagnosis" is made; if above threshold on the screener, a full interview is to be administered.

Empirical data generally have supported the use of screens for identifying persons unlikely to have a personality disorder (e.g., Langbehn et al., 1999; Lenzenweger, Loranger, Korfine, & Neff, 1997). However, two points are important to note. First, the phenomenon is not limited to instruments specifically designed as screeners (e.g., Jacobsberg, 1995; Marlowe, Husband, Bonieskie, & Kirby, 1997), That is, most self-report instruments yield similar results and so could be used for screening purposes as well. Second, the use of either screening or other self-report instruments to identify *positive* cases has been notably unsuccessful in that they tend to yield excessively high numbers of false positives (e.g., Carey, 1994; Guthrie & Mobley, 1994; Lenzenweger et al., 1997). Thus, screeners are best used to screen out cases of no personality disorder in situations in which it would not be feasible to complete a full assessment on the entire sample.

Convergent Validity

Only a few studies have examined the convergent validity of interview-based measures of personality disorder (Hyler, Skodol, Kellman, Oldham, & Rosnick, 1990; Hyler, Skodol, Oldham, Kellman, & Doidge, 1992; Skodol et al., 1991; O'Boyle & Self, 1990). All involved the PDE and SCID-II, either in relation to each other or to clinical assessment, using Spitzer's (1983) LEAD standard. Comparing the two instruments across studies, kappas for "any personality disorder" were .38 to .40, whereas median kappas for specific personality disorders were .35, .46, and .50 (one study was common to these two sets of figures). Between either instrument and the LEAD standard, kappas were .25 and .28 for the PDE in two small-*N* studies and .25 for the SCID-II in one of these two (Skodol et al., 1991).

Clark et al. (1997) discuss a range of issues underlying this poor convergent validity including method variance (global or holistic vs. criterion-based approaches to personality disorder assessment) and differences in conceptualization of disorders, despite the strong influence of the DSM. They note, "without convergent validity in assessment, cumulative science is elusive if not impossible" (p. 211), and so we echo their call for additional research to increase the conceptual clarity of the personality disorder domain. Until a revised conceptualization of personality disorders provides a firmer basis on which to develop more convergent assessment instruments, personality disorder research will remain fragmentary, because instrument-based inconsistent findings will be the rule rather than the exception.

TRAIT-BASED INTERVIEWS

Interviews Focused on Personality Pathology

Four interviews are available for the assessment of pathological personality traits. Each assesses

multiple traits, but one—the Personality Assessment Schedule (PAS; Tyrer, 1988)—is designed to cover the full domain of personality disorder, whereas the others are single-category interviews: the Diagnostic Interview for Borderline Patients (DIB; Gunderson, Kolb, & Austin, 1981), the Diagnostic Interview for Narcissism (DIN; Gunderson, Ronningstam, & Bodkin, 1990), and the Psychopathy Check List—Revised (PCL-R; Hare, 1991). Targeting a specific diagnostic category, the latter interviews are fundamentally different in character from the omnibus diagnostic interviews we have just discussed. First, each is based on a concept of a personality disorder that only partially overlaps with the DSM conceptualization and, second, each assesses its target disorder in far greater depth than any of the omnibus interviews do. This fact is obvious from interview length alone: Most of the omnibus interviews are estimated to require 90–120 minutes (or less if a screener is used) to assess 10–12 personality disorder diagnoses. In contrast, the single-category interviews require up to 120 minutes to assess 20–33 elements of a single disorder.

The DIB and PCL-R both have been used extensively in research, whereas the DIN has been used less widely. Nevertheless, we comment only briefly on each instrument. Clinicians or researchers who are interested specifically in assessing these domains of psychopathology should contact the instrument developers for further information. At the same time, however, it is important to recognize that given the high rate of comorbidity among personality disorders, results based on a particular personality disorder diagnosis likely are not specific to that disorder, but are relevant to other disorders as well (Clark et al., 1997).

Diagnostic Interview for Borderline Patients (Gunderson et al., 1981). The DIB was developed in the 1970s to assess Gunderson's concept of borderline personality, which has influenced, but is not identical with, the DSM concept of this disorder. The 132-item interview yields ratings on 29 summary statements (e.g., one summary statement is "angry, hot-tempered, or sarcastic") that, in turn, are used to rate five areas of functioning: social adaptation, impulsive action patterns, affects, psychosis, and interpersonal relations. The social adaptation section was eliminated in a revision (DIB-R; Zanarini, Gunderson, Frankenburg, & Chauncey, 1989).

Reliability (interrater, test–retest, and internal consistency) of the instrument's total score appears acceptable (> .70), although its temporal stability and internal consistency have not been studied as extensively as its interrater reliability (Kaye & Shea, 2000). Consistent with theory, overlap with DSM borderline personality disorder ranges from modest to moderately strong, and the interview discriminates borderline personality disorder from depression and schizophrenia well. As with other measures of personality disorder, however, its ability to discriminate borderline personality disorder from other personality disorders is modest. A strength of the DIB is its ability to provide a rich clinical picture of severe personality disorder. However, specific interpretation of the area scores is not recommended, as they are of modest reliability (Kaye & Shea, 2000).

Diagnostic Interview for Narcissism (Gunderson et al., 1990). The DIN was developed based on a literature review of prominent characteristics of narcissistic persons as well as the clinical experiences of the authors. The interview consists of 33 statements that yield five scores: grandiosity, interpersonal relations, reactiveness, affects and mood states, and social and moral judgments. Three of the sections (grandiosity, interpersonal relations, and reactiveness) are assessed over a 3-year time frame and affects and mood states over the past year, whereas assessment of social and moral judgments encompasses the previous 5-year period. Ten of the characteristics overlap with the narcissistic personality disorder criteria of the DSM.

Interrater reliability was good for both total score (intraclass coefficient = .88) and section scores (range = .74 to .96) (Gunderson et al., 1990). Internal consistency reliability (Cronbach's alpha) was .81 in a sample of 82 patients. Given the length of the instrument, this represents a moderately heterogeneous set of item (average interitem r = .13). Fourteen of the 33 statements differentiated the patients with and without narcissistic personality disorder, with seven (50%) of the significant items coming from the eight-item grandiosity section (Ronningstam & Gunderson, 1990). Thus, DSM narcissistic personality disorder appears to be more unidimensional than the characteristics measured by the DIN.

Psychopathy Check List—Revised (Hare, 1991). Based on Hare's (1970) modification of Cleckley's (1976) concept of psychopathy, the PCL-R assesses 20 psychopathic characteristics. Factor-analytic studies of the PCL-R (e.g., Hare et al., 1990; Harpur, Hare, & Hakstian, 1989) as well as more recent analyses based on item response theory (Cooke & Michie, 1997) generally have found that these characteristics form two correlated factors: affective and interpersonal features of psychopathy (e.g., glibness or superficial charm and grandiose sense of self-worth) and socially deviant features (e.g., impulsivity and irresponsibility). Ratings are made for lifetime functioning on the basis of both a client interview and review of collateral information. Although considerable clinical judgment is required, trained raters yield reliable scores, and test–retest reliability also is high (Hare, 1991). A 12-item Screening Version of the Psychopathy Checklist—Revised (PCL:SV; Hart, Cox, & Hare, 1995) has been shown to be an effective short form of the PCL-R (Cooke, Michie, Hart, & Hare, 1999).

Correlations of DSM antisocial personality disorder are moderate with PCL-R total scores, low to moderate with Factor 1 (psychopathic personality characteristics) scores, and moderately high with scores on Factor 2 (socially deviant behaviors). At least in forensic settings, antisocial personality disorder is the broader construct, with the vast majority of criminal psychopaths meeting DSM criteria, but only approximately one-quarter of those with antisocial personality disorder meeting criteria for PCL-R psychopathy. Extensive validity data collected primarily in forensic settings over 25 years document relations to outcome following prison release or treatment and to multiple variables related to criminal behavior and criminal history (Hare, 1991).

Personality Assessment Schedule (Tyrer, 1988). Tyrer and colleagues were early proponents of a trait-based approach to assessing personality pathology (Tyrer, Alexander, Cicchetti, Cohen, & Remington, 1979). They also have examined the importance of obtaining information from a collateral source other than the patient (Brothwell, Casey, & Tyrer, 1992; Tyrer, Strauss, & Cicchetti, 1983). The PAS assesses 24 traits (e.g., conscientiousness, aggression, and impulsiveness) that are grouped by cluster analysis into five personality styles: normal, passive–dependent, sociopathic, anankastic (compulsive), and schizoid. Several studies have found good interrater reliability, including cross-nationally (Tyrer et al., 1984), as well as reported validity data comparable to that found with more widely used instruments (e.g., Brophy, 1994; Fahy, Eisler, & Russell, 1993; Tyrer, Merson, Onyett, & Johnson, 1994). The instrument appears to be the only comprehensive interview of personality pathology from a trait-dimensional perspective and so deserves greater attention, especially in the United States.

An Interview Focused on Normal Personality

Structured Interview for the Five-Factor Model of Personality (SIFFM; Trull & Widiger, 1997). The SIFFM is a relatively new instrument and, as an interview designed to assess dimensions of normal personality, appears to be unique. Modeled after the NEO-Personality Inventory—Revised (NEO-PI-R; Costa & McCrae, 1992), the 120-item interview provides scores for all six facets of each of the five domains of neuroticism (N), extraversion (E), conscientiousness (C), agreeableness (A), and openness (O). Somewhat more emphasis was given in the interview to maladaptive aspects of personality compared to the NEO-PI-R (Trull et al., 1998).

Interrater reliability in two studies conducted by the authors was high for both facet (mean intraclass coefficient = .92; range = .71–.98) and domain (mean ICC = .96; range = .94–.97) scores, and alphas for domain scores were acceptable (median = .80; range = .72 for agreeableness to .89 for neuroticism; Trull et al., 1998). However, alphas for facet scores were highly variable, ranging from .31 to .85 (mean = .56), suggesting that interpretation of individual facet scores may be unreliable. Convergent and discriminant validity with both self and peer scores on the NEO-PI-R were generally good for the five domains but, again, variable for facets. Consistent with NEO-PI-R data (Costa & McCrae, 1992), interscale correlations on the SIFFM indicated that the five domains are not as independent as theory would have them. N and E correlated −.54, for example, and only Agreeableness had negligible correlations with all other scores.

Analyses with self-reported personality disorder using the Personality Diagnostic Questionnaire—Revised (PDQ-R) indicated that SIFFM scores contributed significantly to prediction of 10 of 13 PDQ-R scores even after common variance with NEO-PI-R scores had

been removed, which perhaps reflects the SIFFM's increased emphasis on maladaptive aspects of personality. In sum, the instrument appears promising as an alternative method for assessing personality pathology.

DIAGNOSTICALLY BASED SELF-REPORT INSTRUMENTS

As mentioned earlier, there are seven self-report measures designed to assess DSM personality disorder diagnoses. As with the diagnostic interviews, the personality disorder section (Kaye & Shea, 2000) of the American Psychiatric Association's *Handbook of Psychiatric Measures* (Rush et al., 2000) provides basic information on most of these measures. Table 13.3 presents descriptive characteristics of these instruments. All the measures currently are or soon will be available in a DSM-IV version. Again, few psychometric data are available for these revisions, so some caution should be exercised when extrapolating from earlier versions to the newer instruments.

These measures share many important features that are not detailed in the table. Specifically, all the instruments assess the appendixed diagnoses (negativistic and depressive personality disorder) except for the Minnesota Multiphasic Personality Inventory—Personality Disorder Scales (MMPI-PD; Morey, Waugh, & Blashfield, 1985) and the Personality Assessment Inventory (PAI; Morey, 1991). In fact, it is noteworthy that the PAI was developed to assess major clinical constructs that are important for clinical diagnosis, screening for psychopathology and/or treatment planning rather than specific DSM diagnoses. As such, among its 22 scales are 11 clinical scales, only 2 of which measure personality pathology: the Borderline Features and Antisocial Features scales. In this regard, the PAI is likely to be less useful in assessing the full spectrum of personality disorders compared to instruments that were designed explicitly to measure Axis II (Morey & Henry, 1994).

Computer scoring is available for all the measures in Table 13.3, with the exception of the Coolidge Axis II Inventory (CATI; Coolidge & Merwin, 1992) and the MMPI-PD. In addition, the PAI, the Wisconsin Personality Disorders Inventory-IV (WISPI; Klein et al., 1993), and the PDQ-IV (Hyler, 1994) also have computer-administered versions.

TABLE 13.3. Summary of Key Features of Self-Report Instruments Assessing Personality Disorder Diagnoses

Instrument	Primary author	No. of items	Rating format	Collateral form	Admin. (min.)	Total no. of scales	©	Availability
Coolidge Axis II Inventory (CATI)	Coolidge	200	4 pt.	Yes	45–60	18	Yes	Author
Millon Clinical Multiaxial Inventory—III (MCMI-III)	Millon	175	T/F	No	20–30	24	Yes	NCS
Minnesota Multiphasic Personality Inventory— Personality Disorder Scales (MMPI-PD)	Morey	157	T/F	No	60–90[a]	11	Yes[a]	NCS
Personality Assessment Inventory (PAI)	Morey	344	4 pt.	No	40–50	22	Yes	PAR
Personality Diagnostic Questionnaire—4 (PDQ-4)	Hyler	85	T/F	Yes	20–30	14	Yes	NiJo Software[b]
Schedule of Nonadaptive and Adaptive Personality (SNAP)	Clark	375	T/F	Yes	60±15	34	Yes	UMP[c]
Wisconsin Personality Disorders Inventory—IV (WISPI-IV)	Klein	214	10 pt.	No	<60	12	Yes	Author

Note. NCS, National Computer Systems; PAR, Psychological Assessment Resources; UMP, University of Minnesota Press.
[a]In the context of the MMPI(-2); permission must be obtained from NCS and the UMP to administer otherwise.
[b]http://www.pdq4.com
[c]http://www.upress.umn.edu/tests/snap_overview.html

Length

One frequently cited advantage of self-report instruments is their relative efficiency as compared to interviews. In selecting an instrument to maximize efficiency, a potentially critical consideration is the required completion time. There is substantial variability in length and, accordingly, the average administration time of the various measures. Moreover, there is variability in the authors' estimated time of completion. For example, as can be seen from Table 13.3, the shortest measure is the PDQ, at 85 items. Although the authors of both the PDQ and the Millon Clinical Multiaxial Inventory— III (MCMI-III; Millon, Davis, & Millon, 1994) suggest that 20–30 minutes is needed for test administration, with approximately one-half as many items as the MCMI, it is reasonable to assume that the PDQ should require less completion time. Indeed, averaging across estimated times per item (and considering the fact that true–false format items take less time to complete than those using Likert-type ratings), the PDQ completion time is likely an overestimate. However, the potential benefit to efficiency provided by a shorter inventory may be offset by lower reliability and validity with regard to the measured constructs, as a greater number of items will yield higher reliabilities (all other things being equal) and may provide significant incremental validity as well (Widiger & Frances, 1987).

It has been suggested that the PDQ may be particularly useful as a screening instrument, due to its low-to-moderate specificity and high sensitivity coupled with good negative predictive power (Guthrie & Mobley, 1994; Hunt & Andrews, 1992; Hyler et al., 1992). These characteristics, however, are not unique to the PDQ. As described earlier, several of the interviews for personality disorders have screening instruments with these properties. In fact, most self-report measures demonstrate greater sensitivity and less specificity than do structured interviews, with self-report measures often found to produce a higher rate of false positives (Guthrie & Mobley, 1994; Marlowe et al., 1997; Trull & Larson, 1994). In this regard, Loranger (1992) stated that the greatest potential of self-report inventories lies in their utility as screening measures and that, in general, they are unsuitable for making personality disorder diagnoses.

In addition to increased reliability and potential validity, longer measures generally also include other useful indices. For example, the two longest instruments, the PAI (Morey, 1991) and the SNAP (Clark, 1993a), both assess constructs in addition to DSM diagnoses. In addition to the two personality pathology scales, the PAI includes nine other clinical scales, four validity scales, five treatment scales, and two interpersonal scales. The SNAP includes 15 trait and temperament scales and 6 validity scales, in addition to the 13 diagnostic scales. Both instruments allow a fuller characterization of a respondent's clinical picture and response style than do briefer measures.

Method of Construction

An important consideration in selecting a measure to assess personality disorders is the extent to which the content of the instrument corresponds to the DSM personality disorder constructs. For four of the measures discussed here—the CATI, PDQ, SNAP, and WISPI—items were written or selected expressly to assess specific DSM Axis II criteria. In the case of the SNAP, the initial item pool was developed by rational means; items were then retained or eliminated on the basis of empirical correlations with interview-based responses. The WISPI is unique in that items were written to reflect the phenomenology of the disorder being assessed.

On all these instruments, scores are obtained by counting the number of criteria met and/or by summing the diagnostically relevant items. However, the instruments vary on how many items represent each criterion. The high end is anchored by the SNAP, in which two to five items represent each DSM diagnostic criterion (Clark, 1993a). Approximately two items assess each criterion on the CATI, although the number varies with the disorder assessed (Coolidge & Merwin, 1992). The development of the WISPI was not based directly on the DSM but on Benjamin's (1974) SASB model of interpersonal behavior and her conceptions of the DSM Axis II disorders (Benjamin, 1986, 1996a). As with the CATI, approximately two WISPI items assess interpersonal formulations of each DSM criterion (Klein et al., 1993). The PDQ represents the extreme low end, with each item assessing a single criterion.

The PDQ in particular has been criticized because its items and scales were constructed on the basis of face validity in tapping specific diagnostic criteria. This is said to result in a measure that may be more susceptible to invalid responding, with clients easily able to exaggerate or deny the presence of maladaptive personality traits because the targets of assessment are obvious (Widiger & Frances, 1987). Again, however, this criticism is applicable to the other instruments as well; nevertheless, it is important to note that each of the direct-from-DSM measures contains validity scales to flag protocols that reflect extremes of biased responding. For example, the CATI contains two validity scales: One scale, consisting of only three items, was designed to detect individuals who are responding randomly. The other scale was constructed to identify symptom exaggeration or denial (Coolidge & Merwin, 1992). Similarly, the PDQ contains two scales designed to detect random and defensive responding, carelessness, and lying (Hyler, 1994). The SNAP is the most sophisticated instrument in this regard, including five validity scales constructed to indicate the influence of various response sets including carelessness or random responding, two levels of defensive responding and deviant responding, plus a sixth overall index of invalid responding (Clark, 1993a).

In contrast to these criterion-based measures, the content of the remaining instruments' scales overlaps significantly with, but does not fully correspond to, the DSM criteria. These measures provide a global assessment of the personality disorders, without an item-for-item matching with the diagnostic criteria. For example, in constructing the MMPI-PD scales, Morey et al. (1985) employed a rational/empirical strategy of item selection, culling items from the full MMPI item pool (Hathaway & McKinley, 1951) that reflected each diagnosis as a whole. Two sets of scales were developed—one set with overlapping items and another set of nonoverlapping scales. Within the overlapping scales, an item could be designated as representative of more than one disorder, whereas for the nonoverlapping scale each item was placed on the scale for which it was most prototypical.

Similarly, the MCMI provides an holistic assessment of the personality disorders. However, unlike the MMPI-PD scales, which were based on the DSM, the MCMI originally was developed to measure Millon's (1981) diagnostic system. As a result, a frequent criticism of the MCMI has been that it may better reflect Millon's theoretical personality styles than DSM personality disorder diagnoses (Choca, Shanley, Van Denburg, & Agresti, 1992; Flynn, Mc-

Cann, & Fairbank, 1995; McCann, 1991; Widiger, Williams, Spitzer, & Frances, 1985). Reportedly, subsequent revisions to the original inventory have yielded an instrument more closely aligned with the DSM diagnostic system (Millon, 1985; Millon & Davis, 1997). However, the new instrument retains a grounding in Millon's theoretical system. Millon and Davis (1997) describe the MCMI-III as a measure "of the DSM constructs, but more" (p. 84), with the "more" consisting of Millon's theoretical conceptualizations of the Axis II disorders.

Collateral Versions

A final consideration when selecting a self-report instrument is the availability of a collateral (also known as informant) version of the measure. A recurring theme in the personality disorder assessment literature (e.g., Bernstein et al., 1997; Hirschfeld, 1993; Zimmerman, 1994) is the suggestion that individuals with personality disorders may not be accurate reporters of their own problematic thoughts, feelings, and behaviors. However, despite anecdotal evidence of lack of insight in personality disorder patients, we are unaware of any study that has tested this oft-repeated idea empirically using formal assessment. It may be, for example, that personality disorder patients lack insight into the consequences of their behavior or the effects of their behaviors on others but are quite able to report accurately on their behaviors per se.

For normal-range personality, a voluminous literature has revealed that relations between self and peer ratings (as informant or collateral ratings are known in this literature) are quite complex and has helped to clarify the causes of variation in the convergence of self and peer ratings (e.g., Funder, Kolar, & Blackman, 1995; John & Robins, 1994; Ready, Clark, Watson, & Westerhouse, 2000). In contrast, there is little research into this topic in personality pathology, most of which has involved interview-based measures, which introduces the interviewer as additional source of variation (e.g., Bernstein et al., 1997; Brothwell et al., 1992; Zimmerman, Pfohl, Coryell, Stangl, & Corenthal, 1988). Thus, the effect of using collateral information, such as that obtained from a spouse or parent, on the validity of personality disorder assessments derived either from questionnaire ratings or interviews remains unknown. This is clearly an important area of further research. Nevertheless, there is value in multimethod assessment

of any variable, including personality traits, so availability of a collateral rating form may be an asset.

As can be seen in Table 13.3, the CATI, PDQ, and SNAP offer a collateral or informant version. Little has been published using any of these instruments, however. Both the CATI "significant-other form" and the SNAP Collateral Rating Form have been used in one nonpatient study (Coolidge, Burns, & Mooney, 1995, for the CATI; Ready et al., 2000, for the SNAP), with results comparable to those obtained using instruments designed for normal personality. In addition, a version of the SNAP that uses a trait–descriptor format has been developed for use with collateral raters. Harlan and Clark (1999) report on its use in a normal sample and it currently is being tested in patient, community adult, and normal adolescent samples. Use of a version of the PDQ-R modified for informants in a sample of 60 psychiatric patients yielded two reports (Dowson, 1992a, 1992b) that indicated significant correlations between the self and informant versions.

Reliability

In contrast to diagnostically based interviews, which focus on interrater reliability, reliability studies of diagnostically based self-report instruments typically report internal consistency reliabilities (usually Cronbach's coefficient alpha) and, somewhat less frequently, temporal stability. Because the scales of most of these instruments are based directly on the DSM criteria (the Millon instruments are an exception), their internal consistencies are determined to a large extent by those criteria. Table 13.4 shows representative studies of reliability data for those instruments in Table 13.3 that assess the full range of DSM Axis II diagnoses.

Median alphas range from .52 (PDQ-R) to .90 (WISPI). The PDQ-IV scales appear to be somewhat more internally consistent than their predecessors, assuming that they perform in English as they do in Italian. Due to changes in the MMPI, the MMPI-2-PD scales are 0–2 items shorter than the original, but the lower alphas shown in the table are more likely due to restriction of range in the small sample of male prisoners. The WISPI scales have the highest alpha coefficients, which may be, in part, because the scales are longer than those of most other instruments (median = 28 items compared to 22 items for the SNAP and MMPI-PD

TABLE 13.4. Representative Studies of Reliability Data for Diagnostically Based Self-Report Instruments

Measure	Reliability estimates		Sample	Source
	Median	Range		
Internal consistency reliability				
CATI	.76	.68–.87	601 nonpatients	Coolidge & Merwin (1992)
MMPI-PD	.76	.68–.86	475 patients	Morey, Waugh, & Blashfield (1985)
MMPI-2-PD	.66	.56–.81	81 male prisoners	O'Maille & Fine (1995)
PDQ-R	.52	.36–.69	51 patients	Trull (1993)
PDQ-IV	.64	.46–.74	300 Italian patients	Fossati et al. (1998)
SNAP	.78	.53–.90	5 samples; patients and nonpatients	Clark (1993)
WISPI	.90	.84–.96	1,230 patients and nonpatients	Klein et al. (1993)
Short-term test–retest reliability				
CATI	.90	.78–.97	39 students	Coolidge & Merwin (1992)
MCMI-III	.90	.87–.93	Not reported	Craig (1997, citing test manual)
WISPI	.88	.71–.91	80 patients and nonpatients	Klein et al. (1993)
Longer-term test–retest reliability				
MCMI-I/II	.70	.41–.91	16 data sets	Craig (1997)
MMPI-PD	.73	.57–.82	51 patients	Trull (1993)
PDQ-R	.66	.50–.75	51 patients	Trull (1993)
SNAP	.70	.60–.75	56 lower-back-pain patients	Clark (2000)

Note. Internal consistency data not supplied for the MCMI; see text for explanation.

scales, for example) and also because of the mixed nature of the sample on which the coefficient was computed. Moreover, scales with multiple-point rating formats tend to have higher reliabilities than those using a true–false format, so the WISPI and CATI scales (with 10- and 4-point rating scales, respectively) may be more reliable for this reason as well. The MCMI is omitted from this portion of the table because psychometric reports on the MCMI tend to ignore internal consistency (referring the reader to the test manual). Internal consistencies for the MCMI-II scales are reportedly all above .80 (Dyer, 1997, citing the test manual), whereas those for the MCMI-III range from .66 to .90 (Choca & Van Denburg, 1997, citing the test manual).

Test–retest data are presented separately for short and longer retest intervals. Within these subsets, there is little variation between measures, indicating clearly that time is the governing factor rather than instrument. It is also noteworthy that self-report instruments are also prone to unreliability due to measurement error when categorical diagnoses are assessed compared to dimensional scores. For example, the SNAP scales yield both dimensional scores and categorical diagnoses. In the sample of 56 lower back pain patients shown in Table 13.4, for seven personality disorder diagnoses for which at least five patients met criteria either on test or retest, the reliability of the dimensional scores ranged from .66 to .75 with a median of .69, whereas the reliability of the categorical diagnoses ranged from .16 to .88, with a median of .40. For only one diagnosis—borderline personality disorder—was the reliability higher for the diagnosis (kappa = .88) than the dimensional score (.66).

Validity

As mentioned earlier, Clark et al. (1997) recently reviewed the validity of diagnostically based measures of personality disorder, both interview and self-report. Again, we shall cite only their main conclusions here. Median convergence among self-report measures was moderate, with median correlations ranging from

.39 to .68 (grand median = .51). However, convergence between questionnaires and interviews was more modest, with a grand median of .39 (range = .19 to .54). In those studies that reported kappa values, the grand median was .27 in 11 comparisons (range = .08 to .42). To summarize these results, Clark et al. quoted Perry (1992) that for the most part, diagnoses "are not significantly comparable across methods beyond chance, which is not scientifically acceptable" (p. 1645). Degree of convergence was not affected by the version of DSM assessed but did vary according to the scale construction approach of the instrument (i.e., due to method variance). Another source of variation was diagnosis, with some diagnoses (e.g., avoidant personality disorder) evidencing considerably more convergent validity than did others (e.g., obsessive–compulsive personality disorder). As noted earlier, despite the strong influence of the DSM on the field, considerable disagreement still exists regarding the core nature of some personality disorders.

Problems of discriminant validity are equally, if not more, severe, and are revealed by the very high levels of comorbidity across personality disorder diagnoses. Moreover, measures that from the standpoint of convergent validity appear to have superior psychometric properties conversely tend to show poorer discriminant validity (and vice versa). The reason for this is that convergent measures often are correlated because they both tap broad and nonspecific factors of psychopathology, such as negative affectivity (neuroticism). To the extent that this general variance pervades the instruments, they will show poor discriminant validity. Measures that are less saturated with nonspecific pathology will tend to have lower discriminant correlations, but the specific variance tapped by their scales often fails to converge, so they cannot be said to assess the same construct despite the similarity of the scale names or diagnostic labels.

It is impossible to overstate the seriousness of the problems revealed by the poor convergent and discriminant validity of personality disorder measures, and the implications for classification research are profound. That is, when researchers use different instruments (interview or self-reports) to identify individuals with personality disorder—either in general or with a specific diagnosis—they may identify groups of individuals with substantially different characteristics. This virtually guarantees

that research results will not replicate, despite the fact that the groups carry the same diagnostic label or both scored high on scales with similar names. Without replicability, cumulative, critical study of personality disorders cannot occur and we have no possibility of refining our current set of diagnoses.

Conversely, suppose that one research group carries out a study with a set of individuals identified as borderline personality disorder and another research group conducts a study using individuals identified as avoidant personality disorder. Prior research with the measures used in these studies has shown that these diagnoses are approximately 50% overlapping. Clearly, it is inaccurate simply to characterize the results of the first study as relevant to borderline personality disorder and the other to avoidant personality disorder, as if they were unrelated results. Rather, the results of each study are quasi-relevant to those of the other, yet without additional measurement of the personality pathology, it may be impossible to tease apart the precise characteristics that underlie the study results.

Thus, the conceptual adequacy of the DSM constructs and the operationalization of these constructs in the DSM criterion sets are both critical issues. To the extent that existing assessment instruments faithfully reflect the DSM criteria, their convergent and discriminant validity depend on the adequacy with which the criteria represent the underlying constructs. If the criteria validly operationalize the intended constructs and the assessment instruments accurately reflect this operationalization, then we must conclude that the observed overlap among disorders is part of the conceptualization of the DSM personality disorders. However, this is clearly not the case, as evidenced by the efforts of the DSM Axis II Workgroup to distinguish between disorders to the extent possible.

Thus, the data suggest at least three (not mutually exclusive) possibilities: inadequate conceptualization of the basic constructs, a failure of the DSM criteria to represent the underlying constructs adequately, or a failure of existing assessment devices to reflect the criteria accurately. After extended discussion of these and related issues, Clark et al. (1997) concluded "that, while there certainly is room for improvement in both operationalization and instrumentation, it is the conceptualization of the disorders themselves that needs to be reexamined" (p. 214).

TRAIT-BASED SELF-REPORT INSTRUMENTS

Even in the DSM, personality disorders are defined as sets of maladaptive traits. Given this fact, and also the problematic reliability (Zimmerman, 1994) and validity (Clark et al., 1997) of DSM personality disorder diagnoses, many researchers have suggested that assessment of personality pathology should be focused on the fundamental trait dimensions of personality and its pathology rather than on diagnostic categories (Clark, 1990; Clark et al., 1997; Cloninger, 1987; Costa & McCrae, 1990; Eysenck, 1987; Harkness, 1992; Livesley, Jackson, & Schroeder, 1989; Millon, 1987; Siever & Davis, 1991; Telle-

gen & Waller, in press; Tyrer & Alexander, 1979; Widiger, Trull, Hurt, Clarkin, & Frances, 1987). Accordingly, trait-based self-report instruments have been developed specifically to assess personality pathology, whereas other instruments, which were developed to measure normal-range traits, have been applied to personality disorder assessment. Although the instruments developed from these two disparate origins assess overlapping domains (Clark, 1993a; Clark & Livesley, 1994; Schroeder, Wormworth, & Livesley, 1992, 1994), it is reasonable to expect differential coverage of personality dysfunction by these two types of instruments. Table 13.5 summarizes important features of the measures that we review in this chapter.

TABLE 13.5. Summary of Key Features of Self-Report Instruments Assessing Multiple Traits Relevant to Personality Disorder

Instrument	Primary author(s)	No. of items (sets)	Rating format	Collateral form	Admin. (min.)	No. of scales or subscales	©	Availability
Instruments targeting personality pathology								
Dimensional Assessment of Personality Pathology—Basic Questionnaire (DAPP-BQ)	Livesley	290	6 pt.	No	60–75	18	Yes	Sigma Press
Schedule of Nonadaptive and Adaptive Personality (SNAP)	Clark	375	T/F	Yes	60±15	15	Yes	UMP
Personality Psychopathology—Five	Harkness	139/115	T/F	No	60–90[a]	5	Yes	NCS
Inventory of Interpersonal Problems—Personality Disorder scales (IIP-PD)	Pilkonis	47	5 pt.	No	20–30	5	Yes	PC
Instruments targeting normal personality								
NEO Personality Inventory—Revised (NEO-PI-R);	Costa/McCrae	240	5 pt.	Yes	40–50	5/30	Yes	PAR
NEO-Five-Factor Inventory (FFI)		60	5 pt.	No	10–15	5	Yes	PAR
Extended Interpersonal Adjective Scales—Revised-Big 5 (IASR-B5)	Trapnell/Wiggins	124	8 pt.	No	10–15	5	No?	Author?
Personality Adjective Check List (PACL)	Strack	153	CL	No	10–15	11	Yes?	Author?
Tridimensional Personality Questionnaire (TPQ)	Cloninger	100	T/F	No	15–20	3	Yes?	Author?
Temperament and Character Inventory (TCI)	Cloninger	226	T/F	No	35–45	7	Yes?	Author?

Note. NCS, National Computer Systems; PC, Psychological Corporation; PAR, Psychological Assessment Resources; UMP, University of Minnesota Press; CL, checklist; T/F, true/false.
[a]In the context of the MMPI(-2); permission must be obtained from NCS and the UMP to administer otherwise.

As with trait-based interviews, trait-based self-report measures may assess either a single dimension or multiple traits. The decision of which type of instrument to select is largely dependent on the purpose of assessment. A multiscale inventory may be preferred when it is important to assess a range of traits to obtain an overall profile of personality pathology. In contrast, single-scale instruments may be more useful if one is interested in a particular subdomain of personality functioning and is willing either to ignore the problems of comorbidity and discriminant validity or to address them in other ways (Widiger & Frances, 1987).

Instruments Targeting Personality Pathology

Following the advent of Axis II in 1980 and unbeknownst to each other, Livesley and Clark each began developing their respective instruments with the same aim: to assess the components of personality disorders as described in the DSMs without explicitly assessing the DSM diagnoses per se. Interestingly, however, they adopted very different methods in pursuit of this common goal.

Dimensional Assessment of Personality Pathology—Basic Questionnaire (DAPP-BQ; Livesley & Jackson, in press). Livesley first compiled a comprehensive list of trait descriptors and behavioral acts that were characteristic of each DSM-III and DSM-III-R Axis II category. These characteristics were then rated by clinicians as to the prototypicality of the items for the relevant diagnoses (Livesley et al., 1989). After several rounds of data collection and analysis with both normal and patient samples, the result was a 290-item instrument that assesses 18 dimensions of personality pathology. The DAPP-BQ scales are internally consistent—coefficient alphas ranging from .80 to .93—and temporally stable—*r*'s ranged from .82 to .93 (Schroeder et al., 1992). The DAPP-BQ scales have demonstrated good convergence with other self-report measures of personality traits (e.g., Clark, Livesley, Schroeder, & Irish, 1996; Schroeder et al., 1992).

Schedule of Nonadaptive and Adaptive Personality (Clark, 1993a). Clark (1990) compiled criteria culled from DSMs, non-DSM conceptualizations of personality disorders, and selected Axis I disorders that shared features with personality disorders (e.g., generalized anxiety disorder). Clinicians freely sorted these criteria into synonym groups that were then subjected to factor analysis, resulting in 22 consensual criterion clusters. Items were written to assess each cluster. Subsequent rounds of data collection and analysis in both normal and clinical samples yielded 12-trait dimensional scales and 3 higher-order temperament scales. The SNAP scales are internally consistent (alphas ranged from .71 to .92 in both clinical and normal samples) and stable over short to moderate time periods, with 1-week to 2-month retest *r*'s ranging from .68 to .91 (Clark, 1993a). In addition to demonstrating convergence with other trait measures, the SNAP scales have shown strong and systematic correlations with interview-based ratings of personality disorder (Clark, 1993a).

Personality Psychopathology—Five (PSY-5; Harkness & McNulty, 1994). The PSY-5 are a set of personality constructs developed to be relevant to psychopathology and currently measured with items from the MMPI-2 for adults (Harkness, McNulty, & Ben-Porath, 1995) or MMPI-A for adolescents (McNulty, Harkness, Ben-Porath, & Williams, 1997). Two of the dimensions—negative and positive emotionality—have direct counterparts in the five-factor model (FFM; neuroticism and extraversion, respectively). In contrast, aggressiveness, constraint, and psychoticism reflect a combination of higher-order FFM traits; represent more specific, lower-order variance; or tap unique variance not covered by the FFM (Harkness et al., 1995; Trull, Useda, Costa, & McCrae, 1995).

Reliabilities (internal consistency and stability) of the adult MMPI-2 scales were generally high (averaging in the .70s), but variable (ranging from the .40s to the .80s), suggesting that the scales have somewhat different "bandwidths" (Trull et al., 1995). Alphas reported for the adolescent MMPI-A scales were consistently in the .70s in the development samples, but cross-validation is needed and stability has not been studied. The convergent and discriminant validity of the two scale sets in relation to each other also has not yet been studied, but preliminary data suggest that certain scales may tap somewhat different constructs. For example, aggressiveness and negative emotionality scales correlate much more strongly in the adolescent than adult versions, as do constraint and psychoticism.

Correlations with self-report and interview measures of the DSM personality disorders suggest considerable overlapping variance but, somewhat surprisingly, no more (on average) than that between the FFM and DSM (Trull et al., 1995). External validity for the PSY-5 adolescent scales is also encouraging with, for example, correlations of about –.40 between constraint and scales assessing externalizing, drug use, and sexual acting out rated from clinic records (McNulty et al., 1997).

Convergent Validity. Despite disparate developmental processes and origins, the SNAP and the DAPP-BQ shared a similar developmental strategy: They were both constructed from conceptually related lower-order components—traits and behaviors of personality disorder—that were built toward a final, dimensional structure to describe lower-order components of the personality disorder hierarchy. In contrast, the PSY-5 constructs and scales are targeted toward the higher-order level of personality assessment. In two empirical studies, the DAPP-BQ and SNAP demonstrated good convergent and discriminant validity at the level of specific lower-order scales, as well as at the higher-order level of maladaptive personality (Clark & Livesley, 1994; Clark et al., 1996).

Moreover, at the higher-order level, all three instruments have shown strong convergent and discriminant patterns with measures of the FFM (Clark & Livesley, 1994; Clark et al., 1996; Schroeder et al., 1992, 1994; Trull et al., 1995). These convergences indicate, first, that the lower level of personality pathology is more systematic than is generally acknowledged (see also Harkness, 1992) and that these measures, though developed through disparate methodologies, provide broad coverage of the domain. In addition, however, each measure appears to tap additional variance that is not well covered by measures of the FFM.

Inventory of Interpersonal Problems—Personality Disorder Scales (IIP-PD; Pilkonis, Kim, Proietti, & Barkham, 1996). The IIP-PD was constructed from the existing item pool of the Inventory of Interpersonal Problems (IIP; Horowitz, Rosenberg, Baer, Ureño, & Villaseñor, 1988), a 127-item measure developed to assess distress in interpersonal relationships. Pilkonis et al. (1996) identified five subscales (totaling 47 items): Three of these subscales

were based on items that discriminated the presence versus absence of any personality disorder and also served as markers of Cluster B membership. The two additional subscales were created to distinguish patients with any Cluster C diagnosis from all other personality disorders; however, they subsequently demonstrated limited ability to do so. In contrast, the presence versus absence subscales showed good sensitivity in determining the presence of any personality disorder, and Pilkonis et al. (1996) recommended the IIP-PD as a screening measure. A later study (Kim, Pilkonis, & Barkham, 1997) provided further support for the utility of IIP-PD subscales in assessing general personality pathology.

Instruments Targeting Normal Traits

NEO Personality Inventory—Revised (Costa & McCrae, 1992). The NEO-PI-R is arguably the most widely used measure designed to assess the FFM of normal personality. The five robust factors of neuroticism, extraversion, conscientiousness, agreeableness, and openness represent higher-order traits that reflect the broadest dimensions of dispositions or temperaments. The NEO-PI-R provides scores on each of these five domains, as well as on six facets within each domain. Costa and McCrae (1992) report extensive reliability and validity data on the NEO PI-R scales within normal samples. More recently, researchers have advocated the use of the FFM in research and diagnosis of personality pathology (Costa & McCrae, 1992; Widiger, 1993; Widiger, Trull, Clarkin, Sanderson, & Costa, 1994). The NEO-PI (precursor to the NEO-PI-R) has been shown to account for the major dimensions underlying various self-report personality disorder instruments, such as the MCMI-I, the MMPI-PD, and the PAI (Costa & McCrae, 1990, 1992). It is noteworthy, however, that the dimension of openness has consistently demonstrated few significant correlations with variables from these other instruments.

Five-Factor Model Adjective Rating Scales. A number of adjective rating scales are available as measures of the FFM, including Goldberg's (1992) 50- and 100-item scales and John's (1990; John, Donahue, & Kentle, 1991) "Big Five" Inventory. Despite sound psychometric properties and excellent convergent and discriminant validities with other measures of the FFM (Briggs, 1992), however, adjective-based measures of the FFM have not been used extensively in personality disorder research. A minor exception to this statement is the Extended Interpersonal Adjective Scales—Revised—Big 5 (IASR-B5; Trapnell & Wiggins, 1990). This scale is an augmented version of the IAS-R (Wiggins, Trapnell, & Phillips, 1988), which was developed to assess the two domains of the interpersonal circumplex model (ICM), dominance and nurturance. (Researchers have noted that two of the FFM factors, extraversion and agreeableness, can be mapped onto these two dimensions; Costa & McCrae, 1989.) The IASR-B5 retains scales to assess the eight primary dimensions of the ICM, and includes scales created to measure the additional three domains of the FFM—neuroticism, conscientiousness, and openness. The measure has demonstrated excellent internal consistency (alphas ranging from .87 to .94), as well as good convergent and discriminant validity when analyzed with measures of both normal and disordered personality (e.g., NEO-PI-R or MMPI-PD) (Trapnell & Wiggins, 1990; Wiggins & Pincus, 1989, 1994). However, we were unable to locate any studies that reported using the measure in a clinical sample.

Validity of the Five-Factor Model for Assessing Personality Pathology. A frequent criticism of the FFM has been that it may be insufficiently sensitive to clinical problems and inadequate for a complete characterization of personality pathology (e.g., Ben-Porath & Waller, 1992; Clark, 1993b). In fact, Ben-Porath and Waller (1992) suggested that in general, normal personality measures should not be used as stand-alone tests in clinical evaluations because they may not provide clinically relevant incremental information. Costa and Mc-Crae (1992) contested this assertion, arguing that normal personality measures, including the NEO-PI-R, can be useful both in understanding patients' stable characteristics and in guiding treatment decisions.

As noted earlier, there is significant overlap between the constructs assessed by the NEO-PI or its derivatives and measures expressly targeted at personality pathology (Clark & Livesley, 1994; Clark et al., 1996; Schroeder et al., 1992, 1994). Moreover, several studies have documented the utility of the NEO-PI in predicting treatment or other outcomes in depressives (Bagby, Joffe, Parker, Kalemba, & Harkness,

1995), diabetes-related renal disease (Brickman, Yount, Blaney, Rothberg, & De-Nour, 1996), and general outpatient samples (Miller, 1991).

In relation to interview measures of personality disorder, however, instruments designed specifically to assess personality pathology may account for more variance than those targeting only the higher-order dimensions of normal-range personality (e.g., Clark, 1993b). Moreover, aspects of personality pathology may not be well represented by the FFM domains and may need to be added (or facet-level information used) to provide a full representation of the domain, including dependency (Clark et al., 1996; Reynolds & Clark, in press) and dimensions representing aberrant cognitions, deviant thinking, or somatic complaints (Berenbaum & Fujita, 1994; Coolidge et al., 1994; Costa & McCrae, 1990; Montag & Levin, 1994). Conversely, as mentioned earlier, the domain of Openness as assessed in current measures of the FFM does not appear to be a central feature of personality disorder as conceptualized in the DSM.

Quite a few studies have examined correlations between measures of the FFM of personality and the DSM Axis II personality disorders, assessed either via self-report or interview. These studies have used a variety of measures both for the FFM and the DSM personality diagnoses. An intriguing question is how constant relations are between dimensions of the FFM and the DSM personality disorders across different assessment methods and measures. To examine this question, Clark (1998) performed a meta-analysis of 17 studies that reported correlations between an FFM and DSM–personality disorder measure. Five studies assessed the DSM personality disorders by interview; six used a version of the MCMI; and six used one of four other measures. Clark (1998) first examined whether the results differed across these three groups of studies by examining the level and pattern of their FFM–DSM correlations. The overall correlational level of the two sets of self-report studies were similar to each other and both were stronger than the correlations between the FFM and interview-based measures. In terms of correlational pattern, however, although there was good correspondence within each group, the pattern from the MCMI-based studies differed from those using other self-report or interview measures, which yielded similar results. Thus,

Clark computed weighted averages for three groups of studies: five that assessed the DSM by interview, six that used a version of the MCMI, and six that used one of four other measures.

These sets of average correlations were then compared to the set of predictions regarding FFM–DSM relations made by Widiger et al. (1994) based on the criteria and associated features of each disorder as described in the DSM text and the clinical literature. Table 13.6 summarizes the results. Four predictions were completely borne out by data: borderline, avoidant, and dependent personality disorder were all high neuroticism, and avoidant personality dis-

order was low extraversion. This consistency between prediction and data suggests construct validity for both measures and theory. Five additional predictions were borne out by all self-report measures but not by interview: schizotypal personality disorder was high neuroticism, histrionic personality disorder was high—and schizoid personality disorder low—on extraversion, and paranoid and antisocial personality disorder were low on agreeableness. These data suggest that interviews may not be sufficiently sensitive to these particular dimensions in identifying different types of personality pathology.

Four predictions were completely discon-

TABLE 13.6. Summary of FFM–DSM Relations—Theoretical Predictions and Empirical Findings

| FFM score | Diagnosis | Prediction[a] | DSM measure | | |
			MCMI	Other self-report	Interview
		Neuroticism			
High	Paranoid	NO	NO	**YES**	NO
	Schizotypal	YES	YES	YES	**NO**
	Borderline	YES	YES	YES	YES
	Histrionic	**YES**	NO	NO	NO
	Narcissistic	**YES**	NO	NO	NO
	Avoidant	YES	YES	YES	YES
	Dependent	YES	YES	YES	YES
	Obs/Compuls	NO	NO	**YES**	NO
		Extraversion			
High	Histrionic	YES	YES	YES	**NO**
Low	Schizoid	YES	YES	YES	**NO**
	Schizotypal	NO	YES	YES	NO
	Avoidant	YES	YES	YES	YES
		Agreeableness			
High	Dependent	**YES**	NO	NO	NO
Low	Paranoid	YES	YES	YES	**NO**
	Schizotypal	NO	NO	**YES**	NO
	Antisocial	YES	YES	YES	**NO**
	Narcissistic	**YES**	NO	NO	NO
		Conscientiousness			
High	Obs/Compul	YES	YES	NO	NO
Low	Antisocial	YES	NO	YES	NO

Note. Diagnoses in boldface if prediction and results are completely consistent. YES/NO is in boldface if inconsistent with prediction or other results. Based on Clark (1998).
[a]From Widiger et al. (1994).

firmed by all empirical results: Histrionic and narcissistic personality disorder were not high on neuroticism; dependent personality disorder was not high—and narcissistic personality disorder was not low—on agreeableness. This disjunction between prediction and results suggests some conceptual misunderstanding of the FFM in relation to personality disorder.

The MCMI accorded with prediction in one case in which the other measures did not, finding obsessive–compulsive personality disorder high on conscientiousness. Conversely, the other self-report measures alone agreed with prediction that antisocial personality disorder was low on conscientiousness. These results suggest that the way that the MCMI measures obsessive–compulsive personality disorder may be superior but it may miss important aspects of antisocial personality disorder that are tapped by other self-report measures. Moreover, the other self-report measures yielded three unique correlations (high neuroticism for paranoid and obsessive–compulsive personality disorder and low agreeableness for schizotypal personality disorder) that were neither predicted nor found using either the MCMI or interviews. Finally, all self-report measures found low extraversion in schizotypal personality disorder, but this was neither predicted theoretically nor found by interviews. Further data are needed to clarify these inconsistencies.

In any case, these results are generally encouraging with regard to the utility of extending the FFM into the domain of personality pathology. Whereas the criticism of inadequate coverage may need to be addressed by the use of supplementary scales (e.g., dependency and cognitive distortion), and more work is needed both in terms of conceptualization and instrumentation, generic concerns about the appropriateness of the dimensions for characterizing personality pathology appear unfounded. Thus, further development of FFM measures (e.g., to extend measurement of the dimensions to greater extremes of pathology) may be a fruitful direction of future research in this domain.

Personality Adjective Check List (PACL; Strack, 1987). The PACL is an adjective checklist developed by Strack to assess Millon's (1981) theoretical personality types in a normal population. A rational/empirical approach was employed in constructing scales to measure each of Millon's eight basic personalities plus an Experimental scale to assess features of his three severe personality types— borderline, schizotypal, and paranoid. The basic PACL scales have demonstrated acceptable internal consistency (αs range from .76 to .89) and temporal stability, with 3-month test–retest correlations ranging from .69 to .85 (Strack, 1987). However, the Experimental scale, which combines features of three different severe personality types, have consistently demonstrated lower reliabilities (αs and retest r's both in the lower .60s).

Consistent with Millon's theory, the PACL scales were created with item overlap. Scale intercorrelations range from $|.04|$ to $|.64|$. The PACL has demonstrated convergence and discriminant validity with other measures of normal and abnormal personality, including the MCMI-II (Strack, 1987; Strack, 1991; Strack, Lorr, & Campbell, 1990). Again, however, and consistent with Strack's motivation for developing the instrument, we found no studies that had used the PACL in a clinical sample.

Tridimensional Personality Questionnaire (TPQ; Cloninger, Przybeck, & Svrakic, 1991; Cloninger, Svrakic, & Przybeck, 1993) and Temperament and Character Inventory (TCI; Cloninger, Przybeck, Svrakic, & Wetzel, 1994). The TPQ was developed to measure the three higher-order dimensions of Cloninger's (1986) biosocial theory of personality—novelty seeking, harm avoidance, and reward dependence which were postulated to correspond to the underlying genetic structure of personality. In normative data, coefficient alphas ranged from .55 to .85 (median $-$ .72) across four demographic groups of African American and white women and men (Cloninger et al., 1991); 6-month test–retest correlations were .70 (reward dependence), .76 (novelty seeking), and .79 (harm avoidance). The low internal consistency reliability, particularly of reward dependence, was a contributing factor to the revision of the instrument (see later). Consistent with theory, scale intercorrelations are low, but the measure's specificity for demonstrating systematic tridimensional relationships with DSM diagnoses as proposed by Cloninger (1987) is notably weaker (Goldman, Skodol, McGrath, & Oldham, 1994; Starcevic, Uhlenhuth, & Fallon, 1995). Like many self-report measures, the TPQ may be useful as a screening instrument for personality disorders, but convergence with other personality measures has been equivocal, with inconsistent findings (Nagoshi, Walter,

Muntaner, & Haertzen, 1992; Waller, Lilienfeld, Tellegen, & Lykken, 1991; Zuckerman & Cloninger, 1996).

Factor analyses of the TPQ subscales suggested that the persistence component of the reward dependence dimension defined a fourth factor, and the TCI was developed both to incorporate this finding as well as to provide ratings of three additional character dimensions, self-directedness, cooperativeness, and self-transcendence. According to Cloninger's revised psychobiological theory (Cloninger & Svrakic, 1997), the temperament factors are genetically determined and stable throughout life, whereas the character dimensions are hypothesized to mature in response to social learning. As with almost all personality dimensions that have been studied, the temperament factors have been shown to have substantial genetic variability (Stallings, Hewitt, Cloninger, Heath, & Eaves, 1996); genetic analyses for the character scales have not been reported, however.

With the exception of the eight-item persistence factor, which has shown low-to-moderate coefficient alphas, the temperament and character factors have demonstrated good internal consistency (Cloninger, Svrakic, & Przybeck, 1993; Svrakic, Whitehead, Przybeck, & Cloninger, 1993). Moreover, using the SIDP-R as the criterion measure, low self-directedness and uncooperativeness predicted the presence of any personality disorder, as did NEO-PI neuroticism and low agreeableness (self-directedness and neuroticism were correlated −.75; harm avoidance also correlated .71 with neuroticism). Bayon, Hill, Svrakic, Przybeck, and Cloninger (1996) replicated the TCI finding using the MCMI-II as the criterion measure, suggesting that these character factors could be used to screen for personality disorder. Svrakic et al. (1993) further reported that Cluster A, B, and C disorders were differentiated by low reward dependence, high novelty seeking, and high harm avoidance, respectively. However, two subsequent studies, including one by the instrument's authors (Ball, Tennen, Poling, Kranzler, & Rounsaville, 1997; Bayon et al., 1996) have failed to replicate these findings.

Structural Analysis of Social Behavior

The SASB system has not been used widely in personality disorder assessment research, probably because of its complexity and its focus on behavioral transactions rather than personality description. However, illustrations by Benjamin (1987; Benjamin & Wonderlich, 1994) demonstrate its utility in this domain. We include a rather lengthy discussion of the SASB model here in the hopes of stimulating research on this unique system.

The SASB model (Benjamin, 1996a, 1996b) has several conceptual grandparents: Sullivan's (1953) interpersonal psychiatry, Leary's (1957) IPC, and the subsequent literature, including Schaefer's (1965) developmental application. According to the SASB model, the basic structure of social behavior consists of three dimensions: focus of action, affiliation (friendly vs. hostile), and independence versus interdependence. The latter two dimensions (affiliation and [in- vs. inter]dependence) are crossed to form the IPC, but there are two major ways that the SASB model departs from the traditional IPC model.

First, in the SASB model there is not one IPC but three, because the IPC takes a different form for each of three foci of action: What one does (1) with another person as the transitive object (e.g., listen, indulge, blame, or neglect), (2) in relation or reaction to another person (e.g., express to, depend on, defend against, or detach from), or (3) in relation to self (e.g., be pleased with self, practice, feel guilt, or fantasize). For example, blame, appeasement, and guilt are all hostile, interdependent actions, but they are directed, respectively, toward another, in reaction to another, and internally.

Second, an important insight of the SASB model that differs from the traditional IPC is that dominance and submission are complementary rather than opposite. Both dominance and submission occupy the same position on the circumplex: Neutral on the hostile–friendly dimension and extremely interdependent. Where they differ is in the focus of action: Dominance is directed toward another, whereas submission is in response to another. In contrast, opposites share the same focus of action but anchor the two ends of a dimension; thus, the opposite of dominance is emancipation, whereas the opposite of submission is separation.

There are two ways to assess personality pathology using the SASB model: The Intrex Questionnaires (IQs) and coding of on-line or videotaped transactions. The latter requires extensive training and has no standardized stimuli on which the coding is based, so we discuss only the former. The IQs have both short and long forms which provide for 8 and 36 ratings per circumplex, respectively. In both cases the IQs are tailored for a particular use. For example, patients might be asked to complete an IQ with the focus on (1) others (e.g., their therapists, parents, or spouses), (2) their reactions to these others, or (3) their inner selves. With regard to the latter, patients might be asked to rate their "best" and "worst" self. Presumably, a generic form (how do you usually react to other people in general) could be used to elicit data most similar to traditional trait measures.

Single-Domain Measures

Interpersonal Dependency Inventory (IDI; Hirschfeld et al., 1977). The IDI was developed in the 1970s to assess dependency, incorporating conceptions of this construct from object relations theory, attachment theory, and social learning theories (Hirschfeld et al., 1977). Factor-analytic techniques were used to develop three subscales of emotional reliance on another person (ER), lack of social self-confidence (LS), and assertion of autonomy (AA). The authors suggest possible alternatives for deriving whole-scale scores, either summing the three subscale scores or computing scores from an algorithm derived from their mixed normal and clinical samples. However, no published studies have investigated this algorithm, so most researchers have used only subscale scores. Although some investigators have computed whole-scale scores using their own formulas, in the absence of an algorithm incorporating empirically derived weights for each subscale, Bornstein (1994) has suggested that the utility of IDI whole scale scores is severely limited.

The subscales of the IDI have demonstrated good internal consistency, and the ER and LS scales have shown good convergence with other measures of dependency (Bornstein, Manning, Krukonis, Rossner, & Mastrosimone, 1993; Hirschfeld et al., 1977). However, the ER and LS subscale scores also have demonstrated correlations with measures of anxiety and depression that are as strong as those with dependency measures, bringing into question their specificity as dependency measures. In contrast, the AA subscale has not been shown to correlate positively with dependency measures or to demonstrate a systematic pattern of rela-

tions with other measures of personality or psychopathology (Bornstein, 1994).

Narcissistic Personality Inventory (NPI; Raskin & Hall, 1979). Like the IDI, the NPI was developed in the 1970s; it was based on the DSM-III criteria for narcissistic personality disorder. The NPI has a forced-choice format, wherein respondents must select between statements representing a narcissistic and nonnarcissistic feature for each item. According to the authors, the NPI is not a measure of personality disorder but of trait narcissism. Nonetheless, the NPI correlates significantly with the narcissism scale of the MCMI (Auerbach, 1984; Prifitera & Ryan, 1984).

Emmons (1984) examined the internal structure and dimensionality of the NPI and found four moderately correlated factors: exploitativeness, leadership/authority, superiority/arrogance, and self-absorption/self-admiration. Correlations between these factors and scales from several omnibus measures of normal personality (e.g., Sixteen Personality Factor Questionnaire, Cattell, Eber, & Tatsuoka, 1970; Eysenck Personality Inventory, Eysenck & Eysenck, 1968), supported the convergent and discriminant validity of these four NPI factors (Bradlee & Emmons, 1992; Emmons, 1984; Watson, Grisham, Trotter, & Biderman, 1984).

Psychopathic Personality Inventory (PPI; Lilienfeld & Andrews, 1996). The PPI was developed to assess traits of psychopathy (as opposed to antisocial acts) originally in a noncriminal, student population. The PPI includes two validity scales designed to detect malingering and random or careless responding. Eight subscales were developed via factor analysis: machiavellian egocentricity, social potency, cold-heartedness, carefree nonplanfulness, fearlessness, blame externalization, impulsive nonconformity, and stress immunity. Internal consistency of the PPI ranged across samples from .90 to .93, with coefficient alphas of the subscales ranging from .70 to .90 (Lilienfeld & Andrews, 1996). The test–retest correlation across a mean of 26 days was .95, with retest reliabilities for the subscales ranging from .82 to .94. Intercorrelations among the subscales ranged from .00 to .45.

The PPI demonstrated good convergence with other measures of psychopathy as well as with interview and self-report measures of antisocial personality disorder. Moreover, it showed solid discriminant validity with measures of other psychopathological constructs, such as depression and schizotypy, and normal personality traits presumed to be unrelated to psychopathy (Lilienfeld & Andrews, 1996).

Schizotypal Personality Questionnaire (SPQ; Raine, 1991). The SPQ was developed to assess the DSM-III-R criteria for schizotypal personality disorder, with subscales designed to measure each of the diagnostic criteria. The SPQ has demonstrated good internal consistency, with coefficient alphas for the total score ranging from .90 to .91, and alphas for the subscales ranging from .63 to .81. A 2-month test–retest correlation for the SPQ was .82. The instrument showed good convergence with self-report and interview measures of schizotypal personality. In addition, it demonstrated good-to-moderate discriminant validity with measures that may assess traits related to psychosis proneness but are not considered to be features of schizotypal personality (Raine, 1991).

Raine and Benishay (1995) developed a brief, 22-item version of the SPQ (SPQ-B) to be used as a screening instrument for schizotypal personality disorder. The mean internal consistency of the SPQ-B was .76 and the mean test–retest correlation was .90. The SPQ-B showed good-to-moderate convergence with an interview measure of schizotypal personality (Raine & Benishay, 1995).

Schizotypy Questionnaire (STQ; Claridge & Broks, 1984). The STQ was developed to assess various aspects of thinking, attentional, and perceptual disturbances found in schizophrenic patients. The instrument has two subscales that correspond to the DSM-III schizotypal and the borderline personality disorders. As far as we could determine, normative data have not been reported. The STQ scales have demonstrated low-to-moderate convergence with the Psychoticism scale of the Eysenck Personality Questionnaire (Eysenck & Eysenck, 1975) (Claridge & Hewitt, 1987; Claridge, Robinson, & Birchall, 1983). The STQ also has been studied using biological criteria, such as differences in hemispheric functioning (Broks, 1984; Broks, Claridge, Matheson, & Hargreaves, 1984; Rawlings & Claridge, 1984). To the extent that the results are consonant with the left hemisphere dysfunction hypothesis of schizophrenia, they provide support for viewing schizotypal personality disorder as a schizophrenia spectrum disorder.

CONCLUDING REMARKS

Although we have explored a few topics in some detail, such as relations between the FFM of personality and the DSM personality disorders, for the most part this chapter has provided an overview of assessment instruments relevant to the personality disorder domain that can be used clinically and/or in research. We have tried to be inclusive without being exhaustive and to provide comparisons on a range of parameters for widely used instruments, both interviews and self-reports.

Although interviews are the "gold standard" for *diagnosing* personality disorders, they clearly have psychometric limitations that should not be ignored. Conversely, although perhaps of less use for diagnosis per se, self-report instruments clearly have a great deal of validity in the broader assessment of the domain. Several areas deserve further research consideration and development, including (1) deeper exploration of additional methods of personality disorder assessment (e.g., trait-based interviews and use of collateral sources of information), (2) development of self-report measures that better assess maladaptive extremes of personality dimensions, and (3) research that probes the underlying conceptualization of personality and its disorder both in terms of more static factors (e.g., genotypic and phenotypic structure) as well as processes that lead to the development and maintenance of the adaptive and maladaptive patterns of affect, behavior, and cognition which we call personality.

NOTE

1. The Structured Clinical Interview for DSM-IV Axis II Personality Disorders (SCID-II; First, Gibbon, Spitzer, Williams, & Benjamin, 1997) has a self-report version, but we have not included it in this table as it is intended as a screener, not a stand-alone measure. Cloninger also developed an interview for his tridimensional model but we were unable to find any research using it, so we have not included it in the table or discussion.

REFERENCES

American Psychiatric Association. (1980). *Diagnostic and statistical manual of mental disorders* (3rd ed.). Washington, DC: American Psychiatric Press.

Auerbach, J. S. (1984). Validation of two scales for narcissistic personality disorder. *Journal of Personality Assessment, 48,* 649–653.

Bagby, R. M., Joffe, R. T., Parker, J. D. A., Kalemba, V., & Harkness, K. L. (1995). Major depression and the five-factor model of personality. *Journal of Personality Disorders, 9,* 224–234.

Ball, S. A., Tennen, H., Poling, J. C., Kranzler, H. R., & Rounsaville, B. J. (1997). Personality, temperament, and character dimensions and the DSM-IV personality disorders in substance abusers. *Journal of Abnormal Psychology, 104,* 545–553.

Bayon, C., Hill, K., Svrakic, D. M., Przybeck, T. R., & Cloninger, C. R. (1996). Dimensional assessment of personality in an outpatient sample: Relations of the systems of Millon and Cloninger. *Journal of Psychiatric Research, 30,* 341–352.

Benjamin, L. S. (1974). Structural analysis of social behavior. *Psychological Review, 81,* 392–425.

Benjamin, L. S. (1986). Adding social and intrapsychic descriptors to Axis I of DSM-III. In T. Millon & G. Klerman (Eds.). *Contemporary issues in psychopathology* (pp. 599–638). New York: Guilford Press.

Benjamin, L. S. (1987). Use of the SASB dimensional model to development treatment plans for personality disorders: I. Narcissism. *Journal of Personality Disorders, 1,* 43–70.

Benjamin, L. S. (1996a). *Interpersonal diagnosis and treatment of personality disorders* (2nd ed.). New York: Guilford Press.

Benjamin, L. S. (1996b). Introduction to the Special Section on Structural Analysis of Social Behavior. *Journal of Consulting and Clinical Psychology, 64,* 1203–1212.

Benjamin, L. S., & Wonderlich, S. A. (1994). Social perceptions and borderline personality disorder: The relation to mood disorders. *Journal of Abnormal Psychology, 103,* 610–624.

Ben-Porath, Y. S., & Waller, N. G. (1992). "Normal" personality inventories in clinical assessment: General requirements and the potential for using the NEO Personality Inventory. *Psychological Assessment, 4,* 14–19.

Berenbaum, H., & Fujita, F. (1994). Schizophrenia and personality: Exploring the boundaries and connections between vulnerability and outcome. *Journal of Abnormal Psychology, 103,* 148–158.

Bernstein, D. P., Kasapis, C., Bergman, A., Weld, E., Mitropoulou, V., Harvath, T., Klar, H. M., Silverman, J., & Siever, L. (1997). Assessing Axis II disorders by informant interview. *Journal of Personality Disorders, 11,* 158–167.

Blashfield, R. K., Blum, N., & Pfohl, B. (1992). The effects of changing Axis II diagnostic criteria. *Comprehensive Psychiatry, 33,* 245–252.

Bornstein, R. F. (1994). Construct validity of the Interpersonal Dependency Inventory: 1977–1992. *Journal of Personality Disorders, 8,* 64–76.

Bornstein, R. F., Manning, K. M., Krukonis, A. B., Rossner, S. C., & Mastrosimone, C. C. (1993). Sex differences in dependency: A comparison of objective and projective measures. *Journal of Personality Assessment, 61,* 169–181.

Bradlee, P. M., & Emmons, R. A. (1992). Locating narcissism within the interpersonal circumplex and the five-factor model. *Personality and Individual Differences, 13,* 821–830.

Brickman, A. L., Yount, S. E., Blaney, N. T., Rothberg, S. T., & De-Nour, A. K. (1996). Personality traits and long-term health status: The influence of neuroticism and conscientiousness on renal deterioration in Type–1 diabetes. *Psychosomatics, 37,* 459–468.

Broks, P. (1984). Schizotypy and hemisphere function—II. Performance asymmetry on a verbal divided visual-field task. *Personality and Individual Differences, 5,* 649–656.

Broks, P., Claridge, G., Matheson, J., & Hargreaves, J. (1984). Schizotypy and hemisphere function-IV. Story comprehension under binaural and monoaural listening conditions. *Personality and Individual Differences, 5,* 665–670.

Brophy, J. J. (1994). Personality disorder, symptoms and dexamethasone suppression in depression. *Journal of Affective Disorders, 31,* 19–27.

Brothwell, J., Casey, P. R., & Tyrer, P. (1992). Who gives the most reliable account of a psychiatric patient's personality? *Irish Journal of Psychological Medicine, 9,* 90–93.

Carey, K. B. (1994). Use of the Structured Clinical Interview for DSM-III-R Personality Questionnaire in the presence of severe Axis I disorders: A cautionary note. *Journal of Nervous and Mental Disease, 182,* 669–671.

Cattell, R. B., Eber, H. W., & Tatsuoka, M. (1970). *Handbook for the Sixteen Personality Factor Questionnaire.* Champaign, IL: IPAT.

Choca, J., Shanley, L., Van Denburg, E., & Agresti, A. (1992). Personality disorder or personality style: That is the question. *Journal of Counseling and Development, 70,* 429–431.

Choca, J., & Van Denburg, E. (Eds.). (1997). *Interpretive Guide to the Millon Clinical Multiaxial Inventory.* New York: American Psychological Association.

Claridge, G., & Broks, P. (1984). Schizotypy and hemisphere function: I. Theoretical considerations and the measurement of schizotypy. *Personality and Individual Differences, 5,* 633–648.

Claridge, G., & Hewitt, J. K. (1987). A biometrical study of schizotypy in a normal population. *Personality and Individual Differences, 8,* 303–312.

Claridge, G., Robinson, D. L., & Birchall, P. (1983). Characteristics of schizophrenics' and neurotics' relatives. *Personality and Individual Differences, 4,* 651–664.

Clark, L. A. (1989). Depressive and anxiety disorders: Descriptive psychopathology and differential diagnosis. In P. C. Kendall & D. Watson (Eds.), *Anxiety and depression: Distinctive and overlapping features* (pp. 83–129). New York: Academic Press.

Clark, L. A. (1990). Toward a consensual set of symptom clusters for assessment of personality disorder. In J. N. Butcher & C. D. Spielberger (Eds.), *Advances in personality assessment* (Vol. 8, pp. 243–266). Hillsdale, NJ: Erlbaum.

Clark, L. A. (1993a). *Manual for the Schedule for Nonadaptive and Adaptive Personality.* Minneapolis: University of Minnesota Press.

Clark, L. A. (1993b). Personality disorder diagnosis: Limitations of the five-factor model. *Psychological Inquiry, 4,* 100–104.

Clark, L. A. (1998). *The DSM personality disorders and*

the five-factor model of personality: A meta-analysis. Unpublished raw data.

Clark, L. A. (1999). Dimensional approaches to personality disorder assessment and diagnosis. In C. R. Cloninger (Ed.), *Personality and psychopathology* (pp. 219–244). Washington, DC: American Psychiatric Press.

Clark, L. A., & Livesley, W. J. (1994). Two approaches to identifying the dimensions of personality disorder: Convergence on the five-factor model. In P. T. Costa, Jr. & T. A. Widiger (Eds.), *Personality disorders and the five-factor model of personality* (pp. 261–278). Washington, DC: American Psychological Association.

Clark, L. A., Livesley, W. J., & Morey, L. (1997). Personality disorder assessment: The challenge of construct validity. *Journal of Personality Disorders, 11,* 205–231.

Clark, L. A., Livesley, W. J., Schroeder, M. L., & Irish, S. (1996). The structure of maladaptive personality traits: Convergent validity between two systems. *Psychological Assessment, 8,* 294–303.

Cleckley, H. (1976). *The mask of sanity* (5th ed.). St. Louis, MO: Mosby.

Cloninger, C. R. (1986). A unified biosocial theory of personality and its role in the development of anxiety states. *Psychiatric Developments, 3,* 167–226.

Cloninger, C. R. (1987). A systematic method for clinical description and classification of personality variants. *Archives of General Psychiatry, 44,* 573–588.

Cloninger, C. R., Przybeck, T. R., & Svrakic, D. M. (1991). The Tridimensional Personality Questionnaire: U.S. normative data. *Psychological Reports, 69,* 1047–1051.

Cloninger, C. R., Przybeck, T. R., Svrakic, D. M., & Wetzel, R. D. (1994). *The Temperament and Character Inventory (TCI): A guide to its development and use.* St. Louis, MO: Center for Psychobiology of Personality, Washington University.

Cloninger, C. R., & Svrakic, D. M. (1997). Integrative psychobiological approach to psychiatric assessment and treatment. *Psychiatry, 60,* 120–141.

Cloninger, C. R., Svrakic, D. M., & Przybeck, T. R. (1993). A psychobiological model of temperament and character. *Archives of General Psychiatry, 50,* 975–990.

Cohen, J. (1968). Weighted kappa: Nominal scale agreement provision for scaled disagreement or partial credit. *Psychological Bulletin, 70,* 213–220.

Cooke, D. J., & Michie, C. (1997). An item response theory analysis of the Hare Psychopathy Checklist—Revised. *Psychological Assessment, 9,* 3–14.

Cooke, D. J., Michie, C., Hart, S. D., & Hare, R. D. (1999). Evaluating the Screening version of the Hare Psychopathy Checklist—Revised (PCL:SV): An item response theory analysis. *Psychological Assessment, 11,* 3–13.

Coolidge, F. L., Becker, L.A., DiRito, D. C., Durhan, R. L., Kinlaw, M. M., & Philbrick, P. B. (1994). On the relationship of the five-factor personality model to personality disorders: Four reservations. *Psychological Reports, 75,* 11–21.

Coolidge, F. L., Burns, E. M., & Mooney, J. A. (1995). Reliability of observer ratings in the assessment of personality disorders: A preliminary study. *Journal of Clinical Psychology, 51,* 22–28.

Coolidge, F. L., & Merwin, M. M. (1992). Reliability and validity of the Coolidge Axis II Inventory: A new inventory for the assessment of personality disorders. *Journal of Personality Assessment, 59,* 223–238.

Costa, P. T., & McCrae, R. R. (1989). Normal personality assessment in clinical practice: The NEO Personality Inventory. *Psychological Assessment, 4,* 5–13.

Costa, P. T., & McCrae, R. R. (1990). Personality disorders and the five-factor model of personality. *Journal of Personality Disorders, 4,* 362–371.

Costa, P. T., Jr., & McCrae, R. R. (1992). *Revised NEO Personality Inventory (NEO-PI-R) and NEO Five-Factor Inventory (NEO-FFI) professional manual.* Odessa, FL: Psychological Assessment Resources.

Cowdry, R. W., & Gardner, D. L. (1991). Mood variability: A study of four groups. *American Journal of Psychiatry, 148,* 1505–1511.

Dowson, J. H. (1992a). DSM-III-R narcissistic personality disorder evaluated by patients' and informants' self-report questionnaires: Relationships with other personality disorders and a sense of entitlement as an indicator of narcissism. *Comprehensive Psychiatry, 33,* 397–406.

Dowson, J. H. (1992b). Assessment of DSM-III-R personality disorders by self-report questionnaire: The role of informants and a screening test for co-morbid personality disorders (STCPD). *British Journal of Psychiatry, 161,* 344–352.

Dyer, F. J. (1997). Application of the Millon inventories in forensic psychology. In T. Millon (Ed.), *The Millon inventories: Clinical and personality assessment* (pp. 124–139). New York: Guilford Press.

Emmons, R. A. (1984). Factor analysis and construct validity of the Narcissistic Personality Inventory. *Journal of Personality Assessment, 48,* 291–300.

Eysenck, H. (1987). The definition of personality disorders and the criteria appropriate for their description. *Journal of Personality Disorders, 1,* 211–219.

Eysenck, H. J., & Eysenck, S. B. G. (1968). *Manual of the Eysenck Personality Inventory.* San Diego, CA: Educational and Industrial Testing Service.

Fahy, T. A., Eisler, I., & Russell, G. F. (1993). Personality disorder and treatment response in bulimia nervosa. *British Journal of Psychiatry, 162,* 765–770.

First, M., Gibbon, M., Spitzer, R. L., Williams, J. B. W., & Benjamin, L. S. (1997). *User's guide for the Structured Clinical Interview for the DSM-IV Axis II Personality Disorders.* Washington, DC: American Psychiatric Press.

First, M., Spitzer, R. L., Gibbon, M., & Williams, J. B. W. (1995a). The Structured Clinical Interview for the DSM-III-R Personality Disorders (SCID-II): Part I. Description. *Journal of Personality Disorders, 9,* 83–91.

First, M. B., Spitzer, R. L., Gibbon, M., Williams, J. B. W., Davies, M., Borus, J., Howes, M. J., Kane, J., Pope, H. G., Jr., & Rounsaville, B. (1995b). The Structured Clinical Interview for DSM-III-R Personality Disorders (SCID-II): Part II. Multi-site test–retest reliability study. *Journal of Personality Disorders, 9,* 92–104.

Fleenor, J. W., & Eastman, L. (1997). The relationship

between the five-factor model of personality and the California Psychological Inventory. *Educational and Psychological Measurement, 57,* 698–703.

Flynn, P. M., McCann, J. T., & Fairbank, J. A. (1995). Issues in the assessment of personality disorder and substance abuse using the Millon Clinical Multiaxial Inventory (MCMI-II). *Journal of Clinical Psychology, 51,* 415–421.

Fossati, A., Maffei, C., Bagnato, M., Donati, D., Donini, M., Fiorilli, M., Novella, L., & Ansoldi, M. (1998). Brief communication: Criterion validity of the Personality Diagnostic Questionnaire—4+ (PDQ-4+) in a mixed psychiatric sample. *Journal of Personality Disorders, 12,* 172–178.

Funder, D. C., Kolar, D. C., & Blackman, M. C. (1995). Agreement among judges of personality: Interpersonal relations, similarity, and acquaintanceship. *Journal of Personality and Social Psychology, 69,* 656–672.

Goldberg, L. R. (1992). The development of markers of the Big-Five factor structure. *Psychological Assessment, 4,* 26–42.

Goldman, R. G., Skodol, A. E., McGrath, P. J., & Oldham, J. M. (1994). Relationship between the Tridimensional Personality Questionnaire and DSM-III-R personality traits. *American Journal of Psychiatry, 151,* 274–276.

Gough, H. G. (1987). *Manual for the California Personality Inventory.* Palo Alto, CA: Consulting Psychologists Press.

Gunderson, J. G., Kolb, J. E., & Austin, V. (1981). The Diagnostic Interview for Borderline Patients. *American Journal of Psychiatry, 138,* 896–903.

Gunderson, J. G., Ronningstam, E., & Bodkin, A. (1990). The Diagnostic Interview for Narcissistic Patients. *Archives of General Psychiatry, 47,* 676–680.

Guthrie, P. C., & Mobley, B. D. (1994). A comparison of the differential diagnostic efficiency of three personality disorder inventories. *Journal of Clinical Psychology, 50,* 656–665.

Hamilton, J. C., & Shuminsky, T. R. (1990). Self-awareness mediates the relationship between serial position and item reliability. *Journal of Personality and Social Psychology, 59,* 1301–1307.

Hare, R. D. (1970). *Psychopathy: Theory and research.* New York: Wiley.

Hare, R. D. (1991). *The Hare Psychopathy Checklist—Revised Manual.* North Tonawanda, NY: Multi-Health Systems.

Hare, R. D., Harpur, T. J., Hakstian, A. R., Forth, A. E., Hart, S. D., & Newman, J. P. (1990). The Revised Psychopathy Checklist: Descriptive statistics, reliability, and factor structure. *Psychological Assessment, 2,* 228–241.

Hart, S. D., Cox, D. N., & Hare, R. D. (1995). *The Hare Psychopathy Checklist: Screening Version* (1st ed.). Toronto, Ontario, Canada: Multi-Health Systems.

Harkness, A. (1992). Fundamental topics in the personality disorders: Candidate trait dimensions from lower regions of the hierarchy. *Psychological Assessment, 4,* 251–259.

Harkness, A. R., & McNulty, J. L. (1994). The Personality Psychopathology Five (PSY-5): Issues from the pages of a diagnostic manual instead of a dictionary. In S. Strack & M. Lorr (Eds.), *Differentiating normal and abnormal personality* (pp. 291–315). New York: Springer.

Harkness, A. R., McNulty, J. L., & Ben-Porath, Y. S. (1995). The Personality Psychopathology Five (PSY-5): Constructs and MMPI-2 scales. *Psychological Assessment, 7,* 104–114.

Harlan, E., & Clark, L. A. (1999). Short-forms of the Schedule for Nonadaptive and Adaptive Personality (SNAP) for self and collateral ratings: Development, reliability, and validity. *Assessment, 6,* 131–146.

Harpur, T. J., Hare, R. D., & Hakstian, A. R. (1989). Two-factor conceptualization of psychopathy: Construct validity and assessment implications. *Psychological Assessment, 1,* 6–17.

Hathaway, S. R., & McKinley, J. C. (1951). *Manual for the Minnesota Multiphasic Personality Inventory.* New York: Psychological Corporation.

Heumann, K., & Morey, L. (1990). Reliability of categorical and dimensional judgments of personality disorder. *American Journal of Psychiatry, 147,* 498–500.

Hirschfeld, R. M. A. (1993). Personality disorders: Definition and diagnosis. *Journal of Personality Disorders, 7*(Suppl.), 9–17.

Hirschfeld, R. M. A., Klerman, G. L., Gough, H. G., Barrett, J., Korchin, S. J., & Chodoff, P. (1977). A measure of interpersonal dependency. *Journal of Personality Assessment, 41,* 610–618.

Horowitz, L. M., Rosenberg, S. E., Baer, B. A., Ureño, G., & Villaseñor, V. S. (1988). Inventory of Interpersonal Problems: Psychometric properties and clinical applications. *Journal of Consulting and Clinical Psychology, 56,* 885–892.

Hunt, C., & Andrews, G. (1992). Measuring personality disorder: The use of self-report questionnaires. *Journal of Personality Disorders, 6,* 125–133.

Hyler, S. E. (1994). *Personality Diagnostic Questionnaire-IV (PDQ-IV).* New York: New York State Psychiatric Institute.

Hyler, S. E., Skodol, A. E., Kellman, H. D., Oldham, J. M., & Rosnick, L. (1990). Validity of the Personality Diagnostic Questionnaire—Revised (PDQ-R): Comparison with two structured interviews. *American Journal of Psychiatry, 147,* 1043–1048.

Hyler, S. E., Skodol, A. E., Oldham, J. M., Kellman, H. D., & Doidge, N. (1992). Validity of the Personality Diagnostic Questionnaire—Revised (PDQ-R): A replication in an outpatient sample. *Comprehensive Psychiatry, 33,* 73–77.

Jacobsberg, L. (1995). Diagnostic agreement between the SCID-II Screening Questionnaire and the Personality Disorder Examination. *Journal of Personality Assessment, 65,* 428–433.

John, O. (1990). The "Big Five" factor taxonomy: Dimensions of personality in the natural language and in questionnaires. In L. Pervin (Ed.), *Handbook of personality: Theory and research.* New York: Guilford Press.

John, O., Donahue, E., M., & Kentle, R. L. (1991). *The Big Five Inventory—Versions 4a and 54.* Technical Report, Institute of Personality and Social Research, University of California, Berkeley.

John, O., & Robins, R. W. (1994). Accuracy and bias in self-perception: Individual differences in self-enhancement and narcissism. *Journal of Personality and Social Psychology, 66,* 206–219.

Jones, J. K., & Morey, L. C. (1995, August). *Interpersonal stressors and mood variability in borderline personality disorder.* Paper presented at the 101st Annual Meeting of the American Psychological Association. New York, NY.

Kaye, A. L., & Shea, T. M. (2000). Personality disorders, personality traits, and defense mechanisms. In A. J. Rush, H. A. Pincus & M. B. First (Eds.), *Handbook of psychiatric measures* (pp. 713–749). Washington, DC: American Psychiatric Press.

Kim, Y., Pilkonis, P. A., & Barkham, M. (1997) . Confirmatory factor analysis of the personality disorder subscales from the Inventory of Interpersonal Problems. *Journal of Personality Assessment, 69,* 284–296.

Klein, M. H., Benjamin, L. S., Rosenfeld, R., Treece, C., Justed, J., & Greist, J. H. (1993). The Wisconsin Personality Disorders Inventory: Development, reliability, and validity. *Journal of Personality Disorders, 7,* 285–303.

Knowles, E. S. (1988). Item context effects on personality scales: Measuring changes the measure. *Journal of Personality and Social Psychology, 55,* 312–320.

Langbehn, D. R., Pfohl, B. M., Reynolds, S., Clark, L. A., Battaglia, M., Cadoret, R., Grove, W., Pilkonis, P., & Links, P. (1999). The Iowa Personality Disorder Screen: Development and preliminary validation of a brief screening interview for non-antisocial DSM personality diagnoses. *Journal of Personality Disorders, 13,* 75–89.

Leary, T. (1957). *Interpersonal diagnosis of personality: A functional theory and methodology for personality evaluation.* New York: Ronald Press.

Lenzenweger, M. F., Loranger, A. W., Korfine, L., & Neff, C. (1997). Detecting personality disorders in a nonclinical population: Application of a 2-stage procedure for case identification. *Archives of General Psychiatry, 54,* 345–351.

Lilienfeld, S. O., & Andrews, B. P. (1996). Development and preliminary validation of a self-report measure of psychopathic personality traits in noncriminal populations. *Journal of Personality Assessment, 66,* 488–524.

Livesley, W. J., & Jackson, D. N. (in press). *Manual for the Dimensional Assessment of Personality Pathology—Basic Questionnaire.* Port Huron, MI: Sigma Press.

Livesley, W. J., Jackson, D., & Schroeder, M. L. (1989). A study of the factorial structure of personality pathology. *Journal of Personality Disorders, 3,* 292–306.

Livesley, W. J., Schroeder, M. L., Jackson, D. N., & Jang, K. L. (1994). Categorical distinctions in the study of personality disorder: Implications for classification. *Journal of Abnormal Psychology, 103,* 6–17.

Loranger, A. W. (1992). Are current self-report and interview measures adequate for epidemiological studies of personality disorders? *Journal of Personality Disorders, 6,* 313–325.

Loranger, A. W. (1999). *International Personality Disorder Examination Manual: DSM-IV Module.* Washington, DC: American Psychiatric Press.

Loranger, A. W. (1995). *International Personality Disorder Examination Manual: ICD–10 Module.* Geneva, Switzerland: World Health Organization.

Loranger, A. W., Lenzenweger, M. F., Gartner, A. F., Susman, V. L., Herzig, J., Zammit, G. K., Gartner, J. D., Abrams, R. C., & Young, R. C. (1991). Trait-state artifacts and the diagnosis of personality disorders. *Archives of General Psychiatry, 48,* 720–728.

Loranger, A. W., Susman, V. L., Oldham, J. M., & Russakoff, L. M. (1987). The Personality Disorder Examination: A preliminary report. *Journal of Personality Disorders, 1,* 1–13.

Marlowe, D. B., Husband, S. D., Bonieskie, L. M., & Kirby, K. C. (1997). Structured interview versus self-report test vantages for the assessment of personality pathology in cocaine dependence. *Journal of Personality Disorders, 11,* 177–190.

McCann, J. T. (1991). Convergent and discriminant validity of the MCMI-II and MMPI personality disorder scales. *Psychological Assessment, 3,* 9–18.

McNulty, J. L., Harkness, A. R., Ben-Porath, Y. S., & Williams, C. L. (1997). Assessing the Personality Psychopathology Five (PSY-5) in adolescents: New MMPI-A scales. *Psychological Assessment, 9,* 250–259.

Miller, T. R. (1991). The psychotherapeutic utility of the five-factor model of personality: A clinician's experience. *Journal of Personality Assessment, 57,* 415–433.

Millon, T. (1981). *Disorders of personality.* New York: Wiley.

Millon, T. (1985). The MCMI provides a good assessment of DSM-III personality disorders. The MCMI-II will prove even better. *Journal of Personality Assessment, 48,* 450–459.

Millon, T. (1987). *Manual for the Millon Clinical Multiaxial Inventory—II (MCMI-II).* Minneapolis, MN: National Computer Systems.

Millon, T., & Davis, R. D. (1997). The MCMI-III: Present and future directions. *Journal of Personality Assessment, 68,* 69–85.

Millon, T., Davis, R., & Millon, C. (1994). *Manual for the Millon Clinical Multiaxial Inventory—III (MCMI-III).* Minneapolis, MN: National Computer Systems.

Montag, I., & Levin, J. (1994). The five-factor model and psychopathology in nonclinical samples. *Personality and Individual Differences, 17,* 1–7.

Morey, L. C. (1991). *Personality Assessment Inventory.* Odessa, FL: Psychological Assessment Resources, Inc.

Morey, L. C., & Henry, W. (1994). Personality Assessment Inventory. In M. E. Maruish (Ed.), *The use of psychological testing for treatment planning and outcome assessment* (pp. 185–216). Hillsdale, NJ: Erlbaum.

Morey, L. C., Waugh, M. H., & Blashfield, R. L. (1985). MMPI scales for DSM-III personality disorders: Their derivation and correlations. *Journal of Personality Assessment, 49,* 245–256.

Nagoshi, C. T., Walter, D., Muntaner, C., & Haertzen, C. A. (1992). Validation of the Tridimensional Personality Questionnaire in a sample of male drug users. *Personality and Individual Differences, 13,* 401–409.

O'Boyle, M., & Self, D. (1990). A comparison of two

interviews for DSM-III-R personality disorders. *Psychiatry Research, 32,* 85–92.

O'Maille. P. S., & Fine, M. A. (1995). Personality disorder scales for the MMPI–2: An assessment of psychometric properties in a correctional population. *Journal of Personality Disorders, 9,* 235–246.

Perry, C. (1992). Problems and considerations in the valid assessment of personality disorders. *American Journal of Psychiatry, 149,* 1645–1653.

Pfohl, B., Black, D. W., Noyes, R., Coryell, W. H., & Barrash, J. (1990). Axis I/Axis II comorbidity findings: Implications for validity. In J. Oldham (Ed.), *Axis II: New perspectives on validity* (pp. 147–161). Washington, DC: American Psychiatric Association Press.

Pfohl, B., Blum, N., & Zimmerman, M. (1997). *Structured interview for DSM-IV personality (SIDP-IV).* Washington, DC: American Psychiatric Press.

Pilkonis, P. A., Kim, Y., Proietti, J. M., & Barkham, M. (1996). Scales for personality disorders developed from the Inventory of Interpersonal Problems. *Journal of Personality Disorders, 10,* 355–369.

Prifitera, A., & Ryan, J. J. (1984). Validity of the Narcissistic Personality Inventory (NPI) in a psychiatric sample. *Journal of Clinical Psychology, 40,* 140–142.

Raine, A. (1991). The SPQ: A scale for the assessment of schizotypal personality based on DSM-III-R criteria. *Schizophrenia Bulletin, 17,* 555–564.

Raine, A., & Benishay, D. (1995). The SPQ-B: A brief screening instrument for schizotypal personality disorder. *Journal of Personality Disorders, 9,* 346–355.

Raskin, R. N., & Hall, C. S. (1979). A narcissistic personality inventory. *Psychological Reports, 45,* 590.

Rawlings, D, & Claridge, G. (1984). Schizotypy and hemisphere function—III: Performance asymmetries on tasks of letter recognition and local global processing. *Personality and Individual Differences, 5,* 657–663.

Ready, R. E., Clark, L. A., Watson, D., & Westerhouse, K. (2000). Self- and peer-reported personality: Agreement, trait ratability, and the "self-based heuristic." *Journal of Research in Personality, 34,* 208–244.

Renneberg, B., Chambless, D.L., Dowdall, D. J., Fauerbach, J. A., & Gracely, E. J. (1992). The SCID-II and the MCMI: A concurrent validity study of personality disorders among anxious outpatients. *Journal of Personality Disorders, 6,* 117–124.

Reynolds, S. K., & Clark, L. A. (in press). Predicting personality disorder dimensions from domains and facets of the five-factor model. *Journal of Personality.*

Ronningstam, E., & Gunderson, J. G. (1990). Identifying criteria for narcissistic personality disorder. *American Journal of Psychiatry, 147,* 918–922.

Rush, A. J., Pincus H. A. & First, M. B. (Eds.). (2000). *Handbook of psychiatric measures.* Washington, DC: American Psychiatric Press.

Schaefer, E. S. (1965). Configurational analysis of children's reports of parent behavior. *Journal of Consulting Psychology, 29,* 552–557.

Schroeder, M. L., Wormworth, J. A., & Livesley, W. J. (1992). Dimensions of personality disorder and their relationship to the Big Five dimensions of personality. *Psychological Assessment, 4,* 47–53.

Schroeder, M. L., Wormworth, J. A., & Livesley, W. J. (1994). Dimensions of personality disorder and their relationships to the Big Five dimensions of personality. In P. T. Costa, Jr. & T. A. Widiger (Eds.), *Personality disorders and the five-factor model of personality* (pp. 117–127). Washington, DC: American Psychological Association.

Siever, L. J., & Davis, K. L. (1991). A psychobiological perspective on the personality disorders. *American Journal of Psychiatry, 148,* 1647–1658.

Skodol, A. E., Oldham, J. M., Rosnick, L., Kellman, H. D., & Hyler, S. E. (1991). Diagnosis of DSM-III-R personality disorders: A comparison of two structured interviews. *International Journal of Methods in Psychiatric Research, 1,* 13–26.

Spitzer, R. L. (1983). Psychiatric diagnosis: Are clinicians still necessary? *Comprehensive Psychiatry, 24,* 399–411.

Stallings, M. C., Hewitt, J. K., Cloninger, C R., Heath, A. C., & Eaves, L. J. (1996). Genetic and environmental structure of the Tridimensional Personality Questionnaire: Three or four temperament dimensions? *Journal of Personality & Social Psychology, 70,* 127–140.

Standage, K., & Ladha, N. (1988). An examination of the reliability of the Personality Disorder Examination and a comparison with other methods of identifying personality disorders in a clinical sample. *Journal of Personality Disorders, 2,* 267–271.

Stangl, D., Pfohl, B., Zimmerman, M., Bowers, W., & Corenthal, C. (1985). A structured interview for the DSM-III personality disorders: A preliminary report. *Archives of General Psychiatry, 42,* 591–596.

Starcevic, V., Uhlenhuth, E. H., & Fallon, S. (1995). The Tridimensional Personality Questionnaire as an instrument for screening personality disorders: Use in patients with generalized anxiety disorder. *Journal of Personality Disorders, 9,* 247–253.

Strack, S. (1987). Development and validation of an adjective check list to assess the Millon personality types in a normal population. *Journal of Personality Assessment, 51,* 572–587.

Strack, S. (1991). Factor analysis of MCMI-II and PACL basic personality scales in a college sample. *Journal of Personality Assessment, 57,* 345–355.

Strack, S., Lorr, M., & Campbell, L. (1990). An evaluation of Millon's circular model of personality disorders. *Journal of Personality Disorders, 4,* 353–361.

Sullivan, H. S. (1953). *The interpersonal theory of psychiatry.* New York: Norton.

Svrakic, D. M., Whitehead, C., Przybeck, T., & Cloninger, C. R. (1993). Differential diagnosis of personality disorders by the seven-factor model of temperament and character. *Archives of General Psychiatry, 50,* 991–999.

Tellegen, A., & Waller, N. (in press). Exploring personality through test construction: Development of the Multidimensional Personality Questionnaire. In S. R. Briggs & J. M. Cheek (Eds.), *Personality measures: Development and evaluation* (Vol. 1). Greenwich, CT: JAI Press.

Trapnell, P. D., & Wiggins, J. S. (1990). Extension of the Interpersonal Adjective Scales to include the Big Five dimensions of personality. *Journal of Personality and Social Psychology, 59,* 781–790.

Trull, T. J. (1993). Temporal stability and validity of two

personality disorders inventories. *Psychological Assessment, 5,* 11–18.

Trull, T. J., & Larson, S. L. (1994). External validity of two personality disorders inventories. *Journal of Personality Disorders, 8,* 96–103.

Trull, T. J., Useda, J. D., Costa, P. T., Jr., & McCrae, R. R. (1995). Comparison of the MMPI-2 Personality Psychopathology Five (PSY-5), the NEO-PI, and the NEO-PI-R. *Psychological Assessment, 7,* 508–516.

Trull, T., & Widiger, T. A. (1997). *Structured Interview for the Five-Factor Model.* Odessa, FL: Psychological Assessment Resources.

Trull, T., Widiger, T. A., Useda, J. D., Holcomb, J., Doan, B-T., Axelrod, S. R., Stern, B. L., & Gershuny, B. S. (1998). A structured interview for the assessment of the five-factor model of personality. *Psychological Assessment, 10,* 229–240.

Tyrer, P. (1988). *Personality disorders: Diagnosis, management and course.* London, UK: Wright.

Tyrer, P., & Alexander, M. S. (1979). Reliability of a schedule for rating personality disorders. *British Journal of Psychiatry, 135,* 168–174.

Tyrer, P., Alexander, M. S., Cicchetti, D., Cohen, P., & Remington, M. (1979). Reliability of a schedule for rating personality disorders. *British Journal of psychiatry, 135,* 168–174.

Tyrer, P., Cicchetti, D., Casey, P., Fitzpatrick, K., Oliver, R., Balter, A., Giller, E., & Harkness, L. (1984). Cross-national reliability study of a schedule for assessing personality disorders. *Journal of Nervous and Mental Disease, 172,* 718–721.

Tyrer, P., Merson, S. Onyett, S. Johnson, T. (1994). The effect of personality disorder on clinical outcome, social networks and adjustment: A controlled clinical trial of psychiatric emergencies. *Psychological Medicine, 24,* 731–740.

Tyrer, P., Strauss, J., & Cicchetti, D. (1983). Temporal reliability of personality in psychiatric patients. *Psychological Medicine, 13,* 393–398.

Waller, N., G., Lilienfeld, S. O., Tellegen, A., & Lykken, D. T. (1991). The Tridimensional Personality Questionnaire: Structural validity and comparison with the Multidimensional Personality Questionnaire. *Multivariate Behavioral Research, 26,* 1–23.

Watson, D., & Clark, L. A. (Eds.). (1994). Personality and psychopathology [Special issue]. *Journal of Abnormal Psychology, 103*(1).

Watson, P. J., Grisham, S. O., Trotter, M. V., & Biderman, M. D. (1984). Narcissism and empathy: Validity evidence for the Narcissistic Personality Inventory. *Journal of Personality Assessment, 48,* 301–305.

Widiger, T. A. (1993). The DSM-III-R categorical personality disorder diagnoses: A critique and an alternative. *Psychological Inquiry, 4,* 75–90.

Widiger, T. A., & Frances, A. (1987). Interviews and inventories for the measurement of personality disorders. *Clinical Psychology Review, 7,* 49–75.

Widiger, T. A., Mangine, S., Corbitt, E. M., Ellis, C. G., & Thomas, G. V. (1995). *Personality Disorder Interview—IV: A semistructured interview for the assess-*

ment of personality disorders. Odessa, FL: Psychological Assessment Resources.

Widiger, T. A., Trull, T. J., Clarkin, J. F., Sanderson, C., & Costa, P. T. (1994). A description of the DSM-III-R and DSM-IV personality disorders with the five-factor model of personality. In P. T Costa, Jr. & T. A. Widiger (Eds.), *Personality disorders and the five-factor model of personality* (pp. 41–56). Washington, DC: American Psychological Association.

Widiger, T. A., Trull, T. J., Hurt, S., Clarkin, J., & Frances, A. (1987). A multidimensional scaling of the DSM-III personality disorders. *Archives of General Psychiatry, 44,* 557–563.

Widiger, T. A., Williams, J., Spitzer, R., & Frances, A. (1985). The MCMI as a measure of DSM-III personality disorders. *Journal of Personality Assessment, 49,* 366–378.

Wiggins, J. S., & Pincus, A. L. (1989). Conceptions of personality disorders and dimensions of personality. *Psychological Assessment: A Journal of Consulting and Clinical Psychology, 1,* 305–316.

Wiggins, J. S., & Pincus, A. L. (1994). Personality structure and the structure of personality disorders. In P. T. Costa & T. A. Widiger (Eds.), *Personality disorders and the five-factor model of personality* (pp. 73–93). Washington, DC: American Psychological Association.

Wiggins, J. S., Trapnell, P. D., & Phillips, N. (1988). Psychometric and geometric characteristics of the revised Interpersonal Adjective Scales (IAS-R). *Multivariate Behavioral Research, 23,* 17–30.

Zanarini, M. C., Frankenburg, F. R., Chauncey, D. L., & Gunderson, J. G. (1987). The Diagnostic Interview for Personality Disorders: Interrater and test–retest reliability. *Comprehensive Psychiatry, 28,* 467–480.

Zanarini, M., Frankenburg, F. R., Sickel, A. E., & Yong, L. (1996). *Diagnostic Interview for DSM-IV Personality Disorders.* Laboratory for the Study of Adult Development, McLean Hospital, and the Department of Psychiatry, Harvard University.

Zanarini, M., Gunderson, J. G., Frankenburg, F. R., & Chauncey, D. L. (1989). The Revised Diagnostic Interview for Borderlines: Discriminating borderline personality disorder from other Axis II disorders. *Journal of Personality Disorders, 3,* 10–18.

Zimmerman, M. (1994). Diagnosing personality disorders: A review of issues and research methods. *Archives of General Psychiatry, 51,* 225–245.

Zimmerman, M., & Coryell, W. (1989). The reliability of personality disorder diagnoses in a nonpatient sample. *Journal of Personality Disorders, 3,* 53–57.

Zimmerman, M., Pfohl, B., Coryell, W., Stangl, D., & Corenthal, C. (1988). Diagnosing personality disorder in depressed patients: A comparison of patient and informant interviews. *Archives of General Psychiatry, 45,* 733–737.

Zuckerman, J., & Cloninger, C. R. (1996). Relationships between Cloninger's, Zuckerman's, and Eysenck's dimensions of personality. *Personality and Individual Differences, 21,* 283–285.

CHAPTER 14

Personality Assessment in Clinical Practice

K. ROY MacKENZIE

This chapter describes the use of structured assessment procedures for personality disorders in clinical practice. In the broader context of the health care system, measures are helpful in estimating service load and in tracking change over time in relationship to established predictive patterns of change. Measures also have an important role in working with patients, particularly in establishing goals, for focusing the therapeutic process, and contributing to the choice of intervention strategies. Process measures may provide the clinician with an independent source of information about the dynamics of the therapeutic process. In all these contexts, the use of measures must be accompanied by clinically informed judgment.

SYSTEMATIC MEASURES IN HEALTH CARE SYSTEMS

The use of formal measures has rapidly expanded over the last decade. In the United States, the two major accrediting organizations, the Joint Commission on Accrediting Healthcare Organizations (JCAHO) and the National Committee for Quality Assurance (NCQA), have emphasized the importance of collecting service information from patients. The competitive marketplace has tended to emphasize service delivery characteristics related to consumer satisfaction. Unfortunately, satisfaction measures correlate only moderately with measures of clinical outcome (Attkisson & Swick, 1982). Such measures as the number of rings before the phone is answered, the attitude of receptionists, and the delay for receiving an appointment may make receiving health care more pleasant, but they do not necessarily translate into optimum clinical results. However, one result of the implementation of such measures has made the use of patient questionnaires almost universal. Any clinician, whether in a staff position or on a provider panel, will be expected to have some measures related to service delivery routinely completed.

More progressive programs have developed detailed assessment procedures to assist in diagnostic decisions as well as to document clinical change. These are commonly tied to clinical practice guidelines or treatment manuals. For example, protocols for initiating treatment of depression by primary care physicians are common, including indications for referral to specialty consultation. Manual-driven psychotherapies such as cognitive-behavioral therapy, interpersonal psychotherapy, and brief psychodynamic psychotherapy are in wide use. All these encourage the use of brief assessment questionnaires relevant to the population being assessed. One goal of this approach is to address the discrepancy of treatments a patient might receive from different clinicians. A patient diagnosed with an avoidant personality disorder and related social phobia might receive a "not treatable" response in one setting, pharmacotherapy in another, longer-term psychodynamic psychotherapy in a third, a brief psychoeducational group in a fourth, or systematic cognitive coping skill training and exposure to feared situations in a fifth.

The goal of empirically based treatment choices is gradually becoming clearer. However, the discrepancy between controlled clinical trials (efficacy studies) and general clinical practice (clinical effectiveness studies) remains substantial. Most formal research studies systematically reject patients with comorbid conditions, whereas most clinicians find the appearance of a single diagnosis to be uncommon. Major research funding organizations have begun to appreciate the importance of studies of clinical effectiveness in practice settings.

Well-established curves have been developed, many of them based on utilization statistics that antedate the impact of recent managed care programs, regarding the relationship between diagnosis and duration of treatment. This perspective is of direct importance to those treating personality disorders because in general this population is a heavy user of treatment resources. One function of a clinical assessment is to decide how long treatment can be expected to last. The use of formal measures concerning symptom intensity and interpersonal style can contribute to this process.

The enormous databases that are being created in larger clinical service systems offer an unparalleled opportunity to examine patterns of response based on thousands of cases. Although the quality of the data may not be pristine, the power of the numbers allows for identification of reasonable predictors of response. In addition, the clinical setting provides an opportunity for the longer-term follow-up that is essential for understanding the effectiveness of treatment for major personality disorders. As yet, few systems have effectively used the potential of these databases (Burlingame, Lambert, Reisinger, Neff, & Mosier, 1995). The idea of establishing limits on the number of sessions has been met with outrage from the mental health community. However, as treatment services are increasingly being provided through larger service systems or insurance plans, whether private or governmental, it would be irresponsible not to consider utilization factors. The theoretical advantage of a larger patient base is to spread risk over a wider area. Thus increased utilization has an indirect impact on all members. To ignore utilization is to punish those who use the system less frequently.

Dose–Response Curves

One approach to considering service system dynamics is to consider the amount of psychotherapy required to achieve a reasonable clinical outcome, the so-called dose–response ratio (see Figure 14.1). The dose–response curve of the upper line in Figure 14.1 is based on statistically significant improvement (Howard, Kopta, Krause, & Orlinsky, 1986). It is evident that most patients respond quite quickly to formal therapy with over 50% improvement within the first 2 months. The rate of response continues to rise, though at a somewhat slower rate over the next 4 months, so that by the 6-month point there is a 75% response rate. By the end of 2 years the improvement curve has risen slowly to 85%. This curve reflects an impressive response to psychotherapy, better than many medical treatments. The curve suggests that psychotherapy can be conceptualized as occupying three time segments.

1. It is clear that the largest portion of mental health treatment in front-line settings such as mental health clinics or hospital outpatient departments is accomplished in a few sessions, up to 3 months or about 12 sessions. These presentations are often related to acute stressful events.
2. The portion of the curve from 3 to 6 months falls within the usual definition of the intensive time-limited psychotherapies that have been the focus of a number of manual-driven treatments spanning the spectrum through behavioral, cognitive, interpersonal, and psychodynamic models.
3. Statistically speaking, longer-term psychotherapy can be considered to begin after the 6-month point, or about 24 sessions. In fact, relatively few patients actually reach this time marker.

The second dose–response curve is based on more recent analyses identifying clinical recovery in terms of more stringent criteria that require symptom measures to have returned to within a statistically normal range (Kopta, Howard, Lowry, & Beutler, 1994; Kadera, Lambert, & Andrew, 1996;). This curve rises

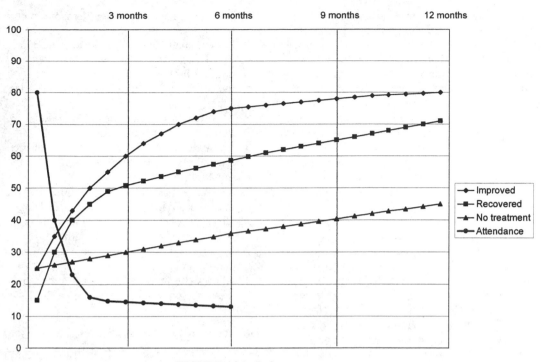

FIGURE 14.1. Dose–response curves.

more slowly but begins to approach the improvement curve by about the 12-month point.

For reference purposes, the third change curve reflects the improvement over time of a nontreated clinical population. This curve begins to approach the treated population toward the 2-year point. Interestingly, the figures for this particular untreated curve are taken from Eysenck's (1952) article which created a storm of controversy with its assertion that patients who receive no treatment recover as much as those receiving formal therapy. This curve is in keeping with other more current sources that track the course of untreated nonpsychotic illness. Eysenck's position was correct only if a time frame of 2 years was applied. In clinical terms, his data indicate a major positive effect of psychotherapy and a substantial relief of morbidity and dysfunction.

Finally, the bottom curve suggests that in practice most patients attend relatively few sessions (Phillips, 1987). By the end of 2 months, most general service systems indicate that only about 20% of those entering will still remain in active treatment. Once this remaining cohort has reached the 6-month point, it is likely that attendance will continue for a longer period. It is worth noting that this curve is based on data

collected prior to the major impact of managed care systems.

These curves constitute a composite picture of change representing many different conditions and severity of dysfunction. Clearly, acute situations related to clear immediate external stress tend to respond quite quickly, whereas long-standing anxiety and depression syndromes respond more slowly, and severe personality disorders longer still. This perspective on the predictable rates of change of a larger clinical population is a useful guide in the development of clinical service programs (Vessey, Howard, Lueger, Kachele, & Mergenthaler, 1994). The curves of Figure 14.1 make no distinction between the modality of service delivery; they include individual, group, and family treatment approaches, and many different models of psychotherapy.

The three time segments just described have interesting implications for the treatment of personality disorders. Few studies are available regarding the Cluster A personality disorders. It is generally felt that the defensive nature of the paranoid personality disorder makes psychotherapy not only difficult but also unlikely to be of benefit. Few reports address the schizoid and schizotypal populations.

Treatment of the severe Cluster B personality disorders, borderline and antisocial personality disorders, typically falls into the longer range of 1 to 2 years. However, quite brief interventions are common in response to acute decompensation. It is also common to have such patients attend formal time-limited treatments with a specific focus (e.g., around skill training and cognitive techniques) or to address specific aspects of interpersonal functioning, often in a group format. Such programs form the basis of most correctional treatment programs. One value of an intensive time-limited approach is to ascertain the patient's capacity to use therapy effectively. This menu of treatment possibilities is increasingly seen as necessary to address the range of disturbance characteristic these disorders. The dose–response curves suggest that ongoing change is increasingly limited beyond the 2-year point. A shift to a maintenance time model might then be instituted with, for instance, a monthly individual or group session. There are no formal studies concerning narcissistic personality disorder and case reports do not present a promising response.

Empirical studies have identified the value of intensive time-limited treatment particularly for the Cluster C avoidant and dependent as well as histrionic personality disorders (Crits-Christoph & Barber, 1991; Laikin, Winston, & McCullough, 1991; Piper, Rosie, Joyce, & Azim, 1996; Safran & Muran, 1998). These are often combined with programs for patients with major neurotic difficulties.

USE OF CHANGE MEASURES IN CLINICAL SETTINGS

Structured assessment techniques may take a variety of forms. It is common in the personality disorders field to use instruments based on diagnostic categories. A closely related application is the measurement of dimensional traits that are believed to underlie the diagnostic categories. The use of symptom measures that may be associated with personality disorder is widespread. Finally, there is increasing recognition of the value of creating target goals that can form the focus for therapeutic work (Battle et al., 1966; Benjamin, 1987; Eells, 1997; Luborsky & Crits-Christoph, 1997; MacKenzie, 1994b; Ryle, 1997). Pfeiffer, Heslin, and Jones (1976) identify 10 benefits of structured assessment:

1. Encourages patient involvement in the treatment process.
2. Fosters open reaction to personal feedback.
3. Clarifies patient goals and facilitates contracting for new behavior.
4. Increases objectivity of measuring patient change.
5. Provides for comparisons of individual patients with normative groups.
6. Facilitates longitudinal assessment of therapeutic change (i.e., before, midpoint, termination, and follow-up).
7. Sensitizes patients and therapists to the multifaceted nature of therapeutic change.
8. Gives patients the sense that their therapist is committed to effective treatment.
9. Improves communication between patients and therapists.
10. Allows the therapist to focus and control therapy more effectively.

Selection of Questionnaires

For clinical use, as opposed to formal research studies, questionnaires should be carefully selected for their relevance to the patient's needs. It is common to cover several areas directly applicable to the general features of personality disorder: symptomatic status, relationship stability, and social functioning. Trait qualities are highly relevant to understanding personality disorders and a measure focusing on these is relevant to an understanding the patient. Some commonly used measures are provided in the list that follows. Above all, only measures that have a solid history of use and with well-documented psychometric properties should be considered. One recent survey of 400 outcome studies found that 422 different questionnaires were used (G. Burlingame, 1999, personal communication). Two-thirds of these were used only once and one-quarter were homemade instruments. The bottom line is to use only widely known measures with established psychometric properties.

- *Symptom questionnaires*
  Outcome Questionnaire (OQ-45.2; Lambert & Burlingame, 1996)
  Symptom Checklist (SCL-90; Derogatis, 1983)
  Brief Symptom Inventory (BSI; Derogatis & Melisaratos, 1983)
  Beck Depression Inventory (BDI; Beck, Mendelson, Mock, & Erbaugh, 1961)

State–Trait Anxiety Inventory (STAI; Spiel-berger, Gorsuch, & Lushene, 1970)

- *Interpersonal functioning questionnaires*

Inventory of Interpersonal Problems (IIP; Alden, Wiggins, & Pincus, 1990; Barkham, Hardy, & Startup, 1996)

Structural Analysis of Social Behavior (SASB; Benjamin, 1993)

- *General social functioning questionnaires*

Social Adjustment Scale (SAS; Weissman & Bothwell, 1976)

Medical Outcomes Study Short Form (SF-36; Medical Outcomes Trust, 1992)

- *Personality traits*

NEO Personality Inventory (NEO-PI; Costa & Widiger, 1994)

Dimensional Assessment of Personality Pathology (DAPP; Livesley & Jackson, 2000)

- *Personality disorder measures*

Structured Clinical Interview for DSM (SCID-II; Spitzer, Williams, & Gibbon, 1987) (includes a screening measure for patient completion)

- *Interview-based measures*

Global Assessment of Functioning Scale (GAFS; American Psychiatric Association, 1994)

Social Adjustment Scale (SAS; Weissman & Bothwell, 1976)

Introducing the Use of Questionnaires

The use of measures should not be done casually. Consideration must be given to the methods used in introducing the questionnaires or scales the clinician wants the patient to complete. The way in which the task is introduced is critical for ensuring compliance and promoting reliable responses. The first step is to legitimize a measurement instrument by explaining its relevance to the patient's clinical problems. A brief explanation of the relevance of areas being tapped in the questionnaires should be given in as direct and open a manner as possible.

"This questionnaire asks you to describe some of the ways you usually relate to others. You described earlier how relationship stresses often trigger your depressions so your answers may help to understand more about how this happens."

A full opportunity should be given to the patient to ask questions or seek further explana-tion. The manner in which the results will be used should also be explained, including confidentiality limits.

The words "research" or "test" should be avoided. Structured assessment tools can legitimately be referred to as one component of the clinical assessment procedure and an opportunity for the patient to describe in a more structured way the issues they are facing. The completion of the questionnaires can be described at the beginning of therapy. The questions are a survey of common issues that may lead patients to think seriously about self and their predicaments in a somewhat objective manner.

Discussing Questionnaire Results with the Patient

The psychotherapy literature has increasingly emphasized the importance of establishing core areas on which the patient and therapist can focus. It is essential that these be developed in a collaborative manner. The formal use of questionnaires can facilitate this process if the results are presented in an optimum manner. Two individual sessions may be adequate for many patients, but in more complex cases the assessment process may extend over several sessions and merge into therapeutic work. It is useful, however, to think of the initial assessment phase as a distinct segment of therapy and to specifically mark its ending following the development of a suitable range of therapeutic objectives. The final discussion of goals follows this general assessment interview or interviews and the completion of questionnaires. Ideally, the therapist and the patient will then be basically in agreement concerning the issues to be addressed.

The clinician needs to structure the focus-setting interview carefully. All clinically relevant information should be reviewed in advance. A clinical stance of neutrality and cognitive clarity is important.

"I'd like to go over the results of the questionnaires that you completed. There should be no surprises here; these are just your own words coming back from the questions. We will go over the printouts of your scores and there is a copy of them for you to take home. Our goal is to try and get a good hold on the most important issues that bring you here for treatment. So let's look at each questionnaire. As you have discovered they deal with several different areas such as symptoms, interpersonal issues and general functioning. What was it like to answer the questions?"

The nature and meaning of questionnaire results are addressed with a direct and open attitude. Some explanation about why a particular scale is included and what it is trying to identify may be helpful.

"The first sheet you completed was the Outcome Questionnaire. It has an overall score and three subscales that deal with your symptoms, your satisfaction with your relationships and your satisfaction with work. Your overall score is 90, which is elevated in keeping with the information from our assessment interview. Your general symptom scale is somewhat lower, just at the edge of what we call a significant level, almost in a usual level. But your interpersonal problem score is quite a bit higher. You are describing your most important problems to be in that area. Does that make sense fore you? I know we talked quite a bit about the tensions you have been experiencing in several areas; your family and also sometimes with your coworkers. The next questionnaire looks at that very area in more detail."

All information is delivered in a tentative manner as ideas to think about, not conclusions to be accepted. It is helpful to base much of the discussion around real-life examples. In this way, the patient can assume a leading role in defining patterns with the clinician available as a technical resource. In the best of circumstances, this will lead to a serious working engagement, with initiative stemming primarily from patient. Once this is established the level of anxiety about being criticized or found "crazy" quickly diminishes. Regular use of the patient's own language in describing his or her behavior, thoughts, and feelings is useful. Technical language needs to be replaced by plain English. The goal is to establish the importance of descriptive patterns, not interpretive understanding. This makes it more palatable to discuss dysfunctional patterns.

"Now let me see if I have this straight. You see yourself as craving a close relationship, a very normal desire. But when the opportunity presents itself you feel very anxious and worry that you might not live up to the oth-

er's expectations. To counteract those thoughts, you might leave without saying anything, or sometimes you might drink too much and feel that you must be making a fool of yourself though nobody has actually told you that. So the underlying issue seems to be your belief that you have nothing to offer. You have connected that pattern to early experiences at home where it seemed you could never do anything right for your father. On the other hand, you describe a positive career and seem to be able to handle yourself satisfactorily in the business environment. So you do have skills, but they don't get applied in all areas. Does that catch the essence of things? Maybe you can give me some more examples of these two patterns: work versus social situations."

Being understood, even if the message is not pleasant, brings relief. Most patients have a partial awareness of their recurrent problematic issues. Aligning with this nascent understanding is a powerful generator of an early therapeutic alliance. It is useful to give the patient a copy of questionnaire results, often with notes, arrows, or additional comments from the interview (see also Ryle, Chapter 19, this volume). Direct connections can be established between the results of the assessment components and the treatment plan that is being developed. The discussion is maintained at a cognitive level, simply trying to be clear about what usually happens in the sequence of events that triggers difficulties.

Different treatment models will emphasize particular types of goals: behavioral, cognitive, relationship patterns, internal conflictual tension, confused self-states. There is some value in translating an understanding of these goals into an integrative language that focuses on the relationship implications. This is an accessible level that patients can quickly understand. The clinician may be conceptualizing the problems in other theoretical terms but virtually all models of psychotherapy involve interpersonal phenomena.

"It is pretty clear from your descriptions that your high level of personal expectations has had a major impact on your life. Your perfectionism seems to have prevented you from carrying out your desire to be more involved with other people and pursue the creative interests you used to have. It also means that you have a lot of trouble delegating work tasks and end up spending a lot of overtime doing things that others could handle. It sounds like some attention to these quality of life issues might make a difference. It's one thing to be a responsible person, but quite another to carry it so far that you can't enjoy your life. Do you think it would be worthwhile to work on some modification of your situation?"

The goal of the review of information, from both clinical data and questionnaires, is to generate a short list of critically important issues that are central to the recurrent difficulties the patient is experiencing. These may be termed "target goals" or "focus areas." Effective goals should meet the following criteria:

1. They are important and relevant to the patient.
2. They should be realistically achievable for the treatment model being offered.
3. They should be realistic for the time frame of treatment.
4. They should be changes the patient can make, not that others have to make.

Such focusing activity is particularly important for time-limited treatment models in which a rapid movement into core areas is needed to counterbalance the limited time.

Assessment material obtained from the patient either verbally or via questionnaire cannot be denied or easily evaded. Patients often experience a sense of relief that issues of which they have been aware as dysfunctional are going to be addressed. An open discussion of descriptive patterns reduces the sense of power imbalance and promotes an early working alliance. A major advantage of this early identification of key issues is that once they have been put into words the therapist can always legitimately and smoothly reintroduce them.

SPECIFIC MEASURES AND THEIR USE

Symptom Measures

Discussion of symptoms is, of course, a standard component of an assessment process. Identifying the actual levels on questionnaire results provides a specific acknowledgement that legitimizes the importance of treatment. A particularly useful aspect of assessment is to explore not just what the symptoms are but what impact they have had on the patient's life. One technique is to prepare a handout with a listing of the DSM-IV features of the identified syndrome. Often patient's do not understand that some of their experiences are in fact recognized as part of a syndrome. For example, a persistently unstable sense of self often associated with chronic feelings of emptiness is characteristic of borderline personality disorder. Patients may be aware only of the sense of chaos they experience and attribute this to the action of others. Hearing this pattern specifically identified provides a cognitive framework within which to locate these experiences, a basic first step toward addressing them. Such discussions also enhance a sense of being understood by the clinician.

"You describe these times when things seem to get out of control. If I understood you correctly, it would often start with you feeling empty and without emotion, maybe numb and a basic sense of not knowing who you are or where you are going. Then something relatively minor would trigger a sense that you have to do something to break out of this, and there's a shift into so much emotion it is hard to manage. These symptoms are common for people like you who have what we call a borderline personality. Getting a good description of what goes on is the first step in getting some control over the pattern."

In a group composed of members with similar diagnostic issues, such a discussion provides a powerful sense of universality that reinforces early development of cohesion.

Interpersonal Measures

This area is of primary concern in the treatment of personality disorders. A measure such as the Inventory of Interpersonal Problems provides a simple but effective picture of eight basic interpersonal dimensions as shown in Figure 14.2 (Alden et al., 1990; Barkham et al., 1996; Horowitz, Rosenberg, Baer, Ureño, & Villaseñor, 1988). The IIP items begin with either "It is hard for me to . . . (be assertive)" or "I am too . . . (controlling)." The eight subscales are organized around two major factors: control/submission (dominance) on the vertical

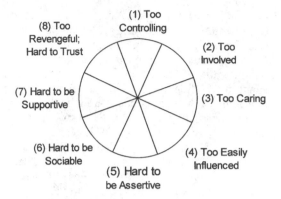

FIGURE 14.2. Scales of the Inventory of Interpersonal Problems.

axis and positive/negative valence (affiliation) on the horizontal axis, forming the interpersonal circumplex. Each of these has logically opposite poles and the circle is filled in with intermediate positions. For example, the combination of a high score on "Too Caring" and "Hard to be Assertive" results in a position of being "Too Easily Influenced," sometimes referred to as the "exploitable" position.

The first step in discussing results with a patient is to review the overall mean item score. This score represents a general level of perceived problems in relationships. If this number is low, below 1.5, the patient is not endorsing significant difficulties in the interpersonal area. If the patient has a diagnosis of personality disorder this presents a fertile opportunity for examining the discrepancy, not in a confrontive manner but in one of benign curiosity regarding the information the patient has personally provided.

"Your overall score on this questionnaire about problems in relationships is relatively low. That seems in contrast to some of the examples you provided earlier concerning your relationships with men. Let's see what that's about. Here is the diagram of your scores."

The next step is to locate the patient's scores on the circumplex diagram. Drawing a pie diagram in the eight segments gives a visual image of the pattern. It is common to find a clustering of high scores in one quadrant or at one pole. For example, a patient experiencing a major problem with assertion may have scores, not only in "Hard to be Assertive" but also in "Too Easily Influenced" (gullible) and "Hard to be sociable" (withdrawn). As a general rule, scores concentrated in the upper right quadrant tend to reflect a more functional adaptation unless they are extremely high. Patients with scores in the lower right quadrant are amenable for psychotherapy because of their propensity for compliance, and agreeableness promotes an early positive therapeutic alliance. Patients scoring in the lower left quadrant are going to have more difficulty engaging in therapeutic work because of their inhibited and distancing style. Finally, patients located in the upper left quadrant are likely to provide the greatest clinical challenge because their negative controlling style makes it difficult to develop a working alliance. Patients with this profile are particularly difficult in group psychotherapy because they have the capacity to shut down group interaction.

An additional perspective revealed in the IIP is the occurrence of high scores in opposite segments. This may be reflected in alternating states producing splitting mechanisms as in borderline personality disorder. Extreme difficulty in relationships related to brittle interpersonal boundaries or internal conflictual tension may be found. The initial therapy strategy is not to resolve these alternatives immediately but, rather, to use the results simply to describe with the patient the recurrent patterns regarding how their interpersonal lives are conducted.

THERAPIST: As you can see on the diagram, you rate yourself down here in the lower right where you are describing yourself as being not very assertive and tending to get too caught up in looking after others. But you also describe yourself in the upper left where you are controlling and critical. These are sort of opposites. Can you tell me more about how you experience these two quite different states of being?

PATIENT: Well, I hadn't thought of it this way before, but I think maybe I can see what I meant. When I get into a relationship, I really go whole hog. That person, and it can be a man or a woman, just fills my whole life. I guess I just sort of take over their lives though in a nice way, I just can't do enough for them. Then it all turns sour. You know I'm thinking right now that I must just burn them out. So they back off or say something a bit critical and I just hit the ceiling. I mean, after all I've been doing for them! So we have a big fight and then I just go all cold, a real ice queen, and nobody can get through to me. I turn into a real bitch. So that's it. Gee, I don't think I've ever quite put it all together like that before. It sounds sort of stupid doesn't it?

The Structural Analysis of Social Behavior (SASB; Benjamin, 1993; see also Chapter 20, this volume) employs assessment procedures that are somewhat more complex, but the complexity adds considerably more detail to interpersonal diagnosis. The basic organization of the SASB INTREX questions consist of eight items also located on a circumplex model like the IIP, but with the vertical axis of Differentiation/Enmeshment. A computer-generated analysis locates the most significant placement on the circle. These eight questions are applied in four directions: "how I act on others" and "how I react to others" as well as "how the other acts" and "reacts toward me." Thus the assessment of a specific relationship entails 32 items. The results of this detailed relationship analysis forms a classical relationship loop that is designed to identify reciprocal patterns that maintain and reinforce the relationship. In addition, a third surface addresses "how I act toward myself," another eight items. This procedure can be applied to a range of significant relationships. The results can be used in the same manner as the IIP but involves a more detailed discussion. The use of diagrams is helpful.

"In this questionnaire you remember how you described each relationship in four different ways describing how both you and your partner acted and reacted to each other. Now let's try and apply your answers. You see yourself as "relying on and trusting" your partner and you see him as being "protecting and nurturing"; these are both strong patterns so in a sense you make a complementary pair. You also treat *yourself* as someone who "needs to be protected" so you are very careful not to get into any situations that might be at all stressful. These patterns keep you feeling relatively safe but seem to be at a price of leading a very insulated life. You describe how you feel your life is boring and empty and that you can't really talk to your partner as an equal. It's as if you are both caught up in a vicious circle and can't get out. These sound like important issues that we can address."

An advantage of the SASB approach is that it does not assume that all relationships take the same form. Indeed, it specifically looks at differences between relationships. It can be effective in picking up a specific relationship style that reveals how early family patterns are reenacted in specific types of adult relationships. Mechanisms of *identification* ("I am just like my father"), *introjection* ("I treat myself just like my father treated me"), and *recapitulation* ("Others will treat me like my father did so I have to be on guard all the time") are described. Because only statistically significant patterns are reported, irrelevant detail is omitted allowing a rapid focusing on core issues.

A woman in her mid-30s presented with recurrent major depression closely connected with the state of her intimate relationships. She either fell quickly into an intense relationship without considering the quality or stability of it or she would find an unavailable man with whom she would carry on an initially exciting romance until it became clear that it would not continue. The ending of these liaisons routinely triggered depression sometimes with suicidal ideation. Increasingly she found herself struggling with her concern that she might never have a family. After the assessment procedures were completed she entered an intensive group program. The group members were asked to develop a relationship schema to discuss in the fourth session, using the SASB idea of a reciprocal relationship loop. She came with a diagram depicting her two patterns in some detail and with considerable anxiety explained them to the group with a mixture of grief and shame. Seeing her patterns written and put into words triggered a deeper appreciation of how they had inhibited her life goals and she was able to continue with effective efforts at change.

Personality Trait Measures

The NEO-PI dimensions of neuroticism, extraversion, agreeableness and conscientiousness identify core aspects of personality disorders (Costa & Widiger, 1994). The DAPP provides a more detailed description of the same terrain (Livesley & Jackson, 2000). An exploration of these scores provides useful information for treatment strategies. Extraversion and agreeableness address interpersonal behaviors similar to the axes of the IIP. For example, high agreeableness patients must address their vulnerability to interpersonal abuse that is associated with the need to become overly involved in helping relationships and their difficulties in personal assertion (a lower-right-quadrant location on the IIP). Low extraversion patients (introvert—lower left quadrant) must challenge their difficulty in expression of self and their disengagement from social contact. High neuroticism patients may need to address self-management strategies before they can effectively use an interpersonal approach. High conscientiousness patients will need to address their self-critical patterns and their tight conntrol over all aspects of life. The question of selection of the most appropriate psychotherapy model for each of the four principal trait dimensions is not fully understood. There is some suggestion that a treatment that is opposite to the style might be more beneficial (Barber & Muenz, 1996; Blatt, 1995). For example, the patient with a high agreeableness style (deferring) might do better with a more constraining treatment such as cognitive-behavior therapy and a patient with a low agreeableness style (autonomous) might do better with a more open and flexible interpersonal approach. These therapeutic questions are not entirely resolved in the empirical literature. The "pushing against the grain" approach mentioned earlier will make early engagement more difficult because of the need to adapt to an unwelcome style of treatment. This may result in higher dropout rates. Many clinicians likely begin where the patient is at, in order to develop a therapeutic alliance, and then move gradually toward the opposite side.

Because traits have considerable genetic loading, these measures have important implications for therapeutic strategies (Livesley, Jang, & Vernon, 1998). The idea of innate traits suggests that therapeutic efforts need to be directed at management of these traits more than interpreting the meaning of the behaviors. This task can be accompanied by a focus on the effects of the particular traits in the patient's relationships. An understanding of trait features arms the clinician to better understand what the patient is experiencing, a helpful quality in developing empathy and a therapeutic alliance. This perspective also encourages a realistic evaluation of how much change can be expected.

Personality Disorder Diagnostic Measures

As with the symptom measures, a formal review of the criteria for a given personality disorder can be productive, perhaps using the re-sults of a self-administered SCID-II (Spitzer et al., 1987) or DSM-IV diagnostic criteria (American Psychiatric Association, 1994). Using written material for this review is helpful in containing affect and maintaining a cognitive and educational stance (Ryle, 1997; see also Chapter 19, this volume). Laying out the features by which patients sabotage their own best interests provides a map on which to plot change. For example, patients with dependent personality disorder must recognize that their efforts to attend to the needs of others, apparently altruistic behavior, masks their excessive need to obtain nurturance and support by covertly controlling others to care for them. This type of discussion must be handled carefully so that patients do not feel that they are being bombarded with pejorative labeling. Regular small debriefing questions regarding how the patient is receiving the information are helpful. A cool, matter-of-fact and somewhat didactic approach will provide some reassurance that the questions are being correctly understood.

SEQUENTIAL CHANGE MEASURES AS A GUIDE TO TREATMENT

Earlier in this chapter several dose–response improvement curves were described. They provide important orienting information about the manner by which most patients change during the course of psychotherapy. Of course, each patient finds his or her own course toward improvement, but most patients do it in about the same way, at least in the same way as others with similar symptoms and difficulties. This concept of predictive improvement curves provides the clinician with guidelines by which to assess the relative standing of a specific patient. For example, one would expect to see clear symptomatic relief emerging within the first four sessions for a patient with a loss-precipitated acute depressive reaction. This is about the same time frame as one would anticipate with the use of an adequate dosage of antidepressive medication. It is perhaps not as clearly appreciated that the same principles apply to the dosage of psychotherapy. No response within the first month of psychotherapy would suggest that the therapeutic approach be reviewed just as one might question the need to adjust medication dosage. The use of sequential measures is more strongly entrenched in behavioral/cognitive models than in interpersonal/psychodynamic models but can be helpful in both.

The application of the dose–response predictive model is somewhat more complex in the treatment of personality disorders. For patients meeting criteria for histrionic and Cluster C personality disorders, the time frame for significant improvement is likely to be measured in several months. But as in the general psychotherapy literature, evidence of early response is predictive of longer-term outcome. A sense of well-being usually emerges early, followed by symptom reduction and then by interpersonal and social application (Howard, Lueger, Maling, & Martinovich, 1993). The other Cluster B personality disorders are likely to show a slower response pattern. While the clinician is usually tracking these stages intuitively, the use of a regular symptom measure such as the OQ-45 (Lambert & Burlingame, 1996), the Beck Depression Inventory (Beck et al., 1961), or the SF-36 (Medical Outcomes Trust, 1992) provides additional alerting information. Such questionnaires may be administered by the receptionist before a session, or at the beginning of the session itself as they take less than 5 minutes to complete. A slow response suggests that a review of strategies is indicated. Is the working alliance as secure as it might be? Are the problems of a more entrenched nature than initially considered? Are there features in the patient's social circumstances that inhibit change? Would the addition of medication be indicated? The questionnaire results do not drive the decisions but simply alert the clinician to a slower than anticipated response rate.

MEASURES OF TREATMENT PROCESS

Using Process Measures in Individual Psychotherapy

A consistent finding in the psychotherapy literature is the centrality of the therapeutic alliance. This has been conceptualized to consist of the *bond* with the therapist, agreement concerning the *goals* of treatment, and a sense of working together on the *tasks* for addressing important issues (Bordin, 1979). This latter component has been labeled the "working alliance" and is the strongest predictor of outcome. Indeed, the quality of the working alliance within the first month of treatment is a robust predictor of eventual outcome, even many months later. It suggests that the therapeutic dyad has established a pattern of acceptable and effective methods for addressing the patient's problems. Several brief measures of the therapeutic alliance are available:

CALPAS: California Psychotherapy Alliance Scales (Gaston & Marmar, 1991)
Helping Alliance (Luborsky et al., 1996)
WAI: Working Alliance Inventory (Horvath & Greenberg, 1989)

The most basic use of an alliance measure would be to administer it at the fourth or fifth session. This is a critical point to assess whether or not the treatment is off to a sound beginning (Horvath & Symonds, 1991). Some clinicians have found it useful to administer one of the brief alliance instruments at each session to serve as a barometer of the alliance over time. The maintenance of the alliance is a central aspect of treatment particularly for personality disorders. No matter what theoretical model is being employed, a constant watch is required in order to immediately identify and address threatened ruptures of the alliance (Safran & Muran, 1998, 2000).

Using Process Measures in Group Psychotherapy

In therapy groups, the concept of the alliance is somewhat more complex than in individual psychotherapy (Fuhriman & Burlingame, 1994). There are three potential ways of conceptualizing the alliance: the alliance among the individual group members, the alliance as reflected in a view of the group as a whole, or the alliance with the group leader or leaders. Available instruments include the following:

GCQ: Group Climate Questionnaire (MacKenzie, 1997): a measure of the whole group atmosphere
CCI: Catharsis, Cohesion, Insight (Fuhriman, Drescher, Hanson, Henrie, & Rybicki, 1986): a measure of the individual's experience in the group.
CALPAS: The individual format has been adapted for use in a group (Gaston & Marmor, 1991): a measure of the individual's experience in the group.
HIM-SS: Hill Interaction Matrix (Hill, 1977). A system for analyzing group process.

Informal studies suggest that the sense of alliance with the other group members might be the strongest predictor of outcome as in the individual literature using the CALPAS measure (MacKenzie & Grabovac, 2001). Most studies have looked at the group as a whole under the general heading of the group climate (using the GCQ or CCI). There is modest evidence that early session measures on the Engaged scale of the GCQ predict better outcome. Groups that have higher levels of reported cohesion appear to have better outcomes. Individual members who endorse higher ratings on the Engaged scale tend to have better outcome (Budman et al., 1989; MacKenzie & Tschuschke, 1993). Few studies have examined the alliance to the group therapist, though one study of training groups found that groups in which members rated the leaders more positively had greater learning scores (MacKenzie, Dies, Coche, Rutan, & Stone, 1987). An interesting aspect of group process measures is the large degree of variation they may reveal among members of the same group. It might be predicted that a measure such as the CALPAS-G, which asks for the individual member's relationship to the group, might be a better predictor of outcome than the GCQ, which asks for a description of the whole group, but only anecdotal evidence is available to support this view. One application of serial group climate measures has been to identify stages of group development (Kivlighan & Goldfine, 1991; Kivlighan & Mullison, 1988; MacKenzie, 1994a; MacKenzie & Tschuschke, 1993; Tschuschke & MacKenzie, 1989). This type of approach has not been adapted to individual psychotherapy, although several individual models emphasize the idea of sequential tasks in the therapy process (e.g., IPT; Weissman, Markowitz, & Klerman, 2000).

REFERENCES

Alden, L. E., Wiggins, J. S., & Pincus, A. L. (1990). Construction of circumplex scales for the Inventory of Interpersonal Problems. *Journal of Personality Assessment, 55,* 521–536.

American Psychiatric Association. (1994). *Diagnostic and statistical manual of Mental disorders.* (4th ed.). Washington DC: Author.

Attkisson, C., & Swick, R. (1982). The Client Satisfaction Questionnaire: Psychometric properties and correlations with service utilization and psychotherapy outcome. *Evaluation and Program Planning, 5,* 233–237.

Barber, J. P., & Muenz, L. R. (1996). The role of avoidance and obsessiveness in matching patients to cognitive and interpersonal psychotherapy: Empirical findings from the treatment of depression collaborative research program. *Journal of Consulting and Clinical Psychology, 64,* 951–958.

Barkham, M., Hardy, G. E., & Startup, M. (1996). The IIP-32: A short version of the Inventory of Interpersonal Problems. *British Journal of Clinical Psychology, 35,* 21–35.

Battle, C. C., Imber, S. D., Hoehn-Saric, R., Stone, A. R., Nash, E. H., & Frank, J. (1966). Target complaints as a criteria of improvement. *American Journal of Psychotherapy, 20,* 184–192.

Beck, A. T., Mendelson, M., Mock, J., & Erbaugh, J. (1961). An inventory for measuring depression. *Archives of General Psychiatry, 4,* 561–571.

Benjamin, L. S. (1987). Use of the SASB dimensional model to develop treatment plans for personality disorders. *Journal of Personality Disorders, 1,* 43–70.

Benjamin, L. S. (1993). *Interpersonal diagnosis and treatment of personality disorders.* New York: Guilford Press.

Blatt, S. J. (1995). The destructiveness of perfectionism: implications for the treatment of depression. *American Psychologist, 50,* 1003–1020.

Bordin, E. S. (1979). The generalizability of the psychoanalytic concept of the working alliance. *Psychotherapy: Theory, Research and Practice, 16,* 252–260.

Budman, S. H., Soldz, S., Demby, A., Feldstein, M., Springer, T., & Davis, S. (1989). Cohesion, alliance and outcome in group psychotherapy. *Psychiatry, 52,* 339–350.

Burlingame, G. M., Lambert, M. J., Reisinger, C. W., Neff, W. N., & Mosier, J. (1995). Pragmatics of tracking mental health outcomes in a managed care setting. *Journal of Mental Health Administration, 22,* 226–236.

Costa, P. T., & Widiger, T. A. (Eds.). (1994). *Personality disorders and the five-factor model of personality.* Washington, DC: American Psychological Association.

Crits-Christoph, P., & Barber, J. P. (1991). *Handbook of short-term dynamic psychotherapy.* New York: Basic Books.

Derogatis, L. R. (1983). *SCL-90: Administration, scoring and procedures manual for the revised version.* Baltimore, MD: Clinical Psychometric Research.

Derogatis, L. R., & Melisaratos, N. (1983). The brief symptom inventory: An introductory report. *Psychological Medicine, 13,* 595–605.

Eells, T. D. (Ed.). (1997). *Handbook of psychotherapy case formulation.* New York: Guilford Press.

Eysenck, H. J. (1952). The effects of psychotherapy: An evaluation. *Journal of Consulting Psychology, 16,* 319–324.

Fuhriman, A., & Burlingame, G. M. (Eds.). (1994). *Handbook of group psychotherapy: An empirical and clinical synthesis.* New York: Wiley.

Fuhriman, A., Drescher, S., Hanson, E., Henrie, R., & Rybicki, W. (1986). Refining the measurement of curativeness: An empirical approach. *Small Group Behavior, 17,* 186–201.

Gaston, L., & Marmar, C. (1991). *Manual of California Psychotherapy Alliance Scales.* San Francisco: University of California.

Hill, W. F. (1977). Hill Interaction Matrix (HIM). The conceptual framework, derived rating scales, and an updated bibliography. *Small Group Behavior, 8,* 251–268.

Horowitz, L. M., Rosenberg, S. E., Baer, B. A., Ureno, G., & Villaseñor, V. S. (1988). Inventory of Interpersonal Problems: Psychometric properties and clinical applications. *Journal of Consulting and Clinical Psychology, 56,* 885–892.

Horvath, A. O., & Greenberg, L. S. (1989). Development and validation of the Working Alliance Inventory. *Journal of Counseling Psychology, 36,* 223–233.

Horvath, A. O., & Symonds, B. D. (1991). Relations between working alliance and outcome in psychotherapy: A meta-analysis. *Journal of Counseling Psychology, 38,* 139–149.

Howard, K. I., Kopta, S. M., Krause, M. S., & Orlinsky, D. E (1986). The dose–effect relationship in psychotherapy. *American Psychologist, 41,* 159–164.

Howard, K. I., Lueger, R. J., Maling, M. S., & Martinovich, Z. (1993). A phase model of psychotherapy: Causal mediation of outcome. *Journal of Consulting and Clinical Psychology, 61,* 678–685.

Kadera, S. W., Lambert, M. J., & Andrew, A. A. (1996). How much therapy is really enough?: A session-by-session analysis of the psychotherapy dose-effect relationship. *The Journal of Psychotherapy Practice and Research, 5,* 132–151.

Kivlighan, D. M., & Goldfine, D. C. (1991). Endorsement of therapeutic factors as a function of stage of group development and participant interpersonal attitudes. *Journal of Counseling Psychology, 38,* 150–158.

Kivlighan, D. M., & Mullison, D. (1988). Participants' perception of therapeutic factors in group counseling: The role of interpersonal style and stage of group development. *Small Group Behavior, 19,* 452–468.

Kopta, S. M., Howard, K. I., Lowry, J. L., & Beutler, L. E. (1994). Patterns of symptomatic recovery in time-unlimited psychotherapy. *Journal of Consulting and Clinical Psychology, 62,* 1009–1016.

Laikin, M., Winston, A., & McCullough, L. (1991). Intensive short-term dynamic psychotherapy. In P. Crits-Christoph & J. P. Barber (Eds.), *Handbook of short-term dynamic psychotherapy* (pp. 80–109). New York: Basic Books.

Lambert, M. J., Burlingame, G. M. (1996). Outcome Questionnaire (OQ-45.2). Washington, DC: American Professional Credentialing Services.

Livesley, J., & Jackson, D. (2000). Dimensional Assessment of Personality Pathology. Port Huron, MI: Sigma Press.

Livesley, W. J., Jang, K. L., & Vernon, P. A. (1998). Phenotypic and genetic structure of traits delineating personality disorder. *Archives of General Psychiatry, 55,* 941–948.

Luborsky, L., Barber, J. P., Siqueland, L., Johnson, S., Najavits, L. M., Frank, A., & Daley, D. (1996). The revised helping alliance questionnaire (HAq-II): Psychometry properties. *Journal of Psychotherapy Practice and Research, 5,* 260–271.

Luborsky, L., & Crits-Christoph, P. (1997). *Understanding transference: The core conflictual realtionship theme method* (2nd ed.). Washington, DC: American Psychological Association.

MacKenzie, K. R. (1994a). Group development. In A. Fuhriman & G. M. Burlingame (Eds.), *Handbook of group psychotherapy: An empirical and clinical synthesis* (pp. 223–268). New York: Wiley.

MacKenzie, K. R. (1994b). Using personality measurements in clinical practice. In P. T. Costa & T. A. Widiger (Eds.), *Personality disorders and the five-factor model of personality* (pp. 237–250). Washington, DC: American Psychological Association.

MacKenzie, K. R. (1997). *Time-managed group psychotherapy: Effective clinical applications.* Washington, DC: American Psychiatric Press.

MacKenzie, K. R., Dies, R. R., Coche, E., Rutan, J. S., & Stone, W. N. (1987). An analysis of AGPA Institute groups. *International Journal of Group Psychotherapy, 37,* 55–74.

MacKenzie, K. R., & Grabovac, A. D. (2001). Interpersonal psychotherapy group (IPT-G) for treatment-resistant depression. *Journal of Psychotherapy Practice and Research, 10,* 46–51.

MacKenzie, K. R., & Tschuschke, V. (1993). Relatedness, group work, and outcome in long-term inpatient psychotherapy groups. *Journal of Psychotherapy Practice and Research, 2,* 147–156.

Medical Outcomes Trust. (1992). *SF-36 Health Survey.* Boston: Author.

Pfeiffer, J. W., Heslin, R., & Jones, J. E. (1976). Instrumentation in human relations training (2nd ed.). La Jolla, CA: University Associates.

Phillips, E. L. (1987). The ubiquitous decay curve: Delivery similarities in psychotherapy, medicine and addiction. *Professional Psychology: Research and Practice, 18,* 650–652.

Piper, W. E., Rosie, J. S., Joyce, A. S., & Azim, H. F. A. (1996). *Time-limited day treatment for personality disorders: Integration of research design and practice in a group program.* Washington, DC: American Psychological Association.

Ryle, A. (1997). *Cognitive analytic therapy and borderline personality disorder.* New York: Wiley.

Safran, J. D., & Muran, J. C. (Eds.) (1998). The therapeutic alliance in brief psychotherapy. Washington, DC: American Psychological Press.

Safran, J. D., & Muran, J. C. (2000). *Negotiating the therapeutic alliance: A relational treatment guide.* New York: Guilford Press.

Spielberger, C. D., Gorsuch, R. L., & Lushene, R. E. (1970). Manual for the State–Trait Inventory. Palo Alto, CA: California Psychologists Press.

Spitzer, R. L., Williams, J. B. W., & Gibbon, M. (1987). Structured Clinical Interview for DSM-III-R (SCID-II). New York: New York State Psychiatric Institute, Biometrics Research.

Tschuschke, V., & MacKenzie, K. R. (1989). Empirical analysis of group development: A methodological report. *Small Group Behavior, 20,* 419–427.

Vessey, J. T., Howard, K. I., Lueger, R. J., Kachele, H.,

& Mergenthaler, E. (1994). The clinician's illusion and the psychotherapy practice: An application of stochastic modeling. *Journal of Consulting and Clinical Psychology, 62,* 679–685.

Weissman, M. M., & Bothwell, S. (1976). The assessment of social adjustment by patient self-report. *Archives of General Psychiatry, 33,* 1111–1115.

Weissman, M. M., Markowitz, J. C., & Klerman, G. L. (2000). *Comprehensive guide to interpersonal psychotherapy.* New York: Basic Books.

PART IV

TREATMENT

CHAPTER 15

Psychosocial Treatment Outcome

WILLIAM E. PIPER
ANTHONY S. JOYCE

This chapter reviews research that has examined the effectiveness of treating personality disorders with psychosocial treatments. There are many different types of personality disorders and psychosocial treatments. Psychosocial treatments differ in both theoretical/technical orientation (e.g., behavioral, cognitive-behavioral, experiential, and psychodynamic) and in modality (e.g., individual, couple, family, group, and milieu). Because personality disorders encompass a broad class of disorders, psychosocial treatments encompass a broad range of treatments, and the many combinations of the two differ in treatment outcomes, it is not possible to provide a simple answer to the question, "Are psychosocial treatments effective with personality disorders?"

Another reason it is not possible to provide a simple answer to the question is that treatment success depends on the particular treatment objectives chosen. According to DSM-IV, a personality disorder is an enduring, pervasive, and inflexible pattern of inner experience and behavior that results in functional impairment and subjective distress. It is characterized by eccentric, dramatic, or fearful clusters of symptoms and behavior that are problematic to both the patients and the people with whom they interact. Accordingly, a considerable range of treatment objectives can be formulated. These include improvements in subjective symptoms

and sense of well-being, isolated dysfunctional behaviors, integrated patterns of behavior, and internal personality structure. Such objectives differ in how difficult they are to achieve. For example, alleviation of subjective distress is usually easier to achieve than modification of integrated patterns of behavior. Thus, conclusions about the effectiveness of treatment can vary considerably depending on the objective.

Given the number of personality disorders, psychosocial treatments, and treatment objectives, it is not surprising that the research literature addresses only a few of the possible combinations. This is particularly true if one considers methodologically strong studies. Conceptual and methodological difficulties limit the value and contribution of much of what is covered in the research literature. Clinical diagnoses rather than standard research diagnoses are often used to define the samples studied. In addition, comorbidity with other personality disorders (Zimmerman & Coryell, 1990) and with Axis I disorders (Docherty, Fiester, & Shea, 1986; Swartz, Blazer, Winfield, 1990; Tyrer, Casey, & Ferguson, 1988; see Dolan, Krueger, & Shea, Chapter 4, this volume) is often high. Sometimes comorbidity is assessed and reported, and sometimes it is not. Thus, personality disorders are often not isolated, which makes it difficult to know which disorders have been studied. Similarly, brief general descriptions of treatments rather than adherence checks of specific manualized treatments are often provided to distinguish the treatments. Multiple psychosocial treatments as well as psychotropic medications are commonly used with patients. Thus, psychosocial treatments are also often not isolated, which makes it difficult to know which treatments have been studied. The consequences of uncertainty regarding which personality disorders and psychosocial treatments have been studied is ironically clear. Findings and conclusions must be regarded as tentative.

One reason that multiple treatments have been used with personality disorders is the belief, which is based on both clinical experience and research evidence, that powerful treatment combinations are required to change integrated patterns of behavior and internal personality structure. By definition, personality disorders are enduring. Evidence documenting the stability of personality disorders comes from several sources. Follow-up studies of patients with personality disorders for periods up to 20 years have indicated stability of traits and persistence of diagnoses (Drake & Vaillant, 1985; Pope, Jonas, & Hudson, 1983; Wolff & Chick, 1980). Also, there is considerable evidence in the literature that treatment of Axis I disorders is less effective if patients also have a personality disorder (Reich & Green, 1991; Reich & Vasile, 1993). Although Tyrer, Gunderson, Lyons, and Tohen (1997) question the generality of this finding and indicate that there are exceptions, they concede that many patients with both an Axis I disorder and a personality disorder are more disturbed after treatment than patients with only an Axis I disorder. Consistent with the evidence for enduring problems are findings from our recent randomized clinical trial of time-limited day treatment (Piper, Rosie, Azim, & Joyce, 1993) that there was minimal evidence of "spontaneous remission" for a large set of outcome variables for patients in the 4-month, wait-list control condition of the clinical trial.

Another contributing factor to the minimal change of patients with personality disorders is that they often resist treatment when it is offered. Although the problematic behaviors of the patients almost always result in negative consequences, the behaviors themselves are usually not experienced by the patient as objectionable but syntonic. Maladaptive personality characteristics often have a long history, and the process of bringing about change is usually slow, gradual, and marked by repetition. Shifts in personality configuration are resisted by force of habit, reinforcing factors within the patient's social and interpersonal environment, and adaptive limitations imposed by temperament (Gunderson, 1989). The patient's ambivalence about change often leads to poor treatment compliance (e.g., lack of involvement, poor attendance, and premature termination). Establishing and maintaining a working alliance become a critical part of the treatment process.

Because strict inclusion of methodologically strong studies and exclusion of others would have limited the present review to only a small number of studies, we have been more inclusive than other recent reviews (Crits-Christoph, 1998; Shea, 1993). In most instances, we searched the literature for approaches to the psychosocial treatment of personality disorders that have undergone at least some empirical scrutiny. Integrated with empirical studies are reports of experienced clinicians and summaries of current clinical theory. Even so, the sampling of the many combinations of personality disorders, psychosocial treatments, and treatment objectives in the present review is limited. The focus is on three areas of the literature. The first section covers treatment approaches that address specific problem behaviors associated with personality disorders (e.g., antisocial acts). The treatment approaches are predominantly behavioral in orientation. The second section considers approaches designed for the treatment of personality disorders in general (i.e., a heterogeneous sample of personality disorders). Along with other approaches, marital, family, and group therapy approaches are considered in this section. The third and final section considers treatment approaches designed and evaluated for specific personality disorders (e.g., borderline personality disorder). Disorder-specific treatments usually offer a definite theoretical rationale, have an extensive history (e.g., therapeutic communities), or use manual guided treatments that have been subject to evaluation. Although the general state of the field is rather primitive in terms of sophisticated, large-scale research studies, there are examples of rigorous evaluations. These are reviewed in the sections that focus on the treatment of personality disorders in general and on specific personality disorders. They tend to represent the state of the art in personality disorder treatment research.

TREATMENTS TARGETING PROBLEMATIC BEHAVIORS

The literature on the behavioral treatment of personality disorders is not extensive, with the exception of juvenile delinquency (Burchard & Lane, 1982). The dearth of efficacy studies is due to several factors (Perry & Flannery, 1989). First, personality-disordered patients are not only difficult to treat but hard to study. Problems associated with comorbid Axis I syndromes, compliance to research protocols, acting-out behavior, and "splitting" of research and clinical personnel are well documented. Second, the psychopathology of personality disorders is seldom focal and discrete, making it difficult to isolate maladaptive behaviors. Third, behavior therapists have shown more interest in target behaviors and symptoms than in psychiatric diagnoses. Finally, behavior therapists have not studied patients' resistance in treatment to the same degree as dynamically oriented therapists have.

The techniques studied are those commonly associated with behavior therapy—that is, relaxation training (Wolpe, 1979), imagery techniques (Cautela, 1979), modeling (Bandura, 1969), token economies and contingency contracting (Allyon & Azrin, 1968), and assertiveness training (Wolpe, 1979). Research indicates that these techniques can be successful with personality disorders. Sloane, Staples, Cristol, Yorkston, and Whipple (1975) reported that short-term behavior therapy was as effective as dynamic therapy and more effective than no treatment for outpatients with neurotic disorders or personality disorders. The following material is organized by behavior problem.

Self-Destructive Impulsive Behavior

Rosen and Thomas (1984) devised a substitute behavior (squeezing a rubber ball) for chronic wrist cutting for three women with borderline personality disorders. On follow-up, all three remained free of wrist cutting. Liberman and Eckman (1981) compared behavior therapy and dynamic therapy for the inpatient treatment of repeated suicide attempters. The therapy consisted of an 8-day combination of individual and group approaches to social skills training, anxiety management (relaxation and imagery), and contingency contracting to improve family relationships. At 36-week follow-up, both treatment groups remained less depressed and suicidal than prior to hospitalization. Behavior therapy

patients showed more improvement across most measures, including full-time employment.

Antisocial and Delinquent Behaviors

Antisocial, impulsive, and undersocialized individuals, particularly incarcerated, juvenile males, have received extensive attention. Shamsie (1981) and Burchard and Lane (1982) concluded that conventional case work, individual therapy, and group and/or family therapy have minimal effectiveness in reducing delinquent behaviors (e.g., truancy, stealing, aggressiveness, and crimes against persons). Behavior modification techniques, such as contingency contracting, may help modify more specific target behaviors (academic performance, cooperation) that are not directly associated with antisocial disorders. However, the evidence does not indicate that treatment gains generalize to life "outside" or that they are associated with reduced recidivism.

Basic Social Skills

Marzillier, Lambert, and Kellett (1976) compared systematic desensitization and social skills training in socially anxious outpatients who had personality disorders or neuroses. Social skills training had a positive effect on the range and frequency of patients' social contacts at termination. Gains were maintained at 6-month follow-up. Neither treatment was successful, however, in reducing social anxiety. Spence and Marzillier (1979, 1981) treated adolescent offenders with a social skills training package that included instructions, modeling, role playing, videotaped feedback, and social reinforcement. Subjects increased eye contact and decreased fidgeting during conversations, but there was no effect on complex social skills, social anxiety, or employability.

Complex Social Skills

Jones, Stayer, Wichlacz, Thomes, and Livingstone (1977) worked with inpatients in the military with behavior or character disorders. In a randomized design, half were discharged back to active service and half were treated in a special open-ward program for 16 weeks. The program involved contingency contracting that targeted specific behaviors. Inappropriate behaviors were extinguished or punished. At 11-month follow-up, positive outcomes were significantly more common in the treated group (80%) than among controls (52%).

Dahl and Merskey (1981) employed an operant behavioral program with involuntarily committed inpatients with personality disorders. The patient and therapist set specific personal, vocational, and educational goals; frequent feedback was given, and successful performance resulted in progression through successive stages. Breaking rules was punished by return to a lower stage. Performance feedback was continued after discharge into the community. Three-quarters of the patients were living independently at 3-month follow-up.

Managing Affects and Affect Expression

Fehrenbach and Thelen (1982) reported that three studies of behavioral treatment demonstrated decreased aggressive outbursts and increased assertiveness among nonpsychotic impulsive adults (Foy, Eisler, & Pinkston, 1975; Frederiksen, Jenkins, Foy, & Eisler, 1976) and college students (Fehrenbach & Thelen, 1981). Combinations of focused directions, assertiveness training, modeling, behavioral rehearsal, and role playing were used.

Conflicting Self-Representations

The existence of "split" self-representations has been regarded as characteristic of a number of personality disorders, including borderline (Kernberg, 1968; Masterson, 1981) and narcissistic (Kohut, 1971). Glantz and Goisman (1990) describe a merging intervention based on relaxation training and imagery techniques as an adjunct to the expressive psychotherapy of 27 patients with Clusters B and C personality disorders. All patients made use of the intervention, and 24 of 27 responded with increased treatment compliance, decreased resistance, and improvement in daily life activities.

Current Status of Behavior Therapy Approaches

Some behaviors associated with personality disorders can be modified with lasting results. The best results appear to be obtained when treatment is individually tailored and the patient and therapist agree on a specific contract. Thus, studies of groups may not provide consistent findings. Patients who are impulsive, ac-

tion oriented, and easily overwhelmed by emotional responses may respond well to the structure provided by behavior therapy. Operant techniques appear to be effective with impulse-ridden patients, perhaps because these approaches provide structure that compensates for the poor attentional functioning.

Behavior changes may not, however, be accompanied by changes in attitudes or beliefs. Moreover, treatment may not generalize across target behaviors, settings, or individuals. Most of the research derives from institutional settings where controls and rewards are easily administered.

TREATMENTS ADDRESSING "PERSONALITY DISORDER"

The review of approaches to the treatment of personality disorder in general is organized according to modality. Individual therapy (psychoanalytic or psychodynamic) is addressed first, followed by marital/family, group (behavioral and psychodynamic), and residential or milieu treatment.

Psychodynamic Psychotherapy and Psychoanalysis

Psychoanalytic approaches to personality disorder began with Reich's (1949) view of character as the chief source of resistance. Alexander and French (1946) proposed shorter approaches to analytic treatment. A host of short-term dynamic therapies have since been developed (Davanloo, 1980; Luborsky, 1984; Malan, 1976; Mann, 1973; Sifneos, 1979; Strupp & Binder, 1984), though none are explicitly oriented to the treatment of personality disorder (Messer & Warren, 1995). Most analytic therapists choose long-term individual therapy or analysis based on the view that short-term methods can treat current problems but not lifelong maldevelopment (Winer & Pollock, 1989). The unique contribution of psychoanalytic theory for the treatment of personality disorder is the emphasis on exploring the relationship between therapist and patient as essential to change in personality structure.

Indications and Contraindications

Which form of analytic treatment to use for the personality-disordered patient is a difficult question. The traditional approach—a neutral analyst dedicated to interpretation of the patient's resistances without recourse to supportive measures—may be unduly depriving for many patients. Modifications by Kernberg (1984) and Kohut (1984) have made analytic therapy possible for many severely personality-disordered patients. Problem solving and supportive measures are central techniques. The therapist is more active in eliciting material, focusing on specific issues, and providing soothing interventions. Medication, marital, group, or family therapy can be profitably combined with insight-oriented individual sessions.

Clinical tradition holds that psychoanalysis and psychodynamic psychotherapy are more effective with the "anxious" cluster of disorders (avoidant, dependent, and obsessive–compulsive). The work of Kohut (1984) has stimulated interest in the psychoanalytic treatment of narcissistic disorders. Kernberg's (1984) views on the "borderline personality organization" and the problems of aggression in more primitive personalities have supported the development of psychoanalytic approaches to the treatment of patients with paranoid and borderline personality disorders. Fewer dramatic advances have occurred with regard to the psychoanalytic treatment of schizoid, schizotypal, or antisocial personality disorders.

Nature and Quality of Available Evidence

No controlled outcome studies of the effectiveness of psychoanalysis as a treatment for personality disorders have been reported, largely due to insurmountable methodological problems. The Menninger project (Kernberg, Coyne, Horwitz, Appelbaum, & Burstein, 1972; Wallerstein, 1986) provided a longitudinal evaluation with severely personality-disordered patients. The study concluded that patients with more ego strength responded better than poorly functioning patients (Luborsky & Spence, 1978). Schlessinger and Robbins (1983), reporting on a follow-up of the analytic treatments, were most impressed not with the resolution of psychic conflicts but with the development of an "identification with the analyzing function of the analyst, as a learned mode of coping with conflicts" (p. 8). Wallerstein (1986) emphasizes the importance of supportive techniques in the Menninger treatments, including those regarded as representative of psychoanalysis. This observation im-

plies that a transference-oriented interpretive focus in the psychoanalytic treatment of patients with personality disorders may require some degree of supportive "holding" on the part of the therapist. The degree of supportive emphasis required is likely a function of personality disorder sensitivity and the patient's ability to work collaboratively with the analyst.

Høglend (1993) compared the outcome of individual dynamic therapy (9–53 sessions) for patients with ($N = 15$) and without personality disorder ($N = 30$). At posttreatment, the Axis II patients showed less improvement than did the non-Axis II patients, but at 4-year follow-up this difference had disappeared. Duration of treatment was directly related to follow-up measures of insight and dynamic change for the Axis II patients.

Monsen and his colleagues (Monsen, Odland, Faugli, Daae, & Eilertsen, 1995a, 1995b) reported outcome findings for 25 outpatients with a range of personality disorders treated in intensive, analytically oriented therapy based on self psychology theory (Kohut, 1971, 1984). The average duration of treatment was 2 years. At posttreatment, clinically and statistically significant decreases in symptomatology as measured by the Minnesota Multiphasic Personality Inventory and Health–Sickness Rating Scale were noted. Patients additionally evidenced dramatic reductions in Axis II pathology. Patients who had received pretherapy diagnoses of paranoid, schizoid, schizotypal, passive–aggressive, or atypical/mixed personality disorder no longer met criteria for diagnosis at posttreatment. The single patient with narcissistic personality disorder retained the diagnosis at termination. Positive changes were also evident on the authors' theoretically relevant measure of affect awareness, tolerance, and expression. Improvements were maintained with a high degree of stability over the 5-year follow-up period. Evidence was also provided at follow-up for improved functioning in intimate relationships and decreased use of social and health services. The indications that patients had achieved structural change and the clinical significance of the improvements supported the authors' confidence in the findings despite the absence of a control condition.

Family Therapy and Couple Therapy

Family therapy and couple therapy are indicated for troubled relationships in which complementarity is evident. Complementarity refers to the "matching" of the interpersonal rigidity of personality disorders, where each party's interpersonal behavior enables and enhances the behavior of the other, leading to stereotyping, lack of flexibility and depth, and a general impoverishment of emotional life (Shapiro, 1989). Since the 1960s, intensive clinical study of the dynamics of personality disorders has suggested that these illnesses are sustained and supported within intimate relationships (Clarkin, Marziali, & Munroe-Blum, 1991).

Research on family and couple treatments for personality disorder is limited. Standard diagnostic categories are often not used and much of this work is based on case studies with the drawbacks of small sample size and clinician bias. Based on a review of available reports, Gurman and Kniskern (1981) drew the following conclusions:

1. The existing evidence from controlled studies of nonbehavioral marital and family therapies for personality disorder suggests that such treatments are often effective beyond chance.
2. Behavioral family therapy shows positive results but appears to be of limited use when severe marital difficulties coexist with deviant child behavior.
3. Among nonbehavioral marital therapies, conjoint treatment is the most effective.

Group Psychotherapy Approaches

Much of the literature describing the group therapy of personality disorders is anecdotal (Leszcz, 1989). Early reports described the therapeutic benefit of adding group therapy to individual psychotherapy with highly resistant patients (Fried, 1954; Jackson & Grotjahn, 1958). Group therapy offered the advantages of (1) confronting resistant, ego-syntonic character traits that arise during group transactions; (2) fostering the integration of strong positive and negative affects; (3) providing *in vivo* demonstration of maladaptive behaviors and a chance to experiment with new and adaptive ones; and (4) reducing the intensity of transference reactions that might occur in individual therapy.

General Evidence for Effectiveness

With the exception of antisocial personality disorder, research into the efficacy of group psychotherapy with personality disorders is limited (Parloff & Dies, 1977). A variety of methodological problems confront the field (Fuhriman & Burlingame, 1994). Investigators often fail to detail the personality disorder diagnoses of their samples. Personality-disordered patients are often mixed with broader samples of outpatients and are rarely studied in homogeneous samples.

Behavioral Approaches. The most frequent behavioral group treatment for personality disorder is social skills training (Bellack & Hersen, 1979). social skills training is generally brief, usually consisting of 6–12 sessions, each lasting 1–2 hours. In social skills training, the group is used as a laboratory for identifying and altering specific maladaptive target behaviors. Techniques such as role play and reinforcement are used to improve interpersonal skills (Argyle, Trower, & Bryant, 1974). Ten weekly sessions of social skills training for patients diagnosed as inadequate personalities resulted in significant improvements in target symptoms, work, and general adjustment (Falloon, Lindley, MacDonald, & Marks, 1977). Similar results were reported for patients diagnosed as avoidant personalities and treated with 12 weeks of social skills training (Stravynski, Marks, & Yule, 1982). Although social behavior shows measurable improvement after social skills training, gains made are often not translated to more intimate situations (Stravynski & Shahar, 1983).

Psychodynamic Approaches. Open-ended, once-weekly psychodynamic group therapy is a common form of treatment for personality disorders. The aims of treatment include clarifying and confronting maladaptive ego-syntonic traits, increasing the capacity to tolerate and integrate one's affect, and learning about the impact of one's behavior on others. What appears to be advantageous is a heterogeneous group, ideally composed of no more than one to two borderline or narcissistic patients and four to six less disturbed patients. Homogeneous groups may exacerbate the pressure toward regression and problematic countertransference reactions on the part of the therapist (Leszcz, 1989).

Both Yalom (1985) and Carney (1972) recommended 1 year as a minimum duration for treatment. In samples that include but are not limited to personality-disordered patients,

35–50% stay in treatment for longer than 2 years (Stone & Rutan, 1984). Clinical observation suggests that the use of concurrent individual therapy (combined or conjoint) can facilitate the retention of certain patients with personality disorder in group therapy and a positive outcome (Bernard & Drob, 1985; Wong, 1980).

In a well-known review of psychotherapy research, Luborsky, Singer, and Luborsky (1975) found group and individual therapy equally efficacious. Bellack (1980) found psychodynamic group therapy more effective than dyadic therapy for personality-disordered patients. In studies that employed diagnostically diverse samples, patients treated with psychodynamic group therapy by experienced clinicians and followed for some time achieved significant and enduring improvement of their long-standing interpersonal problems (Pilkonis, Imber, Lewis, & Rubinsky, 1984; Piper, Debbane, Bienvenu, & Garant, 1984). Malan, Balfour, Hood, and Shooter (1976) were less positive. Studying the outcomes of a mixed sample of neurotic and personality-disordered outpatients treated by group-as-a-whole approaches, they found that few showed marked improvement and, overall, patients who stayed in therapy for more than 2 years fared no better than early dropouts. The authors attributed these negative effects to the infrequent use of individually targeted interventions and the deprivation associated with the therapists' strict group-as-a-whole focus.

Budman, Demby, Soldz, and Merry (1996) conducted a trial of time-limited interpersonal group treatment for personality disorders. Five therapy groups were followed for 18 months (72 sessions) of treatment, with multidimensional change assessed on several occasions. The groups consisted of 9–10 members with a variety of personality disorders from Clusters B and C. Each group had at least two patients with borderline disorder. Of the 49 treated patients, 25 (51%) left prematurely. Eleven of the dropouts had diagnoses of borderline disorder. The authors noted that borderline patients may need "a method of intervention with more structure and intensity than our approach offered" (Budman et al., 1996, p. 374). Patients who continued in treatment showed considerable and steady improvement on most outcome measures.

Despite the occasionally equivocal findings, patients sometimes endorse group therapy. In one study (Gould & Glick, 1976), character-disordered patients highly valued the group therapy they received during their hospitalization. In another, patients with borderline personality disorder ranked a dynamic therapy group as the most important treatment experience during their acute hospitalization (Leszcz, Yalom, & Norden, 1985).

Conclusion

A chief benefit of group psychotherapy is its ability to clarify, elaborate, and confront ego-syntonic personality traits in a less regressive atmosphere than dyadic therapy. In addition, group therapy provides the personality-disordered patient with an opportunity to acquire and practice new methods of interacting.

Milieu Treatment

Milieu treatment comprises modes of outpatient or residential therapy ranging from short-term hospital stays to long-term sheltered community programs. The essence of the milieu approach is the patient's experience of interacting with others in a structured communal setting. Maladaptive behaviors and attitudes are systematically confronted in the context of therapy groups and community meetings involving all members. McGlashan (1989) provided a comprehensive review of the indications for and goals of milieu treatment. Milieu treatments are provided for patients with a range of personality disorders, but most reports concern borderline disorder. Evidence regarding disorder-specific milieu treatments is reviewed in the final section that focuses on specific personality disorders.

General Treatment Considerations

Any standard milieu treatment should feature the following elements: (1) protection; (2) evaluation, diagnosis, and treatment planning; (3) alliance with the patient and family; (4) structured interventions with appropriate limit setting; (5) rehabilitation; and (6) discharge planning, reintegration, and aftercare (McGlashan, 1989). The most effective milieu treatment units are small and have high staff-to-patient ratios and levels of staff–patient interaction; a minority of low-functioning patients; clear and active lines of communication; a task-oriented group focus; and a routine daily schedule of activities to which everyone is expected to adhere (Ellsworth, 1983; Liberman, 1983).

Available Evidence

Day Hospital Approaches. Day hospitals are defined as diagnostic and treatment services for acute patients who would otherwise be treated on inpatient units. Day hospitals also include facilities that support the transition of patients from hospital to outpatient care. Efficacy is usually determined by contrasts with inpatient treatment. The seminal comparative study by Zwerling and Wilder (1964) followed acute psychiatric patients ($N = 189$) assigned to either day hospital or inpatient treatment. The day hospital made use of individual, family, and group modalities in a therapeutic community. Approximately one-third of the entire patient population could be maintained in the day hospital; patients diagnosed with "psychoneuroses and personality disturbances" were more likely to be accommodated. Wilder, Levin, and Zwerling (1966) reported on a 2-year follow-up of the trial. There was no significant difference in readmissions between the two groups. When rehospitalization occurred, the interval between discharge and readmission was longer for day hospital patients. Fewer day hospital patients were actively on medication at the time of discharge. Patients in the day hospital also expressed greater satisfaction and their families rated the treatment as more helpful. The Zwerling and Wilder (1964) sample was a heterogeneous one; that is, not all patients could be regarded as presenting with personality disorder. Nonetheless, the study was one of the first to suggest that partial hospitalization offers a viable treatment alternative to inpatient admission for at least some patients with personality disorders.

Dick, Cameron, Cohen, Barlow, and Ince (1985) conducted a similar comparative trial but were more selective regarding patient inclusion. Patients from a specific diagnostic subgroup (neurotic and personality disorders, adjustment reactions) were randomly assigned to inpatient or day hospital treatment. Both programs used individual counseling, group therapy, activity therapy, and medication. One-fifth of all referrals were capable of admission to either treatment. There were no significant differences in the mean severity of symptoms between day hospital patients and inpatients at any point of assessment. Both groups improved but day hospital patients expressed greater satisfaction with treatment. Costs were lower for day hospital (one-quarter to one-third), although day hospital patients had longer length of stays.

Day Treatment Approaches. Day treatment programs provide more intensive treatment and rehabilitation than is possible in outpatient settings. In addition to symptom reduction, the primary goal is to improve the patient's community functioning. Day treatment programs are generally time limited.

Karterud et al. (1992; see also Mehlum et al., 1991; Vaglum et al., 1990) described a moderate length (4–8 months) day treatment program for patients with severe and chronic personality disorders based on a psychoanalytic object-relations approach. Each day was bracketed by two large group community meetings. Other forms of group and individual therapy, art therapy, and occupational therapy were offered. Ninety-seven consecutive patients were followed prospectively. Three-quarters of the sample were diagnosed as personality disorders, with borderline (35%) or schizotypal (13%) the most frequent. Two patients were hospitalized and two patients made suicide attempts, rates that are substantially lower than commonly reported (Gunderson, 1984). Significant improvement in symptoms of psychological distress was shown for the total sample. Length of stay was directly associated with symptom change. Patients with borderline and other personality disorders showed moderate gains, while patients with schizotypal disorders showed the least improvement.

Piper et al. (1993; Piper, Rosie, Joyce, & Azim, 1996; see also Azim, Chapter 25, this volume) conducted a randomized controlled trial of an 18-week, psychodynamic day treatment program for patients with affective and personality disorders. The sample consisted of 120 patients, matched in pairs on Axis I diagnosis, age, and gender. Each member of the pair was randomly assigned to immediate treatment or a delayed treatment control condition. Seventeen outcome variables addressed symptom severity, interpersonal behavior, self-esteem, life satisfaction, defensive functioning, and individualized treatment objectives. Outcome was monitored before and after the treatment and control periods and at follow-up an average of 8 months after termination. The majority (65%) of the patients were diagnosed with a major depression. Sixty percent of the patients had personality disorders, the most frequent being dependent (22%) and borderline (14%). Treated patients showed greater improvement than controls on 7 of 17 outcome variables, with all areas of functioning except defensive style reflecting significant change. Benefits were maintained over follow-up.

Because of the small and unequal number of patients in each grouping, it was not feasible to analyse the outcome data by personality disorder category or cluster. Presence of a personality disorder was found to be inversely associated with improvement on measures of psychiatric symptomatology. However, this outcome prediction was minor relative to the prediction afforded by two theoretically relevant personality variables, quality of object relations and psychological mindedness. These findings suggest that investigators may be able to identify important patient–treatment matches by considering patient characteristics that have a bearing on the approach to treatment. The patient's Axis II diagnosis may not be the most salient patient variable worth considering.

Conclusion

A number of methodologically sound studies of milieu therapy for personality disorders provide strong evidence of treatment efficacy. Milieu treatments offer a comprehensive intervention "package" and capitalize on the patients' shared group experience. These elements likely work singly and in combination to promote benefit across a range of outcome indices.

DISORDER-SPECIFIC TREATMENT APPROACHES

Cluster A Disorders

Paranoid, schizotypal, and schizoid personality disorders make up the "eccentric" cluster of Axis II. Very little of the treatment literature considers these specific disorders. Most of the recommendations available are based on clinical anecdote rather than empirical study. Patients with paranoid personality disorder are generally regarded as poor candidates for group therapy and intolerant of the intrusive nature of behavioral treatments. "Non-directive cognitive therapy is the initial treatment of choice, trust being required before other procedures can be employed" (Quality Assurance Project, 1990, p. 342). One study of psychoanalytic therapy for patients with schizotypal personality disorder (Stone, 1983) reported little or no change. Open-ended, low intensity supportive psychotherapy to reduce social isolation and encourage affect expression is recommended. The prognosis for schizoid patients is somewhat better. Cognitive therapy and social skills training may assist with self-insight and interpersonal functioning, but more formal behavioral methods appear to be of little use (Quality Assurance Project, 1990). Less severely disturbed schizoid patients may benefit from psychodynamic group therapy if well-prepared and able to establish some intimacy with other members.

Cluster B Disorders

Antisocial Personality Disorder

Treatment for antisocial disorder has been studied for a longer period than for other disorders, partly because of the clear outcome variable of recidivism. The early manifestation of this disorder warrants reference to the group therapy of the delinquent population, although overviews are not very encouraging (Julian & Kilman, 1979; Parloff & Dies, 1977). Whereas outpatient group therapy is probably contraindicated for the unreliable and resistive antisocial personality (Yalom, 1985), treatment in homogeneous groups within institutions and therapeutic communities can lead to positive outcomes (Carney, 1972; Jones, 1983). The most reliable treatments have generally been in an inpatient or court-mandated prison setting (Suedfeld & Landon, 1978) and feature a therapeutic milieu with elements of firm program structure and behavioral control (Stürup, 1968).

Behavioral Approaches. Skills training and modeling approaches addressing particular antisocial behaviors are held to be somewhat effective (Julian & Kilman, 1979). In a meta-analysis of social skills training interventions, however, Corrigan (1991) reports that skill acquisition occurs only while antisocial patients are in treatment and does not generalize to their outside life (Reid, 1985; Taylor, 1986).

Cognitive-Behavioral Approaches. Davidson and Tyrer (1996) evaluated a brief (10-session) cognitive therapy approach using single-case methodology. Two of three patients with antisocial personality disorder reported improvement in target problems, but in neither case were the changes significant. Involvement of family members was found to be crucial to confronting the patient's interpersonal problems.

Valliant and Antonowicz (1991) provided a group cognitive-behavioral treatment to prisoners. The intervention was provided once weekly for 2 hours over 5 weeks. An assessment of pre–post changes on self-report measures revealed improvements in anxiety and self-esteem. More assaultive inmates tended to benefit less.

Psychodynamic Approaches. Reid (1985) offers guidelines for the dynamic therapy of antisocial personality disorder, emphasizing strict adherence to treatment parameters and a rigorous focus on current and here-and-now behavior. Treatment goals should be limited to "symptom relief and defensive restructuring" (p. 834). Woody, McLellan, Luborsky, and O'Brien (1985) conducted a randomized controlled trial of supportive–expressive psychotherapy plus drug counseling, cognitive-behavioral psychotherapy plus drug counseling, and drug counseling alone for 110 opiate addicts. Opiate-dependent patients with antisocial personality disorder and major depression responded to psychotherapy as well as those patients with depression alone. The authors suggest that depression allows the antisocial patient to be amenable to psychotherapy, perhaps due to a heightened tendency to be self-critical. In a follow-up study of the 48 addicts with antisocial personality disorder from the Woody et al. (1985) trial, Gerstley et al. (1989) reported that patients independently regarded as having the capacity to establish a working alliance with their therapist showed significantly better improvement following 24 weeks of therapy. These studies indicate that the common view of antisocial personality as untreatable should be modified. A subgroup of patients with antisocial personality disorder (i.e., those found during "trial therapy" to be able to form a collaborative relationship with the therapist) may indeed receive benefit from engagement in psychotherapy.

Milieu Treatment Approaches. Milieu treatments for antisocial personality disorder draw on elements of inpatient programs such as strict hierarchical structure, patient confrontation, emphasis on assuming responsibility and devel-

oping competence, and parameters that attenuate the patient's manipulative tendencies (Reid, 1985). The therapeutic community at the Henderson Hospital in England (Copas & Whitley, 1976; Whitley, 1970) applied these principles. Patients who benefited had already shown achievement in academic, occupational, and interpersonal areas. Time in treatment was directly associated with improvement; aggressiveness was inversely related to therapeutic change (Copas, O'Brien, Roberts, & Whitley, 1984).

In two popular forms of nonhospital milieu treatment, the community residential program (Reid & Solomon, 1981) and the wilderness experience program (Reid & Matthews, 1980), antisocial behaviors emerging in common daily situations are confronted as part of the treatment. Program completers have shown greater social competence and less recidivism (Reid, 1985). Studies of milieu treatment suggest that reduced recidivism is a function of treatments oriented to coping and adaptation and social supports, both of which mitigate against further engagement in antisocial behavior. Less is known about the patient or treatment variables that are associated with other kinds of outcomes (e.g., symptom improvement and personality change) among patients with antisocial personality disorders.

Borderline Personality Disorder

Borderline personality disorder is by far the most intensively studied of the Axis II categories (Clarkin, Marziali, & Munroe-Blum, 1992). Many factors encourage the study of borderline personality disorder. Characteristic behaviors can frequently put the borderline patient and others at severe risk of harm. Borderline patients tend to be quite heterogeneous in terms of presenting problems and coping style. This wide range of behavior demands that treatment strategies be comprehensive and that therapists have extensive experience (Aronson, 1989). Development of effective treatments for borderline personality disorder can be advantageous for the treatment of other personality disorders, which may present similar behaviors in attenuated form.

Dialectical Behavior Therapy. Linehan (1987) developed a manualized treatment for "parasuicidal" behavior that evolved (Linehan, 1993) into dialectical behavior therapy (DBT) for patients with borderline personality disorder. According to the model, the inability to tolerate strong states of negative affect is central. DBT encourages the patient to accept negative affects without engaging in self-destructive or maladaptive behavior. Behavioral techniques include skills training, contingency management, cognitive modification, and exposure to emotional cues.

The treatment involves both individual and group formats. The group therapy is psychoeducational and teaches interpersonal, distress tolerance, and self-management skills. In individual sessions, the therapist applies directive techniques, (e.g., contingency management and exposure) in concert with supportive techniques (e.g., reflection, empathy, and acceptance). Sessions focus on target behaviors arranged in a hierarchy, which moves through (1) suicidal behaviors; (2) behaviors interfering with the work of therapy; (3) escape behaviors interfering with stability; (4) behavioral skill acquisition (emotion regulation, interpersonal effectiveness, distress tolerance, and self-management); and (5) other specific goals.

In a randomized clinical trial (Linehan, Armstrong, Suarez, Allmon, & Heard, 1991), DBT consisted of 1 hour of individual therapy and 2.5 hours of group therapy per week for a full year. The control condition was "treatment as usual" in the community, generally outpatient individual therapy. However, only about 75% of the control subjects actually received treatment (Hollon & Beck, 1994). This discrepancy would have favored DBT and should be noted as a qualification.

Patients with borderline personality disorder treated with DBT showed greater reductions in symptoms and parasuicidal and dysfunctional behaviors, decreased treatment dropout, fewer and shorter inpatient admissions, and improved work status. No differences were evident on self-reported levels of depression, hopelessness, or suicidal ideation, although scores decreased across treatment for both groups. In a 1-year follow-up, Linehan, Heard, and Armstrong (1993) reported that DBT patients showed significant improvement at 6 months relative to controls on measures of anger and anxiety, social adjustment, and work performance. The differences were less pronounced at 12-month follow-up. No differences were found at follow-up on measures of satisfaction and well-being. In effect, then, DBT patients had improved behaviorally but were "still miserable" (Linehan, Tutek, Heard, & Armstrong,

1994, p. 1775); a single year of DBT, "while beneficial, is not sufficient for this population" (p. 1775). DBT is a useful treatment for helping borderline personality disorder patients achieve behavioral stability and can be used to prepare patients for subsequent involvement in a more intensive psychodynamic treatment (Hurt, Clarkin, Munroe-Blum, & Marziali, 1992).

Other Cognitive-Behavioral Approaches. In the Davidson and Tyrer (1996) case study evaluation of a 10-session cognitive-behavioral treatment described above, all three patients with borderline personality disorder reported improvement in target problems. The authors note that DBT is not particularly applicable to routine clinical practice and, thus, their treatment may be preferable.

Perris (1994) has described a similar treatment model addressing "the restructuring of dysfunctional working models of self and environment" (p. 69). The therapy is augmented with various strategies, tailored to the individual patient, to define a comprehensive treatment package. The average length of stay in treatment is approximately 2 years. In a naturalistic follow-up of 13 borderline personality disorder patients, Perris (1994) reported a low dropout rate (7.7%) and decreases in the frequency of parasuicidal behavior and hospitalization. Improvements in symptoms and social functioning evident at termination were maintained or showed further improvement at 2-year follow-up.

Psychoanalytic Therapy Approaches. Intensive expressive individual psychotherapy of the borderline personality disorder patient was rarely recommended prior to the work of Kohut (1971) and Kernberg (1975, 1984). The demands of a relatively nongratifying analytic approach were regarded as likely to precipitate severe regression, resulting in treatment-threatening acting out and/or a need for hospitalization. The development of modified analytic approaches has been addressed by several clinicians (e.g., Buie & Adler, 1982; Horwitz, 1985; Masterson, 1976; Waldinger, 1987). Two contrasting approaches can be discerned. Theories emphasizing the centrality of intrapsychic conflict (Kernberg) stress the importance of interpretation, particularly of aggressive impulses and the patient's negative transference. In contrast, models based on a presumed deficit in the patient's intrapsychic structure (Kohut) argue that interpersonal learning in a context of supportive "holding" is crucial.

Clarkin, Koenigsberg, et al. (1992) describe a research program on long-term, analytic individual therapy for borderline personality disorder based on Kernberg's approach. It advocates strict therapist neutrality, early and frequent interpretation of primitive transferences, and environmental manipulations to protect the parameters of treatment. The therapy is provided twice weekly, in an open-ended format, and follows a manual (Kernberg, Selzer, Koenigsberg, Carr, & Appelbaum, 1989). The program has yet to progress to a controlled outcome evaluation. The authors have reported a 23% early dropout rate (prior to contracting for therapy) and a cumulative dropout rate of 42% by 12 sessions. Uncontrolled outcome findings for six patients indicated that changes were most likely for behaviors associated with impulsivity. Five of the patients no longer met criteria for borderline personality disorder after 6 months.

Stevenson and Meares (1992) conducted a prospective outcome study of a 12-month, twice-weekly, psychodynamic individual therapy for borderline personality disorder. The therapy was based on a self psychology perspective. Outcome was assessed using a symptom self-report and a set of objective behavioral measures (e.g., time off work, number of medical visits, self-harm episodes, and hospital admissions) for the 1 year prior to and following treatment. The sample of 30 patients showed significant improvement on all measures that was maintained at 1-year follow-up. At follow-up, nine patients (30%) no longer fulfilled diagnostic criteria for borderline personality disorder. In a recent article (Gabbard, 1997), 5-year follow-up findings were summarized, with indications that treatment gains had largely been maintained.

Group Therapy Approaches. The borderline patient can benefit from the unique aspects of group treatment. Horwitz (1980) and Wong (1980) advise concurrent individual treatment. In contrast, Pines (1975) views concurrent individual therapy as unnecessary. Supportive group approaches for borderline personality disorder patients have also been advocated (Kibel, 1980), with the aim of returning the patient to a precrisis level of functioning.

Marziali and Munroe-Blum (1994) describe a group adaptation of interpersonal psychotherapy (Klerman, Weissman, Rounsaville, & Chevron, 1984) for the treatment of borderline personality disorder. Based on the "relationship management" model for borderline patients (Dawson, 1988), the treatment is manualized and consists of 30 90-minute group sessions, weekly for the first 25 weeks and biweekly afterward to termination.

The authors conducted a comparative trial of interpersonal group therapy versus open-ended, individual dynamic psychotherapy (Munroe-Blum & Marziali, 1995). Both were conducted by experienced therapists and monitored for treatment integrity. The findings indicated significant improvement for the total study cohort, but no differences between treatments, on measures of social dysfunction, social performance, and symptomatology. Patient noncompliance or dropout was a notable problem. The overall rate of refusal of treatment or early dropout was 28%, 26% for individual treatment, and 31% for group treatment. The group treatment had better rates of patient attendance (among those who completed therapy), was preferred by the clinicians, and was shown to be more cost-effective than the "as usual" individual therapy.

Residential/Milieu Approaches. Tucker, Bauer, Wagner, Harlam, and Sher (1987) followed 40 patients with severe personality disorder (predominantly borderline personality disorder) for 2 years following treatment in an inpatient therapeutic community. Treatment was long term (mean duration = 8.4 months) and included individual therapy. Self-destructive feelings and associated behaviors decreased markedly. Global functioning showed improvement from pre- to posttreatment, with continued gains at both 1- and 2-year follow-up. Hospital admissions in the 2 years postdischarge were lower compared to an equivalent period before admission.

Dolan, Evans, and Wilson (1992) assessed change in neurotic symptomatology for 62 patients treated in a therapeutic community (see also Copas & Whitley, 1976; Whitley, 1970). The majority (87%) were diagnosed with borderline personality disorder. The average length of stay was 28 weeks. Symptom severity was assessed at preadmission and at 8-month follow-up. Results showed a significant reduction in symptom distress, with 55% of the sample showing reliable improvement. One third (32%) achieved clinically significant change, moving into the "noncase" range on the outcome variable. Only 6.5% showed reliable signs of deterioration.

Hafner and Holme (1996) conducted a prospective outcome evaluation of therapeutic community treatment. The average length of stay for the 48 patients (70% with borderline personality disorder) was 64 days. The sample showed significant decreases in psychiatric symptoms and expressed hostility at discharge, with further improvements evident at 3-month follow-up. Patients regarded the therapy groups as the most helpful component of the program.

Therapeutic community treatment for borderline personality disorder appears to be an effective intervention whether provided short term (Hafner & Holme, 1996) or long term (Tucker et al., 1987). However, realistic expectations of outcome for borderline personality disorder patients are best confined to improvement rather than cure. In reviewing a 15-year follow-up of patients treated at the Chestnut Lodge therapeutic community, McGlashan (1986) indicated that despite clear evidence of improvement, most patients demonstrated evidence of persisting pathology.

Narcissistic Personality Disorder

Nurnberg (1984) notes that there has been no empirical research that "has clearly demonstrated superior efficacy or specificity with any particular modality of treatment" (p. 205) for narcissistic personality disorder. Patients with this disorder commonly present solely for relief of internal distress and rarely for insight or character change. Three functional groupings of the disorder have been outlined (Adler, 1986; Goldberg, 1978; Nurnberg, 1984). The high-level group has good social functioning and receives sustaining gratification from the environment. If in acute crisis, these patients generally respond favorably to time-limited individual therapy (e.g., Horowitz, 1986; Malan, 1976). The middle-level group has severe disturbances in object relations and commonly presents with neurotic symptoms and sexual difficulties. The indicated treatment is analysis or intensive analytic therapy (Kernberg, 1975; Kohut, 1971, 1977). The low-level group exhibits borderline personality organization (Kernberg, 1975) and presents with pronounced ego deficits, poor adaptation, impulsivity, and low frustration tolerance. These patients are considered to be inappropriate for analysis or analytic therapy. A supportive, reality-oriented therapy is required.

Histrionic Personality Disorder

Andrews (1984) has reviewed the principles of clinical treatment for histrionic personality disorder, arguing that effective treatment requires an integration of psychoanalytic and behavioral techniques. Behavioral techniques include the negative reinforcement of histrionic behaviors, positive reinforcement of more effective interpersonal behaviors, and assertiveness training. Analytic techniques emphasize the needed balance between contact and separateness and encourage the direct expression of feelings.

Kass, Silvers, and Abrams (1972) reported on an inpatient behavioral group treatment that targeted specific histrionic behaviors. An operant learning system of individual rewards and contingencies was enforced and supported by the peer group, and the expression of effective, assertive interpersonal behavior was reinforced. Based on a small inpatient sample, significant reductions in symptoms and target behaviors were achieved within 4 to 6 weeks and maintained at 18-month follow-up.

Cluster C Disorders

Cluster C personality disorders tend to be a major focus for treatment research because they are commonly seen by mental health practitioners and tend to have a less problematic course in therapy. This section first considers research on individual therapy for all Cluster C disorders. The following sections briefly consider various approaches to the group treatment of avoidant, dependent, and obsessive–compulsive personality disorders.

Treatment of Cluster C Disorders

Pollack, Winston, McCullough, Flegenheimer, and Winston (1990) conducted a quasi-controlled study of brief adaptational psychotherapy (BAP) for Cluster C disorders. BAP involves a cognitive focus on the major maladaptive interpersonal pattern, with an emphasis on how it is affectively manifest in the transference relationship. The study compared a BAP condition ($N = 15$) to a wait-list control condition ($N = 16$), but assignment to conditions was nonrandom. Control patients were given post-condition assessments after 20 weeks, relative to a mean of 39 weeks for the BAP patients. Results at posttreatment indicated marked improvement on two of three target complaints, symptom severity, and social functioning. At 2.6-year follow-up, treated patients showed continued gains.

In a subsequent randomized trial, BAP was compared with a short-term dynamic psychotherapy (STDP) modeled after Davanloo (1980) and a wait-list control condition. STDP places greater emphasis on confronting defenses and resistance and eliciting affect. The mean duration of treatment in both therapy conditions was 40 weeks; control patients were assessed after 20 weeks and provided with therapy. The team published findings based on 32 Cluster C patients (Winston et al., 1991) at the midpoint of the trial and on 81 patients (Winston et al., 1994) at its conclusion. Treated patients showed significant posttreatment improvement relative to controls on symptoms, social functioning, and target complaints, and there were no differences in outcome between BAP and STDP. At 1.5-year follow-up, gains were maintained or increased. There is some evidence (Winston et al., 1989) that STDP is more effective for patients with an obsessional style (overcontrolled) whereas BAP is more effective for patients with a more histrionic style (undercontrolled).

Hardy et al. (1995) examined the effect of a Cluster C diagnosis on the outcome of one of four approaches to individual treatment for depression: 8-session or 16-session cognitive-behavioral or dynamic–interpersonal therapy. Approximately one-quarter (27) of the sample of 114 had been diagnosed with a Cluster C disorder. At posttreatment and follow-up after dynamic therapy, patients with personality disorder still had significantly greater pathology than did non-personality disorder patients. Following cognitive therapy, however, there was no posttreatment difference between personality disorder and non-personality disorder patients. Treatment length was not found to influence outcome. The findings support the conjecture by Shea, Widiger, and Klein (1992) that patients with personality disorder respond better to more structured cognitive and behavioral treatments.

Avoidant Personality Disorder

Renneberg, Goldstein, Phillips, and Chambless (1990) conducted an uncontrolled evaluation of a four-session intensive behavioral group therapy for avoidant personality disorder ($N = 17$).

Outcome was assessed at posttreatment and 1-year follow-up on measures of social anxiety and functioning, depression, and self-esteem. Significant improvement was observed across all measures. The low dropout rate (< 5%) was attributed to the intensive group format (32 hours over 4 days).

Alden (1989) compared the effectiveness of three group formats (graduated exposure, interpersonal skill training, and intimacy training) to a wait-list control condition for patients with avoidant personality disorder. All patients who participated in the 10-week group program displayed significant improvement relative to controls, but skills training did not prove more effective than graduated exposure alone. Comparisons with norms on the outcome measures indicated that despite significant improvement, the patient's functioning remained within the pathological range. In a subsequent analysis of the same data, Alden and Capreol (1993) hypothesized that different interpersonal problems moderated the response to the various behavioral therapies. Graded exposure was more effective for patients who primarily had problems with mistrust and anger, while intimacy training was more effective for patients who found resisting others' demands to be their major interpersonal problem.

Dependent Personality Disorder

Montgomery (1971) reported on the use of group therapy for difficult clinic patients previously seen individually on a monthly basis. The patients were extremely dependent, frequently demanded medication and magical cures, and often disrupted the clinic's routine with their urgent demands. Marked decreases in the use of psychotropic medication and crisis visits were seen following the group therapy.

Obsessive–Compulsive Personality Disorder

Wells, Glickauf-Hughes, and Buzzell (1990) have outlined a dynamic–interpersonal group therapy approach to the treatment of obsessive–compulsive personality disorder. Treatment goals are to modify a restrictive cognitive style and harsh superego and to increase comfort with affective expression and interpersonal reciprocity. To date, the group has not been subjected to empirical study.

CONCLUSIONS

As indicated in the initial section of this chapter and evident from the preceding sections that have reported specific findings, the literature covers only a small portion of the possible combinations of personality disorders, psychosocial treatments, and treatment objectives. Even if one includes clinical reports and findings from uncontrolled studies along with the relatively small number of methodologically strong studies, one is limited to a piecemeal rather than a comprehensive picture. Nevertheless, some generalizations can be formulated, which should be regarded as tentative until confirmed by future work.

In regard to specific problem behaviors, there is evidence that they can be modified by behavioral techniques, in particular operant methods. However, there are limitations. Often, there is minimal change in associated attitudes and beliefs and minimal generalization across associated behaviors and situations. Much of the success has been restricted to institutional settings. In regard to heterogeneous samples of personality disorders, there are few, if any, controlled studies involving psychoanalysis, individual dynamic therapy, couple therapy, and family therapy. There are a few methodologically strong clinical trials involving group dynamic therapy that have demonstrated significant improvements across a range of outcome variables. The most substantial evidence of improvement for a single treatment involves social skills training, although for a limited range of behavior. There is also substantial evidence for improvement across a range of outcome variables for milieu treatment as represented by day hospital and day treatment programs. These programs capitalize on using a combination of treatments.

In regard to specific disorders, there have been few reports for Cluster A personality disorders. In contrast, there is evidence of positive results from methodologically strong studies for Cluster B personality disorders. Milieu treatment has been successful across a range of outcome variables for both antisocial personality disorder and borderline personality disorder. For antisocial personality disorder, social skills training and cognitive-behavior therapy have met with limited success. The approach known as dialectical behavior therapy, which involves a combination of individual and group treatments, has been effective with a variety of problematic behaviors of borderline personality disorder, although relief for subjective symptoms has been limited. In addition, interpersonal group therapy has been shown to be effective with borderline patients, although the dropout rate may be high. Treatment results for narcissistic personality disorder have not been encouraging and there have been few reports for histrionic personality disorder. In the case of Cluster C personality disorders, there is evidence of success from clinical trials involving time-limited dynamic therapies. Cognitive-behavioral treatment of avoidant personality disorder has met with some success. Finally, there are few outcome reports for dependent personality disorder and obsessive–compulsive personality disorder.

Consistent with the belief that substantial improvements for multiple objectives require powerful treatments, the more impressive results from the more methodologically strong studies tend to involve combinations of treatments (e.g., milieu therapy programs). These treatments typically include group therapies. Group forms of treatment for personality disorders have a number of compelling assets. Maladaptive interpersonal behavior can be demonstrated and examined in the immediacy of the group situation. The patient can receive direct feedback from an entire set of peers. The group situation is particularly conducive to patients who are threatened by the intimacy of the individual therapy situation or who react negatively to authority figures. Peer influence can be powerful. New ways of relating to others can be practiced in the group situation. The patient can also benefit from being helpful to others in the group. An additional advantage associated with group therapies is their potential to be cost-effective, an important asset in today's era of health care reform.

The reality of cost considerations in choosing treatments for personality disorders and the range of treatment objectives that are available indicate that different treatment models can be followed. These range from short-term intermittent treatments to long-term continuous treatments. In the former case, patients with personality disorders can be treated with periodic interventions directed toward crisis resolution and symptom reduction. In the latter case, they can be treated with ongoing interventions directed toward changes in integrated patterns of behavior and internal personality structure. The sequencing of the former followed by the latter is, of course, possible if resources permit. Unfortunately, the absence of studies that have compared such alternatives and the general absence of long-term follow-up data in the literature currently prevent such choices from being made on the basis of evidence.

In addition to highlighting the potential importance of the integration of different therapies in the treatment of personality disorders, the recent review by Crits-Christoph (1998) has cited the potential importance of discovering optimal matches between particular personality disorders and treatments. Although this is a worthy objective, there are only a small number of studies that have, thus far, investigated such matches and that have provided supportive findings. Some were cited in this chapter.

It is also possible that there are optimal matches between personality characteristics and treatments for various personality disorders. Our clinical trial of time-limited day treatment suggested that personality variables such as quality of object relations and psychological mindedness may have this potential (Piper et al., 1996). They were the best predictors of success from a set of seven patient characteristics. Quality of object relations is defined as a person's internal enduring tendency to establish certain types of relationships that range along an overall dimension from primitive to mature. It is assessed by means of a semistructured interview. Quality of object relations was directly related to remaining in the day treatment program and to improvement on two of four basic outcome factors in the study (general symptomatology and target objectives, social maladjustment and dissatisfaction). Psychological mindedness is defined as the ability to identify dynamic (intrapsychic) components of conflict and relate them to a patient's difficulties. It is measured by an interview that focuses on the person's responses to a videotape that portrays a patient–therapist interaction. Psychological mindedness was directly related to working in the program and to improvement on three of the four basic outcome factors (general symptomatology and target objectives, social maladjustment and dissatisfaction, pathological dependency). These two personality variables, which were independent of one another, combined additively or interactively to account for a substantial amount of outcome variation. We believe that their success can be partly attributed

to the relevance of the concepts to the theoretical and technical orientation of the treatment program. The ability to establish meaningful give-and-take relationships (quality of object relations) and the ability to identify important conflictual components (psychological mindedness) likely allowed patients to tolerate the daily interpersonal demands of the program and engage in productive work with patients and staff. Our findings raise the possibility that a dimensional rather than a categorical diagnostic approach to conceptualizing personality disorders (Widiger & Sanderson, 1995) may be more productive in identifying optimal matches between patients and treatments.

In many ways, the investigation of the treatment of patients with personality disorders is at an early stage of development. The questions that need to be addressed and the types of research that are likely to be productive are fairly well-known. Basic questions concerning the optimal matching of treatments and patients are paramount. Thorough descriptions of patients on diagnostic, demographic, personality, and other potentially predictive criteria are crucial. Treatments need to be defined clearly and their integrity assessed. A comprehensive set of reliable and valid outcome criteria needs to be used. Assessment of process variables to identify mechanisms of change is important. Follow-up assessments of patients should be conducted. In comparative trials, steps should be taken to ensure patient equivalence between the conditions to avoid selection bias; this usually means random allocation to conditions. Auxiliary treatments such as medication should be monitored carefully and their relation to outcome investigated. Large samples of patients should be studied to increase statistical power and enhance generalizability. The achievement of these and other methodological objectives requires considerable resources and the persistence of collaborating researchers and clinicians. Mobilizing such resources is a challenge that we must achieve if we wish to make substantial progress in advancing knowledge about psychosocial treatments and personality disorders.

REFERENCES

Adler, G. (1986). Psychotherapy of the narcissistic personality disorder patient: Two contrasting approaches. *American Journal of Psychiatry, 143,* 430–436.

Alden, L. (1989). Short-term structured treatment for avoidant personality disorder. *Journal of Consulting and Clinical Psychology, 57,* 756–764.

Alden, L. E., & Capreol, M. J. (1993). Avoidant personality disorder: Interpersonal problems as predictors of treatment response. *Behavior Therapy, 24,* 357–376.

Alexander, J. F., & French, T. M. (1946). *Psychoanalytic therapy: Principles and applications.* New York: Ronald Press.

Allyon, T., & Azrin, N. (1968). *The token economy.* New York: Appleton-Century-Crofts.

Andrews, J. D. W. (1984). Psychotherapy with the hysterical personality: An interpersonal approach. *Psychiatry, 47,* 211–232.

Argyle, M., Trower, P., & Bryant, B. (1974). Explorations in the treatment of personality disorders and neuroses, by social skills training. *British Journal of Medical Psychology, 47,* 63–72.

Aronson, T. A. (1989). A critical review of psychotherapeutic treatments of the borderline personality: Historical trends and future directions. *Journal of Nervous and Mental Disease, 177,* 511–527.

Bandura, A. (1969). *Principles of behavior modification.* New York: Holt, Rinehart, & Winston.

Bellack, L. (1980). On some limitations of dyadic psychotherapy and the role of group modalities. *International Journal of Group Psychotherapy, 30,* 7–21.

Bellack, A. S., & Hersen, M. (1979). *Research and practice in social skills training.* New York: Plenum Press.

Bernard, H. S., & Drob, S. (1985). The experiences of patients in conjoint individual and group psychotherapy. *International Journal of Group Psychotherapy, 35,* 129–146.

Budman, S. H., Demby, A., Soldz, S., & Merry, J. (1996). Time-limited group psychotherapy for patients with personality disorders: Outcomes and dropouts. *International Journal of Group Psychotherapy, 46,* 357–377.

Buie, D., & Adler, G. (1982). The definitive treatment of the borderline patient. *International Journal of Psychoanalytic Psychotherapy, 9,* 51–87.

Burchard, J. D., & Lane, T. W. (1982). Crime and delinquency. In A. S. Bellack, M. Hersen, & A. E. Kazdin (Eds.), *International handbook of behavior modification and therapy* (pp. 613–652). New York: Plenum Press.

Carney, F. L. (1972). Some recurring therapeutic issues in group psychotherapy with criminal patients. *American Journal of Psychotherapy, 26,* 34–41.

Cautela, J. R. (1979). *Covert conditioning.* New York: Pergamon Press.

Clarkin, J. F., Koenigsberg, H., Yeomans, F., Selzer, M., Kernberg, P., & Kernberg, O. F. (1992). Psychodynamic psychotherapy of the borderline patient. In J. F. Clarkin, E. Marziali, & H. Munroe-Blum (Eds.), *Borderline personality disorder: Clinical and empirical perspectives* (pp. 268–287). New York: Guilford Press.

Clarkin, J. F., Marziali, E., & Munroe-Blum, H. (1991). Group and family treatments for borderline personality disorder. *Hospital and Community Psychiatry, 42,* 1038–1043.

Clarkin, J. F., Marziali, E., & Munroe-Blum, H. (1992).

Borderline personality disorder: Clinical and empirical perspectives. New York: Guilford Press.

Copas, J. B., O'Brien, M., Roberts, J., & Whitley, J. S. (1984). Treatment outcome in personality disorder: The effect of social, psychological and behavioural variables. *Personality and Individual Differences, 5,* 565–573.

Copas, J. B., & Whitley, J. S. (1976). Predicting success in the treatment of psychopaths. *British Journal of Psychiatry, 129,* 388–392.

Corrigan, P. W. (1991). Social skills training in adult psychiatric populations: A meta-analysis. *Journal of Behavior Therapy and Experimental Psychiatry, 22,* 203–210.

Crits-Christoph, P. (1998). Psychosocial treatments for personality disorders. In P. E. Nathan & J. M. Gorman (Eds), *A guide to treatments that work* (pp. 544–553). New York: Oxford University Press.

Dahl, G., & Merskey, D. M. (1981). Clinical patterns in a behavior modification unit. *Canadian Journal of Psychiatry, 26,* 460–463.

Davanloo, H. (1980). *Short-term dynamic psychotherapy.* New York: Jason Aronson.

Davidson, K. M., & Tyrer, P. (1996). Cognitive therapy for antisocial and borderline personality disorders: Single case study series. *British Journal of Clinical Psychology, 35,* 413–429.

Dawson, D. (1988). Treatment of the borderline patient: Relationship management. *Canadian Journal of Psychiatry, 33,* 370–374.

Dick, P., Cameron, L., Cohen, D., Barlow, M., & Ince, A. (1985). Day and full time psychiatric treatment: A controlled comparison. *British Journal of Psychiatry, 147,* 246–250.

Docherty, J., Fiester, S. & Shea, T. (1986). Syndrome diagnosis and personality disorder. In R. Hales & A. Frances (Eds.), *Psychiatric update: American Psychiatric Association annual review* (Vol. 5, pp. 315–355). Washington, DC: American Psychiatric Press.

Dolan, B. M., Evans, C., & Wilson, J. (1992). Therapeutic community treatment for personality disordered adults: Changes in neurotic symptomatology on follow-up. *International Journal of Social Psychiatry, 38,* 243–250.

Drake, R.E., & Vaillant, G. E. (1985). A validity study of Axis II of DSM-III. *American Journal of Psychiatry, 142,* 553–558.

Ellsworth, R. B. (1983). Characteristics of effective treatment milieus. In J. G. Gunderson, O. A. Will, & L. R. Mosher (Eds.), *Principles and practice of milieu therapy* (pp. 87–123). New York: Jason Aronson.

Falloon, F. R. H., Lindley, P., MacDonald, R., & Marks, I. M. (1977). Social skills training of outpatient groups. *British Journal of Psychiatry, 131,* 599–609.

Fehrenbach, P. A., & Thelen, M. H. (1981). Assertive skills training for inappropriately aggressive college males: Effects on assertive and aggressive behaviors. *Journal of Behavior Therapy and Experimental Psychiatry, 12,* 213–217.

Fehrenbach, P. A., & Thelen, M. H. (1982). Behavioral approaches to the treatment of aggressive disorders. *Behavior Modification, 6,* 465–487.

Foy, D. W., Eisler, R. M., & Pinkston, S. (1975). Modeled assertion in a case of explosive rages. *Journal of*

Behavior Therapy and Experimental Psychiatry, 67, 135–137.

Frederiksen, L. W., Jenkins, J. O., Foy, D. W., & Eisler, R. M. (1976). Social skills training to modify abusive verbal outbursts in adults. *Journal of Applied Behavior Analysis, 9,* 117–126.

Fried, E. (1954). The effects of combined therapy on the productivity of patients. *International Journal of Group Psychotherapy, 4,* 42–55.

Fuhriman, A., & Burlingame, G. M. (1994). *Group psychotherapy: An empirical and clinical synthesis.* New York: Wiley.

Gabbard, G. O. (1997). Borderline personality disorder and rational managed care policy. *Psychoanalytic Inquiry Supplement,* 17–28.

Gerstley, L., McLellan, A. T., Alterman, A. I., Woody, G. E., Luborsky, L., & Prout, M. (1989). Ability to form an alliance with the therapist: A possible marker of prognosis for patients with antisocial personality disorder. *American Journal of Psychiatry, 146,* 508–512.

Glantz, K., & Goisman, R. M. (1990). Relaxation and merging in the treatment of personality disorders. *American Journal of Psychotherapy, 44,* 405–413.

Goldberg, A. J. (1978). The psychology of the self: A casebook. New York: International Universities Press.

Gould, E., & Glick, I. D. (1976). Patient–staff judgements of treatment program helpfulness on a psychiatric ward. *British Journal of Medical Psychology, 49,* 23–33.

Gunderson, J. G. (1984). *Borderline personality disorder.* Washington, DC: American Psychiatric Press.

Gunderson, J. G. (1989). Introduction to Section 26 (Personality Disorders). In American Psychiatric Association, *Task force on treatment of psychiatric disorders* (Vol. 3, pp. 2633–2638). Washington, DC: American Psychiatric Association Press.

Gurman, A. S., & Kniskern, D. P. (1981). Family therapy outcome research. In A. S. Gurman & D. P. Kniskern (Eds.), *Handbook of family therapy* (pp. 742–775). New York: Brunner-Mazel.

Hafner, R. J., & Holme, G. (1996). The influence of the therapeutic community on psychiatric disorder. *Journal of Clinical Psychology, 52,* 461–468.

Hardy, G. E., Barkham, M., Shapiro, D. A., Stiles, W. B., Rees, A., & Reynolds, S. (1995). Impact of Cluster C personality disorders on outcomes of contrasting brief psychotherapies for depression. *Journal of Consulting and Clinical Psychology, 63,* 997–1004.

Høglend, P. (1993). Personality disorders and long-term outcome after brief dynamic psychotherapy. *Journal of Personality Disorders, 7,* 168–181.

Hollon, S. D., & Beck, A. T. (1994). Cognitive and cognitive-behavioral therapies. In A. E. Bergin & S. L. Garfield (Eds.), *Handbook of psychotherapy and behavior change* (4th ed., pp. 428–466). New York: Wiley.

Horowitz, M. J. (1986). *Stress response syndromes* (2nd ed.). Northvale, NJ: Jason Aronson.

Horwitz, L. (1980). Group psychotherapy for borderline and narcissistic disorders. *Bulletin of the Menninger Clinic, 44,* 181–200.

Horwitz, L. (1985). Divergent views on the treatment of borderline patients. *Bulletin of the Menninger Clinic, 49,* 525–545.

Hurt, S. W., Clarkin, J. F., Munroe-Blum, H., & Marziali, E. (1992). Borderline behavioral clusters and different treatment approaches. In J. F. Clarkin, E. Marziali, & H. Munroe-Blum (Eds.), *Borderline personality disorder: Clinical and empirical perspectives* (pp. 199–219). New York: Guilford Press.

Jackson, J., & Grotjahn, M. (1958). The treatment of oral defenses by combined individual and group psychotherapy. *International Journal of Group Psychotherapy, 7,* 373–381.

Jones, F. D., Stayer, S. J., Wichlacz, C. R., Thomes, L., & Livingstone, B. L. (1977). Contingency management of hospital diagnosed character and behavior disordered soldiers. *Journal of Behavior Therapy and Experimental Psychiatry, 8,* 333.

Jones, M. S. (1983). Therapeutic community as a system for change. In J. G. Gunderson, O. A. Will, & L. R. Mosher (Eds.), *Principles and practice of milieu therapy* (pp. 177–184). New York: Jason Aronson.

Julian, A., III, & Kilman, P. R. (1979). Group therapy of juvenile delinquents: A review of the outcome literature. *International Journal of Group Psychotherapy, 29,* 3–37.

Karterud, S., Vaglum, S., Friis, S., Irion, T., Johns, S., & Vaglum, P. (1992). Day hospital therapeutic community treatment for patients with personality disorders: An empirical evaluation of the containment function. *Journal of Nervous and Mental Disease, 180,* 238–243.

Kass, D. J., Silvers, F. M., & Abrams, G. M. (1972). Behavioral group treatment of hysterics. *Archives of General Psychiatry, 26,* 42–50.

Kernberg, O. F. (1968). The treatment of patients with borderline personality organization. *International Journal of Psychoanalysis, 49,* 600–619.

Kernberg, O. F. (1975). *Borderline conditions and pathological narcissism.* New York: Jason Aronson.

Kernberg, O. F. (1984). *Severe personality disorders: Psychotherapeutic strategies.* New Haven, CT: Yale University Press.

Kernberg, O. F., Coyne, L., Horwitz, L., Appelbaum, A., & Burstein, E. (1972). Psychotherapy and psychoanalysis: Final report of the Menninger Foundation's Psychotherapy Research Project. *Bulletin of the Menninger Clinic, 36,* 87–195.

Kernberg, O. F., Selzer, M. A., Koenigsberg, H. W., Carr, A. C., & Appelbaum, A. M. (1989). *Psychodynamic psychotherapy of borderline patients.* New York: Basic Books.

Kibel, H. D. (1980). The importance of the comprehensive clinical diagnosis for group psychotherapy of borderline and narcissistic patients. *International Journal of Group Psychotherapy, 30,* 427–444.

Klerman, G. L., Weissman, M. M., Rounsaville, B. J., & Chevron, E. S. (1984). *Interpersonal psychotherapy of depression.* New York: Basic Books.

Kohut, H. (1971). *The analysis of the self.* New York: International Universities Press.

Kohut, H. (1977). *The restoration of the self.* New York: International Universities Press.

Kohut, H. (1984). *How does analysis cure?* Chicago: University of Chicago Press.

Leszcz, M. (1989). Group therapy. In American Psychiatric Association, *Task force on treatment of psychi-*

atric disorders (Vol. 3, pp. 2667–2677). Washington, DC: American Psychiatric Association Press.

Leszcz, M., Yalom, I. D., & Norden, M. (1985). Inpatient group psychotherapy: Patients' perspective. *International Journal of Group Psychotherapy, 35,* 411–433.

Liberman, R. P. (1983). Research on the psychiatric milieu. In J. G. Gunderson, O. A. Will, & L. R. Mosher (Eds.), *Principles and practice of milieu therapy* (pp. 67–86). New York: Jason Aronson.

Liberman, R. P., & Eckman, T. (1981). Behavior therapy versus insight-oriented therapy for repeated suicide attempters. *Archives of General Psychiatry, 38,* 1126–1130.

Linehan, M. (1987). Dialectical behavior therapy: A cognitive behavioral approach to parasuicide. *Journal of Personality Disorders, 1,* 328–333.

Linehan, M. M. (1993). *Cognitive-behavioral treatment of borderline personality disorder.* New York: Guilford Press.

Linehan, M. M., Armstrong, H. E., Suarez, A., Allmon, D., & Heard, H. L. (1991). Cognitive-behavioral treatment of chronically parasuicidal borderline patients. *Archives of General Psychiatry, 48,* 1060–1064.

Linehan, M. M., Heard, H. L., & Armstrong, H. E. (1993). Naturalistic follow-up of a behavioral treatment for chronically parasuicidal borderline patients. *Archives of General Psychiatry, 50,* 971–974.

Linehan, M. M., Tutek, D. A., Heard, H. L., & Armstrong, H. E. (1994). Interpersonal outcome of cognitive behavioral treatment for chronically suicidal borderline patients. *American Journal of Psychiatry, 151,* 1771–1776.

Luborsky, L. (1984). *Principles of psychoanalytic psychotherapy: A manual for supportive–expressive treatment.* New York: Basic Books.

Luborsky, L., Singer, B., & Luborsky, L. (1975). Comparative studies of psychotherapies: Is it true that "everyone has won and all must have prizes"? *Archives of General Psychiatry, 32,* 995–1008.

Luborsky, L., & Spence, D. P. (1978). Quantitative research on psychoanalytic psychotherapy. In S. L. Garfield & A. E. Bergin (Eds.), *Handbook of psychotherapy and behavior change* (pp. 331–368). New York: John Wiley.

Malan, D. H. (1976). *The frontier of brief psychotherapy.* New York: Plenum Press.

Malan, D., Balfour, F. H. G., Hood, V. G., & Shooter, A. M. N. (1976). Group psychotherapy: A long term follow-up study. *Archives of General Psychiatry, 33,* 1303–1315.

Mann, J. (1973). *Time-limited psychotherapy.* Cambridge, MA: Harvard University Press.

Marziali, E., & Munroe-Blum, H. (1994). *Interpersonal group psychotherapy for borderline personality disorder.* New York: Basic Books.

Marzillier, J. S., Lambert, C., & Kellett, J. (1976). A controlled evaluation of systematic desensitization and social skills training for socially inadequate psychiatric patients. *Behavior Research and Therapy, 14,* 225–238.

Masterson, J. F. (1976). *Psychotherapy of the borderline adult: A developmental approach.* New York: Brunner/Mazel.

Masterson, J. F. (1981). *Narcissistic and borderline dis-*

orders: An integrated developmental approach. New York: Brunner/Mazel.

McGlashan, T. H. (1986). The Chestnut Lodge follow-up study: III. Long-term outcome of borderline personalities. *Archives of General Psychiatry, 43,* 20–30.

McGlashan, T. H. (1989). Residential treatment. In American Psychiatric Association, *Task force on treatment of psychiatric disorders* (Vol. 3, pp. 2689–2704). Washington, DC: American Psychiatric Association Press.

Mehlum, L., Friis, S., Irion, T., Johns, S., Karterud, S., Vaglum, P., & Vaglum, S. (1991). Personality disorders 2–5 years after treatment: A prospective follow-up study. *Acta Psychiatrica Scandinavica, 84,* 72–77.

Messer, S. B., & Warren, C. S. (1995). *Models of brief psychodynamic therapy: A comparative approach.* New York: Guilford Press.

Monsen, J. T., Odland, T., Faugli, A., Daae, E., & Eilertsen, D. E. (1995a). Personality disorders: Changes and stability after intensive psychotherapy focusing on affect consciousness. *Psychotherapy Research, 5,* 33–48.

Monsen, J. T., Odland, T., Faugli, A., Daae, E., & Eilertsen, D. E. (1995b). Personality disorders and psychosocial changes after intensive psychotherapy: A prospective follow-up study of an outpatient psychotherapy project, 5 years after end of treatment. *Scandinavian Journal of Psychology, 36,* 256–268.

Montgomery, J. (1971). Treatment management of passive–dependent behavior. *International Journal of Social Psychiatry, 17,* 311–319.

Munroe-Blum, H., & Marziali, E. (1995). A controlled trial of short-term group treatment for borderline personality disorder. *Journal of Personality Disorders, 9,* 190–198.

Nurnberg, H. G. (1984). Survey of psychotherapeutic approaches to narcissistic personality disorder. *Hillside Journal of Clinical Psychiatry, 6,* 204–220.

Parloff, M. B., & Dies, R. R. (1977). Group psychotherapy outcome research, 1966–1975. *International Journal of Group Psychotherapy, 27,* 281–319.

Perris, C. (1994). Cognitive therapy in the treatment of patients with borderline personality disorders. *Acta Psychiatrica Scandinavica, 89,* 69–72.

Perry, J. C., & Flannery, R. B. (1989). Behavior therapy. In American Psychiatric Association, *Task force on treatment of psychiatric disorders* (Vol. 3, pp. 2649–2659). Washington, DC: American Psychiatric Association Press.

Pilkonis, P. A., Imber, S. D., Lewis, P., & Rubinsky, P. (1984). A comparative outcome study of individual, group, and conjoint psychotherapy. *Archives of General Psychiatry, 41,* 431–437.

Pines, M. (1975). Group therapy with difficult patients. In L. R. Wolberg & M. L. Aronson (Eds.), *Group therapy 1975: An overview* (pp. 102–119). New York: Stratton Intercontinental.

Piper, W. E., Debbane, E. G., Bienvenu, J. P., & Garant, J. (1984). A comparative study of four forms of psychotherapy. *Journal of Consulting and Clinical Psychology, 52,* 268–279.

Piper, W. E., Rosie, J. S., Azim, H. F. A., & Joyce, A. S. (1993). A randomized trial of psychiatric day treatment for patients with affective and personality disorders. *Hospital and Community Psychiatry, 44,* 757–763.

Piper, W. E., Rosie, J. S., Joyce, A. S., & Azim, H. F. A. (1996). *Time-limited day treatment for personality disorders: Integration of research and practice in a group program.* Washington, DC: American Psychological Association Press.

Pollack, J., Winston, A., McCullough, L., Flegenheimer, W., & Winston, B. (1990). Efficacy of brief adaptational psychotherapy. *Journal of Personality Disorders, 4,* 244–250.

Pope, H. G., Jonas, M. J., & Hudson, J. I. (1983). The validity of DSM-III borderline personality disorders. *Archives of General Psychiatry, 40,* 23–30.

Quality Assurance Project. (1990). Treatment outlines for paranoid, schizotypal and schizoid personality disorders. *Australian and New Zealand Journal of Psychiatry, 24,* 339–350.

Reich, J. H., & Green, H. I. (1991) Effect of personality disorders on outcome of treatment. *Journal of Nervous and Mental Disease, 179,* 74–82.

Reich, J. H., & Vasile, R. G. (1993). Effect of personality disorders on the treatment outcome of Axis I conditions: An update. *Journal of Nervous and Mental Disease, 181,* 475–484.

Reich, W. (1949). *Character analysis* (3rd ed.). New York: Farrar, Strauss, & Giroux.

Reid, W. H. (1985). The antisocial personality: A review. *Hospital and Community Psychiatry, 36,* 831–837.

Reid, W. H., & Matthews, W. M. (1980). A wilderness experience treatment program for antisocial offenders. *International Journal of Offender Therapy and Comparative Criminology, 24,* 171–178.

Reid, W. H., & Solomon, G. F. (1981). Community-based offender programs. In W. H. Reid (Ed.), *The treatment of antisocial syndromes* (pp. 76–94). New York: Van Nostrand Reinhold.

Renneberg, B., Goldstein, A. J., Phillips, D., & Chambless, D. L. (1990). Intensive behavioral group treatment of avoidant personality disorder. *Behavior Therapy, 21,* 363–377.

Rosen, L. W., & Thomas, M. A. (1984). Treatment technique for chronic wrist cutters. *Journal of Behavior Therapy and Experimental Psychiatry, 15,* 33–36.

Schlessinger, N., & Robbins, F. P. (1983). *A developmental view of the psychoanalytic process: Follow-up studies and their consequences.* New York: International Universities Press.

Shamsie, S. J. (1981). Antisocial adolescents: Our treatments do not work: Where do we go from here? *Canadian Journal of Psychiatry, 26,* 357–364.

Shapiro, E. R. (1989). Family and couples therapy. In American Psychiatric Association, *Task force on treatment of psychiatric disorders* (Vol. 3, pp. 2660–2666). Washington, DC: American Psychiatric Association Press.

Shea, M. T. (1993). Psychosocial treatment of personality disorder. *Journal of Personality Disorders, 7,* 167–180.

Shea, M. T., Widiger, T. A., & Klein, M. H. (1992). Comorbidity of personality disorders and depression: Implications for treatment. *Journal of Consulting and Clinical Psychology, 60,* 857–868.

Sifneos, P. E. (1979). *Short-term dynamic psychothera-*

py: Evaluation and technique. New York: Plenum Press.

Sloane, R. B., Staples, F. R., Cristol, A. H., Yorkston, N. J., & Whipple, K. (1975). *Psychotherapy versus behavior therapy.* Cambridge, MA: Harvard University Press.

Spence, S. H., & Marzillier, J. S. (1979). Social skills training with adolescent offenders. I: Short-term effects. *Behavior Research and Therapy, 17,* 7–16.

Spence, S. H., & Marzillier, J. S. (1981). Social skills training with adolescent offenders. II: Short-term, long-term, and generalized effects. *Behavior Research and Therapy, 19,* 349–368.

Stevenson, J., & Meares, R. (1992). An outcome study of psychotherapy for patients with borderline personality disorder. *American Journal of Psychiatry, 149,* 358–362.

Stone, M. H. (1983). Psychotherapy with schizotypal borderline patients. *Journal of the American Academy of Psychoanalysis, 11,* 87–111.

Stone, W. N., & Rutan, J. S. (1984). Duration of treatment in group psychotherapy. *International Journal of Group Psychotherapy, 34,* 93–111.

Stravynski, A., Marks, I. M., & Yule, W. (1982). Social skills problems in neurotic outpatients. *Archives of General Psychiatry, 39,* 1378–1383.

Stravynski, A., & Shahar, A. (1983). The treatment of social dysfunction in nonpsychotic outpatients: A review. *Journal of Nervous and Mental Disease, 171,* 721–728.

Strupp, H. H., & Binder, J. L. (1984). *Psychotherapy in a new key: A guide to time-limited dynamic psychotherapy.* New York: Basic Books.

Stürup, G. K. (1968). *Treating the "untreatable": Chronic criminals at Herstedvester.* Baltimore: Johns Hopkins University Press.

Suedfeld, P., & Landon, P. B. (1978). Approaches to treatment. In R. Hare & D. Schalling (Eds.), *Psychopathic behavior: Approaches to research* (pp. 347–377). New York: Wiley.

Swartz, M., Blazer, D., & Winfield, I. (1990). Estimating the prevalence of borderline personality disorder in the community. *Journal of Personality Disorders, 4,* 257.

Taylor, P. J. (1986). Psychopaths and their treatment. *Journal of the Royal Society of Medicine, 79,* 693–695.

Tucker, L., Bauer, S. F., Wagner, S., Harlam, D., & Sher, I. (1987). Long-term hospital treatment of borderline patients: A descriptive outcome study. *American Journal of Psychiatry, 144,* 1443–1448.

Tyrer, P. J., Casey, P., & Ferguson, B. (1988). Personality disorder and mental illness. In P. Tyrer (Ed.), *Personality disorders: Diagnosis, management, and course* (pp. 93–104). London: Wright.

Tyrer, P., Gunderson, J., Lyons, M., & Tohen, M. (1997). Special feature: Extent of co-morbidity between mental state and personality disorders. *Journal of Personality Disorders, 11,* 242–259.

Vaglum, P., Friis, S., Irion, T., Johns, S., Karterud, S., Larsen, F., & Vaglum, S. (1990). Treatment response of severe and nonsevere personality disorders in a therapeutic community day unit. *Journal of Personality Disorders, 4,* 161–172.

Valliant, P. M., & Antonowicz, D. H. (1991). Cognitive

behavior therapy and social skills training improves personality and cognition in incarcerated offenders. *Psychological Reports, 68,* 27–33.

Waldinger, R. J. (1987). Intensive psychodynamic therapy with borderline patients: An overview. *American Journal of Psychiatry, 144,* 267–274.

Wallerstein, R. S. (1986). *Forty-two lives in treatment: A study of psychoanalysis and psychotherapy.* New York: Guilford Press.

Wells, M. C., Glickauf-Hughes, C., & Buzzell, V. (1990). Treating obsessive–compulsive personalities in psychodynamic/interpersonal group therapy. *Psychotherapy, 27,* 366–379.

Whitley, J. S. (1970). The response of psychopaths to a therapeutic community. *British Journal of Psychiatry, 116,* 517–529.

Widiger, T.A., & Sanderson, C.J. (1995). Toward a dimensional model of personality disorders. In W. J. Livesley (Ed.), *The DSM-IV personality disorders* (pp. 433–458). New York: Guilford Press.

Wilder, J., Levin, G., & Zwerling, I. (1966). A two-year follow-up evaluation of acute psychotic patients treated in a day hospital. *American Journal of Psychiatry, 122,* 1095–1101.

Winer, J. A., & Pollock, G. H. (1989). Psychoanalysis and dynamic psychotherapy. In American Psychiatric Association, *Task force on treatment of psychiatric disorders* (Vol. 3, pp. 2639–2648). Washington, DC: American Psychiatric Association Press.

Winston, A., Laikin, M., Pollack, J., Samstag, L. W., McCullough, L., & Muran, J. C. (1994). Short-term psychotherapy of personality disorders. *American Journal of Psychiatry, 151,* 190–194.

Winston, A., McCullough, L., Pollack, J., Laikin, M., Pinsker, H., Nezu, A., Flegenheimer, W., & Sadow, J. (1989). The Beth Israel Psychotherapy Research Program: Toward an integration of theory and discovery. *Journal of Integrative and Eclectic Psychotherapy, 4,* 344–356.

Winston, A., Pollack, J., McCullough, L., Flegenheimer, W., Kestenbaum, R., Trujillo, M. (1991). Brief psychotherapy of personality disorders. *Journal of Nervous and Mental Disease, 179,* 188–193.

Wolff, S., & Chick, J. (1980). Schizoid personality in childhood: A controlled follow-up study. *Psychological Medicine, 10,* 85–100.

Wolpe, J. (1979). *The practice of behavior therapy* (3rd ed.). New York: Pergamon.

Wong, J. (1980). Combined group and individual treatment of borderline and narcissistic patients: Heterogeneous versus homogeneous groups. *International Journal of Group Psychotherapy, 30,* 389–404.

Woody, G. E., McLellan, T., Luborsky, L., & O'Brien, C. P. (1985). Sociopathy and psychotherapy outcome. *Archives of General Psychiatry, 42,* 1081–1086.

Yalom, I. D. (1985). *The theory and practice of group psychotherapy* (3rd ed.). New York: Basic Books.

Zimmerman, M., & Coryell, W. H. (1990). Diagnosing personality disorders within the community: A comparison of self-report and interview measures. *Archives of General Psychiatry, 47,* 527.

Zwerling, I., & Wilder, J. (1964). An evaluation of the applicability of the day hospital in the treatment of acutely disturbed patients. *Israel Annals of Psychiatry, 2,* 162–185.

CHAPTER 16

Supportive Psychotherapy

ARNOLD WINSTON
RICHARD N. ROSENTHAL
J. CHRISTOPHER MURAN

Although supportive psychotherapy techniques are more widely used than expressive or insight-oriented techniques, supportive psychotherapy has been under represented in the literature and in psychotherapy research. This has been particularly true in the application and study of supportive therapy in personality disorder. It has been widely held that supportive treatment is only suitable for chronically or severely ill patients and that it is inferior to expressive approaches.

In 1954 Wolberg described supportive therapy as a treatment for "those with good ego strengths who have broken down under the impact of excessively severe environmental pressures and stresses" (p. 101) and also for those "with weak ego structures whose capacities for real change are minimal and who are unable to endure the anxieties inevitably associated with deeper therapy" (p. 101). In 1979, Binstock sounded a stronger negative note:

> Unfortunately, the concept of "support" serves as a ready rationalization for gratifying countertransference wishes to play the role of parent inappropriately. Active efforts to be especially "warm," "giving," "real," "directive," or simply "instructive" convey to the patient that he is especially needful of such efforts. As a result, he feels patronized, infantilized—with the result that he is undermined in his self-confidence and self-esteem, rather than supported. (p. 608)

Franz Alexander (1953) was one of the first to attempt to correct this negative image, stating that *"it is widely but erroneously held that supportive psychotherapy methods require less technical and theoretical preparation than psychoanalysis"* (emphasis added; p. 117). Wallace (1983) summarized the argument that the competent practice of supportive therapy is more difficult than the practice of expressive or uncovering therapy. He wrote that generally, when supportive therapy is indicated,

> the patient's pathology is more severe, there is a wider range of possible responses by the therapist, and it is difficult to decide which response is correct. You cannot wait for the patient to make connections. . . . You must decide . . . now to come down on the side of expressiveness, now of restraint, now to confront his intellectualization or reaction formation, now to support it, now to analyze the transference, now to utilize it as a suggestive or reinforcing lever . . . now to ask him what goes into his question, now to answer it immediately and directly, now to gratify his request for coffee or advice, now to analyze it. (pp. 345–346)

Pinsker, Rosenthal, and McCullough (1991) characterized supportive therapy as "a dyadic treatment which uses direct measures to ameliorate symptoms and maintain, restore, or improve self-esteem, adaptive skills, and psychological function. To the extent necessary to accomplish these objectives, treatment may utilize examination of relationships, real or transferential and both past and current patterns of emotional response or behavior" (pp. 221–222). Change is seen as stemming from learning and from identification with or introjection of an accepting, well-related therapist, not through resolution of unconscious conflicts. Change is not a product of self-understanding or analysis of transference, but rather it is a direct consequence of better self-esteem and improved adaptive skills. Distortions about self and other are corrected by education. Self-understanding, although not central to the treatment, may be pursued to the extent that is supports the accomplishment of patient goals and therapist objectives. By this conceptualization, intellectual insight, although often dismissed as a manifestation of suboptimal therapy, is a satisfactory end point.

RATIONALE

Using a dynamic or analytic framework, supportive psychotherapy can be conceptualized at one end of a continuum with expressive psychotherapy at the other end (Dewald, 1971). In the middle of the continuum is a supportive–expressive approach which combines elements of both supportive and expressive psychotherapy (Luborsky, 1984).

Traditionally, supportive psychotherapy has been used with severely impaired or chronically mentally ill patients, while expressive psychotherapy generally has been indicated for more structurally intact patients with stable and cohesive psychological or ego functions. However, we have treated patients in supportive psychotherapy who improved clinically despite meeting traditional research criteria for expressive treatment. The vast majority of these patients had personality disorder, primarily of the Cluster C type.

The psychopathology of personality disorder involves "an enduring pattern of inner experience and behavior" (American Psychiatric Association, 1994), as manifested in cognition, affectivity, interpersonal functioning, and impulse control. Because supportive psychotherapy is flexible and comprehensive it can be applied to all kinds of psychopathology, including the typical problems of personality disorder. Supportive therapy typically targets dysfunctional thinking, interpersonal conflict and

functioning, affect modulation, and frustration tolerance.

THEORETICAL FOUNDATIONS

It is now widely recognized that the patient–therapist or therapeutic relationship is a key ingredient of psychotherapy (Frank & Frank, 1991). Greenson (1967) suggested that the therapeutic relationship consists of three components: a transference–countertransference configuration, a real relationship, and a working or therapeutic alliance. Whether these components can be clearly separated is open to debate (Greenberg, 1994; Hoffman, 1991), but these constructs are useful in conceptualizing many psychotherapies and in distinguishing supportive from expressive psychotherapy. The transferential relationship in latent or manifest form is the pattern of reflexive attitudes, thoughts, and emotional responses which may be currently maladaptive and directly related to intrapsychic processes from an earlier time in psychosocial development. In expressive psychotherapies, this relationship is deemed to be of paramount importance for revealing conflicts, and therapeutic gain is ascribed to the essentially noncognitive process of working through transferential relationships.

The real relationship is universally recognized and forms the context of all treatment, including expressive therapy. This relationship is manifested in the therapeutic alliance and coexists with, and is to some extent reflective of, the transference relationship. For example, what appears on the surface to be a positive therapeutic alliance may be bolstered, without the patient's awareness, by the fact that dependency needs are gratified in the transference relationship.

In expressive treatment, the real relationship becomes a background or context within which the therapist responds mostly to the transference nature of the interpersonal process. There is a conscious minimization of real information about the therapist in the therapist's statement to the patient. Thus, much of the real relationship and therapeutic alliance depends on the acceptance by the patient of the rules and agreements on the conduct of treatment and its relationship to the therapist.

Supportive psychotherapy, on the other hand, emphasizes the real relationship as reflected in the therapeutic alliance. This process is based on overt mutuality in the conduct of therapy. The relationship between therapist and patient is a mirror of other current relationships. This relationship contrasts to the socially unusual and anxiety-provoking neutral stance of the therapist in expressive treatments. The therapeutic alliance in supportive therapy is supported through the use of accurate empathic responses, validation of feeling states, and attention to detail, but development of transference neurosis is avoided. To that end, there is minimization of focus on transferential material, and "regression in service of ego" is not fostered. The fact that transference is not discussed does not mean that it is not recognized. Negative transference can threaten the alliance and the treatment, so the therapist must be vigilant about recognizing it and dealing with it. With higher-functioning patients, clarification of evidences of negative feelings or thoughts may be productive. With lower-functioning patients, it may be necessary for the therapist to change his stance, as people usually do when talking with someone who is becoming angry or distant.

In brief expressive psychotherapy, development of the transference neurosis is avoided by actively clarifying and confronting defenses and interpreting the transference. Supportive therapy does not confront defenses unless they are maladaptive (primitive projection, splitting, etc.). Although supportive psychotherapy is dynamic in that the therapist pays attention to transference material and recognizes primitive defenses, the therapist's responses are most likely to be within the domain of the real relationship.

Expressive therapies have a primarily intrapsychic focus with respect to the therapist's attention to and interaction with patient material. The therapist and patient look at the conflicts between the patient's mental constructs of id, ego, and superego or, stated in developmental terms, conflict between the inner representations of self and others. The therapist's persistent attention to these conceptual frames during the process of treatment assists the patient in being aware of and then consciously contributing to material with this focus in mind.

In contrast, supportive psychotherapy has a predominately interpersonal focus in that adaptive strategies, coping skills, and anxiety reduction are attended to within a frame of reference that looks at patterns of interpersonal behavior. The relationship between the patient and therapist is used to teach the patient about difficulties in transactions with other people, with the intent of improving the quality of the patient's relationships and diminishing maladaptive personality traits.

Other psychotherapies that are not psychodynamically based use techniques that are largely interpersonal or supportive. For example, cognitive-behavior therapy employs assertiveness training, social skills training, cognitive restructuring, and so on, all of which fit comfortably into supportive psychotherapy. Based on this common use of supportive techniques, Pinsker (1994) suggested another way of conceptualizing supportive therapy using the computer term "shell program." A shell program is one that fits over another program and is easier to use. In the same way supportive therapy can be considered a "shell" that fits over most theoretical orientations. The theoretic constructs of, for example, dynamic or psychoanalytic, cognitive-behavioral, and experiential are different, but they all use supportive techniques. Using a shell approach therefore implies the employment of supportive techniques in a theoretical manner, or that different theoretical orientations can encompass a supportive approach.

In this chapter we are guided by psychoanalytic concepts, but we describe supportive techniques derived from other orientations.

A SUPPORTIVE MODEL OF CHANGE

What constitutes change in supportive psychotherapies has been articulated in a number of different ways. As we have described elsewhere (Hellerstein, Pinsker, Rosenthal, & Klee, 1994; Pinsker & Rosenthal, 1988; Winston, Pinsker, & McCullough, 1986), change in supportive therapy can be understood as learning new adaptive behaviors and skills while ameliorating symptoms and enhancing self-esteem. We have suggested that such change stems from identification with or introjection of an accepting, well-related therapist. Likewise, Wallerstein (1989) has stated that the major operative supportive mechanism is the evocation of a positive dependent transference attachment, which serves as the basis for an enduring "transference cure." Holmes (1995) has seen many borderline patients make great use of the commitment, attention, and concern of supportive technique in psychoanalytic treatment, and he suggests that it is the consequent development of secure attachments that fosters more autonomous functioning in them. Similarly, Buckley (1994) has postulated that a Kohutian empathic–introspective stance is a critical component of effective supportive psychotherapy.

We have also described change in supportive therapy as lasting and substantive because it includes changes in the dynamic structures, in specific intrapsychic configurations, such as defensive operations, thought and affect organization, anxiety tolerance, and ego strength, assumed to underlie and motivate behavior (Rosenthal, Muran, Pinsker, Hellerstein, & Winston, 1999). In the Menninger Psychotherapy Research Project, a naturalistic clinical study, Wallerstein (1989) found lasting and significant structural changes in patients treated with a dynamically based treatment, which although not well defined, was classified as supportive therapy. In the Menninger project, structural change was defined "as changes in specific intrapsychic configurations, in the patterning of defenses, in thought and affect organization, in anxiety tolerance and in ego strength" (p. 203). De Jonghe, Rijnierse, and Janssen (1994) and colleagues have proposed a "post-classical" view of change in supportive psychotherapy, characterized as "growth by experience," which supplants the notion of structural change as solely due to "growth by insight." This perspective invokes a view of change originally sowed by Ferenczi (1932) and later cultivated by Balint (1968), Alexander (Alexander & French, 1946), and Winnicott (1965).

GENERAL PRINCIPLES OF CHANGE

In this section we present some general principles of change that are central to our model of supportive psychotherapy for personality disorders.

Ameliorate Symptoms

Supportive psychotherapy can be characterized by the use of direct measures to ameliorate symptoms, which are described in detail later. Unlike more expressive approaches, which primarily focus on unconscious conflicts and making the unconscious conscious, our supportive approach places primary emphasis on helping patients with their presenting symptoms and complaints.

Minimize Anxiety

Another general principle of supportive psychotherapy is minimizing patients' experience of anxiety and maximizing their sense of control. There are a number of ways that this principle can be fulfilled, and Pine (1984) has described many strategies toward this end. The essence of supportive psychotherapy is not specific supportive techniques but a continuous concern about patient anxiety and a deliberate effort by the therapist to avoid subtle actions that might increase anxiety.

Enhance Self-Esteem

Likewise, the essence of supportive psychotherapy is a continuous concern for patient self-esteem. As we have previously noted (Pinsker et al., 1991), it is interesting how little formal attention has been given to protecting and enhancing self-esteem in psychotherapy. One of the ways in which we encourage supportive therapists in this regard is to watch for questions that have a challenging or critical impact. For example, questions that begin with the word "why" often run the risk of suggesting the meaning, "You shouldn't have done that!"

Respect Defenses

Unlike in expressive forms of psychotherapy, which typically aim to get rid of character defenses so that the core neurosis is exposed, in supportive psychotherapy, adaptive defenses and patient's personal style are generally respected. For example, the individual whose defense is maintaining control over emotions should not necessarily be asked to relax this control, unless there is good reason to believe that lack of expression is a significant problem. Although defenses in general are to be supported, by this we usually mean mature defenses; this support stops when the defense is maladaptive or immature, such as regression, denial, and projection.

Facilitate Adaptive Skills and Psychological Functions

An important principle of supportive psychotherapy involves facilitating the patient's adaptive skills and psychological functions. By adaptive skills, we simply mean almost anything a person does to function more effectively. By psychological functions, we mean ego functions, including reality orientation, defense formation, regulation of affect, and so on. The boundary between adaptive skill and psychological function is not sharply defined. The patient's construal of events reflects psychological function; the action he or she takes in response reflects adaptive skill.

STRATEGIES AND TECHNIQUES

Below is a list of specific techniques used in our model of supportive psychotherapy to fulfill the general principles described previously.

Establishing Definition and Agreement on Tasks and Goals

It is a clear mandate of supportive psychotherapy for the therapist to be explicit about the tasks and goals: that is, the way in which therapist and patient will work, providing a clear rationale, and the direction in which they are headed. Our supportive psychotherapy mandates a meeting of the minds between patient and therapist about the tasks and goals. This mandate echoes Bordin's (1979) definition of the working alliance. We find that it is often helpful, for example, to make explicit how the topic at hand is connected to self-esteem, to a specified adaptive skill or psychological function. This mandate goes a long way toward minimizing the anxiety in the therapeutic situation.

Style of Communication

One way anxiety may be minimized is by the use of a conversational style. We do not mean to suggest that therapy is ordinary conversation but that the interaction between therapist and patient is modeled on conversation rather than interrogation or silent listening. Such conversation differs from normal social conversation in that there is always a clearly defined purpose and focus.

Clarification, Confrontation, and Interpretation

These techniques are often used in supportive psychotherapy, but not with the requirement that the unconscious be made conscious or that full linkages be made with impulses or affects connected with genetic figures. Clarification is used extensively in terms of summarizing, paraphrasing, and organizing the patient's statements without elaboration or inference. Such clarification provides the patient with critical evidence that therapist is actively listening. Confrontation and interpretation, which bring to attention a pattern of behavior or something that the patient is avoiding or not attending to, can be usefully employed within supportive psychotherapy, but with the following considerations: the minimization of anxiety, the maintainance of self-esteem, and the maximization of adaptive functioning. One guiding principle that is often useful with respect to confrontation and interpretation in supportive psychotherapy is one put forth by Pine (1984): Strike when the iron is cold.

Responding to Ventilation

Ventilation may be useful to a patient when a traumatic event is experienced or when something important has been unexpressed. The fact that the therapist has heard the patient's story and is not rejecting may be the essence of support for some. The therapist's active responses may include tracking (indicating the he or she is following the patient), universalizing (making it clear that many people have similar feelings, wishes, or problems), or decatastrophizing (minimizing issues or problems that the patient has exaggerated).

Encouragement

Encouragement may include praise, reassurance, and empathic comments. Most therapists have learned to offer empathic comments as responses to particularly difficult situations (e.g., "That must have been real hard for you."). We try to go further, though, and find opportunities to add words that tell the patient something about him- or herself, but not in a disengenuous way (e.g., "That took a lot of courage!"). The driving force of this strategy is to support self-esteem.

Advice and Suggestion

Advice and suggestion must be factual, related to the therapist's expert knowledge, and limited to the topics of therapy. Advice may be relevant if it is designed to help the patient act in a way that will enhance his or her self-esteem and improve adaptive skills or psychological function. The basis and rationale for the advice must always be stated. It is the therapist's expertise, not his or her authority, that is crucial.

Rationalization

Rationalization can be a legitimate technique if done knowingly and for a good reason. For example, the adult patient who dwells excessively on what her parents did wrong may benefit from a statement such as, "Your parents seem to have been very rigid and cold, but you know, they were doing what the experts taught was the most scientifically correct way to raise children in the 1930s; they may have been doing the best they could."

Reframing and Reattribution

These strategies have often been described within a cognitive-behavioral framework (e.g., Freeman & Simon, 1989). Reframing can be used to assist the patient in diffusing or sidestepping painful affects or negative references, thus enhancing self-esteem. Reattribution typically involves the therapist effecting a more reasonable distribution of responsibility when the patient places sole responsibility for his or her difficulty on self or others.

Modeling

By modeling we refer to the therapist's providing, intentionally or unintentionally, a model of behavior and responsiveness. In a sense, therapists lend their ego to the patient in the course of treatment, by applying their problem-solving skills, affective responsiveness, and knowledge of individual and social behavior to the patient's problem. Another technical issue that can be subsumed under modeling is self-disclosure. As a teacher and role model, the therapist may reveal certain attitudes, ideas, and values. Such disclosure enables patients with severe ego deficits to gradually build more stable and cohesive self and object representations.

Anticipatory Guidance and Rehearsal

Anticipatory guidance allows the patient to move through new situations hypothetically, considering the possible events and ways of responding to them. This allows the patient to become acquainted with the context of the future event, reducing some of the anticipatory anxiety associated with it. Rehearsal further allows the patient to work out more appropriate or novel ways to participate in future events, thus adding to his or her repertoire of adaptive skills.

Developing Alternatives and Problem Solving

These strategies have also been described by cognitive-behaviorial therapists (e.g., Freeman & Simon, 1989). When a patient has alternatives for thinking or behaving, he or she has greater freedom of choice. An anxious style of responding can sometimes be attributed to seeing only one choice rather than many. When an anxious patient can see other options, he or she often assumes a greater sense of control over thoughts and actions. Likewise, educating a patient on how to solve a problem (brainstorming, weighing advantages and disadvantages, etc.) can create a greater sense of mastery.

PROCESS ISSUES INCLUDING COUNTERTRANSFERENCE

Many of the process issues have been elaborated in other sections of this chapter. Thus this section is confined to just a few issues. Typically supportive therapy uses a conversational style, coupled with a high activity level on the part of the therapist. Silence is avoided and the therapist attempts to make the patient feel comfortable by minimizing anxiety. However, at other times especially with personality disorder patients, the therapist may assume an exploratory position, confront maladaptive defenses, engage in relaxation training, teach assertiveness skills, or work on dysfunctional thinking. Therefore, therapists engaging in supportive psychotherapy with patients who have significant personality problems must be flexible and comfortable moving across different technical approaches. Therapists who are rigid and unable to engage difficult patients will have problems with this population.

In this type of therapy, as in others, countertransference issues must be recognized and attended to. Countertransference issues in supportive psychotherapy can be divided into those that particularly relate to the nature of supportive work and common countertransference reactions to the characterological problems of patients with personality disorder. This second category occurs in most psychotherapies and we do not focus on them here.

The first category derives from the nature of supportive psychotherapy. The therapist feels pressure from both the treatment and the patient to "take over" the patient's life to some extent. This can lead to therapist reactions of two types. The first therapist countertransference reaction involves the development of grandiose or arrogant thoughts and is reflected in behaviors toward the patient. Therapists who move into the role of directing or taking over a patient's life might find themselves behaving in a condescending manner and be unwilling to relinquish control over the patient. This could close off or inhibit patient growth and individuation, making the therapist more inclined to hold on to the patient and to not see the indications for termination from treatment. The second therapist reaction would be to defend against the patient's need for direction by becoming frustrated and angry or by withdrawing and distancing from the patient. It is incumbent upon the therapist to consistently monitor his or her feelings and behaviors toward the patient to both prevent untoward behaviors toward the patient and to use countertransference feelings to better understand the character pathology and needs of the patient.

INDICATIONS, CONTRAINDICATIONS, AND EXPECTED RESULTS

The traditional indication for supportive psychotherapy has been the presence of chronic severe mental illness (Drake & Sederer, 1986; Kates & Rockland, 1994), a condition that generally contraindicates uncovering-type treatment. There are also other clinical indications for supportive psychotherapy based on coping with a diagnosis or situation: early sobriety from alcohol or drugs of abuse (Kaufman & Reoux, 1988; O'Malley et al., 1992), acute crisis (Dewald, 1994), acute bereavement in patients with poor ego strength (Horowitz, Marmar, Weiss, DeWitt, & Rosenbaum, 1984), and medical illnesses acute and chronic (Alter, 1996; Markowitz et al., 1995; Massie & Holland, 1990). Diagnostic or situation-specific indications for supportive theerapy are thus described, and there is agreement about the utility

of supportive psychotherapy in these areas, yet there has been little experimental validation through well-controlled randomized clinical trials. There has been little in the way of clinical guidelines to either suggest or reject the use of supportive psychotherapy in patients with personality disorders, yet in everyday clinical practice, this is the type of treatment that most patients with more severe personality disorders have been given in mental health clinics.

As we elucidate later, we believe that there is a broader range of disorders that are amenable to supportive treatment, including personality disturbance. However, in our experience, among the various personality disturbances, help-rejecting complainers and liars and patients with typical problems of hostile dominance do as poorly in supportive psychotherapy as they do in other predominantly dynamic expressive treatments. As such, patients with core psychopathy as a subset of antisocial personality disorder are unlikely to make constructive use of supportive psychotherapy. The controlling and hostile elements of these patients' interpersonal styles most likely interferes with the formation of a solid working alliance and thus precludes the initiation of task oriented treatment.

CLINICAL ILLUSTRATIONS

The two cases presented here briefly illuminate, with historical and clinical data, a graphical representation of change mapped to the Inventory of Interpersonal Problems (IIP; Horowitz, Rosenberg, Baer, Ureno, & Villaseñor, 1988; MacKenzie, Chapter 14, this volume) circumplex model in Figures 16.1 and 16.2, and link the theoretical basis for making specific supportive interventions with specific changes in patients. Interpersonal behavior can be measured based on the circumplex model (Henry, Schacht, & Strupp, 1986, 1990; Kiesler & Watkins, 1989) originally formulated by Leary (1957) and developed subsequently by Benjamin (1974; see Benjamin & Pugh, Chapter 20, this volume), Wiggins (1979), and Kiesler (1983). In the circumplex model, interpersonal behavior and attitudes are mapped on a surface defined by a horizontal "affiliation" axis reflecting with poles of friendliness and hostility, and a vertical "control" axis with poles of dominance and submission. The eight regions between the axes are labeled in this IIP analysis: domineering, vindictive, overly cold, avoidant, nonassertive, exploitable, overly nurturant, and intrusive (Alden, Wiggins, & Pincus, 1990).

Case 1

A 38-year-old separated white man had initial target complaints consisting of being bothered greatly by his silence and withdrawal in dealing with people, severe lack of confidence about decisions made, and chronically low self-esteem. He would become extremely anxious at the workplace, which interfered with his concentration and ability to perform his work as a cashier. He had a history of childhood physical abuse by his distant, domineering, critical, and unpredictable alcoholic father. He believed that his father disliked him. Only at the end of his father's life was the patient able to achieve some degree of closeness with him. He had considered his relationships with his mother and his aunt as warm and close while growing up. He currently felt that the relationship with his mother was cool and strained and that interactions often ended in arguments. He believed that his mother preferred his younger sister's company and was more concerned about her welfare than his. Throughout his life, the patient generally felt inferior to those around him and had always been rejection sensitive with difficulty tolerating criticism. Apparently as a result, he developed an obsequious and distant interpersonal style. However, during his short marriage (3 years), when pressed to the limit of his capacity to contain anger verbally, he would become physically aggressive toward his wife. He also had little interest in sex. He had few friends and was generally aloof in all of his relationships. On screening with the Structured Clinical Interview for DSM-III-R (SCID-I; SCID-II) he met criteria for diagnoses of primary dysthymic disorder and avoidant personality disorder and subthreshold criteria for self-defeating personality disorder. On the subscales of the IIP at intake, he had a prominent concentration of problems in the avoidant, nonassertive, exploitable, and overly nurturant octants, consistent with the initial clinical descriptors and diagnoses (see Figure 16.1).

Conduct of the Treatment

Enhancement of self-esteem, a core principle of supportive psychotherapy, was a focal issue with this patient. The therapist hypothesized that patterns of rejection, criticism, abuse, and impersonal treatment from early caretakers promoted the patient's current expectancy that he would be taken advantage of in interpersonal situations and could not risk advocating for his own needs. The therapist purposely looked for opportunities to support the patient's self-esteem in a way the patient was able to use. This meant reinforcing a sense of empowerment without being perceived by the patient as gratuitous or, as in the case of this rejection-sensitive patient, demeaning. Even approaching the issue with some patients may place the patients in an anxious, self-invalidating state. If it

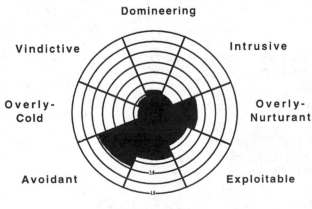

INTAKE

FIGURE 16.1. Scores at intake mapped on the eight circumplex subscales from the 64-item Inventory of Interpersonal Problems.

is hard for the patient to talk about something, consider asking, in a nonchallenging way, "How can we talk about this without increasing your anxiety, or without making you feel that you're being pressured?" (Pinsker & Rosenthal, 1988). The following is a therapy content and process example of how the therapist, using supportive techniques, carefully approached and focused on the issue of the patient's anxiety and experience of inadequacy at work and resulting avoidance of work.

P: I just feel overwhelmed all the time and I don't know how to get out of it, it's confusing . . . [Reiterates one of his chief target complaints.]

T: Maybe we can explore one of those target complaints, your being very anxious at work. [Focuses and clarifies the patient's statement.

P: Jeez, I don't know, it's kinda, you know, too much, and then I feel like an idiot. Like now. And you want an answer. [Becomes anxious, anticipates rejection, experiences decreased self-efficacy.]

T: Maybe there is some way we can discuss this where you don't feel overwhelmed, or pressured into giving an answer. [Gives an empathic suggestion which directly aims to empower the patient. Increasing his sense of control may also reduce or bind anxiety.]

P: Maybe . . . (Sighs.) Okay, let me think about it . . . [Takes on consideration of the problem from a less overwhelmed position.]

This patient's pathological avoidance was predicated on the patient's experience of being overwhelmed by self-doubt, anxiety, and fear of closeness.

P: I can hardly get to work. My supervisor knows I'm, . . . I'm not good at the job (looks away). [States two observations.]

T: So you want to avoid getting there because its so unpleasant for you? [Clarifies empathically.]

P: Yeah (sheepishly). [Agrees.]

T: I'm not clear on what you mean by not good at the job, is it okay with you to tell me how? [Asks if it is tolerable for the patient to clarify his statement.]

P: (nodding) I take too much time with the transactions because it's hard to concentrate. I get distracted. [Elaborates.]

T: Because you're anxious? [Demonstrates knowledge based on his real experience of the patient.]

P: Uh huh.

T: You stated that the supervisor has spoken to you about your performance. [Poses a clarification of the patient's earlier statement.]

P: Well, no, I mean, he hasn't actually said anything, (shrugs) but he must know. [Refutes his earlier observation, reality tests.]

T: People who are self-conscious and upset about a blemish or a pimple are often surprised to find out that they are the only ones who notice! (Smiles.) [Offers a humorous analogy that does not take the patient's actual performance into account.] Even if you were a little slower than some others, it would be unlikely that he knows that you are anxious inside. [Miminizes; supports adaptive defenses.]

P: He's not all that smart.

T: I wonder if you see any other situations where maybe you assume people know more than they really do?

P: Yeah, like, everything! (Laughs.)

The therapist continued to make anxiety-reducing interventions throughout the treatment. The clear focus on maintaining and improving self-esteem through the use of accurate empathic statements, clarifications and rationalizations aimed at increasing a sense of control, and support for adaptive defenses had beneficial results. At follow-up 6 months after the termination of therapy, the patient was bothered only a little by social withdrawal and low confidence in dealing with people. He had become more assertive, less avoidant, and less focused on having to please others. This is mirrored clearly in the diminution of the scores in the avoidant, nonassertive, and overly nurturant octants of the IIP. He was bothered very little by self-esteem problems. Although the concentration of interpersonal problems favored the submissive hemisphere, the entire set is markedly reduced in intensity. In addition, there is a relative shift toward the friendly nurturant side (see Figure 16.2).

Case 2

The second case is a 43-year-old single female freelance music teacher and musician with a

FOLLOW-UP

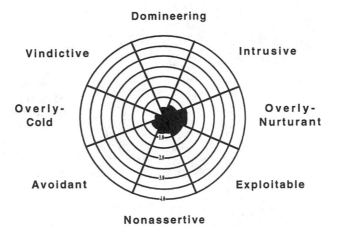

FIGURE 16.2. Scores at follow-up mapped on the eight circumplex subscales from the 64-item Inventory of Interpersonal Problems.

history of atypical depression characterized by symptoms of low energy, overeating and oversleeping, mood reactivity, and sensitivity to rejection and criticism. She was bothered a great deal by her difficulty controlling her weight and inability to complete tasks and to bring plans and ideas to fruition. She remembered feeling "fat" in kindergarten, which she would handle by starting new projects about which she could feel optimistic and good. Typically, the enthusiasm would fade after a time and she would not achieve her goals, a pattern that had persisted into adult life. She attributed her failure to follow through to a fear of exposing too much of herself, as she is sensitive to criticism. She also was quite disturbed by her self- and other-critical behavior. She attributed her being overly critical to parents who were overly critical of each other and her and to having studied music with a critical teacher. She was extremely concerned that she worried too much about her family's and other's reactions to her. She thought that she was not competitive enough with her peers. She believed that she subordinated her own needs in order to maintain attachments, and as a result, was not competitive, especially in her career. She fit SCID-II criteria for simple phobia, personality disorder not otherwise specified, and met subthreshold criteria for dysthymia. About 1 year before treatment began, a former lover had died and she had been grieving since that time. She had a recent 4-year relationship that she described as intense

but very isolating. It ended badly, and the patient found out that he was a serious liar. She described her maternal grandparents as close and nurturing, but her father as distant, awkward, and unable to be intimate with her. She described herself as warm and gregarious in one-on-one situations or at social gatherings with friends but awkward and uncomfortable in work-related group settings with colleagues, worried that she would make a fool of herself. She considered herself a devoted friend. She enjoyed the teaching aspects of her work and the connections she built with her students. She attributed the genesis of her musical career to the development of a crush on her music teacher while learning the flute in junior high school. At intake, she demonstrated a concentration of problems on the IIP subscales in the nonassertive, exploitable, and overly nurturant areas, consistent with her experience of having to sacrifice her needs in order to maintain connections. She had difficulty expressing anger, holding to her position, and competing in a straightforward way, again, consistent with her own description (see Figure 16.3).

Conduct of the Treatment

As in case 1, enhancement of self-esteem is a focal issue here, with emphasis on empowerment and motivation for acting in her own interest. Two other foci are (1) increasing ego functioning, specifically cognitively reframing

INTAKE

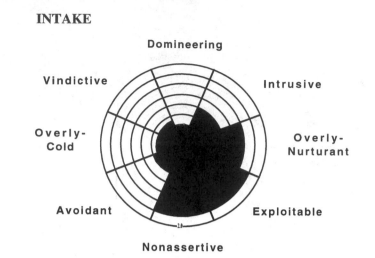

FIGURE 16.3. Scores at intake mapped on the eight circumplex subscales from the 64-item Inventory of Interpersonal Problems.

her perception/expectation that she is or will easily be the subject of ridicule; and (2) development of more adaptive skills, specifically using anticipatory guidance and rationalization to reduce *in situ* anxiety. The therapist hypothesized that an early temperamental vulnerability to dysphoria attendant to real or experienced separation set up interactive patterns which promote the patient's expectation that she dare not risk advocating for her own needs. The therapist looked for opportunities to support the patient's use of accurate estimation of the risk of rejection, while also supporting means by which the patient could reduce her anxiety and negative thoughts about herself. The therapist must support the patient's motivation to pursue her own goals in the face of possible rejection or loss. The real art in this case lay in empowering the patient to risk being more assertive and feeling good about it without the patient feeling "one down" with the therapist.

P: I have another staff meeting this week. I don't even want to show up. [Reiterates one of her chief target complaints.]

T: Maybe we can explore this more, since you've said that this is an example of where you want to be less passive. [Focuses and clarifies from the patient's own statements.]

P: Ughh. I usually just sit there, stewing in my own anxiety. I can hardly look at any one. [Anticipates rejection, experiences decreased self-efficacy.]

T: So, this is maybe where you feel they are looking at you critically? [Joins with her experience, asks an empathic question as a hypothesis.]

P: It sure seems that way—I don't know. I just get so embarrased, like I'm a fake, and they'll find out. [Allows that the criticism by others is anxiously anticipated, but not actually experienced in this case.]

T: . . . and meanwhile you experience yourself as embarrased and not strong. Sitting like that is not good for your self-esteem bacause it confirms your fears . . . [Suggests to the patient that she might be able to manage her her experience of anxiety.]

P: You mean maybe I could do something different in there? [Allows that perhaps they can explore alternatives, in spite of her previous experiences.]

T: One way people use to handle tricky or difficult situations is to rehearse it. Driving a car is complex and makes people anxious when they first get behind the wheel. [Proposes anticipatory guidance. Repetition serves mastery.]

P: But, I never know what someone is going to say, and I always expect the worst, so how can I prepare? [Reiterates an at-risk, anxious position, outwardly focused.]

T: But I'll bet you know pretty much how *you* think and feel, even when no one is talking directly to you (*empathic smile*). [Clarifies and directly supports self-esteem: that he believes the patient has the capacity to change.]

P: (*Pause*) Oh, how I'll handle *ME!* (*Laughs.*) [Gives positive feedback to therapist that she understood the therapist and is willing to look at herself.

T: Can we look at what happens during the meeting? When does your anxiety build up, any particular time or topic? [Focuses patient on tracking her experience more specifically, but allows for her to back off if she feels not ready.]

P: When they start pitching new ideas for teaching, I'm afraid they'll criticize . . .

T: I'm not clear on something. May I ask you to clarify whether this is something you anticipate or something you have generally experienced from the group? [Asks patient in a supportive manner to clarify her experience.]

P: Sure, No, they don't ever get critical because I never offer my ideas. I actually have plenty (*smile*). [Clarifies her experience and reveals her creative side.]

T: So, maybe this is about learning to offer what you think, in spite of the fear? Once people learn to drive, it's far less threatening even though there are real risks . . . [Offers a learning model with a rationalization to help bind anxiety.]

Continued reiteration of the therapist's direct support for the patient's testing reality against anticipated rejection helped her to learn to negotiate tasks that were previously overwhelming for her. Based partly on the therapist's use of reframing and rationalization, and modeling of anticipatory strategies, the patient was able to develop a capacity for positively evaluating her attempts to address high-anxiety situations. She was better able to take some responsibility to reduce her experience of vulnerability as an act of "mental hygiene." At termination she was better able to compete at work and make reasonable demands of those around her, both at work and in her personal life. There was a clear decrease in most areas of interpersonal difficulty, including a reduction in her critical behavior. Brief supportive psychotherapy had a clear impact at follow-up on her overall position with respect to interpersonal space. Though still somewhat reticent and critical, she had become less overly friendly at the expense of autonomy and had become more assertive (see Figure 16.4).

EMPIRICAL EVALUATION OF SUPPORTIVE THERAPY FOR PERSONALITY DISORDERS

Although there has been some research demonstrating the treatment efficacy of supportive psychotherapies (e.g., Conte & Plutchik, 1986; Rockland, 1993; Wallerstein, 1989; Winston et al., 1986), very little has been published on supportive psychotherapy specifically for personality disorders. From our own brief psy-

TERMINATION

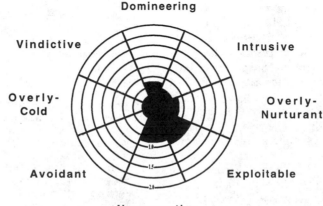

FIGURE 16.4. Scores at termination mapped on the eight circumplex subscales from the 64-item Inventory of Interpersonal Problems.

chotherapy research program, however, we have recently published some preliminary data regarding our supportive psychotherapy model that demonstrate (1) efficacy on various patient-rated measures of symptomatology, presenting complaints, and interpersonal functioning (Hellerstein et al., 1998); (2) change not only at termination of treatment but also sustained change at a 6-month follow-up, (Rosenthal et al., 1999), and (3) efficacy comparable to a short-term dynamic psychotherapy, which was more expressive in nature. The study involved 24 patients who presented with personality disorders that included obsessive–compulsive (5), avoidant (3), dependent (2), narcissistic (2), paranoid (2), self-defeating (2), histrionic (1), and personality disorder not otherwise specified (7), as defined by DSM-III-R (American Psychiatric Association, 1987) and diagnosed (reliably by trained graduate students) by the SCID-II (Spitzer, Williams, & Gibbon, 1987b). Seventeen of the patients also presented with depressive disorders on Axis I on DSM-III-R, four with anxiety disorders, and two with adjustment disorders, according to SCID-I (Spitzer, Williams, & Gibbon, 1987a). Seven patients (29%) dropped out of the supportive treatment, which is consistent with findings from other brief models that we have investigated (Winston, Muran, Safran, Samstag, & Bernbach, 1998). The treatment was generally based on the principles and techniques articulated in this chapter and was 40 sessions in length. Our research has also provided preliminary evidence that the therapeutic alliance as rated by both patient and therapist in our supportive psychotherapy showed stable and high levels across the course of treatment when contrasted with more expressive treatments; this was particularly true in good outcome cases (Hellerstein et al., 1998).

The only other notable exception of empirial evaluation of supportive treatment for personality disorders has been reported by William Piper and colleagues (Piper, Joyce, McCallum, & Azim, 1998). They compared the efficacy of their models of supportive and interpretitive psychotherapy in a sample of 144 outpatients, 60.4% of whom received an Axis II diagnosis: 29.2% avoidant, 24.3% obsesssive–compulsive, 22.2% borderline, and 21.5% paranoid. The results indicated no outcome differences for the two models. The only interesting differences were that quality of object relations had a significant interaction effect and there was a high-

er dropout rate for the interpretative model, which suggests that supportive psychotherapy may be the treatment of choice when considering a wide range of patient types.

CONCLUSION

We believe that supportive psychotherapy is an effective form of treatment for patients with personality disorder. It uses direct measures in a comprehensive and flexible manner to improve self-esteem, adaptive skills, and psychological or ego functions. Additional systematic research, including clinical trials and process investigations, is needed to refine the technique and help determine the most useful approaches for patients with personality disorder.

REFERENCES

Alden, L. E., Wiggins, J. S., & Pincus, A. L. (1990). Construction of circumplex scales for the Inventory of Interpersonal Problems. *Journal of Personality Assessment, 55,* 521–536.

Alexander, F. (1953). Current views on psychotherapy. *Psychiatry, 16,* 113–122.

Alexander, F., & French, T. M. (1946). *Psychoanalytic therapy.* New York: Ronald Press.

Alter, C. L. (1996). Palliative and supportive care of patients with pancreatic cancer. *Seminars in Oncology, 23,* 229–40.

American Psychiatric Association. (1987). *Diagnostic and statistical manual of mental disorders* (3rd ed., rev.). Washington DC: Author.

American Psychiatric Association. (1987). *Diagnostic and statistical manual of mental disorders* (4th ed.). Washington DC: Author.

Balint, M. (1968). *The basic fault.* London: Tavistock.

Benjamin, L. S. (1974). Structural analysis of social behavior. *Psychological Review, 81,* 392–425.

Binstock, W. A. (1979). Prescribing psychotherapy. In A. Lazare (Ed.), *Outpatient psychiatry: Diagnosis and treatment* (pp. 603–611). Baltimore: Williams & Wilkins.

Bordin, E. (1979). The generalizability of the psychoanalytic concept of the working alliance. *Psychotherapy: Theory, Research, and Practice, 16,* 252–260.

Buckley, P. (1994). Self psychology, object relations theory and supportive psychotherapy. *American Journal of Psychotherapy, 48,* 519–529.

Conte, H. R., & Plutchik, R. (1986). Controlled research in supportive psychotherapy. *Psychiatric Annals, 16,* 530–533.

De Jonghe, F., Rijnierse, P., & Janssen, R. (1994). Psychoanalytic supportive psychotherapy. *Journal of the American Psychoanalytic Assocation, 42,* 421–446.

Dewald, P. A. (1971). *Psychotherapy: A dynamic approach* (2nd ed.) New York: Basic Books.

Dewald, P. A. (1994). Principles of supportive psychotherapy. *American Journal of Psychotherapy, 48,* 505–518.

Drake, R. E., & Sederer, L. I. (1986). Inpatient psychosocial treatment of chronic schizophrenia: Negative effects and current guidelines. *Hospital and Community Psychiatry, 37,* 897–901.

Ferenczi, S. (1932). *The clinical diary of Sandor Ferenczi* (J. Dupont, Ed., M. Balint & N. Z. Jackson, Trans.). Cambridge, MA: Harvard University Press.

Frank, J., & Frank, J. (1991). *Persuasion and healing: A comparative study of psychotherapy* (3rd ed.). Baltimore: Johns Hopkins University Press.

Freeman, A., & Simon, K. (1989). Cognitive therapy of anxiety. In A. Freeman, K. Simon, L. Beutler, & H. Arkowitz (Eds.), *Comprehensive handbook of cognitive therapy* (pp. 347–366). New York: Plenum.

Greenberg, L. S. (1994). What is "real" in the relationship? Comment on Gelso and Carter (1994). *Journal of Counseling Psychology, 41,* 307.

Greenson, R. R. (1967). *The technique and practice of psychoanalysis* (Vol. 1). Madison, CT: International Universities Press.

Hellerstein, D. J., Pinsker, H., Rosenthal, R. N., & Klee, S. (1994). Supportive therapy as the treatment model of choice. *Journal of Psychotherapy Practice and Research, 3,* 100–106.

Hellerstein, D. J., Rosenthal, R. N., Pinsker, H., Samstag, L. W., Muran, J. C., & Winston, A. (1998). A randomized prospective study comparing supportive and dynamic therapies: Outcome and alliance. *Journal of Psychotherapy Practice and Research, 7,* 261–271.

Henry, W. P., Schacht, T. E., & Strupp, H. H. (1983). Structural analysis of social behavior: Application to a study of interpersonal process in differential psychotherapeutic outcome. *Journal of Consulting and Clinical Psychology, 54,* 27–31.

Henry, W. P., Schacht, T. E., & Strupp, H. H. (1990). Patient and therapist introject, interpersonal process, and differential psychotherapy outcome. *Journal of Clinical and Consulting Psychology, 5,* 768–774.

Hoffman, I. Z. (1991). Discussion: towards a social-contruetivist view of the psychoanalytic situation. *Psychoanalytic Dialogues, 1,* 74–105.

Holmes, J. (1995). Supportive psychotherapy. The search for positive meanings. *British Journal of Psychiatry, 167,* 439–445.

Horowitz, L. M., Rosenberg, S. E., Baer, B. A., Ureno, G., & Villaseñor, V. S. (1988). Inventory of interpersonal problems: Psychometric properties and clinical applications. *Journal of Consulting and Clinical Psychology,* 885–892.

Horowitz, M., Marmar, C., Weiss, D., DeWitt, K. N., & Rosenbaum, R. (1984). Brief psychotherapy of bereavement reactions. *Archives of General Psychiatry, 41,* 438–448.

Kates, J., & Rockland, L. H. (1994). Supportive psychotherapy of the schizophrenic patient. *American Journal of Psychotherapy, 48,* 543–561.

Kaufman, E., & Reoux, J. (1988). Guidelines for the successful psychotherapy of substance abusers. *American Journal Drug Alcohol Abuse, 14,* 199–209.

Kiesler, D. J. (1983). The 1982 interpersonal circle: A taxonomy for complementarity in human transactions. *Psychological Review, 90,* 185–214.

Kiesler, D. J., & Watkins, K. (1989). Interpersonal complementarity and the therapeutic alliance: A study of relationship in psychotherapy. *Psychotherapy: Theory, Research, and Practice, 26,* 183–194.

Leary T. (1957). *Interpersonal diagnosis of personality.* New York: Ronald Press.

Luborsky, L. (1984). *Principles of psychoanalytic psychotherapy.* New York, Basic Books.

Markowitz, J. C., Klerman, G. L., Clougherty, K. F., Spielman, L. A., Jacobsberg, L. B., Fishman, B., Frances, A. J., Kocsis, J. H., & Perry, S. W. III. (1995). Individual psychotherapies for depressed HIV-positive patients. *American Journal of Psychiatry, 152,* 1504–1509.

Massie, M. J., & Holland, J. C. (1990). Depression and the cancer patient. *Journal of Clinical Psychiatry, 51*(Suppl), 12–19.

O'Malley, S. S., Jaffe, A. J., Chang, G., Schottenfeld, R. S., Meyer, R. E., & Rounsaville, B. (1992). Naltrexone and coping skills therapy for alcohol dependence: A controlled study. *Archives of General Psychiatry, 49,* 881–887.

Pine, F. (1984). The interpretive moment. *Bulletin of the Menninger Clinic, 48,* 54–71.

Pinsker, H. (1994). The role of theory in teaching supportive psychotherapy. *American Journal of Psychotherapy, 48,* 530–542.

Pinsker, H., & Rosenthal, R. N. (1988). Beth Israel Medical Center supportive psychotherapy manual. *Social and Behavioral Sciences Documents, 18,* 2.

Pinsker, H., Rosenthal, R. N., & McCullough, L. (1991). Dynamic supportive psychotherapy. In P. Crits-Christoph & J. P. Barber (Eds.), *Handbook of short-term dynamic psychotherapy* (pp. 220–247). New York: Basic Books.

Piper, W. E., Joyce, A. S., McCallum, M., & Azim, H. F. (1998). Interpretive and supportive forms of psychotherapy and patient personality variables. *Journal of Consulting and Clinical Psychology, 66,* 558–567.

Rockland, L. H. (1993). A review of supportive therapy, 1986–1992. *Hospital and Community Psychiatry, 44,* 1053–1060.

Rosenthal, R. N., Muran, J. C., Pinsker, H., Hellerstein, D. J., & Winston, A. (1999). Interpersonal change in supportive psychotherapy. *Journal of Psychotherapy Practice and Research, 8,* 55–63.

Spitzer, R. L., Williams, J. B. W., & Gibbon, M. (1987a). *Structured Clinical Interview for DSM-III-R (SCID).* New York: New York State Psychiatric Institute, Biometrics Research.

Spitzer, R. L., Williams, J. B. W., & Gibbon, M. (1987b). *Structured Clinical Interview for DSM-III-R personality Disorders* (SCID-II). New York: New York State Psychiatric Institute, Biometrics Research.

Wallace, E. R. (1983). *Supportive psychotherapy, in severe personality disorders: Psychotherapies strategies.* New York: Yale University Press.

Wallerstein, R. S. (1989). The psychotherapy research project of the Menninger Foundation: An overview. *Journal of Consulting and Clinical Psychology, 57,* 195–205.

Wiggins, J. S. (1979). A psychological taxonomy of trait-descriptive terms: The interpersonal domain. *Journal of Personality and Social Psychology, 37,* 395–412.

Winnicott, D. W. (1965). *The maturational process and the facilitating environment.* New York: International Universities Press.

Winston, A., Muran, J. C., Safran, J., Samstag, L. W., & Bernbach, E. (1998). *A comparative analysis of treat-ment efficacy and failure.* Paper presented at the Society for Psychotherapy Research Annual Meeting, Snowbird, Utah.

Winston, A., Pinsker, H., & McCullough, L. (1986). A review of supportive psychotherapy. *Hospital and Community Psychiatry, 37,* 1105–1114.

Wolberg, L. R. (1954). *The technique of psychotherapy.* New York: Grune & Stratton.

CHAPTER 17

Psychoanalysis and Psychoanalytic Psychotherapy

GLEN O. GABBARD

RATIONALE AND THEORETICAL FOUNDATIONS

Although the field of psychoanalysis arose from the study of the discrete neurotic symptoms found in hysteria, in the last 100 years the focus of psychoanalytic treatment has shifted from the symptomatic neuroses to the problems associated with character pathology. This change in focus was foreshadowed as early as 1908 when Freud (1908/1959) wrote his classic paper on anal eroticism and character. Working from a drive–defense model, Freud linked certain character traits, namely, orderliness, miserliness, and obstinacy, with the anal psychosexual stage of development. Whereas neurotic symptoms were viewed as the return of the repressed, he regarded character traits as the end result of the *successful* use of repression and other defenses, particularly sublimation and reaction formation. As he developed the structural model, he expanded his repertoire of defense mechanisms to include identification. His observation that some persons can only give up an object by identifying with it led him to realize that much of character formation in a child is linked to the identification with the child's parents and others.

Karl Abraham (1923/1942) expanded on Freud's work and developed a system of classifying character traits as they related to oral, anal, and genital eroticism. Wilhem Reich (1945) was perhaps the most important early contributor to a psychoanalytic understanding of character. He argued that psychoanalytic technique needed to address the so-called character armor of the patient that was entirely unconscious and ego syntonic. He saw character as stemming from childhood conflicts and the mastery of those conflicts with specific defenses. The patient's style of entering or exiting the office, the body position of the patient on the couch, and the whole style of relating to the analyst all reflected the unique aspects of character that often were not addressed when neurotic symptoms were the analyst's exclusive focus. While neurotic symptoms were viewed as egodystonic compromise formations, the prevailing view of early psychoanalysts was that character traits were ego syntonic. This distinction is often made in contemporary discussions of personality disorders as well—whereas symptoms of anxiety disorders or neuroses may cause distress to the patient, character traits are often regarded as causing distress to others. However, psychoanalytic clinicians would regard this distinction as a generalization that may or may not be valid when considering an individual patient. Many of the symptoms related to character pathology can be a source of considerable distress to the individual patient as well as to others.

Today psychoanalysts and psychoanalytic therapists spend much of their clinical efforts on those who have long-standing patterns of character pathology as the symptomatic neuroses are much less common in practice and often are responsive to other treatment modalities. The psychoanalytic understanding of character has broadened to view character traits as a series of compromise formations between wishes and defenses that oppose those wishes, on the one hand, and constellations of internal representations of self and others, on the other (Gabbard, 2000a). As psychoanalysis has shifted from a drive-dominated paradigm to one geared more to object relatedness, psychoanalysis and psychoanalytic therapy are uniquely situated to address the patient's typical problems in relationships because they are systematically examined as they repeat themselves in the transference–countertransference dimensions of the treatment relationship.

EMPIRICAL EVALUATION

There has been criticism of psychoanalysts (much of it warranted) for not conducting more outcome research on patients with personality disorders, but there are formidable obstacles to the design and implementation of randomized controlled trials. First, the cost of studies that would require 3 to 5 years to complete a single treatment would be prohibitive, especially when funding for research on psychosocial therapies is extraordinarily limited. Second, whereas a dropout rate of 10% is not significant in a 16-week trial of brief therapy, a dropout rate of 10% every 16 weeks over a period of years would reduce the sample size so substantially that statistical analysis would be seriously compromised. Third, experimental controls would be difficult to establish and maintain for a period of years. Fourth, Axis I disorders and intervening life events (deaths, divorces, etc.) would inevitably influence outcomes and produce complications that are not nearly so problematic in brief therapy studies. Fifth, manualization introduces a confounding form of artificiality to the treatment. Therapists involved in these studies have a major problem with adherence to the manual and feel that their

natural flexibility is compromised. Finally, randomization also introduces an artificiality in that self-selection is critical to patients entering psychoanalysis and long-term psychoanalytic therapy, and few would continue in the treatment if they had not selected it themselves. In short, the risk is that the treatment undergoing evaluation might bear little resemblance to the treatment delivered in naturalistic settings.

A number of uncontrolled studies have examined the effect of long-term psychoanalytic psychotherapy on patients with personality disorders. Some focus on process factors, while others focus more on outcome. Still others investigate prognostic factors. Some have used a "pre–post" design in which the patients serve as their own controls.

In the 1950s, the Menninger Psychotherapy Research Project (PRP) was launched as one of the first prospective studies of long-term psychoanalytic psychotherapy for seriously disturbed patients (Kernberg et al., 1972). The study was begun prior to the development of rigorous diagnostic interview schedules. Nevertheless, most observers agree that the majority of the patients in the study, especially those receiving psychotherapy rather than psychoanalysis, would now be diagnosed as suffering from serious personality disorders. Indeed, Kernberg based much of his thinking about the optimal psychoanalytic psychotherapy of patients with borderline personality organization on his findings in the PRP. Forty-two patients were treated by experienced therapists and analysts with a spectrum of modalities, including psychoanalysis, expressive psychotherapy, and supportive psychotherapy.

The 1972 report by Kernberg et al. argued that the patients who were suffering from borderline personality organization made greater improvements with expressive therapy compared to those who received supportive therapy. This conclusion was based on the statistical and quantitative data from the project while excluding much of the rich qualitative data that described in great detail the process between patient and therapist.

Two years after the appearance of the Kernberg report, Horwitz (1974), another investigator in the project, published his own conclusions about the study that examined *all* the available data, both the quantitative and qualitative material, and he arrived at somewhat different conclusions. He felt that many of the patients with borderline ego organization had improved considerably with a predominantly supportive approach. He emphasized the significant role of creating a strong therapeutic alliance with such patients.

Perhaps the most comprehensive report of the study was written by Robert Wallerstein (1986), when he provided a final clinical accounting of the treatment careers of all 42 patients with reports of follow-up stretching over a 30-year span. The major finding of his effort was that most of the treatments, whether psychoanalytic or psychotherapeutic, had been significantly modified during their course in the direction of a more supportive approach. In addition, many of the cases who received predominantly supportive treatment appeared to achieve as much structural change with similar degrees of durability as those who received highly expressive psychotherapy or psychoanalysis. He found that almost all patients in the study received some mixture of supportive and expressive elements in the psychotherapeutic approach and that patients with higher levels of ego strength tended to have better outcomes.

A subsequent group of Menninger researchers further investigated the controversy regarding whether supportive or interpretive/expressive techniques were more effective with borderline patients (Gabbard et al., 1994; Horwitz et al., 1996). In this project, known as the Treatment Interventions Project, the researchers studied audiotaped transcripts of the complete psychoanalytic psychotherapy processes involving three patients with borderline personality disorder treated at the Menninger Clinic. One team of investigators made ratings of the patients' therapeutic alliance in response to specific interventions by the therapist. The other team scored these interventions on an expressive–supportive continuum. They concluded that borderline patients were a heterogeneous group and that no single psychotherapeutic approach is suited to all patients with that diagnosis. In accord with Wallerstein's findings, they noted that typically a mixture of expressive and supportive interventions were used by the therapists. They also stressed that there is little basis for polarizing interpretive and supportive strategies as alternative treatments because they often work synergistically when a mixture of such interventions are used with the same patient. Many patients seem to respond best to transference interpretations after the groundwork has been laid by a series of supportive interventions that help the patient feel understood and that strengthen the therapeutic alliance. All three of the patients had good outcomes as rated by independent judges, even though the three therapies varied considerably in terms of the emphasis on expressive versus supportive interventions.

A reexamination of the original Menninger PRP was conducted by Blatt (1992), and he also found that the psychotherapeutic approach to such patients must be varied based on the nature of the patient's psychopathology. He divided the patient's into two groups: (1) those with *anaclitic* psychopathology, who were more concerned with problems of relatedness than with the development of the self and who employed avoidant defenses such as withdrawal, repression, displacement, denial, and disavowal; and (2) patients with *introjective* pathology, who were more ideational and were primarily concerned with the development and maintenance of a self-concept, with intimate relationships as secondary issue. This group employed the defenses of intellectualization, rationalization, projection, and reaction formation. Blatt noted that the anaclitic group of patients appeared to be much less responsive to insight or interpretation, while gaining considerable value from the quality of the therapeutic relation itself. By contrast, patients in the introjective group appeared to respond with much greater improvement to interpretation and insight.

An Australian study used a "pre post" design to follow 30 patients with DSM-III-R borderline personality disorder prospectively (Stevenson, & Meares, 1992). The patients were first identified and followed for 12 months *prior* to receiving treatment. The same patients then received twice-weekly psychodynamic therapy influenced by the ideas of Winnicott and Kohut for another 12 months. Although the therapy was not manualized, the training therapists were intensively supervised. After termination of the therapy, the same patients were followed for an additional 12 months. Substantial and enduring improvements were observed. Among the statistically significant changes were the following:

1. Prior to therapy, the patients were absent from work an average of 4.7 months per year, whereas following the therapy, the average had declined to 1.37 months per year.
2. The number of self-harm episodes *after* the therapy was one-fourth the level of the pretreatment rates.

3. The number of visits to medical professionals dropped to one-seventh of the pretreatment rates after the psychotherapy.
4. The time spent as an inpatient decreased by half.
5. The number of hospital admissions decreased by 59% after the therapy.

The durability of these changes was confirmed with a 5-year follow-up assessment (Stevenson & Meares, 1995). Most of the outcome measures continued to show declines as compared to the pretreatment rates. The only exception was that the time away from work began to increase over the 5-year follow-up period, but the investigators could not determine how much of that employment difficulty related to the recession that occurred in Sydney during that time period.

The same investigators (Meares, Stevenson, & Comerford, 1999) subsequently published a comparison of their 30 patients with borderline personality disorder to a wait-list control group. The first 30 patients on the waiting list who had been waiting 12 months or more made up the comparison group. These patients had their usual treatments during the waiting period, which included supportive therapy, crisis intervention, and cognitive therapy. The investigators then compared the results of the treated patients with those of the wait-list controls. Of the 30 treated patients, 30% no longer met criteria for borderline personality disorder after 12 months of psychotherapy. The 30 patients on the waiting list for 1 year or more showed no change in diagnosis. Definitive conclusions cannot be drawn from this study because randomization was not employed and the length of time at which follow-up data were collected varied for the wait-list group. Nevertheless, the results are suggestive of substantial gains from the dynamic therapy that was offered.

A team of Norwegian investigators (Monsen, Odland, Faugli, Daae, & Eilersten, 1995a, 1995b) followed 25 outpatients with personality disorders and psychoses in a 7-year prospective outcome study. Twenty-three of the 25 patients were diagnosed as personality disordered at baseline. This group included 28% with borderline personality disorder, 12% with passive–aggressive personality disorder, 12% with dependent personality disorder, and 12% with mixed personality disorder. The rest of the sample included paranoid, avoidant, narcissistic, schizoid, and schizotypal personality disorders.

Each of the patients received long-term psychodynamic psychotherapy based on self psychology and object relations theory with a particular emphasis on interpersonal relations, consciousness of affect, self-image, and parental images. The average length of the psychotherapy was 25.4 months with a mean follow-up period of 5.2 years.

The results at follow-up suggested positive effects of the treatment. At termination fully 72% of the patients with personality disorders no longer met criteria for their Axis II diagnoses. This substantial reduction in psychopathology remained stable when assessed at 5-year follow-up. The areas of improvement included the quality of contact in relationships with friends, the capacity to tolerate intimate relationships, the ability to actually establish such relationships, a reduced usage of ordinary social and health services, and improved global health–sickness ratings.

There is one recent randomized controlled study of psychoanalytic psychotherapy of patients with borderline personality disorder (Bateman & Fonagy, 1999). At the Halliwick Day Unit in London the investigators compared 38 borderline patients in a psychoanalytically oriented partial hospital program to those in a control group. The partial hospital condition consisted of once-weekly individual psychoanalytic psychotherapy, three-times-per-week group psychoanalytic therapy, once-weekly expressive therapy informed by psychodrama techniques, weekly community meeting, meeting with the case coordinator, and medication review by a resident psychiatrist. The control treatment consisted of regular psychiatric review an average of two times a month with a senior psychiatrist, inpatient admission as appropriate, outpatient and community follow-up, no psychotherapy, and medication similar to the partial hospital group.

The investigators found that the treatment group had a clear reduction in the proportion of the sample with suicide attempts in the previous 6 months. That proportion went from 95% on admission to 5.3% at 18-month follow-up. The average length of hospitalization in the control group in the last 6 months of the study increased dramatically, while it remained stable in the treatment group at around 4 days per 6 months. Both self-reported state and trait anxiety decreased substantially in the treatment group but remained unchanged in the control group. Depression scores (as measured by the

Beck Depression Inventory) also significantly decreased in the treatment group. There was a statistically significant decrease in severity of symptoms as measured by the Symptom Checklist-90–Revised at 18 months.

The researchers concluded that the improvement of psychiatric symptoms and suicidal acts occurred after 6 months, but a reduction in frequency of hospital admission and length of inpatient stay was only clear in the last 6 months, indicating a need for longer-term treatment. They also decided that partial hospitalization with psychoanalytic psychotherapy seems to be a promising and cheaper alternative to specialist–inpatient and general psychiatric treatment.

In a subsequent report (Bateman & Fonagy, 2001), patients who had received partial hospitalization treatment not only maintained their substantial gains at 18-month follow-up but also showed statistically significant continued improvement on most measures in contrast to the control group of patients, who showed only limited change during the same period.

Length of Psychotherapy and Outcome

The empirical literature on personality disorders has begun to address the link between the length of psychoanalytic psychotherapy and the outcome. The preponderance of the evidence suggests that while brief dynamic therapies may make some improvements in patients with personality disorders, extended psychotherapy may result in more substantial change.

Winston et al. (1994) randomly assigned 81 patients with a personality disorder diagnosis to one of three groups: short-term dynamic psychotherapy, brief adaptive psychotherapy, or a waiting list. The two psychotherapies lasted 40 weeks. The investigators compared the outcomes of the patients at termination with those of the individuals on the waiting-list for 15 weeks. The patients in the two therapy conditions showed significantly more improvement than the waiting list patients on symptom measures, social adjustment, and target complaints. A follow-up assessment an average of 1.5 years later suggested that the improvements were maintained. The sample of the personality disordered patients included 44% with Cluster C diagnoses, while another 23% had personality disorder not otherwise specified that included some Cluster C features, 22% had Cluster B diagnoses, and 4% came from Cluster A. The investigators noted that most patients with Cluster C conditions, as well as some of those with Cluster B disorders (primarily histrionic patients) responded to either modality. It should be noted, however, that rather broad exclusion criteria were used in this study so that many patients with poor prognoses were not included (Gabbard, 1997d).

Another controlled study, involving 110 male opiate addicts, provided further encouragement for the efficacy of brief dynamic therapies (Woody, McLellan, Luborsky, & O'Brien, 1985). These patients were randomly assigned to either paraprofessional drug counseling or counseling plus professional psychotherapy (the psychotherapy was either brief supportive–expressive or brief cognitive-behavioral in orientation.) Outcome was rated 7 months later, and the researchers found that those who had antisocial personality disorder made significant improvement in their symptoms and employment while also reducing illegal activity and drug use, but *only* if they also had a diagnosis of depression on Axis I. Antisocial personality disorder patients without depression showed little gains from psychotherapy. This report characterizes a relatively select subgroup of antisocial personality disorder patients as capable of benefiting from supportive–expressive psychotherapy, but given the general pessimism for the prognosis of such patients, a result suggesting any improvement whatsoever is impressive.

Although these two studies suggest that some personality-disordered patients may benefit from short-term therapy, many would argue that the 40-week therapy used in the study conducted by Winston et al. (1994) would be considered long term in the current managed care climate. Moreover, studies using more naturalistic designs suggest that most patients with a personality disorder take longer to change than Axis I conditions treated with psychotherapy. Howard, Kopta, Krause, and Orlinsky (1986), using a retrospective chart review method, studied the dose–effect relationship in psychotherapy. They found that 50% of anxious and depressed patients improved in 8 to 13 sessions. By contrast, patients with borderline personality disorder required 26 to 52 sessions to achieve similar levels of improvement. Some of the patients with borderline personality disorder showed no significant improvement until the second year of once-weekly treatment.

The same investigators conducted further research to determine the rapidity of change associated with specific symptom constellations

(Kopta, Howard, Lowry, & Beutler, 1994). Their study examined of 854 psychotherapy outpatients in treatment with 141 psychotherapists who were predominantly psychodynamically oriented. Symptoms were grouped into three distinct classes: (1) chronic distress, (2) acute distress, and (3) characterological. All patients were administered symptom checklists. The typical outpatient needed about 1 year of psychotherapy to have a 75% chance of symptomatic recovery. Those patients with acute symptoms showed an improvement rate of 68% to 98% after 52 once-weekly sessions of psychotherapy. Patients with chronic distress symptoms manifested an improvement rate of 60% to 86% over the same interval. However, when the investigators looked at the patients with characterological symptoms, they found that only 59% improved in that time interval. The researchers concluded that a longer duration of individual psychotherapy appears to be necessary for symptoms embedded in character.

Confirming evidence that patients with personality disorders may take longer to change than those with Axis I conditions was provided by a Norwegian study (Høglend, 1993). In this investigation 48 patients were treated with dynamic psychotherapy that ranged from 9 to 53 sessions. Fifteen of the patients had a personality disorder diagnosis. Of these, eight were avoidant or dependent, while seven were histrionic, borderline, or narcissistic. Other patients in the study suffered from Axis I diagnoses. All patients were provided psychotherapy by psychoanalytically oriented psychiatrists. For those patients with personality disorders, the number of sessions of psychotherapy was significantly related to the acquisition of insight 2 years after therapy and to overall dynamic change 4 years after therapy. This correlation was not found in those patients *without* personality disorders. Significant long-term dynamic changes in patients with personality disorders were observed after treatments that lasted 30 sessions or more. The investigators also found that the patients with Cluster B diagnoses seemed to do as well as those with Cluster C conditions.

Evidence is accumulating that personality disorder patients who can remain in a consistent, stable psychotherapy process over an extended period fare better than those who get in and out of therapy based on the presence or absence of crises in their lives. In the dissertation research of Dr. Lisbeth Hoke (1989), 58 borderline patients were followed for up to 7 years. The borderline personality disorder subjects in this study could be divided into two different groups based on their natural course. The first group (approximately half) had intermittent or inconsistent psychotherapeutic treatments; the second group had consistent psychotherapy over at least 2 years. Those who remained in a stable psychotherapy process showed greater improvement in mood functioning, a decreased need for more intensive psychiatric interventions (e.g., hospitalization, emergency room visits, and day treatment), decreased impulsiveness, and improved Global Assessment Scale scores.

Finally, the Bateman and Fonagy study (1999) suggests that certain aspects of the clinical picture in patients with borderline personality disorder take longer to change than others. Whereas suicidal acts and psychiatric symptoms began to decrease after only 6 months of treatment, the need for inpatient treatment began to drop during the 12- to 18-month period.

Cost-Effectiveness Issues

The Hoke (1989) study underscores an important cost-effectiveness principle in the long-term psychotherapy of personality disorders. In the long run it may be much more cost-effective to provide severe personality disorder patients with regular weekly psychotherapy over a long period than to consign them to periods of brief intermittent therapy which are commonly available under managed care arrangements. By their very nature, borderline personality disorder patients are treatment seekers who will find a way to access the health care system if denied the possibility of extended psychotherapy (Gabbard, 1997a; Gabbard, Lazar, Hornberger, & Spiegel, 1997). The provision of regular weekly therapy greatly diminishes the use of inpatient services, emergency room visits, and treatment by other medical professionals. The Australian study by Stevenson and Meares (1992) shows the same economic impact as the Hoke study—namely, the hospitalization rate dropped dramatically, along with the visits to other specialists and the length of time in the hospital. In a subsequent report (Stevenson & Meares, 1999), the investigators calculated the cost savings inherent in treating borderline patients twice weekly with dynamic psychotherapy. Based on the decrease in hospital treatment alone, the psychotherapy was a good investment. During the 12 months prior to treatment, in Australian dollars, hospital treatment cost $684,346 with a range of $0 to $143,756 per patient. The cost of hospital admissions for the year after treatment was $41,424 with a range of $0 to $12,333 per patient. The average decrease in cost per patient was $21,431 over 12 months. The average cost of therapy per patient was $13,000, representing a savings per patient of $8,431.

Confirming data come from studies using nonpsychodynamic therapies. Linehan, Armstrong, Suarez, Allmon, and Heard (1991) conducted a randomized controlled trial of dialectical behavior therapy with borderline personality disorder patients. After 1 year of group and individual therapy, these patients used significantly less hospitalization than did the control group that received "treatment as usual." The research group calculated that those patients receiving dialectical behavior therapy saved $10,000 per patient per year compared to the control group, largely because of reduced use of hospitalization (Heard, 1994).

When the economic impact of psychotherapy is broadly construed to include work disability, the cost-effectiveness argument can be made even more strongly. For example, in the Stevenson and Meares study, the patients' absenteeism from work was dramatically improved by 1 year of twice-weekly dynamic psychotherapy. These considerations, of course, are primarily applicable to the more severe personality disorders where work functioning is impaired and hospitalization is required. For patients who are reasonably functional at work and do not require hospitalization, the cost-effectiveness argument is much less persuasive.

Overall Evaluation of Empirical Data

In critically evaluating these studies of psychoanalytic therapy with personality-disordered patients, one must remember that the one study using a randomized controlled design had other treatments involved in the partial hospital treatment program. Nevertheless, the core modality in that program was psychoanalytic therapy. Regarding the other studies, without a randomized controlled design, we cannot definitively conclude that the psychotherapeutic intervention *itself* was the reason for the patient's improvement. However, some data suggest that patients with severe personality disorders tend to remain fairly stable over time. In one study

(Vaglum, Friis, Karterud, Mehlum, & Vaglum, 1993), 73 day patients with severe personality disorders were followed over a period of 2.8 years. Only 11% were clearly without serious personality problems at follow-up. Hence substantial improvements would be unlikely without psychotherapeutic efforts.

Moreover, there are a variety of problems with randomized controlled designs that raise questions about their generalizability to clinical work (Gunderson & Gabbard, 1999). Up to 90% of treatment-seeking patients may be excluded from carefully controlled trials because of the large number of inclusion criteria that protect internal validity. Patients with comorbidity, multiple diagnoses, and highly unstable conditions are typically excluded. In addition, patients who have been treatment failures may also be excluded. Those patients who respond to the advertisements for such studies may be better educated and more highly motivated to participate in a study in which they may be randomized to a control condition like a waiting list.

In light of some of these limitations of the randomized controlled trial, Seligman (1996) has suggested that treatments measured in a naturalistic setting, the so-called *effectiveness approach* (as opposed to the *efficacy* model), may yield more useful data. This type of study would involve the kinds of patients typically seen in a clinical setting and would measure multiple outcomes, examining psychotherapy as it is actually practiced rather than using manualized versions that artificially restrict the therapist. The end result is that the patients studied are those seen in actual practice rather than an exclusive subgroup with only one diagnosis, and the treatments are not artificially controlled by the directions in a manual but are flexible and geared to the individual patient.

Historically, psychoanalysts and psychoanalytic therapists have not always approached their work with the empirical rigor of psychotherapists from other persuasions. Gunderson and Gabbard (1999) have outlined several steps that might improve the credibility of psychoanalytic therapies and enhance the empirical rigor of the field. These include a careful definition of the distinguishing features of the treatment, clear identification of indications and contraindications—in other words, which of the personality disorders are most likely to respond to psychoanalytic approaches—systematic collection of case histories in psychoanalytic institute records that reflect successful treatment of diagnosable patients, and the assumption of greater responsibility, conjointly with the patient, for assessing progress in treatment.

Hence an overall evaluation would have to conclude that the paucity of randomized controlled trials of long-term psychoanalytic psychotherapy limits the empirical support for this modality with personality disorders, but that the body of research as a whole is highly encouraging. Some personality-disordered patients appear to make substantial and durable changes with psychodynamic therapy, and with increasing length of the treatment the changes appear to be of greater magnitude. Flexible shifting between expressive and supportive interventions seems to be the key to effective work with the more serious personality disorders, such as borderline personality disorder, and the therapist should be wary of idealizing interpretation as the main instrument of change. Finally, extended psychotherapy of patients with severe personality disorders may ultimately be more cost-effective than brief or intermittent treatments.

A BIOLOGICALLY INFORMED PSYCHODYNAMIC MODEL OF PERSONALITY DISORDER

The psychoanalytic clinician who attempts to treat personality disorders must be biologically and genetically informed. For too long psychoanalytic theory evolved independently of data from the neurosciences and genetic studies of heritability. A heuristically useful starting point is the psychobiological model of personality developed by Cloninger, Svrakic, and Pryzbeck (1993). Within this model, personality is viewed as resulting from a mixture of genetically based temperament and environmentally based character, with each domain contributing approximately 50%. The character variables distinguish whether or not a person is classified as having a personality disorder, whereas the temperament variables are influential in determining the subtype of personality disorder and susceptibility to emotional disorders on Axis I (Cloninger, 1993).

As the other chapter authors in this volume stress, this classification is somewhat controversial. Not all studies in behavioral genetics support the distinction between temperament

and character. Nevertheless, the model is of considerable heuristic value because it reminds the psychoanalyst or psychoanalytic therapist of the need to distinguish which features of personality are likely to respond to psychotherapy and which are not.

A central point emphasized by Cloninger and his colleagues is that the distinction between temperament and character may be essential for effective treatment: "Models that confound temperament and character may lead to therapeutic nihilism because they neglect distinctions crucial for effective treatment" (Svrakic, Whitehead, Pryzbeck, & Cloninger, 1993, p. 999). These investigators include novelty seeking, harm avoidance, reward dependence, and persistence under temperament. The three character variables include self-directedness, cooperativeness, and self-transcendence.

The recognition of the role of biological temperament in personality disorders does not in any way diminish the value of psychotherapeutic approaches to these disorders. On the contrary, this conceptual model allows us to use psychotherapeutic strategies more expertly, often in conjunction with medication. Indeed, as Cloninger's model suggests, character variables distinguish whether or not a personality disorder is present, and therefore the psychotherapeutic approach to those character variables may be crucial in addressing those problems that have led to the diagnosis of personality disorder. Temperament is highly stable over time, even with psychotherapy, while character is malleable and develops throughout adulthood (Svrakic et al., 1993). Antisocial personality disorders, for example, may become more self-directed and cooperative between the ages of 25 and 35, even though the temperament remains pretty much the same (Robins, 1966).

Our advance in knowledge in the area of temperament and character is allowing us to develop the capacity to target certain symptoms such as impulsivity and affective lability with increasingly specific psychopharmacological agents (Coccaro & Kavoussi, 1997; Siever & Davis, 1991), while approaching the patient's problems with self-directedness and cooperativeness psychotherapeutically. These character dimensions readily lend themselves to more typical conceptual terms used by psychoanalysts and psychoanalytic therapists. Specifically, the self-directedness dimension is closely linked to the psychoanalytic constructs of self-representations and ego functions, whereas cooperativeness is easily translatable into internal object relations as they are externalized and manifested in the interpersonal relationships of the individual.

Self-directedness and cooperativeness reflect two fundamental tasks of personality development as defined by Blatt and Ford (1994): (1) the achievement of a stable, differential, realistic, and positive identity; and (2) the establishment of enduring, mutually gratifying relationships with others. These two dimensions evolve in a dialectical and synergistic relationship to one another throughout the life cycle. As noted earlier, patients with character pathology tend to divide into two groups: (1) introjective types, who are primarily focused on self-definition; and (2) anaclitic types, who are more concerned about relatedness.

Psychoanalytic clinicians will find considerable value in thinking about the character dimension of the personality-disordered patient as involving an ongoing attempt to actualize certain patterns of relatedness that reflect wishes in the patient's unconscious. Through the patient's behavior, he or she subtly tries to impose a certain way of responding and experiencing on the clinician. In other words, fixed character traits in the patient may be viewed as playing a role in actualizing an internal object relationship that is part of a wish-fulfilling fantasy in the patient (Sandler, 1981). In this manner the transference–countertransference dimensions of the clinical interaction provide a privileged glimpse of the typical patterns of relatedness that cause difficulties in the patient's outside relationships.

In childhood an individual internalizes a self-representation in interaction with an object representation connected by an affect. This pattern ultimately leads to an internalized set of self- and other-representations in interaction with one another. Rather than relying on concepts such as repetition compulsion, which are intimately linked to outmoded constructs such as the death instinct, psychoanalytic clinicians can understand repetitive patterns of relatedness as efforts to actualize one of these internal object relationships as a way of fulfilling a wish. In this regard, even sadomasochistic relationships involving a "bad" or tormenting object may provide safety and affirmation for a variety of reasons. In other words, for a child who has been abused, a highly conflictual, abusive relationship may be safe in the sense that it is preferable to having no object at all or being abandoned. Many such patients assume that the only way of remaining connected to a significant object is to maintain an abuser–victim paradigm in the relationship. Such relationships are predictable and reliable and provide the patient with a sense of meaning and continuity (Gabbard, 1989). The repetitive interaction seen in personality-disordered patients may reflect actual relationships with real objects in the past, but they may also involve wished-for relationships, such as those often seen in patients with childhood trauma who seek a rescuer. Clinicians who are influenced by the patient's interpersonal pressure to respond in a particular way may unconsciously accept the role in which they have been cast. When this phenomenon occurs, it is often referred to as projective identification (Gabbard, 1995; Ogden, 1979). In other words, the patient may "nudge" the therapist into assuming the role of an abuser in response to the patient's "victim" role. The therapist may then begin to feel countertransference hate or anger and make sarcastic or devaluing comments to the patient.

Alternatively, therapists may ignore the role that is being thrust on them or reject it. Therapists may also defend against the role by assuming an opposite stance. Hence a therapist being "nudged" into an abusive role may become overly kind and empathic as a reaction against the pressure to take on the abuser role. Each clinician will respond differently based on his or her set of internal object relations (Gabbard, 1995). When the role being evoked by the patient is ego dystonic, such as the role of an abusive father or mother, the therapist may well feel that an alien force is taking over and the subjective experience may be something like the following: "I'm not like myself," or "I'm behaving irrationally." On the other hand, if the wished-for interaction that is being actualized is that of an idealized parent who is nurturing and understanding with a needy child, the therapist may experience the role as entirely ego syntonic and may be initially unaware of any countertransference involvement. In any case, a crucial aspect of this conceptual model of character is that the clinician must maintain a free-floating responsiveness (Sandler, 1981) to the patient's provocations as a way of diagnosing and understanding the patient's usual mode of object relatedness outside the treatment situation. One of the principal tasks of the psychoanalyst or the psychoanalytic therapist is to clarify the nature of these unconscious relational patterns and make them understandable to the patient.

This model of character is closely related to the role-relationship model of Horowitz (1988, 1991, 1998). In this theory, person schemas reflect unconscious self–other organizational units. These units are driven by internal motives that lead away from feared outcomes or toward desired ends. Person schemas in this model are belief structures that have both content and form. These schemas may, of course, be filled with conflicting beliefs and desires.

Another major component of character from a psychoanalytic perspective is the particular constellation of defense mechanisms that characterizes the individual patient. Defenses were traditionally regarded as intrapsychic mechanisms designed to prevent awareness of unconscious aggressive or sexual wishes, but the understanding of defense mechanisms has been expanded far beyond Freud's dual-drive theory. We also now understand defenses as preserving a sense of self-esteem in the face of narcissistic vulnerability, ensuring safety when one feels dangerously threatened by abandonment, and insulating one from external dangers through, for example, denial or minimization. As Vaillant and Vaillant (1999) have argued, defenses do not simply alter the relationship between an affect and an idea. They also change the relationship between self and object. They frequently enable the patient to manage unresolved conflicts that exist with important objects in the patient's current life or internal objects from the past that continue to haunt the patient.

Particularly in the realm of personality disorders, defenses are most usefully conceptualized as embedded in relatedness. Vaillant and Vaillant (1999) stress that neurotic symptoms cope with unbearable drive pressures, while the symptoms of personality disorder cope with unbearable people—both from the past and the present. They point out that distinct defense mechanisms are associated with specific personality disorders, and these defenses affect the individual's mode of relatedness. For example, Cluster A patients in the DSM-IV classification, including paranoid, schizoid, and schizotypal personality disorders, typically use projection as a way of disavowing unacknowledged feelings and attributing them to others. Similarly, schizoid individuals may engage in schizoid fantasy as a defense to alleviate their loneliness.

Moreover, while defenses are usually regarded as intrapsychic, they typically emerge in the treatment situation as *resistances* to the process with a strong interpersonal component to them (Gabbard, 2000b; Gill, 1994). In this regard the characteristic fears and hopes associated with a patient's internal object relations and his or her unique constellation of defense mechanisms often work synergistically to create a specific set of transferences that evoke a related set of countertransferences in the therapist.

If one looks at the common defenses associated with obsessive–compulsive personality disorder, for example, one would ordinarily associate this diagnostic entity with several key defensive operations, principally isolation of affect, intellectualization, and reaction formation (Gabbard, 2000b). Powerful affective states are highly threatening to the individual with obsessive–compulsive personality disorder, so these defenses tone down affects and emphasize cognition instead. Hence the defensive repertoire unfolds in the psychoanalytic situation as a careful avoidance of any strong feelings in the patient accompanied by behaviors designed to control the analyst's affective state. Patients with obsessive–compulsive personality disorder may talk about a wide variety of subjects with considerable insight and psychological awareness while also displaying a flattened affect and monotonous vocal intonation. They may conscientiously show up early for every session and pay their bill precisely on time to avoid any possible hint that they may feel aggressive, angry, or resentful toward the analyst. This reaction formation is partially designed to ward off attacks from the analyst, who may unconsciously be regarded as a rather fierce and potentially critical authoritarian figure, and partially to convince the analyst that the patient is essentially a responsible and dutiful person who has transcended any anger in the analytic relationship.

Hence even in an individual of the introjective type, these defenses work in concert with an attempt to actualize a specific wished-for interaction, that of a good, dutiful child who is basking in the glow of an approving parent. In this situation, the wished-for interaction itself can be regarded as a defense against a feared interaction in which the analyst or therapist becomes an embodiment of the patient's harsh and critical superego. In other words, the superego of the ego-psychological structural model becomes translated into a transference fear of a punitive and critical analyst as the patient's internal world becomes externalized in the psychoanalytic or psychotherapeutic setting. Within this conceptual model, character traits represent the final common pathway of instinctual wishes, defenses against those wishes, and ways to elicit responses from significant objects in the environment or in the patient's intrapsychic world.

These characteristic defenses are intimately related to a *third* component of character—cognitive style. Whereas persons with histrionic personality disorder overvalue emotional expression at the cost of careful attention to thinking, the reverse is true for obsessive–compulsive individuals, who try to eradicate affect by being rigid and logical. The lack of spontaneity and flexibility gives them an illusion of control. They dread any situation of uncontrolled emotion. While individuals with histrionic personality disorder respond to questions with impressionistic hunches, individuals with obsessive–compulsive personality disorder focus systematically on detail and logic in an effort to be exact (Shapiro, 1965).

Another implication of this biologically informed psychodynamic model of character is that medications and psychotherapy may work synergistically with patients who have severe personality disorders. Medications such as selective serotonin reuptake inhibitors (SSRIs) and lithium may modify temperamental variables such as impulsivity, temper outbursts, or unmodulated anger, but they are unlikely to change self-concepts or the patient's basic internal object relations. With patients with borderline personality disorder, for example, data suggest that anger and impulsivity are significantly improved with the use of SSRIs (Coccaro & Kavoussi, 1997; Markovitz, 1995; Salzman et al., 1995), which may in turn allow the patient to be more reflective and thoughtful about what is transpiring between the patient and the therapist. Some defenses may become less rigid as a result of pharmacological effects of antidepressants and also contribute to an increase in the patient's observing ego capacity (Marcus, 1990). Certain defensive patterns may also be influenced by genetic factors (Livesley, Jang, Jackson, & Vernon, 1993); thus it is premature to attempt to distinguish environmental and genetic contributions to each discrete defense mechanism (Gunderson, Triebwasser, Phillips, & Sullivan, 1999). On the other hand, clinical experience has repeatedly shown that as

a patient's characteristic patterns of relatedness are analyzed and understood, certain defenses become less necessary. These observations are supported by long-term follow-up studies that demonstrate the malleability of defenses (Perry, 1993; Vaillant, 1993).

To summarize this biologically informed psychoanalytic model, we can conceptualize four basic components of personality:

1. A biologically based temperament.
2. A constellation of internal object relations units that are linked to affect states and externalized in interpersonal relationships.
3. A characteristic set of defense mechanisms.
4. A related cognitive style.

TECHNICAL STRATEGIES AND PROCESS ISSUES

Traditionally psychoanalysis has been conducted four or five times a week with the patient on the couch and with free association as the primary technique. Psychoanalytic psychotherapy is usually conducted one to three times a week and involves face-to-face sessions rather than the use of the couch. However, in discussing technique and process, psychoanalysts have increasingly come to regard psychoanalysis proper and psychoanalytic psychotherapy as occurring on a continuum without an obvious line of demarcation between the two. Weinshel and Renik (1991) recently concluded, "As we hesitantly surrender our illusions concerning the perfectly conducted analysis and the perfect analytic outcome, we also relinquish the fantasy of a crystal clear distinction between psychoanalysis and psychoanalytic psychotherapy" (p. 21).

Wallerstein's (1986) research suggests that psychoanalytic technique occurs on a continuum with psychoanalysis at the most expressive end and supportive psychotherapy at the most supportive end. Nevertheless, he emphasized that at all points on the continuum there is a mixture of supportive and interpretive interventions that are used flexibly according to the patient's needs and capacities.

As a general principle, the more expressively oriented treatments focus more on the patient's transference to the therapist and attempt to provide insight into the meaning of that transference. Supportive therapy is less likely to rely on transference interventions and more likely to focus on extratransference issues. In addition, certain interventions are more closely aligned with expressive work. Figure 17.1 illustrates an expressive–supportive continuum of interventions that reflects specific emphases used at various points along the continuum.

The therapist's technical strategy is inevitably based on a large component of trial and error, in which the therapist carefully notes the patient's response to interpretive efforts. The extent of expressive versus supportive interventions, however, can also be guided by the extent to which the psychopathology is apparently deficit based versus conflict based. Interpretations are generally more suited for conflict-based pathology (Gabbard, 1997b; Killingmo, 1989). Psychopathology that grows out of conflict between intrapsychic agencies or between internal object- or self-representations often is connected with concealed meanings that the therapist attempts to reveal to the patient during the course of the treatment.

On the other hand, patients with deficit-based pathology are often victims of childhood trauma or neglect. They may experience themselves as passive recipients of horrific treatment from others and be entirely uninterested in forming an alliance with the therapist designed to expose concealed meanings. Indeed, they are likely to hear interpretations as accusations, failures of empathy, or attacks. Those patients with severe childhood trauma in particular tend to experience interpretations of the transference as a challenge to their sense of reality (Gabbard, 1997b). For example, if the therapist says, "I think what you are actually feeling towards me is not fear, but anger," the patient may only be aware of the fear and thus feel misunderstood. On the other hand, interventions closer to the supportive end of the continuum, especially empathic validation, may have considerable therapeutic value. Killingmo (1989) referred to these therapist comments as *affirmative* interventions, and he made the observation that "by confirming ex-

actly the way the patient is feeling, the analyst relates to the most urgent need of the patient of deficit, that is the need to feel 'I am' and that 'I have the right to be'" (p. 76). Affirmations of experience allow patients to feel that their reality is being acknowledged.

One caveat is in order when discussing the conflict-versus-deficit axis. Just as expressive-versus-supportive interventions should not be viewed as polarized, neither should one view conflict/deficit as "either/or." Many patients have aspects of both, and adjustments need to made accordingly. As Eagle (1984) has observed, "We are most conflicted in the areas in which we are deprived. . . . [I]t is precisely the person deprived of love who is most conflicted about giving and receiving love" (p. 130).

In parallel with the conflict-versus-deficit and expressive-versus-supportive dimensions of the therapy is a controversy regarding whether insight or the therapeutic relationship itself is responsible for therapeutic change. In the past the therapeutic relationship was denigrated as a therapeutic factor, but the recent literature has shifted to a recognition that insight and the relationship work hand in hand in most psychoanalytic treatments. Pine (1993) made the following observation:

> It is the co-occurrence of the cognitive clarification with an *experience* in the analyst–patient relationship—the actualized contrast to the patient's fantasy and the analyst's noncondemning stance—that produces the maximum therapeutic effect . . . the interpretive factor and the relationship factor are inseparably linked. And, each requires the other. The interpretation can have its maximum effect because the relationship (noncondemning) belies the patient's inner world. (p. 192)

There is a broad consensus in the literature on psychoanalysis and psychoanalytic therapy that the analyst's or therapist's role as a "new object" is crucial for change to take place within the patient. As Cooper (1989) noted:

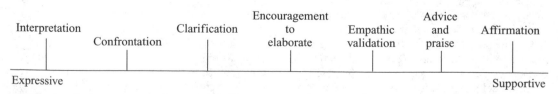

FIGURE 17.1. An expressive–supportive continuum of interventions. From Gabbard (2000, p. 96). Copyright 2000 by American Psychiatric Press. Reprinted by permission.

[The therapist] provides the patient with the experience of living in a different kind of emotional and relational "space"; a "holding" or "facilitating" environment, newly safe and potentially comforting. The analyst, in fact, provides a new emotional experience with another human being, different in essence from the traumatic relationships that were developmentally and genetically at the core of the developing psychopathology. It is of prime significance that the analytic situation is not only a new relational affective experience, but that the transferential meaning of the patient response to this encounter is constantly being interpreted. (p. 12)

Wallerstein's (1986) observations from the PRP provide some empirical support for the notion that both the relationship and insight may be effective change agents in light of the fact that supportive modalities seem to produce durable structural change just as expressive therapies do. Moreover, the work of Blatt (1992) suggests that introjective patients may rely more on interpretation as an agent of change, whereas the anaclitic patients may make use of the therapeutic relationship as the principal means of change.

In addition to the recognition that multiple models of therapeutic action are involved in understanding how people change with psychoanalysis and psychoanalytic psychotherapy, analysts also are reaching consensus that work on the here-and-now interaction supercedes historical reconstruction. Analysts no longer spend most of their time digging for buried relics from the patient's past in the dark recesses of the unconscious. Rather, the focus is on the relationship between analyst and patient as a privileged view of how the patient's past has created certain patterns of conflict and problematic object relations in the present. As Freud noted in his 1914 masterpiece, "Remembering, Repeating and Working Through" (Freud, 1914/1958)what cannot be remembered will be repeated in action in the patient's here-and-now behavior with the analyst. This concept was the original meaning, of course, of *acting out*. The patient's past patterns of internal object relations and the conflicts about those relationships will unfold in front of the analyst's eyes, and no archaeological excavation is necessary to unearth them.

The procedural memories encoded in the nonverbal behavior of the patient are observed and brought into the patient's awareness by the analyst in such a way that the patient ultimately gains a sense of mastery and understanding of what is being repeated in one relationship after another. This process is characterized by Fonagy and Target (1996) as expanding psychic reality by mentalizing or developing reflective function. In developmental terms, a principal mode of therapeutic action is perceiving oneself in the analyst's mind while simultaneously developing a greater sense of the separate subjectivity of the analyst.

However, the conscious mastery of the implicit and repetitive modes of relatedness is accompanied by nonconscious affective and interactive connections that have been referred to by Lyons-Ruth and her colleagues (1998) as *implicit relational knowing*. This knowing may occur in moments of meeting between analyst and patient that are not symbolically represented or dynamically unconscious in the ordinary sense. This notion is based on the mutual regulatory moves in the infant–caregiver relationship as described by Tronick (1989). In other words, some change that occurs in analytic treatment is in the realm of procedural knowledge involving how to act, feel, and think in a particular relational context (Stern et al., 1998). Implied in this conceptualization is the important point that many changes that occur are *outside* planned technical interventions. A shared belly laugh, a teary eye, or a meaningful glance may promote change even though the exchange is entirely spontaneous and not within the therapist's systematic technique.

The model I have described places great emphasis on the transference–countertransference dimensions of the therapeutic dyad. Hence the key strategy for the psychoanalytic therapist with a personality-disordered patient is to pay careful attention to the emerging interaction between the two parties in the dyad. As the patient attempts to actualize a specific interaction, the therapist observes the patient's attitudes toward the therapist as well as the feelings, thoughts, and fantasies he or she attributes to the therapist. Moreover, because countertransference by definition is unconscious, at least initially before it enters the therapist's awareness, the therapist must also monitor subtle forms of enactment (Gabbard, 1995). Minor actions, such as a clenched fist, a change in breathing, and leaning forward or scooting back in one's chair are all examples of almost nonperceptible countertransference enactments that may provide important information for the therapist. Similarly, fleeting feelings or thoughts about the patient may be clues to the type of role in which the therapist has been cast by the patient's projective identification or efforts at actualization. With some forms of personality disorder, such as borderline personality disorder, these provocations may be more extreme and dramatic, and the therapist may literally find himself or herself feeling furious at the patient and wishing to terminate the therapy so he or she will never have to see the patient again. With less dramatic forms of character pathology, such as obsessive–compulsive personality disorder, minor flickers of irritation may be the only sign of the emerging role relationship between patient and therapist.

Because most countertransference responses are jointly constructed by the preexisting internal objects of the therapist in interaction with the projected internal representations of the patient, it is often difficult for therapists to sort out the relative contributions of each member of the analytic couple. Hence therapists must avoid blaming the patient for their own reactions and recognize their own role in creating certain kinds of tensions between the two parties. Similarly, the social constructivist writings in recent years (Gill, 1994; Hoffman, 1991) have led us to recognize that the actual behavior of the therapist is constantly influencing the patient's transference. In this two-person or intersubjective psychology, we can never entirely separate out what we as therapists are initiating versus that which originates in the patient and to which we are reacting. Nevertheless, over time as recurrent patterns of the patient's internal object relations play out again and again, the therapist gradually gets a clearer picture of the origins of the patient's difficulties in relationships outside the transference and can begin to interpret them to the patient. However, it is wise to postpone such interpretation until the therapist has been steeped in the experience for some time and is more comfortable with and clear about the distinction between the patient's and the therapist's contributions to the interaction. It is also helpful when the patient brings in instances of similar interactions in the past and extratransference relationships in the present so that the interpretation can be bolstered with further evidence. An example of such an interpretation is the following: "I often get the impression here that you would like for me to absolve you of any responsibility for your difficulties with others, and it sounds very much like the kind of interaction you had with your

father as a child and currently with your boss at work."

Clearly, a single interpretation rarely resolves a transference issue. The initiation of an interpretive strategy marks the beginning of a prolonged process known as *working through*. Many interpretations will be followed by heightened resistance to uncovering the relevant unconscious themes. As similar patterns emerge in different relationships over time, the therapist persistently calls the pattern to the patient's attention as well as a pattern of resistance that draws the patient's attention away from the underlying issue. Over time, the patient becomes increasingly convinced of the existence of the unconscious pattern the therapist is describing.

IMPLICATIONS FOR ASSESSMENT, INDICATIONS, AND CONTRAINDICATIONS

One implication of this conceptual model for assessment is that a straightforward list of questions, such as those in standard research diagnostic interviews, may not be the best way to diagnose a patient's character pathology. As Westen's (1997) research has demonstrated, clinicians have a different way of diagnosing personality disorders than do researchers. They rely much more on listening to patients describe interpersonal interactions and on the here-and-now interactions in the relationship between the interviewer and the patient to reach their diagnostic conclusions. Other branches of medicine give a good deal of credence to the distinction between signs (i.e., relatively objective observations by the clinician) and symptoms (i.e., subjective reports of the patient), but the same distinction is often forgotten in psychiatry (Gabbard, 1997c). However, important diagnostic information regarding the patient's typical defenses and patterns of object relatedness are readily observable in the manner in which the patient behaves toward the clinician. Some of this behavior is entirely nonverbal. The patient may cross his arms over his chest in a posture of defiance or withholding. The patient may enter and exit the office in a deferential manner with her head bowed and eyes averted from the clinician.

Similarly, the clinician's reactions to the patient may be a gold mine of diagnostic information. As the conceptual model outlined earlier conveys, countertransference is no longer regarded as simply an interference or obstacle but as a source of important information about the patient. Clinicians interviewing a prospective patient must be examining their own responses and forming hypotheses about whether or not their responses might be typical of the reactions of others to the patient. The particular "dance" between patient and clinician may involve many of the same "steps" characteristic of the patient's relationships with parents, lovers, children, coworkers, and so forth.

Direct questions about interpersonal relationships may provoke defensiveness and result in incomplete or superficial information. If the interviewer allows the patient to ramble for a bit before restructuring the interview, however, often extraordinarily useful information will emerge as the patient describes his or her difficulties in love relationships and at work.

Part of the assessment process is also to evaluate the patient's suitability for psychoanalytic therapy. Psychoanalytic clinicians have not always paid sufficient attention to nosology when discussing indications for psychoanalysis or psychoanalytic therapy of patients with personality disorders (Gunderson & Gabbard, 1999). As a general principle, the more neurotically organized personality disorders, such as obsessive–compulsive; avoidant; some histrionic, particularly the higher-level hysterical character (Gabbard, 2000b), and some narcissistic patients, can make use of treatments that emphasize the more expressive interventions such as interpretation and confrontation. Some patients with borderline personality disorder can use highly expressive interventions provided that the therapist pays careful attention to building the therapeutic alliance by empathically validating the patient's experience. This need for validation before offering interpretive interventions is particularly relevant to borderline patients with a history of childhood trauma (Gabbard et al., 1994; Horwitz et al., 1996). Premature interpretation of the projection of an abusive introject into the therapist may be experienced as further persecution from a "bad object." Similarly, patients who have self-defeating or masochistic character pathology may also experience interpretation as a form of criticism or attack that confirms their low self-esteem. Paranoid personality rarely lends itself to an expressive–supportive therapy process because of the patient's fundamental difficulty with trusting the therapist. Some schizoid and schizotypal individuals can be treated with expressive–supportive therapy, provided that the emphasis is on the supportive end of the continuum. It is crucial in such cases to keep one's expectations for change low. Many people with antisocial personality disorder are completely unsuitable for psychotherapy, and it may even be dangerous to attempt to treat them outside an institution (Meloy, 1988). A small subgroup with Axis I conditions involving depression and anxiety may be treatable under some circumstances (Gabbard & Coyne, 1987; Woody et al., 1985).

In addition to the specific personality disorder, the clinician must also assess additional features that bear on the suitability for expressive–supportive therapy. Patients who suffer significantly enough to motivate them to persevere in the face of frustration will do better with an expressive emphasis than those who do not have that capacity. Other considerations that augur well for expressive work are the presence of meaningful relationships, the capacities to sustain productive work, the capacity to think in terms of analogy and metaphor, psychological mindedness, good impulse control, intact reality testing, and reflective responses to trial interpretations (Gabbard, 2000b).

Qualities that contraindicate a psychotherapy with an expressive emphasis are poor impulse control, low intelligence, brain-based cognitive dysfunction, an inability to form a therapeutic alliance, poor reality testing, lack of psychological mindedness, and poor anxiety and frustration tolerance. Also, even a patient who ordinarily might be able to use expressive therapy may be better treated with supportive approaches in the midst of a severe life crisis.

EXPECTED RESULTS AND LIMITATIONS

As suggested in the section on empirical research, most personality-disordered patients who are suitable for and receive extended psychoanalytic therapy or psychoanalysis can expect to derive considerable benefits in their overall functioning, in their symptomatic picture, in object relationships, and in work functioning. A number of follow-up studies (Norman, Blacker, Oremland, & Barrett, 1976; Oremland, Blacker, & Norman, 1975; Pfeffer, 1963; Schlessinger & Robbins, 1974, 1975,

1983) have all concluded that the transferences that unfold in the course of psychoanalytic therapy are not obliterated or resolved. Rather, the patient experiences a degree of mastery and control over them. The unconscious repetitive patterns are understood, and the patient is less at the mercy of the internal conflicts associated with the transference dispositions. Moreover, a consistent finding in the outcome literature is the development of an active self-analytic function, in essence an identification with the analyzing function of the therapist or analyst as an ongoing way to handle new conflicts as they develop.

In the context of the generally successful outcomes of psychoanalytic treatments of personality disorders, we should also be mindful of certain limitations. As noted earlier, the patient's biologically based temperamental disposition is not likely to change radically from psychotherapeutic efforts. Appropriate medication may be necessary as an adjunct in the overall treatment plan. Also, certain behavioral problems may not get the necessary attention they need in a psychoanalytically oriented therapy. In a spin-off project from the PRP, Colson, Lewis, and Horwitz (1985) studied the negative outcome cases. They found a consistent pattern in which the therapist did not set limits on acting-out behaviors of the borderline patients. Instead, the therapist simply interpreted the unconscious meanings of the acting out while the behaviors continued. Hence the psychoanalytic therapist must be active in confronting such behaviors and setting limits on them to avoid this kind of negative outcome. Another limitation of individual psychoanalytic psychotherapy is that important family and marital issues may not be addressed that perpetuate problems in the system in which the patient lives. In many cases of personality disorders, marital or family work concomitant with the individual therapy may be essential. Finally, as with other therapies, the success is likely to be limited with those patients who are not sufficiently motivated to change, who are not curious about why they have the problems they experience, or who cannot collaborate in a therapeutic alliance with the clinician.

REFERENCES

Abraham, K. (1923). Contributions to the theory of anal character. In *Selected papers of Karl Abraham* (pp. 370–392). London: Hogarth Press. (Original work published 1923)

Bateman, A., & Fonagy, P. (1999). The effectiveness of partial hospitalization in the treatment of borderline personality disorder—a randomized control trial. *American Journal of Psychiatry, 156:* 1563–1569.

Bateman, A., & Fonagy, P. (2001). Treatment of borderline personality disorder with psychoanalytically oriented partial hospitalization: An 18-month follow-up. *American Journal of Psychiatry, 158,* 36–42.

Blatt, S. J. (1992). The differential effect of psychotherapy and psychoanalysis with anaclitic and introjective patients: The Menninger Psychotherapy Research Project revisited. *Journal of the American Psychoanalytic Association, 40,* 691–724.

Blatt, S. J., & Ford, T. Q. (1994). *Therapeutic change: An object relations perspective.* New York: Plenum.

Cloninger, C. R. (1993). Commentary. In M. H. Klein, D. J. Kupfer, & M. T. Shea (Eds.), *Personality and depression: A current view* (pp. 61–67). New York: Guilford Press.

Cloninger, C. R., Svrakic, D. M., & Pryzbeck, T. R. (1993). A psychobiological model of temperament and character. *Archives of General Psychiatry, 50,* 975–990.

Coccaro, E. F., & Kavoussi, R. J. (1997). Fluoxetine and impulsive aggressive behavior in personality disordered subjects. *Archives of General Psychiatry, 54,* 1081–1088.

Colson, D. B., Lewis, L., & Horwitz, L. (1985). Negative outcome in psychotherapy and psychoanalysis. In D. T. Mays & C. M. Frank (Eds.), *Negative outcome in psychotherapy and what to do about it* (pp. 59–75). New York: Springer.

Cooper, A. M. (1989). Concepts of therapeutic effectiveness in psychoanalysis: A historical review. *Psychoanalytic Inquiry, 9,* 4–25.

Eagle, M. N. (1984). *Recent developments in psychoanalysis: A critical evaluation.* New York: McGraw-Hill.

Fonagy, P., & Target, M. (1996). Playing with reality: I. Theory of mind in the normal development of psychic reality. *International Journal of Psycho-Analysis, 77,* 217–233.

Freud, S. (1959). Character and anal eroticism. In J. Strachey (Ed. and Trans.), *The standard edition of the complete psychological works of Sigmund Freud* (Vol. 9, pp. 167–175). London: Hogarth Press. (Original work published 1908)

Freud, S. (1958). Remembering, repeating and working-through (Further recommendations on the technique of psycho-analysis II). In J. Strachey (Ed. and Trans.), *The standard edition of the complete psychological works of Sigmund Freud* (Vol. 14, pp. 145–156). London: Hogarth Press. (Original work published 1914)

Gabbard, G. O. (1989). Patients who hate. *Psychiatry, 52,* 96–106.

Gabbard, G. O. (1995). Countertransference: The emerging common ground. *International Journal of Psycho-Analysis, 76,* 475–485.

Gabbard, G. O. (1997a). Borderline personality disorder and rational managed care policy. *Psychoanalytic Inquiry, Supplement,* 17–28.

Gabbard, G. O. (1997b). Challenges in the analysis of adult patients with histories of childhood sexual abuse. *Canadian Journal of Psychoanalysis, 5,* 1–25.

Gabbard, G. O. (1997c). Finding the "person" in personality disorders. *American Journal Psychiatry, 154,* 891–893.

Gabbard, G. O. (1997d). Psychotherapy of personality disorders. *Journal of Practical Psychiatry and Behavioral Health, 3,* 327–333.

Gabbard, G. O. (2000a). Psychoanalysis. In H. I. Kaplan & B. J. Sadock (Eds.), *Comprehensive textbook of psychiatry VI* (Vol. 1, pp. 431–478). Baltimore: Williams &Wilkins.

Gabbard, G. O. (2000b). *Psychodynamic psychiatry in clinical practice* (3rd ed.). Washington, DC: American Psychiatric Press.

Gabbard, G. O., & Coyne, L. (1987). Predictors of response of antisocial patients to hospital treatment. *Hospital and Community Psychiatry, 38,* 1181–1185.

Gabbard, G. O., Horwitz, L., Allen, J. G., Frieswyk, S., Newsom, G., Colson, D. B., & Coyne, L. (1994). Transference interpretation in the psychotherapy of borderline patients: A high-risk, high-gain phenomenon. *Harvard Review of Psychiatry, 2,* 59–69.

Gabbard, G. O., Lazar, S. G., Hornberger, J., & Spiegel, D. (1997). The economic impact of psychotherapy: A review. *American Journal Psychiatry, 154,* 147–155.

Gill, M. M. (1994). *Psychoanalysis in transition: A personal view.* Hillsdale, NJ: Analytic Press.

Gunderson, J. G., & Gabbard, G. O. (1999). Making the case for psychoanalytic therapies in the current psychiatric environment. *Journal of the American Psychoanalytic Association, 47,* 679–703.

Gunderson, J. G., Triebwasser, J. T., Phillips, K. A., & Sullivan, C. N. (1999). Personality and vulnerability to affective disorders. In C. R. Cloninger (Ed.), *Personality and psychopathology* (pp. 3–32). Washington, DC: American Psychiatric Press.

Heard, H. L. (1994, May). Behavior therapies for borderline patients. Presented at the 147th annual meeting of the American Psychiatric Association, Philadelphia.

Hoffman, I. Z. (1991). Discussion: Towards a social constructivist view of the psychoanalytic situation. *Psychoanalytic Dialogues, 1,* 74–105.

Høglend, P. (1993). Personality disorders and long-term outcome after brief dynamic psychotherapy. *Journal of Personality Disorders, 7,* 168–181.

Hoke, L. A. (1989). *Longitudinal patterns of behaviors in borderline personality disorder.* Doctoral dissertation. Boston University Graduate School.

Horowitz, M. J. (1988). *Introduction to psychodynamics: A new synthesis.* New York: Basic Books.

Horowitz, M. J. (1991). *Person schemas and maladaptive interpersonal patterns.* Chicago: University of Chicago Press.

Horowitz, M. J. (1998). *Cognitive psychodynamics: From conflict to character.* New York: Wiley.

Horwitz, L. (1974). *Clinical prediction in psychotherapy.* New York: Jason Aronson.

Horwitz, L., Gabbard, G. O., Allen, J. G., Frieswyk, S. H., Colson, D. B., Newsom, G. E., & Coyne, L. (1996). *Borderline personality disorder: Tailoring the psychotherapy to the patient.* Washington, DC: American Psychiatric Press.

Howard, K. I., Kopta, S. M., Krause, M. S., & Orlinsky, D. E. (1986). The dose–effect relationship in psychotherapy. Special issue: psychotherapy research. *American Psychologist, 41,* 159–164.

Kernberg, O. F., Burstein, E. D., Coyne, L., Appelbaum, A., Horwitz, L., & Voth, H. (1972). Psychotherapy and psychoanalysis: Final report of the Menninger Foundation's Psychotherapy Research Project. *Bulletin of the Menninger Clinic, 36,* 3–275.

Killingmo, B. (1989). Conflict and deficit: Implications for technique. *International Journal of Psycho-Analysis, 70,* 65–79.

Kopta, S. M., Howard, K. I., Lowry, J. L., & Beutler, L. E. (1994). Patterns of symptomatic recovery in psychotherapy. *Journal of Consulting and Clinical Psychology, 62,* 1009–1016.

Linehan, M. M., Armstrong, H. E., Suarez, A., Allmon, D., & Heard, H. L. (1991). Cognitive-behavioral treatment of chronically parasuicidal borderline patients. *Archives of General Psychiatry, 48,* 1060–1064.

Livesley, W. J., Jang, K. L., Jackson, D. N., & Vernon, P. A. (1993). Genetic and environmental contributions of dimensions of personality disorder. *American Journal Psychiatry, 150,* 1826–1831.

Lyons-Ruth, K., & Members of the Change Process Study Group. (1998). Implicit relational knowing: Its role in development and psychoanalytic treatment. *Infant Mental Health Journal, 19,* 282–289.

Marcus, E. (1990). Integrating psychopharmacotherapy, psychotherapy, and the mental structure in the treatment of patients with personality disorders and depression. *Psychiatric Clinics of North America, 13,* 255–263.

Markovitz, P. (1995). Pharmacotherapy of impulsivity, aggression, and related disorders. In E. Hollander & D. J. Stein (Eds.), *Impulsivity and aggression* (pp. 263–287). New York: Wiley.

Meares, R., Stevenson, J., & Comerford, A. (1999). Psychotherapy with borderline patients: I. A comparison between treated and untreated cohorts. *Australia and New Zealand Journal of Psychiatry, 33,* 467–472.

Meloy, J. R. (1988). *The psychopathic mind.* Northvale, NJ: Jason Aronson.

Monsen, J., Odland, T., Faugli, A., Daae, E., & Eilersten, D. E. (1995a). Personality disorders and psychosocial changes after intensive psychotherapy: A prospective follow-up study of an outpatient psychotherapy project, 5 years after end of treatment. *Scandinavian Journal of Psychology, 36,* 256–268.

Monsen, J., Odland, T., Faugli, A., Daae, E., & Eilersten, D. E. (1995b). Personality disorders and psychosocial changes after intensive psychotherapy: Changes and stability after intensive psychotherapy focusing on affect consciousness. *Psychotherapy Research, 5,* 33–48.

Norman, H. F., Blacker, K. H., Oremland, J. D., & Barrett, W. G. (1976). The fate of the transference neurosis after termination of a satisfactory analysis. *Journal of the American Psychoanalytic Association, 24,* 471–498.

Ogden, T. H. (1979). On projective identification. *International Journal of Psycho-Analysis, 60,* 357–373.

Oremland, J. D., Blacker, K. H., & Norman, H. T. (1975). Incompleteness in "successful" psychoanalyses: A follow-up study. *Journal of the American Psychoanalytic Association, 23,* 819–844.

Perry, J. C. (1993). Longitudinal studies of personality disorders. *Journal of Personality Disorders, 7,* 68–85.

Pfeffer, A. Z. (1963). The meaning of the analyst after analysis: A contribution to the theory of therapeutic results. *Journal of the American Psychoanalytic Association, 11,* 229–244.

Pine, F. (1993). A contribution to the analysis of the psychoanalytic process. *Psychoanalytic Quarterly, 62,* 185–205.

Reich, W. (1945). *Character-analysis: Principles and techniques for psychoanalysts in practice and in training.* New York: Orgone Institute Press.

Robins, L. N. (1966). *Deviant children grown up: A sociological and psychiatric study of sociopathic personality.* Baltimore: Williams & Wilkins.

Salzman, C., Wolfson, A. N., Schatzberg, A., Looper, J., Henke, R., Albanese, M., Schwartz, J., & Miyawaki, E. (1995). Effect of fluoxetine on anger in symptomatic volunteers with borderline personality disorder. *Journal of Clinical Psychopharmacology, 15,* 23–29.

Sandler, J. (1981). Character traits and object relationships. *Psychoanalytic Quarterly, 50,* 694–708.

Schlessinger, N., & Robbins, F. P. (1974). Assessment and follow-up in psychoanalysis. *Journal of the American Psychoanalytic Association, 22,* 542–567.

Schlessinger, N., & Robbins, F. P. (1975). The psychoanalytic process: Recurrent patterns of conflict and changes in ego functions. *Journal of the American Psychoanalytic Association, 23,* 761–782.

Schlessinger, N., & Robbins, F. P. (1983). *A developmental view of the psychoanalytic process: Follow-up studies and their consequences.* New York: International Universities Press.

Seligman, M. E. P. (1996). The effectiveness of psychotherapy: The *Consumer Reports* study. *American Psychologist, 50,* 965–974.

Shapiro, D. (1965). *Neurotic styles.* New York: Basic Books.

Siever, L. J., & Davis, K. L. (1991). A psychobiological perspective on the personality disorders. *American Journal Psychiatry, 148,* 1647–1658.

Stern, D. N., Sanders, L. W., Nahum, J. P., Harrison, A. M., Lyons-Ruth, K., Morgan, A. C., Bruschweiler-Stern, N., & Tronick, E. Z. (1998). Non-interpretive mechanisms in psychoanalytic therapy: The "something more" than interpretation. *International Journal of Psycho-Analysis, 79,* 903–921.

Stevenson, J., & Meares, R. (1992). An outcome study of psychotherapy for patients with borderline personality disorder. *American Journal Psychiatry, 149,* 358–362.

Stevenson, J., & Meares, R. (1995, May). *Borderline patients at 5-year follow-up.* Paper presented at the annual Congress of the Royal Australia–New Zealand College of Psychiatrists, Cairns, Australia.

Stevenson, J., & Meares, R. (1999). Psychotherapy with borderline patients: II. A preliminary cost-benefit study. *Australian-New Zealand Journal of Psychiatry, 33,* 473–477.

Svrakic, D. M., Whitehead, C., Pryzbeck, T. R., & Cloninger, C. R. (1993). Differential diagnosis of personality disorders by the seven-factor model of temperament and character. *Archives of General Psychiatry, 50,* 991–999.

Tronick, E. Z. (1989). Emotions and emotional communication in infants. *American Psychologist, 44,* 112–119.

Vaglum, P., Friis, S., Karterud, S., Mehlum, L., & Vaglum, S. (1993). Stability of the severe personality disorder diagnosis: A 2- to 5-year prospective study. *Journal of Personality Disorders, 7,* 348–353.

Vaillant, G. E. (1993). *The wisdom of the ego.* Cambridge, MA: Harvard University Press.

Vaillant, G. E., & Vaillant, L. M. (1999). The role of ego mechanisms of defense in the diagnosis of personality disorders. In J. Barron (Ed.), *Making diagnosis meaningful: Enhancing evaluation and treatment of psychological disorders* (pp. 139–158). Washington, DC: American Psychological Association.

Wallerstein, R. S. (1986). *Forty-two lives in treatment: A study of psychoanalysis and psychotherapy.* New York: Guilford Press.

Weinshel, E. M., & Renik, O. (1991). The past ten years: Psychoanalysis in the United States, 1980–1990. *Psychoanalytic Inquiry, 11,* 13–29.

Westen, D. (1997). Divergences between clinical and research methods for assessing personality disorders: Implications for research and the evolution of Axis II. *American Journal Psychiatry, 154,* 895–903.

Winston, A, Laikin, M., Pollack, J., Samstag, L. W., McCullough, L., & Muran, J. C. (1994). Short-term psychotherapy of personality disorders. *American Journal Psychiatry, 151,* 190–194.

Woody, G. E., McLellan, T., Luborsky, L., & O'Brien, C. P. (1985). Sociopathy and psychotherapy outcome. *Archives of General Psychiatry, 42,* 1081–1086.

CHAPTER 18

Cognitive Therapy

JEAN COTTRAUX
IVY-MARIE BLACKBURN

Life is lived forwards but understood backwards.
—SØREN KIERKEGAARD

Personality can be construed as a stable and individualized pattern of behaviors, emotions, and cognitions that characterize individual responses to environmental cues. Cognitive therapy for personality disorders, first described by Beck, Freeman, and Associates (1990), is a schema-centered psychotherapy based on an information-processing model of psychopathology. In this chapter we review theories, research, and work pertaining to Beckian cognitive therapy and look at the integration of cognitive therapy with behavioral approaches such as cognitive-behavioral therapy and dialectical behavior therapy (Linehan, 1993a).

THEORETICAL MODEL

Early Antecedents

Antecedents to cognitive therapy can be traced at least to Janet's (1889/1998) seminal work "The Psychological Automatism," which described the repressed memories, automatic thoughts, speech, and behaviors associated with fragmentation of personality that follows trauma. This early scientific account of the unconscious inspired Freud's first studies on hysteria (Freud & Breuer, 1895/1956), which led to the topological and hierarchical models of the per-

sonality. Subsequent developments by Anna Freud (1946) and the ego-psychology school (Hartmann, 1958) stressed the importance of adaptation to reality through ego defense mechanisms. These were later reconceptualized by cognitive psychologists as coping cognitive strategies (Monat & Lazarus, 1991).

Perhaps the most powerful influence on the development of cognitive therapy was personal construct theory (Kelly, 1955). According to Kelly, individuals behave as if they were scientists trying to predict events in their lives. They do this by forming hypotheses about the world using personal constructs. These constructs are used to interpret and predict events including interpersonal events involving self or others. The idea of personal construct is similar to the concept of schema as used later in cognitive therapy. Personal constructs are bipolar cognitive structures: Events are classified or anticipated using paired opposites (e.g., bad–good, fair–unfair, and lovable–unlovable). When a construct is used to construe an event, one pole is the conscious or emergent pole and the other is the unconscious or implicit pole. For instance, kindness may be the emergent pole in a verbal communication, but hostility may appear in nonverbal behaviors. The two poles may be recognized by an observer such as a therapist, but they are not part of the patient's awareness.

Constructs vary in stability or permeability. Permeable constructs change readily with experience whereas impermeable constructs are more fixed. Constructs are relatively stable because they influence what is noticed and the way events are interpreted. For this reason they tend to function as self-fulfilling prophecies. Kelly was able to validate some of his ideas about the nature and organization of cognitive structure by using factor analysis, especially the notion of emergent versus implicit pole of the constructs. Pathological personality involves extensive use of maladaptive constructs, the absence of suitable constructs to process personal experience, and a construct system that is impermeable or inflexible.

Schemas and Personality

At the core of the cognitive model is the concept of schema. This concept represents an extension to the domain of psychopathology of the work of cognitively oriented psychologists (Neisser, 1976; Piaget, 1964). Schemas are deep, unconscious cognitive structures seated in long-term memory that give meaning to events. Segal (1988) defined schemas as "organized elements of past reactions and experience that form a relatively cohesive and persistent body of knowledge capable of guiding subsequent perception and appraisals." According to Beck (1967), schemas account for repetitive themes in free associations, automatic thoughts, mental images, and dreams; schemas can be inactive at certain points and activated by environmental cues at other times.

Schemas, like personal constructs, are used to interpret and understand oneself and the world. They are used to impose meaning on events and to control responses from the behavioral, motivational, emotional, attention, and memory systems. Errors or distortions in the ways events are interpreted through the use of dysfunctional schemas or in the way information is processed create cognitive vulnerabilities that predispose to specific disorders.

Alford and Beck (1997) distinguished three levels of cognition: (1) the preconscious or automatic level, which is represented by automatic thoughts; (2) the conscious level; and (3) the metacognitive level which produces realistic, adaptive, or rational responses. Similarly, Cottraux and Blackburn (1995) described three levels to information processing that are relevant to understanding personality disorder (see Figure 18.1). The first level consists of *cognitive schemas* that store postulates and basic assumptions that are used to interpret information. With personality disorder these schemas tend to be maladaptive, having their origin in dysfunctional relationships. Schemas influence the information that is selected for attention. Only information that is consistent with schemas is processed to full awareness. This process is referred to as tunnelization. The second level consists of *cognitive processes or operations*. At this level cognitive distortions occur that include arbitrary inference, selective abstraction, personalization, and overgeneralization. The use of cognitive heuristics instead of hypotheticodeductive thought reflects the preponderance of "top-down" cognitive processes over "bottom-up" processes. Hence assimilation of experience to the content

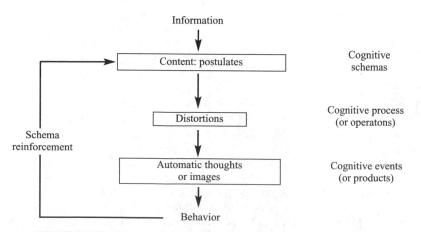

FIGURE 18.1. Information-processing model (Cottraux & Blackburn, 1995).

of a schema predominates over accommodation of a schema to the facts of experience. At the third level, *cognitive processes* translate the deep structure (i.e., the schema) into surface structure, namely, preconscious automatic thoughts. Automatic thoughts are cognitive products or events, operationally defined as inner monologues, dialogues, or images that are not conscious unless the person's attention is focused on them.

The maintenance of schemas is similar to a self-fulfilling prophecy: The schema initiates behaviors that lead to consequences that confirm the schema. For instance, the dysfunctional cognitions about distrust held by a person with paranoia tend to trigger retaliation from other people which confirms the mistrust schema and the general postulate: "All people are potential enemies, if I don't get them first, they'll get me sooner or later." Such a schema may be acquired in early experiences of deception or abuse, familial isolation, intrafamilial paranoia, bellicose adaptation to survival challenges during war, or social conflicts, but it is maintained by the way that it influences attention, the way information is interpreted, and responses made on the basis of this interpretation. Figure 18.1 shows the three levels of cognitions and the reinforcement loop that maintains the schema.

Schemas, Constellations, and Modes

Schemas are stored in long-term memory. The are not conscious but rather latent structures that are triggered by events that recall the interactions that shaped them. Schemas that are oriented toward processing related information are grouped into constellations. These constellations are in turn grouped into modes or subsystems of the cognitive organization that enhance adaptive fitness (i.e., survival, maintenance, or breeding). Hence, Beck, Emery, and Greenberg (1985) described several modes: narcissistic, hostility, fear or danger, dependency, self-enhancing, and erotic. These modes represent the phylogenic underpinnings of personality as shaped by environmental influences. Because most of the events that influence personality are interpersonal and reflect the prolonged influence of significant others during childhood and adolescence, schemas can be activated by trivial everyday events or more dramatic life events related to developmental phases such as professional achievement, loving relationship, dependence/independence problems, separation, social dominance and submission, grief, aging, illness, or adaptation to social and economical circumstances.

Cognitive Shift and Pervasive Effects of Schemas

Schemas associated with personality disorder are more pervasive, enduring, stable, and rigid than schemas underlying Axis I disorders. They also tend to hinder the use of more functional schemas. The prepotency of these maladaptive schemas may result in their generalization over time to situations that are less and less related to the original situations that shaped them. Schemas may also spread from Axis II to Axis I syndromes when personality disorders are associated with Axis I syndromes, leading to an increase in the severity of symptoms. For instance, a schema of dependency will predominate over more healthy schemas and trigger panic attacks (fear of being alone), then agoraphobic avoidance and the search for a protective companion, and eventually depression stemming from the fear of being rejected (see Figure 18.2). This generalization has been referred to as the "cognitive shift."

COGNITIVE APPROACHES TO PERSONALITY DISORDER

The theory underlying cognitive therapy for personality disorders follows the same principles as theories developed for mood and anxiety disorders (Beck, Rush, Shaw, & Emery, 1979; Beck et al., 1985). In this section we briefly review the specific approaches to per-

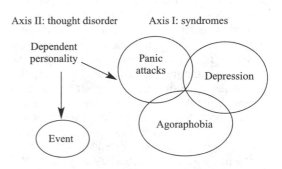

FIGURE 18.2. Preponderance of personality schemas: The cognitive shift.

sonality disorder proposed by Beck et al. (1990) and Young (1990, 1994). We also discuss Linehan's (1993a) dialectical behavior therapy from a cognitive perspective. There are, however, other approaches that warrant mention.

Layden, Newman, Freeman, and Morse (1993) for example, developed a cognitive therapy for borderline personality disorder that incorporated the developmental stages described by Erickson (1963) and Piaget (1952, 1964) into their description of core schemas. They suggest the borderline states may involve a regression to earlier cognitive stages when the patient is confronted with emotional problems. For example, the *sensorimotor* stage (0–2 years), which involves elementary inborn motor responses as sucking and grasping, is characterized by egocentrism, lack of empathy, and lack of object permanence. Regression to this stage may lead to dependency, enmeshment, fear of engulfment, a sense of entitlement, and excessive demands on others. Similarly, the *preoperational* stage (2–7 years) is characterized by self-centering, lack of ability to seriate, magical thinking with confusion between inner and outer world, thought–action fusion, animism, and affective realism. Patients regressed to this stage present vacillations between opposing schemas, emotional reasoning, or magical thinking as opposed to logical thinking. This stage reflects dichotomous thinking and vacillation between opposing poles of schemas. The stage of *concrete logical operations* is characterized by the development of practical logical thinking and appearance of inductive reasoning (7–12 years). Finally, the stage of the *abstract logical operations* is characterized by the development of abstract thinking, hypotheticodeductive reasoning, reasoning in cooperating several factors, meta-thought, and mathematical thoughts (beyond 12 years). The patient with borderline personality disorder may show alteration of logical operations and present lack of inductive and deductive reasoning, inability to see alternatives, lack of meta-thought or theory construction. However, the cognitive regression may be limited. The borderline patient is capable of using logical Piagetian operations when working, for instance, but he or she may regress to a preoperational or sensorimotor stage when faced with emotional problems. The therapist has to be aware of the stage of cognitive regression of the borderline patient to adapt his or her interventions.

Beck's Model

Beck et al. (1990) described a cognitive approach to treating personality based on clinical experience that places greater emphasis on the central role of early schemas or core beliefs than did cognitive models of the affective disorders. This theoretical development takes into account the long-term, rigid, and pervasive psychological dysfunctions shown by patients with personality disorders. They offer a genetic and evolutionary view in which different personality types are considered to reflect alternative behavioral, cognitive, and emotional strategies that were selected over the course of evolution because of their survival value. Due to the variability in the gene pool, however, some individuals show extreme variations in these types or patterns that may have been adaptive for our remote ancestors but which are considered maladaptive in the contemporary world. Some of these strategies lead to personality disorder. Examples of these strategies include excessive help seeking in dependent personality disorder and excessive predatory strategies in antisocial personality disorder. Beck and colleagues view personality disorders as demonstrating typical overdeveloped and underdeveloped strategies. Thus, in dependent personality disorder, help seeking and clinging are over-developed strategies and self-sufficiency is undeveloped (Beck et al., 1990, p. 42).

These phylogenetic programs determine the way individuals process information and their affective, motivational and behavioral reactions. It is assumed that from birth, environmental influences function by increasing or dampening the expression of these innate tendencies. For example, a clinging baby who demands continuous attention may elicit more care and protection from his or her mother than the other siblings. The infant's behaviors are reinforced and may lead to a form of overdependence that persists into adulthood when such behaviors are no longer adaptive.

The innate tendencies described previously may lead to specific belief systems, especially if the individual experiences particular reinforcing events at vulnerable times (usually childhood) or innate tendencies are repeatedly reinforced. These belief structures or schemas fulfill the same role as schemas associated with depression (Beck et al., 1979) but they are more long lasting, pervasive, and generalized than schemas found in Axis I disorders. In a depressed patient, the schema "I am worthless" may apply only to certain aspects of life and will not be active when the patient recovers. Whereas in a patient with personality disorder, the schema "I am worthless" will be more easily triggered and applied to most experiences.

Figure 18.3 describes the way schemas operate in personality disorders. In the example shown, the core schema "I am incompetent" is used to interpret a wide range of experiences. Selective attention to confirming information reinforces the schema and disconfirming evidence is blocked from further processing or distorted. Thus, core schemas are continually reinforced, becoming progressively more rigid and pervasive. Core schemas incorporate conditional schemas or basic assumptions that take the form of "If . . . then . . ." contingencies that are not tested and which lead to behavioral rules or self-injunctions (control schemas) that determine the way individuals function.

In the case of personality disorders, the content of the basic schemas is believed to be limited to five areas: love (e.g., "I am unlovable"), ability (e.g., "I am incompetent"), moral qualities (e.g., "I am an evil person"), normality (e.g., "I am a freak"), and general worth (e.g., "I am worthless"). The different personality

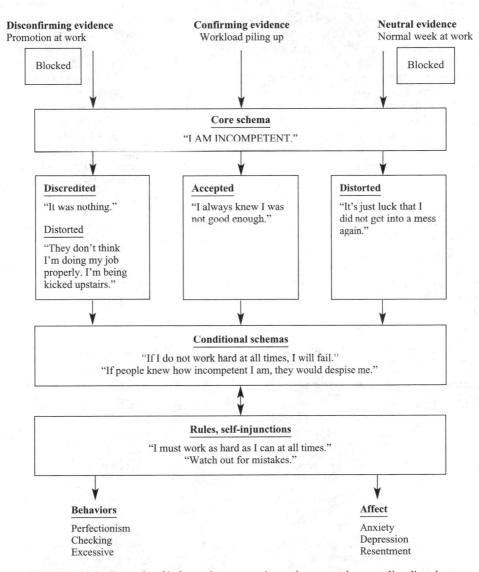

FIGURE 18.3. Example of information processing, schemas, and personality disorders.

disorders are differentiated by the conditional and control schemas the individual developed to cope with his or her core schema. Table 18.1 provides an example of how the core schema "I am unlovable" may lead to different personality disorders.

Young's Theory of Early Maladaptive Schemas

Young (1990; Young & Klosko, 1994; Young & Lindemann 1992), while following the approach of Beck et al. (1990), places greater emphasis to early maladaptive schemas and the processes that contribute to schema inflexibility. Unlike Beck and colleagues, he does not discuss the schemas associated with each DSM-IV personality disorder but, rather, lists typical dysfunctional schemas and attempts to demonstrate how they relate to the individual's developmental history. Young also attaches more emphasis to affects associated to core schemas than does Beck, and hence he advocates the use of interventions to effect emotional change. Of particular interest is Young's explanation of the processes that maintain the rigidity of schemas. He delineates three processes:

1. *Schema maintenance.* The cognitive processes described in Figure 18.1 involving selective attention to confirmatory evidence and the neglect or minimization of contradictory evidence ensure the stability of dysfunctional schema. The persistence of self-defeating behaviors, which may have been adaptive in the past, also contributes to schema maintenance

though repetition of the same negative experiences. For example, the actions of a woman who divorces her violent, alcoholic husband and remarries the same type of individual help to maintain the schema "I am worthless, I cannot do anything right."

2. *Schema avoidance.* Schemas associated with intense negative affects tend to be avoided. A variety of cognitive, affective, and behavioral strategies may be used for this purpose. *Cognitive avoidance* may involve either automatic or volitional attempts to block thoughts and images that trigger schema. Patients may say that they do not want to discuss a particular topic, have forgotten all details of their childhood, and have gone blank, or they may engage in compulsory activities and experiences including depersonalization and derealization. *Affective avoidance* strategies include not having any feelings, feeling empty, engaging in self-harm, or experiencing psychosomatic symptoms. *Behavioral avoidance* strategies are more evident, involving avoidance of situations that may trigger the schema.

3. *Schema compensation.* This involves the occurrence of cognitive and behavioral patterns that are the opposite from those one would predict from the early maladaptive schema that are expected to be present given the patient's developmental history. This concept is similar to the psychodynamic concept of reaction formation. For example, an excessively dependent individual may develop self-protective strategies involving excessive autonomy and a refusal to accept help and advice. Or, an individual lacking self-esteem due to affective deprivation in

TABLE 18.1. Example of Core Schemas, Conditional Beliefs, and Behavioral Strategies in Personality Disorders

Core schema	Conditional schema	Strategies/control schema	Personality disorder
"I am unlovable."	"If I don't do everything people want, they will reject me and I will be alone."	"Keep your wishes to yourself. Make sure to be with others at all time."	Dependent
"I am unlovable."	"If people get to know me they will look down on me."	"Avoid people. Don't let anybody too close."	Avoidant
"I am unlovable."	"If I'm not special, then I'm nothing and nobody will want to know me."	"Use others, behave as if you're the best.	Narcissistic
"I am unlovable."	"If anything goes wrong, they will blame me even if I'm innocent."	"Watch out for others. Keep to the rules."	Paranoid

childhood may develop narcissistic attitudes. Compensation strategies are partially successful attempts to challenge early maladaptive schema, but they may become dysfunctional when overcompensation creates new problems. They also mask core beliefs, making them difficult to identify and modify.

Schema-maintaining processes have evident benefits in that they help patients to avoid pain. However, they also incur costs in terms of their effect on adaptive interpersonal functioning, although these costs are rarely considered. Young (1994) developed the Schema Questionnaire to assess 16 kinds of schemas organized into five problem areas: disconnection and rejection, impaired autonomy and performance, impaired limits, other directedness, and overvigilance and inhibition. Young offers a wealth of clinical experience to support his propositions. The themes he describes are easily recognizable from clinical data, but they probably lack parsimony and need further study to reduce them to basic core themes.

Dialectical Behavior Therapy

Dialectical behavior therapy (Linehan, 1993a) is an eclectic form of psychotherapy that combines group and individual therapy designed specifically to treat patients with borderline personality disorder. The approach uses behavioral techniques such as contingency management, flooding in imagination, problem solving, contracting strategies, and social skills training. Cognitive modification is also used to promote more effective management of affects and impulses and to change the dichotomous thinking style that is said to characterize borderline personality disorder. Emotion relabeling techniques and structured exercises are employed to modify dysfunctional assumptions and beliefs (see Robins, Ivanoff, & Linehan, Chapter 21, this volume, for more details).

A key difference from standard cognitive therapy lies in the use of the concept of "dialectical" to understand pathology and guide interventions. The idea borrowed some of the basic tenets from the Marxist principle that contradictions between social classes are to be solved through a dialectic synthesis that will lead mankind toward a more harmonious society. Applying this approach to psychopathology, Linehan assumed that the patient with borderline personality disorder vacillates between contradictory poles without being able to find a dialectic solution. She speculates that the patient's suffering is often invalidated by a competitive and individualistic social environment which is unable to understand, accept, and fulfill the patient's basic needs for regression and fusion with others. Vacillations typically occur between vulnerability and social invalidation, passivity and apparent competency, and crisis and inhibition of suffering. The therapist's task is to help the patient move from vacillation between these alternative modes to a synthesis. This movement is achieved by helping the patient accept him- or herself prior to change. Acceptance by the therapist of the patient's contradictions is a basic attitude for therapeutic effectiveness. For instance, in the case of suicidal ideas, the therapist is advised not to argue or criticize but, rather, to discuss alternatives without denying the possibility of suicide or its value as a solution to life problems

The therapeutic strategies incorporate mindfulness training—an intervention that combines cognitive and behavioral strategies with Buddhist philosophy. The intent is to redirect attention and promote a sense of distance from emotional turmoil, thereby diminishing tendencies to act out. The patient is invited to differentiate the emotional from the rational mind and to integrate the two to achieve a state of the "wise mind." Meditation is a key technique. Attention to the primary object of observation (breath, sound, thoughts, bodily sensation) is developed through relaxation or Hatha-Yoga. The patient focuses attention on that object and if attention wanders he or she simply notices the event without judgment and returns to the focus of awareness. If fear, anxiety, or pain arises, the patient just observes the feeling as it occurs. To use the Teflon pan metaphor: Experiences come into mind and slip out. When fear, anxiety, or pain subsides, the patient returns to the object of attention. The thinking process itself is observed without personal involvement. Then the patient puts experience into words and may reach the conclusion that thoughts are impermanent mind events, or just passing fancies which are not accurate, and that all thoughts are of equal value. This is obviously a clinical application of Buddha's "Four Noble Truths": (1) life is filled with suffering, (2) the source of suffering is craving, (3) suffering ends when craving ceases, (4) the way to end suffering and craving is the eightfold path, namely, right understanding, right thought, right speech, right action, right livelihood, right effort, right mindfulness and right concentration (Mikulas, 1978).

Unlike standard cognitive behavior therapy, in which dysfunctional beliefs are evaluated and challenged through Socratic discussion, mindfulness training emphasizes the redirection of the patient's attention towards nonconflicted thoughts or feelings. This is an application to psychotherapy of the dialectical principle of "winning through nonresistance" described in Taoist philosophy (Tao Te Ching, 1994).

EMPIRICAL EVALUATION

Cognitive therapy for personality disorders was only introduced in the in the 1990s, hence, evaluation is at an early stage. Nevertheless, early studies are encouraging.

Personality Factors in Cognitive Treatments for Axis I Disorders

Several uncontrolled studies have looked at the effects of personality disorders or traits on cognitive treatment. Two studies on agoraphobia, showed that personality disorder has a negative impact on the outcome (Chambless, Renneberg, Goldstein, & Gracely, 1992; Cottraux, Mollard, Bouvard, & Guerin, 1991). On the other hand, Dressen, Arntz, Luttels, and Sallaerts (1994) found no relation between the presence of personality disorder and outcome for various anxiety disorders. In one study on depression, the personality trait of sociotropy predicted a better outcome with group cognitive therapy whereas autonomy predicted a better outcome with individual cognitive therapy (Zettle, Haflich, & Reynolds, 1992). McKay, Neziroglu, Todaro, and Yaryura-Tobias (1996) in a study on obsessive–compulsive disorder, found that after behavior therapy the mean number of personality diagnoses decreased from 4 to 3. They also found a correlation between the personality change and the decrease of the Yale–Brown Obsessive–Compulsive Scale (Y-BOCS) score.

Tyrer, Seivewright, Ferguson, Murphy, and Johnson (1993) compared a pharmacological treatment, a 6-week abridged cognitive-behavioral therapy program, and a self-management program in various mood and anxiety disorders. The three treatments demonstrated a similar global effectiveness. At 2-year follow-up,

pharmacological treatment had a better effect in patients with comorbid personality disorder. Paradoxically, the two psychological treatments were less effective in patients with personality disorders. However, the psychological treatments were not designed to modify personality problems and the cognitive intervention was less than optimal.

In the National Institute of Mental Health study, Shea et al. (1990) compared four groups: placebo with clinical support, imipramine with clinical support, cognitive therapy, and interpersonal therapy. Globally there was no difference between the three active treatments which were superior to placebo with clinical support condition, at least on some measures. However, patients with higher levels of depression responded better to antidepressants or interpersonal therapy than to cognitive therapy. Seventy-four percent of the patients had a personality disorder. There was a trend for cognitive therapy to have better outcome in patients with personality disorder, but this trend was not significant. Patients without personality disorder did better with the three other therapeutic conditions. This may suggest that a schema-based therapy can do better for patients whose depressive schemas are related to personality disorders. These outcomes are at variance with the pessimism of Mays (1975) and Rush and Shaw (1983), who suggested that cognitive therapy for depression was less effective in patients with personality disorder.

Single-Case Studies

Early evaluations of cognitive-behavioral therapy were based on single-case designs. The first study by Turkat and Levin (1984) and Turkat and Maisto (1985) treated 35 consecutive single cases using behavioral techniques (systematic desensitization, exposure, contingencies management) and cognitive restructuring and self-statement modification. They reported some positive outcomes in patients with narcissistic, avoidant, dependent, and paranoid disorders. Although modest, these results were encouraging. Other authors reported single-case studies of specific personality disorders (Beck, et al., 1990; Cottraux & Blackburn, 1995; Freeman & Dattilio, 1992; Pretzer & Fleming, 1989). Chernen and Friedman (1993), using a repeated measurement single-case design on four subjects showed that behavior led to improvement in personality disorder.

Naturalistic Studies of Group Cognitive-Behavioral Therapy

Three French studies of the use of cognitive-behavioral therapy for various personality disorders, found concomitant effects on Axis I and II disorders and/or personality traits (Cungi, 1995; Fanget and Chambon, 1994; Guérin, Bouvard, Cottraux, & Sechaud, 1994). Improvement was maintained at follow-ups ranging from 6 months to 2 years.

Controlled Studies

Woody, McLellan, Luborsky, and O'Brien (1985) presented a study of 110 patients with drug addictions. They compared three treatment conditions: counseling, counseling plus cognitive therapy, and counseling plus psychodynamic psychotherapy. They studied four subgroups: (1) isolated opiate addiction, (2) opiate addiction plus depression, (3) opiate addiction plus depression plus antisocial personality, and (4) opiate addiction plus antisocial personality. In depressed patients with antisocial personality, cognitive therapy and psychodynamic therapy were both more effective than counseling but demonstrated no difference in their outcomes. Psychopathic personality without concomitant depression was a negative predictor of effectiveness, whatever the treatment. Moreover, in both cognitive and psychodynamic therapy, the quality of the therapeutic alliance and the therapist's strict adherence to the therapeutic model and management were related to outcomes (Luborsky, McLellan, Woody, O'Brien, & Auerbach, 1985).

A controlled study (Linehan, Armstrong, Suarez, Allmon, & Heard, 1991) on borderline patients included 44 patients in two groups and compared dialectic behavior therapy, as described previously, with treatment as usual: supportive or psychodynamic therapies in the community. The group receiving dialectic behavior therapy showed a significantly lower rate of dropouts and parasuicidal behavior. Abuse of medication or street drugs also decreased significantly. Nevertheless, at the end of treatment the two groups did not differ in depression or other symptoms. Change was maintained at a 1-year posttreatment follow-up. At this point there was a significant decrease of pathological anger, suicidal and parasuicidal behaviors, and days spent as inpatients and a better social adjustment (Linehan, Heard, & Armstrong, 1993).

Dialectic behavior therapy is lengthy and relatively expensive, but this is largely outweighed by the cost saved from decreased hospitalization (Heard, 1994).

The effectiveness of group assertiveness training in avoidant personality has been demonstrated in a controlled study by Alden and Capreol (1993), who randomized patients with avoidant personality disorder into four groups: (1) graded exposure, (2) interpersonal skills training, (3) intimacy skills training, and (4) waiting list. Social skills training consisted of blend of cognitive and behavioral techniques. The three active treatments were better than the waiting-list control. Patients having problems with anger and suspiciousness benefited more from exposure therapy. Patients with interpersonal problems related to the feeling of being controlled did better in social skills training, especially in the group receiving intimacy skills training.

Carroll, Rounsaville, Gordon, et al. (1994; Carroll, Rounsaville, Nich, et al., 1994) studied the effects of cognitive-behavioral therapy compared with clinical support, both with placebo or desipramine, in drug addicts. Treatment lasted 12 weeks. The dependent variable was relapse prevention in cocaine addicts followed as outpatients. Forty-nine percent of the patients presented a diagnosis of antisocial personality and 65% had another personality disorder. Cognitive-behavioral therapy demonstrated relapse prevention effects at 1 year after the end of the therapeutic period. Results were similar in patients with antisocial personality and in patients with other personality disorders. No measure of personality change was reported.

GENERAL PRINCIPLES AND MODELS OF CHANGE

Cognitive therapy for personality disorders involves principles similar to those developed to treat Axis I disorders, although some changes are needed to accommodate the distinctive features of these disorders. By definition, personality disorders are pervasive, generalized, and long-standing. Typically they require longer-term treatment than the 12–16 sessions usually required to treat depressive illness. In general, treatment lasts 1 to 2 years although sessions need not be as frequent as they are when treating Axis I disorders. Our experience is that sessions at 3 week intervals are sometimes best. This gives the patient time to collect data and engage in behavioral tests between sessions. This time interval also helps to contain the high level of painful emotions that are often aroused during therapy sessions. The longer treatment time is required because it is often necessary to treat the features of Axis I disorders that are frequently present before addressing longer-term difficulties. This prolonged time allows the patient to achieve a sense of control, to grasp the general model and style of cognitive therapy, and to establish a trusting therapeutic relationship.

The problems encountered in therapy follow from the theoretical foundations described earlier. Personality-disordered patients, unlike most Axis I patients, have difficulty accessing thoughts and images because of their avoidance strategies and difficulty accessing feelings, which is often an even greater obstacle to therapy. The problems they present are multiple and changes in behavior are often resisted, again because of avoidance or because they are so deeply entrenched. Patients often show noncompliance with homework assignments, difficulties can arise in the therapeutic relationship, and therapist motivation may be affected by the slow progress and possible lack of success with similar patients in the past; and patient motivation may be low because of the belief that change is not possible. Termination of therapy may be difficult because as therapy is prolonged, the patient may attribute improvement to regular contacts with the therapist. Continually reviewing termination dates and ensuring that changes are attributed to the patient's own efforts are ways of counteracting excessive dependence.

The general principles for the cognitive therapist who treats patients with personality disorders may be summarized as follows:

1. *Attend to the therapeutic relationship.* Patients are likely to display the same dysfunc-

tional behaviors and attitudes in their relationship with the therapist as they do in their real lives. For example, if the patient exhibits extreme dependence, the therapist must be careful about fostering more dependency by being excessively nurturing; if the patient has problems in setting limits, the therapist needs to be firm regarding timing of interviews or defining acceptable and unacceptable behaviors in the therapy situation; if the patient is mistrustful, the therapist needs to be particularly attentive to fulfilling promises, being on time, and not missing sessions.

2. *Arrange for peer supervision.* Treating personality disorder is difficult and many frustrations are likely to occur during therapy. These problems occur for a variety of reason: the therapist and patient share similar schemas, the therapist attributes lack of progress to his or her ineptitude, and the therapist reacts to problem patient behavior, including noncompliance with homework.

3. *Set realistic standards for therapy.* Beck et al. (1990) identify four different levels of change in therapy, which can be seen as a continuum (see Figure 18.4).

Schema reconstruction is the most ambitious and rarely achieved form of change. It consists of replacing a dysfunctional schema with a new, more adaptive schema. An analogy would be demolishing a building which is no longer functional and replacing it with a totally new building. Building a new schema has been the aim of many therapeutic approaches, particularly psychoanalysis. However, it is often an unattainable goal because of the investment of time required from both patient and therapist. It is, in any case, probably not even a desirable goal to change the schema "I am 100% unlovable" or "I am 100% worthless" to its polar extreme "I am 100% lovable" or "I am 100% worthwhile," which would lead to new problems.

Schema modification is a more achievable goal and it is the usual goal adopted in cogni-

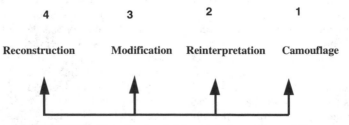

FIGURE 18.4. Four levels of change in schema-focused therapy.

tive therapy. To remain with the architectural analogy, instead of demolishing and rebuilding, aspects of the building are modified to make it more functional. Thus, if the patient believes that he or she is 100% worthless, the aim would perhaps be to decrease this belief to 20–30 %.

Schema reinterpretation does not involve changing the schema, but helping the patient to use the schema in appropriate and adaptive ways. For example, patients with obsessive–compulsive personality disorder may believe that they are "worthless" because they are unable to do their job perfectly and pay full attention to details. Such individuals may be able to use their perfectionism in a job that values attention to details but has no time pressures—say in data analysis, computer programming, or checking the work of others. Or, patients with histrionic personality disorder patient may be encouraged to take a post, which fills their need to be center stage (e.g., teacher, actor, or performer).

Schema camouflage is the least ambitious of goal and may need to be adopted when neither reconstruction nor modification or reinterpretation is possible. The patient can be trained in behaviors that camouflage the maladaptive schema. For example, schizoid patients may be given social skills training to hide beliefs about being "different" or "social misfits." This training may involve encouraging them to look at people when talking to them, saying "good morning" when arriving at the office, smiling, and so on. The building analogy would be simply hiding the worst aspects of a room with a suitable decor.

4. *Careful conceptualization of the case.* It is of primary importance to conceptualize the case in detail before embarking on the treatment of personality disorders. More attention is given to developmental history, especially early experiences in the family and at school, than with Axis I disorders. Sometimes it is helpful to search for particular sayings in the family or particular occasions which were registered by the child as key experiences. For example, a patient remembered his mother saying on numerous occasions, "You have to work harder because you're not as able as your brothers." A young woman remembered her father saying, "Poor Jane, you'll never find a husband because of your looks."

Schemas are often formed at a preverbal developmental stage. It is, therefore, useful to look for mental images or associated sensations to elicit memories. As when formulating Axis I disorders, the therapist looks for common themes in the patient's discourse and records of automatic thoughts, the meaning of events, personal rules, rules for others, typical behaviors, and affective responses. Once the therapist obtains a relatively coherent picture from the patient's developmental history, key experiences and memories, the therapeutic relationship, and basic cognitive therapy methods, he or she tentatively develops a conceptualization and shares it with the patient. Figure 18.5 presents a typical conceptualization. We find a circular model more meaningful than a horizontal model because it shows clearly how the patient is caught in a vicious circle, and several examples obtained from previous discussions can be included in one diagram. Possible methods of change also suggest themselves and can be added to the diagram. The preliminary conceptualization diagram is usually incomplete and to modified after more guided discovery and as therapy progresses. This is a task shared by patient and therapist.

STRATEGIES AND TECHNIQUES FOR CHANGE

Explanation to Patients

The role of schemas in information processing and the factors which maintain the schema need to be carefully discussed with the patient. This discussion engenders hope because it creates the possibility of change. If the patient and the therapist share an understanding of what contributed to the genesis of the problems, then change methods suggest themselves and the belief "I am like this; it is in my genes and therefore I cannot change" can be reevaluated. We find the information-processing model presented in Figure 18.1 invaluable when explaining the role of schema, especially if the model is made specific by incorporating real examples. Padesky (1990) suggests the analogy of self-prejudice as an example of processing bias that can also be used to explain the way a schema influences automatic thoughts and emotions. The patient is asked to give an example of prejudice in a friend or relative which he or she does not share. Through questioning and discussion it can then be demonstrated how prejudiced individuals ignore, minimize, or distort disconfirming information. It can also be

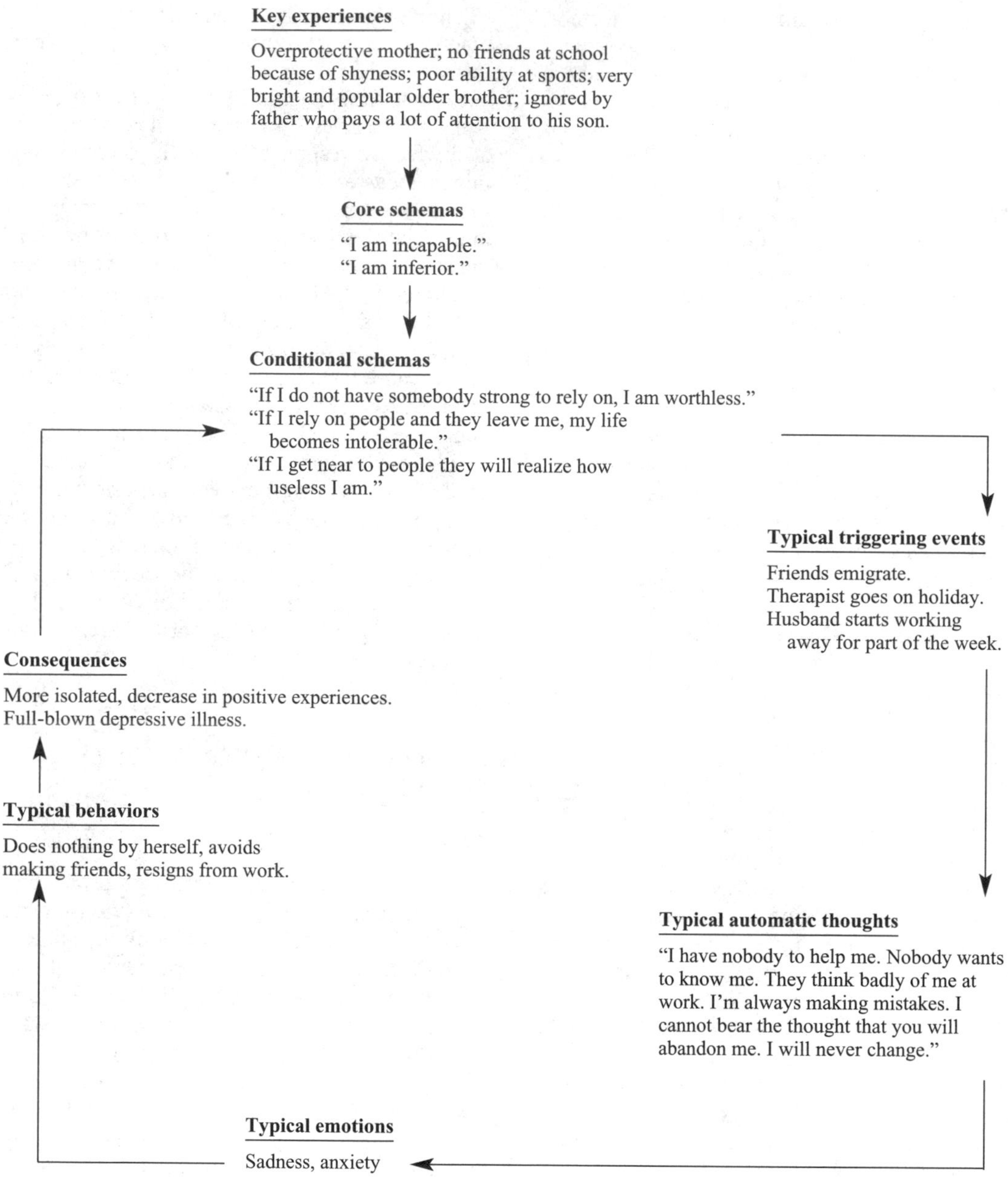

Key experiences

Overprotective mother; no friends at school
because of shyness; poor ability at sports; very
bright and popular older brother; ignored by
father who pays a lot of attention to his son.

Core schemas

"I am incapable."
"I am inferior."

Conditional schemas

"If I do not have somebody strong to rely on, I am worthless."
"If I rely on people and they leave me, my life
    becomes intolerable."
"If I get near to people they will realize how
    useless I am."

Typical triggering events

Friends emigrate.
Therapist goes on holiday.
Husband starts working
    away for part of the week.

Consequences

More isolated, decrease in positive experiences.
Full-blown depressive illness.

Typical behaviors

Does nothing by herself, avoids
making friends, resigns from work.

Typical automatic thoughts

"I have nobody to help me. Nobody wants
to know me. They think badly of me at
work. I'm always making mistakes. I
cannot bear the thought that you will
abandon me. I will never change."

Typical emotions

Sadness, anxiety

FIGURE 18.5. Conceptualization of a case of avoidant and dependent personality disorder.

demonstrated how avoidance strategies maintain the prejudice and how the breakdown of the prejudice requires the person to face a large amount of disconfirming information, to begin to process information in a less biased way, and, most important, to engage in different behaviors to maximize the effects of the new learning experiences. The prejudice model is particularly effective because prejudice is common and

the patient has to decenter (i.e., see the world through somebody else's eyes). This distance often makes the issues clearer.

Another helpful analogy is to compare a dysfunctional schema to looking at oneself through a distorting mirror or wearing distorting glasses. Change involves altering the mirror or lens. Change may also be compared to visiting a foreign land where ways of thinking and behaving are totally different. Young (1990) draws an analogy between early maladaptive schemas and viruses which erupt from time to time to which the patient needs to be immunized. The important point about these analogies is that they help to make the explanation of schemas less abstract and more immediately meaningful.

Therapy is also more likely to be successful after the patient has mastered such basic cognitive therapy concepts as monitoring negative emotions, identification and evaluation of negative automatic thoughts, and identification and modification of dysfunctional behaviors that may be contributing to maintaining problems.

Change Methods

Methods of change are subsumed under four categories: cognitive, behavioral, emotional, and interpersonal (see Beck et al., 1990; Cottraux & Blackburn, 1995; Padesky, 1994; Young, 1990; for more detailed discussion).

Cognitive Methods

These include methods used in brief cognitive therapy for Axis I disorders and additional techniques developed to treat the rigid and pervasive schemas found in personality disorders. It is essential for the therapist to be inductive and nonconfrontational, using guided discovery or Socratic dialogue. The aim is for the patient to begin to process evidence that disconfirms the schema, leading to cognitive, emotional, and behavioral changes.

Defining Negative Schemas. Negative schemas are global and poorly defined and applied erroneously and pervasively. Consider the schema "I am totally worthless." What does it mean to be "totally worthless"? Who is worthwhile and who is worthless? Does the patient have examples of people he or she considers worthwhile or worthless, be it in his or her own life or historical or literary characters? When global schemas are broken down into the idiosyncratic meanings that the patient attaches to them, it becomes easier to apply the revaluation and modification methods described in the other sections.

Examining the Evidence for and against a Schema. Therapist and patient examine all the evidence that the patient has accumulated over the years that lead to the inescapable conclusion found in such schemas as "I am an evil person" or "I am worthless." This evidence is then questioned. For example, are there alternative interpretations of a particular event or of some key person's behaviors or sayings? What processing error is or was the patient making (personalization, magnification, selective abstraction, overgeneralization, arbitrary inference)? Contrary or disconfirming evidence is then reviewed. This process will need several sessions, with appropriate home assignments, as it has to be thorough. As disconfirming evidence will, by definition, have been disregarded or totally blocked, therapist and patient need to be very detailed in their search, to ensure that the same disregarding processes are not continued.

Demonstrating That Invalidating Experiences Have Not Been Considered. Once the foregoing information is gathered, the therapist can refer to the information-processing and prejudice models discussed earlier to demonstrate how contrary evidence has been disregarded, hence reinforcing the validity of the model.

Continuum Method. This is probably the most useful cognitive method, which was first developed for the treatment of personality disorders. Patients are asked to rate on a continuum of 0–100 representing their schema. For example:

0————————————————100
Worthlessness
0————————————————100
Worthwhile

They may then rate others whom they have identified as worthwhile or worthless. When the global schema has been broken into several constituents, these constituents are also represented as continua on which patients can rate themselves and other individuals again. Worthlessness might be broken down as follows:

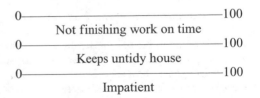

0————————————————100
Not finishing work on time
0————————————————100
Keeps untidy house
0————————————————100
Impatient

It is important to define the poles of the continua carefully to ensure that ratings are not extreme. This method often demonstrates to patients that although they rate themselves at the extreme negative pole on the global continuum, when this is broken down, less negative ratings are made on the detailed continua, and that even individuals whom the patient originally rated as polar opposites (e.g., very worthwhile) do not retain such an extreme positive ratings on the detailed continua. The continuum method is useful in breaking down global thinking and demonstrating bias in information processing. Ratings on the global continuum and detailed continua become standard homework assignments, with ratings being made daily, in the light of evidence that invalidates the schema. This method is also useful in demonstrating that small changes are possible and in establishing realistic goals. When asked to set goals as to where they would like to be on the continuum, patients, in our experience, do not say that they want to be 100% worthwhile. With the process of comparative ratings, most patients opt for about 70–80% of the positive concept.

Reinterpretation of Childhood Experiences. Childhood experiences that may have led to the development of a given schema may be reexamined from the point of view of an adult rather than that of a child. A child does not have the intellectual ability to see the world from other people's points of view, and he or she may make an interpretation of an adult's behaviors and sayings that makes perfect sense to the child but may be erroneous. With careful discussion, the patient may come to form a different and more tolerant view of what a parent has said or done. A different view of parents' motivation and behavior may also be gained by understanding the pressures and influences the parents experienced. The aim is to help the patient to consider that his or her early experiences were not due to an innate deficit but rather are understandable responses to family dynamics or other circumstances external to the individual.

Historical Test of a Schema. This is a version of examining evidence for and against a schema that encompasses the whole life of the patient. For example, if the schema is "I am a bad person," then "badness" would have been there from birth. What evidence is there to con-

firm or disconfirm this. It is important to start with evidence from birth. What evidence, say, from age 0–2, 3–4, 5–10, 11–16, or 17–20 years is there? What does a bad child of 0–2 years do? What is the evidence against? Patients may talk to relatives to obtain evidence; they may read books about child development or look at photo albums. The aim is for the patient to review his or her life in detail to rewrite a more benevolent account. This may require a number of sessions, with very detailed questioning and relevant homework assignments.

Flashcards. Finally, it is useful to encourage the patient to prepare flashcards with statements such as:

"My old belief was. . . ."
"However, I do not believe this any longer, because. . . ."
"My new belief is. . . ."

This flashcard summarizes the main conclusions of therapy and can be used when the old schema threatens to reappear as under highly emotional circumstances. This procedure also prepares the patient for the reemergence of the old schema in particular triggering situations. Old habits die hard and we revert to well-tried old methods when emotionally aroused.

Behavioral Methods

Behavioral methods are essential to modify both conditional and core schemata.

Graded Tasks and Reality Testing. Because avoidant behavioral strategies play an important role in the maintenance of dysfunctional schemata, patients are encouraged to engage in avoided behaviors to test their predictions. The patient who avoids social occasions because of fears of rejection may begin to socialize gradually and record the results. These behavioral experiments need to be carefully planned, predictions must be made, and associated automatic thoughts should be elicited and evaluated.

Acting against Personal Rules. As described earlier, core schemas lead to control schemas and self-injunctions which are adhered to without questions. These rules of conduct can be tested using behavioral experiments that are designed to infringe upon them (e.g., doing a piece of work quicker and less perfectly, saying "no" sometimes instead of always complying with others' demands; talking to people, or not self-harming). The advantages and disadvantages of these rules and the behaviors they entail need to be discussed in sessions and again the new behaviors need careful planning.

Role Plays. Role playing is a helpful way to rehearse the new behaviors, with the therapist acting as model. Through role plays and role reversals, appropriate behaviors can be demonstrated and developed into homework assignments which can be discussed during the following session.

Emotional Methods

Core schemas are highly emotionally charged and formed at a preverbal or prelogical level of intellectual development, making them resistant to purely verbal or behavioral methods of change. Emotional methods of change have been adapted from Gestalt therapy to make changes in implicational as opposed to propositional meanings (Teasdale, 1996).

Psychodrama. Negative schemas that patients attribute to their parents can be erroneous or correct. If the attributions are erroneous, careful examination of various experiences of childhood will demonstrate that less negative interpretations are possible and that the biased conclusions were reached through the thinking of a child and not an adult. In such a case, a reattribution method, as described later, is appropriate. However, if there are real memories of painful experiences, psychodrama can be an effective way to promote change. Various scenes from childhood can be reenacted and restructured. The therapist needs to elicit enough details to know how to play the role of the abusive patient. The therapist then plays the role as harshly as possible and the patient plays him- or herself as a child. Roles are reversed several times until appropriate responses are evoked, the exercise always finishing with the patient playing him- or herself as a child.

The aim is for the adult in the role of child to be able to answer the parent instead of responding as the hurt child who did not have the ability to question the parent's behavior. For example, a patient remembered her mother saying on several occasions that she was "evil" when she had broken a toy or made her younger sister cry. In psychodrama, the adult as a child dares to challenge the mother, to demonstrate that the mother is wrong and that she is not "evil." This method is usually very emotive and requires careful preparation and debriefing. Even reluctant patients get into the role with vigor after practice.

Reattribution of Responsibilities. As indicated in the previous section, a child may have misinterpreted a parent's behavior, leading to the negative self-schema. A useful method to change these attributions is to assign responsibilities using a pie chart. The therapist elicits all possible reasons for the parent's behaviors, including responses to the child's characteristics. In the previous example, the patient may have decided that she was "evil" because her mother was often in tears, often hit her, or ignored her. The therapist elicits all possible reasons for the mother's behavior. These might include the following: mother was depressed, mother had a poor relationship with the child's father, mother had been harshly brought up herself, mother was harassed by bringing up four children, and finally the patient herself was the cause. It is useful to put the patient last on the list to counteract the previous attribution of total responsibility. With careful discussion, the pie is divided into slices of responsibility: say 35% for mother's depression, 30% for relationship with husband, 15% for mother's upbringing, 15% for mother's harassment, leaving 5% for the patient's responsibility. This method questions the global attribution of responsibility to a stable and global characteristic of the self and helps the patient to reappraise early experiences. Following this exercise, a psychodrama can ensue with the patient playing the role of the child discussing with her mother in an assertive but nonaggressive fashion how mother's behavior affected her.

Playing Devil's Advocate. This is another type of role play that is useful to check how reliably the patient's self-image has begun to change. Young (1990) calls this method "point–counterpoint." After explaining the purpose of the exercise, the therapist describes the patient's schema and the patient refutes this idea. Thus, to take the foregoing example, the therapist may say, "Carole, you are an evil person," and the patient counters with arguments to refute the idea. Again, the exercise needs to be repeated several times with role reversals until the patient feels confident in his or her answers. It is evident that this is a rehearsal method which follows considerable amount of previous work.

Interpersonal Methods

Therapeutic Relationship. The importance of the therapeutic relationship in treating personality disorder was stressed earlier. From a cognitive perspective this can be considered a "reparenting" process, with the therapist ensuring that previous maladaptive modes of parenting are not repeated in therapy. These may include overprotectiveness, abusiveness, unreliability, hostility, belittling, lack of respect, and so on. Particular attention needs to be given to emotions triggered in session and to frequent mutual feedback.

Group Therapy. Group therapy is particularly useful to correct unhelpful interpersonal styles. With dialectical behavior therapy, group therapy is used as an adjunct to individual therapy in order to teach social skills, the resolution of conflicts, control of emotions, appropriate reactions to distressing situations, and self-observation. In our experience, four or five joint sessions with a key person in the patient's life are also highly effective.

Consolidation of Therapy

At the end of therapy, several methods may be required to consolidate gains and to train patients in continuing work after active therapy has stopped. The continuum method described earlier can be used throughout therapy. Repeated practice helps to consolidate change. A log of positive experiences kept daily over a long period also helps to maintain a focus on positive, disconfirming evidence. A prediction list can also be used to help the patient to continue to engage in new behaviors. This involves keeping a list of expectations and fears associated with avoided actions that are then evaluated following completion of a new activity in behavioral experiments. This process helps to underscore the lack of validity of the original schema and to reinforce new schema.

PROCESS ISSUES

Several recommendations for implementing a positive therapeutic relationship and an effec-

tive therapeutic process when treating personality disorder have been made by cognitive therapists (Beck et al., 1990; Cottraux & Blackburn, 1995; Layden et al., 1993; Padesky & Greenberger, 1995).

Structuring the Session and the Therapeutic Interaction

Structure is useful because it helps to contain patients' anxiety, disorientation, and confusion and the negative expectations they often have about themselves, the therapist, or the therapy. Having a framework and a formal explanation of the nature of therapy may reduce confusion and create a stable and secure base. A constant length for each session, being on time, and recurrent recapitulations from the therapist helps to create a framework for modifying enduring schemas. This framework may canalize emotional outbursts and reduce the fear of abandonment often found in patients, especially those who have had earlier unsuccessful therapies. Table 18.2 shows the structure for cognitive therapy sessions.

The summary of the session and the elicitation of transference problems should occur at least 10 minutes before the end of the session to allow full consideration. Frequently, issues remain for further discussion and exploration in the next session. To ensure that these issues are not overlooked, the therapist and patient put the unanswered questions or problematic issues on the agenda to be consulted at the beginning of the next session.

Initial Interaction and Schema Elicitation

In some cases, it is important for the therapist to be able to use the initial interview to elicit

---

TABLE 18.2. Cognitive Therapy for Personality Disorder: The Session

1. Agenda: focus on a theme
2. Elicitation of emotions and beliefs
3. Socratic discussion of the schemas
4. Frequent recapitulations and summaries
5. Summary of the session by the patient
6. Feedback on the therapist's interventions; transference and countertransference elicitation and discussion
7. Behavioral experiments to modify the schemas
8. Agenda for the next session

and begin to evaluate the basic personality schema that may manifest itself in a crude and straightforward way in the first interaction. Excerpts from a case study (Cottraux & Blackburn, 1995) exemplify this point.

Theresa, The Busy Businesswoman

Theresa, age 40, consulted after a 2-day assertive training group elsewhere. She said she had been told that she was so unassertive that anybody could take advantage of her. However, she showed herself to be assertive and not at all a social phobic or avoidant person during the interview and psychometric assessment using the Fear Questionnaire. The main features of her personality were anxiety, dramatization, egocentrism, need for important challenges, lofty ideals, and perfectionism in her professional life as a top business executive. But most of all, she argued with the therapist because she would not wait for 2 months before starting therapy. She had decided long in advance that cognitive therapy was the most appropriate treatment for her and that this therapist was the only possible therapist for her. Despite Theresa's flattering interest, the therapist's first intervention was to confront her narcissistic postulate: "If I want something badly, I must have it right now." The therapist used Socratic questioning to explore this schema by asking, "Supposing you were a doctor, what would you do if you had a patient like yourself, demanding to bypass a waiting list." The patient recognized that the waiting list could not be changed unless it was a real emergency. This interaction made it possible for the patient and therapist to agree on a contract and that she would start therapy in 2 months.

At the end of the session, the patient asked the therapist what cognitive therapy was all about. It was easy for the therapist to show that the discussion about the beginning of the therapy had elicited a schema that was frequently active: a schema of entitlement. Confrontation of the schema and a Socratic discussion led to cognitive restructuring and the establishment of a therapeutic alliance based on a mutual agreement respecting both the patient and the therapist. This was indeed cognitive therapy at work.

Subsequent therapy lasted 21 sessions and had a positive outcome. Most of the work centered on the initial schema. The schema of entitlement was a conditional schema compensating an inferiority schema: "I have always been inferior because I am a woman working in a world of machos." Figure 18.6 presents the conceptualization made at the end of Theresa's therapy.

Countertransference

Among the problems encountered in cognitive therapy for personality disorder, although less central than in psychodynamic therapy, countertransference is an important area of inquiry. The fact that therapy is structured does not preclude therapist problems, especially fascination, anger, frustration, sadness, or discouragement. These problems may occur despite the systematic use of feedback at the end of each session to provide an opportunity to discuss the patient's reactions to the therapist's verbal and nonverbal behavior. It does, however, elicit early recognition of negative transference and countertransference, which can be then be used as a therapeutic tool.

Countertransference problems can often be avoided if the therapist takes 5 to 10 minutes after each session to examine his or her own automatic thoughts and to try to understand which schemas have been activated by the patient and uses cognitive restructuring techniques for him- or herself. This also helps to ensure that the therapeutic alliance is developing effectively and that the therapist is maintaining appropriate therapeutic distance. Consultation and supervision are also useful in reducing these problems.

Last but not least, an experienced therapist may have some awareness of the relational traps that are common in treating personality disorder and the role in which he or she is cast by the patient. Although the patient is acting out inflexible relational patterns, the therapist

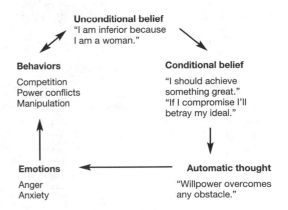

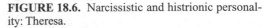

FIGURE 18.6. Narcissistic and histrionic personality: Theresa.

generally has the option of greater relational flexibility than empathy with the problems of the patient. Countertransference may merely be a subjective reflection of the therapist acting out a character in a plot written by the patient's schemas. These roles may be represented by opposing behaviors such as protector versus persecutor, which patients commonly attribute or assign to their therapists. Table 18.3 describes a typical bipolar role in which therapists are commonly cast by patients with various DSM-IV personality disorders. Awareness of these patterns helps to identify the patient's schemas.

Life Scripts, Narratives, and Schemas

The theater metaphor used in the preceding section introduces the concept of life scripts. Most patients' life stories, as told in their narratives, are comparable to literary scripts. Often patients attribute cascades of negative life events provoked by their inflexible schemas to "destiny." Most of the time the life script is hidden (i.e., unconscious) and patients seem trapped in a plot that they do not understand. However, the therapist is able access the global life scripts through specific self-schemas that are more accessible. These schemas may derive from familial, cultural, or subcultural schemas and can be construed as "remakes" of basic screenplays, narratives, or myths (Cottraux & Blackburn, 1995). Figure 18.7 shows the possible relation between life scripts and the patient's narratives.

The practical therapeutic management of pathological life scripts involves several steps.

1. *The therapist should elicit life-scripts through a complete narrative of the life story.*

This narrative helps to draw the therapist's attention to repeated negative events, that may be reminiscent of a "film noir," a "soap opera," or a "tear-jerker." Often, the patient says: "It's the story of my life, it's my destiny." Metaphors and images trigger specific emotions and the narrative generally elicits distress.

2. *Both patient and therapist have to enter into a proper understanding of the life scripts.* At this point the therapist may help the patient to find the hidden meaning of the story. Watching films or reading novels that mirror the patient's life script may help patients understand the plot and stimulate the patients' willingness to accept and change the narrative.

3. *Modifying life scripts requires the use of cognitive techniques discussed earlier.* Change requires a Socratic discussion of the negative and positive consequences of following the script. Consequences of changing the life script are also to be discussed. This is an important point because the patient generally experiences painful feelings of disillusionment that increases resistance to change. A pathological life script is frequently based on self-deceptions that are related to early events that shaped maladaptive schemas. One obstacle to change may be the patient's allegiance to the "author" of the life script who may be a significant other, a supportive figure, or a loved one, dead or alive. This problem is common in cases of child abuse where the patient has divided loyalties: telling the true story to the therapist and keeping allegiance to a fictitious script such "I come from big happy family" or "I am a bad child." The patient can also be torn by allegiance to social or religious groups that contributed to the development of maladaptive schemas. Hence, changing values or criticizing idealized relationships can be construed as betrayal. The

TABLE 18.3. Countertransference and Patient's Problem Areas

Personality	Therapist's casting: Continua	Problem areas
Paranoid	Protector ----------------Persecutor	Trust
Schizoid	Careful supporter -------Intruder	Distance, individuation
Schizotypal	Scientist------------------Wizard	Logical–magical thinking
Antisocial	Judge ---------------------Victim	Violence and law
Borderline	Rescuer ------------------Unreliable person	Competence
Histrionic	Neutral observer --------Seducer/seduced	Lovability and seduction
Narcissistic	Admirer ------------------Critic	Egocentrism and social limits
Avoidant	Lenient ------------------Domineering person	Dominance–submission
Dependent	Attachment --------------Undependable figure	Dependency–abandonment
Obsessive–compulsive	Perfectionist -------------Hedonist	Duty and pleasure

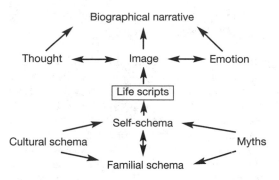

FIGURE 18.7. Life scripts and schemas.

therapist has to acknowledge the difficulty and support the patient through these changes. Cautious role playing using reenactment of the relations with persons of the past, flooding in imagination, and behavioral experiments are all helpful in effecting change.

4. *Specific rescripting techniques.* These techniques have been proposed by several authors and formalized by Arntz and Weertman (1999). They are used for patients with borderline personality disorder who suffered from physical, sexual, or emotional abuse. Rescripting means rewriting the childhood scripts with the patient. The goal is to rebuild early maladaptive self-schemas and the technique is carried out in imagination. There are three phases of mental images presentation. First, the patient imagines the original scene as experienced when he or she was a child. Second, the patient carries out a "rescription": He or she has to imagine the scene viewed from his or her adult perspective. Third, the patient has to imagine that he or she as an adult makes an intervention to protect the child. Then the patient as a child asks for and receives further interventions from the patient as an adult. The session is recorded on audiotape and the patient's homework is to listen to the tape.

IMPLICATIONS FOR ASSESSMENT

Testing the basic hypotheses of cognitive therapy and effective treatment requires a reliable method to assess self-schemas. This assessment is generally conducted in parallel with assessment of DSM-IV personality categories and the major personality traits of psychoticism, extraversion, and neuroticism or the five major factors of personality. The Sociotropy–Autonomy Scale (SAS; Beck, Epstein, Harrison, Emery, 1983), and the Dysfunctional Attitude Scale (DAS; Oliver & Baumgart, 1985; Weissman & Beck, 1978) have been developed to study the schemas underlying depression. Nevertheless, they include some personality schemas. The SAS, for example, assesses social dependence (sociotropy), which is stable between depressive episodes (Moore & Blackburn, 1994). To date only Young's Schema Questionnaire (versions I and II) was developed specifically to assess schemas associated with personality disorder.

The first version of Young's Schema Questionnaire (SQI; Young, 1990) was presented as a clinical checklist of 123 items to study the schemas of personality, but the possibility of a self-rating on a 6-point scale allowed psychometric study. Schemas were grouped into three clusters—autonomy, connectedness, and worthiness—and 15 modes. The autonomy cluster consists of dependence, subjugation, lack of individuation, vulnerability to harm and illness, and fear of losing self-control. Connectedness consists of emotional deprivation, abandonment/loss, mistrust, and social isolation/alienation. Finally, the worthiness cluster involves defectiveness/unlovability, social undesirability, incompetence/failure, guilt/punishment, shame/embarrassment, unrelenting standards, and entitlement/insufficient limits.

The SQI scale has been translated into French and a validation study has been conducted (Mihahescu et al., 1997). Significant differences were obtained in mean scores for patients with only Axis I disorders, patients with an Axis II diagnosis, and control subjects. The SQI score was the highest in patients with personality disorders, reflecting the sensitivity of the scale to Axis II pathology. Principal component analysis identified two factors labeled failure and narcissism.

The revised version of Young's Schema Questionnaire (SQ II; Young, 1994) has 205 items corresponding to 16 kinds of schema groups into five clusters:

1. *Disconnection and rejection.* The expectation that one's need for security, stability, nurturance, acceptance, sharing of feelings, and respect will not be met (schemas: abandonment/instability, mistrust/abuse, emotional deprivation, defectiveness/shame, social isolation/alienation).
2. *Impaired autonomy and performance.* The expectation that because of oneself and the

environment, one will not be able to perform successfully and function independently (schemas: dependence/incompetence, vulnerability to random events, enmeshment/undeveloped self; failure).

3. *Impaired limits.* Deficiency in internal limits, responsibility to others, or long-term goal orientation (schemas: entitlement domination, insufficient self-control/discipline).

4. *Other directedness.* Excessive focus on the wishes, feelings, and responses of others—to gain love and approval (schemas: subjugation, self-sacrifice, approval seeking).

5. *Overvigilance and inhibition.* Excessive control of spontaneous feelings, impulses, and choices—to avoid making mistakes or because of rigid internal rules (schemas: vulnerability to controllable events/negativity, overcontrol, unrelenting standards, punitiveness).

Factor analysis of the scale identified 13 of the 16 hypothesized schemas (Schmidt et al., 1995). Social undesirability, social isolation, subjugation, and entitlement were not identified. Factor analysis of 13 remaining factors yielded a three-factor solution. The three factors were labeled (1) loss of interpersonal relations (abandonment, abuse, emotional deprivation, mistrust, personal defectiveness, emotional inhibition, fear of losing control), (2) social dependence (functional dependence, enmeshment, vulnerability, incompetence/inferiority), and (3) perfectionism (unrelenting standards, self-sacrifice). Insufficient Self-Control had high loadings on each of these three factors. Schmidt and colleagues (1995) also reported on a preliminary analysis on a small sample of patients ($N = 187$) which found that 15 of the 16 factors were present.

The SQ II has good internal consistency and test–retest reliability and shows a significant correlation with the Beck Depression Inventory, the DAS, the scores of depression and anxiety on The Hopkins Symptom Checklist (HSCL-90), and the dimensional global score of a validated personality inventory, the Personality Diagnostic Questionnaire–Revised (PDQ-R). Further research is needed, in both controls and patients, to replicate the factorial structures found by that study. One may also expect studies on the correlation of personality disorder improvement with the modification of the three factors extracted by the factorial analysis of Schmidt, Joiner, Young, and Telch (1995).

INDICATIONS AND CONTRAINDICATIONS

Our earlier review of the clinical and controlled studies on personality disorder testifies to the positive effects of cognitive therapy for a range of Axis II disorders. However, controlled studies have only been reported for the treatment of avoidant personality disorder and borderline personality disorder. Nevertheless the evidence shows that cognitive or cognitive-behavioral therapy had better results than did control conditions. What is needed is a social and therapeutic framework that makes cognitive therapy feasible, such as third-party payments and trained therapists. The main contraindication is low patient motivation. By low motivation we mean that the patient is not aware of interpersonal dysfunctional behaviors and/or is not suffering enough to seek help and to accept a year of therapy. Some patients may be compelled by significant others to seek therapies they do not want. But in our experience most of the patients are coming into therapy with an Axis I problem (depression, anxiety disorder, addiction) triggered by negative life events such as divorce or a professional failure. In cases of both Axis I and II problems, the therapist should help the patient to evaluate the pros and cons of working on Axis II issues. Several strategies may be discussed: for instance carrying out cognitive therapy for personality disorder after a successful approach to the Axis I problem or starting the therapy at the personality level after clarification of the potential benefits with the patient.

EXPECTED OR TYPICAL RESULTS

Dimensional and categorical change can be expected on measures as demonstrated in the part of this chapter dealing with outcome evaluation. But the question is, How much change on the measures is enough to change someone's life? It can be suggested that reconstruction of the schemas is an ambitious goal whose attainment has yet to be proved by any school of psychotherapy. Most of the time, after successful cognitive therapy, the dysfunctional schemas are merely reinterpreted or sufficiently modified to enhance emotional and behavioral adaptation to the familial and work environment. However, once again, hard data are still missing to support clinical evidence. Studies about the change in quality of life after cognitive therapy and its correlation with categorical personality change on DSM-IV are still lacking. Moreover, there are few studies of parallel changes in both Axis I and Axis II pathology. Linehan et al. (1991) is the only author to report significant changes in suicidal behaviors associated with improvement in quality of life (less frequent hospitalizations) after treatment. But there was no difference in change on depression measures when dialectical therapy was compared with the effects of treatment as usual.

LIMITATIONS

The limitations of the cognitive approach to personality disorder cannot be easily determined considering the dearth of hard data and the wide range of personality disorders. From a practical perspective, cognitive therapy requires considerable resources. Trained therapists are required who can follow patients for 1 or 2 years who can manage the transference and countertransference problems common with such patients. Ongoing supervision is also necessary, but such resources are not always available.

Cognitive therapy also requires a highly motivated patient. This is often a problem because the environment deficiencies that led to personality disorder often adversely affect commitment to treatment. The current evidence suggests that patients with Cluster C personality disorders characterized by anxiety, inhibition and moderate levels of depression are the most responsive to cognitive therapy. Linehan's (1993a, 1993b) work with patients with borderline personality disorder suggests that a structured contractual framework is cost-effective, but patients whose impulsivity does not permit them to follow the rules of the therapeutic regimen are not included and therapy is terminated when a patient misses four appointments in a row. It is likely that these patients are the most in need of treatment. This creates practical problems of whether to treat only less severe cases, as in many research studies, and what to do about those who most need help. The problem is especially pertinent with cognitive therapy because it requires high patient motivation, which is often difficult because the environmental deficiencies that led to personality disorder often adversely affect commitment to treatment. Studies are needed to determine the fate of those who are not treated.

A problem in considering wider application of cognitive therapy is uncertainty about how to translate the results of research studies into routine clinical practice. For example, the study by Carroll, Rounsaville, Gordon, et al. (1994) and Carroll, Rounsaville, Nich, et al. (1994) suggested that cocaine users with antisocial personality disorder may benefit from cognitive therapy. But it is difficult to determine how applicable these results are to general clinical situations, especially in a climate of cost containment.

Another potential limitation to cognitive interventions is biological resistance to change. Personality is, in part, the psychological manifestation of character which is biologically determined and less amenable to change through psychological means, unless depression allows some insight, as shown by Woody et al. (1985). A well-intentioned but naive or daring therapist may be confronted with powerful obstacles to change. Mr. Arkadin, the main character of the Orson Welles film *Confidential Report,* who is depicted as the epitome of psychopathic personality, tells the following story: The scorpion wanted to cross a river, so he asked the frog to carry him. "No" said the frog, "No thank you, if I let you on my back, you may sting me, and a sting of a scorpion is death." "Where is the logic of that" replied the scorpion. "Be logical! If I sting you, you will die and I will drown." The frog was convinced to load the scorpion on his back, but just in the middle of the river he felt a terrible pain and realized that the scorpion had stung him. "Logic!" cried the dying frog as he and the scorpion started to drown. "There is no logic in this" said the scorpion, "I know, but I can't help it, it's my character." The message of the scorpion's parable could be that some biologically programmed behaviors, especially impulsive and antisocial behaviors, may be beyond a purely cognitive therapy and may require a combination of psychological and biological treatment administered in a highly structured therapeutic framework.

CONCLUSION

In the last decade, cognitive therapy has provided a model for understanding, conceptualizing, and treating personality disorders. Clinical work has attracted many therapists in several countries and a wealth of clinical data has been gathered and published. We are at the point of moving from clinical work to research designed to establish cognitive therapy as an effective treatment for personality disorder as firmly as it has been established as a treatment for anxiety and mood disorders. To date, only a few controlled studies have been reported, but the results are encouraging. Extensive efficacy, effectiveness, and process studies remain to be conducted. Progress has been made in assessing schemas, but currently available methods of assessment need to be refined and evaluated with larger samples. Moreover, the cognitive model of personality has to be firmly established, especially with regard to the relationship between development and the structure of personality. Research on the relations between biology, education, and personality may provide new insights that will help to define more clearly the role and scope of cognitive therapy. All this represents an exciting new challenge for the future.

REFERENCES

Alden, L. E., & Capreol, M. J. (1993). Avoidant personality disorder: Interpersonal problems as predictors of treatment response. *Behavior Therapy, 24,* 357–376.

Alford, B. A., & Beck, A. T. (1997). *The integrative power of cognitive therapy.* New York: Guilford Press.

Arntz A., & Weertman, A. (1999). Treatment of childhood memories: Theory and practice. *Behaviour Research and Therapy, 37,* 715–740.

Beck, A. T. (1967). *Depression causes and treatment.* Philadelphia: University of Pennsylvania Press.

Beck, A. T., Rush, J., Shaw, B. F., & Emery, G. (1979). *Cognitive therapy of depression.* New York: Guilford Press.

Beck, A. T., Emery, G. & Greenberg, R. L. (1985). *Anxiety disorders and phobias: A cognitive perspective.* New York: Basic Books.

Beck, A. T., Epstein, N., Harrison, R. P., & Emery, G. (1983). *Development of the Sociotropy–Autonomy Scale: A measure of personality factors in psychopathology.* Philadelphia: University of Pennsylvania.

Beck, A. T., Freeman, A., & Associates. (1990). *Cognitive therapy of personality disorders.* New York: Guilford Press.

Carroll, K. M., Rounsaville, B. J., Gordon, L. T., Nich, C., Jatlow, P., Bisighini, R. M., & Gawin, F. H. (1994). Pychotherapy and pharmacotherapy for ambulatory cocaine abusers. *Archives of General Psychiatry, 51,* 177–187.

Carroll, K. M., Rounsaville, B. J., Nich, C., Gordon, L. T., Witrz, L. T., & Gawin, F. H. (1994). One year follow-up of pychotherapy and pharmacoptherapy for cocaine dependence. *Archives of General Psychiatry, 51,* 989–997.

Chambless, D. L., Renneberg, B., Goldstein, A., & Gracely, E. J. (1992). MCMI-diagnosed personality disorder among agoraphobic outpatients: Prevalence and relationship to severity and treatment outcome. *Journal of Anxiety Disorders, 6,* 193–211.

Chernen, L., & Friedman, S. (1993). Treating the personality disordered agoraphobic patient with individual and marital therapy: A multiple replication study, *Journal of Anxiety Disorders, 7,* 163–177.

Cottraux, J., & Blackburn, I. M. (1995). *Thérapies cognitives des troubles de la personnalité* (2nd ed. 1997). Paris: Masson.

Cottraux, J., Mollard, E., Bouvard, M., & Guerin, J. (1991). Facteurs prédictifs des résultats de la thérapie cognitivo-comportementale dans le trouble panique avec agoraphobie. *Journal de Thérapie Comportementale et Cognitive, 1*(1), 4–8.

Cungi, C. (1995). Thérapie en groupe de patients souffrant de phobie sociale ou de troubles de la personnalité. *Journal de Thérapie Comportementale et Cognitive, 5*(2), 45–55.

Dattilio, F. M., & Freeman, A. (Eds.). (1994). *Cognitive-behavioral strategies in crisis intervention.* New York: Guilford Press.

Dressen, L., Arntz, A., Luttels, C., & Sallaerts, S. (1994). Personality disorders do not influence the results of cognitive behavior therapies for anxiety disorders. *Comprehensive Psychiatry, 35,* 265–274.

Erickson, E. H. (1963). *Childhood and society.* New York: Norton.

Fanget, F., & Chambon, O. (1994). Intérêt et efficacité des groupes d'affirmation de soi en cabinet privé. *Journal de Thérapie Comportementale et Cognitive, 4*(4), 116–126.

Freeman, A., & Dattilio, F. M. (Eds.). (1992). *Comprehensive casebook of cognitive therapy.* New York: Plenum.

Freud, A. (1946). *Das Ich und die abweheren mechanismen.* London: Imago Publishing. [*Le moi et les mécanismes de défense.* (A. Berman, French Trans., 1967). Paris: Presses Universitaires de France].

Freud, S., & Breuer, J. (1956). *Etudes sur l'hystérie* (A. Berman, Trans.). Paris: Presses Universitaires de France. (Original work published 1895)

Guérin, J., Bouvard, M., Cottraux, J., & Sechaud, M. (1994). L'affirmation de soi en groupe dans les phobies sociales et les troubles de personnalite: Ètude de 93 cas. *Journal de Thérapie Comportementale et Cognitive, 4*(4), 108–115.

Hartmann, H. (1958). *Ego psychology and the problem of adaptation.* New York: International Universities Press.

Heard, H. L. (1994). Behavior therapies for borderline patients. In *CME Syllabus and Proceedings Summary,* 147th annual meeting of the American Psychological Association, Washington, DC.

Janet, P. (1998). *L'automatisme psychologique.* Paris: Editions Odile Jacob. (Original work published 1889)

Kelly, G. (1955). *A theory of personality. The psychology of personal constructs.* New York: Norton.

Layden, M. A., Newman, C. F., Freeman, A., & Morse, S. B. (1993). *Cognitive therapy of borderline personality disorder.* Boston: Allyn & Bacon.

Linehan, M. M. (1993a). *Cognitive-behavioral treatment of borderline personality disorder.* New York: Guilford Press.

Linehan, M. M. (1993b). *Skills training manual for treating borderline personality disorder*. New York: Guilford Press.

Linehan, M., Armstrong, H., Suarez, A., Allmon, D., & Heard, H. (1991). Cognitive-behavioral treatment of chronically parasuicidal borderline patients. *Archives of General Psychiatry, 48,* 1060–1064.

Linehan M., Heard, H., & Armstrong, H. (1993). Naturalistic followup of behavioral treatment for chronically parasuicidal borderline patients. *Archives of General Psychiatry, 50,* 971–974.

Luborsky, L., Mc Lellan, T., Woody, G., O'Brien, C., & Auerbach, A. (1985). Therapist success and its determinants. *Archives of General Psychiatry, 42,* 602–611.

Mays, D. T. (1975). Behavior therapy with borderline personality disorder: One clinician perspective. In D. T. Mays & C. M. Franks (Eds.), *Negative outcome in psychotherapy and what to do about it*. New York: Springer.

McKay, D., Neziroglu, F., Todaro, J., & Yaryura-Tobias, J. A. (1996). Changes in personality disorders following behavior therapy for obsessive–compulsive disorder. *Journal of Anxiety Disorders, 10*(1), 47–58.

Mihahescu, G., Séchaud, M., Cottraux, J., Velardi, A., Heinze, X., Finot, S. C., & Baettig, D. (1997). Le questionnaire des schémas cognitifs de Young: Traduction et validation préliminaire. *L'Encéphale, 23,* 200–208.

Mikulas, W. L. (1978). Four noble truths of Buddhism related to behavior therapy. *Psychological Record, 28,* 59 67.

Monat, A., & Lazarus, R. S. (1991). *Stress and coping: An anthology*. New York: Columbia University Press.

Moore, R. G., & Blackburn, I. M. (1994). The relation of sociotropy and autonomy to symptoms, cognitions and personality in depressed patients. *Journal of Affective Disorders, 32,* 239–245.

Neisser, U. (1976). *Cognition and reality*. San Francisco: Freeman.

Oliver, J. M., & Baumgart, E. P. (1985). The dysfunctional attitude scale: Psychometric properties and relation to depression in an unselected adult population. *Cognitive Therapy and Research, 9,* 161–167.

Piaget, J. (1952). *The origins of intelligence in childhood*. New York: International Universities Press.

Piaget, J. (1964). *Six études de psychologie*. Paris: Gonthier, Médiations.

Padesky, C. A. (1990). Schema as self prejudice. *International Cognitive Therapy Newsletter, 6,* 1617.

Padesky, C. A. (1994). Schema change processes in cognitive therapy. *Clinical Psychology and Psychotherapy, 1*(5), 267—278.

Padesky, C. A., & Greenberger, D. (1995). *Clinician's guide to mind over mood*. New York: Guilford Press.

Pretzer, J., & Fleming, B. (1989). Cognitive behavioral treatment of personality disorders. *The Behavior Therapist, 12,* 105–109.

Rush, A. J., & Shaw, B. F. (1983). Failure in treating depression by cognitive therapy. In E. B. Foa & P. G. M. Emmelkamp (Eds.), *Failures in behavior therapy* (pp. 212–228). New York: Wiley.

Schmidt, N. B., Joiner, T. E., Young, J. E., & Telch, M. J. (1995). The schema questionnaire: Investigation of psychometric porperties and the hierarchichal structure and measure of maladaptive schemas. *Cognitive Therapy and Research, 19*(5), 295–321.

Segal, Z. (1988). Appraisal of the self schema: Construct in cognitive models of depression. *Psychological Bulletin, 103,* 147–162.

Shea, M. T., Pilkonis, P. A., Beckham, E., Collins, J. F., Elkin, I., Solsky, S. M., & Docherty, J. P. (1990). Personality disorders and treatment outcome in the NIMH Treatment of Depression Collaborative Research Program. *American Journal of Psychiatry, 147,* 711–718.

Tao Te Ching. (1994). *The new translation* (Man-Ho Wok, M. Palmer, & J. Ramsay, Trans.) Shaftesbury, Dorset, UK: Elements Books.

Teasdale, J. D. (1996). Clinically relevant theory: Integrating clinical insight with cognitive science. In P. M. Salkovskis (Ed.), *Frontiers of cognitive therapy*. (pp. 26—47). New York: Guilford Press.

Turkat, I. D., & Levin, R. A. (1984). Formulation of personality disorders. In H. E. Adamson & P. B. Sutker (Eds.), *Comprehensive handbook of psychotherapy* (pp. 502–520). New York: Plenum.

Turkat, I. D., & Maisto, S. A. (1985). Personality disorders: Application of the experimental method to the formulation and modification of personality disorders. In D. H. Barlow (Ed.), *Clinical handbook of psychological disorders* (pp. 502–570). New York: Guilford Press.

Tyrer, P., Seivewright, N., Ferguson, B., Murphy, S., & Johnson, A. L. (1993). The Nottingham study of neurotic disorder. Effect of personality status on response to drug treatment, cognitive therapy, and self-help over two years. *British Journal of Psychiatry, 162,* 219–226.

Weissman, A., & Beck, A. T. (1978). *Development and validation of the Dysunctional Attitude Scale*. Paper presented at the annual meeting of the Association for Advancement of Behavior Therapy, Chicago.

Woody, G. E., McLellan, T., Luborsky, L., & O'Brien, C. P. (1985). Sociopathy and psychotherapy outcome. *Archives of General Psychiatry, 42,* 1081–1086.

Young, J. E. (1990). *Cognitive therapy for personality disorders: A schema focused approach*. Sarasota, FI: Professional Resource Exchange.

Young, J. (1994). *Cognitive therapy for personality disorders: A schema focused approach* (rev.). Sarasota, FL: Professional Resource Exchange.

Young, J. E., & Klosko, J. S. (1994). *Reinventing your life*. New York: Penguin Books.

Young, J. E., & Lindemann, M. D. (1992). An integrative schema-focused model for personality disorders. *Journal of Cognitive Psychotherapy. An International Quarterly, 6*(1), 11—23.

Zettle, R. D., Haflich, J. L., & Reynolds, R. A. (1992). Responsivity to cognitive therapy as a function of treatment format and client personality dimensions. *Journal of Clinical Psychology, 48*(6), 787–797.

CHAPTER 19

Cognitive Analytic Therapy

ANTHONY RYLE

THE DEVELOPMENT AND MAIN FEATURES OF COGNITIVE ANALYTIC THERAPY

Cognitive analytic therapy (CAT) originated, as its name suggests, in the integration of psychodynamic and cognitive ideas. There were two main sources for this integration. One was the use of repertory grid techniques to investigate aspects of structure and change in patients who received psychodynamic therapy (summarized in Ryle, 1975). The experience of demonstrating how patients could be described using the two different theoretical frameworks provoked an interest in the development of a common language and a theoretical and practical integration of psychotherapy models (Ryle, 1982). The other influence was the attempt to devise ways to describe the goals of dynamic therapy in terms permitting outcome research. A study of the notes of completed therapies revealed that most had concentrated on one or two key issues and that these had been evident in the first session in most cases. Moreover, these issues could be highlighted by describing the repeatedly used unsuccessful strategies. The reasons for nonrevision became the focus and led to the recognition of three general patterns, namely, (1) *traps,* in which negative assumptions generate acts which elicit consequences evidently confirming the assumptions; (2) *dilemmas,* in which the apparent options for action, including relating to others and self-management, are conceived of in terms of limited, polarised choices; (3) *snags,* in which appro-

priate goals are abandoned or dismantled as if unacceptable to others or the self.

THE PROCEDURAL SEQUENCE MODEL AND BASIC COGNITIVE ANALYTIC THERAPY PRACTICE

The subsequent development of CAT involved the development of a theoretical model based on the idea of the procedural sequence as the appropriate unit of description. In this model, aim-directed action is described in terms of the following recurrent sequence:

1. The context is appraised.
2. The possibility of action and the likely efficacy and consequences of available action plans are considered.
3. The selected plan is enacted.
4. The aim and the means are evaluated in the light of the perceived consequences and are confirmed or revised.

The early reformulation of patients' difficulties in terms of the model, carried out with their full involvement and culminating in the creation of a written, agreed account, proved to have a powerful therapeutic impact. *Early, collaborative descriptive reformulation* became one defining characteristic of CAT. This took the form of (1) a letter from the therapist summarizing an understanding of the patient's history and how current procedures had been derived from it; this letter was discussed and revised as necessary; (2) a summary description of current target problems and of the underlying damaging or restricting target problem procedures was agreed upon; in time this description was supplemented by the construction of *sequential diagrams* of the main recurrent patterns.

USE OF THE MODEL IN TIME-LIMITED OUTPATIENT PSYCHOTHERAPY

The further development of the model was accelerated by the need to provide a psychotherapy service for an inner-city population of about 170, 000. The number of trained staff grew over a 10-year period from none to a small number of part-time workers (equivalent to one full-time worker), all of whom were involved in the supervision of trainees drawn from social work, occupational therapy, nursing, psychology and psychiatry. As between 120 and 160 patients were referred annually it was clearly important to deliver the minimum sufficient intervention, and, influenced by Mann (1973), a predetermined time limit of 12–16 sessions was introduced. Apart from the later availability of group therapy, all those referred by psychiatrists or general practitioners who attended for assessment were offered CAT.

This experience was encouraging in that the model proved to be an effective, supportive framework for trainee therapists, only a minority of whom had had any prior therapy training. It proved to be a satisfactory intervention for more than two-thirds of patients, including those with personality disorders.

DIFFERENTIATION AND DEVELOPMENT OF THE COGNITIVE ANALYTIC THERAPY MODEL

The original integration of separate theories was followed by a process of differentiation from these sources and by the introduction of ideas drawn from other sources. A full account of this evolution will be found in Leiman (1994) and Ryle (1995).

Theoretical extension involved the fuller integration of object relations ideas in the *procedural sequence object relations model* (PSORM; Ryle, 1985). The procedures of concern to psychotherapists are those controlling interpersonal action and self-management. In seeking a relationship, an individual attempts to find or elicit an appropriate response from the other, an idea expressed in the concept of the *reciprocal role procedure* (RRP). An individual's *repertoire* of RRPs is derived from early interactions with caretakers and other children and will both maintain relationships with others and organize self-management. The "building blocks" of the self are hence derived from interactions with others. This model is parallel to the ideas proposed within psychoanalysis by Ogden (1983) but is differentiated by its emphasis on the actual experiences of the infant and child as opposed to innate unconscious fantasy. It is a model close to that proposed by Mead and to the ideas of Vygotsky and his followers on the social formation of mind; these ideas and those of Bakhtin have been influential in the later developments of CAT as described in Ryle (1991) and as elaborated by Leiman (1992, 1994, 1995, 1997, 2000).

THE COGNITIVE ANALYTIC THERAPY MODEL OF PERSONALITY FORMATION

A model of personality must encompass the full complexity of being human. In the account presented here, the emphasis is on the areas of main concern to psychotherapists, namely, the social and psychological. Biological factors are, of course, important, but the discontinuities between animals and humans are of particular significance to our understanding of personality. Our biological evolution over the past 4 million years has selectively favored characteristics adapted to the parallel evolution of complex, flexible social forms, notably through great increases in brain size and in the ability to communicate (Donald, 1991). As a result, the human infant is *biologically adapted to be socially formed.* The human genotype has flourished with negligible change through widely differing historical epochs and cultures because it allows each individual to learn from, be formed by, and contribute to the particular culture into which he or she is born.

This formation takes place from birth. The child is born into a world of meanings and, as physical maturation proceeds, acquires its knowledge of physical and social reality through its own active curiosity in a context of, and with a commentary by, its caretakers and others. The observational studies of recent years have documented the intense interactions of the child with those around. Vygotskian ideas introduce a perspective on these observations, above all by challenging the "monadic" assumptions which still underpin most current theories. The view that the child is an individual arising *sui generis* who then proceeds to build up theories about, and representations of, self and other through separate systems of information processing concerned with knowledge and feeling is rejected. The individuality of the child is created and shaped within the relationships with others and knowledge about the world is internalized through the signs and meanings developed with caretakers. The child does not store representations to which a mayonnaise of meaning is applied; affects and cognitions, meanings and facts, and the definitions of self and other are acquired in the course of actively engaging with others whose own meanings also reflect and transmit those of the wider culture.

The developmental perspective of CAT, with its focus on reciprocal roles, was clarified and sharpened by these Vygotskian ideas and by the work of Bakhtin with its emphasis on the continuities between external and internal dialogue. It receives empirical support from studies of child development (Boyes, Giordano, & Pool, 1997; Oliviera, 1997). The dialogical self is conceived of as made up of "conversations" between past and present "voices" rather than as a battleground between warring internal "objects" conveying innate and conflicted instinctual forces. The stability of self-processes, while to some extent maintained by the traps, dilemmas, and snags described in early CAT, is more generally a result of the early (preverbal) acquisition of the major procedural patterns defining self–other relationships and of the fact that individuals generally seek out those who are seen to reciprocate (and hence appear to confirm) their role procedures.

The CAT model does not contain a replica of the dynamic unconscious of psychoanalysis and does not consider unconscious conflict as universal or as central to the understanding of neurotic phenomena. In the course of their formation, *all* role procedures are, in psychoanalytic terms, compromise formations, in which action takes into account desire, reality, and the (external or internalized) reactions of others. The main procedural patterns are laid down

early and continue to operate without awareness. In this view, the unconscious is largely shaped (before speech) by social forces rather than by innate fantasies (see Burkitt, 1995). Damaging, restricted, and avoidant procedures, which are often accompanied by symptoms, result from the internalization of neglecting, harsh, critical or conditional voices, the source and content of which may or may not be known by the individual.

Apart from restating repression and other ego defenses as reflecting harsh internalized reciprocal role procedures, CAT emphasizes another form of unconsciousness, namely, the extent to which people show little awareness of the nature of their own enacted procedures. This is particularly the case in relation to the broader patterns which determine or limit the range of day-to-day acts. Once described, these patterns become readily recognized.

In clinical practice, descriptions of personality and its disorders must be based on identifying the repertoire of reciprocal roles. In arriving at descriptions of these roles, the aim is to create the highest-level, most general account on the assumption of a hierarchical structure whereby lower-order "tactical" procedures operate within the terms of higher-order "strategic" procedures.

In practice, descriptions that combine *sequential* elements with developmentally derived *structural* considerations can be best expressed diagrammatically. In constructing such diagrams, the first step is to list, in the core of the diagram, the main *reciprocal role repertoire*. This is a heuristic device. Enacted role procedures are traced on procedural loops which describe actions and consequences. In most cases problematic procedures end up by returning to and reinforcing the core procedural pattern. Such diagrams make it clear how each described role may be enacted by the subject and how others may be recruited to reciprocate. The form of the diagram provides guidance to therapists in resisting pressures to collude with negative procedures and makes patients aware of, and hence able to reflect, on the nature and consequences of their procedures. Figure 19.1 provides an example of a sequential diagram. The patient was a health professional with a history of elective mutism in childhood who had contrasting reciprocal role patterns derived from his parents. Giving care in the hope of receiving care generated resentment and withholding and perceiving others to be critical led

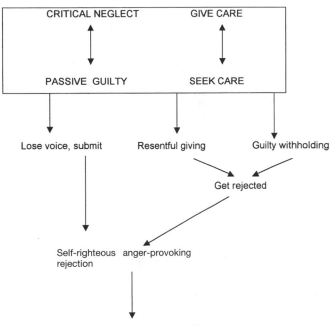

FIGURE 19.1. Sequential diagram of a depressed health professional.

to submission (with an occasional return of a literal inability to speak). The overall result was a continuing sense of unmet emotional needs and depression.

In Vygotsky's account, learning takes place on two planes, the first external and the second, involving some transformation, internal. Learning takes place in the zone of proximal development, which is defined as the area in which the child has the potential capacity to learn if given appropriate assistance by a more experienced other. The internalization of such learning involves the provision and mutual development of signs. As the developing child explores the world, the parent or teacher provides a "scaffolding."

Learning involves the internalization of the meanings accorded to physical and social reality and to the scaffolding which—whether enabling, restricting, prescriptive, or unsupportive—will contribute to the emerging sense and definition of the self. The content and the terms of the "conversation" or relationship between child and others will be repeated internally as between different voices within the self and will also continue to shape and be shaped by continuing patterns of relating to others. In this sense the self is dialogic and permeable. The CAT emphasis on reciprocal roles and on the

scaffolding created during the reformulation process represent the application of Vygotskian understandings to the process of therapy.

THE COGNITIVE ANALYTIC THERAPY "MULTIPLE-SELF-STATES MODEL" OF BORDERLINE PERSONALITY DISORDER

There are several problems with the concept of borderline personality disorder.

1. The majority of the features contributing to the diagnosis refer to instability or variability but provide no satisfactory understanding of the underlying processes and structures. Explanations in terms of "ego weakness" are somewhat tautological. The psychoanalytic concept of splitting is more explanatory but is frequently seen to reflect internal and innate rather than environmental and experiential processes.

2. The concept of comorbidity seems an inappropriate way to describe the normal association with borderline personality disorder of other diagnoses in both Axis I and II. The disease model cannot be transferred crudely to personality deviations, and the evidence points to there being a common underlying set of causes

of various forms of damage and distortion in individual development.

3. Fonagy and Target (1997) see the inability to reflect on the psychological states of self and other as a fundamental cause of borderline personality disorder. They seem to accept that the capacity to generate inferences and predict behaviors and form a 'theory of mind' on the basis of unobservable mental states is an innate capacity. The Vygotskian account of personal formation through the internalization of external dialogue offers a more plausible and parsimonious explanation of the child's acquisition of understandings of self and others, understandings which include intentionality.

Origins of the Cognitive Analytic Therapy Model

In constructing diagrams with less disturbed patients, it is usually possible to identify two or three key reciprocal role procedures which constitute the core of the diagram from which the various enacted problematic procedures can be seen to be generated, as in Figure 19.1. In devising these diagrams, both historical and current relationships and the emerging transference are considered, and patients may need to carry out self-monitoring in order to trace their sequences through and to identify how they end up by reinforcing the existing system. Transitions between the roles are usually smooth and appropriate. In working with more disturbed patients, however, it became evident that this reformulation process was often undermined by the confusions and discontinuities experienced by patients and induced in the therapist. The practical solution to this confusion came with the recognition that these patients were operating discontinuously from one or other of a number of separate procedural systems and that transitions between these were often sudden and evidently unprovoked. Only when these separate *self-states* (partially dissociated reciprocal role patterns) were identified and described could their appearances and disappearances be traced. This development of practice contributed to a clarification of the phenomenology of borderline personality disorder.

Figure 19.2 provides an example of a *self-states sequential diagram* of a borderline patient. The diagram shows how the RRP derived from early experience are still reenacted in relation to self and to others and how the original child role of needy victim may be transformed to a placatory coping mode. Seeking care can

also lead to a switch to an idealizing–idealized relationship (a self-state), which, in due course, ends in disappointment. This experience and repeated neglect or abuse from others may lead to the recontacting of the original unmanageable feelings, marked "X" on the diagram, which may result in expressed rage (against self or others), in dissociative symptoms, or in a switch to the "zombie" role in a third self-state.

The Multiple-Self-States Model

The CAT multiple-self-states model (MSSM; Ryle, 1997a, 1997b) is consistent with the clinical evidence of partial dissociation between RRPs and with the known associations between gross neglect and abuse in childhood and adult borderline personality disorder. It offers explanations of much of the phenomenology of borderline personality disorder, of the high comorbidity rates, and of patients' inadequate self-reflective capacity. The magnitude of these effects will vary according to the degree of genetic predisposition. The model describes three forms of disorder.

Extreme Roles

The characteristic damaging patterns of self-management and relationships with others and the associated Axis I conditions, notably depression and eating disorders, reflect a damaging, restrictive, and often extreme repertoire of RRPs. These either repeat in some form the patterns experienced in childhood, typically *abusing/neglecting in relation to deprived and victimized and/or revengeful,* or they represent partially dissociated patterns developed as alternatives to the usually avoided unmanageably intense feelings. Typical patterns are submissive placation, perfectionist striving or affectless coping, all liable to be accompanied by depression and somatization, in relation to abusive demands from self and others.

Partial Dissociation

Different RRPs are located in different self-states. In normal subjects, RRPs are less separate and are mobilized in ways appropriate to the context and the individual's intentions, through the operation of largely unconscious *metaprocedures*. In borderline personality disorder, in contrast, state switches occur abruptly and often inappropriately and in the absence of

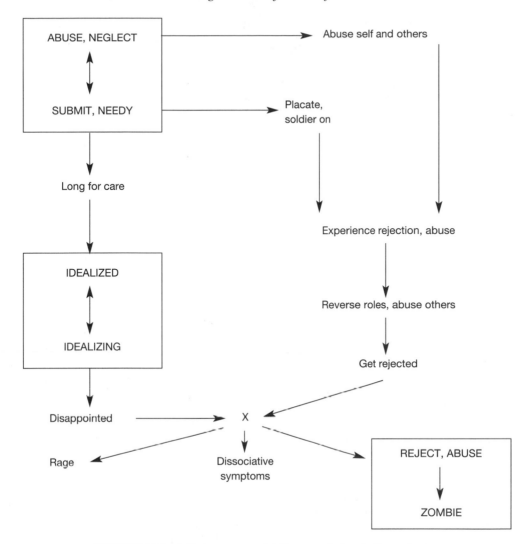

FIGURE 19.2. Self states sequential diagram of a borderline patient.

evident provocations; such switches reflect the inadequate development and/or the traumatic disruption of the metaprocedural system. Over time, behavior may be governed and experience interpreted by any of the different reciprocal role patterns in the disrupted system. Some particular roles may be perceived, sought, or provoked in the other but seldom or never enacted by the self. This is a way of describing the process of projective identification, as described by Sandler (1976) and Ryle (1994); it is usually described in relation to negative roles and their affects but may apply equally to idealized roles. The variable and intermittent presence of many borderline personality disorder features can be understood as reflecting the fol-

lowing phenomena: (1) *response shifts* within a given RRP (e.g., from submissive to rebellious in relation to controlling), (2) role reversals (e.g., from victimized to abuser to abuser to victimized), or (3) self-state shifts (e.g., from ideally cared for in relation to perfect caring to abusive in relation to abandoning).

In clinical work, a more fine-grained form of diagram may be of value, namely, Leiman's "dialogic sequence analysis" (Leiman, 1997). This is especially helpful in the case of those borderline patients who, during tense phases evoked by therapy or difficult situations, may show rapid switches between states (described as "whirlpooling" by one therapist). In such instances, each segment of the account is described in terms of the particular reciprocal roles involved. As in the previous examples, switches may be the result of response shifts, role reversals, or self-state shifts.

Stability of the sense of self is generally dependent in part on the ability to elicit reciprocation from others of the roles being offered. The dissociated self-states of borderline personality disorder are unstable and have, in most instances, a single dominant RRP, often involving extreme behaviors, and the attempts to elicit confirmation are correspondingly intense. This feature accounts for the powerful countertransference feelings elicited by patients with borderline personality disorder.

Deficient Self-Reflection

The capacity for self-reflection is impaired in borderline personality disorder for two reasons. The kinds of parenting or substitute care experienced in childhood have usually involved inconsistency, such as alternations of affection and abuse or of care and abandonment, combined with disinterest in the child's subjective experiences. No model of concern has been internalized and access to language conveying feeling may be limited. Also, such capacity for self-reflection as has developed is not continuous, due to the disruption of awareness by state switches. Such switches tend to occur at the precise moment at which the current role procedure cannot accommodate nonreciprocation or a new event, that is, at the moment when procedural revision would be particularly valuable. The common failure of borderline personality disorder patients to learn from experience and to take responsibility for their acts can be attributed to these switches between states, in some of which memory of other states may be considerably impaired.

RESEARCH EVIDENCE FOR THE MULTIPLE-SELF-STATES MODEL

As explained earlier, the MSSM was derived in part from the elaboration of self-states sequential diagrams, as illustrated in Figure 19.2. Bennett and Parry (1998) tested the ability of such jointly produced self-states sequential diagrams to identify the themes emerging in early therapy sessions. Judges were required to match the self-states sequential diagrams of an individual patient with a number of borderline therapies ana-lyzed by the Core Conflict Relationship Theme (CCRT; Luborsky & Crits-Christoph, 1990) and the Structural Analysis of Social Behavior— Cyclic Maladaptive Pattern (SASB-CMP; Schacht & Henry, 1994). Highly accurate matching was achieved and this finding was repeated on three subsequent cases (D. Bennett, personal communication, 1998). Further support for the MSSM comes from a study by Golynkina and Ryle (1999) of 20 borderline personality disorder cases. The states identified by these patients and their therapists in the early sessions constituted the elements in a repertory grid (the States Grid); these were rated against constructs concerned with sense of self and other and describing the dominant mood and the degree of access to, and control of, emotion. Most patients could carry out the task in relation to all their states, despite impaired access to memory in some instances. Analysis of the grids demonstrated that all the patients made meaningful discriminations between their states and that in many cases both poles of an identified RRP were described. The states described by different patients showed many similarities. Thus all patients identified states derived from their early internalization of reciprocal role patterns of, for example, *abusing neglect in relation to victim or to rebel,* and most showed some relating to patterns of *ideally caring to ideally cared for* and of either *soldiering on* or *affectless coping in relation to abandoning or threatening.*

THE PRACTICE OF COGNITIVE ANALYTIC THERAPY WITH BORDERLINE PATIENTS

Selection and Assessment

Identifying Borderline Patients

Different services will see borderline patients differing in terms of severity and associated problems, and the extent to which the diagnosis is made also varies widely. Only a minority of borderline patients are referred to psychotherapy services and in many cases they will be considered too disturbed for the available therapists. Many patients with borderline personality disorder are seen in primary care settings, and some of them will be referred to general psychiatric settings for the treatment of depression or anxiety or somatization; in both settings the personality disorder is frequently undiagnosed or consists of no more than the label "difficult patient."

Others are seen after self-harm or in relation to substance abuse or in forensic settings. While a severe case of borderline personality disorder will usually provide clear evidence of the diagnosis in the form of self-destructive behaviors and numerous unhelpful encounters with clinical and possible forensic agencies, less severely disturbed patients may present themselves, at least initially, in compliant, coping modes and the diagnosis may be missed. In CAT, outpatient practice screening questions describing shifts between distinct and often extreme states have proved useful in this respect.

Indications and Contraindications

The great majority of patients referred for outpatient CAT and who attend for assessment will be accepted for treatment. Given that deficient self-reflection is a characteristic of the condition, patients are *not* expected to arrive with established "psychological mindedness"; developing this will be a main focus of the therapy. During the early sessions a few patients will prove unable to work in this way, either because of continuing substance abuse or because of the overwhelming severity of their disturbance, (manifest, for example, in massive and extreme state shifts or disruptive psychotic episodes) or because their social context is too threatening or violent to allow any therapeutic work to be done. A past history of unsuccessful interventions is not usually considered a contraindication, partly because such interventions have frequently been inadequate or inappropriate and partly because attendance for assessment may indicate a greater willingness and ability to engage than was previously the case.

There are, however, some contraindications to outpatient CAT. Most patients with borderline personality disorder have experienced loss of control of anger and many have done physical harm to themselves and others. Any patients with high violence potential must be carefully screened in relation to the treatment setting. Patients who might be successfully treated in secure inpatient or forensic settings could be unsuitable for treatment in primary care or outpatient clinics. Similarly, outpatient treatment may be unsafe for some patients who have intense suicidal preoccupations or whose acts of self-harm are severe.

Another contraindication is a high level of current substance abuse. Ideally, total withdrawal should precede psychotherapy, for outcome is significantly worse in patients continuing to abuse alcohol or cannabis, even if use is intermittent and controlled. But total withdrawal cannot always be achieved. Combining CAT with treatment of addiction or linking it with withdrawal programs may be useful (see Leighton, 1997) and may be a way of avoiding the paradox of requiring these patients to recover before they can receive treatment.

Some borderline patients have accompanying Axis I conditions, which may be life threatening or may need treatment before therapy is possible. An example would be anorexia nervosa, but even here management and treatment within a CAT framework may be helpful (Bell, 1999; Treasure & Ward, 1997). In general, accompanying somatic or mood disorders would not be a contraindication to CAT and would not be the primary focus of therapy. Determining which procedure or self-state is associated with the symptom or which potential procedure the symptom seems to have replaced allows therapy to be focused on the issues of personality integration and on high-level interpersonal and self-management procedures. When such treatment is effective direct treatment of the symptoms is usually unnecessary.

Medication

At the time of the assessment, current prescribed medication or the need for medication in those patients not receiving any should be reviewed. Prescribing and management are best in the hands of someone other than the therapist, preferably a psychiatrist with a special interest in personality disorders who would be able to admit for inpatient care should it become necessary. The use of minor tranquilizers is seldom indicated and is potentially harmful in borderline patients given their proneness to addiction. In patients prone to enter states with intense paranoid or other psychotic features, antipsychotic medication may be helpful, preferably taken only when the symptoms are present. Antidepressant medication, while of uncertain impact on the depression of borderline patients, is sometimes of value and occasionally has marked effect on mood, which in turn may reduce borderline symptoms.

Contracting

When patients are accepted for therapy it is helpful to provide an overall idea of the nature of the therapy and its frequency (weekly) and probable duration (usually 24 weeks). Clear expectations about attendance and notification of canceled sessions (by both patient and therapist) should be spelled out. Particular features such as homework assignments should be described and, if intended, agreement to audiotaping should be sought. Such contracts, as well as offering a model of clarity and openness, mean that departures from the contract during the therapy can be taken as manifestations of the patient's procedures and used therapeutically.

The Reformulation Phase

During the first session the therapist describes the overall nature of the therapy and explains that the first phase is concerned with getting a sense of what it is like to be the patient and giving the patient a chance to see what is being offered. The first 4 to 6 sessions will culminate in the collaborative creation of a written and diagrammatic reformulation. For the therapist, the process of reformulation needs to start right away; in most cases hints of the main themes will be evident in the first half of the first session from the stories told and the patient's demeanor. The style could be called active empathic listening; while leaving the agenda to the patient for much of the time, the therapist refers every detailed event to the broader pattern of which it might be an example. Either as the story unfolds or at the end of each session the therapist proposes links between historical events, current relationships, and transference manifestations in the form of general descriptions from which models of damaging role procedures will be derived in due course.

Self-State Sequential Diagrams

As the main concerns are interpersonal and intrapersonal processes, individual reports or events can usually be seen as exemplifying particular patterns of interaction such as *caring–cared for, rejecting–rejected, controlling–submitting, controlling–rebelling, threatening–avoiding, and abusing–abused,* and in this way a summary *repertoire of RRPs* can be assembled.

In borderline patients each role will be experienced as a discrete state, usually described in terms of mood or affect and often extreme. Further inquiry and homework by the patient identifies the accompanying sense of self and oth-

ers, the degree to which affect is accessed or controlled, and the accompanying symptoms of each experienced state. This process also leads to the identification of the reciprocal to each role or state (frequently this too is a recognizable state, but in some cases it is not experienced, being always elicited from others). It should be recalled that *self-states* are theoretical constructs describing partially dissociated reciprocal role patterns, whereas states are subjectively experiences associated with particular roles. The concept of the self-state brings into focus, for both therapist and patient, the fact that each role or state is a response to a real, perceived, or internalized reciprocal.

Once the self-states have been identified in this way, careful observation and self-monitoring can identify the particular procedures generated from each role (these will either be direct enactments of the role or defensive or symptomatic replacements) and the provocations of state switches. Some such switches may be responses to events, but many appear to be unprovoked. Priority will be given to recognizing the states and procedures leading to self-harm or to therapy-threatening behaviors. The final product will be a *self-states sequential diagram* as shown in Figure 19.2.

Reformulation Letters

The diagrammatic reformulation of the patient's current procedural repertoire is a paradigmatic exercise; it is preceded or accompanied by a letter offering a narrative reformulation which is presented by the therapist and refined in discussion. These letters are the therapist's account of his or her understanding of the patient's life and problems. Their form involves a brief summary of key past experiences and of how the patient coped with them and a description of how current patterns represent either repetitions of early ones or the persistence of the alternatives developed as coping methods which now are themselves problematic. These alternatives are identified as representing separate, alternating sources of experience and action. The aims of therapy are the revision of these patterns and the integration of the different self-states. The ways in which the negative patterns are or may be manifest in the therapy relationship are outlined. These letters are usually experienced as profoundly moving by patients, and the experience of the joint work involved in forming the diagram is also a new and valued one for most patients with borderline personality disorder. With the completion of this reformulation phase the agenda shifts from reformulation to recognition and revision—the three R's of CAT.

Active Therapy: Recognition and Revision

Change in CAT involves the enlargement of the patient's capacity for accurate self-reflection. This capacity is achieved through a combination of the formal, cognitive task of learning to recognize and block the damaging automatic procedures with the experience of a respecting and noncollusive relationship with the therapist. Recognition involves self-monitoring and diary keeping; it is based on clear, accurate working diagrams, often color coded, which are used continually by the patient to identify the moments at which damaging procedures are triggered or enacted. At times the emphasis may be on particular procedures (e.g., those threatening to life or therapy), but usually the patient keeps a day-to-day diary of disturbing experiences or acts and learns to locate them on the diagram. Maintaining the noncollusive relationship involves the therapist's use of the diagram to avoid or correct acts or comments which constitute reciprocation and reinforcement of the patient's negative procedures. It is also helpful to challenge the patient's interpretations of events when they are based on the negative patterns described in the diagram.

These activities provide a framework of understanding which is containing while permitting an emotionally intense relationship. This process is seldom smooth, however, for the experienced safety may lead to the patient's greater awareness or memory of early terror and abuse. Patients not only contact or amplify memories of past abuses but may, in response to disappointments or the prospect of termination, enact negative procedures or enter negative self-states in the therapy. The recognition of these negative states allows therapists to offer responses aiding their mitigation and assimilation. Suggesting or probing for memories of abuse is not part of CAT practice; if such memories are accessed it is important to grant to the patient the right to control the pace or to keep silent. In general, patients go as far as they feel safe to go, and procedural change is often achieved without exploration of all that has been forgotten. But therapists may find themselves on a knife edge, poised between being experienced as intrusive on the one hand and indifferent on the other—a dilemma which is best shared with the patient.

The Model of Therapist Interventions

CAT is not a manualized therapy, but an "ideal model" of intervention has been defined and empirically developed using Task Analysis by Bennett (Bennett, Parry, & Ryle, 2000). Coding how therapists had responded to threats to the alliance on the basis of this model showed that therapist adherence to the model had been significantly higher in successful therapies. Thus in rating audiotapes of good-outcome cases it was found that therapists had recognized 80% of threats and resolved about 80% of them, whereas in poor-outcome cases only 30% of examples were recognized. Moreover, it was found that more experienced therapists scored higher than less experienced ones and that supervised trainees improved their scores through time. This work suggests that specific CAT techniques have had a positive impact in the short term, and that this was reflected in better overall outcomes.

The empirically refined model describes a sequence of responses which can be made in relation to new enactments in the therapy relationship or to narratives. Adherence may involve repetitions and tangents but eventually interventions go through the stages summarized next. It will be noted that these stages parallel the overall shape of a CAT therapy.

1. *Acknowledgment* of the event or report, which to be full involves . . .
2. *Exploration,* on the basis of which . . .
3. *Explanation and linking* will be worked at. Linking may involve noting resemblances to other events or stories but crucially, in CAT, will involve locating the particular instance, whether a reported or an enacted (transference) one, in relation to a more general, higher order procedural description or to the relevant self-state. This will involve a process of . . .
4. *Negotiation* and the achievement of . . .
5. *Consensus.* Linking becomes real to the extent that the patient fully understands and participates in the process. Both understanding (e.g., "I can see that that is how it is; I had not realized that before . . .") and emotional responses are involved.

6. Sometimes a more *general explanation* may be offered, for example, of how procedural patterns are formed and maintained, or of how the recognition of them may introduce a new possibility of choice. It may also be helpful to offer an understanding of the sadness involved in realizing the degree to which aspects of life have been closed off in the past.

7. In the course of these stages, as a result of feeling contained by the explanations, the patient may contact hitherto *unassimilated feelings;* this is usually accompanied with relief even when the feelings themselves may be largely of grief and anger.

8. When the main issues have been examined in this way on a number of occasions and recognition is fairly securely established, the possible *"exits" from the system* can be considered. This involves exploring—in the therapy or in relation to other situations—what might replace the damaging procedures and how greater integration might be achieved. Except in the case of dangerous procedures, this stage should be postponed until reliable recognition is established. One patient described this as having the diagram "burnt on his brain."

Common therapeutic errors derive from inadequately clear or incomplete diagrams and from the failure to link reported events and in-session enactments to the diagram. Such linking depends on the construction of a good diagram; any significant event which cannot be located on the diagram must lead to its revision. In the early stages of therapy the patient and therapist may collude in not including on the diagram some area of shared difficulty; supervision can be of particular importance in recognizing this.

There should be no conflict between the "cognitive" and "affective" elements in the therapy because clear descriptions and understandings make feeling safer and because the understandings sought are those concerned with experienced and expressed feelings (or their suppression). Therapists doing CAT need to take every opportunity to suggest links with the higher-level, more general understandings encapsulated in the diagram, but trainees coming from dynamic or Rogerian backgrounds often prefer to remain in a passive reflective mode, illustrating Oscar Wilde's comment that it is easier to have sympathy with suffering than sympathy with thought. Others may distance themselves from the disturbing emotional experience provoked by being caught up in the turmoil of their patients, by being busy with the formal tasks and bits of paper involved in CAT, or by focusing on the treatment of more familiar specific symptoms and behaviors. Generally, therapists may be invited into every role described on the diagram and only vigilance will prevent inadvertent collusion. There are few therapists, however experienced, able to avoid being drawn in to some collusive responses by some patients. During training—and preferably later—supervision offers the best safeguard and the most effective form involves the analysis of audiotapes or videotapes of sessions. Therapists cannot bring to supervision issues they have not recognized.

Within the overall framework, some specific interventions may be of value; any technique aimed at procedural revision and integration may be employed provided its relevance to the overall aims is clear. Thus, for example, behavioral programs to revise identified procedures, role playing to explore RRPs and the use of drawing or writing as alternative expressions and sources of self-reflection may all be helpful. The overall aim, however, remains the achievement of continuing awareness across states. Linked with this, the internalization of the therapy relationship as a model of a different reciprocal role patterns is crucial. Ultimately, the detailed "techniques" employed in CAT enable therapists to maintain a respecting human relationship with disturbed and disturbing patients.

Termination and Follow-Up

Termination of therapy with deprived and damaged patients is always difficult; the use of predetermined time limits and reference to termination from the beginning does not make it easy but does prevent regressive dependency. These patients cannot ever be given enough to compensate for their early lacks and hurts, but an intense time-limited therapy can offer a powerful experience and a manageable disappointment from which real change and more realistic hopes can stem.

For this to happen, the patient needs to take away an accurate memory which neither denies disappointment nor devalues what was achieved. The common return of symptoms during late sessions should be expected and calmly contained by therapists, with links to the reformulation and to earlier losses being kept in mind. At the penultimate or last session a "good-bye letter" is prepared and discussed with the patient, who is invited to write a similar evaluation. The therapist's letter should briefly summarize, accurately and without bland optimism, what has been achieved in relation to the problems and problem procedures described in the reformulation, should note anger or disappointment (which may or may not have been expressed), should suggest a continuing use of the reformulation tools and "allow" a good memory of the work done together, and should indicate what remains to be done. Follow-up meetings are usually arranged at 1, 2, 3, and 6 months. The assessment of further needs at that time, or earlier if there are still pressing difficulties, is best carried out by the assessment team or the referring unit, as therapists may have difficulty in making objective judgments at this stage. As far as possible the full follow-up period should elapse before further therapy is arranged in order to allow the patient the experience of discovering how much he or she has achieved.

THE EVIDENCE BASE OF COGNITIVE ANALYTIC THERAPY

Studies of process and of borderline personality structure have been reported previously, providing evidence for the accuracy of the model and for the specific impact of CAT treatment methods. A naturalistic outcome study designed to describe the impact of outpatient CAT on borderline personality disorder and to identify pretherapy variables associated with outcome has been completed (Ryle & Golynkina, 2000) and a randomized controlled trial of 24 sessions of CAT plus 4 follow-ups compared to "business as usual" is currently under way.

The naturalistic study described 37 patients meeting standardized diagnostic criteria. Of these, one was referred out for inpatient care and 3 for treatment of persistent substance abuse. Two moved away before completing treatment. Of the remaining 31, 4 dropped out of treatment. The remaining 27 cases were assessed 6 months after termination, at which time half no longer met diagnostic criteria for borderline personality disorder. Mean scores for the whole sample on inventories measuring depression, general symptoms, and interper-

sonal difficulties fell significantly, the changes being greater in those no longer borderline; these patients were also more likely to be in some kind of employment and in a stable relationship and less likely to report episodes of out-of-control violence. Half of those still borderline showed some improvement by the other criteria. Half the sample were discharged from further care at this 6-month follow-up. Retesting 18 months after termination showed further reduction in scores in the two-thirds successfully followed up.

Age, gender, childhood abuse history, previous treatment, current medication, impulsivity, and pretherapy questionnaire scores were not predictive of treatment response. Less successful outcome was predicted by a greater severity of borderline features, a poor occupational history, and a past history of self-cutting and alcohol abuse.

THE WIDER ROLE OF COGNITIVE ANALYTIC THERAPY

Although the model was developed in the context of individual psychotherapy, it is being increasingly applied in other treatment modes and settings. Duignan and Mitzman (1994) reported the impact of a CAT-based time-limited group containing two borderline patients. Dunn and Parry (1997) reported the use of CAT reformulation as a basis for case management in a small inpatient unit for severely disturbed borderline patients. Kerr (1999) described the use of CAT understandings in the management of a disruptive borderline patient and introduced the notion of contextual reformulation to demonstrate parallels between the patient's procedures, problems within the staff group, and difficulties between the unit and other agencies. Kerr (2000) has also proposed a theoretical model of therapeutic communities drawing on Vygotskian ideas. Pollock and Belshaw (1998) describe the use of CAT in forensic settings.

Only a small minority of patients with personality disorders receive psychotherapy, but most spend some time in contact with psychiatric, forensic, or social agencies. In the absence of clear, shared understandings, staff are all too easily drawn into unhelpful or actively collusive relationships with borderline patients. The theoretical model on which CAT is based emphasizes the permeability of the individual self and the crucial influence of the social and personal context provided. The collaborative ethos can be extended beyond individual therapy to other settings, and the jointly fashioned tools, notably diagrams, are accessible to staff and patients as a basis for the maintenance of a humane, respecting working relationship. In a comprehensive service CAT could provide an economical and effective intervention for less severe cases and could contribute to longer-term management involving day hospital, therapeutic community, and other inpatient care. By its provision of adequately detailed understandings of the intrapsychic and interpersonal procedures of each individual patient, CAT reformulation can ensure that specific therapeutic inputs (e.g., behavioral programs or art therapy) are offered in ways supportive of the overall objective of aiding integration.

SUMMARY: THE DISTINGUISHING FEATURES OF COGNITIVE ANALYTIC THERAPY FOR BORDERLINE PERSONALITY DISORDER

Although it shares features with other approaches, CAT has developed a distinct theory and specific methods. In regard to theory, the emphasis on the formation and maintenance of personality functioning through the understandings and activities shared with others offers a revision of object relations theories, with an emphasis on actual experience and socially derived meanings as opposed to fantasy. This underlies the central importance accorded to the provision of a noncollusive therapy relationship. The MSSM describes the structural features of borderline personality disorder which are derived from trauma-induced partial dissociation. The effect of treatment is understood to be due to the influence of the therapy relationship and to the creation within it of clear written and diagrammatic descriptions which represent, in Vygotskian terms, jointly elaborated interpsychological tools which, in due course, are internalized. The explicit framework provided by reformulation provides a safety within which an active and intense therapeutic relationship can be maintained, even by relatively inexperienced trainee therapists. The time-limited intervention is cost-effective and provides enough therapy for less severely disturbed patients. The reformulation of individual patients can provide a containing ba-

sis for management in longer-term treatments and for coordinated care planning in institutional settings. Finally, CAT is accumulating an expanding evidence base.

FURTHER READING

The description offered in this chapter is, of necessity, brief and may convey too technical a flavor. A full account of the CAT method applied to treating borderline personality disorder and a discussion of its relation to other approaches is found in Ryle (1997a) and case histories are provided in Ryle and Beard (1993) and Dunn (1994).

REFERENCES

Bell, L. (1999). The spectrum of psychological problems in people with eating disorders. *Journal of Clinical Psychology and Psychotherapy, 6,* 29–38.

Bennett, D., & Parry, G. (1998). The accuracy of reformulation in Cognitive Analytic Therapy: A validation study. *Psychotherapy Research, 8*(1), 84–103.

Bennett, D., Parry, G., & Ryle, A. (2000). *Deriving a model of therapist competence for the resolution of alliance threatening transference enactments. a) Model development. b) Verification phase.* Manuscript in preparation.

Boyes, M., Giordano, R., & Pool, M. (1997). Internalisation of social discourse: A Vygotskian account of the development of young children's theories of mind. In B. D. Cox & C. Lightfoot (Eds.), *Sociogenic perspectives on internalization.* Mahwah, NJ: Erlbaum.

Burkitt, I. (1995). *Social selves: Theories of the social formation of personality.* London: Sage.

Donald, M. (1991). *Origins of the modern mind.* Cambridge, MA. Harvard University Press.

Duignan, I., & Mitzman, S. (1994). Change in patients receiving time-limited cognition analytic group therapy. *International Journal of Short-Term Psychotherapy, 9,* 151–160.

Dunn, M. (1994). Variations in cognitive analytic therapy technique in the treatment of a severely disordered patient. *International Journal of Short-Term Psychotherapy, 9,* 83–92.

Dunn, M., & Parry, G. (1997). A formulated case plan approach to caring for people with borderline personality disorder in a community mental health service setting. *Clinical Psychology Forum, 104,* 19–22.

Fonagy, P., & Target, M. (1997). Attachment and reflective function: Their role in self-organisation. *Development and Psychopathology, 9,* 679–700.

Golynkina, K., & Ryle, A. (1999). The identification and characteristics of the partially dissociated states of patients with borderline personality disorder. *British Journal of Medical Psychology, 72,* 429–445.

Kerr, I. B. (1999). Cognitive analytic therapy for borderline personality disorder in the context of a community mental health team: individual and organisational psychodynamic implications. *British Journal of Psychotherapy, 15,* 425–438.

Kerr, I. B. (2000). Vygotsky, activity theory and the therapeutic community; a further paradigm? *Therapeutic Communities, 21*(3), 151–164.

Leighton, T. (1997). Borderline personality and substance abuse problems. In A. Ryle (Ed.), *Cognitive analytic therapy and borderline personality disorder: The model and the method.* Chichester, UK: Wiley.

Leiman, M. (1992). The concept of sign in the work of Vygotsky, Winnicott and Bakhtin: Further integration of object relations theory and activity theory. *British Journal of Medical Psychology, 65,* 209–221.

Leiman, M. (1994). The development of cognitive analytic therapy. *International Journal of Short-term Psychotherapy, 9*(2–3), 67–82.

Leiman, M. (1995). Early development. In A. Ryle (Ed.), *Cognitive analytic therapy: Developments in theory and practice.* Chichester, UK: Wiley.

Leiman, M. (1997). Procedures as dialogic sequences: A revised version of the fundamental concept in cognitive analytic therapy. *British Journal of Medical Psychology, 70,* 193–207.

Leiman, M. (2000). Ogden's matrix of transference and the concept of sign. *British Journal of Medical Psychology, 73,* 385–400.

Luborsky, L., & Crits-Christoph, P. (1990). *Understanding transference: The CCRT method.* New York. Basic Books.

Mann, J. (1973). *Time-limited psychotherapy.* Cambridge, MA: Harvard University Press.

Ogden, T. H. (1983). The concept of internal object relations. *International Journal of Psychoanalysis, 64,* 227–241.

Oliviera, Z. M. R. (1997). The concept of role in the discussion of the internalisation process. In B. D. Cox & C. Lightfoot (Eds.), *Sociogenic perspectives on internalisation.* Mahwah, NJ: Erlbaum.

Pollock, P., & Belshaw, T. (1998). Cognitive analytic therapy for offenders. *Journal of Forensic Psychiatry, 9,* 629–642.

Ryle, A. (1975). *Frames and cages.* London: Sussex University Press.

Ryle, A. (1982). *Psychotherapy: A cognitive integration of theory and practice.* London: Academic Press.

Ryle, A. (1985). Cognitive theory, object relations and the self. *British Journal of Medical Psychology, 58,* 1–7.

Ryle, A. (1991). Object relations theory and activity theory: A proposed link by way of the procedural sequence model. *British Journal of Medical Psychology, 64,* 307–316.

Ryle, A. (1994). Projective identification: A particular form of reciprocal role procedure. *British Journal of Medical Psychology, 67,* 107–114.

Ryle, A. (Ed.). (1995). *Cognitive analytic therapy: Developments in theory and practice.* Chichester, UK: Wiley.

Ryle, A. (1997a). *Cognitive analytic therapy and borderline personality disorder: The model and the method.* Chichester, UK: Wiley.

Ryle, A. (1997b). The structure and development of borderline personality disorder: A proposed model. *British Journal of Psychiatry, 170,* 82–87.

Ryle, A., & Beard, H. (1993). The integrative effort of reformation: Cognitive analytic therapy with a patient with borderline personality disorder. *British Journal of Psychology, 66,* 249–258.

Ryle, A., & Golynkina, K. (2000). Effectiveness of time-limited cognitive analytic therapy of borderline personality disorder: Factors associated with outcome. *British Journal of Medical Psychology, 73,* 197–200.

Sandler, J. (1976). Countertransference and role-responsiveness. *International Review of Psychoanalysis. 3,* 43–47.

Schacht, T. E., & Henry, W. P. (1994). Modelling recurrent relationship patterns with structural analysis of social behaviour: The SASB-CMP. *Psychotherapy Research, 4,* 208–221.

CHAPTER 20

Using Interpersonal Theory to Select Effective Treatment Interventions

LORNA SMITH BENJAMIN
CHRISTIE PUGH

Despite the evolution of huge numbers of different therapies that are effective in one context or another, a group of individuals remains who fail to respond to treatment no matter what the approach. A substantial number of these people qualify for the DSM-IV (American Psychiatric Association, 1994) label "personality disorder." "The personality disorders constitute one of the most important sources of long-term impairment in both treated and untreated populations. Nearly one in every 10 adults in the general population, and over one-half those in treated populations, may be expected to suffer from one of the personality disorders" (Merikangas & Weissman, 1986, p. 274). Any comorbid clinical syndromes, such depression or anxiety, are likely to be more intense and longer lasting if accompanied by personality disorder (Shea, Glass, Pilkonis, Watkins, & Docherty, 1987). Even biochemistry brings little relief to a chronically tormented and sometimes tormenting group. Even biochemistry does not reliably bring relief to this chronically tormented and sometimes tormenting group. These facts make it clear that finding an effective approach to the treatment of personality disorder is both important and difficult.

In today's empirically driven world, the clinician is exhorted just to get to the bottom line—manage those destructive behavioral patterns. However, many personality-disordered individuals are not about to be "managed." Thus, the current affection for empirically validated therapies (EVTs) leads third-party payers to disallow payments for treatment of personality disorder on the grounds that they are "untreatable."[1] Benjamin (1997) has argued that treatment of a personality disorder cannot be investigated under the typical 6- to 12-week EVT protocol. These problems necessarily require longer-term treatment. Despite its greater duration, longer-term therapy can be cost-effective if the measure of outcome includes total system costs: rehospitalizations, maintainance on medications, other medical costs, lost days at work, well-being, and so on. The idea is that if the personality disorder is treated rather than managed, the problems can remit greatly and permanently. Unfortunately, the methods of the many practitioners who are effective in this arena but who do not participate in research protocols have not been codified and documented. It therefore is important to describe more precisely and to document effectiveness whenever it is found in the treatment of personality disorder.

We argue that treatments that directly address cause (whether or not the practitioner is aware of the mechanism) are more likely to be successful than treatments that simply address symptoms. By analogy to internal medicine, a fever is more likely to remit if treated by a method that addresses its cause (e.g., antibiotic) than if treated only symptomatically (e.g., aspirin). A treatment of personality disorder will be more successful if the intervention addresses underlying causes rather than consequent symptoms or behaviors. This perspective immediately points to the need for a theory of cause in order to choose effective treatment.

Benjamin, an interpersonal psychologist, has suggested that the maladaptive patterns of personality disorder can be explained by the theory (Benjamin, 1993, 1996b) that "Every psychopathology is a gift of love" (Benjamin, 1993, p. 1). Briefly, the argument is that the relentless destructiveness so characteristic of personality disorder has strikingly direct connections to patterns learned in relation to early loved ones, or "attachment objects." The interpersonal or intrapsychic "repetition compulsion" represents nothing more or less than unconscious attempts to follow the "old rules." Behaving in ways that are consistent with early settings (usually the family of origin) has the unconscious purpose of pleasing and reconciling with an important early person or persons (mother, father, big brother, uncle). This theory holds that rather than hate and destruction or desire for power and superiority, love and attachment organize human (as well as infrahuman primate) behaviors. This chapter presents the reasoning and selected related empirical literature that support this theory.

Benjamin's (1996a, 1996b) case formulation method proposes that the problem behaviors seen at intake almost always reflect one or more of three copy processes in relation to early attachment objects. The connections are as follows: (1) Be like him or her (identification); (2) act as if he or she is still there and in charge (recapitulation); (3) treat yourself as did he or she (introjection). The parallels may not be at all apparent "to the naked eye." The key to seeing the connections between the problem patterns of personality disorder in adulthood and early important relationships is the lens offered by Structural Analysis of Social Behavior (SASB; Benjamin 1974, 1984). This model systematically describes interactions with key figures, past and present, in terms of (1) interpersonal focus (other, self, introjection), (2) love and hate, and (3) enmeshment and differentiation. Using the SASB lens, even the most outra-

geously self-destructive behaviors can be seen as repetitions of patterns with important persons. For example, the self-mutilating individual with borderline personality disorder may be recreating a particular version of incest that involved pleasure and pain, helplessness and power, and loneliness and intimacy (Benjamin, 1996a, Chap. 5). The motivation to continue such early patterns, to "do it" as if that early important person still prevailed, is, at base, a wish for reconciliation and validation by (the internalized representations of) early important person(s). In the example, the hypothesis would be that the individual with borderline personality disorder in circumscribed and sometimes unconscious ways loved and still loves her sexual abuser and wants to "make it right" or "make it have been better" with him or her.

The individual responds not to the "real" object but to his or her perception of that person as it has been internalized. Those portrayals are named Important Persons and their Internalized Representations (IPIRs). The use of SASB to describe the original patterns of interaction and their interpersonal and intrapsychic representations in adulthood essentially codifies Bowlby's (1977) description of "internal working models." Shafer (1968) provides an excellent presentation of a psychoanalytic perspective on the variety of possible relationships with internal models. The most important treatment implication of the present analysis is that the underlying attachment must be consistently addressed in therapy until the wish for reconciliation and validation from the driving internalizations is given up. Benjamin has argued that normal and pathological adaptations follow exactly the same mechanisms (Benjamin, 1973, 1974, 1995, 1996b; Henry, 1994). The difference is that normal individuals have copied normal models whereas disordered individuals have had to cope with deviant models. Usually normal individuals function in a region of interpersonal space described by the SASB model as friendly: moderately enmeshed and moderately differentiated. The points on the SASB model that describe these normal positions are called the Attachment Group (AG) of behaviors.[2] These normal baseline patterns of interaction are usually "good" in the sense that they are associated with pleasant affects, good health, lasting relationships and satisfaction

The goal of therapy is to give patients or clients the option of functioning mainly in "good" interpersonal space, that is, in the AG of interpersonal positions. Therapy is viewed as an interpersonal and intrapsychic learning experience that involves (1) learning what your patterns are, where they came from, and what they are for; (2) deciding whether to give up the early wishes and fantasies that drive the behaviors, and change; and (3) learning new patterns (Benjamin, 1996a, 1996b). Deciding "what they are for" and "whether to give up the associated wishes and fantasies" has largely to do with unearthing and working with thoughts, feelings, and actions in relation to the IPIRs.

Any and all known therapy approaches and modes can be relevant to this process. A given intervention is correct if it conforms to one or more of the following five steps, each of which is consistent with the present description of therapy as a learning process.

1. Collaborate against "it" (i.e., the problem patterns and the wishes that sustain them).
2. Learn about patterns, where they are from and what they are for.
3. Block maladaptive patterns.
4. Enable the will to change.
5. Learn new patterns.

These five steps or stages are roughly sequential, though sharp deviations can be observed. Nonetheless, appreciation of the fundamentally sequential nature of the steps is helpful. For change to occur, the patient or client must contract to work on the underlying problem. Then, he or she must understand what needs to be worked on. Next, the patient must decide to and be willing to endure the pain of letting go of old hopes and to put the necessary effort into the change process. Finally, the patient or client must practice new and unfamiliar ways of being, without any guarantees that he or she will like normality any better than the old ways. Reconstruction of personality requires substantial effort and force of will on the part of both the patient or client and the therapist.

A probable reason that the personality disordered are regarded as "untreatable" is that modern interventions should not be attempted until step 5. After the will to change has been fully engaged (step 4), it is possible to teach new patterns using behavioral technologies such as cognitive-behavioral therapy, assertiveness training, affective expression, communication skills training, social skills training, and parenting training. If the will to change has not been enabled, such efforts to teach new patterns are likely to fail. Individuals with personality disorder can change only if they will give up old hopes and fears in relation to IPIRs. The will to stay attached to old internalizations and the associated problematic patterns is the cause of the personality disorder. Only if it is addressed effectively can personality disorder remit.

Benjamin (2000) describes clinical techniques that can facilitate each of the five therapy steps in treating individuals with personality disorder. The most important and the most difficult is step 4, enabling the will to change. The goal of the approach is to help patients develop stable and marked improvement in their ways of relating to themselves and to others. If step 4 can be mastered, the goal is within reach. We believe the resulting reconstructive interpersonal changes lead to greater productivity and satisfaction as well as to fewer overall requests of the health care system.

The purposes of this chapter are (1) briefly to sketch this approach that seeks to transform the underlying wishes that organize (cause) personality disorder before trying to facilitate change and (2) to review empirical evidence in support of the perspective. The topics to be covered include (1) review of the SASB model and assessment instruments that can be used to operationalize important aspects of therapy process and content as well as internalized representation of attachment objects and current relationships, (2) review of related developmental theory and empirical evidence, (3) case demonstration of how the SASB model can connect early attachments and pathological patterns of adult disorder, (4) review of treatment implications and related empirical evidence, and (5) comments on future developments.

STRUCTURAL ANALYSIS OF SOCIAL BEHAVIOR

The SASB (Benjamin, 1974, 1984, 1996b) provides a method for operationalizing therapy-relevant interpersonal and intrapsychic concepts. Therapists or researchers can use the model to quantify patients' perceptions of themselves and others, to make clear connections between past experience and current problem patterns, to organize and measure the interpersonal process that takes place within the therapy session, and more. Among other things, there is strong convergence among process, treatment, and outcome measures (Henry, 1996). Assessments can be made at any stage by participant self-ratings or by objective observer ratings, all within the same metric.

Historical Antecedents

The roots of the SASB model are found in the early efforts of psychotherapists and personality and developmental theorists to understand psychopathology objectively and interpersonally. The most influential precursors were Harry Stack Sullivan, Henry Murray, Timothy Leary, Earl Shaefer, and Harry Harlow.

Harry Stack Sullivan (1953) emphasized anxiety avoidance as a basic motivation and interpreted it interpersonally. The power of the mothering object lay in her ability to relieve anxiety. Sullivan believed that interpersonal interactions with the mother and later with others deeply affected the psyche. He described the process of introjection as treating the self as did the "good mother and the bad mother" (Sullivan, 1953). Even the severe and bizarre disorder of schizophrenia was described as a fundamentally human process by Sullivan (1962).

Murray (1938) made one of the earliest attempts to apply scientific method to psychoanalytic concepts. Along with many colleagues of diverse persuasion, Murray conducted exhaustive studies of 51 normal male college students. The theoretical work product was a long list of basic human needs, arranged in hierarchies. Timothy Leary (1957) arranged selected needs from Murray's list around horizontal and vertical axes to form a circle. A circular arrangement of categories is now known as a circumplex (Guttman, 1966). There have been several variations on the circumplex originally proposed by Leary, but all define the horizontal axis in terms of love versus hate. By so doing, they incorporate aspects of Freud's proposal that sexuality and aggression (id) as basic human motivations. The Leary-based circumplexes define the vertical axis in terms of Dominance versus Submission. This practice incorporates Adler's belief that "the psyche has as its objective, the goal of superiority" (Adler, 1955, p. 289). Nobody, however, has claimed that its "opposite," submission, is a universal driver.

The circumplex models provide that behaviors can be described in terms of the underlying dimensions defined by their axes. In the case of the Leary-based models, behaviors that fall in between the poles of love and control represent graded combinations of love and control (e.g., responsible and hypernormal; Leary, 1957). Behaviors between the poles of control and attack represent combinations of those poles (e.g., competitive–narcissistic). Circumplex order provides that behaviors next to each other are most highly correlated, and similarity decreases as the distance that separates the items increases. Following this logic, items on opposite sides of the circumplex are maximally dissimilar and are called opposites (e.g., love vs. hate).

While models based on Leary's circumplex oppose dominance with submission, Schaefer's (1965) model of parenting behaviors provided a vertical axis that ranged from control to autonomy-giving. Both the Leary type of circumplex models and Schaefer's model have been confirmed by factor analysis of self-ratings (Schaefer, 1965; Wiggins, 1982).

Structure of the SASB Model

Benjamin suggested a resolution to the question of how the opposite of dominance could both be submission (according to Leary) and emancipation (according to Schaefer). SASB (Benjamin, 1974) presented in Figure 20.1, includes two interpersonal surfaces.

As is the case in the Leary-based circles, the SASB model places love and hate on the horizontal axis for each surface of the model. The first surface is devoted to prototypically parent-like behavior that focuses on another person (e.g., **PROTECT**, located at 4 o'clock). The second surface shows prototypically child-like behavior that focuses on the self in relation to another person (e.g., TRUST, also located at 4 o'clock). The parentlike surface used Schafer's definition of the vertical axis: **EMANCIPATE** was placed opposite **CONTROL**. On the childlike surface, the vertical dimension placed SUBMIT at one pole, and SEPARATE at the other.

On the SASB model, **CONTROL** and SUBMIT are located at the same position in interpersonal space (6 o'clock), but they differ in focus. Focus is the dimension that distinguishes the three surfaces. Focus on other (e.g., **CONTROL**) involves a transitive action focused on, directed toward another person. Focus on self (e.g., SUBMIT) is an intransitive reaction, a condition, or a state of the self. In terms of English grammar, focus on other requires a direct object (I **CONTROL** you) whereas focus on

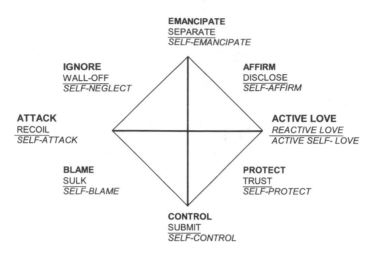

FIGURE 20.1. Simple cluster version of the SASB model. Labels in **bold** print describe actions directed at another person (parent-like focus). The underlined labels describe reactions to another person's (perceived) initiations (child-like focus). Adjacent boldface and underlined labels describe complementary pairings. Labels in *italics* show what happens if a person treats him- or herself just as important others have treated him or her (introjected focus). From Benjamin (1996a, p. 55). Copyright 1996 by The Guilford Press. Reprinted by permission.

self implies an indirect object (I <u>SUBMIT to</u> you). Benjamin (e.g., 1979) suggests the combination of **CONTROL**/<u>SUBMIT</u> can be interpreted as maximal enmeshment, whereas the combination of emancipate/separate is a good description of differentiation. In sum, the two interpersonal surfaces (other, self) of the SASB model describes interpersonal interactions in terms of love versus hate and enmeshment versus differentiation.

When two members of a dyad focus on the same person with comparable amounts of love–hate and of enmeshment–differentiation, they are in complementary relation. If one **CONTROLs** and the other <u>SUBMITs</u>, they match their positions in interpersonal space. No opposition is involved. One position "pulls" for the other. Similarly, <u>TRUST</u> and **PROTECT** are complementary. <u>TRUST</u> makes **PROTECT** more likely and **PROTECT** makes <u>TRUST</u> more likely. The cluster model, shown in Figure 20.1, provides a description of eight complementary pairings. Complementarity is an important predictive principle for the study of social interaction in the developmental process, in therapy process, and elsewhere (Benjamin, 1974; Carson, 1969; Kiesler, 1996; Sullivan, 1953).

In addition to providing a resolution to the question of how **CONTROL** could have two "opposites" (**EMANCIPATE**/<u>SUBMIT</u>), the

SASB model offers full articulation of the many possible forms of differentiation, a concept that is recognized as important by developmental and family researchers as well as psychoanalytic theorists (Olson, 1996).

Predictive Principles

The SASB model offers several predictive principles that are useful in tracking links from attachment objects to adult personality. The main predictive principles are introjection, complementarity, similarity, opposition, and antithesis. It is not possible to know which predictive principle will apply in any given instance. Nonetheless, the model does mark a limited array of possibilities likely to emerge in any given SASB codeable interpersonal context.

Introjection

The SASB model encompasses Sullivan's notion of introjection with a third, or intrapsychic, surface (Figure 20.1). This surface represents what happens if one treats oneself as one has been treated. For example, the introjection of parental **CONTROL** results in *SELF-CONTROL*. In this example, both the developmental antecedent, shown on the first surface, and the consequent, shown on the third surface, are located at 6 o'clock. Similarly, Figure 20.1 suggests that one who has been **PROTECT**ed is likely to *SELF-PROTECT*. The cluster model articulates eight theoretical antecedents to eight different types of self-concept. It is important to note that this description of introjection is only one aspect of self-concept. All three copy processes affect the self-concept, and introjection is but one of them.

Consider the concept of "low self-esteem. " This concept is associated with not being "valued" by important others, whereas feeling valued promotes a positive self-concept. In Figure 20.1, important aspects of low and high self-esteem are shown by the respective positions, *SELF-BLAME* (7:30 o'clock) and *SELF-AFFIRM* (2:30 o'clock). These are the theoretical consequences of perceived **BLAME** (7:30 o'clock) and **AFFIRM** (2:30 o'clock). Articulation of the introject can be helpful in predicting responses in therapy and elsewhere. For example, a SASB-informed clinician knows that a patient who tends to blame him- or herself is likely to see others as blaming and also to be quick to **BLAME** others. For example, the patient might say, "You are not helping me at all." The therapist should not counter with, "You are resisting this treatment." To avoid enhancing poor self-concept, the therapist does well to avoid complementing or returning patient attacks and, instead, to affirm the patient in a way that builds collaboration and strength. For example, in this case, the therapist might say, "It is easy to see why you would see me as completely useless, given your history. But I wonder if we could look together at the possibility that your expectations might be interfering with your ability to find something useful in what we are working on here."

Introject change is an important index of outcome in interpersonal psychotherapy, and therapist behaviors are directly linked to patient introject change (Henry, Schacht, & Strupp, 1990; Rudy, McLemore, & Gorsuch, 1985). There is some SASB-based evidence that patients' internalizations of the therapist's actions toward them are consistent with the specific changes in introject that occur over the course of therapy (Quintana & Meara, 1990).

Complementarity

Complementarity on the friendliness/hostility dimension has been well documented in all circumplex models. The vertical dimension has not fared so well when Leary-style circumplex-

es provide the measures (Orford, 1986). Investigations using complementarity as defined by the SASB model (discussed earlier) have consistently been empirically supported in both the horizontal and vertical dimensions (Benjamin, 1994; Gurtman, in press).

As is the case with introjection, prediction based on complementarity can be useful in therapy with personality disordered patients. For example, a person with histrionic personality disorder might engage in any of a number of behaviors that amount to coercive dependency ("I can't handle this and I must have an extra appointment today"). These can be characterized by a complex SASB code **CONTROL** plus <u>TRUST</u>. A complementary response from the therapist or spouse would be to provide compliant nurturance ("OK. I can see you after my last appointment today"). The complementary complex SASB code is <u>SUBMIT</u> plus **PROTECT**. Note that both elements of the initial complex code are matched by their theoretical complements (<u>SUBMIT</u>/**CONTROL** and **PROTECT**/<u>TRUST</u>) in this example. That is not at all unusual in practice. There is a strong draw for the therapist to do what is expected and inadvertently to enable a basic problem pattern (the coercive dependency). The exchange might better be used to help the patient recognize this pattern in his or her interpersonal relationships and relate it to its origins. For example, rather than agreeing to the extra appointment right away, the therapist might say, "Let's look again at your wish to have the extra appointment. Can you relate it at all to what we have been talking about?" Perhaps the patient can discover a connection: "Daddy would take care of whatever she needed—but only if he was around." Awareness of the activation of an old habit could bring the patient closer to giving up the self-weakening wish to have things be the way they used to be. This should contribute to strengthening the will to change and to a better outcome. In a related study, Henry, Schacht, and Strupp (1986) showed that therapists who were unable to resist the draw to hostile complementarity had poorer outcomes.

If, in relation to a spouse or important others, like the therapist, the patient maintains the position that was complementary to the attachment object, the patient implements the copy process of Recapitulation. In this example, the patient continues her habit of making a dominant male take care of her. She is recapitulating the relationship with her father.

Similarity

The principle of Similarity is shown when the SASB codes for one person are the same as for another. For example, if the parent is described by **BLAME** (Figure 20.1), and the patient behaves the same way in relation to her husband, she implements the principle of Similiarity in relation to the parent. The principle of Similiarity describes the copy process of Identification. If the patient **BLAME**s his blaming mother, he invokes the principle of Similarity. If he **BLAME**s his spouse, he invokes the copy process of Identification. He is taking the pattern learned in relation to an attachment object and implements it elsewhere.

Opposition

The principle of Opposition is shown at 180-degree angles in Figure 20.1. Sometimes people develop in reverse image of the attachment object. For example, if the parent was quite negligent (**IGNORE** on Figure 20.1), the grown-up version of the child will be protective (**PROTECT** is located opposite **IGNORE** in Figure 20.1). A pattern of opposition is illustrated by the observation that many overprotective, highly enmeshed mothers themselves have a history of abandonment and neglect. They seem to be trying to make sure their child does not suffer their own history, and so they do the opposite of their parent. Unfortunately, they often overcorrect and pass along a new problem. Opposition can be a manifest in any of the three copy processes. In this example, the overprotective mother is copying her own mother in an oppositional manner. She may feel she is "different," but the fact that her behaviors are exact 180-degree opposites and not contingent upon her child's reaction connect her to her attachment object in her own relations as a parent.

Antithesis

The principle of Antithesis is manifest when one person gives the complement of the opposite. For example, the passive–aggressive individual likely has a history of punitive overcontrol (Benjamin, 1996a, Chap. 11). These individuals specialize in the complement of the opposite of **CONTROL**, namely, SEPARATE. Antithetical points differ in focus and are located at 180-degree angles. An example of antithesis is found in a popular couple therapy intervention that asks partners to disclose their own feelings rather than to blame and try to change the other. Note that in Figure 20.1, DISCLOSE is the antithesis of **BLAME**, By providing the antithesis of **BLAME**, partners draw for its opposite, **AFFIRM**. If the suggestion is followed, the partners stop the blaming war and begin to listen to each other and to disclose in meaningful ways. The cluster version of the SASB model details 16 different types of antithetical behaviors.

Antithethetical behaviors also can be seen in any of the three copy processes. For example, if the patient's father was fiercely overcontrolling, suppose the patient maintained an antithetical position of SEPARATE from the father. If the patient now is very separate from his wife, he recapitulates the relationship with his father. On the other hand, if he overcontrols his wife, he identifies with his father. Suppose now that the patient was very submissive to his overcontrolling father but now is quite separate from his wife. He is recapitulating the opposite of his early pattern and showing the antithesis to his father's position.

The presence of the three surfaces, each showing a horizontal axis that ranges from love to hate, and vertical axes that describe relations among dominance, submission, and emancipation, makes the SASB model quite a bit more complex relative to others (Carson, 1994). However, the complexity provides a substantial number of clinical advantages, including the ability to describe differentiation well and to define predictive principles and copy processes that have direct and helpful clinical implications.

The Intrex Questionnaires

Formal research coding or informal on-line clinical coding is only one of the available methods of measurement using the SASB model. The Intrex questionnaires (Benjamin, 1984) can generate self-ratings or observer ratings. The questionnaires contain items that directly reflect the interpersonal behaviors on each point of the SASB model. Raters are asked to indicate the degree (ranging from 0 to 100) to which the items are seen as true for each rated relationship.

Like the SASB model itself, the Intrex questionnaires are available in varying levels of resolution. The short, medium, and long forms provide increasingly detailed information about a person's patterns. The reliability and validity of the questionnaires is described in detail in the user's manuals for the respective forms.[3] An Intrex-based assessment of a psychotherapy patient provides information about the patient's patterns in past and current important relationships, as well as the characteristic ways in which the patient treats him- or herself. The Intrex report includes a description of possible connections among the patient's early social relationships and his or her self-concept. In other words, the Intrex output offers hypotheses about connections among the patient's "object relations."

These questionnaires differ from most traditional assessment measures in some important ways. First, they directly measure perceptions of interpersonal and intrapsychic interactions and of significant others in interpersonal relationships. Most traditional self-report techniques, including those that ask about relationship functioning, only ask the rater to describe him- or herself in relationships. By failing to assess the perception of other, they lose important information. A related point is that the questionnaires are used to understand the patients differently in different relationships. Whereas most approaches view the patient's behaviors as indicative of "traits," the SASB-based approach is consistent with the interpersonal perspective that patient's behaviors vary by interpersonal context. One normally does not behave with a spouse as with a colleague or a child or a parent. Also, the Intrex questionnaires provide results in language that relates directly to what happens in interpersonal psychotherapy. For example, patients easily understand SASB-coded reflections based on the output: "Your mother was controlling and blaming, and it appears that you see your supervisor in the same way." This means that assessment results are directly clinically useful—they do not need to be translated into any other "language."

SASB and Personality Disorder

Benjamin (1996b) has shown that SASB codes of the DSM-IV definitions of personality disorder provide descriptions that can reduce overlap among categories and provide testable etiological hypotheses and useful treatment suggestions. The process may be reversed. One can assess a patient's baseline interpersonal positions on the SASB model and make a DSM diagnosis by comparing the interpersonal style to the SASB codes of the respective DSM personality disorders. For example, a person likely to meet DSM-IV criteria for obsessive–compulsive personality disorder is likely to tell narratives indicative of inconsiderate control of others (**CONTROL** plus **IGNORE**). He or she probably also will show deference to authority and moral causes that is fundamentally unsociable (SUBMIT plus WALL-OFF). Finally, he or she will embrace perfectionism that precludes a balanced self-concept (*SELF-CONTROL* plus *SELF-NEGLECT*).

Another SASB-informed approach to diagnosis is the Wisconsin Personality Inventory (WISPI; Klein et al., 1993), a self-report questionnaire that assesses whether the patient meets criteria for one or more DSM-IV (American Psychiatric Association, 1994) personality disorders. SASB was used to elicit endorsement of DSM items based on wording from the perspective of the client (rather than the observer). For example, consider DSM-IV criterion 5 for the category of narcissistic personality disorder: "has a sense of entitlement, i.e., unreasonable expectations of especially favorable treatment or automatic compliance with his or her expectations" (p. 661). The corresponding WISPI item is: "I really get irritated when others fail to assist me in my very important work" (p. 661). A patient with narcissistic personality disorder is unlikely to endorse the "objective" behavior of the DSM-IV item, especially as it implies that his or her expectations are "unreasonable" (i.e., don't make sense). The WISPI item addresses the criterion through the phenomenology of the narcissistic personality disorder patient, and does so specifically enough that it is more likely to be endorsed by patients with narcissistic personality disorder than by other groups of personality-disordered patients.

REVIEW OF RELATED DEVELOPMENTAL THEORY AND EMPIRICAL EVIDENCE

The underlying assumption behind the present approach to therapy is that the maladaptive patterns of personality disorder are organized and maintained by wishes that relations with early attachment objects could have been or somehow could be better—the unrecognized wish that things will work out if only the patient can do things as he or she is "supposed to." The personality-disordered patient repeats old patterns and lives out old prophesies in an attempt to realize the fantasied reconciliation. The individual follows old rules in order to maintain "psychic proximity" to the internalized loved one. The connections to the early attachment objects are rather straightforward when seen through the SASB lens. Again, they are, quite simply: Be like him or her; Act as if he or she is still there and in control; Treat yourself as did he or she. The treatment implications of this analysis are equally simple in concept but not in practice: Recognize the connections and give up the fantasy; grieve the loss of what never was and never will be. In other words, personality pathology is a direct consequence of habits and wishes associated with persisting attachments. It cannot remit until those wishes are changed.

Research on the importance of attachment is cascading through the literature. Several disciplines are engaged in the discovery process, including developmental psychology, developmental neurology, social psychology, clinical psychology, cognitive neuroscience, and psychiatry. Baumeister and Leary's (1995) perspective from social psychology is particularly broad and gives a good overview of the breadth and importance of attachment research. Two branches of this literature are especially relevant to the present context. One is the vast array of studies that suggest that attachment has far-reaching effects. The other is the quite new discipline of developmental neurology. Each is briefly reviewed.

Developmental Stages

The analysis of developmental stages begins with the "attachment" phase. Freud, Erickson, and Mahler, named the first stage, respectively, the oral stage; trust versus mistrust; and (autism and) symbiotic stage. Despite important differences, all three theorists thought of the beginning as a time of intense closeness between the mother and infant. The well-tended infant experiences nurturance, comfort, and protection from the primary caregiver. Bowlby (1969) detailed at length how neonatal and infantile reflexes converge to maximize the chances for a good attachment. This vital process is coded on the SASB model within the AG. If the attachment does not go well, many untoward consequences, discussed later, follow.

As the infant grows, an "opposing" need for independence emerges. Freud (1949) named

the second stage the "sadistic–anal stage, because satisfaction is then sought in aggression and in the excretory function" (p. 11). Erikson (1959) marked the second stage as a time of conflict between autonomy versus shame and doubt. Mahler (1968) also tagged independence as the issue at the second stage. She described separation–individuation in terms of subphases: hatching, practicing and rapprochement. Bowlby and Mahler emphasized that the infant's confident and successful individuation and development of a secure sense of self are dependent on having a secure attachment object to return to during times of distress. If the attachment is not secure, the individuation phase may be characterized by clinginess and overly tentative exploration, or a tendency to remain altogether outside the proximity of the parent.

Bowlby (1977) detailed a "dance" between attachment and independence that is crucial to the development of a separate but secure and well-socialized self. A host of psychiatric disorders are thought to be related to failure to negotiate this second stage successfully. Difficulties stemming from the second stage are related to differentiation failure and reflect either too much enmeshment or too much distance. These problems can be coded on the vertical axis of the SASB model, which defines enmeshment and differentiation. In sum, the horizontal axis of the SASB model depicts attachment versus disrupted attachment (DAG). The vertical axis details enmeshment versus differentiation.

The first two developmental stages, according to these psychoanalytic theorists, reflect the idea that attachment orients the person toward other human beings and then differentiation helps the person define him- or herself separately from others. According to many, the process involves balancing opposites. According to the SASB-based description of interpersonal space, however, the process merely involves two orthogonal (independent) thrusts, each of which must occur to fully articulate interpersonal space. Affiliation and autonomy appear at 90 degrees rather than at 180-degree angles on the SASB model. The distinction is not "academic." In other words, it matters. Because affiliation and autonomy appear at right angles on the SASB model, they can jointly define a space that is called "friendly autonomy." If they were at opposite ends, the dimensions of affiliation and autonomy could not conjointly define any space. Placed as they are, the two axes describe friendly autonomy, an important part of normative, "healthy" space. The psychological meaning of the observation that love and independence are orthogonal rather than opposite is that the child can be well attached and well differentiated without any tension. A strong attachment (noncontrolling love) easily permits friendly separation and conflict-free reunion. If there is conflict about self definition within a relationship, it must exist because one or both participants want to control the other. Control and permission for autonomy are opposites and are associated with conflict and ambivalence. In contrast, according to SASB theory, good attachment and good self-definition are perfectly compatible.

Bowlby's (1969) monograph on the importance of attachment relied primarily for supporting evidence on observations of mother–infant behaviors in various cultures and on field studies of primate behavior. Strongly supportive laboratory data were provided by Harlow's laboratory studies of infant monkeys separated from their mothers at varying ages from birth. The association in monkeys between attachment disruption (by social isolation) and depression, poor social skills, and nearly nonexistent parenting skills was demonstrated by an extraordinary collection of studies directed by Harry Harlow. For example, Bowlby's earlier writings about attachment focused on depression that results from separation from the attachment object. A relatively succinct review of the early laboratory studies related to depression in monkeys is offered by McKinney, Suomi, and Harlow (1973). Their findings resoundingly supported Bowlby's ideas about attachment and loss. Another series of studies from Harlow's laboratory confirmed Bowlby's thesis that attachment is primary, and not dependent on the mother's ability to nurture.

Ainsworth and Wittig (1969) presented a standardized laboratory test for humans that subjected infants and toddlers to the stress of separation from their mother while in an unfamiliar situation (the Strange Situation test). The responses observed during repeated separations and upon reunion led to classification of infants based on their attachment type. Systems of classification vary somewhat, but the Ainsworth group originally suggested three categories of attachment: secure, avoidant, and ambivalently attached. Although this paradigm and the measures that followed are known as studies of attachment, the method clearly as-

sesses both attachment and differentiation. It holds that how the child separates or fails to separate from the mother, and how he or she behaves during reunion, defines the quality of the attachment. The massive literature built on the Strange Situation assessment repeatedly shows that attachment (and differentiation) has both short- and long-term effects on the development of personality. Some examples follow.

Attachment behaviors demonstrated in children between the ages of 1 and 2 years predict later sociability with other children and unfamiliar adults, behavioral problems, and effectiveness of emotional regulation. Reviews of this impressive literature have been prepared (Ainsworth, Blehar, Waters, & Wall, 1978; Greenberg & Speltz, 1988; Richters & Waters, 1991). Insecure attachment relationships place children at risk for a wide variety of behavioral problems during the preschool years (Greenberg, Speltz, DeKlyen, & Endriga, 1991) and beyond (Sroufe, Egeland, & Kreutzer, 1990; Elicker, Englund, & Sroufe, 1992). Toth and Cicchetti (1996) have suggested that "insecure attachment relationships and the resulting negative representational models of the self and the self in relation to others may be a central mechanism contributing to the emergence of disturbances in children who have been maltreated" (p. 34). For example, maltreated toddlers with insecure attachment relationships talk less about themselves, their feelings, and their activities than do other toddlers (Beeghly & Cicchetti, 1994). Also, such toddlers display neutral or negative reactions on recognizing themselves in a mirror, in contrast to the positive responses displayed by most children (Schneider-Rosen & Cicchetti, 1991).

The impact of early attachment experiences is now also being measured in adults, and adult representations of their own attachment experiences have been linked to the attachment behaviors displayed by their own infants, preschoolers, and school-age children (Cowan, Cohn, Cowan, & Pearson, 1996; Deklyen, 1996; Fonagy, Steele, & Steele, 1991). Recent findings also support links between adolescents' and adults' representations of their attachment relationships and specific Axis I and II psychiatric disorders, psychopathology in general, and responsiveness to psychotherapy (Rosenstein & Horowitz, 1996; van IJzendoorn & Bakermans-Kranenburg, 1996).

Some data support the idea that patterns in early relationships with the primary caregiver drive expectations for future social interactions. Children with nonoptimal relationships with primary caregivers are more likely to develop similar relationships with peers and teachers, whereas those with optimal relationships are somewhat more flexible (Toth & Cicchetti, 1996). In fact, only 11% of the children in this sample with a nonoptimal parent–child relationship formed positive relationships with peers or teachers. Even more startling was the report that only 2% formed positive relationships with both peers and teachers.

Longitudinal studies show that a large number of individuals with histories of insecure attachment, abuse experiences, or other problems in early relationships never require clinical treatment. We believe the impact of developmental experience, traumatic or not, can be traced directly through the three named copy processes as illustrated below. If the child is attached to the abuser, he or she will be far more seriously harmed than if not. There would be little wish to copy patterns in relation to someone who does not "matter." How the child experiences an abusive episode and what he or she learns learns from it about self and others matters far more than the category of the event itself. This line of thinking means that searches for generic traumatic marker events, like sexual or physical abuse, will not "explain" adult personality disorder. Others (Paris, 1997; Rutter, 1989; Zanarini & Frankenburg, 1997) also have argued that developmental events must be viewed with consideration of predispositions, the larger context in which events occurred, and the specific meaning that the events had for the child and his or her relationships with significant others. Toth and Cicchetti (1996) found that patterns of relatedness in childhood are better predictors of behavior than simple consideration of abuse status.

Having reviewed theory and data related to attachment (and, implicitly, the ability to separate while remaining attached), it is appropriate to comment briefly on whether there are any subsequent important developmental stages. For later years, Bowlby's emphasis remains on attachment and the dance with independence (Bowlby, 1969). Freud and Mahler marked different subsequent issues. The third stage in development is one of reconciliation and rapprochement, according to Mahler. Freud describes an Oedipal stage wherein the little boy wants to marry his mother and the girl her father. A perhaps oversimplified view of what Freud said is that there is a fair amount of internal conflict that stems from these wishes.

The SASB model provides a testable hypothesis about what is important about this third developmental stage. The SASB-based operationalization of the new development is that the third stage adds understanding about focus on others. Developmental data (Benjamin, 1974, p. 404) suggest that child-like (intransitive) focus is well integrated from earliest infancy. By contrast, parent-like focus (transitive) is nonexistent during the earliest months and becomes progressively better integrated through the years. The coefficient of internal consistency for focus on others is near zero at birth. Babies are rated near zero on nearly all parent-like (focus on other) behaviors. As they develop, the parent-like domain begins to fill in and integrate. Its coefficient of internal consistency shows rather rapid increases in magnitude over the first 2 years. By 3 years of age, the approximate time of rapprochement, the magnitude of the coefficient of internal consistency for focus on other begins to level off. However, it is not until ages 7 to 9 that focus on other actually reaches adult levels of integration. In sum, according to data based on the SASB model, the third stage marks the arrival of the ability to show parent-like, as well as child-like interpersonal focus. For example, the 3- to 4-year-old begins to **PROTECT** his mother as well as to TRUST her. He or she can assume **CONTROL** and **BLAME** too, especially if the family models those patterns frequently. The 3-year-old also knows how to **IGNORE** or to **AFFIRM** the attachment object.

The preceding discussion suggests that important aspects of clinical and folk wisdom can be summarized by appeal to the SASB model and data. The first task is to develop a good attachment (horizontal axis of the SASB model). The next is to define a separate self in relation to attachment objects (vertical axis of the SASB model). The third is to discover focus on other to add to the present-at-birth focus on self. When these tasks are complete, the child has a grasp of the basic dimensions of interpersonal space. Subsequent development will let the child combine those basic understandings to maintain or change patterns of personality throughout the life cycle. The argument is not that everything important about personality is determined by age 3. There is plenty of opportunity for imbalances to develop and to be corrected after the first three stages. The thesis is that the three main issues (attachment, differentiation, balance of focus) should be defined by that time. If they are not, serious subsequent psychopathology may result. The reason is straightforward: Subsequent stages will tend to reflect, even consolidate, early patterns. Subsequent stages necessarily draw on the earliest skills and abilities. If something basic is missing (attachment, differentiation, balance of focus), the result cannot be normative. Under the reasoning that earlier stages affect later ones, but not vice versa, it would appear that failure at the first, attachment, would have the most serious consequences. Data previously above support that reasoning.

Developmental Neurology

Having considered the evidence that early attachment experiences have profound and lasting effects on social behavior, the next question is: What is the mechanism? Eisenberg (1995) and Schore (1996) have provided overviews that include evidence demonstrating that early attachment experiences have a major influence on social behavior in general and the central nervous system development in particular. The neurological argument frequently is drawn by appealing to simpler systems. For example, Eisenberg notes that in the postnatal environment, infants must receive visual stimulation in order for visual structures in the occipital cortex to properly develop. Abnormal stimulation produces structural abnormalities and functional impairments that are directly related to experience. If one eye is covered or blurred, the unimpaired eye will develop proportionally more occular dominance columns than will the impaired eye. Conversely, extra stimulation of developing systems can have a positive impact on structure and function. Expanding inquiry to other systems, Eisenberg notes that in rodents, enriched stimulation has been demonstrated to lead to improved function as well as increased density of neurons and concentration of neurotransmitters. Animal and human studies have also demonstrated that adult brains can undergo functional, if not structural, reorganization in response to such physical changes.

   Direct evidence of a connection between attachment and neurobiology in primates is summarized by Kraemer's (1992) psychobiological model of attachment. His model is based on important differences in neurochemistry between laboratory monkeys with good maternal attachments and those without. Focusing specifically on personality disorder, Figueroa and Silk (1997) as well as Sabo (1997) reviewed the literature to find links between early trauma/abuse, and the "possible biological disturbances and clinical picture of borderline personality disorder (BPD). They suspect involvement of autonomic nervous system reactivity and hypothalamic–pituitary–adrenal axis in borderline personality disorder. They note that responses to stress differ depending on individual histories, and, for some cases, abnormally high reactivity is displayed only in response to specific triggering events. Sabo (1997) concludes that a variety of research studies show that stress may be regulated by physiological derivatives of attachment and caregiving.

Conclusions Based on Empirical Evidence from These Two Domains

The empirical studies of the far-reaching impact of attachment experiences on behavior, self-concept, and neurological development are consistent with the present hypotheses about the development and maintenance of personality disorder. These literatures establish that early patterns are important and begin examination of possible mechanisms for the transmission of the effects. The literature review does not clearly prove the existence of internal working models. Nor does it establish that patterns of personality disorder are related specifically to early attachment objects via one or more of the three copy processes. Toward that end, the next section presents a case history that is highly representative of hundreds of diagnostic interviews with psychiatric inpatients. It was the consistency of results with those interviews, processed via the SASB lens, that led Benjamin to the copy process IPIR theory.

CASE DEMONSTRATION OF IPIR THEORY

Case Formulation Method

Benjamin's (1993, 1996b) argument, "Every Psychopathology Is a Gift of Love" holds that the relentless destructiveness so characteristic of personality disorder has a strikingly direct connection to patterns learned in relation to early loved ones, or "attachment objects." This belief is reflected directly in the case formulation method (Benjamin, 1996c). Problem behaviors seen at intake are related via one or more of three copy processes to early attachment objects. The key to seeing the connections between the problem patterns of personality disorder in adulthood and early important relationships is the lens offered by SASB.

The procedure for identifying the connections is well operationalized (Benjamin, 1996b, 2000). Briefly, the assessment interviews are divided into two parts. The first covers material that might be found in a well-organized standard medical survey and includes presenting problems, current stresses, responses to stresses, conscious self-concept, current diagnoses, and current treatment. The second part seeks information that helps organize and understand the medical presentation. The method is to assess the patient in interpersonal context, both present and past. For each key relationship, there is a systematic evaluation of input (what is the patient doing/what is happening), response (how does the patient respond), and impact on self-concept (how does this relationship/event affect the self-concept). Key figures are identified by the patient's stream of consciousness. The people patients mention when asked at the beginning of the interview: "What do you want and need?" are more than likely key figures. The patient's affect and flow of conversation will soon identify the key figures. Even so, toward the end of the assessment, the interviewer needs to ask about categories of relationship that were not covered in the free-flowing part of the interview. The standard list to be covered by the end of the assessment is spouse, children, employers, coworkers and friends, mother or mother figure, father or father figure (including surrogates), religious and other salient institutions, and other (rapist, important babysitter, former therapist, etc.).

Perhaps the most important feature of this interview is that for all relationships, there must be specific examples to illustrate the characteristic patterns. If the patient says, "My father sexually abused me," the interviewer knows almost nothing. This statement must be pursued with questions such as "Will you say more about how he did that?; Can we discuss a specific episode?" Only if the exchanges are extremely concrete and evaluated in remembered context can SASB codes be made. For example, sexual abuse can take place in a nearly infinite variety of contexts and can have as many different impacts. One has to know exactly what happened to this individual and what he or she learned about the world and him- or herself from it.

This systematic assessment of current and past social perceptions, based on specific examples that can be SASB coded, will reveal the copy processes. Often the very words that are mentioned when describing important others will be noted to have been applied to the self or important others earlier in the interview. After the copy processes (be like her; act as if she is still there and in charge; treat yourself as did she) have been identified and linked to the presenting problems, treatment implications are drawn. The general idea is always the same: The wishes in relation to the attachment objects must be given up so that new motivations and behaviors relevant to the current adult life have a chance to emerge. The case formulation sets up the treatment planning so that interventions will consistently support the patient in the direction of giving up the old fantasies. Without such a case formulation, usual and customary therapy interventions are at risk for enabling rather than changing problem patterns.

For example, suppose the patient is identified with an angry blaming parent and rages on in therapy sessions, meanwhile unconsciously wanting reconciliation with the internalization of the parent. In this case, facilitating expression of anger at that parent probably exacerbates the patient's problem. Her blaming style is not serving her well and yet her therapy is supporting, even encouraging, it. Here, the "generic" therapy intervention of facilitating expression of affect is likely to be iatrogenic. The result will be no change, and this individual will join the ranks of those with an "untreatable" personality disorder. However, the conclusion that the person is "untreatable" might better be replaced by the thought that the therapy is not "treating" properly. Treatment of the untreatable requires a relevant case formulation that effectively directs the choice of each intervention.

Case Example

This 42-year-old man had been depressed and on disability for several months. He believed that his boss had conspired to get rid of him and he was consulting a lawyer to see if he had legal recourse. The issue was his uncontrolled attacks of rage, which had included attacks on one particular child but not the others. The latter had been contained for a number of years, but the anger when on the job remained unchecked. He was fond of alcohol, and during his binges he often became suicidal. During one of these episodes, his family managed, with the help of police, to bring him to the hospital. His worst stress at the time of the interview was the recent death of an aunt to whom he had a special attachment. Much against his will and hers, she had been placed in a nursing home, where she failed to thrive and died shortly thereafter. His response to his unenviable situation was to drink, rage, and be depressed. The patient's conscious self-concept included the following statements: "I am crazy when regular; I have rage attacks; I do drink sometimes but I do not remember what I do. I can dissociate from reality. But mostly, I am very logical and kind. I love my family." His current diagnosis was major depressive disorder and alcohol dependence. He was referred for assessment of Axis II complications. There was strong evidence of brain damage and associated dysfunction (e.g., performance IQ was far below his reasonably high verbal IQ), but a stroke had been ruled out by medical tests. His current treatment was Paxil.

The case formulation interview quickly centered on his father, whom he described in the same terms he used to describe himself: "crazy when regular." This man would rage unpredictably and the specific targets of his rage were his mother (for alleged infidelity) and the patient. The father never attacked any of the other children. The attacks on the patient usually would include full-strength fisticuffs to the head. But there were other forms of threat too. For example, the father shot the patient's pet cat and threw it in the trash, allegedly because the cat might scratch the patient. The father also frequently called the patient stupid.

Identification with the father was reflected in the fact that, like his father, the patient had earned the title of "ogre" in his own marital family. Like his father, he targeted one particular child for abuse. Like his father, the patient accused his wife of infidelity. And he offered the same unusual description for his father and himself: "I am crazy when regular." The patient recapitulated his relationship with his father by being paranoid in relation to male authorities (the boss at work). He introjected his father's messages with his suicidality and his thoughts of himself as stupid. Staff agreed that, given the history, it was likely that the brain damage

was the consequence of chronic blows to the head.

A second key figure was the mother, whom the patient described as "kind and logical." She had often been knocked out by the father's beatings. When the father had an affair, she divorced him and then became severely depressed and neglected the children. She became alcoholic and the children were moved to the home of a relative until she remarried quite a bit later. The patient identified with the mother in that he was "kind and logical." Like her, as an adult he was nonfunctional because of severe depression and alcoholism. It appeared that he experienced his current ineffective "protection" of his aunt as a recapitulation of helplessness he had felt as he filed to protect his mother from his father.

The treatment implications of this case analysis, as usual, are to give up the underlying wishes to become closer to the father by being like him, acting as if he were still in control, and treating himself as did his father. For the precipitating problem of rage attacks, the case formulation suggests that he should be helped to mobilize his rage at his father in service of being different rather than being like him. For example, the patient could learn to say, when he feels himself becoming angry, "I don't want to be like him. I hate what he did to me. I will not do that to others. I will be better than him. This family tradition will stop right here." In relation to his devotion to alcohol, the patient will need to let go of his attachment to his nonfunctional alcoholic mother. Her neglect of him, and his of his own family as well as himself, needs to be rejected by the patient as acceptable. In the longer term, the patient will need to work through his strong feelings of fear, rage, and loneliness, especially in relation to his father and his mother. New perspectives can emerge from revisiting childhood helplessness and from developing compassion for oneself. In the supportive and deeply understanding therapy environment, patients can change and leave the old rules and wishes and associated patterns behind.

If therapy interventions center consistently on such attachments and their connections to the current problem patterns, these "untreatable" cases become treatable. Any and all therapy interventions from any school of therapy are relevant to this process, provided they conform to one of the five correct therapy steps discussed in the next section. Once the attachments are grieved, usual and customary interventions (skills training and the like) can become quite useful.

Relevant Research Data

The SASB Intrex data provide evidence in support of the copy processes. A scan of the output for individual psychiatric inpatients often suggests that some aspect of the patient's problems are related to a pattern with attachment objects. For example, a hostile introject would be suggested by high ratings for *SELF-BLAME*; If one of the parents was rated high on **BLAME**, one could reason that the self-blame represented internalization of the criticism of that parent. Patients often will say they can "hear" the voice of that parent when asked to "listen" to what they tell themselves when they are feeling guilty. Similiarly, withdrawal from spouse, shown as high ratings for WALL-OFF, could represent recapitulation of a pattern with a parent, where the ratings of WALL-OFF were equally high. Large numbers of individuals have informally confirmed the existence of such copy processes on viewing their output from the Intrex questionnaires.

The existence of copy processes also can be shown by several methods of formal analysis. Table 20.1 illustrates one way. Using canonical R in a sample of 184 psychiatric inpatients, the eight clusters for introject at worst were predicted ($p < .000$) from the eight clusters for "mother focused on me" ($R^2 = .555$). Table 20.1 shows that each of the clusters in the Introject at worst were predicted at a highly significant level by subjects' recollection of "Mother focused on

me." Results were equally powerful when using ratings of "Mother focused on me" to predict "I focus on my significant other when we are at our worst" ($R^2 = .541$, $p < 0.000$). This association between experienced focus from mother and practiced focus on spouse reflects the principle of similarity and the copy process of identification. The connection between recalled maternal focus and subsequent focus on spouse was not nearly so strong when the marital relationship was at its best. It may be that the interpersonal version of copying (identification) becomes more powerful in the worst (regressed) state than when the adult is in the best state. A more complete examination of data in support of copy processes in a normal as well as in this inpatient sample will be presented elsewhere.[4]

Dickenson (1997) asked 370 undergraduates to rate themselves on a measure of personality disorder (Personality Diagnostic Questionnaire; by Hyler et al., 1988), the Adult Attachment Questionnaire (AAQ; Bartholomew & Horowitz, 1991), and the SASB Intrex. Three groups were identified: subjects having narcissistic traits and dependent traits and subjects having no personality disorder. Among other things, Dickenson found partial support for Benjamin's (1996b) predictions for parental representations in these two groups. Compared to controls, both analogue groups had less affiliative self-representations and representations of themselves with their parents. "Distinctions between the NPD and DPD analogues arose in their parental representations and adult attachment styles, with the NPD analogues recalling responding to their parents with less submission and approaching current relationships with greater dismissiveness" (p. 34).

Clinicians have long argued that statistical significance does not necessarily establish clinical significance. The practitioner wants to understand at the $N = 1$ level. SASB data do allow comprehension at that level as subjects view the computer analysis of their own interpersonal history. Similiarities, complementarities, and introjections often are apparent to the rater viewing his or her results.

TABLE 20.1. Test of Introjection by Predicting "My Introject at Worst" from Perceptions of "Mother Focused on Me" by 183 Psychiatric Inpatients

Variable	F	p
Self-Emancipate	3.751	.000
Self-Affirm	5.617	.000
Self-Love	7.325	.000
Self-Protect	5.222	.000
Self-Control	3.078	.003
Self-Blame	2.851	.005
Self-Attack	2.767	.007
Self-Neglect	2.097	.038

Note. Using canonical correlation, the eight clusters for introject at worst were predicted ($p < .000$) from the eight clusters for "Mother focused on me." $R^2 = .555$.

REVIEW OF TREATMENT IMPLICATIONS AND RELATED EMPIRICAL EVIDENCE

Treatment that is directed by IPIR theory centers on the need for the patient to give up the wish for reconciliation and validation from the IPIRs. The goal of therapy is to give patients or clients the option of functioning mainly in "good" interpersonal space (i.e., in the SASB Attachment Group of interpersonal and intrapsychic positions). Therapy is viewed as an interpersonal and intrapsychic learning experience that involves consistent implementation of five steps:

1. Collaborate against "it" (i.e., the problem patterns and the wishes that sustain them).
2. Learn about patterns, where they are from, and what they are for.
3. Block maladaptive patterns.
4. Enable the will to change.
5. Learn new patterns.

A review of empirical studies that relate to these respective five steps follows.

Collaboration

"The concept [of collaboration] focuses on the importance of the client and therapist forming a partnership against the common foe of the client's debilitating pain" (Horvath & Greenberg, 1994, p. 1). Collaboration is a core feature of current conceptualizations of the therapeutic relationship (Bordin, 1979), and its significance has been supported by factor-analytic studies (Hatcher & Barends, 1996). The therapeutic relationship itself relates powerfully to psychotherapy outcome (for reviews, see Horvath & Symonds, 1991; Orlinsky, Grawe, & Parks, 1994). "Confident collaboration" indicates the degree to which patients are confident in and committed to a process that feels promising and helpful. This relationship has a forward-looking, vital quality—the absence of this positive, purposeful relationship is associated with less effective work and less progress (Hatcher & Barends, 1996). Horvath and Symonds (1991) performed a meta-analysis that linked three core aspects of the therapy alliance to therapy outcome: collaboration, mutuality, and engagement.

This literature is consistent with the idea that the patient or client and the therapist must work well together as they both focus on problem patterns. That perspective is concretized in SASB coding by "dividing" the therapy patient or client into "two referents." One referent is the healthy, conscious part of the patient that comes to therapy and wants to change (the

Growth Collaborator). The other referent is the older, more regressive part that wants to remain loyal to the old rules and ways and wishes and fears (the Regressor Loyalist). Helpful therapy process will support the Growth Collaborator and block and attempt to transform the Regressor Loyalist. Helpful therapy need not always be friendly; nor does it have to be simple (noncomplex). In fact, skilled therapists know how to be complex and hostile in service of the five therapy steps. For one example, therapist-generated double-binds (Humphrey & Benjamin, 1986) can be helpful if they block the Regressor Loyalist and support the Growth Collaborator. Such sophisticated but fully operationalized tracking of different interventions for different aspects of the patient can enrich understanding of the complicated enterprise of psychotherapy.

Learning about Patterns

"Learning about your patterns, where they are from, and what they are for" resembles the *American Heritage Electronic Dictionary* (1993) definition of insight as "1. The capacity to discern the true nature of a situation; penetration. 2. The act or outcome of grasping the inward or hidden nature of things or of perceiving in an intuitive manner." The present approach holds that the function of such insight is to help the patient or client gain a perspective that may enhance the will to stop being so loyal to the problem patterns and the attachments that inspired them. Seeing as an adult "how it was" as a child helps one distance from the situation and make more informed judgments and choices. Patients usually are not aware of the connections between their current problems and their early attachments but do intuit them. This conclusion is supported by the fact that at the end of the consultative interviews described previously, patients often can, sometimes reluctantly, draw the connections between their current problems and the patterns they showed with early attachment figures. Typically, they are quite upset by the experience as they also affirm that it is very important and valuable to them. Often their defenses then take over, and by the next day staff report that many patients have "forgotten" about that aspect of the interview.

Studies of insight in the literature have been disappointing. Crits-Christoph, Barber, Miller, and Beebe (1993) concluded: "More work on the reliability and particularly the validity of in-struments designed to assess the various types of insight is needed" (p 419). Crits-Christoph directs a therapy research center that focuses in part on Luborsky's (1984) proposal that therapy is best conceived and researched in terms of core conflict relationship themes (CCRTs). A CCRT includes wishes and fears, the perceived responses of others, and the patient or client's consequent reaction. A series of well-designed and carefully analyzed studies from this group have greatly enhanced understanding of many aspects of dynamic psychotherapy. For exam-ple, Crits-Christoph (1998) and colleagues have established that therapy narratives do include consistent CCRTs in relation to significant peo-ple, and that these themes (more than one) are often reflected in the therapy relationship (Con-nolly et al., 1996). The QUAINT, a SASB-based coding system, is used to describe com-ponents of the CCRT.

For studies of therapist accuracy, an important component of insight, CCRTs within the patient narratives are compared to CCRTs reflected in therapist speech. Findings reveal that therapist accuracy about wishes and perceived responses of others is significantly related to treatment outcome, even after controlling for effects of the therapeutic alliance. Therapist accuracy also is related to the development of the therapeutic al-liance itself (Crits-Christoph, Barber, & Kur-cias, 1993). Furthermore, low therapist accuracy is significantly related to dropout in cognitive-behavioral therapy (Crits-Christoph, Cooper, & Luborsky, 1988). It seems that across schools of therapy, it is possible to identify CCRTs (inter-personal patterns and associated wishes and fears), and that therapist accuracy is vital to ther-apy success. This same group of researchers has recently developed a measure of self-under-standing of interpersonal patterns (SUIP; Con-nolly et al., 1999) which shows substantial promise as a measure of step 2, learning about patterns. Patients acknowledge relevant prob-lem patterns from a list and rate the selected pat-terns on a 4-point scale ranging from "I recog-nize I feel and act this way with a significant person in my life, but I don't know why" to "I can clearly see that I feel and act this way be-cause of past relationship experiences." This measure shows good reliability and promises to provide a way to study insight, defined as pat-tern recognition that is linked to past important relationships (attachments).

Blocking Maladaptive Patterns

Clinicians working with aggressive and self-de-structive populations are at times faced with the need to set limits on their patients' behaviors. This need, which often arises in relation to per-sonality disorder, conflicts with the widespread psychotherapy norm to avoid taking control. Limit setting seems antithetical to principles of psychoanalytic or client-centered therapy. In general, it is likely to be viewed as disrespectful and power-centric on the part of the therapist. There are few studies of blocking interventions or limit setting in therapy (Pam, 1984; Rosen-heck, 1995), perhaps because taking control is seen as "bad" within the therapy culture.

An exception to this trend to eschew control in therapy is in the treatment of substance abusers. For example, 69 heroin-addicted indi-viduals at a methadone maintenance clinic were randomly assigned membership in one of two treatment groups. An "unstructured" group re-ceived methadone (and other center services) whether or not the addicted individuals contin-ued to use heroin. A "structured" group con-tracted to receive methadone contingent upon the results of the individuals' weekly urine tests. Outcome of the structured group was sig-nificantly better than the unstructured group in terms of heroin abstinence and program reten-tion (McCarthy, 1985). A series of studies on the treatment of inpatient alcoholics used con-tracts in which social "reinforcers," including job counseling, marital and family counseling, and participation in a social group of recover-ing alcoholics, were made contingent upon ces-sation of alcohol abuse (Azrin, 1976). The sub-jects in the treatment groups demonstrated striking, statistically significant improvements over treatment-as-usual controls in total time spent drinking, unemployed, out of the home, and institutionalized (as assessed at 6 months following discharge from the program). Chil-dress, McLellan, and O'Brien (1985) reviewed the literature and concluded that approaches that demanded compliance by contingency management were successful. Control can achieve symptom remission in this population. Unfortunately, these authors also reported that "behaviors tend to revert to baseline when con-tingencies are removed" (p. 955). This failure of the effect to persist is a serious problem. The present perspective would suggest that the ef-fect did not persist because it was not interpersonal and there was no attachment to another person (e.g., therapist) or group that would encourage the introjection of therapy **CONTROL** to result in *SELF-CONTROL*.

A second area in which blocking interventions are acknowledged and studied is in the treatment of borderline personality disorder. Most approaches to this colorful group involve written or verbal contracts with patients regarding the course of action that will be taken when they threaten or display dangerous behaviors (Kernberg, Selzer, Koeningsberg, Carr, & Applebaum, 1989; Linehan, 1993; Waldinger & Gunderson, 1987). In a book devoted to the subject of treatment contracts with patients with borderline personality disorder, Yeomans, Selzer, and Clarkin (1992) describe the use of the contract to create a safe, holding climate within which the patient's intense affective states and internal dynamics can emerge. Clinician researchers such as Linehan and Kernberg and collaborators provide empirical evidence that their approaches overall are effective in stopping problem patterns in individuals with borderline personality disorder, but the specific role of the therapist's limit setting has not been dissected from the overall context. It is reasonable to assume, however, that the limit-setting component of these treatment approaches is important in helping people with borderline personality disorder contain their destructive acting out.

Enabling the Will to Change

Defined as "the perceived desire for therapeutic involvement by participants in the patient role," there is mixed support for the association between motivation and psychotherapy outcome, and strong support for the association between the related concept of "engagement" (Hoglend) and outcome (for a review, see Orlinsky et al., 1994). Exactly what comprises "motivation" (or engagement) in psychotherapy in general is unclear.

In research on addictions, motivational theory has been defined more precisely. Prochaska, DiClemente, & Norcross, (1992) have identified "transtheoretical" stages of change: precontemplation, contemplation, preparation, action, and maintenance. They suggest that interventions should vary, depending on the patient's stage of change. For example, it does not make sense to choose action-oriented behavior change interventions for patients who are still

at the precontemplation stage. They do not even recognize a problem and have essentially no motivation to change. Telling them how to take action does not make sense. On the other hand, those who are already in an action stage are less likely to benefit from insight-oriented interventions which also are assumed by these researchers to enhance motivation.

The most widely cited study from the Prochaska group is about smoking cessation. Success was related to the stage patients were in before treatment. Just as one would expect, the least change was from those in the precontemplation stage, and the most change was observed in those in the action stage. Unfortunately, the processes that result in a patient's attaining a particular level of motivation or readiness for change have not been clearly identified. The use of this research appears to be confined to identifying who is most likely to benefit from a therapy program.

How does one motivate a person to give up old ways and try new ones? Sadly, this vital question is rarely directly addressed in the empirical literature. The most relevant efforts, again, are found in the treatment of substance abusers. Here, confrontation is widely thought to be essential. The enemy is "denial," and only when the patient admits the problem will he or she change. Confrontation motivates change, it is thought. Miller, Benefield, and Tonigan (1993) compared progress in problem drinkers under three treatment conditions: confrontational, client-centered and wait-list control. Clients in the directive–confrontational group displayed significantly more arguing, interrupting, ignoring, and denying of problems. The more the therapist confronted, the more the client drank at 1-year follow-up. This study contradicts the popular belief that confrontation is helpful. Instead, results suggests that confrontation is counterproductive. Perhaps therapist confrontation is like spanking: the instigator (therapist) is rewarded with a sense of control, but the intervention is, at best, ineffective. As positive alternatives, Miller (1985), lists some noncontrolling interventions that do seem to motivate change. These include video or role-played feedback (involving the patient when drunk) combined with the presence of specific, attainable goals and providing voluntary choices. Therapist characteristics matter too. Empathy and expectance of success help motivate change. Hostility does not.

Learning New Patterns

This stage can be facilitated by many of the therapy interventions that comprise modern behavioral "technology." Once patients or clients have given up the old wishes and fantasies that have kept them faithful to their maladaptive patterns, change is comparatively easy. Personality-disordered individuals who have given up old wishes and fears can make good use of all training techniques including lessons in thinking logically (cognitive-behavioral therapy), assertiveness skills, communications skills, socialization skills, relationship skills, parenting skills, and more. Empirical literature on the effectiveness of these interventions with selected populations is vast. A good example is a study by Kendall and Southam-Gerow (1996), who used cognitive-behavioral therapy to treat anxiety-disordered youth. They provided learning in the role of cognition and self-talk, the use of problem-solving and coping skills to manage anxiety, the use of self-evaluation and self-reinforcement strategies, and more. Symptom change was significant compared to a control group and gains were maintained at 3-year follow-up. At that time, subjects still recalled the steps to take when they felt anxious, but most interestingly, the therapy relationship was most often identified by subjects as being important to their change. That finding is consistent with the present perspective: The therapist or therapy group becomes a new IPIR, and the subjects follow the new "rules." If the new "rules" are principles of cognitive-behavioral training or assertiveness and the like, so much the better! Parent training can be effective too. However, parent training is less likely to have a sustained impact in single-parent homes if the mother is depressed, if socioeconomic status is low, or if there is alcoholism in the immediate family (Webster-Stratton, 1990). Again, one might reason that internalization of new learning is less likely when other factors interfere with attachment to the trainers, not to mention with implementation of the new learning. Depression is associated with withdrawal (WALL-OFF), the opposite of the tendency to take in and learn (TRUST). Lack of money can cause enormous stresses that fatally distract from new learning. Alcoholism frequently is associated with chaos and power struggles, leaving little inclination for gentle and steady, helpful parenting behaviors.

It is widely recognized that personality-disordered clients have not been particularly responsive to behavioral technologies. The reason has correctly been identified as lack of motivation. However, the "diagnosis" of personality-disordered individuals as untreatable has put the entire burden on the trait of motivation, which allegedly resides solely within the individual. This must be the reasoning that allows insurance managers to be so dismissive of psychotherapy for personality disorder. However, the addiction research literature has suggested that motivation for change probably is the interactive result of the stage of the patient and specific therapy interventions. The key to successful treatment of personality-disordered people likely is to enable the will to change, to help these people become, as Prochaska et al. (1992) would say: "action oriented." The therapist's burden is heavy but bearable.

COMMENTS ON CURRENT AND FUTURE DEVELOPMENTS

Treatment under the present reconstructive model is necessarily longer term. Systematic validation of the worth of this particular version of long-term psychotherapy must eventually emerge. The current priority is to show how to implement each of the five steps and validate that they are effective in treatment of personality-disordered individuals. Benjamin (1996a) outlined a method for understanding how the specific (SASB coded) developmental learning model can be related to specific patterns characteristic of personality disorder. Benjamin sketched treatment suggestions related to each of the five steps. A second monograph (Benjamin, 2000) discusses in detail and provides clinical examples of each of the five steps. Once that book is completed, there will be an effort to use a formal research protocol to validate the approach with personality disordered individuals.

In the meantime, a wide variety of studies are under way that approach a number of related but circumscribed issues. For example, Pugh (1999) is pursuing the idea that therapist intervention must be tailored carefully to context. Smith (2001) is using the SASB Intrex to assess inpatients in terms of their recalled relations with early attachment objects and current significant others. The central purpose is to develop a more precise understanding of the connection between specific developmental interpersonal learning and adult personality disorder.

Moore (1998) had 60 alcoholics rate their self-concept and their relationship with their significant other person on the SASB Intrex questionnaires. The assessments were directed to recalled state just before drinking and to what was hoped for when drinking. Preliminary results suggest that individuals with different disorders have differing hopes for what alcohol will do for them. For example, those rating high on the WISPI obsessive–compulsive personality disorder scale wish for an *increase* in attack and control from their spouse. This is consistent with Benjamin's (1996b) statement that obsessive–compulsive traits are learned in an environment of hostile control, and that pathology is driven by regressive wishes.

Cushing and Benjamin (1999) provided the first in a series of analyses of a SASB-coded data base of previously depressed mothers (and matched controls) interacting with their toddlers in the Ainsworth "Strange Situation."[5] The hope is to identify at a microscopic level, the SASB-coded attachment behaviors and relate them to the depressive status of the mother as well as to the child's subsequent adjustment.

Critchfield and Pincus are independently using a data base of 183 psychiatric inpatients to study the copy processes. Rothweiler is conducting a methodological study that will independently replicate or revise Benjamin's earlier studies of the structure of the SASB and apply the same methodologies to the best available single circumplex (Wiggins, 1982). Sandor (1995) has demonstrated that cocaine and heroin addicts have well-articulated "relationships" with their drug of choice, as assessed by Intrex ratings. Both show highly organized attachment to their drug of choice. Schloredt (1995) has studied hardy victims of abuse in a college population. Her study supports the idea that abuse experiences must be interpreted in context and the effects have much to do with the victim's interpersonal experience of the abusing attachment object. What matters in abuse is what it teaches him or her about self and others.

Strand (1995) asked imprisoned sexual abusers to rate their object relations on the Intrex and discovered an amazing amount of affection for (attachment to) the abusers. Their view of their prey resembled their own positions as victim. Strand's data clearly support the hypothesis that pathological patterns are gifts of love, testimonials to the rules and ways of early abusers.

The plan is to facilitate the publication of these studies and to continue studying the hypotheses about development of interpersonal and intrapsychic patterns of psychopathology in general and personality disorder in particular. Newer studies will focus more on methods of effectively encouraging and formally documenting therapeutic change, based on the thesis that every psychopathology is a gift of love.

NOTES

1. Benjamin recently received the following e-mail to that effect from a former student, now practicing privately: "I had an extended discussion with a representative of managed care today about the efficacy of treating Axis II disorders. He claimed there is no evidence that they are treatable."
2. Benjamin (1974) called this "the happy hour" in relation to the full SASB model. In Benjamin (1995), the idea was related to the cluster model and called the Attachment Group (AG). With Benjamin's permission, Henry used an early draft of that paper as the basis of his similar view of normality (Henry, 1994).
3. The University of Utah owns and distributes SASB technology, including the Intrex questionnaires. Interested professionals can write to Intrex, Department of Psychology, University of Utah, 390 South, 1530 East, Salt Lake City, UT 84112.
4. These sets were arbitrarily selected for this chapter. Other comparisons have not yet been made. Thorough analysis of the copy processes will require inspecting within-subject correlations as well as between-subject comparisons. There are several methods that deserve exploration. A proper examination of the copy processes will be presented elsewhere, probably in collaboration with Ken Critchfield and/or Aaron Pincus, both of whom have copies of this data set.
5. The data base was generated by Gelfand, Benjamin, Schloredt, and Callaway and was supported by the Depression Research Branch of the MacArthur foundation, David Kupfer, director.

REFERENCES

Adler, A. (1955). Individual psychology, its assumptions and results. In C. Thompson, M. Mazer, & E. Witenberg (Eds.), *An outline of psychoanalysis* (rev. ed., pp. 283–297). New York: Modern Library.

Ainsworth, M., Blehar, M., Waters, E., & Wall, S. (1978). *Patterns of attachment*. Hillsdale, NJ: Erlbaum.

Ainsworth, M. D. S., & Wittig, B. A. (1969). Attachment and exploratory behavior of one-year-olds in a strange situation. In B. M. Foss (Ed.), *Determinants of infant behavior* (Vol. 4, pp. 111–136). London: Methuen.

American Heritage Electronic Dictionary (3rd. ed.). (1993). Wordstar International. Based on *American Heritage Dictionary* (1992). New York: Houghton.

American Psychiatric Association. (1994). *Diagnostic and statistical manual of mental disorders* (4th ed.). Washington, DC: Author.

Azrin, N. H. (1976). Improvements in the community-reinforcement approach to alcoholism. *Behaviour Research and Therapy, 14,* 339–348.

Bartholomew, K., & Horowitz, L. M. (1991). Attachment styles among young adults: A test of a four-category model. *Journal of Personality and Social Psychology, 61,* 226–244.

Baumeister, R. F., & Leary, M. R. (1995). The need to belong: Desire for interpersonal attachments as a fundamental human motivation. *Psychological Bulletin, 117,* 497–529.

Beeghly, M., & Cicchetti, D. (1994). Child maltreatment, attachment, and the self system: Emergence of an internal state lexicon in toddlers at high social risk. *Development and psychopathology, 6,* 5–30.

Benjamin, L. S. (2000). *Interpersonal reconstructive therapy (IRT).* Manuscript in preparation.

Benjamin, L. S. (1973). A biological model for studying individual differences. In J. Westman (Ed.), *Individual differences in children* (pp. 379–412). New York: Wiley Interscience.

Benjamin, L. S. (1974). Structural Analysis of Social Behavior. *Psychological Review, 81,* 392–425.

Benjamin, L. S. (1979). Structural analysis of differentiation failure. *Psychiatry: Journal for the Study of Interpersonal Processes, 42,* 1–23.

Benjamin, L. S. (1984). Principles of prediction using Structural Analysis of Social Behavior. In R. A. Zucker, J. Aronoff, & A. J. Rabin (Eds.), *Personality and the Prediction of Behavior* (121–173). New York: Academic Press.

Benjamin, L. S. (1993). Every psychopathology is a gift of love. *Psychotherapy Research, 3,* 1–24

Benjamin, L. S. (1994). SASB: A bridge between personality theory and clinical psychology. *Psychological Inquiry, 5,* 273–316.

Benjamin, L. S. (1995) Good defenses make good neighbors. In H. R. Conte & R. Plutchik (Eds.), *Ego defenses: Theory and measurement.* New York: Wiley.

Benjamin, L. S. (1996a). *Interpersonal diagnosis and treatment of personality disorders.* New York: Guilford Press.

Benjamin, L. S. (1996b). An interpersonal theory of personality disorders. In J. F. Clarkin & M. F. Lenzenweg (Eds.), *Major theories of personality disorder* (141–220). New York: Guilford Press.

Benjamin, L. S. (1996c). Introduction to the special section on Structural Analysis of Social Behavior (SASB). *Journal of Consulting and Clinical Psychology, 64,* 1203–1212.

Benjamin, L. S. (1997). Personality disorders: Models for treatment and strategies for treatment development. *Journal of Personality Disorders, 11,* 307–324.

Bordin, E. S. (1979). The generalizability of the psychoanalytic concept of the working alliance. *Psychotherapy: Theory, Research, and Practice, 16,* 252–260.

Bowlby, J. (1969). *Attachment and loss. Volume I. Attachment.* London: Tavistock.

Bowlby, J. (1977). The making and breaking of affectional bonds. *British Journal of Psychiatry, 130,* 201–210, 421–431.

Carson, R. C. (1969). *Interaction concepts of personality.* Chicago: Aldine.

Carson, R. C. (1994). Reflections on th SASB and the assessment enterprise. *Psychological Inquiry, 5,* 317–335.

Childress, A. R., McLellan, A. T., & O'Brien, C. P. (1985). Behavioral therapies for substance abuse. *International Journal of the Addictions, 20,* 947–969.

Connolly, M. B., Crits-Christoph, P., Demorest, A., Azarian, K., Muenz, L, & Chittams, J. (1996). Varieties of transference patterns in psychotherapy. *Journal of Consulting and Clinical Psychology, 64,* 1213–1221.

Connolly, M. B., Crits-Christoph, P., Shelton, R. C., Hollon, S., Kurtz, J., Barber, J. P., Butler, S. F., Baker, S., & Thase, M. E. (1999). Reliability and validity of a measure of self-understanding of interpersonal patterns. *Journal of Counseling Psychology, 46,* 472–482.

Cowan, P. A., Cohn, D. A., Cowan, C. P., & Pearson, J. L. (1996). Parents' attachment histories and children's externalizing and internalizing behaviors: Exploring family systems models of linkage. *Journal of Consulting and Clinical Psychology, 64,* 53–63.

Crits-Christoph, P. (1998). The interpersonal interior of psychotherapy. *Psychotherapy Research, 8,* 1–16.

Crits-Christoph, P., Barber, J. P., & Kurcias, J. S. (1993). The accuracy of therapists' interpretations and the development of the therapeutic alliance. *Psychotherapy Research, 3,* 25–35.

Crits-Christoph, P., Barber, J. P., Miller, N. E., & Beebe, K. (1993). Evaluating insight. In N. E. Miller, L. Luborsky, J. P. Barber, & J. P Docherty (Eds.), *Psychodynamic treatment research: A handbook for clinical practice* (pp. 407–422). New York: Basic Books.

Crits-Christoph, P., Cooper, A., & Luborsky, L. (1988). The accuracy of therapists' interpretations and the outcome of dynamic psychotherapy. *Journal of Consulting and Clinical Psychology, 56,* 490–495.

Cushing, G., & Benjamin, L. S. (1999, May). *The effect of maternal depression on mother–infant complementarity defined by SASB.* Paper presented to the Society for Research in Interpersonal Processes. Madison, WI.

DeKlyen, M. (1996). Disruptive behavior disorder and intergenerational attachment patterns: A comparison of clinic-referred and normally functioning preschoolers and their mothers. *Journal of Consulting and Clinical Psychology, 64,* 357–365.

Dickenson, K. A. (1997). *Comparison of parental representations and attachment styles in young adults with narcissistic and dependent personality disorder features.* Master's thesis, University of Pennsylvania.

Eisenberg, L. (1995). The social construction of the human brain. *American Journal of Psychiatry, 152,* 1563–1575.

Elicker, J., Englund, M., & Sroufe, L. A. (1992). Predicting peer competence and peer relationships in childhood from early parent-child relationships. In R. D. Parke & G. Ladd (Eds.), *Family–peer relationships: Modes of linkage* (pp. 77–106). Hillsdale, NJ: Erlbaum.

Erikson, E. H. (1959). Identity and the life cycle. *Psychological Issues, 1,* 1–171.

Figueroa, E., & Silk, K. R. (1997). Biological implications of childhood sexual abuse in borderline personality disorder. *Journal of Personality Disorders, 11,* 71–92.

Fonagy, P., Steele, H., & Steele, M. (1991). Maternal representations of attachment during pregnancy predict the organization of infant–mother attachment at age one. *Child Development, 62,* 891–905.

Freud, S. (1949). The development of the sexual function. In *An outline of psychoanalysis.* New York: Norton. (Reprinted 1955 in C. Thompson, M. Mazer, & E. Wittenberg (Eds.), *An outline of psychoanalysis* (pp. 9–13). New York: Modern Library.

Greenberg, M. T., & Speltz, M. L. (1988). Contributions of attachment theory to the understanding of conduct problems during the preschool years. In J. Belsky & T. Nezworski (Eds.), *Clinical implications of attachment* (pp. 177–218). Hillsdale, NJ: Erlbaum.

Greenberg, M. T., Speltz, M. L., DeKlyen, M., & Endriga, M. C. (1991). Attachment security in preschoolers with and without externalizing problems: A replication. *Development and Psychopathology, 3,* 413–430.

Gurtman, M. B. (in press). Interpersonal complementarity: Integrating interpersonal measurement with interpersonal models. *Journal of Counseling Psychology.*

Guttman, L. C. (1966). Order analysis of correlation matrices. In R. B. Cattell (Ed.), *Handbook of multivariate experimental psychology* (pp. 439–458). Chicago: Rand McNally.

Hatcher, R. L., & Barends, A. W. (1996). Patients' view of the alliance in psychotherapy: Exploratory factor analysis of three alliance measures. *Journal of Consulting and Clinical Psychology, 64,* 1326–1336.

Henry, W. P. (1994). Differentiating normal and abnormal personality: An interpersonal approach based on the Structural Analysis of Social Behavior. In S. Strack & M. Lorr (Eds.), *Differentiating normal and abnormal personality* (pp. 316–340). New York: Springer.

Henry, W. P. (1996). Structural Analysis of Social Behavior as a common meteric for programmatic psychopathology and psychotherapy research. *Journal of Consulting and Clinical Psychology, 64,* 1263–1275.

Henry, W. P., Schacht, T. E., & Strupp, H. H. (1986). Structural analysis of social behavior: Application to a study of interpersonal process in differential psychotherapeutic outcome. *Journal of Consulting and Clinical Psychology, 54,* 27–31.

Henry, W. P., Schacht, T. E., & Strupp, H. H. (1990). Patient and therapist introject, interpersonal process, and differential therapy outcome. *Journal of Consulting and Clinical Psychology 58,* 768–774.

Høglend, P. (1996). Motivation for brief dynamic psychotherapy. *Psychotherapy and Psychosomatics, 65,* 209–215.

Horvath, A. O., & Greenberg, L. S. (1994). Introduction. In A. O. Horvath & L. S. Greenberg (Eds.), *The working alliance: Theory, research, and practice* (pp. 1–9). New York: Wiley.

Horvath, A. O., & Symonds, B. D. (1991). Relation between working alliance and outcome in psychotherapy: A meta-analysis. *Journal of Counseling Psychology, 38,* 139–149.

Humphrey, L. L., & Benjamin, L. S. (1986). Using Structural Analysis of Social Behavior to assess critical but elusive family processes: a new solution to an old problem. *American Psychologist, 41,* 979–989.

Hyler, S. E., & Rieder, R. O., Williams, J. B. W., Spitzer, R. L., Hendler, J., & Lyons, M. (1988). The Personality Disgnostic Questionnaire: Development and preliminary results. *Journal of Personality Disorders, 2,* 229–237.

Kendall, P. C., & Southam-Gerow, M. A. (1996). Long-term follow-up of a cognitive-behavioral therapy for anxiety disordered youth. *Journal of Consulting and Clinical Psychology, 64,* 724–730.

Kernberg, O. F., Selzer, M. A., Koeningsberg, H. W., Carr, A. C., & Applebaum, A. H. (1989). *Psychodynamic psychotherapy of borderline patients.* New York: Basic Books.

Kiesler, D. J. (1996). *Contemporary interpersonal theory and research: Personality, psychopathology, and psychotherapy.* New York: Wiley.

Klein, M. H., Benjamin, L. S., Rosenfeld, R., Treece, C., Husted, J., & Greist, J. H. (1993). The Wisconsin Personality Disorders Inventory: I. Development, reliability, and validity. *Journal of Personality Disorders, 7,* 285–303.

Kraemer, G. W. (1992). A psychobiological theory of attachment. *Behavioral and Brain Sciences, 14,* 1–28.

Leary, T. (1957). *Interpersonal diagnosis of personality: A functional theory and methodology for personality evaluation.* New York: Ronald Press.

Linchan, M. (1993). *Cognitive-behavioral therapy for borderline personality disorder.* New York: Guilford Press.

Luborsky, L. (1984). *Principles of psychoanalytic psychotherapy: A manual for supportive–expressive treatment.* New York: Basic Books.

Mahler, M. S. (1968). *On human symbiosis and the vicissitudes of individuation.* New York: International Universities Press

McCarthy, J. J. (1985). Limit setting on drug abuse in methadone maintenance patients. *American Journal of Psychiatry, 142,* 1419–1423.

McKinney, W. T., Suomi, S., & Harlow, H. (1973). Methods and models in primate personality research. In J. Westman (Ed.), *Individual differences in children* (pp. 265–287). New York: Wiley.

Merikangas, K. R., & Weissman, M. M. (1986). Epidemiology of DSM-III Axis II personality disorders. In A. J. Frances & R. E. Hales (Eds.), *American Psychiatric Association annual review* (vol. 5). Washington, DC: American Psychiatric Association.

Miller, W. R. (1985). Motivation for treatment: A review with special emphasis on alcoholism. *Psychological Bulletin, 98,* 84–107.

Miller, W. R., Benefield, R. G., & Tonigan, J. S. (1993). Enhancing motivation for change in problem drinking: A controlled comparison of two therapist styles. *Journal of Consulting and Clinical Psychology, 61,* 455–461.

Moore, A. M. (1998). *Why people drink: An interpersonal analysis.* PhD dissertation, University of Utah, Salt Lake City, UT.

Murray, H. A. (1938). *Explorations in personality.* New York: Oxford University Press.

Olson, D. H. (1996). Clinical assessment and treatment

interventions using the family circumplex model. In F. W. Kaslow (Ed.), *Handbook of relational diagnosis and dysfunctional family patterns* (pp. 59–80). New York: Wiley.

Orford, J. (1986). The rules of interpersonal complementarity: Does hostility beget hostility and dominance, submission? *Psychological Review, 93,* 365–377.

Orlinsky, D. E., Grawe, K., & Parks, B. K. (1994). Process and outcome in psychotherapy—noc'h einmal. In A. E. Bergin & S. L. Garfield (Eds.), *Handbook of psychotherapy and behavior change* (4th ed., pp. 270–376). New York: Wiley.

Pam, A. (1994). Limit setting: Theory, techniques, and risks. *American Journal of Psychotherapy, 48,* 432–440.

Paris, J. (1997). Childhood trauma as an etiological factor in the personality disorders. *Journal of Personality Disorders, 11,* 34–49.

Prochaska, J. O., DiClemente, C. C., & Norcross, J. C. (1992). In search of how people change: Applications to addictive behaviors. *American Psychologist, 47,* 1102–1114.

Pugh, C. (1999). *Affirmation in psychotherapy: The specific operation of a common therapy process.* PhD dissertation, University of Utah, Salt Lake City, UT.

Quintana, S. M., & Meara, N. M. (1990). Internalization of therapeutic relationships in short-term psychotherapy. *Journal of Counseling Psychology, 37,* 123–130.

Richters, J. E., & Waters, E. (1991). Attachment and socialization: The positive side of social influence. In M. Lewis & S. Feinman (Eds.), *Social influences and socialization in infancy* (pp. 185–213). New York: Plenum.

Rosenheck, R. (1995). Substance abuse and the chronically mentally ill: Therapeutic alliance and therapeutic limit-setting. *Community Mental Health Journal, 31,* 283–295.

Rosenstein, D. S., & Horowitz, H. A. (1996). Adolescent attachment and psychopathology. *Journal of Consulting and Clinical Psychology, 64,* 244–253.

Rudy, J. P., McLemore, C. W., & Gorsuch, R. L. (1985). Interpersonal behavior and therapeutic progress: therapists and clients rate themselves and each other. *Psychiatry: Journal for the Study of Interpersonal Process, 48,* 264–281.

Rutter, M. (1989). Pathways from childhood to adult life. *Journal of Child Psychology and Psychiatry, 30,* 23–51.

Sabo, A. N. (1997). Etiological significance of associations between childhood trauma and borderline personality disorder: Conceptual and clinical implications. *Journal of Personality Disorders, 11,* 50–70.

Sandor, C. (1995). *Interpersonal analysis of cocaine and heroin use.* PhD dissertation, University of Utah, Salt Lake City, UT.

Schaefer, E. S. (1965). Configurational analysis of children's reports of parent behavior. *Journal of Consulting Psychology, 29,* 552–557.

Schloredt, K. (1995). *Child maltreatment: An applica-*

tion of interpersonal theory. PhD dissertation, University of Utah, Salt Lake City, UT.

Schneider-Rosen, K., & Cicchetti, D. (1991). Early self-knowledge and emotional development: Visual self-recognition and affective reactions to mirror self-image in maltreated and nonmaltreated toddlers. *Developmental Psychology, 27,* 481–48

Schore, A. N. (1996). The experience–dependent maturation of a regulatory system in the orbital prefrontal cortex and the origin of developmental psychopathology *Development and Psychopathology, 8,* 59–87.

Shafer, R. (1968). *Aspects of internalization.* New York: International Universities Press.

Shea, M. T., Glass, D. R., Pilkonis, P. A., Watkins J., & Docherty, J. P. (1987). Frequency and implications of personality disorders in a sample of depressed outpatients. *Journal of Personality Disorders, 1,* 27–42.

Smith, T. (2001). *Specific psychosocial perceptions and specific symptoms of personality and other psychiatric disorders.* Unpublished PhD dissertation study, University of Utah, Salt Lake City, UT.

Sroufe, L. A., Egeland, B., & Kreutzer, T. (1990). The fate of early experience following developmental change: Longitudinal approaches to individual adaptation in childhood. *Child Development, 61,* 1363–1373.

Strand, J. (1995). *Interpersonal construals of pedophiles.* PhD dissertation, University of Utah, Salt Lake City, UT.

Sullivan, H. S. (1953). *The interpersonal theory of psychiatry.* New York: Norton.

Sullivan, H. S. (1962). *Schizophrenia as a human process.* Washington, DC: William Alanson White Psychiatric Foundation.

Toth, S. L., & Cicchetti, D. (1996). Patterns of relatedness, depressive symptomatology, and perceived competence in maltreated children. *Journal of Consulting and Clinical Psychology, 64,* 32–41.

van IJzendoorn, M. H., & Bakermans-Kranenburg, M. J. (1996). Attachment representations in mothers, fathers, adolescents, and clinical groups: A meta-analytic search for normative data. *Journal of Consulting and Clinical Psychology, 64,* 8–21

Waldinger, R. J., & Gunderson, J. G. (1987). *Effective psychotherapy with borderline patients: Case studies.* New York: Macmillan.

Webster-Stratton, C. (1990). Long-term follow-up of families with young conduct problem children: From preschool to grade school. *Journal of Clinical Child Psychology, 19,* 144–149.

Wiggins, J. S. (1982). Circumplex models of interpersonal behavior in clinical psychology. In P. C. Kendall & J. N. Butcher (Eds.), *Perspectives in personality* (Vol. 1). Greenwich, CT: JAI Press.

Yeomans, F. E., Selzer, M. A., & Clarkin, J. F. (1992). *Treating the borderline patient: A contract-based approach.* New York: Basic Books.

Zanarini, M. C., & Frankenburg, F. R. (1997). Pathways to the development of borderline personality disorder. *Journal of Personality Disorders, 11,* 93–104.

—◆—

CHAPTER 21

Dialectical Behavior Therapy

CLIVE J. ROBINS
ANDRE M. IVANOFF
MARSHA M. LINEHAN

RATIONALE FOR THE TREATMENT

The Borderline Patient in Treatment

Clinicians experienced in treatment of borderline personality disorder typically report that progress often is difficult and outcomes relatively modest. In addition, the behaviors of some patients with borderline personality disorder at times generate extreme stress in clinicians. Among the most stressful aspects of the work of mental health clinicians are suicide attempts by patients, suicide threats by patients, and anger expressed toward the therapist. Patients with a diagnosis of borderline personality disorder probably are the most likely to engage in a constellation of all three of these behaviors. Because working with borderline patients frequently is stressful, dialectical behavior therapy (DBT) requires that all therapists doing any part of this treatment work only as part of a treatment team that provides support, guidance, and continuing education.

According to DSM-IV, to be diagnosed with borderline personality disorder, an individual needs to demonstrate five or more out of nine criteria that reflect "a pervasive pattern of instability of interpersonal relationships, self-image, and affects, and marked impulsivity" (American Psychiatric Association, 1994, p. 654). In DBT (Linehan, 1987, 1993a), it is helpful to organize these nine criteria into five areas in which the individual is dysregulated: emotions, interpersonal relationships, sense of self, impulsive and suicidal behaviors, and cognition.

Emotion Dysregulation

DBT proposes that emotion dysregulation is the core dysregulation that drives the others. DSM-IV refers to "affective instability due to a marked reactivity of mood" (p. 654). The criteria do not mention the frequent co-occurrence of major depressive disorder (about 50%; Gunderson & Elliott, 1985). In our experience, many patients with borderline personality disorder have both chronic moderate to severe depression as well as being very labile and extreme in their experience and expression of emotions, covering the gamut from rage to terror to deepest melancholy. There are also those who appear to meet criteria both for borderline personality disorder and bipolar type II disorder, both disorders for which this particular symptom is relevant. The second criterion related to emotion regulation is "inappropriate, intense anger or difficulty controlling anger" (p. 654). This certainly is one of the criteria most likely to get a clinician thinking about this diagnosis. However, in our experience, more than half the patients with this diagnosis have a greater problem with *underexpression* of anger. Some oscillate between the two extremes, whereas others stay mostly polarized. Few are able to achieve an appropriate synthesis of assertive responding. DBT proposes that despite its singling out in DSM, anger holds no special place among the range of emotions. Borderline patients are proposed to have difficulty controlling emotions of all kinds, both "negative" ones, such as anger, fear, sadness, shame, and envy, and often "positive" ones, such as joy and love.

Interpersonal Dysregulation

DSM-IV describes "frantic efforts to avoid real or imagined abandonment" (p. 654). In our experience, these efforts often are associated with an actual history, or current ongoing experience, of actual abandonment. Concerns over abandonment are almost universal among patients with this diagnosis, and some make frantic efforts to avoid it. Abandonments are just one part of "a pattern of unstable and intense interpersonal relationships characterized by alternating between extremes of idealization and devaluation" (p. 654). The intense need for close relationships and their frequent absence in many of these patients' lives conspire to lead to an idealization of those who are helpful, admired, or otherwise positively valued. The therapist may hear early in treatment that he or she is "the only therapist who has really understood me and been able to help me like this." This may well be a valid expression of the patient's experience at that time. However, the experienced therapist knows that there is a good chance that at some time he or she may disappoint or thwart the patient, possibly in a serious way, and be seen as a villain, a fool, an uncaring automaton, or inept. To deal with the ups and downs in the valence and the closeness of the relationship, the therapist needs not only a consultation team but also a theory that helps put objectionable or stressful behavior into a context of understanding. In DBT, it is proposed that a core emotional dysregulation leads the individual to depend on others to an unusual degree to help regulate his or her emotions.

Self-Dysregulation

DSM-IV describes "markedly and persistently unstable self-image or sense of self" and "chronic feelings of emptiness" (p. 654). The DBT model suggests that feelings of emptiness also reflect difficulties with a sense of self. Pa-

tients frequently are unsure of their goals, direction, and values. They also have little belief in themselves or sense that they have anything inside. There is one aspect, however, in which these patients' self-image often is quite stable, and that is as being "bad" or "defective." This core self-image often persists long after some of the more overt dysregulated behaviors have significantly improved. The instability of many aspects of self-image may be a consequence of the extreme peaks and valleys of mood experienced by the person, and their associated extreme behaviors.

Behavioral Dysregulation

In DSM-IV, borderline patients are described as demonstrating both "impulsivity in at least two areas that are potentially self-damaging (e.g., spending, sex, substance abuse, reckless driving, binge eating)" and "recurrent suicidal behavior, gestures, or threats, or self-mutilating behavior" (p. 654). Borderline patients tend to engage in extreme behaviors that often have negative consequences for them. In our experience, these sometimes are, and sometimes are not, impulsive. Sometimes they are quite planned. Either way, they are high-priority behaviors to change. DBT looks at these behaviors from a functional point of view and suggests that their function often is to change emotional experience. They therefore also often result from the basic core problem of emotion dysregulation. Whether they cut or burn themselves, binge and purge food, use drugs or alcohol, or engage in other "impulsive" behaviors, patients almost always report that they feel better in the context of the behavior or immediately after the behavior. Combating this built-in reinforcement contingency for the most serious of the individual's maladaptive behaviors is one of the major challenges facing the therapist. In addition to typically chronic suicidal ideation, related affects, and expectations, these patients may engage in overt parasuicide, which is any act of deliberate, intentional self-injury. Self-injury could range the gamut anywhere from the most minor scratch or blow to the patient's own head all the way to the most medically serious, 100% intended, suicide attempt (i.e., anything short of suicide). Terms such as suicide "gestures" imply a particular motive (i.e., communication) for the suicidal behavior, and this motive often is inferred by clinicians, we believe, with little or no evidence. Communication sometimes is, and sometimes is not, the intention. In DBT, we prefer to assess intent rather than assume it and prefer a term such as "parasuicide," which is neutral with regard to intent and free of value judgment. Also avoided are such terms as "manipulative." Therapists and others may feel manipulated, but one must be careful not to infer intent from effect. Borderline patients frequently are poor manipulators in the sense of being able to subtly achieve an outcome, as the term implies. More problematic is that perceiving one's patient as "manipulative" does make it more likely that one will have difficulty working with this person, because liking a patient probably is essential to staying the course needed for the patient to achieve a life worth living. Understanding what drives such "crazy" and sometimes scary behavior as parasuicide can help the therapist to tolerate it while it is occurring and to maintain the basic compassion and respect for patients that is necessary to help them change.

Cognitive Dysregulation

The final criterial symptom of borderline personality disorder in DSM-IV is "transient, stress-related paranoid ideation or severe dissociative symptoms" (p. 654). Under stress, a minority of patients seem to become temporarily paranoid, to dissociate more, or to have mood-congruent auditory hallucinations, often of a self-critical nature. DBT suggests that extreme emotions lead to distorted cognition in all individuals, including these symptoms in the extreme. When these episodes occur, the level of stress for both patient and therapist is increased enormously, and the therapist needs to consider hospitalization and other high-intensity treatment options.

Dialectical Behavior Therapy: An Overview

Behavior therapy has a long and productive history of empirically researched treatments for a wide range of adult and child disorders, but what is *dialectical* behavior therapy? It is an integration of behavior therapy with other perspectives and practices that includes, most notably, principles and practice of Zen and an overarching dialectical philosophy that guides the treatment. The treatment, developed by Marsha Linehan (1987; 1993a) evolved over almost 20 years of work with chronically suicidal

women. It is rooted firmly in the principles and practices of behavior therapy and cognitive therapy, including a strong emphasis on systematic ongoing assessment and data collection during treatment; operational definitions of clearly defined target behaviors; a therapist–patient relationship that emphasizes collaboration, orienting the patient to the treatment, and education of the patient; and the use of any standard cognitive and behavioral treatment strategies. But it also has a number of distinctive characteristics that have emerged partly in response to characteristics of this patient population. One of these is an emphasis on dialectics. The fundamental dialectic with this population is the need for both acceptance and change. The therapist needs to fully accept the patient as he or she is and at the same time to persistently and insistently push for and help the patient to change. The therapist also tries to develop and strengthen an attitude of acceptance toward reality on the part of the patient as well as the motivation and ability to change what can be changed. This dialectic both flows from and is addressed by the integration of behavior therapy with Zen practice, Rogerian practice, and others. The therapist also needs to think in a dialectical fashion, not becoming polarized but seeing the value of opposing points of view and finding appropriate syntheses.

The treatment rests on the dialectic of two core sets of strategies: validation strategies and problem-solving strategies. Behavior therapy has emphasized problem solving but has had little to say about validation or acceptance. DBT also involves a dialectic of communication style between a reciprocal, warm, genuine interpersonal style and a more irreverent style and a dialectic in case management between consultation to the patient regarding how to manage his or her environment on the one hand and direct environmental intervention by the therapist on the other. DBT was developed to address the issues that lead therapists of not only behavioral but also other theoretical orientations to frequently get stuck, go down blind alleys, and in some cases even contribute to serious, even fatal, deterioration in the patient's well-being. DBT does not particularly emphasize the role of the patient's motivational factors (e.g., resistance) in understanding the difficulty these patients have in changing. Rather, it recognizes that they almost always are seriously deficient in a wide spectrum of interpersonal, emotion regulation, distress tolerance, and other skills. However, the behavior therapist who attempts to treat the borderline patient by a relatively structured sequence of skills acquisition and practice, as one might do with some patients who have depressive or anxiety disorders, quickly discovers that the patient's emotional sensitivity necessitates presenting skills, and problem solving in general, within a context in which the patient feels understood and validated, particularly with regard to his or her emotions and motives.

Conducting skills training in individual therapy with borderline patients is frequently almost impossible because of the recurrent chaos and crises of their lives, so that at every session some new behavior or situation may need to be dealt with. Linehan therefore decided to separate skills training into a separate component of the treatment, typically in a group format, to free up the individual psychotherapist for helping patients manage crises, reinforce the use of skills, and deal with motivational issues that interfere with their using the skills they have. Thus, it is assumed that patients not only have skills deficits but typically also do not use the skills they have. In DBT, the term "motivational" refers to emotions, cognitions, or reinforcement contingencies that interfere with skilled behavior. The therapist's job therefore becomes one of helping the patient overcome inhibitions, change beliefs and thinking styles, and rearrange reinforcement contingencies for adaptive and maladaptive behavior. The treatment therefore targets both improvement in skills and adequate attention to these several motivational factors that can interfere with them.

EMPIRICAL EVIDENCE

DBT is the only outpatient psychotherapy for which there is evidence of efficacy from a randomized controlled trial (Linehan, Armstrong, Suarez, Allmon, & Heard (1991). Linehan, Tutek, Heard, and Armstrong (1994) reported that DBT had significantly greater effects over 1 year than treatment as usual (TAU) in the community, for chronically parasuicidal women, on frequency and medical severity of self-injury, on frequency and duration of hospitalizations, and treatment dropout rates. Patients in DBT also had greater decreases in the experience and expression of anger and improvements in social role functioning. These ef-

fects endured over a 6- and 12-month follow-up period (Linehan, Heard, & Armstrong, 1993).

The first study by independent investigators to replicate effects of DBT did find superiority to TAU on several important variables. Koons et al. (in press) compared DBT with TAU in a Veteran's Administration clinic treating 20 women veterans who met criteria for borderline personality disorder. After 6 months of treatment, compared with TAU, patients in DBT reported significantly greater reductions in suicidal ideation, hopelessness, depression, and anger expression. In addition, only patients in DBT demonstrated significant decreases in number of parasuicide acts, anger experienced but not expressed, and dissociation. Patients in both conditions reported decreases in depressive symptoms and number of borderline personality disorder criteria and did not improve in anxiety.

It appears that this treatment can be conducted effectively at another site by a different research therapy team and thus can be disseminated. It now becomes important to compare DBT with other manualized or otherwise disseminated treatments. Bateman and Fonagy (1999) recently reported the only other evidence from a randomized study of a psychosocial treatment for borderline personality disorder. A long-term psychodynamically oriented partial hospitalization program produced significantly better outcomes than outpatient medications and clinical management alone.

THEORETICAL FOUNDATION OF DIALECTICAL BEHAVIOR THERAPY

Two bodies of theory provide the foundation for DBT: (1) a biosocial theory of borderline personality disorder, which helps the therapist to understand the patient's behaviors, and to know both how he or she needs to change and what he or she needs to learn; and (2) the core treatment principles, drawn from behavior therapy, Zen, and dialectics, which inform the therapist how to help bring about those changes.

A Biosocial Theory of Borderline Personality Disorder

In developing a theory of the etiology and maintenance of borderline personality disorder, Linehan was mindful of several requirements:

(1) that it be compatible with current empirical data; (2) that it be practical, guiding the therapist in what to do when interacting with the patient; and (3) that it engender in the therapist an attitude of effective compassion that will help him or her to stick with the patient through difficult times. The core of the biosocial theory is that borderline personality disorder results from a series of transactions over time of a person factor, namely, a dysfunction of the emotion regulation system, with an environment factor, referred to as the invalidating environment. The individual who displays extreme emotional reactions will tend to elicit invalidation of his or her experiences and behavior from others who have difficulty understanding their degree of intensity. The experience of being persistently invalidated, in turn, tends to increase emotional dysregulation and decrease learning of emotion regulation skills.

Emotion Dysregulation

Emotional regulation difficulties can occur because of a combination of two factors: an inherent emotional vulnerability and difficulty in modulating emotions. If the individual had little emotional vulnerability, or had emotional vulnerability but also good skills at modulating emotions, he or she would not behave in the ways that lead to this diagnosis.

Emotional vulnerability may, in part, be biologically determined as temperament. The emotionally vulnerable person has low thresholds, rapid emotional reactions, and high-level reactions. High levels of emotion, in turn, dysregulate cognitive processing, as they do for everyone. Unfortunately, most borderline patients spend much of their time in a state of high arousal and thus are cognitively dysregulated. Emotional vulnerability also usually entails a slow return to baseline levels, which contributes to a high sensitivity to the next emotional stimulus.

Difficulty modulating emotions is also a challenge for the borderline patient. Basic research has found several tasks to be important for emotion modulation. These tasks include the ability to reorient attention, to inhibit mood-dependent action, to change physiological arousal, to experience emotions without escalating or blunting them, and to organize one's behavior in the service of external, non-mood-dependent goals. These all are skilled behaviors that can, to a large degree, be learned. They are skills that most borderline patients, for whatever reason, have not learned. An important aspect of the treatment therefore is teaching skills.

The Invalidating Environment

The primary characteristic of an invalidating environment is that private experiences (emotions and thoughts), as well as overt behaviors, "are often taken as invalid responses to events; are punished, trivialized, dismissed, or disregarded; and/or are attributed to socially unacceptable characteristics" (Linehan & Kehrer, 1993, p. 402). In addition, although emotional communication may be ignored or met by punishment, high-level escalation may result in attention, meeting of demands, and other types of reinforcement. Finally, an invalidating environment may oversimplify the ease of meeting life's goals and problem solving. Certain behaviors of the emotionally vulnerable "difficult" child's behavior may elicit these types of responses from the environment. Some possible consequences of pervasive invalidation include difficulties in accurately labeling emotions, effectively regulating emotions, and trusting one's own experiences as valid. By oversimplifying problem solving, such an environment does not teach problem solving, graduated goals, or distress tolerance but, instead, teaches perfectionistic standards and self-punishment as a strategy to try to change one's behavior. Finally, reinforcement of only escalated emotional displays teaches the individual to oscillate between emotional inhibition and extreme emotional behavior.

This model is presented as not only a model of etiology but also a model of maintenance of borderline personality disorder behaviors and current transactions. Therapists need to be aware of the likelihood that they will have a tendency to respond to the patient in invalidating ways. In keeping with the emphasis that the model places on invalidation as a causal influence, validation is one of the two core sets of DBT strategies. Much of the behavior of the patient is invalid from many perspectives. All behavior can be valid from some perspectives, however. The therapist needs to make a conscious effort to locate and acknowledge the island of validity in the possible sea of invalidity of the patient's behavior (a dialectical approach) so that the patient, feeling understood and accepted, is able to move toward more skillful behavior.

Core Treatment Principles Underlying Dialectical Behavior Therapy

The three areas of knowledge from which DBT draws most of its treatment principles are behavior therapy, Zen, and dialectical philosophy.

Behavior Therapy

By principles of behavior therapy, we primarily mean principles of learning. DBT assumes that many maladaptive behaviors, both overt and private (thoughts, feelings) are learned and therefore can, in principle, be replaced by new learning. Three primary ways in which organisms learn are through (1) modeling, which involves learning through observation of others; (2) operant conditioning, which refers to learning an association between a behavior and its consequences; and (3) respondent conditioning, which involves learning about an association between two stimuli. All three processes are central to understanding and changing maladaptive behavior.

When consequences follow a behavior and result in a subsequent increase or decrease in that behavior, these are the operant (instrumental conditioning) processes of reinforcement and punishment, respectively. When previously reinforced behavior is no longer reinforced, the behavior will decrease, a process called extinction. These principles are widely known and frequently employed systematically by parents, teachers, and others but often are not considered by therapists in relation to patient behaviors and therapist–patient interactions. Therapists need to avoid unwittingly reinforcing maladaptive behaviors by, for example, providing greater attention to patients when they engage in this behavior than when they do not, or punishing or failing to reinforce fledgling efforts toward more adaptive behavior because the behavior still falls so far short of the mark. Therapists also need constantly to be looking for opportunities, moment to moment, to deliberately and contingently provide interpersonal and other consequences to the patient's behavior.

In respondent (classical) conditioning, two stimuli become associated, so that the natural response to one becomes a learned response to the other. After being raped in a dark alley, being near a dark alley may provoke a full-force fear response. Positive but maladaptive associations may also be learned in this way, such as

an association between the sight or feel of a knife used previously in self-injuring and emotional relief.

Before trying to change a behavior, it is essential first to fully understand what variables currently are maintaining the behavior. This understanding is arrived at through a behavioral analysis, which is a detailed, step-by-step analysis of the sequence of the antecedents of the behavior, the behavior itself, and its consequences. We describe later in more detail how this is done in a clinical context.

Zen

The introduction of principles from Zen practice into DBT came about largely because of the strong need for patients to develop an attitude of greater acceptance toward a reality that is often painful. Other spiritual traditions also provide valuable teachings on issues related to acceptance, but Zen particularly has developed methods for this. Some of the most vital Zen principles and practices central to DBT are the importance of being mindful to the current moment, seeing reality without delusion, accepting reality without judgment, letting go of attachments that cause suffering, and finding the middle way. Zen is also characterized by the humanistic assumption that all individuals have an inherent capacity for enlightenment and truth, referred to in DBT as wise mind.

Dialectics

Dialectics refers to a process of synthesis of opposing elements, ideas, or events, the thesis and the antithesis. Individuals with borderline personality disorder usually are nondialectical in their thinking and behavior, exhibiting extreme polarized beliefs and actions. Modeling and directly teaching more balanced, synthesized, and dialectical patterns of thinking and behavior are overarching strategies used by DBT therapists. In addition, a dialectical world view pervades the treatment. In dialectical philosophy, reality is viewed as whole and interrelated and at the same time as bipolar and oppositional, as in the opposing forces of subatomic particles. Reality is in continuous change as its components transact with one another. This world view is consistent with the transactional, systemic nature of the biosocial theory, and with a view of the patient and therapist as being in a dialectical relationship, transacting in ways that will inevitably lead to changes in both. Dialectical philosophy also is applied in the balance of treatment strategies that are heavily change oriented with others that are heavily acceptance oriented, as we discuss in detail later. Balancing treatment does not mean watering down strong oppositions but frequently the firm embracing of both, and rapid movement from one type of strategy to another. The quality of mindfulness in the therapist is essential for this speed and flow and needs to be developed by the therapist him- or herself deliberately practicing mindfulness (Lynch & Robins, 1997; Robins, in press). Finally, dialectical philosophy informs the treatment goals and skills taught in DBT, including the change-oriented goals of improving emotion regulation and interpersonal relationship effectiveness and the more acceptance-oriented goals of learning mindfulness and the ability to tolerate distress. Patients need to learn to accept as much as they need to change. Learning to accept is, of course, a change in itself.

ASSUMPTIONS ABOUT PATIENTS AND TREATMENT

Grounded in learning theory, meditational practices, and a dialectical philosophy as described previously, several assumptions about therapy and about patients inform DBT practice. These assumptions reflect the belief that the lives of suicidal, borderline individuals are unbearable as they are currently being lived, as well as the balance between acceptance (e.g., "patients are doing the best they can," "patients want to improve," and "patients cannot fail in DBT") and change (e.g., "patients may not have caused all of their own problems, but they have to solve them anyway" and "patients need to do better, try harder, and be more motivated to change"). Assumptions about therapy conduct and process directed to the therapist illustrate a therapeutic system that applies similar principles to both patient and therapist. These premises guide therapeutic "world view" and behavior, validating therapists' need for support and the realities of failure.

TREATMENT STAGES AND TARGETS

DBT consists of five stages: pretreatment and four active treatment stages—control, order,

synthesis, and transcendence. Treatment goals are hierarchical within stages and determine the treatment agenda within and across sessions; each session agenda is based on the client's behavior since the last session. It is the therapist's responsibility to remain mindful of treatment goals and to ensure that client treatment activities are directed toward creating a life worth living.

Pretreatment

During this stage, orientation to the philosophy and structure of the treatment occurs, and the patient commits to change, agreeing on the goals of treatment. These goals are clearly prescribed. If a patient is currently engaging in suicidal or other self-harm behaviors, he or she must agree that reducing or eliminating such behavior is the first priority. Patients must also agree not to kill themselves while they are in DBT. Although the coexistence of suicidal behaviors and desire to live is dialectically understood within DBT, treatment cannot progress beyond this target until it is under control. Obtaining explicit patient agreement is necessary prior to full participation in treatment; in settings in which patients may be reluctant to commit themselves to DBT goals, ongoing pretreatment may be used to focus on commitment-enhancing strategies.

Although sometimes difficult, respect and flexibility for the patient's stated priorities and goals are important. Becoming committed may entail numerous steps. Evaluating the pros and cons of commitment to treatment offers a good starting point and identifying patient expectations and hopes (and lack thereof) about treatment effects can be useful in developing counterarguments to obstacles that periodically arise in treatment. Playing the devil's advocate by framing arguments against commitment may strengthen a tentative agreement if the arguments posed are just slightly weaker than those posed by the patient for change. Borrowed from social psychology, the "foot in the door" and "door in the face" techniques can be used to elicit initial commitment to work toward a vague but favorable goal, "Wouldn't you like to be happier with your life?" Realistic appraisal of difficulty requiring greater commitment must be introduced gradually. A variant of "foot-in-the-door" is highlighting prior commitments and connecting them to current agreements, renegotiating if warranted and focusing on the patient's choice to commit while acknowledging realistic consequences of not committing. Finally, basic principles of shaping, building on small steps toward larger commitments, and the strong use of encouragement and reinforcement round out commitment-enhancing strategies.

Stage 1

For patients who enter treatment with severe behavioral dyscontrol, such as self-injury or substance abuse, DBT focuses on current behavior and on movement from severe behavioral dyscontrol to behavioral control. Suicidal, self-harm, and other life-threatening behaviors, including harm to others, are primary targets addressed through increasing basic capacities (self-control and connection to therapy) necessary to function in treatment. The goals of Stage 1 include attaining a reasonable (immediate) life expectancy, a connection to help givers, stability, and control of action. Patients and therapists make explicit agreements when they enter this phase, designed to enhance a strong sense of goodwill, moral and ethical behavior, and a commitment to the work of treatment. Although they cannot anticipate the specific interpersonal issues that may arise between patients with borderline personality disorder and their therapists, the agreements provide a collaborative and reciprocal context in which to address these issues.

The primary targets of Stage 1 are (1) decreasing behaviors involving self-harm, suicide, or violence toward others; (2) decreasing therapy-interfering behaviors; (3) decreasing quality-of-life-interfering behaviors; and (4) increasing behavioral skills needed to make life changes (i.e., core mindfulness skills—the ability to focus thought and thinking—distress tolerance, emotion regulation skills, and interpersonal effectiveness skills). These skills are described in more detail later.

During Stage 1 of standard DBT, treatment occurs in several modes: individual psychotherapy, group skills training, telephone consultation, and team meetings. The assumption is that it is frequently difficult for the individual therapist to conduct a structured sequence of skills training because of the frequent crises that need to be addressed in individual sessions, yet the patient usually is deficient in needed skills. Skills training therefore occurs in a setting in which it can be the primary focus, freeing the individual therapist to focus on the motivational (i.e., reinforcement, attitudinal, and emotional) difficulties that interfere with the use of skills and to help patients enact skillful behavior in their natural environment.

Individual Therapy

Weekly diary cards are used to collect ongoing information about target problems. Targets listed on the standard cards may be individually tailored as needed but generally include suicidal behavior and self-harm; suicidal ideation and urges; prescription, over-the-counter, and illicit drug use; binge eating; and general misery level. On the flip side is a checklist of DBT skills to mark as used during the week. Reviewed at the beginning of each individual session, the presence or absence of target problems since the last session identifies priorities for that session agenda.

Patient self-monitoring via diary cards has a number of advantages over traditional memory-based narrative recall as it provides feedback and data unavailable through other means; when completed by the patient between sessions, it may also increase the accuracy of reported events. Structurally, the diary card provides temporal detail about the relationship between dysfunctional behaviors and daily fluctuations in anxious or depressed mood (intensity of anxious or depressed mood tied to imminent self-harm or suicidal behavior, level of mood that can be tolerated without resorting to self-harm or suicidal behavior, etc.). Group skills training and treatment planning meetings in some settings also make use of the diary cards; they provide an efficient and portable means of collecting standard patient data related to functioning and progress.

All direct self-harm, suicide crisis behavior, intrusive or intense suicidal ideation, images or communications, and significant changes in ideation or urges to self-destruct are addressed in individual therapy immediately following their occurrence. Self-harm, regardless of lethality or intent, is never ignored; these behaviors are good predictors of future lethal acts, can cause substantial harm, and, as primary DBT targets, must be brought under control before treatment can progress.

Behavioral or "chain" analysis is the standard tool for analyzing dysfunctional behavior. It also provides the framework for generating solutions to such behavior. Behavioral analysis identifies the problem and then the internal (cognitive, affective, sensory) and external (social, contextual, physical environment) events preceding and causing the problem (antecedents and precipitants). Finally, the consequences of engaging in the target behavior are examined, for the client and for the environment. Once the behavioral chain is clarified, the task becomes "solution analysis," identifying potential resources and obstacles for solving the problem, using one or more of four change strategies: (1) skills training addressing capability deficits that interfere with more adaptive responses, (2) contingency management strategies addressing the reinforcement that may support problematic behavior, (3) cognitive modification procedures addressing faulty beliefs and assumptions interfering with problem-solving capabilities, and/or (4) exposure-based strategies to address anxiety, shame, or other emotional responses that interfere with adaptive problem-solving attempts. Behavioral analyses may take 10 minutes or the majority of an entire session.

Skills Training

DBT assumes that many of the problems experienced by patients who are chronically suicidal, self-harm, or engage in other behaviors characteristic of borderline personality disorder result from a combination of motivational problems and behavioral skill deficits; that is, they never learned the necessary skills to regulate painful affect. For this reason, DBT emphasizes skills building to facilitate behavior change and acceptance. In standard DBT, four skills modules are taught sequentially in weekly psychoeducational skills training groups. The four skills training modules directly target the behavioral, emotional, and cognitive instability and dysregulation of borderline personality disorder: mindfulness, interpersonal effectiveness, emotion regulation, and distress tolerance. Each module takes approximately 8 weeks to complete, except mindfulness skills, which take about 2 sessions and are repeated between each of the other modules. These skills are described in detail in a skills training manual (Linehan, 1993b). Groups use a standard behavior therapy skills-building format and procedures: didactic instructions, modeled examples, coached rehearsal of new skills, feedback, and homework assignments.

Working in tandem, simultaneous group and individual treatments create dedicated time to learn much needed skills and a separate context for coached individual application. This allows individual therapy attention to priority target behaviors as well as other crisis issues borderline patients frequently bring to session without the pressure to also teach skill fundamentals. When skills are taught in group, the individual therapist may deal with current crises and serve as skills coach, encouraging transfer and generalization of skills to individual patient situations.

Group skills training has several advantages over individual skills training. Skills are practiced with group members engaged in the same tasks and members learn from each other; skills practice is coached by an expert skills trainer; group membership often decreases real isolation and increases patients' sense of feeling understood. Socially phobic patients or those who must begin skills training in individual sessions are moved to group skills training as soon as possible.

Mindfulness is a psychological and behavioral translation of meditation and contemplation skills taught in Eastern and Western spiritual practices. The goal of this module is to increase attentional control, nonjudgmental awareness, and sense of true self while decreasing identity confusion, emptiness, and cognitive dysregulation. Three primary states of mind are presented: reasonable mind (logical, analytical, problem solving), emotion mind (creative, passionate, and dramatic), and wise mind (the integration of both reasonable and emotion mind). Wise mind involves intuition and knowing what is right beyond reasoning and beyond direct experience. This synthesis of reasonable mind and emotion mind enables appropriate responses; one responds as needed given the situation.

Group members first learn to simply observe and then to describe external and internal stimuli. Suicidal behaviors are regarded as a response of emotion mind; that is, while the results may feel positive in the short term, they are negative in the longer term, leading to other painful states or events. Particularly among individuals with impulse control difficulty or those who use drugs or alcohol, acknowledging and labeling affective states is a major goal. Fully entering experiences, or "participating" is the next mindfulness skill. Finally, patients learn that these acts are most useful when performed nonjudgmentally, onemindfully, and effectively. Although these may sound like lofty Zen goals for patient mindfulness, the basic principles are expressed simply for learning and practice.

Distress tolerance focuses on the ability to accept both oneself and the current environmental situation in a nonevaluative manner. Goals of this module include reducing impulsive behaviors, suicide threats, and all self-harm. Distress tolerance is useful in situations in which nothing can be immediately done to change the environment; for example, when the patient, alone in his or her apartment at 3 A.M., begins thinking the series of thoughts that leads to intense suicidal ideation or self-harm and is trying to resist the urge to engage in such behavior. Incorporating both change and acceptance strategies, distress tolerance targets modulation to the point of tolerance rather than the amelioration of distress. Accepting reality and therefore painful experience as a part of life (i.e., "radical acceptance") figures prominently, as do lists of distracting and soothing activities that convey the notion of myriad paths to tolerance. Activity-oriented distraction toward improving the moment, sensory self-soothing and consideration of the advantages and disadvantages of distress tolerance are strategies within this module.

Interpersonal effectiveness is similar to standard interpersonal problem solving and assertion training. Goals include reducing interpersonal chaos and fears of abandonment. Skills taught include effective strategies for asking for what one needs and saying no to requests. The ability to do this skillfully requires awareness of desired objectives whether related to a specific outcome, to relationship development or maintenance, or to building and sustaining self-respect. Effectiveness is defined as obtaining the changes or objectives one wants. Developing clarity about expected and reasonable outcomes of interpersonal situations is a challenging task for many patients. As part of improving skills, strategies and procedures for analyzing and planning interpersonal situations and for anticipating outcomes can decrease emotional vulnerability and invalidation.

Emotion regulation is defined as the ability to (1) increase or decrease physiological arousal associated with emotion, (2) reorient attention, (3) inhibit mood-dependent actions, (4) experience emotions without escalating or blunting, and (5) organize behavior in the service of external non-mood-dependent goals.

The goals of emotion regulation are to decrease labile affect, including excessive anger. Skills begin with identifying and labeling current emotions by observing and describing events that prompt emotions directly or through one's interpretations of such events, the physiological responses, expressive behaviors, and aftereffects of emotions. In addition, the adaptive functions of emotions are discussed. The focus on describing, labeling, and understanding primary emotional states is followed by strategies for reducing vulnerability to painful emotions and steps for increasing positive emotions. Patients identify the emotions that precipitate dysfunctional behavior, explore the functions emotions serve, and learn to monitor the specific vulnerabilities (e.g., sleep, eating, alcohol or drug use) that lead to dysregulation. Building in positive, goal-oriented, competence-enhancing experiences also helps strengthen resistance to the emotion mind that precedes dysfunctional behavior. Finally, methods for regulating emotions, including nonjudgmental awareness and acceptance and acting opposite to the urge associated with the emotion, are discussed and rehearsed.

Although these four modules are taught as independent skills sets, avoidance of repetitive dysfunctional behavior such as suicidal behavior, binge eating, or drug use may involve the use of two or more skills, determined by the individual's behavioral chain leading to the event. Mindfulness practice and the need to observe, describe, and let pass by (i.e., accept or tolerate) individual emotional experiences are underscored as prerequisites to implementing change strategies in each of the modules.

Telephone Consultation

Between-session contact is an integral component of DBT and serves three functions: (1) to provide skills coaching *in vivo* and to promote skills generalization, (2) to promote emergency crisis intervention in a contingent manner, and (3) to provide an opportunity to resolve misunderstandings and conflicts that arise during therapy sessions, instead of waiting until the next session to deal with the emotions. Patients are taught early in treatment to call their individual therapist for the foregoing reasons; the inability to do so is viewed as therapy-interfering behavior and becomes a target. If patients are reluctant to call, planned calls are prescribed. The therapist may begin by asking the noncalling patient to call at a specific time and leave a message on an answering service; asking for coaching and resolving interpersonal conflicts are approximated and shaped over time. Typical skills coaching situations include those when the patient is not certain which skill to use or feels the skill is inhibited.

DBT patients are strongly encouraged to call before suicidal crises, or at least before they harm themselves; once self-harm has occurred, they are told they cannot phone their therapist for 24 hours afterward. Consistent with viewing the therapist as coach for adaptive behavior, this contact must occur prior to any direct self-harm. If the patient has already engaged in such behavior, the therapist does not provide supportive contact to the patient for 24 hours, limiting whatever contact may occur to management of safety. This provides reinforcement for adaptive coping and realistic consequences after the fact (i.e., "What help can I give you after you've already decided to hurt yourself?") for dysfunctional behavior.

Consultation Team

DBT is best viewed as a treatment system in which the therapist applies DBT to patients while the supervisor and consultation team simultaneously apply DBT to the therapist, similar to several other models of psychotherapy supervision. Because DBT was developed to treat emotionally distressed, demanding, and often difficult patients, and because working with suicidal, borderline patients can be extremely trying for therapists, supervision and consultation were included as components of the original treatment model. Over time, this dual application has gained critical salience as we have learned how essential the treatment system is in sustaining effective engagement of the therapist and effective delivery of the treatment. Consultation to the therapist has several purposes, most important, ensuring that the clinician remains in the therapeutic relationship and remains effectively in that relationship. Without ongoing supervision or consultation, clinicians working with this patient population can become extreme in their positions, blame the patient and themselves, and become less open to feedback from others about the conduct of their treatment. The consultation team functions to provide support to the therapist and to cheerlead efforts to maintain movement and balance. Validation of the therapist's reactions, feelings,

and experiences in working with this extremely difficult population is combined with reciprocal communication and irreverence. The team also functions to improve treatment integrity or accuracy; therapist behavior that deviates from the model is noted and corrective actions are suggested.

In addition to the functions described previously, the consultation group also evaluates treatment development and implementation with each patient. Is the treatment formulation consistent with the data on this individual? Is the hierarchy of target behavior priorities being followed? Is progress being made? Although no particular structure is required for the consultation group, most meet weekly for 1 to 2 hours. Leadership may be rotating, shared, or stable, and in rural settings consultation groups have even been held by telephone conference, supplemented by session audiotapes mailed to all members. The agenda is set at the beginning of each meeting and covers patient updates, therapist difficulties, and observation and discussion of videotaped treatment segments. Information is also exchanged between skills trainers and individual therapists.

Stages 2–4

If Stage 1 may be thought of as guiding the patient to a state of quiet desperation (beginning from one of loud desperation), then Stage 2 is to raise the patient from unremitting emotional desperation (Koerner & Linehan, 1997; Linehan, 1999). Stage 2 DBT addresses posttraumatic stress syndrome and may include "uncovering" and reexperiencing prior traumatic or emotionally important events. It is important that this work not occur before the patient has the emotion regulation and distress tolerance skills needed to process the most emotionally arousing experiences he or she has had. When therapists focus on these issues with a patient who still engages in serious maladaptive behaviors to cope with emotions, the patient often resorts to these behaviors and may become a serious suicide risk. When the patient is more prepared for such work, posttraumatic responses targeted include the distortion or denial of the facts of trauma, self-invalidation and stigmatization, denial or avoidance of traumatic cues, and a dichotomous response style. Goals include the ability to experience emotions in a nontraumatizing manner and increased sense of connection to the environment. Although patients might enter Stage 2 with suicidal ideation and strong wishes to be dead, they are not in Stage 2 if they are engaging in direct self-harm, buying guns for suicide, hoarding pills, or making other concrete plans for suicide. Stage 3 treatment focuses on moving problems in living to the level of ordinary happiness and unhappiness, thereby attaining an acceptable quality of life. Targets include self-respect and achievement of individual goals through the synthesis of prior DBT learning tasks. Developing an ongoing sense of connection to self, others, and to life is emphasized as patients work toward mastery, self-efficacy, and a sense of personal morality. Stage 4, a recent addition (Linehan, 1999), addresses the lingering sense of incompleteness that plagues some individuals even after the resolution of problems in living. The goals of Stage 4 include developing the capacity for sustained joy by integrating past, present, and future and self and others and accepting reality as it is. Functionally this includes expanded awareness of oneself, of the past to present, and of the self to others.

DIALECTICAL BEHAVIOR THERAPY STRATEGIES

Overview

Confronted with the enormity of change that a borderline patient must accomplish to attain a life worth living, and the patient's high level of distress, a therapist may focus relentlessly on change strategies, targeting the patient's thoughts, interpersonal behaviors, motives, abnormal biology, emotional reactivity, and intensity. This approach, however, runs the risk of recapitulating the invalidating environment and often contributes either to the patient feeling misunderstood and angry or to increased self-invalidation, perfectionistic standards, and hopelessness. Either way, little behavioral change is likely to occur. Alternatively, the therapist may focus primarily on validating the patient's pain and on helping the patient to accept his or her problems, including parasuicide, frequent hospitalization, and interpersonal chaos. Once again, the invalidating environment is recreated, as the patient's experience that his or her life is intolerable and desperately needs to change is not addressed. In DBT, change and acceptance strategies are woven together, integrated throughout the treatment, always in an effort to achieve a dialectical balance.

A therapist doing DBT therefore strives to balance the use of both acceptance strategies and change strategies. Balance involves movement between polarities as much as it does finding a middle way. DBT strategies are identified on four levels, each representing a particular acceptance/change dialectic. In core strategies, the key dialectic is between validation (acceptance) and problem solving (change). In communication-style strategies, it is between a reciprocal style (acceptance) and an irreverent one (change). In case management strategies, it is between intervening in the environment for the patient (acceptance) and being a consultant to the patient (change). The case is also managed in a dialectical manner through the therapist consultation meetings. In addition, there is an overarching set of strategies that, because they use the conflict of the polarity to achieve synthesis, are termed "dialectical strategies."

Dialectical Strategies

The most fundamental dialectical strategy is *balancing* all the other treatment strategies, as the needs of patient and situation constantly shift. Another is *entering the paradox,* where, much as in a Zen koan, the therapist simply highlights the constant paradoxes of life without attempting to explain them, modeling and teaching "both this and that" rather than "this or that." Another dialectical strategy is the use of *metaphor*. When collaboration has broken down, when the patient is feeling hopeless, or in many other situations, teaching, persuading, and making a point through metaphor often can be far more powerful than direct or literal communication. Borderline patients seem particularly to respond well to metaphor, and a helpful metaphor may be revisited in a variety of ways over the course of treatment. In the *devil's advocate* strategy, the patient's statement of commitment is strengthened by the therapist's producing arguments for the opposing point of view, a strategy akin to some paradoxical interventions. The dialectical strategy of *extending* borrows a concept from the martial art aikido. The partner's blow is not opposed but, rather, flowed with and pulled beyond its intended target. For example, the patient's statement "If I don't get X . . . I may as well kill myself" might be met with "This is very serious. How can we talk about X, when your life is on the line. Perhaps we should think about hospitalization." The strategy *wise mind* refers to the belief, and communication to the patient, that each person has inherent wisdom and knowledge of what is best for them in each situation and can learn to attend to it once emotional dysregulation is controlled. Making *lemonade out of lemons* is a dialectical strategy of making the best of a difficult situation, always remembering that to make lemonade one also needs sugar (validation). In *allowing natural change,* the therapist accepts that nature and the patient's world are constantly changing and therefore makes no special effort to shield the patient from change in the treatment parameters or the environment. In *dialectical assessment,* the therapist continuously seeks to understand the patient in a situational context, constantly asking, "What is left out?"

Core Strategies: Validation and Problem Solving

Validation

In light of the important role assigned to invalidation in the biosocial theory underlying DBT, and the frequency of self-invalidating behavior on the part of borderline patients, it is natural that validation is one of the primary strategies employed by the DBT therapist. Before being helped by another person to solve a problem, most of us need to feel that the problem and our responses to it are acknowledged and understood by the other person. This need may be particularly strong in persons diagnosed with borderline personality disorder. Thus, validation by the therapist serves an important function of facilitating problem solving. It may also function at times to strengthen patterns of self-validation and to combat self-invalidation, as well as to strengthen the therapeutic relationship or to reinforce clinical progress. By validation, we refer to communicating to the patient that his or her responses do make sense in the current context. This of course raises the issue of how one can validate seemingly invalid behaviors such as self-injury, substance abuse, and many others that create difficulties in the patient's life and lead to this diagnosis. It does not make sense and is not clinically indicated to validate the invalid. However, there are many ways in which a behavior can be valid at the same time that there may be other ways in which it is invalid. For example, self-injury may be valid (i.e., understandable) in the sense that it serves a function for the individual, whether this be communicative or emotion regulation. In other words, the patient has had a reinforcement history that has strengthened this behavior. Because all behaviors occur for a reason, or are caused, in this sense all behavior is valid. On the other hand, this behavior is not valid with respect to its effectiveness for reaching the individual's ultimate goals in life. At some points in therapy, it may make perfect sense to validate self-injury in the sense of communicating to the patient that it is understandable why the patient engages in this behavior. This is not the same as communicating approval of the behavior, and such validating statements can and usually should be coupled with statements that it is essential to learn and practice new behaviors that are more appropriate to the individual's long-term goals. In addition to overt behaviors, it is particularly important that the therapist validate internal private behaviors such as thoughts and feelings. For example, suppose that a patient has a date with a person who calls to cancel the date, saying that he or she will call back later to find another time. The patient's interpretation may be that he or she is being rejected once more and that this is because the other person finds the patient undesirable. The therapist can validate that the emotional response of disappointment or dejection makes perfect sense and that, given the patient's history of rejection, his or her interpretation also is understandable. At the same time, the therapist might point out that the patient's interpretation goes far beyond the data and that it is quite possible that it involves a distortion of the facts. Thus, even when the patient appears to be engaging in cognitive distortion, a common consequence of being emotionally dysregulated, the therapist can search for what is true and valid in the patient's response. This can be at times like searching for a nugget of gold in a bucket of sand.

Validation can occur at a number of levels. The most basic level involves simply unbiased listening and observing. The therapist's alertness and attention to detail, particularly his or her nonverbal behavior, implicitly communicates to the patient that he or she is important and that his or her communication is worth listening to and taking seriously. This is a good example of the fact that validation does not always have to involve an explicit verbal statement but can at times be more implicit. The second level of validation involves accurate reflection of the patient's communications. This is a point emphasized by Carl Rogers and other client-centered therapists and is probably a core activity of skilled therapists of any theoretical persuasion. Accurate reflection, summarizing, and paraphrasing communicate to patients that they have been understood. A more advanced level of validation involves articulating unverbalized emotions, thoughts, and behavior patterns. If the therapist says, "I see I made you angry," or "If I were in that situation, I'd be really mad," this communicates that the therapist understands the situation so well that the patient did not even have to communicate his or her reaction. Of course, this is only experienced as validating if the therapist's inference is correct: otherwise it is likely to be experienced as invalidating. In DBT, therapists do not articulate high-level inferences that stray far from the observable data. A fourth level of validation is in terms of the patient's past learning history or biological dysfunction. For example, the therapist might state, "I think it is understandable that you often find it difficult to focus because of your diagnosed attention-deficit disorder," or "It makes sense that you would have difficulty trusting me, as I am a man and you have been treated very badly by men in the past." However, this last example also illustrates that implicit in the therapist's statement is the notion that the patient's reaction involves a distortion (i.e., is a transference reaction). At times it may be more helpful to validate in terms of the present context or normative functioning such as "It makes sense that you would be having difficulty trusting me. After all, we have only met a few times and it usually takes some time for most people to come to trust their therapist." The highest level of validation described in DBT is "radical genuineness." This involves the therapist responding as his or her natural self rather than with role-prescribed behavior. It involves the willingness to be direct and to share one's own reactions to the patient. As we describe later, certain stylistic aspects of both reciprocal communication and irreverent communication involve radical genuineness. A good rule of thumb is to respond to the patient's statements and behavior as one would to those of one's sibling or good friend. This involves not treating the patient as overly fragile but, instead, as able to tolerate one's natural reactions. It therefore validates the patient's strength.

Problem Solving

Problem-solving strategies are the primary change strategies in DBT directed toward changing target behaviors. The elements of such problem solving can, for purposes of exposition, be divided into a number of steps, though in actual practice these steps are not likely to be followed in linear fashion but rather interwoven. First, the behavior to be addressed must be fully understood. Such understanding involves a behavioral analysis, which we describe more fully later. As a number of instances of a particular behavior are analyzed, the therapist and patient together arrive at some insights about what factors maintain the behavior. This then leads naturally to generating and evaluating various possible solutions. These solutions usually involve some combination of learning new skills, changing the reinforcement contingencies that may maintain a behavior, reducing inhibitions that interfere with more skillful behavior by conducting graduated exposure to cues that elicit the emotional response, and/or identifying and modifying maladaptive cognitive styles and content. Simply arriving at what would seem to be a helpful solution is not enough, however. It is, of course, also essential that the patient actively work toward the solution. This may require the therapist to employ didactic strategies in which he or she is in the role of teacher. This may involve teaching about principles of behavior change; what is known about biological bases of depression, sleep, and so on; or interpersonal relationships. The patient also needs to be clearly oriented to his or her role and expected behaviors, not only in the treatment as a whole but with regard to particular solutions generated for specific target behaviors. Finally, it is important to elicit an explicit verbal commitment from the patient to engage in the specific behaviors suggested by the solution analysis. Although such an explicit commitment does not guarantee that the behavior will occur, it does enhance the probability.

Behavioral Analysis. One of the key characteristics of behavior therapy that differentiates it from most other approaches is its use of behavioral analysis strategies. The goal of a behavioral analysis is to understand the factors that lead to, or maintain, the problem behavior. Rather than focusing on broad personality constructs or developmental antecedents, the focus is on first defining and describing the target behavior in an explicit and detailed manner and then attempting to understand the behavior in its current context by means of a chain analysis. A chain analysis involves examining the behavior in relation to both its immediate antecedents and its consequences in as much detail as possible. In DBT, we typically try to identify a prompting event, something external to the patient that precipitated the chain of events. For example, a patient may have chronic suicidal ideation, but at some times it is more severe. This and other problem behaviors are tracked on a daily basis by the patient on a diary card, which is given to the therapist early in each therapy session. If the therapist notices that suicidal ideation is markedly stronger on a given day during the past week, he or she might inquire about precipitating events. The patient may initially be unable to identify what led to this increase. A useful strategy may then be to pinpoint more exactly the point at which the urge increased. For example, how strong was the urge when the patient awoke in the morning? How was the patient feeling during the afternoon or the evening? When a prompting event has been identified, it may even turn out not to be a major event but, simply, the last straw that was enough to push the patient to a higher level of suicidal ideation, or to actual self-injury, substance abuse, or other behavior. It is also often helpful to identify vulnerability factors that may have preceded the prompting event, and it is always helpful to establish the links in the chain that led from the prompting event to the actual problem behavior. These links may involve thoughts that the patient had about the event, feelings associated with those thoughts, subsequent behaviors, reactions to those behaviors by others and by the patient him- or herself, and so on. The therapist also inquires about consequences of the problem behavior, including its affective consequences for the patient, interpersonal responses of others, and environmental changes that resulted. This may help to identify possible reinforcing factors and to provide the therapist with opportunities to highlight negative consequences. In conducting a chain analysis, the object is to develop a chain with as many links as possible. The more links in the chain, the more places there are that something different could occur. Perhaps the patient needs to avoid certain situations in which this type of prompting event is likely, or perhaps he or she needs to develop greater skills in changing that situation, or in tolerating it. Or, perhaps changes are indicated at the level of cognitive interpretations. Or, at the very last link prior to the actual behavior, the patient could engage in one or more distress tolerance strategies that would help him or her to tolerate the urge to engage in the behavior without doing so.

Problem-Solving Procedures. Once a "behavior in situation" has been analyzed and understood and possible solutions evaluated by the therapist and patient, implementing those solutions may require some combination of four sets of behavior therapy procedures: skills training, contingency management, cognitive modification, and exposure. If the patient simply does not know how to behave more skillfully, skills training is indicated. If, however, the patient knows what to do but is punished or not reinforced for doing so, or is reinforced for doing otherwise, contingency management is called for. If skilled behavior is impeded by the patient's beliefs, attitudes, and thoughts, cognitive modification procedures may be helpful. If the patient is unable to act more skillfully because of strong emotional reactions, exposure procedures that allow those reactions to habituate may be useful.

Skills-Training Procedures. These procedures can teach new skills and also facilitate use of learned but unused skills. Skills acquired need to be strengthened and to generalize across situations. The individual therapist and skills trainers may help the patient acquire skills by direct instruction, by modeling, such as by thinking out loud in front of the client, or by self-disclosing his or her own use of skilled behaviors, and particularly through role play and behavior rehearsal. Fledgling skills then need to be strengthened by further in-session behavior rehearsals and imaginal practice, as well as *in vivo* practice. Any small movements toward more skilled behavior on the patient's part need to be noticed and promptly reinforced by the therapist, even though this means reinforcing still unskilled behavior (shaping). Skills are also strengthened by direct feedback and coaching from the therapist, conveyed in a nonjudgmental manner focused on performance rather than inferred motives. Borderline patients are particularly sensitive to critical feedback, yet such feedback often needs to be given, so it is best to surround it with positive feedback. Skills generalization is enhanced by *in vivo* behavior rehearsal assignments and also by between-session telephone consultation. Other skills generalization procedures might include having the patient tape-record the therapy session for later review. Hearing the session again may strengthen learning, lead the patient to new insights, and provide an opportunity for learning to occur in the home context where it is often most needed. Changing the environment to one that reinforces skilled behavior may also be necessary, such as by having the patient make public commitments or by the therapist meeting with the patient and his or her spouse or family.

Contingency Management Procedures. The therapist tries to arrange for target-relevant adaptive behaviors to be reinforced, and for target-relevant maladaptive behaviors to be extinguished through lack of reinforcement or, when this does not work, the use of punishment. The primary reinforcer used by the DBT therapist is his or her behavior in relationship to the patient. The therapist observes and consciously directs, in a contingent manner, his or her warmth versus coolness, closeness versus distance, approval versus disapproval, presence and availability versus unavailability, and other dimensions of his or her behavior in the relationship. Some may question whether this is a "manipulative" therapeutic relationship. In fact, our natural responses in all relationships function as consequences that do influence others' behavior. The main difference here is the intended beneficiary of the use of contingencies (usually the patient) and their more deliberate application. For the therapeutic relationship to be used contingently, it must be highly valued by the patient. The DBT therapist works hard to establish a strong therapeutic relationship, to "get money in the bank" in order to have it to spend, by developing an attachment between therapist and patient that is mutual and genuine.

The therapist also attends to contingencies outside the therapeutic relationship that may need to change. Suggesting to patients that their maladaptive behavior may be maintained by reinforcement can be experienced as invalidating. "Are you saying that I injure myself in order to get into the hospital?" the patient may respond. It is helpful to discuss with patients how reinforcement works regardless of intent or awareness, and that even unintended consequences influence behavior.

Reinforcement and punishment are defined by their effects on behavior, which can only be determined by experience with a particular patient and behavior. Although praise is a reinforcer for most people, some borderline patients feel embarrassed, fear raised expectations, or for some other reason find praise aversive. The therapist then would need to expose the patient to praise and make it reinforcing by repeatedly pairing it with a reinforcer (respondent conditioning). For most patients, therapist relationship behaviors that are reinforcing include expression of approval, interest, concern and care, liking or admiring the patient, reassurance regarding the dependability of the relationship, direct validation, being responsive to the patient's requests, and increasing attention from, or contact with, the therapist. Therapists need to take care that they do not engage in these behaviors immediately following some maladaptive behavior of the patient, whereas it may be their natural urge to do so.

Withholding, or arranging for the nonoccurrence of, reinforcers that previously followed a behavior may gradually extinguish it, but behaviors on an extinction schedule typically show a "burst" in responding before they decrease. If the therapist then backs down and provides a reinforcer, he or she will now have reinforced an increased intensity of the behavior. Battles should therefore be picked wisely, so to speak, and targets for extinction guided by the hierarchy of targets. It is also essential to help the patient find another response that will meet with reinforcement, and to soothe and validate the patient regarding the emotional effects of being on an extinction schedule.

Punishment is used with great care in behavior therapy because it can lead to strong emotional reactions that interfere with learning, strengthen a self-invalidating style, and fail to teach specific adaptive behavior. Nonetheless, it is sometimes necessary or helpful, usually when high-priority behavior is still occurring and is reinforced primarily by consequences that are not under the therapist's control, so that extinction cannot be used. Examples are the affect regulation that frequently accompanies self-injury and inpatient psychiatric admissions that may reinforce such behavior for some patients. The most common punishers in DBT are the therapist's disapproval, confrontation, or reduction in therapist availability. With emotionally sensitive individuals, disapproval needs to be mild in order to be most effective. Care must be taken to punish specific behaviors rather than the person, and to observe the distinction between punishment and punitiveness. Support from the consultation team helps a therapist to avoid expressing vindictive or hostile feelings under the guise of being therapeutic. Other punishment procedures used in DBT include overcorrection (doing the reverse behavior or undoing the effects of the behavior and going beyond that), taking a "vacation from therapy" in which access to the DBT individual therapist is made contingent upon some commitment or change in behavior and, as a last resort, termination from therapy. Although a strong commitment to therapy is required of both patient and therapist, just as in a marriage, it is also the case that not all marriages work out and not all therapies do either. This rare event in DBT generally can be avoided by appropriate attention to the "observing limits" procedures, to which we now turn.

Observing Limits Procedures. Contingency management procedures are applied in DBT not only to behaviors that interfere with the patient's life but also to those that interfere with the therapist's life. Therapists strive to be aware of their own limits and to take responsibility for being clear with the patient about these limits and the consequences for moving beyond them. This is a somewhat different concept from "setting limits," which typically is viewed as something for the good of the patient, to help him or her "establish boundaries," rather than for the good of the therapist. DBT takes a dialectical stance, viewing boundaries as essentially context driven and relational. A patient's distressed call in the middle of the night may be unacceptable to me, whereas such a call from my best friend may not be. This is because my personal limits are different in each situation, not because the act of calling is in itself pathological. People often need what others are not willing to give. Rather than feeling guilty for attending to one's own needs rather than just the good of the patient, DBT therapists must observe their own limits to prevent the burnout and dropout from treatment that otherwise are likely. The content of these limits is not defined by DBT but is that which is natural to this therapist, with this patient, at this time, and in this situation. Because there are no rules on which to fall back, the therapist needs to be self-aware, receptive to feedback from the consultation team, and assertive with the patient. Limits are often unknown until they are closely approached. Common areas for therapists to observe and to set limits with patients are frequency or utility of telephone calls, suicidal behavior, aggressive behavior, and sporadic attendance or other nonengagement in the treatment. We have found that when one's own limits are clearly delineated and described as something about one's self rather than patient pathology or what is best for the patient, and the behaviors that cross these limits are clearly specified in a nonjudgmental way, many battles over how the patient "should" behave can be resolved or avoided.

Cognitive Modification Procedures. DBT differs from cognitive therapy by placing a less central emphasis on cognition. Instead, thoughts, beliefs, assumptions, and expectations are seen in DBT as just one category of behaviors that influence, and are reciprocally influenced by, transactions with emotional processes, overt behavior, and environmental factors. DBT also differs from cognitive therapy in its emphasis on first validating the wisdom in the patient's cognitions. This helps decrease the likelihood that the patient will interpret the cognitive model as "It's all in your head," or "It's your own fault. Just change your attitude," which the patient typically has heard incessantly. In general, however, all the standard cognitive therapy procedures are consistent with, and may be used in, DBT. The therapist stays alert for distortions of cognitive content and style. Content refers to negative automatic thoughts and maladaptive beliefs, attitudes, or schemas, frequently concerning self as worthless, defective, unlovable, and vulnerable, and others as excessively admired, despised, or feared. Problems of cognitive style in borderline personality disorder include dichotomous thinking (splitting) and dysfunctional allocation of attention (ruminating, dissociating, etc.). The therapist tries to help patients to change these contents and styles by (1) teaching self-observation through mindfulness practice and written assignments; (2) identifying maladaptive cognitions, as when conducting a behavioral analysis, and by pointing to nondialectical thinking; (3) generating alternative more adaptive cognitive content and style in session and for homework assignments; and (4) developing guidelines for when patients should trust versus suspect their own interpretations, as self-validation is often also a goal. The concept of wise mind can be useful here. In a state of strong emotion, our cognitive processes are more likely to be distorted. If a particular thought still seems to be true when examined in a calmer state, it is more likely to be realistic.

DBT recognizes a special case of cognitive modification, *contingency clarification procedures*. It is extremely important that the patient understand the contingencies that currently operate in his or her life, including in the therapeutic relationship, and see how his or her behaviors are influenced by them. It is particularly helpful with borderline patients to have clear rules, which the patient nonetheless may have difficulty learning or following. Consistent use of contingencies and clear communication are the best response to this.

Exposure Procedures. One of the greatest successes of behavior therapy has been the treatment of many anxiety disorders. The core of these treatments involves repeated exposure to the anxiety-provoking stimulus or situation, while ensuring that the normal escape or avoidance response does not occur. This basic approach is extended in DBT to other emotions such as guilt, shame, and anger. When these emotions are problematic in themselves, lead to dysfunctional avoidance behavior, inhibit the use of skills, or are associated with posttraumatic stress disorder symptoms, exposure procedures may be useful. During Stage 2 of treatment, when maladaptive behaviors are under control, more structured protocols for posttraumatic stress disorder may be developed, but, typically, exposure and response prevention are done more informally. Space precludes a detailed description, but the primary steps are (1) to orient the patient, often using a story or metaphor that teaches the basic phenomenon of habituation; (2) to provide nonreinforced exposure, meaning exposure that does not meet with an outcome that could reinforce the emotional response; (3) to block action and expressive tendencies associated with the problem emotion, especially behavioral or cognitive avoidance; and (4) to enhance the patient's control over exposure as much as possible, such as by graduating intensity, as it is easier to tolerate aversive events when one experiences one's self as having some control.

Most of the change strategies used in DBT (and some of the acceptance strategies) can be viewed as involving emotional exposure. This exposure occurs when scrutinizing the patient's recent behavior and experience in a behavioral analysis; in skills training, such as practicing behaviors in interpersonal situations that gener-

ate discomfort; in contingency strategies by exposure to therapist disapproval or approval that may set off feelings of shame or fear, anger, or pride; and in mindfulness practice, where the object may be to observe, in a nonjudgmental manner, the ebb and flow of one's thoughts or feelings. A thorough understanding of the importance of exposure for changes in emotional behavior can therefore help the therapist to take advantage of the innumerable opportunities that present themselves during all aspects of therapy sessions to work directly on patient's emotional reactions using the principle of graduated exposure.

Stylistic Strategies

Reciprocal Communication

Reciprocal communication is the modal stylistic strategy in DBT and is used to convey acceptance and validation and to reduce the inherent power differential between patient and therapist. Characterized by interest, genuineness, warm engagement, and responsiveness, it requires the therapist to take the patient's agenda and wishes seriously and to respond directly to the content of the communications rather than interpreting or suggesting that either the content or the intent of the patient's communication is invalid. As an example, the patient who states, "Today I really, really wish I were dead," might be replied to with, "I'm sorry to hear that. You must feel pretty awful," rather than, "Let's get back to how you're going to talk with your family tonight." Therapists are encouraged to use self-involving self-disclosures such as pointing out the effects of the patient's behavior on the therapist in a nonjudgmental manner (e.g., "When you stare out the window instead of looking at me, it makes me think you don't want to work on these problems and I feel like I'm working harder than you"), and letting patients know where they stand (e.g., "I'm having a hard time feeling like we're getting much done here today"). Personal self-disclosures are used to validate and model coping and normative responses (e.g., "Once I realized that acting angry would not get the lecturer to stop talking, I just threw myself into one-thing-in-the-moment participating by listening and felt better almost right away," or "I've got to admit I'd be pretty miserable if I were in your shoes right now").

Irreverent Communication

Irreverent communication involves a direct, confrontational, matter-of-fact, or "off-the-wall" style. Used to move the patient from a rigid stance to one that admits uncertainty and therefore promotes the potential for change, irreverent communication can be beneficial when the therapist and patient are stuck or at an impasse. In addition to introducing an offbeat or potentially humorous moment, it may also occur when the therapist pays closer attention to indirect rather than direct communications. For example, when a patient says, "I am going to kill myself!" the therapist might irreverently respond, "But I thought you agreed not to drop out of therapy!" In another example, the patient who challenged, "You just put up with me because you're paid to put up with me," received the following response, "Do you think there's enough money in the world to pay me for *this*?" Clearly, care is taken in observing the effects of irreverent communication, to avoid misuse and alienating the patient.

Whereas reciprocal communication is expected in most psychotherapies, irreverence is not included in most psychotherapy training, nor is it part of all therapists' natural communication styles. Our experience has been, however, that it is possible to learn irreverence by paying close attention to peers who are naturally irreverent, culling their behavior for responses that might fit or be tailored to fit, and then practicing such responses in personal life and consultation group until they become genuine.

Case Management Strategies

Case management strategies in DBT are important for enhancing skills generalization. More broadly defined than the traditional notion of case management, these strategies include consultation to the patient, environmental intervention, and consultation to the therapist. In addition to their broad application, DBT case management strategies fundamentally differ from other models of patient case management due to a strong reliance on social learning theory and primary emphasis on methods that teach the patient consistently within the biosocial framework and dialectic philosophy. The primary role of the therapist is to consult to patients about how to manage their social or professional networks, *not* to consult with the network about how to manage the patient. This skills-building focus fosters belief in the clients' ability to learn more effective ways of intervening in their own environments. Advocacy for its own sake is regarded as neither empowering nor helpful, but as iatrogenic to skills acquisition.

DBT case management helps the patient manage the physical and social environment to enhance overall life functioning and well-being. These strategies function as guidelines for applying the DBT core strategies to the environment outside the client–therapist relationship. The therapist coaches the patient in effective interaction with the environment, working to generalize skills. If the patient does not possess the requisite skill for effectively intervening in the environment and the situation requires immediate resolution, the therapist acts as advocate and model, interacting with other professionals on behalf of the patient but only in the patient's presence.

Consultation to the Patient

Consultation to the patient strategies begin by orienting the patient and the patient's social network to the approach, advising and coaching the patient about how to manage other professionals, and consultation about the management of other members of the interpersonal network. Other professionals are given general information about the treatment program but are not told how to treat the patient, nor are they given details or other treatment information without the patient present. Patients learn self-advocacy via skills training and therapists perform case management tasks *only* when the patient truly lacks the skill and cannot learn it quickly enough to prevent an immediate adverse outcome. Dialectically, patients are regarded as able to learn more effective ways of intervening in their own environment while the therapist remains responsible for (1) knowledge of effective environmental intervention and (2) carrying these out should the cost of not doing so prove prohibitive.

Environmental Intervention

Environmental intervention strategies include providing information to others independent of the patient, patient advocacy, and entering the patient's environment to provide assistance. Direct environmental intervention by the therapist is approved only under conditions when the short-term gain is worth the long-term loss in learning. Examples of conditions requiring direct intervention include (1) when the patient is unable to act on his or her own and the outcome is very important (e.g., the suicidal, depersonalizing patient who cannot tell her family she needs them to stay with her); (2) when the environment is intransigent and high in power (e.g., an application for social services that will automatically be denied without professional involvement); (3) when patient life risk or substantial risk to others is probable (e.g., high suicidality or risk of child abuse); (4) when direct intervention is the humane thing to do and will cause no harm; that is, it does not substitute passive for active problem solving (e.g., meeting with patients outside ordinary settings in a crisis); (5) when the patient is a minor (Linehan, 1993a).

Consultation to the Therapist

Consultation to the therapist in the consultation team is the final component of DBT case management and has been previously described. Its purpose is to enhance the therapist's capabilities and motivation to stay within the treatment frame. Prominent within this model is acknowledging that those treating patients with borderline personality disorder need support and ready feedback on their work. The consultation team meeting is the primary means through which this occurs, a group committed to keeping consultation agreements and providing dialectical balance for each other.

THE THERAPEUTIC RELATIONSHIP IN DIALECTICAL BEHAVIOR THERAPY

Therapeutic relationship issues have been touched on throughout this chapter. In this section, we highlight some of the ways in which DBT's approach to the therapeutic relationship is most evident or receives particular emphasis.

Theoretical Foundation

In DBT, an important function of theory is to help the therapist understand and deal with the effects of common borderline personality disorder behaviors on therapists. The biosocial theory is intended to influence therapists' attitudes. Its concept of the invalidating environment

leads naturally to the emphasis on validation strategies in the treatment, and the overarching position of dialectics leads to a therapeutic relationship that pays attention to dialectics, balance, and rapid movement back and forth on the teeter-totter on which the therapist sits with the patient.

Treatment Targets

Problematic interactions in the therapeutic relationship are directly targeted for change in DBT. These include a variety of therapy-interfering behaviors of both therapist and patient, which are a priority second only to life-threatening and self-injurious behaviors. The secondary targets of DBT, such as self-invalidation by the patient and emotion dysregulation, frequently show up in session in response to interactions between patient and therapist. These interactions are analyzed collaboratively and modified when possible. Finally, DBT pays attention particularly to in-session behavior probably to a far greater extent than behavior therapies in general.

Modes of Treatment

Each mode of therapy has its own set of parameters for the therapeutic relationship. Relatively unique to DBT is the use of planned telephone or other consultation availability between sessions, which tends to generate a different type of therapeutic relationship than is prescribed in some treatments. DBT also emphasizes another therapeutic relationship, that between the therapist and the consultation team, which provides the support and guidance that is so helpful in this work.

Treatment Strategies

Every strategy suggests some form of therapeutic relationship, but we highlight several here. The dialectical strategy of *allowing natural change* to occur is different from emphasizing the need for structure and consistency in the treatment of borderline patients. At the level of core validation strategies, a good therapeutic relationship is seen in DBT as having healing qualities of its own for many patients, even though usually not sufficient for the goal of a life well worth living. The emphasis on validation itself, and particularly the use of cheerleading strategies, also sets DBT apart from some other treatments. Finally, the position of radical genuineness, largely being one's natural, rather than role-defined, self, leads to a different type of therapeutic relationship from a more formal, reserved, or superior stance.

Many of the core behavioral strategies also suggest aspects of the therapeutic relationship as central and sometimes different from other approaches. These include therapist as detective, conducting behavioral analyses, therapist as model, therapist as teacher, therapist as reinforcer/punisher, and therapist as exposure stimulus, as when the patient is exposed to threatening topics that he or she usually avoids.

At the level of stylistic strategies, the therapist quite deliberately varies his or her interpersonal style. Reciprocal and irreverent styles are poles apart both in the therapist's behavior and in their impact on the therapeutic relationship.

Therapist Characteristics

DBT, done well, requires the ability to behave and relate in a number of often highly contrasting ways. Because most of us tend to have our strengths toward one end of most dimensions, each therapist has to be aware of the polar oppositions that he or she also needs to strengthen in his or her repertoire. The primary dimension on which DBT therapists strive to maintain dialectical balance is the dialectic of acceptance and change. An excessive orientation toward either is therapy-interfering behavior, yet strength in both may require development by the therapist, with the help of the team. Other variants of this acceptance/change dialectic are nurturing and taking care of the patient on the one hand and a benevolent demandingness of the patient on the other, and a compassionate flexibility regarding treatment parameters on one hand and a nonmoving centeredness about treatment principles on the other.

IMPLICATIONS FOR ASSESSMENT

Evaluation of whether or not an individual meets criteria for borderline personality disorder is best accomplished by means of a structured diagnostic interview, such as the Structured Clinical Interview for DSM-IV (First, Gibbon, Spitzer, Williams, & Benjamin, 1996) or the Personality Disorders Examination (Loranger, 1988). However, simply establishing a diagnosis is of limited utility for dialectical be-

havior therapy, and possibly for any psychotherapy. More important is to know the specific patterns of behavior that are creating difficulty for this particular individual, and what its maintaining variables are. Assessment in DBT therefore emphasises day-to-day monitoring of target behaviors and in-depth behavioral analysis of them within therapy sessions, as described earlier. We have found the completion of diary cards to be absolutely essential for successful treatment, and the therapist is advised to continue having the patient complete them even when he or she is doing considerably better and may not have had any suicidal, substance-abusing, or other high-priority target behaviors in some time. Although borderline patients often will not lie to their therapists, they frequently omit to mention the occurrence of such behaviors if they are not specifically asked about and/or monitored. Another implication flowing from the biosocial theory, and from a dialectical view of assessment, is that it is at times helpful to learn as much as possible about the patient's social context, including bringing in family members and significant others, for collateral information and to better understand these relationships. The patient's behavior is seen as frequently occurring within an interpersonal context, including that of the therapeutic relationship, and the state of that relationship, including the therapist's own contribution to it, is in need of ongoing assessment.

INDICATIONS AND CONTRAINDICATIONS

DBT was developed for treatment of chronically suicidal women with borderline personality disorder. It has now been shown to be effective in improving the lives of not only this population (Linehan et al., 1991) but also borderline women who are not necessarily parasuicidal (Koons et al., in press). In addition, our clinical experience and that of others suggests that it may be a useful treatment approach with other populations with which it has yet to be empirically tested. There is no reason to think that the treatment would be unsuitable for men with borderline personality disorder. Randomized studies recently completed support the efficacy of DBT for patients with both borderline personality disorder and drug dependence (Linehan et al., 1999) and for alcohol/drug dependence with or without borderline personality disorder (van den Bosch, 1999). Nonrandomized controlled trials suggest the efficacy of DBT for suicidal adolescents (Miller, Rathus, Linehan, Wetzler, & Leigh, 1997; Rathus & Miller, 1999), for binge eaters (Telch, Agras, & Linehan, 2000; Wiser & Telch, 1999), and for families in which one member is diagnosed with borderline personality disorder (Fruzzetti, Hoffman, & Linehan, in press), and DBT has been adapted for use in inpatient settings (Barley et al., 1993), day treatment programs (Simpson et al., 1998), correctional facilities (McCann, Ball, & Ivanoff, 2000), and for treatment of depressed elders (Lynch, 2000). It is not clear for whom this treatment might be contraindicated.

Expected Results

Our clinical experience suggests a wide range of outcomes from DBT. Some patients may remain in the first stage of treatment for years. At the other extreme, some patients who initially are engaging in frequent self-injurious behavior may bring it under control rapidly, may have few therapy-interfering behaviors, and may make rapid progress. In one recent study (Koons et al., in press) at the end of 6 months of treatment, only 3 out of 10 patients in DBT still fully met criteria for the disorder, and the mean number of criteria met dropped from 6.8 to 3.6. We feel this is a clinically significant change after a relatively brief (for this population) period of treatment. The majority of patients with borderline personality disorder can be expected to have most serious Stage 1 target behaviors under reasonably good control within a year or two but are likely to continue to need further treatment, perhaps periodically throughout the lifespan. There are few data to predict who is most likely to do well or improve more quickly. The Linehan et al. (1991) study indicated that being younger was a predictor of poorer outcome. A small pilot project, reported in Linehan (1993a, p. 25), suggested that adding a DBT skills-training group to non-DBT individual therapy did not improve the outcomes of that therapy.

Limitations

Although this treatment shows great promise, its efficacy so far has only been demonstrated in three randomized studies (Linehan et al., 1991; Linehan et al., 1999; Koons et al., in press). More research of various kinds is clearly needed. One need is simply more replication of the basic treatment effect for borderline patients. A second need is to conduct dismantling studies that try to identify components of the treatment that are essential or most important. A third type of study is to compare DBT to other plausibly effective treatments, including other standardized psychotherapies and medications, singly and in combination. Finally, as noted previously, this treatment is being extended to other populations, and empirical studies are needed to determine the boundaries of its effectiveness. It is our hope that continuous evolution of DBT and development of other treatments will lead to significant improvements in the lives of those we describe as having borderline personality disorder.

REFERENCES

American Psychiatric Association. (1994). *Diagnostic and statistical manual of mental disorders* (4th ed.). Washington, DC: Author.

Barley, W. D., Buie, S. E., Peterson, E. W., Hollingsworth, A. S., Griva, M., Hickerson, S. C., Lawson, J. E., & Bailey, B. J. (1993). The development of an inpatient cognitive-behavioral treatment program for borderline personality disorder. *Journal of Personality Disorders, 7,* 232–240.

Batemen, A., & Fonagy, P. (1999). Effectiveness of partial hospitalization in the treatment of borderline personality disorder: A randomized controlled trial. *American Journal of Psychiatry, 156,* 1563–1569.

First, M. B., Gibbon, M., Spitzer, R. L., Williams, J. B. W., & Benjamin, L. (1996). *User's guide for the Structured Clinical Interview for DSM-IV Axis II Personality Disorders.* New York: Biometrics Research Department, New York State Psychiatric Institute.

Fruzzetti, A. E., Hoffman, P. D., & Linehan, M. M. (in press). *Dialectical behavior therapy with couples and families.* New York: Guilford Press.

Gunderson, J. G., & Elliott, G. R. (1985). The interface between borderline personality disorder and affective disorder. *American Journal of Psychiatry, 142,* 277–288.

Koerner, K., & Linehan, M. M. (1997). Case formulation in dialectical behavior therapy for borderline personality disorder. In T. D. Eells (Ed.), *Handbook of psychotherapy case formulation* (pp. 340–367). New York: Guilford Press.

Koons, C. R., Robins, C. J., Tweed, J. L., Lynch, T. R., Gonzalez, A. M., Morse, J. Q., Bishop, G. K., Butterfield, M. F., & Bastian, L. A. (in press). Efficacy of dialectical behavior therapy in women veterans with borderline personality disorder. *Behavior Therapy.*

Linehan, M. M. (1987). Dialectical behavior therapy: A cognitive-behavioral approach to parasuicide. *Journal of Personality Disorders, 1,* 328–333.

Linehan, M. M. (1993a). *Cognitive-behavioral treatment of borderline personality disorder.* New York: Guilford Press.

Linehan, M. M. (1993b). *Skills training manual for treating borderline personality disorder.* New York: Guilford Press.

Linehan, M. M. (1999). Development, evaluation, and dissemination of effective psychosocial treatments: Stages of disorder, levels of care, and stages of treatment research. In M. D. Glantz & C. R. Hartel (Eds.), *Drug abuse: Origins and interventions* (pp. 367–394). Washington, DC: American Psychological Association.

Linehan, M. M., Armstrong, H. E., Suarez, A., Allmon, D., & Heard, H. L. (1991). Cognitive-behavioral treatment of chronically parasuicidal borderline patients. *Archives of General Psychiatry, 48,* 1060–1064.

Linehan, M. M., Heard, H. L., & Armstrong, H. E. (1993). Naturalistic follow-up of a behavioral treatment for chronically parasuicidal borderline patients. *Archives of General Psychiatry, 50,* 971–974.

Linehan, M. M., & Kehrer, C. A. (1993). Borderline personality disorder. In D. H. Barlow (Ed.), *Clinical handbook of psychological disorders: A step-by-step treatment manual* (2nd ed., pp. 396–441). New York: Guilford Press.

Linehan, M. M., Schmidt, H. I., Dimeff, L. A., Craft, J. C., Kanter, J., & Comtois, K. A. (1999). Dialectical behavior therapy for patients with borderline personality disorder and drug dependence. *American Journal on Addictions, 8,* 279–292.

Linehan, M. M., Tutek, D. A., Heard, H. L., & Armstrong, H. E. (1994). Interpersonal outcome of cognitive behavioral treatment for chronically suicidal borderline patients. *American Journal of Psychiatry, 151,* 1771–1776.

Loranger, A. W. (1988). *Personality Disorder Examination (PDE) manual.* Yonkers, NY: DV Communications.

Lynch, T. R. (2000). Treatment of elderly depression with personality disorder comorbidity with dialectical behavior therapy. *Cognitive and Behavioral Practice, 7,* 468–477.

Lynch, T. R., & Robins, C. J. (1997). Treatment of borderline personality disorder using dialectical behavior therapy. *Journal of the California Alliance for the Mentally Ill, 8*(1), 47–49.

McCann, R. A., Ball, E. M., & Ivanoff, A. M. (2000). DBT with an inpatient forensic population: The CMHIP Forensic model. *Cognitive and Behavioral Practice, 7,* 447–456.

Miller, A. L., Rathus, J. H., Linehan, M. M., Watzler, S., & Leigh, E. (1997). Dialectical behavior therapy adapted for suicidal adolescents. *Journal of Practical Psychiatry and Behavioral Health, 3,* 78–86.

Rathus, J. H., & Miller, A. L. (1999). *Dialectical behavior therapy for suicidal adolescents: A pilot study.* Manuscript submitted for publication.

Robins, C. J. (in press). Zen principles and mindfulness practice in dialectical behavior therapy. *Cognitive and Behavioral Practice.*

Simpson, E. B., Pistorello, J., Begin, A., Costello, E., Levinson, H., Mulberry, S., Pearlstein, T., Rosen, K., & Stevens, M. (1998). Use of dialectical behavior therapy in a partial hospital program for women with borderline personality disorder. *Psychiatric Services, 49,* 669–673.

Telch, C. F., Agras, W. S., & Linehan, M. M. (2000). Group dialectical behavior therapy for binge eating disorder: A preliminary uncontrolled trial. *Behavior Therapy, 31,* 569–582.

van den Bosch, L. M. C. (1999, November). A study of the effectiveness of dialectical behavior therapy in the treatment of substance and non-substance abusing women in Holland. In C. J. Robins (Chair), *Dialectical behavior therapy for multi-problem patients: Findings from controlled studies.* Symposium conducted at the meeting of the Association for Advancement of Behavior Therapy, Toronto, Canada.

Wiser, S., & Telch, C. F. (1999). Dialectical behavior therapy for binge eating disorder. *Journal of Clinical Psychology, 55,* 755–768.

CHAPTER 22

———◦⟫◦⟨◦———

Psychoeducational Approaches

ANA M. RUIZ-SANCHO
GEORGE W. SMITH
JOHN G. GUNDERSON

Changes in the mental health field and greater society have made psychoeducational (PE) interventions for the treatment of personality disorders indispensable. This chapter presents an overview of such treatments and identifies critical issues specific to personality disorders that make such programs specially challenging.

Psychoeducational treatments have not yet been fully standardized. Due to space constraints, we briefly mention the reported work of clinicians who have begun to incorporate an educational format to assist the families and patients with a personality disorder, and describe two of the most developed programs in detail. In addition, we cite "non-PE" treatment programs that include a PE (i.e., didactic) component. For heuristic purposes we have chosen to refer separately to psychoeducation directed at families and psychoeducation for patients with personality disorder, although rationales, goals, and therapeutic mechanisms are frequently similar for the two populations, and some programs include both the patient and his or her relatives.

RATIONALES FOR PSYCHIATRIC PATIENT AND FAMILY PSYCHOEDUCATION

Changes in Mental Health: The Needs

Though patients and their families have always profited by education about mental illnesses, the delivery of clinical care in the past has rarely offered explanations about the nature, prognosis, causes, and treatment possibilities of a given condition to patients and their significant others. Patients and families were often kept out of the treatment planning process, open discussions about the illness were generally avoided, and decisions were made unilaterally.

Recent changes in the health system have involved a shift from hospital-based treatment toward community-based treatment, with an increased responsibility for the care of patients by the families. This shift has increased the burden of families as well as forcing patients themselves to be more responsible for their own care.

Social and economic changes have also fostered a change in the relationship between patients, families, and professionals in the health system. The once stratified doctor–patient (and family) relationship is now more of an egalitarian consumer–provider relationship that introduces the role of active decision maker for patients and their families. Families and patients are not just passive recipients of help but consumers who select and evaluate the treatments that they receive. Therefore, patients and families can be expected to be more able to define their own needs and to advocate for better services. Any effort aimed to provide a better understanding of a patient's illness is an efficient way to help patients and their families so they will be better prepared to make decisions about their treatment options.

As part of the modern renaissance in Western society of "antistigma" attitudes toward the mentally ill and other disenfranchised groups, the psychiatric profession is now more aware that patients and their families have strengths and resources (Solomon & Draine, 1995). As a result, professionals are now more active in enhancing patients and families' behavioral responses to the illness. Families and patients themselves become active participants in treatment and indispensable elements for change and improvement.

Finally, managed care companies' cost-reduction policies favor standardized treatments whose effectiveness is clinically and financially established. The extensive empirical support for PE interventions in the treatment of Axis I disorders is an important precedent for attempting to implement such strategies in the treatment of personality disorders.

Patient and Family Education: The Theory

Educational concepts entered the mental health field with the development of psychiatric rehabilitation. Rehabilitative approaches begin with seeing psychiatric illnesses as chronic conditions that handicap and/or disable patients from optimal psychosocial functioning in society and make patients more vulnerable to everyday stresses. Improving patients' competency, actively involving the patient in his or her own care and working with his or her strengths, instilling hope, and training social skills are all important elements of the psychiatric rehabilitation model (Lamb, 1994).

In light of the long-term psychosocial dysfunction attached by definition to personality disorders and the available research on the long-term outcome of personality disorders (Perry, 1993), the psychiatric rehabilitation model appears an appropriate model to guide our interventions with personality-disordered patients. The application of the psychiatric rehabilitation model encompasses redirecting the focus from diagnosis towards role dysfunction, changing clinicians' attitudes toward patients and their families, and targeting our interventions toward acquiring skills and fostering environmental change (Links, 1993).

Patient and family education has been addressed from two different perspectives: the PE and educational perspective (Hatfield, 1994). The term "psychoeducational" was first used by Anderson, Hogarty, and Reiss (1980). The basic assumption was that family behavior played an important role in patient functioning and that families could be trained to create environments in which relapse could be reduced. The PE model focuses on what the family can do for the benefit of the patient (i.e., what he or she needs to remain stable). Family burden and family perceptions of problems and needs receive limited attention. Researchers measured the impact of PE interventions in terms of relapse prevention. Because families with high levels of expressed emotion (EE) defined as criticism, hostility, or overinvolvement were predictive of patient relapse, the goal of family psychoeducation was to reduce EE and thereby increase family coping skills (Hatfield, 1994).

"Educational" principles focus on the well-being of the family itself. The education movement found its impetus in the results of a series of studies conducted to determine the effect of highly disturbed family members on the well-being of the rest of the family. The movement stresses that the family is worthy of help apart from its role in caring for a mentally ill relative. Families' reactions are viewed as natural responses to a devastating experience. The goal of educational programs is to disseminate information and teach coping skills using didactic teaching methods, often in a classroom format (Hatfield, 1994).

In practice, most treatment models combine information, skill training, and support in a single intervention and use a balanced approach that addresses both the patient's and families' well-being. Thus we use the terms "educational" and "psychoeducational" interchangeably.

Because they were first developed, several PE approaches have been well studied and have proven successful in the treatment of patients with schizophrenia (summarized by Goldstein, 1995) and bipolar illness (Goldstein & Miklowitz, 1994; Honig, Hofman, Hilwig, Noorthoorn, & Ponds, 1995). Psychoeducational family interventions have an additive role to the regular maintenance of antipsychotic medication in diminishing the risk of relapse in the treatment of schizophrenia. Relapse rate dropped an average of 40% in the group that received psychoeducation compared to those who received regular antipsychotic maintenance (Goldstein, 1995). McFarlane, Link, Dushay, Marchal, and Crilly (1995) and McFarlane, and Lukens, et al. (1995) have published the most remarkable reduction in relapse risk for schizophrenia. The relapse rate was less than half the expected rate for patients receiving individual treatment and medication.

The results have been replicated although the results are not so remarkable for intervention with families of bipolar patients and depression. A more recent development has been the expansion of such programs for the treatment of other psychiatric illnesses such as posttraumatic stress disorder (Benham, 1995), trauma-related disorders (Allen, Kelly, & Glodich, 1997), dual disorders (psychiatric/substance abuse) (Ryglewicz, 1991), and multiple personality disorder (Porter, Kelly, & Grame, 1993).

The independent effect or additive value of the several components of PE interventions (education, enhanced communication and problem-solving skills, support, increased self-efficacy) is not yet clearly established. However, previous experiences in using PE models on other major psychiatric disorders offer a strong precedent for attempting to develop similar programs for the treatment of personality disorders.

Personality Disorders and Patient/Family Education

New Diagnosis: Limited Clinical and Empirical Knowledge

Despite the added recognition given to personality disorders by placing them on a separate axis in the official nomenclature in 1980 (DSM-III; American Psychiatric Association, 1980), and the remarkable advances in knowledge about them since then, these conditions remain shrouded with questions and controversies. Even among experts, personality disorders are controversial diagnostic entities—one example being the open and ongoing discussion about whether they are best conceptualized as dimensions or categories (Frances, 1982; Gunderson, Links, & Reich, 1991; Livesley, Schroeder, Jackson, & Jang, 1994). Research is still too limited to draw definitive conclusions about causality or prognosis, and there is little controlled clinical examination about how these people are best treated. In addition, personality disorders may not be seen as mental disorders, due to the often blurred boundaries between normal traits or personality styles and "disordered" personality. Personality style is "your way of being, of becoming, and of meeting life's challenges" (Oldham & Morris, 1990, p. 17). When a personality style is inflexible, maladaptive, and repetitive, we speak of personality disorder.

Hence, although controversy stimulates interest and fosters research on personality disorders, it hinders the development of educational curricula and the implementation of PE programs in clinical practice. The controversial nature of personality disorders and the still limited knowledge also explain the lack of recognition in clinical practice. People suffering from personality disorders usually present with high degrees of comorbidity with other diagnostic entities—mostly depression, substance abuse, eating disorders, and anxiety disorders. Clinicians who focus on symptoms may see personality problems as secondary and not deserving attention.

Some clinicians are reluctant to conceptualize patients as personality disordered because it means "labeling" the person. Instead, patients with traits that conform to a personality disorder are often conceptualized as "difficult," "untreatable," or "resistant" individuals. This rather moralistic perspective may unintentionally (and ironically) lead to the stigmatization of patients and their families. In our opinion, clinicians' resistance to name the "personality disorder" might at times reflect countertransference reactions (Ruiz-Sancho & Gunderson, 2000). In contrast to what might be expected, patients and their families usually welcome hearing the personality disorder specifically labeled.

Both the denial of the patient's problems as a real (personality) disorder and lack of agreement among professionals have an impact on the nature of the interaction between patient/family and the mental health system. It is common for patients and families to find that different professionals subscribe to different views and attitudes and may even be ignorant about or hostile to viewpoints that differ from their own. Families and patients are left perplexed and wondering about these poorly explained conditions that surely affect their everyday life and can at times carry serious morbidity and functional impairment (Mitton & Links, 1996).

The Nature (vs. Nurture) of the Disorder

Most PE curricula for the treatment of Axis I disorders such as schizophrenia are based on the "illness" or "brain disease" model; the etiology is thought to be predominantly in the neurophysiology of the brain, and at least partial remediation is expected from psychopharmacological intervention (McFarlane & Dunne, 1991). An important consequence of such an approach is that families are not viewed as inherently dysfunctional and are exempted from any causal role in their mentally ill relative's disorder. Personality disorders, however, are not usually conceptualized as brain diseases for which family functioning is insignificant. Psychoeducational contents must therefore differ from those used for Axis I disorders such as schizophrenia, bipolar disorder, and depression. Although etiological theories for personality disorder agree that certain inborn vulnerabilities put people at risk for developing a personality disorder, other factors (developmental, familial) are presumed to be necessary in their ontogeny. Psychoeducational material attempts to convey a complicated message: Families are not to be blamed, but the family environment may have contributed to the disorder.

Another consequence of using an illness model is that it suggests that patients suffering from a personality disorder are passive and hopeless victims of a disease and therefore they cannot be (or become) responsible for their problematic behaviors. Psychoeducational models of personality disorder should communicate the idea that patients with personality disorder are "handicapped" but not "disabled." In other words, patients have deficits or impairments that influence their behavior, but these deficits or impairments do not completely override their ability to control or to learn how to control their behavior.

The Lack of Insight into Having a Disorder

Another characteristic of personality disorders that makes them different from most Axis I disorders is that whereas the latter are based on symptoms (i.e., sources of distress), personality disorders are frequently ego syntonic and may not cause subjective distress. While some personality-disordered patients report painful inner experiences, most others do not even agree that they have pathology (Paris, 1996). In contrast, the maladaptive traits that typically define patients with a personality disorder usually manifest in their interpersonal relationships. Although it seems relevant, there is little known about the impact that individuals with personality disorders have on others.

Personality Disorders as a Group Are Heterogenous

As noted, it is unclear whether personality disorders as a group can be partitioned into distinct categories. Although there are common characteristics among them, patients with personality disorders are different from each other and display different degrees of functional and clinical impairment, burden, and subjective suffering. Developing and implementing a treatment program for such heterogeneous groups of patients with diverse needs and degrees of treatability is an impossible task. The amount of clinical and empirical attention given to the various personality disorders is highly variable. Borderline personality disorder has been by far the most studied of all personality disorders, but findings about it cannot be safely extrapolated to any other personality disorder.

PSYCHOEDUCATIONAL APPROACHES FOR FAMILIES

Background and Rationales

Most theories of the development of personality psychopathology and the derivative research efforts have assumed that personality disorders are significantly influenced by a disturbed and pathogenic family environment. The functionally deficient, pathogenic role that has been assigned to families has had a negative impact on the relationship between families and clinicians. Some clinicians attempt to involve families in family therapy in which family disagreements and conflicts are discussed and feelings are expressed. This approach sees the family system as pathological and the patients as the primary symptom carrier. Most clinicians, however, have been generally reluctant to approach families at all and have been especially wary about involving them (particularly parents) as collaborators in their treatment programs. These clinicians have failed both to invoke and to use families as important resources, as well as to see them as potentially in need of help themselves. This tendency to "vilify" families has specifically represented an important drawback in the treatment of borderline personality disorder (Gunderson, Berkowitz, & Ruiz-Sancho, 1997).

Contemporary researchers accept that personality disorders have a negative impact on the family and social system surrounding the individual. Hence, clinicians now tend to approach families with a more balanced attitude that attends to their needs and invokes them as allies in treatment while neither directly blaming them for nor exempting them from responsibility for the origin of psychopathology.

The empirical evidence provided by the only study that measured the impact of borderline personality disorder and schizotypal personality disorder pathology on patients and their families (Schulz et al., 1985), shows that families have to deal with the same issues as relatives of patients with other chronic mental or physical disorders. Families indicated that having a borderline relative was slightly more burdensome than having one with a serious physical illness. They felt that the greater burden was correlated with antisocial acts such as drunkenness, substance abuse, absenteeism, and promiscuity. Unemployment and dependency were experienced as significant burdens for both the families and the patients. In addition, families with a borderline or schizotypal member felt excluded from the therapeutic process and in some cases felt they were being blamed, either directly or by inference, for the patient's disorder.

Another important issue that families have to confront is the grief implicit in accepting a loved one's psychiatric difficulties. Grief is a shared reaction with other mental disorders, but families of people with personality disorders can find it more difficult to accept that their relative with a personality disorder cannot live up to the expectations they have held for that person and/or their relationship with him or her. For some personality disorders, such as borderline personality, the grief may be especially aggra-

vated by the fact that the observable traits fluctuate and by the selective and changeable nature of the patient's difficulties and symptoms.

Mitton and Links (1996) surveyed the needs of a sample of 15 family members in relation to patients with personality disorder. Patients had been referred to a specialized clinic for the outpatient treatment of personality disorder. All respondents expressed a wish to be informed about different aspects of their relative's illness. More than half the sample (67%) expressed their need for professional assistance for themselves regarding the patient and interest in the development of a support group (60%). Not every family member (only 66%) believed their relative had a psychiatric disorder. Most family members believed their relative's main problem was depression (80%).

In a recent study, Gunderson and Lyoo (1997) assessed the problems experienced by 21 adult borderline patients and their parents (N = 40). Both parents and their offspring pointed out that minimal or poor communication was the major problem that burdened them. Other major problems were conflict and anger in family interactions. In addition, parents rated the patient's suicidality and self-destructiveness as serious problem.

In our own clinical experience with families of borderline patients the following questions are nearly universal: how to react to self-destructive behavior or life-threatening behaviors, what functions can reasonably be expected from their relative, or whether certain annoying or disturbing behaviors are or are not willful. Our work with such families makes clear that families of individuals with personality disorders are very appreciative of the staples of all PE approaches:

- Information about the nature of the condition; its origins, course, and likely prognosis; and the available treatments and their indications.
- Practical guidelines and management strategies to cope with everyday interactions and behaviors that are disruptive to family life. Families need to learn how to deal with intense feelings and how to respond with understanding and compassion rather than defensiveness.
- Support, as families benefit from being treated in an accepting and tolerating environment in which their feelings can be understood and validated.

Finally, a fundamental rationale for the psychoeducation of families of patients with personality disorder is the influence of family interactions on the present course of the patient's illness. Families are usually witness to the ongoing difficulties, failures, and limitations of their relative with personality disorder. We believe families usually play a key role in creating or perpetuating a maladaptive pattern interaction. Because people with personality disorder have special vulnerabilities that make them less able to tolerate particular situations, the way that families react to their relative with personality disorder (although it may be quite natural and appropriate) might inadvertently complicate the situation. Through a better understanding of the disorder, families will be able to learn and modify their responses to the maladaptive behaviors of their relative with personality disorder.

Common Goals and Variations among Approaches

Clinicians working from the PE paradigm are using and adapting models that have proven to be helpful with other mental disorders, such as schizophrenia. As in other areas in the arena of personality disorder, literature on psychoeducation has been led by the efforts devoted to borderline personality disorder.

Table 22.1 presents a summary of the general characteristics of personality disorders for PE curricula.

Common *goals* of family psychoeducation about personality disorder include the following:

1. Providing a theoretical framework that allows families and patients to make sense of

difficult interactions and dysfunctional behaviors.
2. Providing a place where families can have their feelings ventilated and validated.
3. Educating about life stresses and specific situations that make people with personality disorder more vulnerable to decompensation and prone to crisis in extreme situations.
4. Assisting families to acquire coping behaviors and attitudes that can help improve not only the individual with a personality disorder but the family's quality of life.
5. Supporting families in tolerating and dealing with the difficult behaviors of the relative with personality disorder, including periods of diminished functioning, while at the same time helping them to set limits on those behaviors that are disruptive to family life or abusive. At times the treatment might involve supporting families through life decisions like divorce or asking son/daughter to leave the house.

Variations among approaches include the following:

• Family-oriented PE interventions might follow different theoretical traditions. Some interventions might be purely PE (traditionally focus on altering negative attributions about patient illness, teaching coping skills, and providing support). In contrast, other programs, such as those based on systems models, may retain educational elements but tend to see the family as a system in which the patient's symptoms express dysfunctional family relationships. This maladaptive family pattern of function might be reinforcing the patient's symptoms.

• Some programs may be disorder relevant—that is, specifically designed to focus on a specific personality disorder—while some clinicians prefer to provide general information about personality disorders and later address the specific need of individual families.

• Approaches can vary as well in the family members who receive the treatment and whether the program includes the patient–relative in their design. Some might be primarily designed only for parents, spouses, or might involve any family members including siblings or other close relatives. Most PE models for schizophrenia or bipolar disorder have allowed, but not required, the participation of the patients themselves. The presence of some patients with

---

TABLE 22.1. Psychoeducational Contents

• Personality disorders are long-standing, rigid, and inflexible patterns of being in the world.

• Personality disorders will manifest in the interpersonal field.

• Patients with personality disorders typically display a lack of insight.

• Patients with personality disorders are handicapped but not disabled.

• Other comorbid conditions (e.g., depression, substance abuse, anxiety disorders) are very frequent.

a personality disorder (e.g., borderline personality disorder) might be expected to be disruptive at times due to these patients' reactivity and wish for attention.

Experience in the implementation of PE interventions with spouses of bipolar patients shows that there are differences in the response styles of families of origin versus couples and that spouses have different needs from families of origin. Goldstein and Miklowitz (1994) have pointed out that among families of origin, themes of disappointment (born out of failed hopes for the patient offspring) and worries about the future are central. Spouses more readily accept the idea that their communication skills need improvement, but there is the implicit understanding that if the patient fails to show improvement, the spouse may terminate the relationship.

• Regarding individual (one-to-one) family versus multiple-family-group (MFG) approaches, experience in PE interventions for the treatment of schizophrenia and bipolar illness has showed that the implementation of such programs in the group format might have better outcomes. McFarlane (1990) argues that the MFG brings such additional therapeutic elements as the expansion of the family's social network and numerous possibilities of interfamily interactions (e.g., cross-family linkage) to the ordinary PE format.

Proposed Models

Family psychoeducation is rapidly growing in use, but thus far there is little evidence to support the benefits (Mitton & Links, 1996). To our knowledge, the only approach undergoing standardization and empirical testing is the psychoeducational multifamily group (PE/MFG) for families of borderline patients developed at McLean Hospital.

The McLean Psychoeducational and Multiple Family Group

The McLean PE/MFG is an adaptation of the program developed by McFarlane (1990) for the families of patients with schizophrenia. The treatment is disorder relevant, addressing the problems that are specific to borderline personality disorder and the difficulties that families most commonly encounter when dealing with this disorder. It is a PE approach for families that seeks to alter the course of the illness by changing family environment (Berkowitz & Gunderson, 1997). In this approach, borderline personality disorder is viewed as a disorder involving deficits that result from the interaction of multiple risk factors. The deficits—affect and impulse dyscontrol, dichotomous thinking, and intolerance of aloneness—are seen as limitations that might be overcome with long-term treatment or rehabilitative strategies.

Families are engaged as allies in the treatment and the interventions are directed at helping family members develop new strategies to better cope with the problems that their relative with borderline personality disorder presents for them. The approach is proactive and practical, and contains the therapeutic elements of psychoeducation, problem solving, and MFG.

We have developed guidelines to help families become less crisis oriented, maintain stable patterns and consistency, and create a "cooler home environment" (Table 22.2). The 15 guidelines are handed out to families and referred to as the tools for problem solving in every phase of the treatment.

The guidelines advise patients and families to shift expectations to a slower pace of progress with small and attainable goals, along with stressing the importance of keeping things cool in the face of conflict. The guidelines advise families on ways of dealing with crisis and

---

TABLE 22.2. McLean Psychoeducational Program: Family Guidelines

- Go slowly. Recovery takes time. Lower your expectations.
- Family environment
- Enthusiasm and disagreements are normal. Tone them down.
- Maintain family routines as much as possible. There's more to life than problems, so don't give up the good times.
- Managing crises
- Don't ignore threats of self-destructiveness. Express concern. Discuss with professionals.
- Listen. Don't get defensive in the face of criticism. However unfair, say little. Allow yourself to be hurt.
- Addressing problems: Collaborate and be consistent.
- Limit setting: Be direct but careful.

Note. Adapted from Berkowitz and Gunderson (1997). Adapted by permission of the authors.

recommend that any threat of self-destructiveness should never be ignored. We encourage families about not keeping secrets about self-destructive acts (i.e. talking openly with the ill relative and making sure professionals know). Our guidelines advise listening patiently to angry accusations and not getting angry in return. We encourage families to discusss problems when their relative is not angry and when other family members are not upset. The guidelines address the need for negotiation and collaboration when solving problems and point out the undermining nature of parental inconsistencies. The guidelines offer principles for limit setting: The goal is to be firm and direct, avoid the use of unnecessary hostility, and use ultimatums as a last resort. We advise giving ultimatums when they can and will be carried through, not as a form of manipulation.

The McLean PE/MFG treatment has two phases: the "joining" and the MFG phases. The joining phase consists of one to five PE individual sessions and a halfday PE workshop. This joining phase helps families understand their patient relative's illness and creates an alliance for joining a biweekly MFG.

At the joining sessions one of the co-leaders of the group meets with a single family. The main focus is on establishing a working relationship with the family. We obtain a history of the difficulties and try to gain an understanding of the particular conflicts and stresses within the family that will become the focus of subsequent therapeutic work. The therapist's stance of empathically listening to the family's presentation helps to establish the alliance. Frequently these families present as frustrated, skeptical, and distrustful because of past encounters with the health care system. When the therapist demonstrates to families positive regard, interest, and concern, the family's fear of criticism eases and their interest, in the treatment is heightened. We also provide each family with PE reading materials. Relatives are told about the nature of the treatment and its goal.

The joining sessions are then followed by a halfday workshop attended by about 20 relatives of patients. The workshop (WS) is informal and includes bagels or doughnuts and coffee, and people are encouraged to become acquainted. We start with a didactic presentation with slides on phenomenology, epidemiology, course, etiology, and treatment of borderline personality disorder. Each section is followed by questions and discussion. We explain the hardships facing the relative and present our rationale for adopting new methods for coping with conflict. We introduce our guidelines for families in the second part of the WS. Finally, we role-play an MFG session: We invite the family to identify a recent problem, review the problem, and identify possible "solutions" to it, and then we ask all of the families to evaluate the relative merits of these solutions.

After the WS, the MFG begins. The purpose of the MFG meetings is to teach families how to apply the communication skills and coping guidelines to their everyday interactions. The group consists of about six families and two leaders and meets for 1½ hours every 2 weeks. The group is tightly structured. Each meeting always starts with a 10-minute period in which members socialize and are not allowed to talk about problems in their families. By encouraging family members to put away their concerns temporarily, we convey the message that there is more to life than problems, and that keeping their normal routines and leisure activities is essential for them to be able to help their relative. We then start with a go-around. Each family takes a turn and briefly updates the group about their current situation and latest difficulties in their dealing with the family member who has borderline personality disorder. At the end of the go-around the leaders select a small, discrete problem, especially one similar to problems shared by other families. Large, long-standing, abstract problems are avoided. The problem is written on a large board and we encourage members to brainstorm ways of handling it. Every suggestion is written down, no matter how inadvisable or humorous it may be. We get a list of 6 to 10 solutions and then we ask everyone to evaluate the pros and cons. The family is asked which of these are they going to implement, and the details of a plan are refined. At the next meeting, the family will be asked to give a report of what happened at the beginning of the go-around. Finally, we close again with a social chat. The optimal duration of the MFG is not yet established. Our experience suggests that for most families the more natural termination time is about 18 months.

Preliminary data concerning the feasibility of using this treatment show that most patients and family members welcome the opportunity to participate in this type of program. The rate of patient/family refusals (17.1%) is lower than the reported rates in PE groups for families of schizophrenics (mean = 47%) and similar to the

19.2% reported by McFarlane for PE/MFG for schizophrenics. The rate of dropouts (26%) was lower than that reported in schizophrenia (mean = 37%; 30% in McFarlane's PE/MFG) as well.

Preliminary data on the effectiveness of the PE/MFG indicate that this type of intervention has a range of positive effects. After 1 year, parents believed they knew more about borderline personality disorder and they uniformly reported improvements by feeling less burdened and specifically less concerned about suicidality and unpredictability. Overall group means indicated that parents had much better communications and less conflict with their borderline offspring. On relational measures from the borderline patients' perspective, they felt less troubled by parental efforts to control them, less angry at their parents, and much more aware of separation anxieties. We interpreted this to show that the PE/MFG helps patients with borderline personality disorder who initially project their resistance to separation onto their parents and internalize or "own" this aspect of themselves.

Another result involved the coordination of baseline EE (expressed emotion) scores and subsequent course. Five of 11 parents decreased their levels of criticism, whereas 2 increased their criticisms. In all instances these changes were in accord with what the PE/MFG leaders perceived to be clinically desirable. Of note, high baseline levels of EE did not predict a poor course for the offspring with borderline personality disorder. High levels of overinvolvement seem to be a positive predictor (Vuchetich, Fogler, Hooley, & Gunderson, 2000).

The PE/MFG approach is appropriate to the early phases of a long-term treatment, when containment is unnecessary but the patients with borderline personality disorder still require unusually high levels of support and structure.

CLINICAL VIGNETTE

The parents of a 16-year-old girl with borderline personality disorder were frustrated about their daughter's plans for the summer. She had attended summer school during July, and insisted that she have the month of August to relax before starting school again in September. One parent was insistent that she go to summer camp and the other adamant that she get a job. They asked for the group's help during the problem-solving exercise to resolve their dilemma.

The group discussion focused on realistic expectations for the summer, reminded them that they were getting along with their daughter much better than in the spring. Given that the daughter was actually functioning well, the group suggested that the daughter's request for a month off was not unreasonable. Both parents were reluctant to relinquish their view of what would have been optimal but agreed with the reframing of expectations for the summer and went along the daughter's request. The remainder of the summer proceeded uneventfully, and the daughter resumed school in September.

Adaptations of the Dialectical Behavior Therapy

Dialectical behavior therapy (DBT) is a manualized cognitive-behavioral therapy developed by Linehan for chronically suicidal patients with borderline personality disorder which includes a coordinated individual and group format (Linehan, Armstrong, Suarez, Allmon, & Heard, 1991). DBT has an important educational accent: One major component of DBT is skill training and the application of DBT requires the education of the patient on the basic principles behind the therapy. Although DBT was initially designed for treatment of individuals with borderline personality disorder, clinicians are now developing adaptations for the patient's relatives. The favorable results reported by Linenhan et al. (1991) for the individual modality raise hopes that DBT might be a very valuable treatment for patients with borderline personality disorder and their families.

New York Hospital/Cornell Medical Center—Westchester Division in White Plains "Family Partnership." Perry Hoffman (1997) has developed a form of family therapy in which borderline patients and members of their family participate together in a MFG format. The treatment has two major goals: to provide education about borderline personality disorder and to assist family members in acquiring effective coping and problem-solving strategies. By including relatives, it is hoped that the generalization of the skills taught in DBT will be maximized by creating an environment that reinforces skilled behaviors.

Montefiore Medical Center (Bronx, New York). Miller, Rathus, Linehan, Wetzler, and

Leigh (1997) at the Adolescent Depression and Suicide Program have adapted DBT for the treatment of suicidal adolescents. Their program incorporates a multifamily skills-training group that includes the adolescents and at least one family member. Because adolescent patients usually reside in their "invalidating environment," parental involvement is seen as a necessary element for the treatment of these patients. Additional modifications made in this program include shortening the length of the treatment to 12 weeks, simplifying the language used, and reducing the number of skills taught.

PSYCHOEDUCATIONAL APPROACHES FOR PATIENTS

Background and Rationales

Although standard psychiatric care always includes patient education, we refer in this section only to those structured, organized efforts to provide educational services for persons with personality disorders. As with families, patient education is a new area in the field of personality disorders. Only one study (Schulz et al., 1985) has measured the educational needs of patients with these conditions. The study included 31 patients identified as having borderline personality disorder, schizotypal personality disorder, or both, as well as 35 family members. Patients were interviewed about their views about the etiology of the disorder and the burden that created on the family unit. The results show that borderline personality disorder and schizotypal personality disorder patients know little about the disorders. Half the patients attributed the cause of their disorder to chemical imbalance, and 48% said they did not know what might have caused the disorder. Although patients indicated that borderline personality disorder and schizotypal personality disorder caused a similar burden on the family as a severe physical illness (e.g., diabetes and cancer), they were frequently unaware of the extent of the impact of their behaviors on their relatives. Although limited, this study illustrates patients' lack of knowledge about their own difficulties.

Following are rationales that we believe underscore the usefulness of PE interventions for patients with personality disorder:

1. Supports the patient's right to know.
2. Increases awareness and motivation for treatment.
3. Enrolls the patient as active participant in the treatment and decision making.
4. Enhances adherence to treatment protocols.
5. Is a source of validation of feelings.
6. Invokes patient strengths and increases a sense of mastery and competence.

Proposed Models

Iowa Systems Training for Emotional Predictability and Problem-Solving Program

At the University of Iowa, Nancy Blum and Bruce Pfohl have adapted and revised a systems approach to the treatment of borderline personality disorder originally developed by Bartels and Crotty (1992). This is a cognitive-behavioral skills-training approach that seeks to provide both the individual with borderline personality disorder and relatives and significant others—the "reinforcement team"—with a common language that allows them to clearly communicate about the disorder and the techniques for managing it. The Iowa Systems Training and Emotional Predictability and Problem-Solving (STEPPS) program understands borderline personality disorder as a disorder that might be characterized as a defect in the individual's internal ability to regulate emotional intensity. An active interplay between the underlying vulnerability—the emotional intensity disorder (Bartels & Crotty, 1992)—and the social environment of the patient with borderline personality disorder may, over time, create the syndrome we think of as a serious case of borderline personality disorder.

The program has evolved since it began 3 years ago. Currently the program includes two phases: the STEPPS program—a 17-week entry-level group program—and the STAIR-WAYS program—a 1-year advanced group program (Pfohl, personal communication).

At the STEPPS program, patients participate in 17 weekly group meetings of 2 hours that follow a classroom format. The group consists of two trainers and 6 to 10 trainees. Each week is organized around a skill which is the focus of the session. The training is composed of three steps: awareness of borderline personality disorder, emotion management and training, and behavior management training. Awareness of borderline personality disorder educates the patient trainee with borderline personality disorder about the disorder. Although the full recognition by the patient that an illness is at the core of the problem is not necessary, such recognition by the patient trainee helps effectively use the skills to be taught. The materials used in this stage include a review of the DSM-IV criteria for borderline personality disorder and the introduction of Young's schema focused approach to personality disorder (Young, 1994). The schema questionnaire is used to help trainees identify their own individual schemas and to see the relationship between the disordered pattern of feelings, thoughts, and behaviors that comprise the DSM criteria and their cognitive schemas. The emotion management and training describes and teaches skills that aid the patient in managing the cognitive and emotional effects of the illness. The skills assist the patient in predicting the course of an episode, anticipating stressful situations, and building confidence in their ability to manage the disorder. The behavior management training outlines behavioral skills that the patient must master to keep disordered behaviors under control (e.g., eating/sleep behaviors) during crisis periods.

A typical class session begins with trainees completing the Borderline Estimate of Severity over Time (BEST). This is a self-report measure that allows patients to rate the intensity of their thoughts, feelings, and behaviors over the past week. The BEST uses a 5-point scale in which "1" is feeling calm and at ease and "5" is feeling out of control. Trainees are expected to keep track on a daily basis and to summarize the percent of time spent at each level during the previous week at each level (1–5) of an Emotional Intensity Continuum. Along with the weekly review of the Emotional Intensity Continuum is a review of the Skills Monitoring Card which lists the skills being taught and allows trainees to indicate which skills they used in the previous week. After reviewing the previous week's homework assignment, the remainder of the session is devoted to introducing the material for the current lesson.

Relatives and significant others are encouraged to participate in the program and a special session is held that includes them. The optimal treatment system is one in which, in addition to the weekly skills training provided by the treater teachers, the patient with borderline personality disorder receives skills and behavior reinforcement from all members of the treatment system personnel, including family and friends.

Although the recommended setting for the STEPPS program is an outpatient group, the approach is adaptable to other treatment settings such as partial hospitalization, day-treatment programs, residential facilities, and substance abuse treatment programs.

Patients who have completed the 17-week cycle either go on to the STAIRWAYS program or, if appropriate, repeat the STEPPS program.

STAIRWAYS[1] is a 1-year program consisting of biweekly meetings. (STAIRWAYS is an acronym that stands for Setting Goals, Trusting and Taking Risks, Anger Management, Impulsivity Control, Relationship Behaviors, Writing a Script, Assertiveness Training, Your Choice: Victim or Volunteer, Schemas Revisited.) The goal is to reinforce and extend the skills learned during the STEPPS program. Handouts are provided at each session which are added to the notebook.

Other Educational Approaches: The Menninger Clinic Attachment Perspective

At the Menninger Clinic, Jon G. Allen (1995) approaches education of the patient with borderline personality disorder from an attachment theory perspective. Allen suggests that the core problem of borderline personality disorder is the inability to establish secure attachment relationships. He organizes his explanation around the first DSM-IV criterion—the fear of abandonment. The patient's inability to establish a "secure base" explains abandonment fears and his or her lifelong need for security. Other symptoms, such as intense and unmanageable affects (anger, depression, anxiety, feelings of emptiness) and "tension relieving" behaviors (self-destructive and impulse acts) are understood as coming from that fear.

Explaining the dynamics of borderline personality disorder from the attachment perspective diminishes the stigma attached to the diagnosis and helps the patient to accept him- or herself. In addition, it encourages the patient with borderline personality disorder to meet the challenge of developing secure attachments and using them effectively to regulate emotion.

USE OF OTHER RESOURCES FOR PSYCHOEDUCATIONAL PURPOSES

Mental Health Organizations/ Self-Help Groups

Hatfield (1987) has summarized the different ways self-help groups provide therapeutic benefit to their members:

1. Members serve as role models to each other.
2. Help giving is reciprocal and inherently therapeutic.
3. Self-help groups provide opportunities for learning.

Since they first started, support and advocacy groups of families with mentally ill relatives, such as the National Alliance for the Mentally Ill (NAMI), have provided support and education for families, advocated for better services, and funded and encouraged research in mental illness. These organizations have traditionally referred to mental illness in a restricted sense to mean "biologically" caused disorders which are seriously disabling (e.g., schizophrenia). Although personality disorders have been generally excluded from the list of disorders that have deserved advocacy groups' attention, growing recognition of the public health significance and clinical relevance of personality disorders seems to be taking place among such organizations.

In addition, new consumer groups are forming whose primary interests are to provide education about personality-disorders, to support families of personality-disordered patients, and to advocate for the development and increase of clinical programs for the treatment of these conditions. The New England Personality Disorder Association (NEPDA) was founded recently in Boston. NEPDA is primarily interested in providing education and increasing public awareness about personality disorders, especially borderline personality disorder. NEPDA sponsors a monthly lecture series in which local experts on personality disorder are invited to present and discuss both clinical aspects and research developments on personality disorders. Other NEPDA activities include producing educational brochures and a book club for patients with borderline personality disorder, family members, and clinicians who meet monthly to discuss readings concerning person-

ality disorders. NEPDA is hoping to expand its competencies. A recent project is development of a Web site.

NEPDA's initiative has been followed in Maine and Vermont. A similar organization has formed in New York. Ideally the expansion of these groups will assist a neglected population and create a mental health climate that fosters clinical services and research.

Books and Other Printed Material

In the last decade, several publications about borderline personality disorder written in an easily accessible language have been published for laypeople.

Mitton and Links (1996) provide a complete list of reading materials about different aspects of personality disorders which briefly summarizes the contents of the suggested books. Other valuable sources of information are articles written by leading specialists and published in nonprofessional journals and magazines. We particularly recommend a recent issue devoted to borderline personality disorder in the *Journal of the California Alliance of the Mentally Ill* (1997).

At McLean we have prepared an unpublished manuscript given to families that briefly summarizes the diagnosis, course, etiology, and treatment of borderline personality disorder. Nancy Blum and Bruce Pfohl at the University of Iowa have developed an educational brochure for family and friends of patients with borderline personality disorder.

Audiovisual Material

Hyler and Schanzer (1997) have recently reported on their experience in using videotaped commercial movies in teaching students, medical trainees, and residents about borderline personality disorder and the value of this resource for the psychoeducation of patients and their families. While warning about the limitations and risks of using commercial videos, they demonstrate how various films might be used to illustrate different aspects of DSM-IV borderline personality disorder diagnostic criteria. At McLean we use tapes that contain information on diagnosis, course, etiology, and treatment of borderline personality disorder to teach families about the disorder.

The Internet

The Internet is a rapidly expanding source of information and support for personality-disordered patients, their families, and their loved ones. Clinicians offer a wide range of services over the 'net (i.e., general information on specific DSM criteria for individual personality disorders, practical advice on psychopharmacology). Patients also create and maintain Web sites that are creative offerings of information and support for a cyber community of other recovering patients. Most of the major support groups and mental health agencies also have Web sites that provide useful information and "links" to other sites where the patient, spouse, family member, or clinician may access a variety of support and informational services (Fogler & Gunderson, 2001).

PSYCHOEDUCATION: PRESENT STATUS AND FUTURE DIRECTIONS

The development of PE interventions for personality-disordered individuals is still at an early stage. Such development has been fostered by recent changes in the health system and demonstrated usefulness of these interventions in managing Axis I disorders.

Professionals who work with these families still need to rely on clinical experience and teaching. Although in its early stages, clinical and empirical efforts are being devoted to adapt models (including rationales and methodology) that have proven useful in treating of Axis I disorders. Future developments should take into consideration the specific characteristics of personality disorders. A better understanding about the origins of personality psychopathology will offer material for the elaboration of PE curricula that are particularly relevant to personality disorders. Meanwhile, it is important to keep in mind the limitations of what can be taught. As in other areas in the arena of personality disorder, literature in the field of psychoeducation has been led by the efforts devoted to borderline personality disorder. However, the findings and clinical experience about borderline personality disorder may not be safely extrapolated to any other personality disorder.

Both patients with a personality disorder and their families share with patients suffering from other psychiatric illnesses and their relatives the need for education, support, and improved coping skills. To guide our PE interventions, more effort should go into evaluating the needs of family members and the problems they encounter in their transactions with their family member with a personality disorder. This effort must be extended to the evaluation of patients' needs for education and patient's perception of their problems and those of their family. Convincing empirical evidence is needed on the effectiveness of PE interventions for individuals with personality disorders.

Research on the use of PE interventions in schizophrenia and other disorders such as bipolar illness and depression is based on the theoretical construct of EE. Most outcome results have been measured in terms of relapse prevention. Further research needs to be undertaken to establish the relevance of the EE construct to personality disorders. In addition, it needs to be determined whether outcome variables used to measure the effectiveness of PE interventions for Axis I disorders need to be modified for personality disorders. Such measures should evaluate both changes in the patient's clinical symptoms and functional level and in the family environment (i.e., communication and type and quality of interactions). Equally important outcome variables might be measures of patient and family satisfaction, stress level, or knowledge learned and assimilated.

Attention should be paid to factors related to recruitment, engagement, and retention of families and patients in PE treatment programs. These factors are important because they affect the feasibility of such programs and identify who is likely to benefit from them.

A further step will be to answer more specific questions such as the type and format that will be most efficacious and cost-effective. Recent clinical experiences and preliminary empirical results that we have summarized support the potential value of PE interventions in the management of this difficult patient population and their families.

ACKNOWLEDGMENTS

This work is supported by Grant No. MH53515-02 from the National Institute of Mental Health. Ana M. Ruiz-Sancho's work has been supported, in part, by a fellowship awarded by the Academic Council of the Real Colegio Complutense.

NOTES

1. A treatment manual for group leaders is being developed by the authors. At the present time, a supplemental packet for the STEPPS program, used in conjunction with the Bartels and Crotty (1992) manual, may be ordered from Blum and Pfohl, Dept. of Psychiatry, 1942 JPP, University of Iowa Hospital, Iowa City, Iowa, 52242.

REFERENCES

Allen, J. G. (1995). Explaining "borderline personality disorder" to patients. *Treatment Today, 7*(3), 37, 39.

Allen, J. G., Kelly, K. A., & Glodich, A. (1997). A psychoeducational program for patients with trauma-related disorders. *Bulletin of the Menninger Clinic, 6*(2), 222–239.

American Psychiatric Association. (1980). *Diagnostic and statistical manual of mental disorders* (3rd ed.). Washington, DC: Author.

Anderson, C. M., Hogarty, G., & Reiss, D. J. (1980). Family treatment of adult schizophrenic patients: A psychoeducational approach. *Schizophrenia Bulletin, 6,* 490–505.

Bartels, N., & Crotty, M. (1992). *The borderline personality disorder skill training manual.* Winfield, IL: E.I.D. Treatment Systems.

Benham, E. (1995). Coping strategies: A psychoeducational approach to post-traumatic symptomatology. *Journal of Psychosocial Nursing, 33*(6), 30–35.

Berkowitz, C., & Gunderson, J. G. (1997). *Psychoeducational treatment of borderline personality disorders in multiple family groups: A manual.* Unpublished manuscript.

Fogler, J., & Gunderson, J. G. (2001). Borderline personality disorder: A guide to psychoeducation resources. (Appendix). In *Borderline personality disorder: A clinical guide* (pp. 451–453). Washington, DC: American Psychiatric Press.

Frances, A. (1982). Categorical and dimensional systems of personality diagnosis: A comparison. *Comprehensive Psychiatry, 23*(6), 516–527.

Goldstein, M. J. (1995). Psychoeducation and relapse prevention. *International Clinical Psychopharmacology, 9*(5), 59–69.

Goldstein, M. J., & Miklowitz, D. J. (1994). Family intervention for persons with bipolar disorder. In A. B. Hatfield (Ed.), *New directions in the treatment of the mentally ill* (pp. 23–35). San Francisco: Jossey-Bass.

Gunderson, J. G., Berkowitz, C., & Ruiz-Sancho, A. M. (1997). Families of borderline patients: A psychoeducational approach. *Bulletin of the Menninger Clinic, 61*(4), 447–457.

Gunderson, J. G., Links, P. S., & Reich, J. H. (1991). Competing models of personality disorders. *Journal of Personality Disorders, 5,* 60–68.

Gunderson, J. G., & Lyoo, I. (1997). Family problems and relationships for adults with borderline personality disorder. *Harvard Review of Psychiatry, 4,* 272–278.

Hatfield, A. B. (1987). Social support and family coping. In A. B. Hatfield & H. P. Lefley (Eds.), *Families of the mentally ill: Coping and adaptation* (pp. 191–207). New York: Guilford Press.

Hatfield, A. B. (1994). Family education: Theory and practice. In A. B. Hatfield (Ed.), *New directions in the treatment of the mentally ill* (pp. 3–11). San Francisco: Jossey-Bass.

Hyler, S. E., & Schanzer, B. (1997). Using commercially available films to teach about borderline personality disorder. *Bulletin of the Menninger Clinic, 61*(4), 458–468.

Hoffman, P. D. (1997). A family partnership. *Journal of the California Alliance for the Mentally Ill, 8,* 52–53.

Honig, A., Hofman, A., Hilwig, M., Noorthoorn, E., & Ponds, R. (1995). Psychoeducation and expressed emotion in bipolar disorder: Preliminary findings. *Psychiatric Research, 56,* 229–231.

Journal of the California Alliance for the Mentally Ill. (1997). *8,* 1–82.

Lamb, H. R. (1994). A century and a half of psychiatric rehabilitation in the United States. *Hospital and Community Psychiatry, 45*(10), 1015–1020.

Linehan, M. M., Armstrong, H. E., Suarez, A., Allmon, D., & Heard H. L. (1991). Cognitive-behavioral treatment of chronically parasuicidal borderline patients. *Archives of General Psychiatry, 48,* 1060–1064.

Links, P. S. (1993). Psychiatric rehabilitation model for borderline personality disorder. *Canadian Journal of Psychiatry, 38*(Suppl. 1), 35–38.

Livesley, W. J., Schroeder, M. L., Jackson, D. N., & Jang, K. L. (1994). Categorical distinctions in the study of personality disorder: Implications for classification. *Journal of Abnormal Psychology, 103*(1), 6–17.

McFarlane, W. R. (1990). Multiple family groups and the treatment of schizophrenia. In M. I. Herz, S. J. Keith, & J. P. Docherty (Eds.), *Handbook of Schizophrenia: Vol. 4. Psychosocial treatment of schizophrenia* (pp. 167–189). Amsterdam, The Netherlands, Elsevier Science.

McFarlane, W. R., & Dunne, E. (1991). Family psychoeducation and multifamily groups in the treatment of schizophrenia. In *Directions in psychiatry, 11*(20). New York: Hatherleigh.

McFarlane, W. R., Link, B., Dushay, R., Marchal, J., & Crilly, J. (1995). Psychoeducational multiple family groups: Four-year relapse outcome in schizophrenia. *Family Process, 34,* 127–144.

McFarlane, W. R., Lukens, E., Link, B., Dushay, R., Deakins, S. A., Newmark, M., Dunne, E. J., Horen, B., & Toran, J. (1995). Multiple-family groups and psychoeducation in the treatment of schizophrenia. *Archives of General Psychiatry, 52,* 679–687.

Miller, A. L., Rathus, J. H., Linehan, M. M., Wetzler, S., & Leigh, E. (1997, March). Dialectical behavior therapy adapted for suicidal adolescents. *Journal of Practical Psychiatry and Behavioral Health, 3,* 78–86.

Mitton, J. M., & Links, P. S. (1996). Helping the family:

A framework for intervention. In P. S. Links (Ed.), *Clinical assessment and management of severe personality disorders. Clinical practice* (no. 35, pp. 195–218). Washington, DC: American Psychiatric Press.

Oldham, J. M., & Morris, L. B. (1990). *Personality self-portrait. Why you think, work, love, and act, the way you do.* New York: Bantam Books.

Paris, J. (1996). *Social factors in the personality disorders. A biopsychosocial approach to etiology and treatment.* New York: Cambridge University Press.

Perry, J. (1993, Spring). Longitudinal studies of personality disorders. *Journal of Personality Disorders, 7*(Suppl.), 63–85.

Porter, S., Kelly, K. A., & Grame, C. J. (1993). Family treatment of spouses and children of patients with multiple personality disorder. *Bulletin of the Menninger Clinic, 57*(3), 371–379.

Ruiz-Sancho, A. M., & Gunderson, J. G. (2000). Families of patients with borderline personality disorder: A review of the literature. In O. F. Kernberg, B. Dulz, & V. Sachsse (Eds.), *Handbook of borderline personality disorder* (pp. 771–791). Stuttgart: Schattauer-Verlag.

Ryglewicz, H. (1991). Psychoeducation for clients and families: A way in, out, and through in working with people with dual disorders. *Psychosocial Rehabilitation Journal, 15*(2), 80–89.

Schulz, P. M., Schulz, S. C. H., Hamer, R., Resnick, R. J., Friedel, R. O., & Goldberg, S. C. (1985). The impact of borderline and schizotypal personality disorders on patients and their families. *Hospital Community Psychiatry, 36,* 879–881.

Solomon, P., & Draine, J. (1995). Subjective burden among family members of mentally ill adults: Relation to stress, coping and adaptation. *American Journal of Orthopsychiatry, 65*(3), 419–427.

Vuchetich, J. P., Fogler, J. M., Hooley, J. H., & Gunderson, J. G. (2000). *Expressed emotion in family members of borderline women: Effects on course of illness.* Unpublished manuscript.

Young, J. (1994). *Cognitive therapy for personality disorder: A schema-focused approach.* Sarasota, FL: Professional Resource Press.

CHAPTER 23

⟨⟩⬦⟨⟩

Pharmacotherapy

PAUL MARKOVITZ

Most discussions of personality disorders center on the learned components of personality and the psychotherapeutic methods available to help individuals develop alternative ways of viewing and dealing with the world. Emerging studies indicate that personality disorders may be minimally learned and instead may be part of the way an individual is hard-wired at the time of conception. If this is the case, psychotherapy aimed at minimizing personality disorders would be only partially effective in the majority of patients. Using a medical model, therapy would be better given after the biological cause of the behavior is treated and would serve as a means of rehabilitation. Few pharmacological studies have been conducted in patients with personality disorders over the past 10 years, yet the cost and acuity of these disorders clearly places a stress on society. This chapter reviews studies involving pharmacotherapy of personality disorders and elaborates on details of treatment not available in other published studies.

Clinical trials suggest that many personality characteristics are associated with neurochemical anomalies of the central nervous system. The biochemistry of abnormal personality is well documented in a number of studies (Coccaro, Berman, Kavoussi, & Hauger, 1996; Coccaro, Kavoussi, Hauger, Cooper, & Ferris, 1998; Hollander et al., 1994; Fuente et al., 1994, 1997; Fuente & Mendlewicz, 1996; Martial et al., 1997; McBride et al., 1994; Pine et al., 1996; Stein et al., 1996; Unis et al., 1997;

Verkes, Pijl, Meinders, & Van Kempen, 1996; Verkes et al., 1998). These biochemical data suggest that abnormal neurochemistry is associated with behavioral changes, and potentially that some of our personality arises from these underpinnings. These findings suggest that many behavioral traits called personality may be biologically ordained and not learned. Even if personality arises from learned components, which in turn leads to neurochemical changes, restoring the central nervous system to a more optimal/normal biochemistry should always be a treatment option. Ultimately, the greater the number of credible options offered to a patient to be well, the higher his or her chances of recovery. Restoring the central nervous system to a more normal neurochemical state makes good clinical sense.

There are many difficulties in assessing the efficacy of pharmacotherapies for personality disorders. First, not all patients diagnosed with any single personality disorder have the same behavioral characteristics (Torgersen, 1994). There are different types of borderline personality disorder, for example, just as there are different types of diabetes, asthma, depression, or hypertension. No single pharmacotherapy should be expected to work in all forms of an illness. Delineating symptomatic behaviors which predict the response of one agent over another is an important consideration in future studies. Second, comorbid behaviors and illnesses can greatly affect response rates to pharmacotherapies. Ongoing alcohol and drug abuse will hamper response rates to pharmacotherapy, yet many of the patients treated in clinical practice will have substance abuse problems. Comorbid depression, anxiety, or psychosis can affect medication options available to the clinician, as certain medications can worsen psychosis or anxiety initially. Insight and motivation to change are also key components and are covered elsewhere in this text. Third, it is difficult to assess change in personality. We can monitor changes in anxiety, socioeconomic status, schooling, criminal activity, depression, and a host of other behaviors, but it is difficult to convey the true change taking place in a personality disorder that has been successfully treated. For example, is an individual with borderline personality disorder changed if the individual no longer meets criteria for the disease? If so, for how long must the individual be symptom-free? Because little work exists that does anything other than speak of acute changes in characterological behaviors, there are no set guidelines available for measuring change in personality-disordered patients. Finally, diagnostic criteria change so frequently, it is difficult to compare patients with borderline personality disorder from studies in 1986 (DSM-III) to patients with the same illness using different diagnostic criteria in 1990 (DSM-III-R) or 1997 (DSM-IV). Nonetheless, there is a substantial body of data linking certain diagnoses and behaviors to medication responsivity.

This chapter reviews the pharmacotherapy of personality disorders diagnosed using DSM criteria, and treated pharmacologically. Studies primarily are done based on the frequency with which these patients present for treatment. Thus, borderline personality disorder, antisocial personality disorder, schizotypal personality disorder, and avoidant personality disorder are the major disorders studied. They are all reviewed here. Second, there is a discussion of using behavioral clusters instead of DSM diagnoses to determine treatment. DSM criteria are groupings of behaviors that have evolved over time as a means of categorizing what is seen clinically to describe personality. Data are emerging that appropriate pharmacotherapy choices may be better selected by using behavioral clusters that differ from DSM diagnoses. This latter idea provides a simpler mode of choosing pharmacotherapy but an even less structured method of conveying what one is treating.

BORDERLINE PERSONALITY DISORDER

The vast majority of personality disorder studies have been done in patients with borderline personality disorder, and the vast majority of the chapter centers on this diagnosis. Borderline personality disorder is frequently accompanied by anxiety, depression, psychosis, hostility, impulsivity, mood lability, chaotic social situations, substance abuse, and poor treatment outcome. Borderline personality disorder is the most common of the personality disorders seen in clinical practice, and the aforementioned behaviors are often amenable to pharmacological intervention. Virtually all medications used to treat borderline personality disorder are used to treat the symptoms which they are known to affect (lithium in mood swings, neuroleptics for psychosis, etc.). Regardless of the medications investigated, the size of the studied populations is extremely small based on the prevalence of borderline personality disorder and its cost of treatment to society. The treatment of borderline personality disorder is reviewed next by pharmacological action of medications utilized.

Lithium

Lithium use in borderline personality disorder was based on its ability to help stabilize mood swings in bipolar patients. It was hypothesized that this same effect might be seen in borderline personality disorder. Rifkin, Quitkin, Carillo, Blumberg, and Klein (1972) studied the effects of lithium in 21 patients meeting criteria for emotionally unstable character disorder, a diagnostic precursor to borderline personality disorder. Behavioral improvement was seen in 67% (14 of 21) of the patients studied, whereas only four patients showed improvement on placebo. Both manic-like behaviors and depressive behaviors were reduced. A prospective open trial by the same group (Rifkin, Levitan, Glaewski, & Klein, 1972) showed that one-third of the group improved with lithium, one-third stayed the same, and one-third worsened. This may reflect the heterogeneity of the emotionally unstable character disorder diagnosis and indicates that some patients do benefit statistically from treatment. Goldberg has reported on the use of lithium in patients diagnosed with borderline personality disorder, and his results also show benefits for some patients (Goldberg, 1989).

A review of the foregoing papers, however, indicates that lithium is at best only partially effective for even those patients showing statistical improvement. Affective instability continues on lithium although the intensity and frequency are decreased. Likewise, for many patients the side effects of lithium are so severe that they do not take the medication (Rifkin, Levitan, et al., 1972). These side effects include diarrhea, weight gain, tremor, mental slowing, physical slowing, and polyuria. Most important, few if any patients have a resolution of all the biologically driven symptoms of their borderline personality disorder with lithium. The threat of impulsive overdosage is also high in borderline personality disorder, and lithium's lethality must also be considered. Based on its incomplete efficacy, poorly tolerated side-effect profile, and lethality in overdose, lithium should be considered a second-line pharmacotherapeutic intervention in borderline personality disorder.

Anticonvulsants

The majority of studies using anticonvulsants in borderline personality disorder consist mainly of reports lacking placebo control. Jonas (1967), Stephens and Shaffer (1970), Mattes (1990), Barratt, Kent, Bryant, and Felthous (1991), and Stein, Simeon, Frenkel, Islam, and Hollander (1995) have presented cases demonstrating the efficacy of anticonvulsants in patients with probable or definite borderline personality disorder. Gardner and Cowdry (1986b) showed the beneficial effects of carbamazepine in borderline personality disorder in a double-blind placebo-controlled cross-over trial. Of the four medications (alprazolam, tranylcypromine, trifluoperazine, and carbamazepine) investigated, carbamazepine proved the most beneficial, with 11 of 15 patients opting to remain on or return to carbamazepine therapy at the study's conclusion. Although the medication did not eliminate behavioral dyscontrol, it markedly diminished the severity of this behavior. Unfortunately, three patients noted the development of severe melancholic depression while on carbamazepine (Gardner & Cowdry, 1986a).

Carbamazepine may be effective for treating affective instability and behavioral dyscontrol accompanying borderline personality disorder but inappropriate for patients with comorbid depression. Lethargy is a common side effect of carbamazepine, as is induction of liver hepatic oxidative enzymes and dermatological reactions (Elphick, 1989). This group of medications is only partially effective in borderline personality disorder (Gardner & Cowdry, 1989) and probably not a first-line choice for treating borderline personality disorder.

Benzodiazepines can be looked at as both antiepileptic agents or anxiolytics. Although some early reports suggested efficacy of benzodiazepines (Faltus, 1984; Vilkin, 1972) Gardner and Cowdry (1985) showed these agents to be detrimental in the treatment of borderline personality disorder. The data for use or nonuse of these agents remains modest, but they are probably best avoided in a group prone to substance abuse, overdose attempts, disinhibition, and depression.

Naltrexone

Two reports (McGee, 1997; Sonne, Rubey, Brady, Malcolm, & Morris, 1996) suggest that the opiate antagonist naltrexone may be effective in some patients with borderline personality disorder. The data indicate a decrease in self-injury when these agents are used, albeit none of the patients ($N = 6$ in total) were on naltrexone alone. No mention is made of the effects of the drug on depression or anxiety, nor is there any longitudinal data on efficacy beyond the acute treatment phase of 3 weeks. Further studies are needed, but the idea of using this relatively benign agent to acutely manage self-injury in some patients needs to be investigated further.

Neuroleptics

Past reviews have only looked at standard neuroleptics. This chapter discusses the use of the newer atypical antipsychotics and their potential mode of action. Open studies suggest that the newer agents may be much more effective than the older antipsychotics in borderline personality disorder.

Typical Antipsychotics

Neuroleptic use in borderline personality disorder was initially rationalized as being useful because data supported neuroleptic efficacy in impulsive–aggressive acts and psychosis. A number of open trials were published that described the beneficial effects of neuroleptics in borderline patients (Brinkley, Beitman, &

Friedel, 1979; Leone, 1982; Serban & Siegel, 1984; Teicher et al., 1989). Two double-blind placebo-controlled trials were also conducted and published simultaneously (Goldberg et al., 1986; Soloff et al., 1986b). Goldberg et al. (1986) showed statistical efficacy of modest doses of thiothixene (8.7 mg/day average dosage) in outpatients with borderline personality disorder with brief psychotic episodes. Patients without brief psychotic episodes did not benefit from thiothixene. Psychosis, obsessionality, phobic anxiety, and ideas of reference were reduced in the psychotic patients. The neuroleptic did not reduce anger or hostility as measured by the Hopkins Symptom Checklist—90 (HSCL-90) in either psychotic or nonpsychotic patients. No longitudinal studies were conducted in any of the patients.

Soloff et al. (1986b) showed acute efficacy of haloperidol in inpatients with borderline personality disorder. The average daily dosage of medication (7.2 mg/day haloperidol) was higher in neuroleptic equivalents than in the Goldberg study, but this might be secondary to the patients in the Soloff study being ill enough to require inpatient treatment. The statistical improvement seen in the Soloff study was much more robust than that of the Goldberg study and showed improvement on all 10 of the HSCL-90 scales. This study also showed haloperidol to be as effective as amitriptyline in treating depressive symptoms in borderline patients, and much better than amitriptyline in treating behavioral dyscontrol and rage/anger.

Longitudinal studies, however, have shown that the gains on haloperidol are temporary (Cornelius, Soloff, Perel, & Ulrich, 1993; Soloff et al., 1993). Patients receiving haloperidol had a much higher drop-out rate than placebo during treatment (64% vs. 28%) and showed so little functional benefit over placebo that the investigators concluded that the use of neuroleptics longitudinally was of little value.

Cowdry and Gardner (1988) used trifluoperazine and saw some statistical improvement in rejection sensitivity, suicidality, and anxiety compared to placebo. They noted no change in the behavioral dyscontrol plaguing their patients. These authors believed the trifluoperazine was minimally beneficial in the acute treatment of borderline personality disorder.

Typical neuroleptics may help some patients with borderline personality disorder with psychotic symptoms acutely, but overall they do not resolve the impulsivity, suicidality, self-injury, dysphoria, and anxiety components of the illness. Borderlines do not tolerate typical neuroleptics based on the high dropout rates seen in acute trials (39% in Soloff, George, Nathan, Schulz, & Perel, 1986a, and 54% in Goldberg et al., 1986) or longitudinal trials (64% in Cornelius et al., 1993). Typical neuroleptics also have many potentially harmful side effects, including tardive dyskinesia, lethargy, weight gain, mental slowing, akathisia, tremor, and galactorrhea. At best, these drugs should be looked at as a short-term intervention in patients with borderline personality disorder with psychotic symptoms. Their overall efficacy in controlling aggression, impulsivity, anxiety, and suicidality is not supported by any of the controlled trials to date.

Atypical Antipsychotics

Atypical antipsychotics have neuroleptic-like activity at the dopamine-2 (D_2) receptors, and also antagonize serotonin-2 (5-HT_2) receptors. Typical antipsychotics lack this 5-HT_2 binding property. 5-HT_2 receptor abnormalities has been implicated in anxiety, depression, psychosis, and suicidality, Thus agents binding to this receptor could cover many of the symptom clusters seen in borderline personality disorder. Two studies, both open, and two case reports provide data on the use of atypical antipsychotics in borderline personality disorder.

Frankenburg and Zanarini (1993) described the use of clozapine in 15 patients with borderline personality disorder. The authors also note that every patient had a comorbid psychotic disorder using DSM-III-R criteria. Only seven of the patients had schizotypal personality disorder. The group mean length of clozapine treatment was 4.2 ± 2.1 months, with an average dose of 253.3 ± 163.7 mg/day. The authors candidly noted that all patients had troubling side effects, including sedation, weight gain, nausea, and dizziness. The Brief Psychiatric Rating Scale (BPRS) improved in 12 of 18 areas statistically, albeit the patients remained ill. Even in those areas showing improvement the response was only partial. The results of this open trial are encouraging and suggested that clozapine-like medications might prove effective in patients with borderline personality disorder with psychotic symptoms. They are discouraging in the area of side effects, which inevitably lead to poor compliance.

A similar study by Benedetti, Sforzini,

Colombo, Maffei, and Smeraldi (1998) conducted over 16 weeks investigated the effects of clozapine in 12 inpatients with borderline personality disorder. Patients were stabilized on clozapine and followed as outpatients. The length of stay in hospital was 20.3 ± 7.2 days. Clozapine dosage ranged from 26 to 100 mg/day with an average daily dosage of 43.8 ± 18.8 mg/day, which is about 16% of the clozapine dosage used in the Frankenburg and Zanarini (1993) study. The patients showed meaningful improvement in a number of measures including the BPRS, the Hamilton Depression Scale (HAM-D), the Global Assessment of Function (GAF), impulsivity, affective instability, suicidality, and physical fights. Side effects included sedation, hypersialorrhea, and a decreased white blood cell count in six patients which never reached a level of clinical concern. This open trial showed encouraging longitudinal improvement in a difficult patient population. It may well be that the Frankenburg and Zanarini (1993) study used too high a dosage of clozapine, and many of the side effects described could be minimized or even eliminated by lowering the dosage of clozapine.

Risperidone use in borderline personality disorder is limited to two case reports (Szigethy & Schulz, 1997; Khouzam & Donnelly, 1997). The case report by Szigethy and Schulz (1997) involved a patient with borderline personality disorder with comorbid dysthymia. She was also receiving 300 mg/day of fluvoxamine in conjunction with 1 mg of risperidone. The report noted improvement in energy and mood. Khouzam and Donnelly (1997) noted decreased self-injury in a patient treated with 4 mg/day of risperidone who had failed to respond to typical antipsychotics, tricyclic antidepressants, selective serotonin reuptake inhibitors (SSRIs), and mood stabilizers. This patient was continuing to show gains 11 months after the initiation of treatment.

In all cases reported involving risperidone or clozapine, the improvements noted in the studies may arise not from the atypical antipsychotic per se but the 5-HT$_2$ antagonism properties of the medication. The atypical antipsychotics are thought to work through antagonism of both D$_2$ receptors and 5-HT$_2$ receptors. The available data using standard neuroleptics, agents which work through D$_2$ antagonism, show little effect in borderline personality disorder. It is possible that the advantages noted with both clozapine and risperidone arise from the 5-HT$_2$ antagonism of these drugs. This would also suggest that agents which act through antagonism of 5-HT$_2$ receptors would be potentially efficacious in some patients with borderline personality disorder. A second possibility is that the combination of D$_2$ and 5-HT$_2$ antagonism leads to the improvements seen in borderline personality disorder. This could be tested by using a 5-HT$_2$ antagonist in a placebo-controlled trial compared to an atypical antipsychotic. Whatever the mode of action, the initial studies with atypical antipsychotics are encouraging and indicate that these agents might be of benefit in some patients with borderline personality disorder with psychotic features.

Antidepressants

Nefazodone

Nefazodone is an antidepressant which likely mediates its effects through 5-HT$_2$ antagonism (Narayan et al., 1998; Taylor et al., 1995). An open trial by Markovitz and Wagner (1997a) investigated the used of nefazodone in 57 patients (25 females and 32 males) with borderline personality disorder. The average age of patients was 40.1 ± 28.7 (range = 14 to 66), with a trial length of 40.1 ± 28.7 weeks (range = 3 to 99 weeks). The Diagnostic Interview for Borderlines (DID) Personality Scale score was 7.8 ± 1.3 with a minimum score of 7 necessary for inclusion in the study. The average daily nefazodone dosage was 508.8 ± 142.4 mg/day and all the medication was administered at bedtime. Responsivity was assessed through changes in Clinical Global Impression (CGI) scores, self-injury, suicidality, somatic complaints, and elimination of borderline personality disorder as a diagnosis for 4 months or longer. All areas showed statistically significant changes. Reductions in some somatic symptoms were not unexpected based on prior studies with serotonin re-uptake inhibitors (SSRIs; Markovitz, 1995; Markovitz & Wagner, 1996) but somewhat surprising in that symptoms related to receptors other than the 5-HT$_2$ showed improvement (Table 23.1).

Thirty-six patients (63%), demonstrated response to nefazodone. Side effects to nefazodone included sedation, dry mouth, constipation, and palinopsia. Only five patients (9%) discontinued the study because of side effects to the medication. Thirty patients (53%) had

TABLE 23.1. Somatic Syndrome Reductions in Borderline Personality Disorder Treated with Nefazodone (*N* = 57)

Syndrome	Baseline	Posttreatment	Improved
Headache	29	14*	52%
Migraines	10	5**	50%
Fibromyalgia	21	9*	57%
Irritable bowel syndrome	21	10*	52%
Neurodermatitis	16	5*	69%
Tempomandibular joint syndrome	16	5*	69%
Premenstrual syndrome	15	4*	73%

*Note. *p = .0001; **p = .015*

been on one or more prior trials of psychotropic medications. Half of these patients (*N* = 15, 26%), were using SSRIs prior to nefazodone and discontinued these medications because of sexual dysfunction. Eight of these 15 patients met response criteria on nefazodone. No patients using nefazodone reported sexual dysfunction as a side effect.

This open trial needs to be replicated in a double-blind placebo-controlled trial, but the findings do support a role for the 5-HT$_2$ receptor in the treatment of some patients with borderline personality disorder. This 5-HT$_2$ antagonism may be the mechanism by which atypical antipsychotics (e.g., risperidone and clozapine) mediate their effects. Because typical neuroleptics are ineffectual longitudinally in borderline personality disorder, it is unlikely the D$_2$ antagonistic effect of these drugs is causing the responsivity. More likely is the antagonism of 5-HT$_2$ receptors, as these receptors are associated with behaviors that are common in borderline personality disorder, such as depression and suicidality (McBride et al., 1994). Because patients with borderline personality disorder will need to remain on drug treatment longitudinally, and sexual dysfunction is the primary reason they discontinue treatment with SSRIs, this type of drug may have advantages. Further, the cost of nefazodone treatment is markedly less than the cost of an atypical antipsychotic agent. On the negative side, nefazodone seems to be largely ineffectual in patients with borderline personality disorder with comorbid obsessive–compulsive symptoms (Markovitz & Wagner, 1997b).

Tricyclic Antidepressants

The use of tricyclic antidepressants (TCAs) in borderline personality disorder has been fairly

well investigated in both open and placebo-controlled trials. Open trials by Fink, Pollack, and Klein (1964) and Klein (1967, 1968) showed some benefit in a group of patients who would likely be labeled as borderline personality disorder in many cases today. Placebo-controlled trials were initiated by Soloff et al. (1986b) and these showed a modest improvement in some patients with borderline personality disorder treated with amitriptyline. Soloff et al. (1986a) also found that many of their patients had a paradoxical effect to amitriptyline with an increase in hostility and affective instability. The high lethality of these drugs in overdosage, mild to moderate improvement in only a subset of patients, weight gain, sedation, dry mouth, and interactions with alcohol make this group of medications largely ineffectual in borderline personality disorder as a short- or long-term pharmacological treatment option.

Monoamine Oxidase Inhibitors

Treatment with monoamine oxidase inhibitors (MAOIs) is problematic in borderline personality disorder. The overall benefit to patients is minimal (Cowdry & Gardner, 1988; Gardner & Cowdry, 1989), and the side effects are severe. Overdosage, hypotension, weight gain, poor sleep, drug interactions, and interaction with alcohol and other drugs of abuse make these agents a poor choice for most patients. The reversible MAOIs, however, if studied in this group, may turn out to be a highly effective treatment option. Unlike standard MAOIs, these agents inhibit only MAO-A, and have a side effect profile similar to a serotonin reuptake inhibitor (SRI) or a serotonin and noradrenaline reuptake inhibitor (SNRI). They are nonlethal in overdosage, have minimal drug–drug interactions, and do not require close monitoring. They also cause reduction in carbohydrate craving, and this has provided a good means of checking the adequacy of dose. No studies are yet available on these agents in borderline personality disorder, but mechanistically they are very promising

Selective Serotonin Reuptake Inhibitors

The selective serotonin reuptake inhibitors in borderline personality disorder have been the most promising group of medications for borderline personality disorder studied over the past 10 years. Initial open trials of fluoxetine (Coccaro, Astill, Herbert, & Schut, 1990; Cornelius, Soloff, Perel, & Ulrich, 1991; Markovitz, Calabrese, Schulz, & Meltzer, 1991; Norden 1989) all gave positive results in reducing a number of symptoms clusters seen in these patients. Every study showed a decrease in depression, anxiety, and self-injury when evaluated. The Markovitz study (Markovitz et al., 1991), but not the Cornelius study (Cornelius et al., 1991), showed a reduction in both hostility and psychotic symptomatology based on changes in the Hopkins Symptom Checklist (HSCL). This could have been secondary to the difference in dosage in the two studies. The former study used 80 mg/day of fluoxetine in all patients and the latter study used 20–40 mg/day of fluoxetine in all patients. Higher dosages of fluoxetine may be required to eliminate certain symptoms in borderline personality disorder. None of the four studies discussed side effects and compliance.

Three controlled trials of fluoxetine in patients with borderline personality disorder have been conducted (Coccaro & Kavoussi, 1997; Markovitz, 1995; Salzman et al., 1995). Salzman showed that fluoxetine at doses of up to 60 mg/day (no mean dosage provided in the paper) was effective in reducing aggression in mild to moderate patients with borderline personality disorder. The patients had a DIB-R (Zanarini, Gunderson, Frankenburg, and Chauncey, 1989) average score of about 7, indicating a high probability of a borderline personality disorder diagnosis. The authors, however, excluded patients with suicidal ideation, a history of prior psychiatric hospitalizations, self-injury, or comorbid Axis II diagnoses of clinical significance. None of the patients included in the trial had any current substance abuse or other significant Axis I problems. The authors noted a fairly high placebo response rate, but the data still

indicated significant improvement in depression and anger in the fluoxetine group. Because of the mild nature of the illness in their patient cohort, the author's cautioned against generalizing the data to significantly ill patients with borderline personality disorder.

Markovitz (1995) reported on the interim analysis of fluoxetine use in a more ill group of patients with borderline personality disorder and the final data set (Markovitz & Wagner, 1997b) showed that the group had a DIB score average of 9.0 ± 1.1, and contained 11 chronically self-injurious patients. The patients in the double-blind placebo-controlled study were randomized to either 80 mg/day of fluoxetine ($N = 16$) or placebo ($N = 15$). Current substance abuse or inability to comply with the study visits were the only exclusion criteria. Entry requirements included (1) a DIB score of 7 or higher (DIB 9.0 ± 1.1 for the group), (2) diagnosis of labile disorder from the Schedule for Affective Disorders and Schizophrenia, (3) diagnosis of borderline personality disorder based on meeting the required criteria from the Structured Clinical Interview for DSM-III-R Personality Disorders (SCID-P; Spitzer, Williams, Gibbon, & First, 1990), and (4) unanimous consensus by two blinded clinicians and two raters. All patients provided written informed consent to participate in the study.

Tables 23.2–23.4 show Axis I, II, and III diagnoses. The heterogeneity of diagnoses likely represents a series of behaviors biologically

TABLE 23.2. Axis I Diagnoses in Borderline Personality Disorder Patients Treated with Fluoxetine or Placebo ($N = 31$)

Axis I diagnoses	Current	Lifetime
Major depression	16	18
Bipolar disorder		
Type I	2	2
Type II	7	7
Generalized anxiety disorder	14	25
Obsessive–compulsive disorder	9	11
Panic disorder	6	10
Drug abuse or dependence	8	12
Alcoholism	9	11
Somatization disorders	3	4
Eating disorders	5	5
Social phobia	3	4
Dysthymia	7	16
Total Axis I Diagnoses	89	125
Diagnoses/patient	2.9	4.0

TABLE 23.3. Axis II Diagnoses in Borderline Personality Disorder Patients Treated with Fluoxetine or Placebo (N = 31)

Axis II diagnoses	Patients with diagnosis
Borderline	31
Paranoid	23
Dependent	21
Histrionic	21
Self-defeating	20
Compulsive	18
Avoidant	17
Schizotypal	14
Passive–aggressive	12
Narcissistic	10
Antisocial	9
Schizoid	0
Total diagnoses	196
Diagnoses/patient	6.3

linked to a common cause. Thus, the comorbid findings of borderline personality disorder, depression, panic, migraines, and irritable bowel could be explained by these diagnoses representing a behavioral state arising from the same biological cause. This would be analogous to patients with a strep throat having malaise, fever, diarrhea, and irritability. The latter four symptoms arise from the strep infection and resolve if the underlying cause is treated. This model further suggests that any of the symptoms listed in Tables 23.2–23.4 are biological equivalents when they co-occur. Thus, migraines and irritable bowel are no different biologically than the depression or panic with which they co-occur. This biochemistry underlying this concept has been reviewed previously (Markovitz, 1995).

On all measures used in the study, the active group, but not the placebo group, showed clini-

TABLE 23.4. Axis III Diagnoses in Borderline Personality Disorder Patients Prior to Treatment with Fluoxetine or Placebo (N = 31)

Syndrome	No. with syndrome	Percent with syndrome
Premenstrual syndrome (N = 22)	18	82
Cluster headaches/migraines	17	55
Irritable bowel syndrome	15	48
Fibromyalgia	7	23
Neurodermatitis	7	23
Sleep apnea	7	23

cal response. This lack of statistical improvement in the placebo group differed from the Salzman study. The high DIB score in the Markovitz study indicated a more ill patient cohort, and this group may have a lower placebo response rate. Every rating scale analyzed in the fluoxetine group showed a statistically better outcome than the placebo group ($p \leq$ .0005). These measures included the HAM-D, HAM-A, SCL-90-R, Beck Depression Inventory, and Global Assessment Scale. Not only did the data indicate clinically meaningful improvement, but the slope of the graphs also indicates a trend for ongoing improvement with fluoxetine.

Self-injury changes were also assessed during the trial. To qualify as self-injurious, it was decided that patients needed to harm themselves through cutting, burning, and so on, at least one time weekly for 6 weeks prior to trial entry. Nine patients on active medication (56%) and two on placebo (15%) were self-injurious. No patients who were not self-injurious developed self-injury during the trial. Because of the small size of the study, high dropout rate, and unequal distribution of self-injurious patients between the placebo and active group, no statistical analysis was possible. Clearly, however, the data did suggest that fluoxetine decreased self-injurious behavior. Over the course of the 14-week trial, self-injury did not change in the placebo group (14 positive responses of the 14 time points). The fluoxetine group showed a reduction in self-injurious behavior (8 of 53 possible time points).

The authors noted some potential problems with the study. Dropout rates were high for the fluoxetine treatment group, as only 9 of 16 patients (56%) completed all 14 weeks of the trial. This high dropout rate may be occurring for a number of reasons. Sexual dysfunction (N = 4) was the major reason for discontinuing treatment. The illness severity of this particular patient group studied likely also contributed to the high dropout rate in a lengthy study for this patient population. While the overall rating scores were similar in both groups, there were more self-injurious patients in the fluoxetine group. This may have inadvertently selected for a subset of patients potentially more likely to respond to fluoxetine. There also was significant comorbid Axis I and III pathology in the two treatment groups (Tables 23.1 and 23.3), and this may have also selected for a cohort more likely to respond to fluoxetine. Finally, the data set is relatively small, albeit the changes with fluoxetine were large and there was no placebo effect. The data strongly suggest that fluoxetine at 80 mg/day is effective in many patients with borderline personality disorder presenting for clinical treatment.

Coccarro and Kavoussi (1997) presented data on 40 patients with impulsive–aggressive behavior treated with fluoxetine or placebo (*N* = 27 fluoxetine, 13 placebo). The patients had a number of personality disorders, and borderline personality disorder was present in 13 of the 40 subjects (33%). No separate analysis was done for the patients with borderline personality disorder; thus it is difficult to assess fluoxetine's specific impact on impulsive aggression in borderline personality disorder. Nonetheless, the data presented unequivocally showed that fluoxetine decreased impulsive–aggressive behavior in patients who had this characteristic, and this characteristic is common to patients with borderline personality disorder.

Just as important as the decrease in impulsive–aggressive behavior symptomatology is the idea that diagnoses used clinically may be less satisfactory in predicting outcome than the behaviors that make up the diagnoses. Any DSM diagnosis may serve as a generalized way of classifying certain behaviors which may or may not be related or clinically relevant. Borderlines with impulsive–aggressive behaviors may respond to a different subset of medications and/or psychotherapy than borderlines with predominantly rejection sensitivity, schizotype, or dysphoria. For example, the literature contains numerous examples of treating egosyntonic versus ego-dystonic character disorders. The latter are easier to treat because of the dysphoria they engender and the desire to rid oneself of a dysphoric experience. Patients with borderline personality disorder exist across a broad spectrum. Certain subtypes may respond favorably to one medication but not another. As long as we are dependent on nosology for classification, as opposed to a biological marker, it is unlikely that we will be able to predict responsivity to medications. Through their studies, Coccarro et al. (1996, 1997, 1998) are providing a biological basis for the prediction of clinical outcome.

Sertraline

No controlled trials of sertraline in borderline personality disorder have been published. Kavoussi, Liu, and Coccaro (1994) reported on four patients treated with sertraline who had borderline personality disorder and Markovitz (1995) reported on a small open trial of sertraline in 23 patients with borderline personality disorder. The results were similar in both studies.

Kavoussi et al. (1994) showed that sertraline could diminish the impulsive aggression seen in personality-disordered patients, many of whom had borderline personality disorder. The Markovitz (1995) trial looked at the efficacy of sertraline in borderline personality disorder. Twenty-three patients were begun on 50 mg/day of sertraline, and the dosage increased to at least 200 mg/day. Eleven of the 23 patients responded (48%) based on decreases in self-injurious behavior, suicidality, and depression. The most common predictor of a positive response to sertraline was reduction in carbohydrate craving. This occurred in 10 of the 11 patients showing a response to sertraline. The 12 patients not responding to 200 mg/day of sertraline had their daily dosage increased by 100 mg/day every week until the carbohydrate craving was reduced. Six of the 12 patients showed a statistically significant level of improvement based on decreases in self-injury, depression, and suicidality. Thus, 74% (17 of 23) showed improvement. All 23 of the sertraline-treated patients were followed over a 12-month-or-longer period, and the showed no loss of efficacy based on changes in depression, self-injury, or suicidality.

The data suggested that a certain serum level of sertraline might be necessary to achieve response, and that this level correlates with reduction in carbohydrate craving. To test this hypothesis, 207 patients with borderline personality disorder with poor or no response to 200 mg/day of sertraline were entered in a trial to assess the significance of serum levels of sertraline and responsivity. Prior to increasing their dosage of medication, peak serum levels of sertraline were measured 6 to 8 hours after the dosage of medication. It should be pointed out that these nonresponsive patients came from a larger data set of 757 patients, 550 of whom (73%) had shown a 50% or more improvement with sertraline. The poor response group of 207 had their serum levels of sertraline monitored after they responded or failed to respond to higher doses of sertraline.

When the 207 individuals were investigated for reasons for prior nonresponsivity, it was found that 72 failed because of side effects from the medication (35%), 39 failed because of noncompliance (19%), and 96 failed because of lack of efficacy (46%). For the entire group, the ratio of smokers to nonsmokers was 1 to 2. The response failures due to side effects and failures due to noncompliance were approximately 1 to 2, smokers to nonsmokers. When failure to respond because of lack of efficacy was investigated, the ratios flipped. There were twice as many smokers as nonsmokers who failed to respond, which suggested that in some cases, cigarette use may have a negative impact on outcome.

From the total group of 207 patients, 187 gave written informed consent and agreed to take amounts of sertraline above the recommended dosage of 200 mg/day to help control their borderline personality disorder and have serum sertraline levels monitored. Forty-eight of the 187 patients (26%) responded to increased dosages of sertraline. The responders in the group took statistically similar dosages of sertraline compared to the nonresponders (304.7 ± 101.5 mg vs. 288.4 ± 98.3 mg), but the serum levels of the responders were statistically higher (202.9 ± 51.1 ng/ml vs. 151.8 ± 102.4 ng/ml, $p < .03$). Once again, a positive response was accompanied by a reduction in carbohydrate craving. It may be that serum sertraline levels of 200 ng/ml or higher are needed to treat borderline personality disorder. Why such a large amount of medication is required is unclear. Even the 200-mg/day dosage of sertraline is above the amount routinely used to treat depression, and any dosage over 200 mg/day is above the recommended amount. Yet, lower doses of medication do not help most individuals with borderline personality disorder. Further studies are needed to assess whether peak serum levels of sertraline are useful in predicting responsivity to the drug. Although not all patients will respond to sertraline regardless of the serum level, it is probable that a certain serum level of medication is necessary to prompt a response.

Venlafaxine

Venlafaxine works as both a serotonin and noradrenaline reuptake inhibitor (SNRI) and at higher dosages also as a dopaminergic reuptake inhibitor. The medication is unique in this spectrum of action. Only one open trial has been published on the efficacy of venlafaxine in borderline personality disorder (Markovitz & Wagner, 1996), and the results were encouraging. Forty-five patients with borderline personality disorder were openly treated with venlafaxine over a 12-week period and 39 of the patients (86.7%) completed all 12 weeks of the trial. The patients had a DIB score of 8.8 ± 1.2, and an average age of 35.0 ± 10.3. The average daily dosage of venlafaxine was 315.2 ± 95.8 mg/day (range 200 to 400 mg/day).

HSCL-90 scores were reduced from 125.5 ± 56.9 to 74.6 ± 54.9 ($p < .0005$) with all 10 subscales showing statistically similar reductions. Somatic symptoms were also reduced for the group from a total of 102 of the listed syndromes (Table 23.4) to 56 ($p < .001$). This reduction in somatic complaints corresponded to the reduction seen in the SCL-90 somatization subscale from 13.2 ± 10.0 to 8.5 ± 9.1 ($p < .0005$). Self-injurious behavior was eliminated in five of the seven patients presenting with this problem. Sexual dysfunction was surprisingly low occurring in only 3 of the 39 patients (8%), and 2 of the patients who had sexual dysfunction prior to the trial had resolution of the sexual dysfunction once they were on medication. Side effects were discussed and overall were minimal. Eleven of the patients in the trial had been treated with fluoxetine, sertraline, or paroxetine without benefit or side effects (sexual dysfunction in eight), which made these treatments unacceptable to the patient. Eight of these patients responded to venlafaxine (73%).

ANTISOCIAL PERSONALITY DISORDER

Few medication trials have been done in this personality cohort despite its frequency and impact on society. Patients with antisocial personality disorder have little dysphoria associated with their actions, and little motivation to take medications unless their situation dictates an advantage in doing so. Sheard, Marini, Bridges, and Wagner (1976) studied aggressive behaviors in prisoners treated double-blindedly with either placebo or lithium. The lithium group showed a marked decrease in major infractions and the placebo group none. Interestingly, the number of minor infractions increased in the lithium-treated group suggested that there was a dampening of aggression but not elimination. Tupin et al. (1973) followed up on an earlier Sheard study with a 10-month open trial of lithium in prisoners and documented decreases in violent acts, less need for surveillance, patient reports of less anger, and improved ratings by the hospital staff. Side effects and Axis II diagnoses were not presented in either study. Although it could be argued that the chosen individuals suffered from antisocial personality disorder based on their imprisonment and types of crimes committed, no antisocial personality disorder diagnosis had been made.

Coccaro et al. (1997) and Markovitz (1995) both presented data in their patient cohort where a portion of treated patients had comorbid antisocial personality disorder. Coccaro showed a decrease in impulsive aggression but did not comment on the effects of treatment on the antisocial personality disorder diagnosis. Markovitz et al. (1991) did not comment on either the behavioral changes or elimination of the diagnosis. Considering the prevalence of antisocial personality disorder and its negative impact on society, pharmacological studies in this group are clearly warranted. Ongoing use of medications in this patient cohort will probably be futile as the afflicted individuals have little dysphoria associated with their illness and little motivation to change or take medications.

SCHIZOTYPAL PERSONALITY DISORDER

Schizotypal personality disorder is rarely seen as the primary reason for treatment in a clinical setting, but it occurs frequently as a comorbid finding with other Axis I and II diagnoses. Schizotypal personality disorder can also present across a fairly wide spectrum of behaviors. Some individuals with schizotypal personality disorder appear almost schizophrenic in their beliefs and behaviors. They have eccentric beliefs which can appear to be delusional, bizarre dress, stereotypical movements, and poor social skills. These patients are frequently called schizophrenic and are treated with antipsychotics. At the other end of the schizotypal personality disorder behavioral spectrum are individuals who are more obsessive–compulsive in their beliefs and behaviors. There are so few reports about treatment of schizotypal personality disorder, that none of the authors have even tried to differentiate between these two subgroups of schizotypal personality disorder to show whether there are any

differences in comorbidity and treatment outcome. Hymowitz, Frances, Jacobsberg, Sickles, and Hoyt (1986) conducted a small open study in patients with schizotypal personality disorder, and showed that neuroleptics are effective in reducing the schizotype. No comment was made about compliance, side effects, or longitudinal outcome.

Much like neuroleptics in borderline personality disorder, there may be an acute response to these agents in schizotypal personality disorder, but long-term efficacy is doubtful. Neuroleptics have obvious side effects, and individuals are unlikely to take them secondary to how the neuroleptics make them feel.

In the Markovitz et al. (1991) open-label study of fluoxetine in borderline personality disorder, the patients were divided into three groups. Schizotypal personality disorder occurs comorbidly in 40–60% of patients with borderline personality disorder, and in the study, patients were divided according to the presence of little, moderate, or high levels of schizotypal personality disorder comorbid with the borderline personality disorder. Group 1 was predominantly borderline personality disorder in behavior. Group 2 was roughly equally comorbid for borderline personality disorder and schizotypal personality disorder. Group 3 was more strongly schizotypal personality disorder in character than borderline personality disorder. All three groups showed clinically meaningful improvement, and group 3 showed the most improvement as a percentage of change from baseline. This was very surprising as many of the patients with schizotypal personality disorder in this group were more schizophrenic-like in behavior than obsessive. No explanation was offered for why these patients not only responded to antidepressant treatment but did proportionately better than the other two groups. Perhaps the high incidence of comorbidity with depression and borderline personality disorder selected for a group of patients more likely to respond to SSRIs. Parsimoniously, the schizotype may be better viewed as an obsessive–compulsive behavior and thus it more likely to respond to SSRIs. What the study does strongly suggest, however, is that no single behavior can predict responsivity to a medication group. Clinically, the use of neuroleptics, either atypical or typical, is repugnant to most patients. Not only can outcome be measured in reductions in psychosis, but it must also be measured in terms of quality of life, functioning, and side effects. Good clinical practice should be based on the use of the least repugnant treatment for the patient. Psychotic behaviors, in and of themselves, do not necessarily justify the use of neuroleptics, as indicated by the excellent response to fluoxetine in this trial.

AVOIDANT PERSONALITY DISORDER

Avoidant personality disorder has been gaining increasing notoriety because of ongoing trials in social anxiety disorder. Between 70 and 85% of patients with social phobia have concomitant avoidant personality disorder. Studies using paroxetine, sertraline, fluoxetine, venlafaxine, brofaromine (a reversible MAOI), and substance P antagonists have all shown efficacy in reducing social anxiety. No comments were made on reductions in avoidant personality disorder in any of the studies. If, however, the diagnoses of social anxiety and avoidant personality disorder are viewed as a parsimonious behavioral grouping, it is logical to assume they flow from the same chemical cause. Treating the aberrant chemistry is imperative if inroads are to be made in treating the behaviors flowing from it. If avoidant personality disorder is a logical personality construct flowing from a chemistry giving rise to social avoidance, even a perfect neurochemical intervention will be only a start. The afflicted individual will have established a behavioral pattern based on a pathological learning model generated by the faulty neurochemistry. It will be essential to both restore the chemistry and concomitantly provide therapy that will teach the individual how to respond in a more socially acceptable manner. As with the other cases presented, the more options provided a patient to improve, the better. Nothing is lost by providing both biological and psychological interventions. It is logical to assume, however, that if there is an underlying biological disorder causing the social anxiety, and it is not addressed, the social phobia will likely not improve.

TREATMENT STRATEGIES

Personality disorders in any individual are better viewed as clusterings of neurochemically mediated behavioral maladaptations than as discrete diagnoses. An individual with border-line personality, histrionic personality, and schizotypal personality likely has a single disease with the aforementioned behavioral symptom clusters. It is likely that the neurochemical anomaly causing the personality problems arises from a single flaw. The chances of an individual having two or more chemical maladaptations at the same time is low. Thus, treatment should consist of linking all symptoms into a single illness arising from this biological flaw and providing treatment to correct the flaw. This idea differs from the cause-and-effect paradigm commonly used in psychiatry and psychological practices. For example, it is often assumed that some type of trauma could cause the emergence of borderline personality disorder, which in turn can lead to comorbid anxiety, depression, somatic complaints, and other personality disorders. A better scientific viewpoint is that the same chemical which gives rise to borderline personality disorder will also cause anxiety, depression, somatic complaints, and personality disorders including borderline personality disorder. The idea of parsimony of diagnoses is the key concept.

Continuing with borderline personality disorder as an example, there are approximately three Axis I, five Axis II, and three Axis III concomitant diagnoses for each patient studied in the double-blind, placebo-controlled trial of fluoxetine by Markovitz et al. (1991; Tables 23.2–23.4). Each of these diagnoses would be better viewed as a symptom of a single disease state. Much like a person has fever, achy joints, nausea, chills, and malaise with a streptococcal infection of the throat, an individual has depression, panic, borderline personality, histrionic personality, migraines, premenstrual syndrome, and so on, with whatever the biological condition is that causes these symptoms. In the past, we have tended to treat the psychiatric illness by the most strongly represented symptom. If depression is the primary symptom, the assumption is made that the character problems, anxiety problems, and somatic problems are all secondary to the depression. This would be akin to choosing a different medication for the streptococcal infection based on whether there are chills, rigors, nausea, and so on. The cause of the malaise or fever or chills is the strep infection. Regardless of the symptoms present, an antibiotic is needed to treat the infection. All the symptoms make up variables of the disease state. Analogously, in patients with personality disorders, treatment is probably best based on all the symptoms present and picking a medication that best addresses them all.

There are few studies that address pharmacotherapy of personality disorders, let alone which symptom cluster groups respond best to which medications. If anything, the literature is becoming more confused in this respect. Part of the confusion arises from looking at a single behavioral symptom, say, impulsivity, and using a medication to treat this behavior. Just as a fever can arise from many biological causes, so can impulsivity. Should impulsivity with aggression be treated differently than impulsivity with panic attacks? Clearly, some causes of any disease are common and some rare, but one must still look at the context of the behavior to decide on the best treatment. Certain symptoms are hierarchically more important and dictate treatment choices. Thus, the following caveats are also important to consider before choosing a pharmacological intervention.

First, a patient will likely need to be on a medication chronically. Side effects are the most important consideration to be made before a medication is even started. As an example, while the serotonin reuptake inhibitors are effective in borderline personality disorder-like conditions, they have a tremendous amount of sexual dysfunction, making long-term compliance difficult. Not all patients experience this particular side effect, but it will reduce efficacy via reduced compliance in those affected. Sexual dysfunction on fluoxetine, as an example, was the primary reason for dropping out of the study in the Markovitz et al. (1991) placebo-controlled fluoxetine trial (data not shown). Although the sexual dysfunction passes for many individuals after 4 to 8 weeks, most patients stop the medication prior to this because of the sexual dysfunction. It is imperative to know the side effects of the medications and to clearly discuss them with the patient so that rational changes can be made. All too often patients will not return for follow-up because of a side effect to a medication and will subsequently discontinue the medication without discussing the situation with the clinician. The extra few minutes spent discussing these side effects early on saves time and transference issues later on. Other considerations to discuss with patients include SSRIs and SNRIs precipitating short-term weight loss but long-term weight gain. Both groups of medication seem to lose effect in some patients over time ranging from 2 to 12 months. Nefazodone can cause daytime sedation and lethargy. Atypical antipsychotics can cause sedation, mental slowing, and weight gain. Second, health care in the world is in a period of transition at this time. Cost of all health care delivery from start to finish is now severely limited. Each patient has a certain quanta of resources available to him or her. Treatments offering roughly equipotent outcomes will not be considered equal if one is cheaper than another. If a pharmacological intervention can be given at half the price of another with equally good results, the cheaper intervention will leave more funds for psychotherapy, social interventions, and so on. Third, all illnesses evolve over time. Diabetics develop different complications of their illness longitudinally, sickle cell anemia causes ongoing sequelae, and so forth. The clinician should assume that any treatment will need to be continually reviewed and changed to meet the ongoing needs of a patient. The more difficult a medication is to manipulate, the less flexibility a clinician will have in making these changes. Thus, the effects of the medication on its own metabolism, interactions with other pharmacological agents, interactions with alcohol, and ease of stopping the medication need to be considered. With these thoughts in mind, I offer the following paradigms to guide treatment for specific personality disorders.

Borderline Personality Disorder

Patients with borderline personality disorder will need to be on medications longitudinally. Much like depression, reductions in effective dosages result in relapses. Thus, it is imperative to use a medication that minimizes side effects. There is a world of difference between being statistically better and feeling well. Clinicians should always choose a medication that addresses all the patient symptoms with as few short- and long-term side effects as possible. In this regard, antidepressants will always be preferable to lithium and antiepileptic drugs, which in turn are superior to the antipsychotics.

If the patient displays pathology consistent with borderline personality disorder, only one important question needs to be addressed at the outset. Does the individual have obsessive–compulsive behaviors? If he or she does not, nefazodone at $\geq$ 500 mg should be considered as it has minimal sexual dysfunction and low cost and is effective as a once-a-day bedtime dose (Markovitz, 1997a). The nefazodone is particularly effective in nonobsessive patients with borderline personality disorder with insomnia. Somatic complaints such as migraines, irritable bowel, fibromyalgia, and premenstrual sydrome should all improve within a few weeks of achieving an effective dosage. Likewise, carbohydrate craving, if present, should be reduced or eliminated with adequate pharmacotherapy. The reductions in somatic complaints and carbohydrate craving will all occur before the dysphoria and mood swings associated with borderline personality disorder resolve. It is helpful to the clinician to see these reductions as it is predictive of medication efficacy. Likewise, these positive changes can be pointed out to the patient early in the treatment to help with compliance and to generate optimism on the patient's part. Because nefazodone appears to be fairly specific for illness arising from 5-HT$_2$ anomalies, it may not be as broad spectrum as the SSRIs and SNRIs. In clinical practice, about 30% of patients started on this medication benefit and continue to use it longitudinally (2 years or longer).

If the patient has obsessive–compulsive behaviors, an SSRI or SNRI is indicated. In theory, all these medications should work equally well, but in practice, this is not the case. Some patients may become sedated on one medication (paroxetine) and not on another (sertraline), even though they are from the same class of medications. Other individuals can become agitated on the same medications. Overall, our clinical data suggest that higher rates of sedation as a side effect occur as paroxetine > fluvoxamine > venlafaxine > fluoxetine > sertraline. Although sedation is often a desirable side effect in the acute phase of treatment, it is an undesirable problem longitudinally and is best avoided. Sexual dysfunction, as previously mentioned, is the number-one reason for noncompliance with treatment. Venlafaxine seems to have about half as much sexual dysfunction as the SSRIs. This could be secondary to the higher dosages of venlafaxine used in patients with borderline personality disorder, as it becomes a noradrenergic and dopaminergic reuptake inhibitor at higher dosages, and medications which increase either of these neurotransmitters have been shown to reduce sexual dysfunction. Finally, one should always pick the best pharmacological intervention but should assume at the same time that his or her choice will fail and need to be changed. About half the time, the first choice will work, but for the other 50% changes will need to be made. The agent used as a first choice should have as few drug–drug interactions and withdrawal problems as possible for this reason. In this respect, sertraline and venlafaxine are easier to use than the other agents. What clinically happens most often in treatment failures is that the patient has a partial response. If the initial agent is removed, the patient's condition will deteriorate back to baseline. Sertraline and venlafaxine allow an individual to add on another agent without fear of drug–drug interactions, so the initial gains are not lost. If the patient shows responsivity to the second agent, the first can be tapered without the patient relapsing. Overall, these drugs have close to a 50% response rate in longitudinal usage. Venlafaxine may be the most effective agent in this group because of its multimodal methods of action.

The choice of agents is somewhat reminiscent of rheumatology and the use of nonsteroidal anti-inflammatory drugs (NSAIDs) to treat arthritis. Although all the NSAIDs work, one may fit an individual better than any of the others. This is an important area for the clinician to pay attention. Fine tuning the SSRIs, SNRIs, or other medications will enhance compliance and outcome.

The dosages of medications used in borderline personality disorder are higher than those used for depression. The following dosages were found to be effective in patients. Fluoxetine ($N = 212$) is invariably ineffective under 80 mg/day. Sertraline patients ($N = 757$) average a daily dosage of 325 mg, which in turn corresponds to a serum level of 180 ng/ml. About half the patients did well on 200 mg/day and the other half required higher amounts (see above). Venlafaxine-treated patients with borderline personality disorder ($N = 337$) also averaged a daily dosage of about 325 mg. Most of these patients were initially started on the immediate-release venlafaxine. The sustained-release formulation can be substituted on a mg-per-mg basis with no falloff in efficacy. Fortunately, side effects of sedation, agitation, nausea and sexual dysfunction all seem to be less with the sustained release formulation. This is likely due to the lower peak serum levels of medication. Nefazodone ($N = 143$) dosages in borderline personality disorder averaged approximately 517 mg given as a bedtime dosage.

None of the aforementioned medications are toxic in overdosage; thus this is not an issue with any of them. Correct dosage, however, is an issue. It is unclear why such high levels of these medications are necessary to work in borderline personality disorder. Whereas serotonin levels are discussed in this chapter as a possible means of viewing many of the pathological behaviors linked to borderline personality disorder, lower levels of SSRIs and SNRIs would correct this imbalance. Clinically, the best predictor of response that I have seen is reduction in carbohydrate craving in my patients. One could argue that this is a symptom of an atypical depression, which it is, but many patients with borderline personality disorder also have carbohydrate craving. It is best to push the oral dosage of medication until carbohydrate craving is eliminated. The idea of using a single dosage of a SSRI or SNRI is a marketing idea, not a scientific one. The available data show better resolution of borderline personality disorder with higher dosages of medications. If there are qualms about pushing the dosage to the levels described, one can always measure a serum sertraline level. The amount of medication in the blood stream is the determinant of adequacy of dosage. This number provides a clear means of measuring how much medication is in the body. Concomitantly, venlafaxine, nefazodone, fluvoxamine, and fluoxetine are all metabolized through the same enzymatic system as sertraline ($IIIA_4$). If sertraline is rapidly metabolized, all these other agents will also be rapidly metabolized, and higher dosages will also be needed of these agents.

Lithium is poorly tolerated in patients with borderline personality disorder and is rarely a consideration because of compliance issues and side effects. Likewise, antiepileptic drugs will be poorly tolerated longitudinally in this group, and in the vast majority of patients lead to depressive episodes, just as they do in bipolars. This may arise from an increased transport of tryptophan to the central nervous system by the antiepileptic drugs which causes a depletion of serum tryptophan. This results in carbohydrate craving, weight gain, and ultimately depression from the low tryptophan levels.

Neuroleptics in borderline personality disorder have not proven as effective in my practice. Patients do not tolerate the side effects of these agents, such as mental slowing, weight gain, and lethargy. More important, they do not seem to work in near as broad a cohort as SSRIs and SNRIs. Soloff et al. (1993) has shown convincingly that typical neuroleptics are not beneficial longitudinally for the vast majority of patients.

Atypical agents have been largely unstudied, but based on their mechanism of action they will likely be poorly tolerated longitudinally. Patients feel poorly on these medications. Because they are probably mediating their action via $5-HT_2$ antagonism, the same mechanism by which nefazodone works, it makes more sense to use nefazodone first. The latter agent has many fewer side effects and is markedly cheaper. Atypical antipsychotic agents may be beneficial in some patients but will probably be relegated to a third- or fourth-line medication for all the reasons listed.

Antisocial Personality Disorder

There is no data available that show actual changes in antisocial personality disorder over time. Clinically, patients are more likely to seek treatment either for comorbid behaviors accompanying the antisocial personality disorder or by court order. Our trials with fluoxetine and sertraline in patients with borderline personality disorder with comorbid antisocial personality disorder indicated that the antisocial personality disorder did not change very much but the other accompanying behaviors did. Guidelines are similar for antisocial personality disorder as they are for borderline personality disorder. Sexual dysfunction is more of an issue in this group. Nefazodone has proven to be a well-tolerated medication that dampens impulsivity, helps with sleep and anxiety problems, and is beneficial for many in decreasing anger and rage. Lethargy and sedation are the primary side effects in this group.

If nefazodone fails, venlafaxine is usually tried next. If obsessionality is present this is always a first-choice medication because it addresses the chemistry and has the fewest side effects of agents that are effective. As in borderline personality disorder, venlafaxine probably has the widest spectrum of efficacy and highest response rates. Side effects are less well tolerated in this patient cohort. Studies are under way to analyze the effects of a comorbid antisocial personality disorder diagnosis on pharmacotherapy choices, compliance, and outcomes.

Schizotypal Personality Disorder

Although this disorder is viewed as a schizophrenia–spectrum disorder, there is minimal treatment data to back up this assertion. As pointed out earlier, the better tolerated a medication, the better one's chances for successful treatment. Viewing the schizotypal personality disorder as a symptom of a larger illness is the key. One or more of concomitant obsessive–compulsive behaviors, anxiety, somatic complaints, or depression would all argue for the use of an antidepressant to treat the illness. Before an antipsychotic is used, one should also consider an agent such as nefazodone for its coverage of the 5-HT$_2$ receptor. Atypical antipsychotics may be of benefit in this group but have not been studied. Because the SSRIs, SNRIs, and nefazodone seem to work and are well tolerated, they should be used first.

In those patients requiring antipsychotics, lower dosages than those used to treat schizophrenia seem to be effective. Many of the patients use them on an as-needed basis to treat brief psychotic episodes or periods of high anxiety. A few patients have clearly benefited from the use of atypical antipsychotics, but the data are still sparse. They do hold promise from a mechanistic standpoint, but side effects may preclude their tolerability and cost their widespread use.

Avoidant Personality Disorder

Agents effective in treating social anxiety will also be beneficial to patients with avoidant personality disorder. Currently, venlafaxine, paroxetine, sertraline, fluoxetine, and fluvoxamine have been studied and shown to reduce social anxiety. The symptoms accompanying the avoidant personality disorder will dictate which treatment option is selected. Because of the high level of anxiety in these patients, less stimulating antidepressants may be preferred to decrease the initial agitation seen when antidepressants are first started. No trials looking at avoidant personality disorder specifically have yet been published, but it would be logical to use fluvoxamine, venlafaxine, or paroxetine because of their lower rates of agitation. No data on dosages of these agents for treating the avoidant personality disorder are available. Like borderline personality disorder compared to depression, it could take higher dosages of medication to treat avoidant personality disorder than social anxiety. Following the comorbid reductions in carbohydrate craving or somatic complaints, if they are present, will likely prove a good indicator of adequacy of dose.

DISCUSSION

The foregoing data suggest that much of what we call personality is actually biochemically driven. This should not be surprising based on the large number of biological studies indicating neurochemical anomalies in many of the personality disorders. Although the question whether the changes occurred because of a genetic cause, an environmentally driven phenomena, or a reaction to a social phenomena is open, the presence of neurochemical flaws in many patients with personality disorders is clear. Our goal as clinicians is to provide the best possible treatment for remedying the aberrant behaviors that make up a personality disorder. Both biological studies and pharmacological trial data are pointing to the benefits of pharmacotherapy in the treatment of personality disorders. Although there are no data showing the benefits of combined pharmacotherapy and psychotherapy in patients with personality disorders, it is reasonable at this time to suggest that combination therapy is better than psychotherapy or pharmacotherapy alone. The more pressing issue is what types of both to use in which patient groups. This in turn raises the question whether personality disorders should be diagnosed and addressed directly or whether clinicians should only attempt to treat problematic behaviors (e.g., impulsivity and aggression) along with comorbid Axis I and III problems believed to arise from the same biological cause. If the biochemistry of the disorder forces an individual to behave in a dysphoric or unacceptable manner, it would make sense to address the underlying biochemistry before one attempted to do psychotherapy. This would be akin to a medical model for treating a broken leg. The bone break (primary physical problem/neurochemical imbalance) causes a behavioral problem (atrophy of muscles while the broken bone is casted/poor social adaptation) which requires physical therapy (psychotherapy) to alleviate the atrophy once the bone is healed. Thus the ordering of interventions may also be very important.

Patients, after successful pharmacotherapy, continue to behave in much the same fashion they did prior to medication intervention. They display better sleep, decreased aggression, decreased impulsivity, improved affective control, and better mood parameters. The medications do not change a patient's understanding of the world. At best they change the patient's ability to learn to understand it differently. It is also possible, that the ability to change is limited, regardless of how aggressive the pharmacotherapy and psychotherapy are administered in a willing subject. Individuals may become hardwired for a number of reasons over time and unable to change. Brain synapses can be formed over time and remain relatively fixed. Likewise, if an individual has learned to understand his or her world through an antisocial point of view, this may be the only way he or she can process new information. The individual can only understand this new information and frame it from an antisocial perspective. In these cases I have found that all therapies are best used to help maximize an individual's potential with his or her current personality construct, as opposed to making changes to a different personality/behavioral construct.

The term "personality disorder" is used in such a disparaging manner in many clinical practices that labeling a patient with an Axis II diagnosis is tantamount to calling the patient irreparable. Yet, personality disorders may be the most important variable in predicting outcome (Shea et al., 1990). The biological underpinnings of personality suggest that many of these behaviors are not learned but preordained. The vast numbers of afflicted individuals—borderlines in psychiatric hospitals, antisocial personality patients in jails—indicates a need to find ways to help these individuals. The aforementioned studies provide a starting point for treating these individuals and future research efforts. Successful work in this area will reduce what is currently an economic and criminal burden on society and a terrible illness for those afflicted patients.

ACKNOWLEDGMENTS

Special thanks to Sue Wagner for her thoughtful discussions on the paper and key contributions as a collaborator over the years and to Ginger Mallette for unwavering support and feedback over the course of this chapter's writing.

REFERENCES

Barratt, E. S., Kent, T. A., Bryant, S. G., & Felthous, A. R. (1991). A controlled trial of phenytoin in impulsive aggression [letter]. *Journal of Clinical Psychopharmacology, 11,* 388–389.

Benedetti, F., Sforzini, L., Colombo, C., Maffei, C., &

Smeraldi, E. (1998). Low-dose clozapine in acute and continuation treatment of severe borderline personality disorder. *Journal of Clinical Psychiatry, 59,* 103–107.

Brinkley, J. R., Beitman, B. D., & Friedel, R. O. (1979). Low dose neuroleptic regimens in the treatment of borderline patients. *Archives of General Psychiatry, 36,* 319–326.

Coccaro, E. F., Astill, J. L., Herbert, J. L., & Schut, A. G. (1990). Fluoxetine treatment of impulsive aggression in DSM-III-R personality disorder patients. *Journal of Clinical Psychopharmacology, 10,* 373–375.

Coccaro, E. F., Berman, M. E., Kavoussi, R. J., & Hauger, R. L. (1996). Relationship of prolactin response to d-fenfluramine to behavioral and questionnaire assessments of aggression in personality-disordered men. *Biological Psychiatry, 40,* 157–164.

Coccaro, E. F., Kavoussi, R. J., Trestman, R. L., Gabriel, S. M., Cooper, T. B., & Sievers, L. J. (1997). Serotonin function in human subjects: Intercorrelates among central 5-HT indices and aggression. *Psychiatry Research, 73,* 1–14.

Coccaro, E. F., & Kavoussi, R. J. (1997). Fluoxetine and impulsive aggressive behavior in personality-disordered subjects. *Archives of General Psychiatry, 54,* 1081–1088.

Coccaro, E. F., Kavoussi, R. J., Hauger, R. L., Cooper, T. B., & Ferris, C. F. (1998). Cerebrospinal fluid vasopressin levels: Correlates with aggression and serotonin function in personality-disordered subjects. *Archives of General Psychiatry, 55,* 708–714.

Cornelius, J. R., Soloff, P. H., Perel, J. M., & Ulrich, R. F. (1991). A preliminary trial of fluoxetine in refractory borderline patients. *Journal of Clinical Psychopharmacology, 11,* 116–120.

Cornelius, J. R., Soloff, P. H., Perel, J. M., & Ulrich, R. F. (1993). Continuation of pharmacotherapy of borderline personality disorder with haloperidol and phenelzine. *American Journal of Psychiatry, 150,* 1843–1848.

Cowdry, R. W., & Gardner, D. L. (1988). Pharmacotherapy of borderline personality disorder: Alprazolam, carbamazepine, trifluoperazine, and tranylcypromine. *Archives of General Psychiatry, 45,* 111–119.

Elphick, M. (1988). Clinical issues in the use of carbamazepine in psychiatry: A review. *Psychological Medicine, 19,* 591–604.

Faltus, F. J. (1984). The positive effects of alprazolam in the treatment of three patients with borderline personality disorder. *American Journal of Psychiatry, 141,* 802–803.

Frankenburg, F. R., & Zanarini, M. C. (1993). Clozapine treatment of borderline patients: a preliminary study. *Comprehensive Psychiatry, 34,* 402–405.

Fink, M., Pollack, M., & Klein, D. F. (1964). Comparative studies of chlorpromazine and imipramine: I. Drug discriminating patterns. *Neuropsychpharmacology, 3,* 370–372.

Fuente, J. M. D., Goldman, S., Stanus, E., Vizuete, C., Morlan, I., Bobes, J., & Mendlewicz, J. (1997). Brain glucose metabolism in borderline personality disorder. *Journal of Psychiatric Research, 31,* 531–541.

Fuente, J. M. D., Lotstra, F., Goldman, S., Biver, F., Bidaut, A. L. L., Stanus, E., & Mendlewicz, J. (1994).

Temporal glucose metabolism in borderline personality disorder. *Psychiatry Research: Neuroimaging, 55,* 237–245.

Fuente, J. M. D., & Mendlewicz, J. (1996). TRH stimulation and dexamethasone suppression in borderline personality disorder. *Biological Psychiatry, 40,* 412–418.

Gardner, D. L., & Cowdry, R. W. (1985). Alprazolam-induced dyscontrol in borderline personality disorder. *American Journal of Psychiatry, 142,* 98–100.

Gardner, D. L., & Cowdry, R. W. (1986a). Development of melancholia during carbamazepine treatment in borderline personality disorder. *Journal of Clinical Psychopharmacology, 6,* 236–239.

Gardner, D. L., & Cowdry, R. W. (1986b). Positive effects of carbamazepine on behavioral dyscontrol in borderline personality disorder. *American Journal of Psychiatry, 143,* 519–522.

Gardner, D. L., & Cowdry, R. W. (1989). Pharmacotherapy of borderline personality disorder: A review. *Psychopharmacology Bulletin, 25,* 515–523.

Goldberg, S. C. (1989). Lithium in the treatment of borderline personality disorder. *Psychopharmacology Bulletin, 25,* 550–555.

Goldberg, S. C., Schulz, S. C., Schulz, P. M., Resnick, R. J., Hamer, R. M., & Friedel, R. O. (1986). Borderline and schizotypal personality disorders treated with low-dose thiothixene vs. placebo. *Archives of General Psychiatry, 43,* 680–686.

Hollander, E., Stein, D. J., DeCaria, C. M., Cohen, L., Saoud, J. B., Skodol, A. E., Kellman, D., Rosnick, L., & Oldham, J. M. (1994). Serotonergic sensitivity in borderline personality disorder: Preliminary findings. *American Journal of Psychiatry, 151,* 277–280.

Hymowitz, P., Frances, A. J., Jacobsberg, L. B., Sickles, M., & Hoyt, R. (1986). Neuroleptic treatment of schizotypal personality disorder. *Comprehensive Psychiatry, 27,* 267–271.

Jonas, A. D. (1967). The diagnostic and therapeutic use of diphenyl-hydantoin in the subictal state and non-epileptic dysphoria. *International Journal of Neuropsychiatry, 3* (Suppl.), 21–29.

Kavoussi, R. J., Liu, J., & Coccaro, E. F. (1994). An open trial of sertraline in personality disordered patients with impulsive aggression. *Journal of Clinical Psychiatry, 55,* 137–141.

Khouzam, H. R., & Donnelly, N. J. (1997). Remission of self-mutilation in a patient with borderline personality during risperidone therapy. *Journal of Nervous and Mental Disease, 195,* 348–349.

Klein, D. F. (1967). Importance of psychiatric diagnosis in prediction of clinical drug effects. *Archives of General Psychiatry, 16,* 118–126.

Klein, D. F. (1968). Psychiatric diagnosis and a typology of clinical drug effects. *Psychopharmacologia, 13,* 359–386.

Leone, F. N. (1982). Response of borderline patients to loxapine and chlorpromazine. *Journal of Clinical Psychiatry, 43,* 148–150.

Markovitz, P. J. (1995) Pharmacotherapy of impulsivity, aggression, and related disorders. In D. Stein & E. Hollander (Eds.), *Impulsive aggression and disorders of impulse control* (pp. 263–287). Sussex, UK: Wiley.

Markovitz, P. J., Calabrese, J. R., Schulz, S. C., & Meltzer, H. Y. (1991). Fluoxetine in borderline and schizotypal personality disorder. *American Journal of Psychiatry, 148,* 1064–1067.

Markovitz, P. J., & Wagner, S. (1996). Venlafaxine in the treatment of borderline personality disorder. *Psychopharmacology Bulletin, 31,* 773–777.

Markovitz, P. J., & Wagner, S. (1977a, May 20). *An open trial of once versus twice daily nefazodone* (abstract NR222). Paper presented at the American Psychiatric Association annual meeting, NR222, San Diego, CA.

Markovitz, P. J., & Wagner, S. (1997b, June 24). *Pharmacotherapy of borderline personality disorders* (abstract). Paper presented at International Society for the Study of Personality Disorders, Vancouver, British Columbia, Canada.

Martial, J., Paris, J., Leyton, M., Zweig-Frank, H., Schwartz, G., Teboul, E., Thavundayil, J., Larue, S., Kin, N. M., & Nair, N. P. V. (1997). Neuroendocrine study of serotonin function in female borderline personality disorder patients: A pilot study. *Biological Psychiatry, 42,* 737–739.

Mattes, J. (1990). Comparative effectiveness of carbamazepine and propranolol for rage outbursts. *Journal of Neuropsychiatry and Clinical Neuroscience, 2,* 159–164.

McBride, P. A., Brown, R. P., DeMeo, M., Keilp, J., Mieczkowski, T., & Mann, J. J. (1994). The relationship of platelet 5-HT$_2$ receptor indices to major depressive disorder, personality traits, and suicidal behavior. *Biological Psychiatry, 35,* 295–308.

McGee, M. D. (1997). Cessation of self-mutilation in a patient with borderline personality disorder treated with naltrexone. *Journal of Clinical Psychiatry, 58,* 32–33.

Narayan, M., Anderson, G., Cellar, J., Mallison, R. T., Price, L. H., & Nielson, J. C. (1998). Serotonin transporter-blocking properties of nefazodone assessed by measurement of platelet serotonin. *Journal of Clinical Psychopharmacology 18,* 67–71.

Norden, M. J. (1989). Fluoxetine in borderline personality disorder. *Progress in Neuropsychopharmacology and Biological Psychiatry, 13,* 885–893.

Pine, D. S., Waserman, G. A., Coplan, J., Fried J. A., Huang, Y. Y., Kassir, S., Greenhill, L., Shaffer, D., & Parsons, B. (1996). Platelet serotonin 2A (5-HT$_{2A}$) receptor characteristics and parenting factors for boys at risk for delinquency: A preliminary report. *American Journal of Psychiatry, 153,* 538–544.

Rifkin, A., Levitan, S. J., Glaewski, J., & Klein, D. F. (1972). Emotionally unstable character disorder—A follow-up study. Description of patients and outcome. *Biological Psychiatry, 4,* 65–79.

Rifkin, A., Quitkin, F., Carrillo, C., Blumberg, A. G., & Klein, D. F. (1972). Lithium carbonate in emotionally unstable character disorder. *Archives of General Psychiatry, 27,* 519–523.

Salzman, C., Wolfson, A. N., Schatzberg, A., Looper, J., Henke, R., Albanese, M., Schwartz, J., & Miyawaki, E. (1995). Effects of fluoxetine on anger in symptomatic volunteers with borderline personality disorder. *Journal of Clinical Psychopharmacology, 15,* 23–29.

Serban, G., & Siegel, S. (1984). Response of borderline

and schizotypal patients to small doses of thiothixene and haloperidol. *American Journal of Psychiatry, 141,* 1455–158.

Shea, M. T., Pilkonis, P. A., Beckham, E., Collins, J. F., Elkin, I., Sotsky, S. M., Docherty, J. P. (1990). Personality disorders and treatment outcome in the NIMH treatment of depression collaborative research program. *American Journal of Psychiatry, 147,* 711–718.

Sheard, M. H., Marini, J. L., Bridges, C. L., & Wagner, E. (1976). The effect of lithium on impulsive–aggressive behavior in man. *American Journal of Psychiatry, 133,* 1409–1413.

Soloff, P. H., George, A., Nathan, R. S., Schulz, P. M., & Perel, J. M (1986a). Paradoxical effects of amitriptyline on borderline patients. *American Journal of Psychiatry, 143,* 1603–1605.

Soloff, P. H., George, A., Nathan, R. S., Schulz, P. M., Ulrich, R. F., & Perel, J. (1986b). Progress in pharmacotherapy of borderline disorders. *Archives of General Psychiatry, 43,* 691–697.

Soloff, P. H., Cornelius, J. R., George, A., Nathan, S., Perel, J. M., & Ulrich, R. F. (1993). Efficacy of phenelzine and haloperidol in borderline personality disorder. *Archives of General Psychiatry, 50,* 377–385.

Sonne, S., Rubey, R., Brady, K., Malcolm, R., & Morris, T. (1996). Naltrexone treatment of self-injurious thoughts and behaviors. *Journal of Nervous and Mental Disease, 184,* 192–195.

Spitzer, R. L., Williams, J. B. W., Gibbon, M., & First, M. B. (1990). *Structured Clinical Interview for DSM-III-R Personality Disorders.* Washington, DC: American Psychiatric Press.

Stein, D. J., Hollander, E., DeCaria, C. M., Simeon, D., Cohen, L., & Aronowitz, B. (1996) m-chlorophenyl piperazine challenge in borderline personality disorder: Relationship of neuroendocrine response, behavioral response, and clinical measures. *Biological Psychiatry, 40,* 508–513.

Stein, D. J., Simeon, D, Frenkel, M., Islam, M. N., & Hollander, E. (1995). An open trial of valproate in borderline personality disorder. *Journal of Clinical Psychiatry, 56,* 506–510.

Stephens, J. H., & Shaffer, J. W. (1970). A controlled study of the effects of diphenylhydantoin on anxiety, irritability, and anger in neurotic outpatients. *Psychopharmacologia (Berlin.), 17,* 169–181.

Szigethy, E. M., & Schulz, S. C. (1997). Risperidone in co-morbid borderline personality disorder and dysthymia. *Journal of Clinical Psychopharmacology, 17,* 326–327.

Taylor, D., Carter, R., Eison, A., Mullins, U., Smith, H., Torrente, J., Wright, R., & Yocca, F. (1995). Pharmacology and neurochemistry of nefazodone, a novel antidepressant drug. *Journal of Clinical Psychiatry, 56* (Suppl. 6), 3–11.

Teicher, M. H., Glod, C. A., Aaronson, S. T., Gunter, P. A., Schatzberg, A. F., & Cole, J. O. (1989). Open assessment of the safety and efficacy of thioridazine in the treatment of patients with borderline personality disorder. *Psychopharmacology Bulletin, 25,* 535–549.

Torgersen, S. (1994). Genetics in borderline conditions. *Acta Psychiatrica Scandinavica, 89* (Suppl. 379), 19–25.

Tupin, J. P., Smith, D. B., Clanon, T. L., Kim, L. I., Nugent, A., & Groupe, A. (1973). The long-term use of lithium in aggressive prisoners. *Comprehensive Psychiatry, 14,* 311–317.

Unis, A. S., Cook, E. H., Vincent, J. G., Gjerde, D. K., Perry, B. D., Mason, C., & Mitchell, J. (1997). Platelet serotonin measures in adolescents with conduct disorder. *Biological Psychiatry, 42,* 553–559.

Verkes, R. J., Pijl, H., Meinders, E., & Van Kempen, G. M. J. (1996). Borderline personality, impulsiveness, and platelet monoamine measures in bulimia nervosa and recurrent suicidal behavior. *Biological Psychiatry, 40,* 173–180.

Verkes, R. J., Van der Mast, R. C., Kerkhof, A. J. F. M., Fekkes, D., Hengeveld, M. W., Tuyl, J. P., & Van Kempen, G. M. J. (1998). Platelet serotonin, monoamine oxidase activity, and [^{3}H]paroxetine binding related to impulsive suicide attempts and borderline personality disorder. *Biological Psychiatry, 43,* 740–746.

Vilkin, M. I. (1972). Comparative chemotherapeutic trial in treatment of chronic borderline patients. *American Journal of Psychiatry, 120,* 1004.

Zanarini, M. C., Gunderson, J. G., Frankenburg, F. R., & Chauncey, D. L. (1989). The revised diagnostic interview for borderlines: Discriminating BPD from other axis II disorders. *Journal of Personality Disorders, 3,* 10–18.

PART V

TREATMENT MODALITIES AND SPECIAL ISSUES

CHAPTER 24

—=✦=—

Group Psychotherapy

K. ROY MacKENZIE

This book addresses a variety of models of psychotherapy. Group psychotherapy, on the other hand, is a modality. The small interactive group format is a vehicle through which a variety of therapeutic models can be delivered. Psychoanalytic groups and psychoeducational groups are at opposite ends of the spectrum in terms of level of focus and therapeutic technique. However, both must be taken into account in the management of the social milieu of the group and its impact on the members. Group psychotherapy must inevitably address the nature of the interpersonal patterns of the members if only to maintain the integrity of the treatment process. Because personality pathology is primarily reflected in interpersonal phenomena, the group format would seem to be particularly appealing as a treatment approach.

This chapter focuses on the impact of "groupness" both as a necessary component to the treatment approach and also as a major factor modulating the application of various psychotherapy models delivered through a group format. In particular, it addresses how the presence of personality-disordered patients affects the basic structural components of group functioning; describes several models that have been developed to treat personality disorder, many of which are of relatively recent origin; and considers strategies and techniques that are helpful for this population.

Group psychotherapy has developed in parallel with individual psychotherapy over the last half century. For much of that period, group psychotherapy was primarily conceptualized as longer-term treatment with a gradual turnover of group membership based mainly on psychodynamic or interpersonal process-focused models applied to a broad range of conditions. However, this has radically changed and the use of a range of group models is now common. Cognitive-behavioral models for a variety of personality disorders have been adapted for use in groups. Psychoeducational groups are now prevalent, often as the first stage in a treatment program. Intensive time-limited formats of 4–6 months have also been on the ascendance. The field of group psychotherapy has been split with these developments. Therapists employing longer-term process-oriented groups tend to view the shorter formats as mere band-aid solutions that do not do justice to the power of the group process. Those implementing targeted briefer formats cannot see the point of general process learning when there are clear symptoms to be addressed as quickly as possible to return the patient to normal functioning. In addition, the field is still bedeviled by beliefs that groups are a second-rate therapy, an image reinforced by distorted media presentations of chaotic sessions.

ADAPTING GROUP PSYCHOTHERAPY FOR USE WITH PERSONALITY DISORDERS

Personality disorder is defined and diagnosed on the basis of interpersonal functioning, primarily through deficits or excesses of particular patterns as they are enacted with others. Recent reports have identified heritable dimensions underlying virtually all the major, and most of the minor, interpersonal traits (Jang, McCrae, Angleitner, Riemann, & Livesley, 1998; Livesley, 1998; Livesley, Jang, & Vernon, 1998). The intensity of expression of these heritable dimensions is influenced by interpersonal experiences, especially those of a persistent nature in early age. The group situation provides a unique context in which interpersonal phenomena can be enacted within a boundaried space. Rather than the artificial relationship of individual therapy with its built-in hierarchical structure, the group provides an opportunity for a more naturalistic expression of interpersonal proclivities.

The study of interpersonal phenomena focuses on human transactions, not on the behavior of individuals per se. Sullivan (1953), building on the work of Cooley (1912) and Mead (1934), articulated this with his belief that a person's self-system is above all interpersonal in both its development and its current evolving contents. Much of the personality disorder literature has dealt with either intrapersonal or specific behavioral events of the individual. This tends to diminish an appreciation of how deeply personality is embedded in dyadic and group transactions (Anchin & Kiesler, 1982). A major access to understanding the interpersonal style of an individual is to identify the distinct covert and overt responses the person elicits or "pulls" from others. This leads to the concept of circular rather than linear causality. Each action/thought/feeling of the individual has both an antecedent stimulus and a resultant effect on the nature of the interaction.

Interpersonal theory applied to individual therapy emphasizes the importance of understanding the reciprocal patterns being enacted between patient and therapist. This has tended to be applied particularly to the internal response the therapist experiences from actions of the patient. Somewhat less focus has been directed at the implicit messages the therapist may be sending to the patient. The question in interpersonal therapy becomes "what is happening between us," not "what underlying dynamics are driving the behavior."

The frame of the encounter traditionally establishes the reciprocal role positions in individual therapy. Characteristically the therapist is in a dominant role of knowledge and influence, while the patient is in a receptive mode seeking relief. No matter how egalitarian the therapist may be, the role structure exerts a significant influence on the nature of the interaction. The group psychotherapy situation is markedly different. Initially the therapist may be seen as the "leader" and the knowledgeable expert. However, as an interactive process emerges, the transactions among the members assume an increasingly important component of the group experience. Intermember interactions will develop in response to the relationship between each of the members. In an eight-member group, this amounts to a possible total of 28 relationships, not counting those with the therapist or cotherapy dyad.

Because by definition personality pathology is revealed through interaction, group psychotherapy provides a unique opportunity to examine the core features of the syndrome. The presence of a real-life quality promotes spontaneity and lower guardedness that more closely mimics how the individuals function in everyday life. This includes the opportunity to try out new behaviors that have been seen as too risky to attempt in personal relationships outside. The group can also provide challenge and encouragement that has less of the demand quality of a therapist intervention.

The group situation therefore provides a real and complex opportunity for multiple unique relationships through which the individual member may demonstrate his or her repertoire of interactional capacities. These relationships are relatively free of the status imbalance found in the individual therapy context. Several advantages of a group approach have been identified (Budman, Cooley, et al., 1996; MacKenzie, 1997; Marziali & Munroe-Blum, 1994; Vaillant, 1992). Table 24.1 lists some of these advantages.

The empirical literature regarding personality disorder is itself in disorder. The current DSM-IV categorical diagnostic approach has poor established validity and therefore forms a weak underpinning for empirical studies (Livesley, 1998). Comorbid Axis I and Axis II conditions are the norm, making it unrealistic to strive to find personality disorders without

TABLE 24.1. Possible Advantages of Group Psychotherapy for Treatment of Personality Disorders

1. The role of the leader is less central in group psychotherapy than in individual therapy. There is a greater egalitarian atmosphere with a clear expectation that many of the benefits of treatment will come from the member-to-member interactions. Thus the intensity of transference attachment to the leader is diluted and therefore may be more accessible to constructive management.

2. The group is better able to absorb the assault of immature projections that frequently overwhelm the efforts of the individual therapist.

3. Patients can be more tolerant and accepting when input is received from other members in contrast to that received from the high status of the leader.

4. Members can engage in altruistic, supportive, and empathic behaviors with each other that enhance a sense of self-worth and self-esteem.

5. The patient has the opportunity to engage in many different roles within the diversity of the group membership and to see a variety of behaviors in other members that encourages an objective view of interpersonal characteristics.

6. Group pressure may help to prevent some types of acting out behavior as well as to influence the use of prosocial behaviors.

7. Members may be able to see themselves in a more objective manner through seeing others in the group describing or enacting the same sorts of behaviors.

comorbid features. Even with the current categories, few studies of efficacy have been conducted. The majority of papers regarding personality disorders deal only with dyadic therapy despite the fact that there is no substantial evidence for the superiority of individual psychotherapy. Impaired interpersonal functioning is the hallmark of all the personality disorders, suggesting that a modality such as group psychotherapy that emphasizes interpersonal phenomena would make most sense in approaching treatment choice.

IMPACT OF PERSONALITY DISORDER ON ASPECTS OF GROUP STRUCTURE

The general processes of psychotherapy are found in the group setting. The challenge to the group therapist is to adapt these processes to the group environment. A basic theoretical position of the group therapist is to consider therapy as being delivered through the group process. Failure to adhere to this requirement dilutes the impact of the treatment and provides an opportunity for group-level resistance to undercut therapeutic work. The higher the level of personality pathology in the group, the greater the likelihood of this occurring. The complex interpersonal environment of the group stimulates expression of characteristic interpersonal patterns along with the associated affect. At one level, this is an advantage because the presence of dysfunction is evident and can be descriptively identified within the group at an early point. At the same time the behavior must be managed, especially in the early group, in order to contain behavioral excesses that might impede group development (Klein, Orleans, & Soule, 1991; Pines & Hutchinson, 1993).

The initial task in beginning a new group is to develop a sense of "groupness," of the individual's sense of connection to the group. Initially this usually takes the form of a sense of general membership that is centered on the leader. Later this expands into relationships with individual members. The therapist is in a position to promote the development of the basic building blocks for group creation. These strategies are not unique to groups for personality disorders. However, the likelihood of intense interpersonal reactions within the group makes it particularly important that careful attention is paid to the structural aspects of the group. The early phase of the group is the most vulnerable to disruption.

PLANNING A GROUP

There is a wide range of possibilities in implementing group psychotherapy. The decisions about the basic structure of the group require careful consideration. The first choice is between a time-limited group or an open-ended group with rotating membership. Examples exist in the personality disorder literature across a wide range of options. These begin with skill-focused groups that use cognitive and behavioral strategies. In general, these are of a brief nature (8–12 sessions is common) and are characterized by a relatively high degree of process control. An agenda is followed and structured tasks and homework assignments are common.

Such groups are frequently found as part of a comprehensive treatment approach, often during the earlier stages of the treatment plan. The next grouping format would be in the time-limited 4–6-month range. These tend to be of an interpersonal or psychodynamic nature. More ambitious goals are sought in terms of overall interpersonal functioning. These groups are commonly developed for Cluster C and histrionic personality disorders, often with an attendant Axis I diagnosis such as depression or eating disorder. Longer-term slow, open groups are generally reserved for Cluster B diagnoses where the membership of any one member would be in the 1–2-year range. Cluster A diagnoses will be distributed according to the level of dysfunction.

Time-limited groups have the advantage of a tight focus that is given extra intensity by the clearly stated end point. They do require rapid involvement in the group and the capacity to apply the group experience to outside situations from an early point. Thus they present a challenge for Cluster B problems but are commonly used for Cluster C problems. They may also be seen as a starting point to test the individual's capacity to use a group approach. Referral to a longer-term group could follow. Open-ended longer-term groups have the advantage of an established working atmosphere into which the new member can be absorbed. This provides an opportunity for the newer members to model on senior members and to learn from others how to maximize their benefits from the group experience.

GROUP COMPOSITION

A widely used practice is to form groups on the basis of common diagnostic categories. For example, manuals are available for cognitive-behavioral therapy (CBT) depression groups or interpersonal therapy (IPT) binge eating groups. Such groups provide the opportunity to employ specific strategies relevant to the diagnosis. Such approaches are required by research-granting bodies and are convenient for larger service systems where a front-end diagnostic label can determine the treatment course. However, this approach fails to take into account many other aspects of selection. For example, a subset of patients with major depression present with an intensification of a negative controlling interpersonal style that can

effectively shut down a group despite therapeutic efforts.

Historically, membership in open-ended groups has been based on the "level of functioning," or "capacity to interact" based on the assumption that this would promote an rapid working atmosphere. One implicit goal has often been to select out major personality disorders. The last decade has seen a major increase in group programs designed specifically for the personality-disordered population, particularly in programs for borderline personality disorder. There have been no systematic studies of whether it is advantageous to cluster such patients in a common group or to dilute the groups with a mixture of more interpersonally functional members.

Azim, Piper, Segal, Nixon, and Duncan (1991) found a significant predictor variable to be a measure of quality of object relations (QOR) based on a structured interview. In a study of individual psychotherapy, QOR was a strong predictor of therapeutic alliance and outcome. Patients with a lower level of interpersonal functioning on this measure demonstrate difficulty in responding constructively to interpretative interventions. They also have a higher dropout rate in psychodynamically oriented groups. In the day treatment program discussed later, QOR predicted higher dropout rate, symptom reduction, and social maladjustment.

A reasonable case can be made for the use of homogeneous groups to treat borderline personality disorder as described in a following section. There are numerous reports of high dropout rates of borderline patients in general therapy groups (Budman, Demby, Soldz, & Merry, 1996). The challenges that these patients present are probably best handled by clinicians with special interest and expertise. This conclusion is based not only on better outcome and lower attrition but also on consideration of the degree to which patients with borderline personality disorder can impede the work of a group. The group clinician always assumes a dual responsibility for both individual members and also the group membership collectively. Few empirical reports are available for other Cluster B syndromes. Clinical wisdom suggests that narcissistic disorders would also fall into the category of specialized groups, perhaps combined with patients with borderline personality disorder.

Antisocial and psychopathic individuals are generally treated in a corrections format which has a major focus on addressing the crime cycle and relapse prevention strategies. Although these approaches may have relevance for a broader patient population, the nature of the criminal material sets them apart from routine clinical work.

There are numerous clinical reports regarding groups designed for severe chronic neurotic problems and a mix of Cluster C and histrionic personality disorders. Personality pathology is frequently found as a comorbid condition with Axis I syndromes, especially anxiety, depression, and eating disorders. The empirical literature follows the clinical in being unclear as to the relative responsiveness of the personality disorder per se. Most report an overall general level of improvement for both components. The question of group composition is therefore unresolved regarding these Cluster C syndromes. Most patients are referred for the Axis I diagnosis and bring with them the characterological features.

The development of large service systems provides an environment in which group programming may be effectively implemented. The large flow of patients receiving a systematic assessment can be used to place patients in a range of groups at an early point. This requires the careful development of appropriate types of groups and clear acceptance criteria.

PRETHERAPY PREPARATION AND EARLY STRUCTURE

A consistent empirical literature documents the value of systematic preparation of members for the group experience. Novice group members frequently bring inaccurate and often quite unrealistic ideas about what will happen in a therapy group and how they can act to benefit maximally from the experience. Various methods have been tested with more or less equivalent results, suggesting that it is the implementation of a systematic process that is more important than the details (Bednar, Melnick, & Kaul, 1974; Kaul & Bednar, 1994).

1. *Written handout.* The simplest model to prepare patients for group is to provide a brief handout describing how groups work and how to get the most out of the experience. For example, one four-page handout (MacKenzie, 1997) contains the sections listed in Table 24.2. This handout is given to the member to read at home

TABLE 24.2. Patient Information Handout

1. Do groups really help people? A brief outline of the empirical literature.

2. How group therapy works: the concept of learned interpersonal patterns and a mention of the common types of groups.

3. Common myths about group therapy: not a second-rate treatment, no forced confessions, the value of being with others with similar problems, the therapist in control of process, understandable apprehension about being accepted. These are all common fears of a new group member.

4. How to get the most out of group: get involved, group as a "living laboratory," talk of your inner reactions, think of nonverbal messages, learn from the group experience itself.

5. Common stumbling blocks: anxiety is normal, the leader keeps the group focused but does not provide pat answers, emotions are normal and can be expressed, after the excitement of initial sessions there may be a letdown, negative thoughts or anger can be talked about, outside application is important, do not act on group advice without thinking hard about it.

6. Group expectations: confidentiality is very important, attendance and punctuality are important for the group as well as for you, extragroup socializing (yes or no depending on the type of group), how between-session contacts with the leader will be handled, no alcohol or drugs before sessions.

and then is reviewed briefly with the member individually before the group begins. Questions and concerns are elicited and specific discussion around "myths" and "expectations" are covered.

2. *A formal structured training session* (Piper, Debbane, Garant, & Bienvenu, 1979; Piper, Debbane, Bienvenu, Garant, 1982). This would include didactic material as in the handout but supplemented with simple communication exercises that get people to talk to each other.

3. *Videotaped examples of group interaction that are discussed* (Hilkey, Wilhelm, & Horne, 1982). This provides both a modeling opportunity as well as an innocuous introduction to talking together.

4. *Specific training in communication style* using role induction films, laboratory communication exercises, and detailed exercises in specific behaviors such as assertiveness or affect display.

5. *Structured group activities in early sessions.* One model (MacKenzie, 1998) begins the first session with a formal go-around regarding target goals, the second session with a detailed discussion of DSM-IV symptoms of the presenting disorder, with an emphasis on the impact of life adjustment, and the third session with another go-around based on written target goal sheets prepared from the individual initial assessment interviews. Thus the content is focused on the therapeutic targets from the beginning but is handled in a structured way that reduces anxiety. Regular debriefing questions concerning how members are experiencing the group interaction are helpful in dampening anxiety and detecting members who are experiencing greater problems. By the end of the first three sessions the members are interacting more openly without the inhibiting effects of performance anxiety associated with silences and unknown expectations.

The most important goal of pretherapy preparation and initial structure is to achieve a lower rate of early group dropout. Across a spectrum of different types of groups, most premature terminations occur in the first six sessions and reflect a failure of integration into the group milieu. If the new members can be retained within the group, they have an opportunity to be exposed to supportive elements that will draw them toward a sense of group membership. Personality-disordered patients are likely to have particularly strong expectations regarding negative events, and the opportunity to discuss these with the therapist individually can be quite helpful. This discussion is also helpful in building an alliance with the patient by allowing the patient to vent his or her concerns and to receive factual answers. This initial bond with the therapist may make the difference between an early dropout and a successful course of treatment.

GROUP COHESION

The concept of the therapeutic alliance has proven of value in the individual psychotherapy literature (Bordin, 1979). Early measures of the alliance are robust predictors of eventual outcome (Gaston, 1990; Horvath & Symonds, 1991). Strategies to repair ruptures in the alliance lead to better outcome (Safran & Muran, 1996, 1998).

The concept of group cohesion is the closest analogue to the therapeutic alliance, particularly that aspect of the alliance referred to by the more general term "therapeutic bond." Cohesion is reflected in such terms as "group morale" and "esprit de corps." It has not been easy to develop satisfactory measures for such a construct. Despite these technical problems the notion of evaluating a sense of "groupness," attraction, or vitality seems intuitively sensible. The therapeutic factors of universality, acceptance, and altruism interact with the development of cohesion. "Cohesion" appears to be a useful term for describing the whole group, not specifically the individual members. The members of cohesive groups are characterized by a commitment to the goals of the group, a need to belong, and identification with each other in a compatible manner. Cohesive groups have lower dropout rates, better attendance, less tardiness, higher participation, and less inhibited affect. Cohesive groups are also characterized by higher levels of challenging, confronting, and risk-taking behaviors.

The currently most widely used measure of cohesion is the Group Climate Questionnaire (GCQ; MacKenzie, 1983) completed by the group members. In particular, the engaged scale on this instrument reflects an atmosphere of belonging and participating that is analogous to the concept of the *working alliance* in the individual literature. Budman et al. (1987) developed an observer Group Cohesiveness Scale consisting of five global dimensions. The use of this scale has been limited, although acceptable interrater reliability has been reported. The California Psychotherapy Alliance Scale (CALPAS) has a group version that focuses on the relationship between the individual member and the group (Gaston, 1991; Gaston & Marmar, 1991). This makes it a truly group-focused instrument.

The relatively small number of reports using cohesion/alliance process measures in psychotherapy groups suggests that the same general results apply: Early measures predict outcome and threatened ruptures need to be addressed (Budman et al., 1989; Kivlighan & Goldfine, 1991; Kivlighan & Mullison, 1988; MacKenzie & Tschuschke, 1993).

Groups for personality-disordered members are prone to process disruption. This may occur at a blatant level but also at a more subtle level of withdrawal or covert messages that are not necessarily acknowledged. Subgrouping may also pose a problem. One might argue that the most important task for the therapist in a personality disorders group is to maintain a reasonably solid cohesive atmosphere. This may expose the members to what is for them a unique environment of stability, predictability, and acceptance. The members of a cohesive group are accepting of one another, supportive, and inclined to form meaningful relationships in the group. They will be more likely to express and explore themselves and their issues. These processes are associated with increased self-esteem and a sense of greater mastery for members over themselves and their interpersonal world. The use of process measures can provide an additional avenue for understanding the experience each member is having in the group. For example, a member consistently rating his sense of commitment low on the CAL-PAS is giving a warning of difficulty; as is a consistent rating of the group as low on the Engaged scale of the GCQ.

GROUP NORMS

Groups can be described according to the implicit or explicit interactional rules they follow (Bond, 1983; MacKenzie, 1979). By definition, personality disorders tend to be ruled by arbitrary, idiosyncratic, or constantly shifting rules in their relationships. These shifting rules will be almost immediately reflected in their group interactions. The group arena allows, in fact invites, members to demonstrate their interpersonal patterns. The group leader will need to be as active as necessary to shape these normative structures into productive channels. By addressing the whole group, the leader can establish guidelines that do not appear to be specifically directed at any one member and therefore can be accepted by all. Many norms are shaped subtly by nonverbal reactions and through choices made about what aspect of the interaction to reinforce. This norm building and maintaining process provides a major component toward developing a group that itself becomes the agent of change. Table 24.3 lists some constructive norms. As groups develop a positive normative structure they become to an increasing extent self-monitoring and self-regulating. An ongoing open group has the task of recruiting new members into the group's normative structure.

It is clear from the items in Table 24.3 that

TABLE 24.3. Constructive Group Norms

1. On-time and regular attendance is expected.
2. Communication goes in all directions, not predominantly through the leader.
3. Interaction is fluid, generally not lengthy on one person at a time, a "take turns" model.
4. Active participation is expected.
5. There is a nonjudgmental acceptance of others.
6. The members see the group as basically supportive and safe.
7. Self-disclosure is anticipated.
8. An interest in understanding one's self is expected.
9. There is an eagerness for change.
10. Risk taking with new behaviors is rewarded.
11. Identifying problematic aspects of others does not involve uncharitable criticism.

personality-disordered patients will find many opportunities to challenge normative expectations. That is why it is important that norms be clearly enunciated. The individual member has the opportunity to learn from interactions with specific other members but also with the collectivity of the group. The group is often seen as a more neutral zone in which to establish a working threshold without the intensity that accompanies individual relationships. The process of accommodating to the group norms is a prosocial experience that has important value in social adaptation outside the group itself.

SOCIAL ROLE

A familiar phenomenon in groups is the emergence of an individual in a strong role pattern that is somewhat uncharacteristic of him or her (MacKenzie, 1997). Individuals who experience this sometimes describe themselves as being drawn into behaving differently by playing a role that seemed outside their control, so-called role suction. Two common roles are becoming the spokesperson for the group while other members remain silent or behaving in such a way as to be the scapegoat and target of group anger. Both may be understood as a response for the collective need within the group for a strong leader or a mechanism to contain negative feelings respectively.

THE GROUP AS A WHOLE

A unique advantage of the group approach is the evocative properties of the whole group for triggering family-of-origin themes (Kernberg, 1975b; Scheidlinger, 1974, 1983) that have an impact beyond that of the individual group relationships. This affectively charged atmosphere may create times in a group when rather deep attachment issues become vocalized, centering around issues of dependency, abandonment/aggression, or isolation. Members often reflect on such times as providing a particularly important triggering function for their psychotherapeutic work.

GENERAL EVIDENCE REGARDING EFFICACY OF GROUP PSYCHOTHERAPY

There is a large data base confirming the global effectiveness of individual psychotherapy across many diagnostic categories and treatment models (Howard, Kopta, Krause, & Orlinsky, 1986; Howard, Lueger, & Schank, 1992; Howard, Lueger, Maling, & Martinovich, 1993). Reliable change curves indicate that most therapeutic gains are found in the first 6 months of treatment with an improvement rate of approximately 75% and a recovery rate of 60–65%. Improvement then continues but at a much slower rate over a 2-year period. The curve for major personality disorders is lower, rising to around 50% by the end of the first year of treatment (Kopta, Howard, Lowry, & Beutler, 1994; Kolden & Howard, 1992). These figures are based on cumulative data within which there are undoubtedly many subpopulations in regard to response rate. However, they do indicate in general terms the temporal rates of change.

There is a smaller but still substantial empirical data base concerning the use of group psychotherapy. The landmark Smith, Glass, and Miller (1980) meta-analytic report reviewed 475 psychotherapy studies and found an average effective size of 0.85. Approximately half of the studies in this sample used a group format. There was no difference in effect size between the individual and group studies. Further meta-analytic studies were conducted by Toseland and Siporin (1986) and Tillitski (1990), again finding no difference according to modality. Rockland (1992) suggests that the patients with more severe borderline personality disorder with marked splitting operations, or those who have demonstrated minimal response to extensive individual treatment, would be candidates for group psychotherapy. This is another example of difficult patient populations, such as substance abusers or criminals, being preferentially treated in groups.

Two recent studies selected only research reports that met quite stringent quality criteria. Piper and Joyce (1996) reviewed 86 articles from 1983–1994. Of the 50 reports that included time-limited group therapy versus a control comparison, 48 found significantly greater benefit for the therapy condition. Of six studies that directly compared individual and group methods, all six found no difference.

McRoberts, Burlingame, and Hoag (1998) reviewed 23 studies that reported individual and group results within the same study. The subjects had to exhibit clinical problems typically treated by mental health professionals. Studies had to use either matching or random assignment to groups. Outcome variables had to be amenable to calculation of effect size. Studies of children or adolescents and inpatient settings were excluded. There was no difference in overall effect size between individual and group formats. When individual psychotherapy was compared with wait-list controls within the same study, it was significantly effective with an effect size of 0.76. For group psychotherapy, the effect size was 0.90. This means that individual patients fared better on average than 78% of wait-list patients, and that group therapy patients fared better on average than 82% of wait-list patients. These results are comparable to previous meta-analytic reviews.

McRoberts et al. (1998) also identified seven previous meta-analytic studies comparing individual and group treatment. Five of these found no difference in outcome. Two studies found a better outcome for individual therapy. On further examination of these two reports, it was noted that a number of the group studies used a form of cognitive-behavioral therapy that was based on predetermined treatment interventions with no attempt to incorporate or capitalize on the unique properties deemed therapeutic to the group format as a cost-effective vehicle. They could be described as "individual treatment in the presence of others."

The empirical literature provides solid support for the effectiveness of group psychotherapy. Across a broad range of models and target populations, outcome figures appear to be equal to individual therapy. This is reassuring and for practical purposes suggests that it is unlikely that group treatment for personality disorders would be inferior. However, the two most recent and sophisticated meta-analytic reviews described previously included only a small number of studies dealing with major personality disorders: Piper and Joyce (1996) found two studies and McRoberts et al. (1998) only one.

GROUP MODELS FOR BORDERLINE PERSONALITY DISORDER

The majority of empirical studies related to personality disorders deal with borderline personality disorder. The same is true in the group literature. Several specific group psychotherapy models have been developed for the treatment of severe personality disorder. All have detailed operational manuals and all have been validated with satisfactory outcome measures. Each model is unique in terms of specific techniques, but all share a number of common features. These developments represent a significant advancement in the treatment of a pervasive and debilitating illness with significant mortality. Borderline personality disorder also accounts for a sizable component of the intensive inpatient and day treatment service load. Each model is described here in some detail along with evidence for its effectiveness.

Interpersonal Group Psychotherapy

The choice of "interpersonal" for the title of this model is accurate but can also be misleading as there are several distinct treatment applications based on interpersonal orientation each with its own unique application characteristics. The interpersonal group psychotherapy (IGP) model employs a special version of interpersonal psychotherapy that focuses specifically on the therapist's management of the treatment relationship. In addition, close attention is paid to the nature of the patient's current relationships and the social contextual features of the manifestations of the disorder itself. Etiology is assumed to be multifactorial with uncertain links to the development of effective treatment. The core of the technique was initially developed by Dawson (1988) and manualized by

Dawson and Macmillan (1993) for use in individual therapy under the label "relationship management." The group therapeutic application evolved through a decade of progressively more complex clinical research at McMaster University culminating in a major study (Marziali & Munroe-Blum, 1995; Munroe-Blum & Marziali, 1995). Details of the model are contained in a book/manual *Interpersonal Group Psychotherapy for Borderline Personality Disorder* (Marziali & Munroe-Blum, 1994).

The 110 subjects who met the criteria for borderline personality disorder diagnosis according to Gunderson's Diagnostic Interview for Borderlines (DIB; Gunderson, 1984) were randomly allocated to either the experimental group treatment or a comparison condition consisting of psychodynamic individual psychotherapy that emphasized the developmental genesis of the disorder. This model was chosen as being the typical approach for outpatient treatment of borderline personality disorder and the model most reported in the literature (Kernberg, 1975a; Waldinger & Gunderson, 1987). However, this was not "treatment as usual," although the individual psychodynamic treatment is the most commonly used model for borderline personality disorder. Of the 110, 79 subjects accepted treatment. The individual therapy component was provided by senior clinicians experienced in treating borderline personality disorder with sessions once or twice a week. Audiotaped recordings of the individual sessions indicated that the therapists used traditional psychodynamic strategies of interpretation, confrontation, and exploration, among others.

There was no difference in terms of diagnosis or comorbid conditions between those who accepted and those who refused treatment. Therapists in both treatments had equal levels of experience. Standardized process and outcome measures were used, plus a free-form account from subjects concerning what factors they felt did or did not help. The group treatment consisted of 25 weekly sessions, followed by 5 biweekly sessions. A research assistant trained to use IGP strategies followed most subjects for several weeks prior to beginning treatment during the phase of collecting adequate members for randomization to a group. Treatment system contact therefore stretched over close to 1 year. Assessments were made at 6, 12, 18, and 24 months (i.e., 1-year follow-up).

The treatment trial found that borderline patients achieved significant benefit from both forms of treatment. Outcome was measured through patient self-reports of depression, general symptoms, and social adjustment. An interview-based measure, the Objective Behavioral Index, included hospitalizations, suicide attempts (including severity), problems with the law, substance abuse, impulse control, house moves, psychotherapy, and use of mental health services (Marziali, Munroe-Blum, & McCleary, 1999). Table 24.4 shows the effect size for the various measures, indicating a major response that is comparable with that reported in the general psychotherapy literature despite the difficult patient population.

The group model used approximately half the contact hours of the individual model, resulting in significant cost-effectiveness. The imposition of a firm time boundary was found to be paradoxically settling because there was no ambiguity as to when the group would end, providing a sense of predictability and therefore safety.

All study therapists were highly experienced. Therapists in the group model reported greater satisfaction than those in individual therapy. Their anxieties at starting treatment with a new patient with borderline personality disorder were lower. The fact that a shared state of confusion was an expected dimension of the treatment allayed many of their fears about being in a room with a group of impulsive, demanding patients. They felt able to establish a therapeutic alliance with each member. The individual therapists were often unaware of why their patients terminated treatment and felt the treatments had not been completed. In addition, the authors report that the group model created a more tolerant and less stigmatizing atmosphere toward the management of patients with borderline personality disorder. They attribute this to the emphasis the model places on understanding the therapists' subjective reactions and the view that these patients share a universal need for care, respect, and empathy.

The core of the relationship model on which the IGP group is based centers on the accurate alignment of the therapist with the state of the patient. The therapists are trained to monitor the meaning of group member interactions within the context of the patients' expectations of the therapists. During the early phase of therapy, there is no other reality but that presented by the patient. The therapists' task is to understand the often garbled messages being sent to them, particularly in regard to the patient's expectations of the therapist. To be misunderstood is to suffer abandonment and rejection. Reality-oriented interpretations or clarifications will obstruct this task. Extensive exploration of early childhood experiences is not helpful and distracts from the focus on current immediate emotions and mental states. Similarly, education and advice from either the therapist or members is discouraged. The group is designed to support a therapeutic context in which the borderline patient is able to replicate problematic interpersonal behaviors without having to resort to "fight" or "flight" measures. The members find it easy to identify with each other and with their common problems and can thus provide an understanding and supportive sustaining force.

Particular efforts are exerted to identify the point at which "derailment" of the alliance has occurred so that it can be immediately addressed. A failure in proper alignment is commonly followed by a group response of anxiety, hopelessness, or rage. It was found that a general phenomena emerged later in treatment characterized by a mourning process focused on giving up wished-for fantasies embedded in interpersonal relations. The eventual goal of treatment is to decrease the negative interpersonal transactions characteristic of the patient with borderline personality disorder. In this way, a more benign aspect of the self in relationship to others can be developed.

TABLE 24.4. Outcome Effect Sizes

	OBI	HSCL	BDI	SAS	SU
Termination	0.09	0.74	0.76	0.52	
1-year follow-up	0.77	1.10	1.14	0.57	0.54

Note. OBI, Objective Behavioral Index; HSCL, Hopkins Symptom Checklist; BDI, Beck Depression Inventory; SAS, Social Adjustment Scale; SU, service utilization (hospitalization and *all* mental health visits).

Areas of Interest

1. The IGP model requires specialized training and careful monitoring. Therapists must be prepared to examine openly their individual subjective reactions to each member and to the group process. Regular meetings of therapists are helpful to provide a forum for continuing

learning and for processing difficult situations. Therapists probably self-select for this type of therapy, but service directors need to be aware of the strains of the work and match these with the suitability of the clinician.

2. Some 31% of the group therapy patients dropped out within the first five sessions. This is considerably higher than the 15% to 20% commonly cited in the general group literature but lower than the dropout rate generally found with patients with borderline personality disorder. The authors suggest a limited number of individual sessions during the initial period to address this. Budman, Demby, et al. (1996) found this technique helpful in a group format for personality disorders.

3. A subgroup of patients adopting "pseudo-competent" roles appeared less able to benefit from the IGP format as applied. They may be quite helpful with suggestions and ideas to others but had difficulty addressing their own difficulties.

4. The IGP model handles early group phenomena differently than most time-limited approaches. The general group literature reports that positive effects are found with pretherapy preparation and through being clear about areas on which to focus, setting target goals, setting contracts, and giving pretherapy information about groups. The IGP model specifically does not provide such services. Instead, the patient is given every opportunity to reject treatment and has the option of meeting with the therapists prior to beginning the group, when they might receive a brief written outline of the group if they wish.

5. The Objective Behavioral Index assesses a range of behaviors including service utilization and level of seriousness of self-harm episodes. The 1-year follow-up change is impressive. All symptom measures indicated highly significant improvement. This broad a range of improvement is not usually found in borderline personality disorder studies.

6. The IGP model incorporates many features typically found in psychodynamic and interpersonal therapies and is therefore comfortable for many clinicians. It is different from the IPT model of Klerman, Weissman, Rounsaville, and Chevron (1984) in that there is a major focus on the relationship with the therapist. Its unique feature is the intense focus on maintaining the therapeutic alliance and understanding the importance of the sensitivity of the therapist's role in this.

Dialectical Behavior Therapy

Dialectical behavior therapy (DBT) was also developed specifically for the treatment of borderline personality disorder (Linehan, 1993; Linehan, Armstrong, Suarez, Allmon, & Heard, 1991; Linehan, Heard, & Armstrong, 1993). This complex model uses a weekly 2½-hour group psychosocial skills training session and an individual psychotherapy session. In addition, it is recommended that the leaders of both of these treatments meet regularly, preferably weekly, to coordinate their therapeutic efforts. Treatment is expected to last about a year. Various applications have been developed from the theoretical base of the model for use in briefer applications, especially inpatient units and day treatment programs.

As in IGP, the therapeutic relationship is considered central to effective treatment. The alliance is centered around acceptance of a treatment philosophy based on a dialectical world view. This perspective is associated with the ancient theories of Eastern philosophy that stress the fundamental interrelatedness or wholeness of reality. The immediate and larger contexts of behavior are important in understanding the interrelatedness of individual behavior patterns. These ideas are augmented with current feminist theory that emphasizes the impact of the larger culture on the developmental experiences of women. The basic goals are to learn self-regulation skills and skills at influencing the environment.

The dialectic focus emphasizes that reality is not static but composed of opposing forces (thesis vs. antithesis). All propositions contain their own oppositions. The goal is to find a way to move to a synthesis. This has parallels to the theories of the psychodynamic conflict model: "I wish, but . . ." (Book, 1998; Luborsky & Crits-Christoph, 1997). The patient with borderline personality disorder is seen is continually stuck in three tensions:

1. Need to accept self as is versus need to change.
2. Getting what you need interpersonally versus losing what you need if you become more competent.
3. Maintaining personal integrity and validating one's own views of the problem versus learning new skills that will help to emerge from suffering.

Fundamental reality is seen as change and

process rather than content and structure. The individual and the environment are continuously changing. Therapist and treatment also change over time.

Emotional dysregulation is considered the core defect in borderline personality disorder, resulting in high sensitivity to emotional stimuli, an intense response to emotional stimuli, and a slow return to baseline emotional state. These features result in faulty emotional regulation as revealed through difficulty in inhibiting inappropriate behavior to emotions, in organizing the self for concerted action, in soothing physiological arousal, and in refocusing attention in presence of strong emotion. The origins of the disorder are considered to lie in temperamental features leading to emotional dysregulation accompanied by an invalidating family environment that augments rather than soothes the dysregulation. The borderline individual's inner experience is seen as having been continuously invalidated and emotional expression, especially negative affect, is inhibited. It is speculated that these phenomena are particularly evident in societies that promote individualism. The invalidation at a personal level may be echoed in societal experiences that negate or inhibit the female role. The emotional dysregulation results in repeated self-harm to obtain transient relief, elicitation of strong responses from environment (family and clinicians), and development of an unstable sense of self through the lack of consistency or predictability.

The application of these theoretical ideas is grounded in the standard practices of cognitive therapy. These are based on a framework of ongoing assessment, data collection, clear treatment targets, maintaining a collaborative working relationship, and establishing mutual treatment goals. Techniques include problem solving, exposure, skills training, contingency management, and cognitive modification. Dysfunctional behaviors are reframed as part of a learned problem-solving repertoire. All problematic behaviors are subject to analysis, beginning with behaviors that are lower in the hierarchy and progressing to more distressing behaviors. Fear-inducing situations must be confronted. Basic tasks focus on identifying alternative behaviors and applying these in the therapy situation and to outside circumstances.

DBT differs from the usual cognitive therapy approach in several ways. There is a constant effort to validate current emotional, cognitive, and behavioral responses, including validation of emotional desperation. These need to be addressed in the moment. Closely parallel is the importance of addressing therapy-interfering behaviors of the client and reinforcing behaviors of the therapist. This brings into focus the immediate process of the therapy in a manner that is much closer to the interpersonal/psychodynamic model. The maintenance of the therapeutic relationship is essential. All these produce a more active focus on the interaction between therapist and patient than would be normally be found in CBT. Finally, the theme of dialectic tensions that must be resolved through a process of acceptance is a unique feature of the DBT model. This theme includes an acceptance of one's self and one's world, a component of Zen philosophy.

The group session is typically 2½ hours. Groups generally have six to eight members. This session may be broken into two shorter sessions focusing on presenting new material and reviewing homework, respectively. This format was, at least in part, developed to ensure that there is a consistent focus on skill building and understanding and mastering the basic material of DBT. The group format makes it easier to stay on target with the session plan. Ideally, the group provides the material and the individual therapist focuses on reinforcing the basic strategies and their application in the patient's daily life as well as promoting motivation. Skills are applied initially to problems of general daily functioning and may not be applied to acute suicidal situations for some time. Discussion of suicidal issues is not encouraged in the skills group as shaping must begin with lower-intensity issues and individual therapists must appreciate this and keep their focus largely on skill application, not more extensive interpersonal topics. If a group is not available for some reason the skills training can be given individually, preferably with a different therapist. It is emphasized that the group format provides an important socialization experience and is the preferred format.

The group sessions deal with four modules. The first of these is a brief module on mindfullness skills. This module is then reapplied at the beginning of each of the following three modules. The other modules, about eight sessions each, deal with emotion regulation skills, interpersonal effectiveness skills, and distress tolerance skills. These are repeated twice in the year of treatment. The mindfullness and distress tolerance modules are seen as the basic foundation and are sometimes the main material presented in inpatient/day treatment programs.

Individual skill training is difficult because the constantly changing issues in the patient's life are constantly intruding. The therapist must be active and directive. The group provides a steadier environment. It important that the leader is highly committed, in order to keep the members motivated to apply the skills and to bring their experiences into the group session. Indeed, the decision to separate the skills teaching from the focus on application in the individual sessions was in part based on the value of having two approaches to reinforce involvement.

Open groups are preferred, though turnover will be slow because of the length of treatment and the small group size. It was found in preliminary studies that closed groups could deviate more easily from the task and evolve into more active group process. New members quickly pick up the expectation that skills are to be learned. Coping with the changing membership also provides an experience in dealing with change and the trust issues involved. Although all members meet borderline personality disorder disorder criteria and parasuicidal acts, they otherwise may be quite diverse.

Areas of Interest

1. If the full program is instituted, it would comprise an individual session (60 minutes), a group session (150 minutes), a supervision/consultation meeting (120 minutes), and allowance for chart work (30 minutes) for a total of 5 hours per week with the majority of the time involving two therapists. In addition, 24-hour access to a clinician is provided. This makes DBT an intensive and cost-intensive program.

2. The format of the skills training portion of the DBT model is very clear. However, the overall structure of the treatment program becomes problematic outside a funded research setting. It would seem likely that the supervision/consultation meeting would be the first to suffer in a private practice context, resulting in a clear possibility of significant splitting between formats. The manual is clear about the need to be alert to such possibilities, but the implementation details are complex.

3. DBT clearly employs some useful, perhaps powerful, strategies. Many of these are being implemented piecemeal in a variety of programs with the validation of the author. For example, inpatient programs may apply only the mindfulness and distress tolerance modules with or without an individual component. It is unclear what should be considered a standard DBT treatment package model. Dismantling studies that assess the relative value of the various components would be welcome.

4. A group format was chosen to deliver the skills training portion of the model because the group can provide normative pressures to keep a clear focus on the didactic task. There are rather firm guidelines to keep on task and assume that the application task is going to be amplified by the individual therapy. However, a group of borderline patients is a challenge for the most experienced group psychotherapists. The predictable problems are identified in the manual, including group contagion around suicidal ideation, the need for the therapists to read nonverbal cues fast and accurately, misinterpretation of therapist interventions, insensitive comments among the members creating a group crisis, problems in handling negative feelings about the therapist or the group, and the pressure experienced by the group therapists from the suction of group emotion. The relatively loose nature of group boundary issues through regular use of nongroup clinical contacts with individual therapists and a 24-hour access line further complicates consistent management. This is a daunting but realistic list of issues common to any group with seriously dysfunctional members. In a long-term group with members with borderline personality disorder, group process cannot be ignored or handled in a superficial manner. Direct attempts to impose process structure in the service of mastering the clearly defined therapeutic tasks are not likely to be effective. Close attention to boundary issues and management of whole group responses involving splitting and projective identification mechanisms is likely to be required. If DBT is to be widely used outside carefully controlled academic circumstances, it is predictable that group-shattering incidents can be anticipated. These comments are not directed at the model itself. From the perspective of a group psychotherapist, the implementation of the theoretical principles of the model stand in danger of being undercut by failure to attend to basic group mechanisms as outlined earlier in this chapter.

5. The author identifies the problem faced by a group member who is making progress but

in doing so must differentiate him- or herself from the other group members. Therapists conducting longer-term groups generally see this in the opposite direction—older group members being helpful in supporting new members and indoctrinating them into a positive working atmosphere. This issue does, however, raise the question of closed or open groups. The advantage of a closed group is that members can move through the program as a unit and thus provide stage-appropriate support, challenge, and motivation for each other.

6. Linehan speculates about the possibility of a follow-up group experience to maintain improvement and to continue to apply the principles of DBT. There is also speculation about the individual therapy portion being replaced by a group format. This would simplify the model considerably and might offer the prospect of a controlled use of group process to integrate skills training material within the group itself as well as provide the opportunity to share experiences in applying the skills outside.

7. It is recommended that the group be led by cotherapists, certainly in keeping with the usual practice of longer-term group psychotherapy with severely dysfunctional members. The suggestion that there be a primary leader and a (secondary) co-leader would be problematic from the standpoint of group dynamics. The description of the leader as the "bad guy" who reinforces group norms and the co-leader as the "good guy" who empathizes and aligns with the members is of particular concern. Such a role imbalance would be considered an error in most groups, inviting a splitting process that would exert considerable pressure on the therapists to be pulled off a position of neutrality. Perhaps the descriptions in DBT material are overly graphic. The idea that therapists may have different roles is understandable, but a process to be kept continually under careful consideration so that the cotherapists are seen as a well functioning dyad with clear acknowledgement of their complementary activities. All co-led groups must struggle with the projections of group expectations and postgroup debriefings are essential for identifying subtle shifts and devising corrective actions.

The IGP and DBT models raise many interesting issues that will likely continue to be refined over time. Because these two studies are the most sophisticated in the group treatment of

borderline personality disorders, it is worth looking more closely at their comparative features. Both are designed with a clear theoretical rationale for the borderline personality disorder population. Both models place major emphasis on the features of the therapeutic alliance. The DBT emphasis on validating current emotional, cognitive, and behavioral responses is echoed in the IGP efforts to accurately understand what interpersonal issue the patient is seeking to satisfy or resolve in their interaction with his or her therapist.

Although both use a group format, there is a great difference in how the group process is applied. DBT manages group events only if they are getting in the way, whereas IGP focuses consistently on the group experience of the members. Both entail the supportive group factors of universality, acceptance, and altruism, as well as vicarious learning from other members. DBT sees skill learning as the important process; IGP views interpersonal learning as the key. The general psychotherapy appreciation of the central role of common factors would certainly apply to both. The broadening application of DBT in a variety of formats suggests that it might be better considered as a technique more than a therapy model per se. Although the same might perhaps be said for IGP, the technique is more intensely integral to the group format.

Process studies are needed of these two promising models with measures of behaviors, symptoms, syndromal features, and service utilization to gauge just how much they have in common. From the written material available, I would suggest that the group format may not be used to its fullest value in delivering the DBT material. Reviewing these two models has highlighted the issue of therapist match. DBT group therapists need to be enthusiastic about skills training or they will sabotage the treatment. IGP therapists must see the learning potential of group interaction and be comfortable in wading into it. The outcome achieved by both models is substantial, although the IGP format appeared to result in a broader range of improvement. IGP is also less complex and much closer to traditional interpersonal/psychodynamic techniques providing a more user-friendly and cost-effective approach.

It should be noted that these two studies used different technical comparison formats. The IGP used an intensive individual psychotherapy for the comparative approach. The DBT study used "treatment as usual" in the community, with 75% of control sample receiving no active treatment at all. In the psychotherapy empirical literature, virtually all active-treatment comparison studies yield relatively small differences, as is true in the pharmacotherapy literature. Thus the findings of a difference in the DBT study and no difference in the IGP study are not surprising.

Cognitive Analytic Therapy

The cognitive analytic therapy (CAT) model has evolved over the last 10–15 years from the empirical studies using repertory grid techniques conducted by Anthony Ryle (1995, 1997) in London. It has created considerable interest in the United Kingdom and Europe but is virtually unknown in North America. Like IGP and DBT, it was developed for the treatment of severe personality disorders particularly borderline personality disorder. CAT is an attractive model for psychodynamic therapists wishing to practice brief, structured therapy and also for cognitive therapists wishing to develop skills in using the therapeutic relationship.

The approach is an integration and extension of ideas and methods used in different, conventionally opposed, theoretical approaches. The main sources are as follows:

- *From psychoanalysis:* Concepts of conflict, defense, object relations, and countertransference. However, the theory is restated in cognitive terms and the therapist's interventions are more active and various than in psychoanalytic therapies.
- *From personal construct theory:* A focus on how people make sense of their world ("man as scientist") and on common sense, cooperative work with patients. However, more attention is paid to the organization of action as well as to cognitive construing.
- *From cognitive-behavioral approaches:* The step-by-step planning and measurement of change, teaching patients self-observation of moods, thoughts and symptoms. However, attention is not confined to visible behaviors and consciously accessible thoughts.
- *From developmental and cognitive psychology and artificial intelligence:* An information-processing model of how experience and actions are organized is proposed, with emphasis on the recurrent sequences of re-

lated mental (internal) and behavioral (external) processes.

CAT is a time-limited model of 24 weeks for patients with borderline personality disorder. The assessment focus is on the identification of problematic interpersonal transactions using a number of specially developed techniques. This material is then displayed in schematic diagrams that are used systematically in each session and applied by the patient. The goal is to detect patterns that do not work but are hard to break. These are descriptively clustered under the mechanisms of traps, snags, and dilemmas. For example, a dilemma might be as follows: "Either I'm involved with others and feel engulfed, taken over or smothered; or I stay safe and uninvolved but feel lonely and isolated." The parallels with both IGP and DBT are evident. After several assessment sessions, the therapist develops a "reformulation" letter to the patient that describes past experiences and their impact on the patient, the procedures developed to cope, and the nature of target problems and predicts how these might emerge in the therapy itself. This letter is read by the therapist in the session and each member recieves a copy of his or her letter to take home. Dissent is invited and a joint process of revisions is undertaken. This extended assessment process is designed to build a working alliance by accurately identifying central issues, but the written and diagrammatic process also helps to contain and soothe while minimizing regression.

The main features of the therapy are that it is active, integrated, and focused. A wide range of therapeutic methods may be combined, but the defining characteristic is the emphasis placed on the formulation and the sharing with the patient of dense descriptions of the procedures which maintain their problems. Procedures are linked sequences of mental and behavioral processes which serve as repeatedly used guidelines for purposive action. They operate mostly outside conscious awareness. Problems are caused by the persistent, unrevised use of ineffective procedures, and therapy aims to identify and revise such procedures. The constant use of the diagrams in sessions helps prevent the therapist from colluding by adopting a reciprocal role to the patient's problematic role. Although interpretations are not used, the diagrams clearly have an explanatory goal.

At the final session both therapist and patient write a formal letter describing their experience in the therapy sessions by way of saying good-bye. There is encouragement for both parties to identify possible disappointments, sadness, or anger, so that a realistic, not idealized, picture is presented. A follow-up session is scheduled in 3 months. This focuses on the target problems and the patient's continued awareness of the problematic procedures.

No randomized clinical trial has as yet been conducted with CAT. In a series of 31 carefully diagnosed patients with borderline personality disorder the dropout rate was 13% and 50% attended all sessions. At follow-up, 50% no longer met borderline personality disorder criteria and 44% were judged not to require further treatment; 26% were considered to have no change or were worse. Standard measures of symptoms showed considerable decrease with the follow-up mean scores below a level of clinical significance.

Areas of Interest

1. The use of CAT in a group context has been described in informal contributions to the CAT newsletter, but no formal group outcome studies have been performed. The model is included here because it is a carefully developed model designed specifically for borderline personality disorder that shows promise as an effective time-limited treatment. It incorporates a number of unique strategies as well as parallels to IGP and DBT techniques.

2. The use of CAT in individual therapy entails a close tracking of the interaction between therapist and patient. Such interaction would be somewhat diluted in a group. The use of written materials compensates for this dilution to some extent. In addition, the group context provides a larger range of possible interactions to use as examples of interactional procedures.

3. The extended assessment process that culminates in a "reformulation" letter could be conducted prior to the start of the group and used in early group sessions as an avenue of introduction.

Experiential Group Psychotherapy

The experiential group psychotherapy (EGP) model is based on the widely used group techniques described by Yalom (1995) as modified by Budman and Gurman (1988). The principle therapeutic experience is focused on the nature of the relationships that develop among the members. This process orientation includes many psychodynamic concepts, but these are applied to interpersonal issues, not couched in intrapsychic interpretative statements. The relationship to the therapist may be explored. The group environment is seen as a microcosm of outside-of-group issues, and there is recognition of the importance of the interpersonal transactions within the group.

Individual assessment sessions are used to establish a focus with a particular interest in how the individual's problems connect with the theme of the group. Either in the individual session(s) or in a single pregroup workshop, the members are oriented to the group and the ways in which they can most effectively use it. Maintaining a solid state of group cohesion is central, and the perspective of evolving themes related to group development is used. In each stage the issues of focus, cohesion, and more general existential issues are described. Termination is seen as particularly important for its power to deal with consolidation of learning and tolerance of separation. A follow-up interview is usually planned.

This model uses a closed group composed of 9–10 members meeting weekly for 90 minutes for about 70 sessions (18 months). No randomized clinical trial has been reported. Outcome has been reported for five groups with a total of 49 members with a range of personality disorders, not solely borderline personality disorder (Budman, Demby, et al., 1996). The results are not broken down by diagnosis, except that patients with borderline personality disorder were significantly more likely to drop out. The overall dropout rate was 51%, though much of this was because one group had major problems and was discontinued. A portion of the dropout effect may have been related to members losing their medical coverage after being laid-off because of a major recession. For those who completed treatment, symptoms, self-esteem, and social functioning all improved throughout treatment. Overall, there was a modest drop in the number of personality-disorder criteria on the Personality Disorder Examination (Loranger, Susman, Oldham, & Russakoff, 1988).

Areas of Interest

1. The empirical data base for this model is meager and the lack of data concerning those with a borderline personality disorder diagnosis makes any treatment outcome conclusions pre-

mature. The overall dropout rate was 51% and was still about 40% for the four groups that survived. The authors do not give figures for how many of the patients met full borderline personality disorder criteria and how they fared except that they were statistically more likely to be in the dropout category. This is unfortunate, because it has been an established practice to include patients with borderline personality disorder in a group with patients with neurotic problems (Pines & Hutchinson, 1993). This is based on the belief that the less disturbed members can act as a holding environment and contain the borderline personality disorder as well provide a model for managing stress through less turbulent behavior. This model has demonstrated that patients with borderline personality disorder are less likely to complete than patients without borderline personality disorder, but there is little empirical data concerning more subtle aspects of the combination approach.

2. This program is modeled on a well-established interpersonal model of group psychotherapy. It was not designed specifically for the borderline personality disorder population but has generally been assumed to be appropriate for them though with obvious technical difficulties. Many of the general principles of this model are included in the IGP model described earlier, where they provide an important perspective on managing the group effectively. These principles are not as evident in the DBT model.

Psychodynamic Group Psychotherapy

Psychodynamic group psychotherapy (PGP) shares much in common with both the Marziali and Munroe-Blum (1995) and Budman, Demby, et al. (1996) models. The difference lies in a greater use of individually focused formal intrapsychic interpretive interventions rather than a focus on interpersonal events as well as a longer-term time frame. Shaskan (1957) provided the first article to discuss in-depth group psychotherapy with borderline personality disorder. Longer-term psychodynamic group psychotherapy has probably been the modal approach for group psychotherapy over the last 50 years, largely related to Yalom's (1995) influential text. There have been few empirical studies of this model, but there is an extensive clinical literature.

The use of a combination of individual sessions and group sessions both administered by the same therapist, so-called combined therapy, has been recommended by therapists espousing both an interpretive and supportive psychodynamic model (Gans, 1990; Horwitz, 1980, 1987; Kernberg, 1975b; Kernberg, Selzer, Koenigsberg, Carr, & Appelbaum, 1989; Porter, 1993). Roller and Nelson (1991, 1999; Wong, 1980) suggest caution with this approach because of the likelihood of therapist burnout. They recommend conjoint therapy with two different therapists, emphasizing the importance of close collaboration and communication between them.

The psychodynamic group literature has tended to recommend the practice of including only up to three or four patients with borderline personality disorder in a group with predominantly chronic neurotic difficulties. The list of possible advantages of group psychotherapy (see Table 24.4) is largely derived from the psychodynamic group literature. There is a clinical impression that the therapeutic process can be accelerated in groups compared to individual therapy (Gabbard, 1995; Glatzer, 1962). This perception is thought to be related to the diffusion of relationship experiences compared to the intensity of the sole relationship found in individual work. Supportive relationships within the group that allow a gradual incorporation of less polarized relationship patterns can balance negative relationships. The borderline patient's ability to verbalize internal emotional states and fantasies may help the work of the group. The group is seen as an opportunity to display and address multiple sources of transference, countertransference, and resistance. Because of the fragmentation characteristic of patients with borderline personality disorder, the group provides a "hall of mirrors" (Foulkes, 1975) within which various split-off parts can be recognized and eventually integrated.

A major theoretical issue concerns the balance between psychodynamic interventions directed at the individual member or directed at the group-as-a-whole. Various authors (Azima, 1993; Bion, 1959; Kernberg, 1975b; Roth, Stone, & Kibel, 1990; Scheidlinger, 1974) have described the power of regressive emotional pulls to stimulate the activation of early object relationship themes, particularly in the early group. These bring with them developmentally early levels of anxiety at an early point in treatment relating to the inherent dangers of close relationships. The group-as-a-whole approach makes the assumption that all or most of the group is resonating to the same thematic material and that identifying this material will aid the group in addressing their common issues.

During early stages in the group, most therapists advocate the avoidance of interpretive interventions (Kohut, 1971). Simple empathic statements identifying and aligning with the patient's state are helpful. Even inactive participants should be allowed to enter the group process at their own rate assisted by the therapist providing supportive elements of empathy and understanding. Questions may be answered in a direct manner, a conversational style resembling "the average expectable environment." Horwitz (1977) suggests that identification of the individual member's contribution to group-centered conflict should take precedence over group-level interpretations. All these ideas reflect strategies to deal with the problems of engaging the borderline patient in the group process.

Yalom (1995) emphasizes the use of interpretive interventions that focus primarily on current group events. Past experiences and relationships are seen as important primarily because of the light they shed on understanding present behaviors. This ahistoric "here-and-now" interactional focus is to be differentiated from the application of more traditional uncovering psychoanalytic techniques in the group format.

The development of group cohesion versus idealization may pose a management problem (Stone & Whitman, 1977; Wong, 1979). Cohesion is based on each member seeing the group as a number of individuals collaborating around common tasks. This is analogous to the working alliance in individual psychotherapy. Idealization, on the other hand, carries the risk of an unrealistic distortion of the group environment. It may also lead to exposing areas of developmental arrest and the sense that others exist only to gratify personal needs. This may be reflected in an exhibitionistic quality and monopolization. The therapist must tread a difficult path between providing adequate empathy to retain the member while trying to help the group understand the function the behavior has for the individual, a function others may also be experiencing.

In groups, most confrontations occur between members. This has the advantage of coming from peers rather than more intensely invested parental transference figures. Group consensus can also be a further impetus for self-examination and change. The therapist must be alert to intercept excessive blaming or ill-motivated attacks. The therapist is also in a position to identify and align with the affective response that the target person is experiencing as well as to identify efforts to change.

Stone and Gustafson (1982) describe several dilemmas facing the therapist that must be addressed in psychodynamic group psychotherapy with severe personality disorders.

1. The narcissistic patient may idealize the therapist in order to achieve a sense of safety, whereas a borderline patient may use idealization to mask envy and rage toward the leader. Therefore the idealizing group may leave the angry patient in a false position while a common group attack on the leader leaves the idealizing patient without security. The therapist is therefore caught between opposing theoretical options for intervention.

2. The traditional cool thoughtfulness of the analytic stance may trigger an array of responses in the group members. Some may see it as a reassuring counterbalance to their own sense of turmoil. Others may view it as coldness or implying potential abandonment and seek greater empathy. Still others may be suspicious of the leader and see only "phony empathy." The therapist here again must address varying responses to varying members.

3. Empathic alignment is an important general technique with the borderline patient. However, in the group context, therapists must share interventions with all group members. Therefore, it is inevitable that members will from time to time feel that they are not receiving enough from the therapist, or that others are receiving more.

Areas of Interest

1. Perhaps the most interesting issue arises in regard to groups designed specifically for borderline personality disorder versus those that include only a smaller minority of members with more severe problems. The usual clinical impression is that those members who meet personality disorder criteria require more time and have a less satisfactory outcome. However, few papers include the use of specific diagnostic criteria. Certainly clinical reports suggest that many longer-term psychodynamic groups contain a number of patients with personality

disorders, but these tend to be primarily Cluster C diagnoses. As more patients are being treated within larger service systems, the question of group composition becomes an important issue. A larger system provides an opportunity to develop groups for such special patient populations as severe personality disorders. As this chapter attests, a variety of models are now available for consideration.

2. Piper et al. (1991) and Piper and Duncan (1999) have found a consistent predictor in the QOR measure. Patients scoring low on this measure do poorly with a formal psychodynamic interpretative approach. Mixed psychodynamic groups have historically tended to be quite interpretive in nature. This would suggest that if mixed groups were employed, an approach that stays firmly on the supportive end of the supportive–expressive continuum would be in order.

3. If the results of IGP and DBT can be maintained, then significant cost-effectiveness can be achieved within a year or less of treatment. Some of the psychodynamic literature recommends considerably longer treatment duration. The special attention to the quality of the alliance that is at the core of IGP is quite compatible with the general psychodynamic emphasis on supportive alliance-building techniques for borderline personality disorder.

4. Unfortunately, there is a dearth of empirical evidence to support the effectiveness of longer-term psychodynamic group psychotherapy and also the relative value of either individual versus group or combined treatment in this mode (Leszcz, 1992a, 1992b).

5. In a review of this area, Higgit and Fonagy (1992) suggest that "there is no compelling evidence available to recommend group therapy over individual therapy other than those deriving from economic and practical considerations." This blatant bias is customary regarding the use of groups. A more accurate interpretation of the clinical literature would be that individual and group modalities appear to be equally effective and that groups provide greater cost-effectiveness—presumably not an evil benefit.

SELECTIVE DIAGNOSTIC POPULATIONS

Avoidant Personality Disorder

Avoidant personality disorder is a syndrome characterized by a pervasive fear of criticism, humiliation and rejection, and a long-standing pattern of social anxiety and withdrawal. Avoidant personality disorder is commonly associated with a diagnosis of social phobia and often with a concurrent depressive syndrome (Turner, Beidel, Dancu, & Keys, 1986). Schizotypal features may also be found.

Social phobia has been the principal diagnostic target in most investigations, with a general recognition that social phobia comorbid with avoidant personality disorder results in a slower response (Barber, Morse, Krakauer, Chittams, & Crits-Christoph, 1997; Brown, Heimberg, & Juster, 1995; Feske, Perry, Chambless, Renneberg, & Goldstein, 1996; Van-Velzen, Emmelkamp, & Scholing, 1997). Three explanatory models have been developed: a skills-deficit model that results in anxiety and therefore withdrawal; a conditioned-anxiety model that leads to avoidance; and a cognitive-inhibition model in which negative attributions to a social context results in avoidance. Cognitive therapy, exposure *in vivo*, and social skills training have shown the most promise (Emmelkamp & Scholing, 1990; Gelernter et al., 1991; Heimberg & Juster, 1995; Hope, Heimberg & Bruch, 1995).

One of the most thoroughly studied treatments is cognitive-behavioral group therapy (CBGT; Heimberg, Juster, Hope, & Mattia, 1995). This is a multicomponent package including (1) training in cognitive coping skills, (2) multiple exposures to simulations of feared situations in session, (3) homework assignments for exposure to feared situations, and (4) use of cognitive coping skills in conjunction with exposures. CBGT has been evaluated in several studies and found to be more effective than attention–placebo treatment after 12 weeks. Patients continued to do well at 4.5- to 6.25-year follow-up.

A major randomized control study has recently been reported (Heimberg et al., 1998). Four treatment conditions were applied: phenelzine with 30-minute weekly management sessions; placebo pill with weekly sessions, cognitive-behavioral group therapy administered in 12 sessions of 2½ hours each to groups of five to seven patients, and a control educational–supportive group for 12 sessions.

In the first two sessions of CBGT, patients are taught to identify negative automatic thoughts (ATs), to observe the association between anxiety and ATs, to challenge logical errors in ATs, and to formulate rational alternatives. Thereafter, they confront increasingly difficult feared situations (first in the session and then in real life) while applying cognitive skills. When patients work on their personal target situations, a standard sequence is followed: (1) identification of ATs, (2) identification of logical errors in ATs, (3) disputation of ATs and formulation of rational responses, and (4) establishment of behavioral goals. Patients practice cognitive skills while completing behavioral tasks (e.g., conversing with another group member or giving a speech). Goal attainment and use of cognitive skills are reviewed. Behavioral "experiments" are used to confront specific reactions to the exposure. Patients are given assignments for exposure to real-life situations between sessions and instructed to complete self-administered cognitive restructuring exercises before and after.

In the control treatment, an educational–supportive group therapy, topics relevant to social phobia (e.g., fear of negative evaluation and conversation skills) was presented and discussed. Weekly handouts outline the agenda for the next session and pose questions for patients' consideration. Written responses are brought to the sessions and serve as a basis for discussion. Supportive group therapy is conducted in the second half of sessions 2 through 12. Therapists do not instruct patients to confront feared situations.

Attrition was the same in CBGT as in the medication condition. Completers and dropouts had similar demographic features and pretest measures. Group cohesion was the same in CBGT and educational–supportive group therapy. Follow-ups revealed significant differences on all measures except measures of the avoidant personality disorder syndrome itself.

Both phenelzine therapy and CBGT seem to be effective for social phobia. Compared to the pill placebo and attention–placebo conditions, both active treatments were associated with higher rates of response after 12 weeks. At this global level of response, the two active treatments produced equivalent outcomes. Seventy-seven percent of patients receiving phenelzine and 75% of patients undergoing CBGT who completed treatment (65% and 58% of enrolled patients, respectively) were classified as responders, significantly more than for placebo use or attention–placebo. Although rates of response to phenelzine therapy and CBGT were similar after 12 weeks, the pattern of response was different: 80% of 12-week phenelzine re-

sponders reached that threshold after 6 weeks, whereas only 48% of 12-week CBGT responders did so.

Areas of Interest

1. This comprehensive study provides solid evidence for the effectiveness of a psychosocial intervention for social phobia. However, medication achieved faster response and a lower level of anxiety symptoms. Avoidant personality disorder symptoms did not change although behavior did. Further details regarding the impact specifically on those patients meeting criteria for avoidant personality disorder are awaited, along with longer-term follow-up information.

2. Major depression was an exclusion item for entry into the study. In clinical practice, depression at some level is almost a routine comorbid condition.

3. The results of this study would be compatible with the practice of combining a pharmacological component and a brief course of CBGT. Further investigations with longer term follow-up data would be helpful.

4. This study is rather unique in that a creditable group therapy model was employed. This model was highly structured and avoided the core therapeutic ingredients of the active treatments. But the cohesion measures suggest that it was truly an interactive group. Such a control condition is an important feature, reinforcing the therapeutic power of the specific techniques being used. The findings are somewhat at odds with the common factor literature and deserve further investigation.

Antisocial Personality Disorder

Most studies of antisocial behavior are found in the forensic and corrections literature. Treatment has characteristically been delivered in a group format with a predominance of behavioral and cognitive models accompanied by psychoeducational modules. A common program mix might include the topics listed in Table 24.5. The corrections literature has provided evidence for the effectiveness of these types of programs (Andrews & Bonta, 1994; Barbaree, Seto, & Maric, 1996: Dwyer & Rosser, 1992; Grossman, Martis, & Fichtner, 1999; Losel, 1996; Nouwens, Motik, & Boe, 1993; Rice, Harris, & Cormier, 1992; Wexler, DeLeon, Thomas, Kressel, & Peters, 1999).

The construct of psychopathy, as tradition-

TABLE 24.5. Modules in Corrections Programs

1. Personal autobiography
2. Criminal autobiography
3. Rational-emotive behavior therapy
4. Anger management
5. Thinking errors/violence fantasies (cognitive-behavioral therapy)
6. Communication skills
7. Human relationships and sexuality
8. Crime cycle
9. Empathy
10. Relapse prevention
11. Substance use
12. Discharge plan

ly defined by Cleckley (1976), focuses on predatory personality characteristics such as superficial charm, lack of remorse or shame, and a chronically unstable and antisocial lifestyle. Hare has operationalized this construct with the 20 item Psychopathy Checklist—Revised (PCL-R; Hare, 1991; Hare, Harpur, 1990). The PCL-R incorporates two factors:

Factor 1: predatory personality characteristics related to interpersonal and affective style (e.g., grandiosity, manipulativeness, and lack of remorse or empathy) drawn from Cleckley's clinical conceptualization.

Factor 2: antisocial behavior (e.g., parasitic lifestyle, impulsivity, and irresponsibility) reflecting the DSM-IV criteria for antisocial personality disorder.

The empirical literature suggests that psychopaths, as defined by the PCL-R, respond at a significantly lower level to therapeutic interventions than do nonpsychopathic offenders. For example, Hart, Kropp, and Hare (1988) found that the probability of remaining out of prison during the first year of supervised release was directly related to PCL-R scores. Twenty-four percent of those with low scores violated the condition of release, 49% of those with medium scores, and 65% of those with high PCL-R scores. Harris, Rice, and Cormier (1991) found that psychopaths had double the rate of violent offences over a 10-year period. Extensive research indicates that PCL-R scores predict general, violent, and sexual relapse

(Grann, Langstroehm, Tengstroem, & Kullgren, 1999; Hare, 1993, 1996; Hare, McPherson, & Forth, 1988; Quinsey & Walker, 1992; Rice & Harris, 1995; Serin, 1993, 1996; Serin, Peters, & Barbaree, 1990). Approximately 20% of the forensic population have elevated scores on the PCL-R (Gacono & Hutton, 1994).

A modest literature (and a widespread belief) suggests that psychopaths do not have the capacity to respond to treatment programs. In particular, concern has been expressed that process-oriented groups are simply another playground within which the psychopath can hone manipulative skills (Harris et al., 1991; Ogloff, Wong, & Greenwood, 1990). The groups that have been described in this manner are characterized by low levels of leader focusing and control, in some cases using inmate leaders, and with poor attention to maintaining group boundaries. There is a suggestion that such groups may actually result in a worsening of pychopathic behaviors. These reports have been widely used as a rationale to avoid any group programs that contain an emphasis on the group process. This is unfortunate because these groups bear little resemblance to a properly run group program that maintains a focus on criminogenic factors.

The more technical question of the capacity of the psychopath to respond to intensive treatment has not been adequately answered in the empirical literature. The DSM-IV criteria for antisocial personality disorder do not cover most of the items of the PCL-R, including only two of the eight criteria used to define Factor 1 that describes the characterological features of the psychopath. Factor 1 is the strongest predictor of future criminal behavior even though it contains in the items no specific reference to criminal behavior per se. Only three of the nine criteria for Factor 2 are included in the DSM-IV criteria. As noted previously, the PCL-R can reliably predict criminal behavior. The relatively minor overlap between the PCL-R and DSM-IV criteria for antisocial personality disorder suggests that studies using antisocial personality disorder criteria must be considered of dubious value (Cunningham & Reidy, 1998; Hare, Hart, & Harpur, 1991). The PCL-R emphasis on characterological features is very much in keeping with the broader personality disorder literature.

A recent study examined demographic and outcome information on 171 male federal violent and sexual offenders who participated in a unique intensive treatment program between 1990 and 1994 (MacKenzie et al., 1999). As noted earlier, most corrections programs use only cognitive-behavioral and psychoeducational programming. No studies have reported results of the concomitant use of a semistructured interpersonal integrative module. This module is designed to maintain a focus on crime cycle-related behavior in several ways: as it is expressed in past history including family of origin, as it is demonstrated in the group, and as it relates to the role of affect in the crime cycle.

The program, located in the Correctional Service of Canada (CSC) Pacific Regional Health Center, is an intensive treatment program that addresses an offender's criminogenic factor domain by structuring treatment approaches to focus on the integration of adaptive coping skills. The 8-month program is built around a series of cognitive-behavioral and psychoeducational modules. In parallel with the modules, an integration module provides an opportunity to amplify and apply the other modular material. The modules are sequenced to move from factual learning to applied behavior while the integration module moves in a parallel manner into more intense interactional application with a deepening focus on the meaning of the crime cycle and relapse prevention. This combination uses two complementary methods to maintain a focus on criminal behavior. The CBT modules provide a focus through a controlled and structured process in a sequential presentation of material relevant to criminal behavior. The integration module provides a focus through a consistent tracking and reinforcing of relevant interactional patterns that apply in both the personal and criminal history of the offender as well as his behavior in the group. Thus the offender is exposed to two complementary learning modalities of gradually increasing intensity, both dealing with aspects of the criminal behavior. A related goal is to address the mechanism of splitting off of affect that may contribute to committing violent acts.

The technical goal is to create an environment in which the offender can develop a cognitive and affective appreciation of the destructive nature of his personal and criminal patterns as an internal replay of early experiences. This progression of the integrative module atmosphere promotes a deeper approach to the personal autobiography module and even more

specifically to the crime cycle and empathy modules. It provides a guided process for an active and personalized focus for addressing criminogenic factors. Much of this work is conducted between the members with the assistance of active focusing activities by the therapists.

The integrative module has a clear structured component, but the method of applying this component is different than that used in the other modules. The modules are structured around firm process control as they follow manual-driven guidelines. The integrative module structure is applied through active therapist interventions to maintain a focus on interpersonal behaviors relevant to their criminogenic patterns. The relational focus encourages active recognition of dysfunctional interpersonal behaviors and the connections of these to earlier experiences so that they can be addressed in the present context. The "real" experiences in the module also provide an opportunity to experience strong affective responses that serve both to identify issues and also to provide motivation for change.

A reasonably cohesive group environment promotes an openness to self that encourages taking the risk of revelation of areas of perceived personal vulnerability. This process promotes deeper exploration of the nature of criminal behavior and its consequences. The goal is to develop a more integrative sense of self that will support higher levels of self-efficacy and a sense of enhanced mastery over criminogenic patterns and more adaptive coping. This process builds on the earlier modules that have developed more adaptive cognitive mechanisms and applied interpersonal skills. The focus on the experience of relationship to others and to self also addresses the importance of interpersonal triggers for recidivism. Dealing directly with affective states in the module interaction provides a specific application for material from the modules, which is directed at addressing limited coping skills in which violence is seen as the only route to managing affective responses.

The offense history of the violent and sexual offenders treated in the CSC program is extensive. The mean age at first contact with correctional system is 19 years. Thirteen percent of the offenders had been convicted of one federal offense before the index offense and 57% had been convicted of two or more federal offenses. Retrospective Psychopathy Checklist scores based on pretreatment file information were correlated with postrelease follow-up information from the national offender management system data base. PCL-R scores were based on a thorough review of pretreatment file information. Total PCL-R scores can range from 0 to 40, and for this study a score of 30 or more warranted classification as a psychopath, in accordance with standard practice. Interrater reliability of three independent trained raters was monitored on an ongoing, random basis and found to be excellent ($r = .90$; $p < .001$).

Ninety-seven subjects from the total sample have been released into the community and therefore have had the opportunity to reoffend. The overall recidivism rate is considerably better than the usual recidivism curves for this group of serious criminals. This study will continue to follow these released offenders over time.

One study does not establish the validity of a treatment model, but these results with a substantial sample size are most encouraging. Further studies are required to establish the value of a treatment program that combines traditional modules focused on criminogenic factors with an intensive interpersonal module

Mixed Syndromes

There are few empirical data regarding the application of group psychotherapy to specific Cluster C syndromes and virtually none for Cluster A (Sanislow & McGlashan, 1998).

Characterological features commonly accompany treatment-resistant depression. Comorbid dysthymia is common which frequently brings with it avoidant, obsessive–compulsive and dependent features. A recent effectiveness study with 59 patients using an 18-session group format of interpersonal therapy (IPT-G) found an overall satisfactory effect size of 0.71 at termination and 1.1 at 4-month follow-up (MacKenzie, 1999). However, no formal assessment for personality disorder was used in this study. Subjects with marked schizoid and avoidant traits did less favorably.

Similarly, a series of studies of impulsive eating behaviors, bulimia nervosa, and binge eating have found a favorable response to 16-week CBT and IPT group formats (Castonguay, Pincus, Agras, & Hines, 1998; Davis, McVey, Heinmaa, Rockert, & Kennedy, 1999; Garner & Garfinkel, 1997; Nevonen, Broberg, Lindstroem, & Levin, 1999; Wilfley, Frank, Welch,

Spurrell, & Rounsaville, 1998). This patient pool also frequently contains significant personality traits, particularly borderline phenomena with bulimia nervosa and avoidant patterns with binge eating. The clinical literature reports that patients with such a comorbid presentation are less likely to have a full response to treatment. Both depression and compulsive eating disorders have a high prevalence rate. A systematic investigation of the role of personality traits and personality disorders is sorely needed in both.

It is unusual for a patient to have a single personality diagnosis. This reflects the inherent weakness of the Axis II categorical diagnostic system that contains many areas of overlapping symptoms. Benjamin (1993) has proposed an alternative approach that circumvents these problems. Her system, the Structural Analysis of Social Behavior (SASB), could be considered a generic tool for managing personality dimensions. The SASB structural model is based on a melding of the interpersonal circle (Leary, 1957) and the circumplex model developed by Schaefer (1965). In essence, the result is a triaxial system consisting of love versus hate, dominance versus submission, and psychological control-versus-psychological autonomy giving. These three dimensions account for a major portion of the variance in interpersonal behavior. The control vs. autonomy dimension reflects the importance of differentiation in the maturing process. The SASB therapist will systemically identify the patient's behavior in terms of these dimensions and purposefully respond in a manner that will not reinforce the dysfunctional pattern being displayed. For example, a patient with a tendency to positive but dependent attachment patterns would fall into the "relying on, trusting" quadrant of SASB that tends to elicit "protecting and nurturing" responses from others. These would reinforce the dependent pattern. The SASB therapist would respond in a relatively neutral, affirming manner that emphasizes a message of freeing up and autonomy while carefully avoiding overt helping behaviors. The SASB model provides a comprehensive range of such reciprocal patterns. Clearly, each personality category has typical patterns that would be in focus for these process-identifying efforts. The model is particularly effective at helping therapists avoid countertransference responses that reinforce maladaptive patterns. The SASB model has been built through many therapy process studies that indicate the validity of the theoretical basis. Formal treatment outcome studies are now required that would link interpersonal pattern changes with symptoms and overall level of functioning.

DAY TREATMENT PROGRAMS

Most of this chapter has been devoted to group models as the single treatment modality. Group psychotherapy is also an integral part of many mental health service programs: inclusion as a service component in inpatient wards, day hospitals, partial hospitalization, evening hospitals (McCallum & Piper, 1999), and day treatment programs (DTPs). Such programs are primarily designed for patients in severely dysfunctional states or patients with a psychotic illness, and to some extent personality disorders during a phase of acute decompensation. DTPs are the most common multimodality format for elective treatment of personality disorders.

The use of intensive DTPs for treatment of severe personality disorders has a lengthy history (MacKenzie & Pilling, 1972). These generally consist of 4–5 days a week with involvement in a series of groups with specialized features. DTPs typically contain a mix of interpersonal–psychodynamic theory along with influences from systems theory, milieu theory, social learning theory and biological psychiatry.

Piper, Rosie, Joyce, and Azim (1996) provide a comprehensive review of the 18-week Edmonton program that represents a particularly well-developed model for such programs. This reference includes a major survey of the DTP literature. The authors calculate that the service provides the equivalent of about 1 year's individual therapy for each patient. The compressed time frame provides an intense therapeutic atmosphere that is helpful in moving patients quickly into a working alliance. The provision of an array of groups provides a multivariate model that addresses the patient's therapeutic needs on various levels. In the course of each week, patients will participate in a variety of large and small process-oriented and structured groups. Table 24.6 lists these groups. This list represents a comprehensive application of day program scheduling. The Edmonton program can accommodate 40 patients with 10 staff members. Various DTPs will have components of such a list incorporated into their programs in relationship to the needs of the patient population.

The Edmonton program has reported a detailed empirical analysis of outcome using a randomized wait-list control group matched on diagnosis, age, and gender. Sixty percent of the patients met criteria for personality disorder, almost all from Clusters B and C. Fifty percent received diagnoses of both an affective disorder and a personality disorder. A sophisticated selection of outcome measures was used. The treated patients were significantly improved compared to the control patients in all four areas measured: interpersonal functioning, symptoms, life satisfaction, and self-esteem. Control patients showed no evidence of spontaneous re-

TABLE 24.6. Spectrum of Day Treatment Program Groups

Phase I (weeks 1–6)	Phase II (weeks 7–12)	Phase III (weeks 13–18)
Large psychotherapy group	Large psychotherapy group	Large psychotherapy group
Government group	Government group	Government group
Communications group	Personal relations group	Personal relations group
Daily living seminar I	Daily living seminar II	Daily living seminar II
Self-awareness group	Small group	Small group
Projectives group	TV group	Reentry group
	Life skills group	Life skills group
		Vocational group
Action group I	Action group II	Action group II
Exercise group	Exercise/relaxation group	Exercise group
Social outing activity	Social outing activity	Social outing activity
Recreation activity	Recreation activity	Recreation activity
Patient evaluation meeting	Patient evaluation meeting	Patient evaluation meeting

mission during the 18-week wait-list delay but did improve significantly during the treatment phase. Eight-month follow-up showed maintenance of gains and further improvement in ratings of target goal severity. Mean effect size for 19 outcome variables was 0.71; effect size for 7 core measures was 1.18. These are substantial effect sizes indicating that for the core measures, treated patients exceeded 87% of control patients. These data are well within the overall range of psychotherapy outcome despite being a population with serious and long-standing psychiatric disorders. An interesting finding was that the most powerful predictive variables were two personality characteristics: Psychological Mindedness (McCallum & Piper, 1990) and QOR (Piper & Duncan, 1999). Presence of a personality disorder was a weak predictor. Level of symptomatic distress was not a predictor of outcome.

Karterud (1992) described a 4–8-month DTP. Of the 97 patients reported in the study, about three-quarters had personality disorder diagnoses, mainly borderline personality disorder and schizotypal, and the remainder severe chronic neurotic disorders. There were few hospitalizations or suicide attempts and the dropout rate was 23% mainly from the PD patients. There was significant overall improvement with borderline personality disorder, other personality disorders showed moderate gain, and schizotypal behavior showed the least improvement. The authors emphasize that the mix of borderline personality disorder with neurotic disorders creates a balanced therapeutic community beneficial to both subgroups.

Areas for Consideration

1. Intense programs such as these raise the question of the relative value of overall duration of treatment for personality-disordered patients. The Karterud study found that outcome improved with more time, in this case between 4 to 8 months. The Edmonton program provides about the same amount of hours as a 1-year weekly individual psychotherapy. However, there is a clinical sense that change takes time, particularly for long-entrenched patterns, and usually is quoted at a year or more. Where does the optimum balance lie in terms of intensity and duration for DTPs? How important is elapsed time compared to the number of therapeutic hours? Would it be better to have fewer hours a week but longer duration? These are unanswered questions for now.

2. DTPs provide a good survey of the many uses that can be made of the group format. The coexistence of intensive small group psychotherapy presented back to back with highly structured groups seems entirely acceptable to patients, who change their mode of interaction quickly from one group to the next. This allows the impact of the program to apply at many levels of functioning. This is congruent with the current emphasis in the personality disorder literature that techniques focusing on self-management skills can be combined in individual therapy with psychological self-exploration (Livesley, 2000). The DBT model uses a highly structured group for skills training and less structured individual psychotherapy for details of application. Various other combinations could be developed such as two groups a week, one structured and one process oriented. The interesting question is how much we can learn from a fully developed day treatment model that can be applied to a less intensive format. This might have major significance in returning patients to a work environment at the earliest opportunity while still providing an intensive multimodal treatment program.

3. It needs to be emphasized that a complex DTP requires skilled and experienced leadership. The variety of programs and staff present multiple opportunities for boundary stresses. The Edmonton program, in fact, describes a time when there was major splitting between the value attributed to action-oriented groups such as psychodrama and insight-oriented groups. Most DTPs emphasize a flattened staff hierarchy and an expectation that patients will assume a significant role in the treatment process. This role must be balanced with the importance of maintaining reasonably stable intra- and intergroup boundaries. The judicious use of authority is required. Regular program management meetings with all staff are necessary and need to include the opportunity to review intrastaff tensions.

4. In an atmosphere of funding restrictions, there may be pressure to admit a broad range of patients into a single DTP. This often involves mixing treatment of personality disorders with schizophrenic rehabilitation. Such a recommendation reflects a failure to appreciate the goals of treatment. The personality disorder population needs skills training but primarily focused on interpersonal patterns, along with an opportunity for a more introspective component. The schizophrenic population requires skills of daily living and a primarily supportive

atmosphere. In fact, as described by the "expressed emotion" literature (Butzlaff & Hooley, 1998), an intrusive psychotherapy approach is likely to be harmful. A clear definition of the target population is required.

5. DTPs have been found useful in decreasing the need for inpatient care and for reducing subsequent use of intensive treatment services. Paradoxically, funding for such programs has been decreasing as these programs are replaced by quite brief and less comprehensive approaches. The capacity to generate more accurate utilization statistics now available should provide a data base to document these results in large general-service systems. This may eventually force a reconsideration of the role DTPs for selected target populations by demonstrating significant cost-effectiveness.

6. It is not clear in the literature what ingredients have the most therapeutic impact in an integrated multimodal program such as the DTP. This issue has two main questions. What are the central and universal components required for an effective program? Would streaming be useful to tailor the program to major subcategories of patients? For example, would subprograms based on interpersonal patterns for patients who have inhibitory features (i.e., nonassertive/dependent) and another for those with activation features (i.e., controlling/critical) be indicated? Or a special self-management stream for those with the major affective dyscontrol issues of borderline personality disorder? The goal would be more precise targeting based on assessment dimensions. The danger would be an interference in the nonspecific power of the large group.

SUMMARY

This chapter has reviewed the application of group psychotherapy to a diverse range of diagnoses and treatment settings. In all these, the basic principles concerning management of a group environment are important. The group process provides a powerful, nonspecific supporting, challenging, and motivating environment. This is analogous to the working alliance in individual psychotherapy but has a broader range of features. In addition to these common factors, specific applications may use the group process for specified pattern recognition or intervention strategies. The chapter has identified a number of group models for application to specific personality disorders. It is no longer appropriate to speak simply of prescribing group psychotherapy. As in the individual psychotherapy literature, specific models are now available to augment the general benefits of group psychotherapy.

REFERENCES

Anchin, J. C., & Kiesler, D. J. (Eds.) (1982). *Handbook of interpersonal psychotherapy.* New York: Pergamon Press.

Andrews, D. A., & Bonta, J. (1994). *The psychology of criminal conduct.* Cincinnati: Anderson.

Azim, H. F. A., Piper, W. E., Segal., P. M., Nixon, G. W. H., & Duncan, S. C. (1991). The quality of object relations scale. *Bulletin of the Menninger Clinic, 55,* 323–343.

Azima, F. (1993). Group psychotherapy with personality disorders. In H. L. Kaplan & B. J. Sadock (Eds.), *Comprehensive group psychotherapy* (pp. 393–406). Baltimore: Williams & Wilkins.

Barbaree, H. E., Seto, M., & Maric, A. (1996). Effective sex offender treatment: The Warkworth Sexual Behavior Clinic. *Forum on Correctional Research, 8,* 13–15.

Barber, J. P., Morse, J. Q., Krakauer, I. D., Chittams, J., & Crits-Christoph, K. (1997). Change in obsessive–compulsive and avoidant personality disorders following time-limited supportive–expressive therapy. *Psychotherapy, 34,* 133–143.

Bednar, R. L., Melnick, J., & Kaul, T. J. (1974). Risk, responsibility, and structure: a conceptual framework for initiating group counseling and psychotherapy. *Journal of Counseling Psychology, 21,* 31–37.

Benjamin, L. S. (1993). *Interpersonal diagnosis and treatment of personality disorders.* New York: Guilford Press.

Bion, W. R. (1959). *Experiences in groups and other papers.* New York: Basic Books.

Bond, G. R. (1983). Norm regulation in therapy groups. In R. R. Dies & K R. MacKenzie (Eds.), *Advances in group psychotherapy: Integrating research and practice.* (pp. 171–189). New York: International Universities Press.

Book, H. (1998). *How to practice brief psychodynamic psychotherapy: The core conflictual relationship theme model.* Washington, DC: American Psychological Association.

Bordin, E. S. (1979). The generalizability of the psychoanalytic concept of the working alliance. *Psychotherapy: Theory, Research and Practice, 16,* 252–260.

Brown, E. J., Heimberg, R. G., & Juster, H. R. (1995). Social phobia subtype and avoidant personality disorder: Effect on severity of social phobia, impairment, and outcome of cognitive-behavioral treatment. *Behavior Therapy, 26,* 467–486.

Budman, S. H., Cooley, S., Demby, A., Koppenaal, G., Koslof, J., & Powers, T. (1996). A model of time-effective group psychotherapy for patients with personality disorders: The clinical model. *International Journal of Group Psychotherapy, 46,* 329–355.

Budman, S. H., Demby, A., Feldstein, M., Redondo, J., Scherz, B., Bennett, M. J., Koppenaal, G., Daley, B. S., Hunter, M., & Ellis, J. (1987). Preliminary findings on a new instrument to measure cohesion in group psychotherapy. *International Journal of Group Psychotherapy, 37,* 75–94.

Budman, S. H., Demby, A., Soldz, S., & Merry, J. (1996). Time-limited group psychotherapy for patients with personality disorders: Outcomes and dropouts. *International Journal of Group Psychotherapy, 46,* 357–377.

Budman, S. H., & Gurman, A. S. (1988). *Theory and practice of brief therapy.* New York: Guilford Press.

Budman, S. H., Soldz, S., Demby, A., Feldstein, M., Springer, T., & Davis, S. (1989). Cohesion, alliance and outcome in group psychotherapy. *Psychiatry, 52,* 339–350.

Butzlaff, R. L., & Hooley, J. M. (1998). Expressed emotion and psychiatric relapse: A meta-analysis. *Archives of General Psychiatry, 55,* 547–552.

Castonguay, L. G., Pincus, A. L., Agras, W. S., & Hines, C. E. (1998). The role of emotion in group cognitive-behavioral therapy for binge eating disorder: When things have to feel worse before they get better. *Psychotherapy Research, 8,* 225–238.

Cleckley, H. (1976). *The mask of sanity.* St. Louis: Mosby.

Cooley, C. H. (1912). *Human nature and the social order.* New York: Scribner.

Cunningham, M. D., & Reidy, T. J. (1998). Antisocial personality disorder and psychopathy: Diagnostic dilemmas in classifying patterns of antisocial behavior in sentencing evaluations. *Behavioral Sciences and the Law, 16,* 333–351.

Davis, R., McVey, G., Heinmaa, M., Rockert, W., & Kennedy, S. (1999). Sequencing of cognitive-behavioral treatments for bulimia nervosa. *International Journal of Eating Disorders, 25,* 361–374.

Dawson, D. F. (1988). Treatment of the borderline patient, relationship management. *Canadian Journal of Psychiatry, 33,* 370–374.

Dawson, D. L., & Macmillan, H. L. (1993). *Relationship management of the borderline patient: From understanding to treatment.* New York: Brunner/Mazel.

Dwyer, S. M., & Rosser, B. R. S. (1992). Treatment outcome research: Cross-referencing a six-month to ten-year follow-up study on sex offenders. *Annals of Sex Research, 5,* 87–97.

Emmelkamp, P. M. G., & Scholing, A. (1990). A behavioral treatment for simple and social phobics. In G. D. Burrows, R. Noyes, & G. M. Roth (Eds.), *Handbook of anxiety* (Vol. 4, pp. 327–361). Amsterdam: Elsevier.

Feske, U., Perry, K. J., Chambless, D. L., Renneberg, B., & Goldstein, A. J. (1996). Avoidant personality disorder as a predictor for treatment outcome among generalized social phobics. *Journal of Personality Disorders, 10,* 174–184.

Foulkes, S. H. (1975). *Group-analytic psychotherapy: Method and principles.* London: Gordon & Breach.

Gabbard, G. O. (1995). *Psychodynamic psychiatry in clinical practice.* Washington, DC: American Psychiatric Press.

Gacano, C. B., & Hutton, H. E. (1994). Suggestions for the clinical and forensic uses of the Hare Pschopathy Checklist—Revised (PCL-R). *International Journal of Law and Psychiatry, 17,* 303–317.

Gans, J. S. (1990). Broaching and exploring the question of combined group and individual therapy. *International Journal of Group Psychotherapy, 40,* 123–137.

Garner, D. M., & Garfinkel, P. E. (Eds.). (1997). *Handbook of treatment for eating disorders* (2nd ed.). New York: Guilford Press.

Gaston, L. (1990). The concept of the alliance and its role in psychotherapy: Theoretical and empirical considerations. *Psychotherapy, 27,* 143–153.

Gaston, L. (1991). Reliability and criterion-related validity of the California Psychotherapy Alliance Scales—Patient version. *Psychological Assessment: A Journal of Consulting and Clinical Psychology, 3,* 68–74.

Gaston, L., & Marmar, C. (1991). *Manual of California Psychotherapy Alliance Scales.* San Francisco: University of California Press.

Gelernter, C. S., Uhde, T. W., Cimbolic, P., Arnkoff, D. B., Vittone, B. J., Tancer, M. E., & Bartko, J. J. (1991). Cognitive-behavioral and pharmacological treatments of social phobia: A controlled study. *Archives of General Psychiatry, 48,* 938–945.

Glatzer, H. I. (1962). Handling narcissistic problems in group psychotherapy. *International Journal of Group Psychotherapy, 12,* 448–455.

Grann, M., Langstroem, N., Tengstroem, A., & Kullgren, G. (1999). Psychopathy (PCL-R) predicts violent recidivism among criminal offenders with personality disorders in Sweden. *Law and Human Behavior, 23,* 205–217.

Grossman, L. S., Martis, B., & Fichtner, C. G. (1999). Are sex offenders treatable? A research overview. *Psychiatric Services, 50,* 349–361.

Gunderson, J. G. (1984). *Borderline personality disorder.* Washington, DC: American Psychiatric Press.

Hare, R. D. (1991). *The Hare Psychopathy Checklist—Revised.* Toronto: Multi-Health Systems.

Hare, R. D. (1993). *Without conscience.* New York: Simon & Schuster.

Hare, R. D. (1996). *Psychopathy: A clinical construct whose time has come. Criminal Justice and Behavior, 23,* 25–54.

Hare, R. D., Harpur, T. J., Hakstian, A. R., Forth, A. E., Hart, S. D., & Newman, J. P. (1990). The revised Psychopathy Checklist: Reliability and factor structure. *Psychological Assessment: A Journal of Consulting and Clinical Psychology, 2,* 338–341.

Hare, R. D., Hart, S. D., & Harpur, T. J. (1991). Psychopathy and the DSM-IV criteria for antisocial personality disorder. *Journal of Abnormal Psychology, 100,* 391–398.

Hare, R. D., McPherson, L. M., & Forth, A. E. (1988). Male psychopaths and their criminal careers. *Journal of Consulting and Clinical Psychology, 56,* 710–714.

Harris, G. T., Rice, M. E., & Cormier, C. A. (1991). Psychopathy and violent recidivism. *Law and Human Behavior, 15,* 625–637.

Hart, S. D., Kropp, P. R., & Hare, R. D. (1988). Performane of male psychopaths following conditional release from prison. *Journal of Clinical and Consulting Psychology, 56,* 227–232.

Heimberg, R. G., & Juster, H. R. (1995). Cognitive behavioral treatments: Literature review. In R. G. Heimberg, M. R. Liebowitz, D. H. Hope, & F. R. Schneier (Eds.), *Social phobia: Diagnosis, assessment and treament* (pp. 261–309). New York: Guilford Press.

Heimberg, R. G., Juster, H. R., Hope, D. A., & Mattia, J. I. (1995). Cognitive behavioral group treatment for social phobia: Description, case presentation and empirical support. In M. B. Stein (Ed.), *Social phobia: Clinical and research perspectives* (pp. 293–321). Washington, DC: American Psychiatric Press.

Heimberg, R. G., Liebowitz, M. R., Hope, D. A., Schneier, F. R., Holt, C. S., Welkowitz, L. A., Juster, H. R., Campeas, R., Bruch, M. A., Cloitre, M., Fallon, B., & Klein, D. F. (1998). Cognitive behavioral group therapy vs phenelzine therapy for social phobia: 12 week outcome. *Archives of General Psychiatry, 55,* 1133–1141.

Higgit, A., & Fonagy, P. (1992). Psychotherapy in borderline and narcissistic personality disorder. *British Journal of Psychiatry, 161,* 23–43.

Hilkey, J., Wilhelm, C., & Horne, A. (1982). Comparative effectiveness of videotape pretraining versus no pretraining on selected process and outcome variables in group therapy. *Psychological Reports, 50,* 1151–1159.

Hope, D. A., Heimberg, R. G., & Bruch, M. A. (1995). Dismantling cognitive-behavioral group therapy for social phobia. *Behavior Research Therapy, 33,* 637–650.

Horvath, A. O., & Symonds, B. D. (1991). Relations between working alliance and outcome in psychotherapy: A meta-analysis. *Journal of Counseling Psychology, 38,* 139–149.

Horwitz, L. (1977). A group-centered approach to group psychotherapy. *International Journal of Group Psychotherapy, 27,* 423–439.

Horwitz, L. (1980). Group psychotherapy for borderline and narcissistic patients. *Bulletin of the Menninger Clinic, 44,* 281–299.

Horwitz, L. (1987). Indications for group psychotherapy with borderline and narcissistic patients. *Bulletin of the Menninger Clinic, 51,* 248–260.

Howard, K. I., Kopta, S. M., Krause, M. S., & Orlinsky, D. E. (1986). The dose–effect relationship in psychotherapy. *American Psychologist, 41,* 159–164.

Howard, K. I., Lueger, R., & Schank, D. (1992). The psychotherapeutic service delivery system. *Psychotherapy Research, 2,* 164–180.

Howard, K. I., Lueger, R. J., Maling, M. S., & Martinovich, Z. (1993). A phase model of psychotherapy: Causal mediation of outcome. *Journal of Consulting and Clinical Psychology, 61,* 678–685.

Jang, K. L., McCrae, R. R., Angleitner, A., Riemann, R., & Livesley, W. J. (1998). Heritability of facet-level traits in a cross-cultural twin sample: Support for a hierarchical model of personality. *Journal of Personality and Social Psychology, 74,* 1556–1565.

Karterud, S. (1992). Day hospital therapeutic community treatment for patients with personality disorders: An empirical evaluation of the containment function. *Journal of Nervous and Mental Disease, 180,* 238–243.

Kaul, T. J., & Bednar, R. L. (1994). Pretaining and structure: Parallel lines yet to meet. In A. Fuhriman, G. M. Burlingame (Eds.), *Handbook of group psychotherapy: An empirical and clinical synthesis* (pp. 155–188). New York: Wiley.

Kernberg, O. (1975a). *Borderline conditions and pathological narcissism.* New York: Jason Aronson.

Kernberg, O. (1975b). A systems approach to priority setting of interventions in groups. *International Journal of Group Psychotherapy, 25,* 251–275.

Kernberg, O. F., Selzer, M. A., Koenigsberg, H. W., Carr, A. C., & Appelbaum, A. H. (1989). *Psychodynamic psychotherapy of borderline patients.* New York: Basic Books.

Kivlighan, D. M., & Goldfine, D. C. (1991). Endorsement of therapeutic factors as a function of stage of group development and participant interpersonal attitudes. *Journal of Counseling Psychology, 38,* 150–158.

Kivlighan, D. M., & Mullison, D. (1988). Participants' perception of therapeutic factors in group counseling: The role of interpersonal style and stage of group development. *Small Group Behavior, 19,* 452–468.

Klein, R. H., Orleans, J. F, & Soule C. R. (1991). The axis 11 group: Treating severely characterologically disturbed patients. *International Journal of Group Psychotherapy, 41,* 97–115.

Klerman, G. L., Weissman, M. M., Rounsaville, B. J., & Chevron, E. S. (1984). *Interpersonal Psychotherapy of depression.* New York: Basic Books.

Kohut, H. (1971). *The analysis of the self.* New York: International Universities Press.

Kolden, G., & Howard, K. (1992). An empirical test of the generic model of psychotherapy. *Journal of Psychotherapy Practice and Research, 1,* 225–236.

Kopta, S. M., Howard, K. I., Lowry, J. L., & Beutler, L. E. (1994). Patterns of symptomatic recovery in time-unlimited psychotherapy. *Journal of Consulting and Clinical Psychology, 62,* 1009–1016.

Leary, T. (1957). *Interpersonal diagnosis of personality.* New York: Ronald Press.

Leszcz, M. (1992a). Group psychotherapy of the borderline patient. In D. Silver & M. Rosenbluth (Eds.), *Handbook of borderline disorders* (pp. 435–469). Madison, CT: International Universities Press.

Leszcz, M. (1992b). The interpersonal approach to group psychotherapy. *International Journal of Group Psychotherapy, 42,* 37–62.

Linehan, M. M. (1993). *Cognitive-behavioral treatment of borderline personality disorder.* New York: Guilford Press.

Linehan, M. M., Armstrong, H. E., Suarez, A., Allmon, D., & Heard, H. L. (1991). Cognitive-behavioral treatment of chronically parasuicidal borderline patients. *Archives of General Psychiatry, 48,* 1060–1064.

Linehan, M. M., Heard, H. L., & Armstrong, H. E. (1993). Naturalistic follow-up of a behavioral treatment of chronically parasuicidal borderline patients. *Archives of General Psychiatry, 50,* 971–974.

Livesley, W. J. (1998). Suggestions for a framework for

an empirically based classification of personality disorder. *Canadian Journal of Psychiatry, 43,* 137–147.

Livesley, W. J., Jang, K. L., & Vernon, P. A. (1998). Phenotypic and genetic structure of traits delineating personality disorder. *Archives of General Psychiatry, 55,* 941–948.

Livesley, W. J. (2000). A practical approach to the treatment of borderline personality disorder. *Psychiatric Clinics of North America, 23,* 211–232.

Loranger, A. W., Susman, V. L., Oldham, J. M., & Russakoff, L. M. (1988). *Personality Disorder Examination (PDE) manual.* Yonkers, NY: DV Communications.

Losel, F. (1996). Effective correctional programming: what empirical research tells us and what it doesn't. *Forum on Correctional Research, 8,* 33–37.

Luborsky, L., & Crits-Christoph, P. (1997). *Understanding transference: The core conflictual realtionship theme method* (2nd ed.). Washington, DC: American Psychological Association.

MacKenzie, K. R. (1979). Group norms: Importance and measurement. *International Journal of Group Psychotherapy, 29,* 471–480.

MacKenzie, K. R. (1983). The clinical application of a group climate measure. In R. R. Dies & K. R. MacKenzie (Eds.), *Advances in group psychotherapy: Integrating research and practice* (pp. 159–170). New York: International Universities Press.

MacKenzie, K. R. (1997). *Time-managed group psychotherapy: Effective clinical applications.* Washington DC: American Psychiatric Press.

MacKenzie, K. R. (1998). The alliance in time-limited group psychotherapy. In J. D. Safran & J. C. Muran (Eds.), *The therapeutic alliance in brief psychotherapy* (pp. 193–215). Washington DC: American Psychological Press.

MacKenzie, K. R. (1999). *Anti-depression interpersonal psychotherapy groups: Preliminary effectiveness data.* Paper presented at the Society for Psychotherapy Research Conference, Braga, Portugal.

MacKenzie, K. R., Brink, J., Hills, A. L., Jang, K., Livesley, J., Smiley, W. C., & McHattie, L. (1999). *Group treatment outcome for psychopathic inmates.* Paper presented at the annual conference of the American Psychiatric Association, Washington, DC.

MacKenzie, K. R., & Pilling, L. F. (1972). An intensive therapy day clinic for out-of-town patients with neurotic and psychosomatic problems. *International Journal of Group Psychotherapy, 22,* 352–363.

MacKenzie, K. R., & Tschuschke, V. (1993). Relatedness, group work, and outcome in long-term inpatient psychotherapy groups. *Journal of Psychotherapy Practice and Research, 2,* 147–156.

Marziali, E., & Munroe-Blum, H. (1994). *Interpersonal group psychotherapy for borderline personality disorder.* New York: Basic Books.

Marziali, E., & Munroe-Blum, H. (1995). An interpersonal approach to group psychotherapy with borderline personality disorder. *Journal of Personality Disorders, 9,* 179–189.

Marziali, E., Munroe-Blum, H., & McCleary, L. (1999). The Ojective Behavioral Index: A measure for assessing treatment response of patients with severe personality disorders. *Journal of Nervous and Mental Disease, 187,* 290–295.

McCallum, M., Piper, W. E. (1990). The psychological mindedness assessment procedure. *Psychological Assessment: A Journal of Consulting and Clinical Psychology 2,* 412–418.

McCallum, M., & Piper, W. E. (1999). Personality disorders and response to group-oriented evening treatment. *Group Dynamics: Theory, Research, and Practice 3,* 3–14.

McRoberts, C., Burlingame, G. M., & Hoag, M. J. (1998). Comparative efficacy of individual and group psychotherapy: a meta-analytic perspective. *Group Dynamics: Theory, Research, and Practice 2,* 101–117.

Mead, G. H. (1934). *Mind, self and society.* Chicago: University of Chicago Press.

Munroe-Blum, H., & Marziali, E. (1995). A controlled trial of short-term group treatment for borderline personality disorder. *Journal of Personality Disorders, 9,* 190–198.

Nevonen, L., Broberg, A. G., Lindstroem, M., & Levin, B. (1999). A sequenced group psychotherapy model for bulimia nervosa patients: A pilot study. European Eating Disorders Review 7, 17–27.

Nouwens, T., Motik, L., & Boe, R. (1993). So you want to know the recidivism rate. Forum on Correctional Research 5, 22–26.

Ogloff, J. R., Wong, S., & Greenwood, A. (1990). Treating criminal psychopaths in a therapeutic community program. *Behavioral Sciences and the Law 8,* 181–190.

Piper, W. E., Azim, H. F. A., Joyce, A. S., McCallum, M., Nixon, G. W. H., & Segal, P. S. (1991). Quality of object relations versus interpersonal functioning as predictors of therapeutic alliance and psychotherapy outcome. *Journal of Nervous and Mental Disease, 179,* 432–438.

Piper, W. E., Debbane, E. G., Bienvenu, J. P., & Garant, J, (1982). A study of group pretraining for group psychotherapy. *International Journal of Group Psychotherapy, 32,* 309–325.

Piper, W., Debbane, E., Garant, J., & Bienvenu, J. (1979). Pretraining for group psychotherapy. *Archives of General Psychiatry, 36,* 1250–1256.

Piper, W. E., & Duncan, S. (1999). Object relations theory and short-term dynamic psychotherapy: findings from the Quality of Object Relations Scale. *Clinical Psychology Review 19,* 669–686.

Piper, W. E., & Joyce, A. S. (1996). A consideration of factors influencing the utilization of time-limited, short-term group therapy. *International Journal of Group Psychotherapy, 46,* 311–328.

Piper, W. E., Rosie, J. S., Joyce, A. S., & Azim, H. F. A. (1996). *Time-limited day treatment for personality disorders: Integration of research design and practice in a group program.* Washington DC: American Psychological Association.

Porter, K. (1993). Combined individual and group psychotherapy. In A. Alonso & H. I. Swiller (Eds.),

Group therapy in clinical practice (pp. 309–341). Washington, DC: American Psychiatric Press.

Quinsey, V. L., & Walker, W. D. (1992). Dealing with dangerousness: Community risk management strategies with violent offenders. In D. V. Peters, R. J. McMahon, & V. L. Quinsey (Eds.), *Aggression and Violence throughout the lifespan* (pp. 244–262). Newbury Park, CA: Sage.

Rice, M. E., & Harris, G. T. (1995). Violent recidivism: assessing predictive validity. *Journal of Consulting and Clinical Psychology, 63,* 737–748.

Rice, M. E., Harris, G. T., & Cormier, C. A. (1992). An evaluation of a maximum security therapeutic community for psychopaths and other mentally disordered offenders. *Law and Human Behavior 16,* 399–412.

Rockland, L. H. (1992). *Supportive therapy for borderline patients: A psychodynamic approach.* New York: Guilford Press.

Roller, B., & Nelson, V. (1991). *The art of co-therapy: How therapists work together.* New York: Guilford.

Roller, B., & Nelson, V. (1999). Group psychotherapy treatment of borderline personalities. *International Journal of Group Psychotherapy, 49,* 369–385.

Roth, B. E., Stone, W. N., & Kibel, H. D. (Eds.) (1990). *The difficult patient in group: Group psychotherapy with borderline and narcissistic disorders.* Madison, CT: International Universities Press.

Ryle, A. (Ed.) (1995). *Cognitive analytic therapy.* New York: Wiley.

Ryle, A. (1997). *Cognitive analytic therapy and borderline personality disorder.* New York: Wiley.

Safran, J. D., & Muran, J. C. (1996). The resolution of ruptures in the therapeutic alliance. *Journal of Consulting and Clinical Psychology, 64,* 447–458.

Safran, J. D., & Muran, J. C. (Eds.) (1998). *The therapeutic alliance in brief psychotherapy.* Washington, DC: American Psychological Press.

Sanislow, C. A., & McGlashan, T. H. (1998). Treatment outcome of personality disorders. *Canadian Journal of Psychiatry 43,* 237–250.

Schaefer, E. S. (1965). Configurational analysis of children's reports of parent behavior. *Journal of Consulting Psychology, 29,* 552–557.

Scheidlinger, S. (1974). On the concept of "mother-group." *International Journal of Group Psychotherapy, 24,* 417–428.

Scheidlinger, S. (1983). *Focus on group psychotherapy.* New York: Basic Books.

Serin, R. C. (1993). Diagnosis of psychopathology with and without an interview. *Journal of Clinical Psychology 49,* 367–372.

Serin, R. C. (1996). Violent recidivism in criminal psychopaths. *Law and Human Behavior 20,* 207–217.

Serin, R. C., Peters, R. D., & Barbaree, H. E. (1990). Predictors of psychopathy and release outcome in a criminal population. *Psychological Assessment: A Journal of Consulting and Clinical Psychology 2,* 419–422.

Shaskan, D. A. (1957). Treatment of a borderline case with group analytically oriented psychotherapy. *Journal of Forensic Sciences II,* 195–201.

Smith, M. L., Glass, G. V., & Miller, T. I. (1980). *The benefits of psychotherapy.* Baltimore: Johns Hopkins University Press.

Stone, W. M., & Gustafson, J. P. (1982). Technique in group psychotherapy of narcissistic and borderline patients. *International Journal of Group Psychotherapy, 32,* 29–47.

Stone, W. N., & Whitman, R. M. (1977). Contributions of the psychology of the self to group process and group therapy. *International Journal of Group Psychotherapy, 27,* 343–359.

Sullivan, H. S. (1953). *The interpersonal theory of psychiatry.* New York: Norton.

Tillitski, C. J. (1990). A meta-analysis of estimated effect size for group vs. individual vs. control treatments. *International Journal of Group Psychotherapy, 40,* 215–224.

Toseland, R. W., & Siporin, M. (1986). When to recommend group treatment: A review of the clinical and group literature. *International Journal of Group Psychotherapy, 36,* 171–201.

Turner, S. M., Beidel, D. C., Dancu, C. V., & Keys, D. J. (1986). Psychopathology of social phobia and comparison to avoidant personality disorder. *Journal of Abnormal Psychology 95,* 389–394.

Vaillant, G. E. (1992). The beginning of wisdom is never calling a patient a borderline. *Journal of Psychotherapy Practice and Research 1,* 117–134.

Van-Velzen, C. J. M., Emmelkamp, P. M. G., & Scholing, A. (1997). The impact of personality disorders on behavioral treatment outcome for social phobia. *Behavior Research and Therapy 35,* 889–900.

Waldinger, R., & Gunderson, J. G. (1987). *Effective psychotherapy wih borderline patients.* Toronto: MacMillan.

Wexler, H. K., DeLeon, G., Thomas, G., Kressel, D., & Peters, J. (1999). The Amity prison TC evaluation: Reincarceration outcomes. *Criminal Justice and Behavior 26,* 147–167.

Wilfley, D. E., Frank, M. A., Welch, R., Spurrell, E. B., & Rounsaville, B. J. (1998). Adapting interpersonal psychotherapy to a group format (IPT-G) for binge eating disorder: Toward a model for adapting empirically supported treatments. *Psychotherapy Research 8,* 379–391.

Wong, N. (1979). Clinical considerations in group treatment of narcissistic disorders. *International Journal of Group Psychotherapy, 29,* 325–345.

Wong, N. (1980). Combined group and individual treatment of borderline and narcissisic patients: Heterogenous vs. homogenous groups. *International Journal of Group Psychotherapy, 30,* 389–404.

Yalom, I. D. (1995). *The theory and practice of group psychotherapy* (4th ed.). New York: Basic Books.

CHAPTER 25

Partial Hospitalization Programs

HASSAN F. AZIM

Partial hospitalization has been offered as day, evening/night, but rarely weekend programs. It will be advanced in this chapter that partial hospitalization has been one of the effective treatment modalities for persons suffering from personality disorders. Yet, until recently, there has been a paucity of reports on the subject in general. Two interacting reasons have been suggested for such benign neglect: a history of a lack of classificatory clarity and underutilization. The former consists of a combination of a lack of operational definitions and a common language for communication, and thus an insufficiency of the research findings. This lack of clarity has prevailed until a member of my team proposed a clarification that has since been adopted in the literature (Rosie, 1987). Three main categories of partial hospitalization were identified. *Day hospitals* proper have been serving two functions: an alternative to inpatient care or a transitional service between inpatient and outpatient or community care (step-down units). *Day care* is a modality characterized by offering time-unlimited maintenance and rehabilitation for patients suffering from persistent, severe, and disabling illness, including personality disorders. In contrast, day treatment programs provide time-limited intensive combination of treatment, habilitation (see later), and rehabilitation to patients with relatively higher psycho-social functioning than the two other forms (Azim, 1993). The other reason

has been the historical underutilization of partial hospitalization programs, particularly in the United States, a country with the highest levels of concentration, openings, and closures of day hospitals than any other. This issue of underutilization has been so ubiquitous that there is hardly any publication on partial hospitalization that does not include comments on this issue.

Economic factors have been proposed as the determinant agents of this phenomenon. Thus, whereas inpatient psychiatric care has traditionally been fully covered and has consumed 70% of all mental health expenditures in the United States (Kiesler, 1982), only 20–25% of all patient charges for partial hospitalization are covered by insurance, public or private. Furthermore, the cost of partial hospitalization, like that of home care and outpatient psychiatry, has been subjected to copayment by the patients and their families. In addition to these discriminatory practices and inequitable coverage of partial hospitalization, the programs themselves have contributed to underutilization. There has been a tendency to be remiss in attending to the sensibilities of the referring sources, inevitably leading to a perception of elitism and hence to a decline in admissions. (Rosie, Azim, Piper, & Joyce 1995). Patients' living arrangements, the distance between the patients' residence and the treatment site, and the need for transportation and other instrumental factors all play a role. Moreover, for decades hospital administrators had no incentives to use innovative and less costly alternatives such as partial hospitalization, in favor of the more economically rewarding policies of keeping the oversupply of their beds fully occupied (Herz, Ferman, & Cohen, 1985). Such practices continued despite the assertion that 70–90% of patients treated as inpatients may benefit from partial hospitalization (Schene & Gensons, 1986). Ideally, recent health reform efforts should stem this tide. Many studies have documented a general acceptance, a higher level of satisfaction, and a less objective and subjective burden experienced by partial hospitalization patients and their families, in comparison to inpatients (Lystad, 1958; Odenheimer, 1965; Washburn, Vannicelli, Longabaugh, & Scheff, 1976).

Clinician bias against partial hospitalization has been attributed to such factors as lack of knowledge and training and the lower level of remuneration compared to inpatient care, leading to a disinclination by clinicians to refer patients and, more importantly, less interest in working in partial hospitalization settings. (For a fuller review of underutilization, see Piper, Rosie, Joyce, & Azim, 1996.)

It is perhaps instructive that the drive behind inaugurating the first modern-day hospital in 1946 at the Allan Memorial Institute of Psychiatry of McGill University in Montreal was not the obvious cost-effectiveness of partial hospitalization. The explicit intention of its innovator, Dr. Ewin Cameron, was to give expression to his conviction that psychiatric patients do not need to stay in bed and do not have to remain in the hospital until they are well (and in fact they often do not get well if we try to make them stay), and that in addition to the patient, the family unit and the general social setting are required to be attended to (Cameron, 1947). By any measure, this was revolutionary then, still is, and has hardly been heeded even today, notwithstanding the advocacy for a biopsychosocial model.

The nefarious effects of the marketplace morality on the utilization of partial hospitalization can be demonstrated by its reverse. There are reports from countries such as Canada and the Netherlands documenting full or even overutilization of such programs, all thanks to the grace of the social responsibility that made the Canadian and Dutch universal health care systems what they have been until recently (Piper et al., 1996; Schene, van Lieshout, & Mastboom, 1988; Whitelaw & Perez, 1987). A literature search yielded reports on only two partial hospitalization programs in the United States that had enjoyed full utilization. In both cases, funding was uncharacteristically stable and not copayment-dependent (Glenner & Glenner, 1989; Sternquist, 1991).

DAY-HOSPITAL PROGRAMS

The first modern-day hospital in North America was organized as a day hospital program. Such programs as inpatient services offered intensive treatment, including somatic interventions in the form of insulin coma and subcoma, sedatives, hypnotics, and electroconvulsive therapy. The length of stay usually varied from a few days to a few weeks. This stay was often supplemented by psychosocial therapy, sometimes in a different setting (Cameron, 1947; Dickey, Berren, Santiago, & Breslau, 1990). According to Cameron "the day hospital [was] thought of as extending and supplementing the work of the [inpatient unit]. It may be that for certain categories of patients at least, it will eventually take its place; but at present the Day Hospital . . . [has been] operated in association with [an inpatient service]" (Cameron, 1947). Thus the day hospital proper has served two functions: (1) an alternative to inpatient care and (2) a transitional service between inpatient and outpatient or community care. More recently, the latter has been resurrected under the rubric of step-down units. The admission criteria have been primarily exclusionary ones: serious potential for harm to self or others, active substance abuse, and cognitive impairment. However, the potential of seriously harming self or others depends in part on the perceptions of the referring source, the day-hospital staff and the patient's relatives (Creed, Black, & Anthony, 1989). These criteria cannot be more challenging than in the case of patients suffering from personality disorders who characteristically exhibit impulsivity, paranoid thinking, compulsivity, and parasuicidal tendencies. A better understanding of the psychodynamics of these behaviors has been on the rise during the last two decades. In addition there has been accumulated evidence for the effectiveness of the selective reuptake ihhibitors (SRIs), anticonvulsants, and neuroleptics (Koenigsberg, 1993) in the treatment of the manifestations of personality disorders. It therefore seems more possible than ever and even desirable to treat these patients in a day-hospital program during a crisis. An alternative would be to transfer the patient to a step-down setting after as short an inpatient admission as possible. If this is done at the onset of the illness, the personality disordered might be spared a career of a revolving inpatient readmissions, eventually leading to invalidism. Such recurrent episodes of promised tender loving care followed by perceived abandonment at the time of discharge are often experienced as a traumatic recapitulation of their past. By contrast, the day hospital staff should offer an explicit contract to provide crisis intervention, limited to hours or days, with an emphasis on forging a follow-up plan worked out with the patient and the significant others on admission. It is at this crucial juncture of the disorder's trajectory that a thorough assessment of the patient's level of functioning and disability should be done in order to make informed and individually tailored decisions regarding follow-up. A failure to do so can only lead to dire and costly consequences: the patient reliving abandonment and neglect, the family feeling more helpless and hateful toward the patient, and the setting of a pattern of recurrent crises and heroic interventions. The availability of the two other forms of partial hospitalization (day care and day treatment programs) could meet the needs of the majority of the personality-disordered beyond crisis interventions.

Research on Day-Hospital Programs

Early studies of day-hospitalization programs beginning in the 1960s concentrated on comparing inpatient treatment as usual with day hospitalization, or with brief inpatient admissions followed by day hospitalization. At that time, information was not readily available regarding the suitability of the individual patient to a specific partial hospitalization approach. However, by the late 1970s accumulated empirical evidence and unintended research findings showed that patients suffering from neurotic and personality disorders had benefited more from the new modality than had those suffering from psychosis. Generalizations from the relatively more rigorous investigations could not be arrived at because of the lack of precision in describing adequately the patient populations or the programs' structures. To complicate matters further, studies often combined elements of day hospitalization, day care, and day treat-

ment. Nevertheless, some tentative conclusions emerged. Most studies found that day hospitalization was as efficacious as inpatient treatment and more cost-effective, resulted in better social functioning and employment record in the community, and was perceived by the patients and their families as less burdensome and more satisfying. The general conclusion was that day hospitalization should be considered a distinct rather than an alternative modality for specific patient populations (Bowman, Shelley, Sheehy-Skeffington, & Sinanan, 1983; Dick, Sweeney, Crombie, 1991; Fink, Longabaugh, & Stout, 1978; Kris, 1965; Penk, Charles, & Van Hoose, 1978; Piper, et al., 1996; Stefansson & Petursson, 1989; Zwerling & Wilder, 1964).

DAY CARE AND SUPPORTIVE TREATMENT PROGRAMS

Day care offers long-term maintenance and rehabilitation to patient populations suffering from persistent, severe, and disabling disorders. Originally such services catered to patients with schizophrenic disorder. Gradually the use of day care was extended to persons who suffer from schizoaffective, affective, and personality disorders, often in the same program. As better understanding of the varied needs of these different populations emerged, and as the sophistication of the treatment increased, more specialized services were designed to treat specific disorders. Day care for patients with personality disorders also became known as supportive treatment programs. Regardless of the label, the target populations share severe and persistent symptoms and dysfunctions characterized by long duration and requiring time-unlimited care. The protracted nature of personality disorders has been demonstrated in two recent studies. A meta-analysis of all the outcome studies of psychotherapy for patients with personality disorders that used systematic means of making the diagnoses; incorporated valid outcome measures; and allowed for the calculation of magnitude of effect was reported. The authors were able to calculate that with treatment, 11.57% of patients remitted each year, so that by 8.33 years, no patient had a diagnosis of a personality disorder. This finding contrasted with five natural history studies of borderline personality disorder resulting in a remission rate of 3.7% per year, necessitating 24 years for 100% total remission. (Banon, Perry, & Ianni,

1995). This is not surprising given the etiology of personality disorders. History of early neglect and/or abuse and lack of fit between parents and infant interact with genetic factors to produce such enduring difficulties. It has therefore been encouraging that the last decade has witnessed an expansion of the empirical and research evidence of the effectiveness of the supportive therapies (Piper, McCallum, Joyce, Azim, & Ogrodniczuk, in press; Piper, Joyce, McCallum, & Azim, 1998; Rockland, 1989; Wallerstein, 1986). This has led to a higher regard for the modality and its practice.

Supportive treatment programs for personality disorders are usually in the form of group therapy. The assignment of the individual patient to a specific group has to be determined by the patient's level of psychosocial functioning, the patient's current level of disability, and also the quality of the patient's object relations (Azim, Piper, Segal, Nixon, & Duncan, 1991), notwithstanding any Axis I disorder. Program–therapist match has also been shown to be of equally vital importance and consequence. Neither patients nor their therapists appear to do well in a day care program staffed with highly trained therapists, particularly those with doctorate degrees (Klein, 1974). In contrast, appropriately trained occupational therapists, nurses, and social workers have been found to be far better suited for the tasks and the unique demands of these programs.

Certain psychodynamic principles and their application in supportive treatment programs sets them apart from the traditional therapies.

1. An awareness of the destructiveness of therapeutic zeal to "cure or kill." The therapists have to spell out to the patients at the outset that full remission is not the main goal of the program and therefore discharging the patient is not a consideration. In fact, both therapists and patients have to be aware that the tenure of any individual patient in the day care program might very well exceed that of any particular therapist.

2. Time-unlimited care is provided and institutional transference is fostered as a means of undoing the consequences of early abuse, neglect, and abandonment.

3. Patients are encouraged but not required or coerced to attend the program regularly. It has to be expected that the constant availability of the program will be tested out by many patients.

4. The crucial therapeutic role of this constancy is the eventual reduction or elimination of the need to resort to self-damaging or threatening behaviors as tokens for repeated hospital admissions.

5. Patients usually fall in two major categories: those who attend for long periods even if irregularly and others who elect to report only during periods of perceived need (Misunis, Feist, Thorkelsson, & McAuley, 1990).

6. Recognition that a primary need of this patient population is not only to be understood but also to feel understood by the therapy team. Self-understanding in the form of insight is at best not helpful and at worst destructively experienced as blame, aggression, seduction, rejection, or abandonment. Patients themselves might arrive at very significant insights on their own and they often do, but it is the competent, skillful, knowledgeable, and above all, secure therapist who can endure abstaining day in and day out from making technically correct interpretations (Steiner, 1993; Piper et al., 1998) that could prove to be potentially destructive.

7. Meticulous attention is paid to powerful countertransference reactions evoked in the therapists and explored in regular supervision and staff–staff relations meetings (Azim, 1993; O'Kelly & Azim, 1993; Piper et al., 1996).

Research on Day Care Programs

There are few reports of day care programs, usually descriptive in nature, but none were dedicated to the study of personality disorders (Stein & Test, 1980; Misunis et al., 1990). The Stein and Test investigation was an evaluation of their day care program featuring " assertive psychosocial work" in comparison to inpatient care. At the 14-month end-point life of the program, the overall results of the experimental group were encouraging. It showed that the readmission rate of day care patients was 6% compared to 58% for the inpatients. The experimental population also spent significantly more time in sheltered employment, had more contact with friends, enjoyed higher satisfaction with their lives, and showed better functioning on 7 of 13 items on nurse rating scale and better compliance in taking medication compared to the control group. Most significantly, the withdrawal of funding leading to discharging the patients did lead to the loss of the posttherapy gains when the patients were reassessed at 28-month follow-up.

A few years ago, I inaugurated a supportive treatment program at the Psychiatric Outpatient Services of Lions Gate Hospital in North Vancouver, based on all the previously mentioned principles. Depending on their individual needs, some patients were assigned to more than one supportive group (e.g., attending the three-groups-per-week supportive treatment program and also a dual-diagnosis group). Occasionally a supportive group patient expressed a wish, usually tinged with anxiety, to be transferred to one of the more intensive, expressive, and insight-oriented groups available at the outpatient services. Following an exploration and assessment regarding the level of personality integration and psychosocial functioning, the patient was reassigned if deemed appropriate.

I then wanted to evaluate the impact of the supportive groups on the use of all medical–surgical and psychiatric services. Because health care coverage in Canada is universal and provided by a single payer, the provincial government, extensive data are collected routinely. I obtained the aggregate costs of health care for the first 100 consecutive patients who met an arbitrary end-point criterion of attendance of eight sessions. In accordance with the treatment contract, the eight groups could have been attended in anything from a few weeks to many months. Costs were obtained for all hospitalizations and attendance at emergency rooms and physicians' offices for the year before attending the first group, for the year after attending one group, and for the year after the eighth group for all patients. The preliminary figures (on 93 patients) indicated that the cost of acute care, reflecting the number of days in hospitals had declined 64% and physician billings by 39%. The total cost was reduced by only 39%, reflecting an appropriate increase in the utilization, adherence to, and thus cost of medications. Of note was the finding that the costs in the year after attending the first group had de-

creased by 27%. It was speculated that this finding represents a response of the patient population to the intent to treat and more specifically to the attention-placebo effect of the time-unlimited nature of the offered contract. These findings require replication and longer-term follow-up. The study was limited by the lack of a treatment-as-usual control group with random assignment. Nevertheless, the results are promising and suggest that support groups play a useful role in the long-term care of patients with serious personality disorders. Eighteen months later, I repeated the study. The extant results are based on $N = 134$. The reduction in expenditures in the year following the first group was not realized. The total cost of health care expenditures in the year prior to the first group was \$1,973,926 (in Canadian funds), divided between \$1,299,517 for females ($N = 77$) and \$574,408 for males ($N = 57$). This was reduced to \$691,837, \$434,568, and \$257,269, respectively during the year after the attendance of the eighth group, or a decrease of 66.55%, 61.80%, and 64.95% respectively (Table 25.1). Of note is the equivalent effectiveness of the modality for both genders. The average number of patients per group was 10–15. The approximate cost of conducting a group was \$100. This translated into a saving of almost \$10,000 per patient at the 1 year endpoint following the eighth group.

DAY TREATMENT PROGRAMS

In contrast to day hospitalization and day care, day treatment programs provide an intensive combination of time-limited treatment, habilitation, and rehabilitation to personality-disordered patients whose levels of social functioning, impulse control, quality of object relations (Azim et al., 1991), psychological mindedness, and motivation for change are commensurate

TABLE 25.1. Total Cost of Utilization of Health Services by Users of the Supportive Group (in Canadian Dollars)

Gender	Year before attending first group	Year after attending eighth group	Decrease	Percent decrease
Females	\$1,299,517	\$434,568	\$864,949	66.6%
Males	\$ 674,408	\$257,269	\$417,139	61.8%
Total	\$1,973,925	\$691,837	\$1,282,088	65.0%

Note. Figures are not collected for nonsubsidized cost of medications.

with the rigors of the modality. The availability of external social support also plays a crucial role in terms of adherence and outcome (Table 25.2). The relative emphasis on treatment, habilitation, and rehabilitation varies across day treatment programs. The goal of *treatment* is to help a patient to attain a syndromal remission of a psychiatric disorder(s). This goal involves symptom relief and the acquisition of insight and positive changes in life functioning. *Habilitation* is a concept rarely addressed in the psychiatric literature. The *Compact Edition of the Oxford English Dictionary* (1971) defines "habilitation (also abilitation) as the action of enabling or endowing with ability or fitness; capacitation, qualification" (p. 1235). Habilitation plays a particularly significant role in the care of personality disorders because of the early and persistent nature of the patterns which characterizes these disorders. Successful habilitation is revealed, for example, in de novo experiences of a sense of liberation, peace of mind, healthier conceptual and perceptual options, less reactivity, and particularly freedom from compulsivity and impulsivity. In short, habilitation leads to a never before experienced sense of mastery over one's being, self-control, and the acquisition of a newly found self-agency. Significantly, this experience is usually ushered by a salutary process of grieving over what could have been but never was and mourning the wasting of one's life. Besides treatment and habilitation, *rehabilitation* is also an ingredient of day treatment programs that is designed to help the patients achieve a functional remission: accept the reality of the disorder, adapt to some of its consequences, and achieve optimal social functioning. An important aspect of rehabilitation for many patients in day treatment is the emphasis on and availability of treatment for comorbid substance abuse. A study of the prevalence of substance abuse in 137 inpatients with a DSM-III diagnosis of borderline personality disorder was 67% (Dulit, Fyer, Haas, Sullivan, & Frances, 1990). A more recent study found that close to 60% of persons diagnosed with substance use disorders also suffer from personality disorders (Skodol, Oldham, & Gallaher, 1999). Considering the secretiveness and the tendency to minimize, if not to resort to denial by patients of both sets of disorders, the aforementioned figures should be considered as conservative. Substance abuse disorders have to be addressed simultaneously or prior to admission because the continued use of substances compromises the effectiveness of pharmacotherapy and the ability to benefit from group work. These patients possess a penchant for attributing their substance abuse disorders to the comorbid psychiatric disorders and press for receiving treatment only for the latter, which needs to be firmly declined.

The characteristics of a highly structured day treatment program have been detailed in Azim (1993) and Piper et al. (1996). Such a program usually incorporates the tenets of therapeutic community, group dynamics, psychodynamics, family dynamics, organizational dynamics,

TABLE 25.2. Distinguishing Features of the Three Subtypes of Day Hospitals

Features	DHP	DCP	DTP
Length of stay	Brief	Time unlimited	Time limited (weeks–months)
Patients' psychosocial functioning	Variable	Relatively low	Relatively high
Goal	Symptom relief	Support, symptom relief, rehabilitation, improved community tenure	Symptom relief, insight, habilitation, rehabilitation, improved relations
Interventions	Pharmacotherapy; ECT; individual group, and family	Supportive and family work, pharmacotherapy group therapy	Treatment, habilitation and rehabilitation groups, pharmacotherapy
Disposition	OPD, DCP, DTP	12-step programs, DTP, DHP, lifetime contracts	Family therapy, pharmacotherapy, follow-up group, DHP, DTP

Note. DHP, day-hospital program; DCP, day care program; DTP, day-treatment program; ECT, electroconvulsive therapy; OPD, outpatient department.

general systems theory, and biological psychiatry.

Like the other two types of partial hospitalization, day treatment programs can be distinguished by the length of stay. Whereas day hospitals offer a brief stay to resolve a critical phase, and day care offers a time-unlimited contract, day treatment programs stipulate a time-limit, be it the same for all patients or individually tailored. Decades of experience taught me that 18-week duration is optimal for significant relief of symptoms, improved social adjustment, and acquisition of insight. Furthermore, my research findings support this conclusion.

More than 30 years of personal experience in organizing, developing, and leading day treatment programs in Montreal, Edmonton, and now Vancouver, as well as presenting, observing, and consulting, also taught me what follows.

Conceptual Issues

Tom Main (1946) coined the term "therapeutic community." It was the result of his experience as an army psychiatrist during World War II. He noticed wide variations in the sickness rates between battalions under similar combat conditions. He came to the conclusion that differences in the culture and the quality of human relations in each battalion were the determining factors (Main, 1975). Following the war, psychiatrists such as Main, Bion, and Jones applied their observations and war experiences to the organization of psychiatric units for veterans and exprisoners of war. Their new techniques were sometimes referred to as milieu therapy. A social anthropologist, Robert Rapoport, studied the Social Rehabilitation Clinic established in 1946 by Jones (Rapoport, 1980). He delineated four principles as the cornerstones of the approach: democratization, permissiveness, communalism, and reality confrontation. Each concept has gone through periods of misunderstanding and misapplication on the road to its transformation into modern usage. Thus democratization is now reflected in the deliberate flattening of the hierarchy among the staff and between the staff and the patient population. Permissiveness now entails therapeutic tolerance for the expression of affects, thoughts, and actions considered to be deviant by social standards. Communalism denotes the highly structured group interaction nature of

the programs. Reality confrontation has evolved into an environment of inquiry and sharing of feedback.

What was sometimes forgotten, often with disastrous consequences, was that the major aim of these four principles was the enhanced undertaking of responsibility by all concerned: patients as well as every level of the staff's traditional hierarchy. They were developed in part in response to the then prevailing excesses of power issues in mental hospitals. Power signifies self-serving and coercive actions over others, inevitably leading to competitive and destructive group processes. By contrast legitimate authority implies the exercise of leadership towards the achievement of collective goals (Buckley, 1967; Rosie et al., 1995). However, the adoption of a laissez-faire abdication of authority and responsibility by the staff of some early experiments resulted in a pseudo-democracy in which patients voted on the admission, the management, and the discharge of other patients. Such practices contributed to underutilization and bias against day treatment programs and even to the demise to some of these programs. Such a state of affairs was epitomized in an article entitled "The patient–staff community meeting: A tea party with the mad hatter" (Klein, 1981). Notwithstanding these struggles, it is ironic that it is often forgotten that many modern organizational theory and management courses are merely a repackaging of these early contributions by the proponents of social psychiatry toward the recognition of issues of power in human relations and in the emotional climates of organizations. It is also worth noting that the psychiatric day hospitals have spearheaded day treatment and day surgery for other medical and surgical subspecialties.

Curbing the powers while increasing the responsibilities, of patients and staff alike and the judicious exercise of the treaters' authority are vitally important, particularly in any program designed for the treatment of patients with personality disorders. The therapists in these programs operate more generically as mental health professionals and less as members of their particular disciplines. This underscores the organizational imperative that day treatment programs utilizing a milieu therapy approach be administratively structured as discrete self-managed programs internally responsible for budgeting, training, supervising, and evaluating their staff members. This is necessary to diminish the negative consequences of multiple loyalties and splitting among the staff members. Psychiatric partial hospitalization has become a model for today's movement to organize all hospital services as self-managed programs. Day treatment programs can be either free-standing or integrated with other psychiatric services, both outpatient and inpatient.

The major contribution of psychoanalysis to day treatment programs has been the attention to the powerful transference–countertransference manifestations that typically occur in these programs. As many as 30 patients and 10 staff members have been known to attend large and small therapy groups (Rosie & Azim, 1990), thus creating a multitude of transference and countertransference reactions. Patients experience positive and negative transference reactions not only toward staff members and each other but also toward each group, as well as toward the program as a whole, and can span the whole spectrum of transferential manifestations including but not restricted to idealization and devaluation. The role of hate in the transference and countertransference interactions in the treatment of this patient population cannot be emphasized enough (Frederickson, 1990; Groves, 1978). Used judiciously, the differences in each person's transference–countertransference reactions can contribute to reality testing and to a realization of the extent to which individual perceptions tend to be poignantly vicarious.

Cameron (1947) cited family dynamics and family involvement in his earliest writings on day hospitals. Some present day treatment programs, including mine, stipulate in the pretreatment contract that the patient consents to at least one family assessment during the course of treatment. Depending on the patient's life situation, this may include any and all members of the nuclear and/or extended family and any other person considered a significant other. Babes in arms and on occasion pets are included, and their nonverbal responses to the ebb and flow of the nuances of the prevailing affects are always a source of fascination if not awe. In response to some patients' suggestions, long-distance and overseas conference calls for family members who are unable to attend have been instituted successfully. At times, following the assessment, family treatment was found to be indicated and was offered concurrent with and/or at follow-up. Recommendations of psychiatric assessments and treatment for other

family members are sometimes judiciously and sensitively made and referrals arranged as indicated. One of the most rewarding aspects of the family meetings has been the astute and forthright contribution by young children as well as the benefits accrued to them, as a result of the parents' increased awareness. The inevitable defensive apprehension of the patients prior to the family meeting over the inclusion of their young is usually rendered manageable by the sharing of the anxieties before, and the relief following, the previously held family assessments of fellow patients. The goals of the family meetings have to be limited to the better understanding of the family dynamics without getting sucked into them, to provide psychoeducation and to be supportive to all parties. The treaters have to make every effort not to foster the fear of the expectation of the assignment of blame to any family members.

As mentioned earlier, biological methods of treatment were a mainstay of the early day hospitals. During the last decade, psychopharmacology has widened the scope of day hospital programs, making it possible to treat patients who would have been previously excluded due to the severity of their symptoms and character traits. The daily groups provide an opportunity to evaluate valuable subjective responses to different medications and to understand the interaction of psychodynamics, group dynamics, and pharmacodynamics. Here again, shared experiences, encouragement, and assurances by fellow patients have such an invaluable effect on the fostering, receptivity, and adherence to pharmacotherapy in patients who are notorious for having difficulties in adhering to all therapeutic interventions. The intensity of the program also allows, when necessary, for the introduction of extreme dosages and unusual combinations in otherwise pharmacologically treatment-resistant cases (Geagea, 1999), such as may be required for patients who had suffered severe and persistent mixed Axis I and Axis II diagnoses (e.g., symptoms of a double depression in association with varying degrees of paranoid, borderline, and obsessive compulsive–personality traits or disorders and substance abuse disorders). The fact that rates of drug metabolism differ significantly among the members of the same ethnic group by a factor of up to 10 and among ethnic groups by a factor of 100 has not been adequately appreciated (Lin, Polaud, Smith, Strickland, & Mendosa, 1991). As a result, patients, their families, pharmacists, and family physicians tend to feel alarmed by the dosages required by some patients in order to achieve full remission. Recently and at long last there is a growing awareness of the difference between drug use in controlled drug trials and pharmacotherapy in real-life situations. Studies involve highly selected patients and physicians who have consented to take part in such research activity. Compliance is closely monitored if not sometimes coercively reinforced. The purpose of these studies is to establish the efficacy of the drug (i.e., its best achievable result under ideal conditions). This could very well be at variance of the effectiveness of the medication as actually used in clinical practice, as is the case in day programs. Reliance is put on SRIs for the control of the symptoms of anxiety, depression, and obsessive–compulsive disorder; on anticonvulsants for mood stabilization and control of aggression and anxiety; and on trazodone and doxepine for sleep normalization.

Program Description

Partially based on firsthand observation, Karterud (1993) wrote:

> John Rosie and Hassan Azim (1990) described an unusually well structured day treatment program for nonpsychotic patients. Each day, Monday through Friday, started with the community meeting; which assembled about 50 patients and staff members and which lasted for an hour. The primary task of the meeting, as Rosie and Azim described it, was similar to that of small group psychotherapy:
>
> > "Dialogue is encouraged, expression of affect is supported, dreams are welcomed and emotionally laden material from other groups is introduced. Exploration of relationships within the groups in the here-and-now is commonplace. Transference interpretations are made, usually by the therapists, occasionally by patients. . . . Group-as-a-whole interventions are generally restricted to those occasions when such processes are seen to be significantly affecting the group work. Individual patients are encouraged to do as much individual work as they seem to be ready for at the time."
>
> Another impressive aspect of that well-designed day treatment program was that its efficacy was scientifically proved by a controlled clinical trial. (p. 605)

A description of the same program was later elaborated on in further detail by Azim (1993) and Piper et al. (1996). The process and content of every group in the program were featured in the latter. Figure 25.1 is a schematic representation of the relative emphasis on the treatment, habilitation and rehabilitation domains.

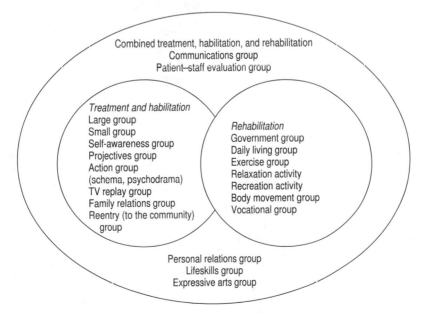

FIGURE 25.1. Schematic representation of a day-treatment program.

Staff Issues

Attention to staff issues is critical in these programs. Comprehensive day treatment programs are labor intensive. Three-to-one patient-to-staff ratio is desirable in view of the intensity of the program. The staff members have to be almost constantly able to negotiate the contradictions if not the paradoxes inherent in working in day treatment programs. Thus the staff have to weigh the exercise of therapeutic tolerance against the need for limit setting; fostering closeness among the patients yet actively discouraging and interpreting the destructiveness of subgrouping; expecting the patients to share whatever they become aware of yet censuring attacking and advice giving; being least restrictive while attending to the enhancement of safety; fostering assertiveness by all players that has to be associated with the containment of emotional explosion and adherence to mindful interactions; promoting group-as-a-whole processes and dynamics and at the same time keeping in focus the ultimate goal of treating the individual in the group; increasing the freedom of action of the individual but only in tandem with a rise in one's own responsibility; and advancing the program cohesion while being heedful of the context in which the program is funded and the community served.

Assuming the role of a leader of such an intensive program for the treatment of personality disorders is not for the fainthearted. The leader needs to possess organizational skills and has to be well versed not only in individual, group, family, and institutional dynamics but also in psychopharmacology. It is also important for the leaders to be able to contain the ever-present pressures of persecutory anxiety within themselves in relation to the program's staff and to the powers that be. This has been possible to accomplish by holding weekly staff–staff relations meetings. Here, the leader should model openness without burdening staff with unnecessary self-disclosure. The leader should also make every effort to invite and encourage the staff members to express any and all grievances toward the leadership and to facilitate supportive confrontation toward each other (O'Kelly & Azim, 1993). The overarching task of the leader has to be the meticulous maintenance of the boundary between the legitimate attention to the here and now of the work situation on the one hand and the dangerous descent into therapy on the other. In these meetings, flight into discussing patients or bringing up administrative issues has to be identified and referred back to other weekly meetings devoted to one and to the other. To the extent that staff–staff relations meetings succeed in unearthing covert staff conflicts, the incidence of patients' parallel collective disturbances is kept at bay. However, the latter are inevitable and their resolution usually requires emergency staff–staff relations meetings followed by large group meetings. (For details, see Azim, 1993; O'Kelly & Azim, 1993; Rosie & Azim, 1990.)

Research on Day Treatment Programs

The early studies that appeared in the 1970s shared many of the limitations mentioned in the section "Research on Day Hospital Programs." MacKenzie and Pilling (1972) conducted a prospective study of 100 consecutive patients suffering from neurotic or psychosomatic disorders in a day treatment program and reported that 69% of the patients showed improvement in symptoms, interpersonal relations, and work and social functioning on clinical assessments. Most maintained their gains at 6-month follow-up.

Subsequently, a study by Dick et al. (1991) reported the important finding that day treatment was more effective than outpatient care for patients with more severe anxiety and depression, while the less severe cases benefited more from outpatient treatment.

More relevant to personality disorders was the study by Karterud et al. (1992). The program explicitly combined a therapeutic community organizational structure and a psychoanalytic object relations orientation to treat severe personality disorders. The majority of the 97 consecutive admissions were diagnosed with borderline and schizotypal personality disorder. The authors reported gains that were moderate for the former and less favorable for the latter population.

To my knowledge, the only prospective study of the outcome of a day treatment program using a randomized treatment-versus-control design was done at my day treatment program in Edmonton and was reported by Piper and colleagues (Piper, Rosie, Azim, & Joyce, 1993; Piper et al., 1996). The study was designed to avoid the methodological weaknesses of earlier studies, including small sample size, selection bias, lack of randomization, minimal control of variables, lack of standard outcome measures, and poorly defined programs. All the patients referred to this program were asked to participate in the project, which lasted from January 1989 to December 1990. Ninety-five percent of these patients consented to join the study. The selection criteria were long-term psychiatric problems that led to psychosocial dysfunction, ability to engage in group work, motivation for intensive therapy, and age 13 and older. Exclusion criteria were current psychotic disorders, need for inpatient hospitalization, suicidal and homicidal threat, severe intellectual impairment, current substance abuse, and participation in another ongoing treatment. The control condition chosen was a wait-list delay. The average waiting period to admission prior to launching the study, the delay period, and the treatment-as-usual length-of-stay in the program were all the same: 18 weeks. Before being assigned to immediate treatment or the delay condition, the patients were assessed by the clinical staff for Axis I and Axis II diagnoses according to DSM-III-R (American Psychiatric Association, 1987) criteria. Independent assessors used various interview schedules and questionnaires and outcome variables. The 17 outcome variables tapped the following areas: interpersonal functioning, psychiatric symptomatology, self-esteem, life satisfaction, defensive functioning, and the level of the patient's treatment objectives. Subjects were then matched in pairs according to lifetime diagnosis and gender and randomly assigned to either immediate treatment or delay condition. No statistical difference in the use of medications, mostly antidepressants, was found.

Outcome variables were administered at the end of the treatment and delay periods and again at follow-up point of 8 months on average after completion of treatment (Table 25.3). Eighty women and 40 men comprised the 120 patients who completed the treatment and control conditions. Diagnostically, 78% had lifetime diagnoses of major depression, 60% of personality disorder, and half a combination of both.

The results showed that treated patients had attained significantly greater improvement than the control group on the following seven variables: social dysfunction, family dysfunction; interpersonal behavior, mood level, life satisfaction, self-esteem, and individualized goals of treatment as measured by an independent assessor, while the measure of adaptive defenses approached significance. Another set of analyses revealed that compared to pretreatment, the patients showed significant improvement in 11 variables. By contrast, at the end of the wait period, the patients showed significant improvement in only one variable (treatment objectives severity as assessed by the patient). Thus there was little evidence of spontaneous remission in the control group.

At follow-up, 16 of the variables demonstrated maintenance of results while one (target severity as assessed by patients) showed further improvement. While statistical significance of results such as the ones reported so far address probabilities, measuring the magnitude of effect directly expresses the size of the effect that one variable (here treatment) has on another (here outcome). The study measured the effect size for each of the 17 outcome variables. The magnitude varied considerably from .10 to 1.96. In terms of outcome, the mean size was .71, indicating that the average treated patient exceeded about 76% of the patients in the control group. When applied only to the seven variables in which significant differences were found, the mean magnitude effect was 1.18, implying that the average treated patient surpassed 87% of the patients in the control group.

The limitations of the study include the lack of comparison with other forms of treatment and attention–placebo activities. Another limiting factor is that the program was evaluated as a whole; therefore, it was not possible to determine the relative contributions of the particular components of the program. A dropout rate of 37%, comparable to findings reported in the literature, prevailed and the subjects were replaced by matched patients.

Together, the results are notable, especially when the treatment-resistant nature, the long duration, and the burden on the patients, their families, and the social and medical systems are taken into consideration. Ninety percent of the subjects had previous psychiatric treatment and 43% had been hospitalized, all with few benefits.

Later, Bateman and Fonagy (1999) reported the results of their randomized controlled trial on the effectiveness of a partial hospitalization program for the treatment of patients suffering from borderline personality disorder. The control group received psychiatric care as usual. Each population was comprised of 19 patients. The program was psychoanalytically oriented and the partial hospitalization patients received on a weekly basis a combination of individual

TABLE 25.3. Design for the Day Treatment Program Study

Patients	18-week period	18 (or 36)-week period	36-week period
Matched on diagnosis, age, gender	Immediate DTP	Follow-up period	—
	Wait-list control period	Delayed DTP	Follow-up period

and group therapy, and psychodrama, and also attended a weekly community meeting. The total number of hours of care was approximately seven, spread over five days. The average length of stay was 1.45 years, and attendance at the psychotherapy sessions was 62%. The results showed statistically significant superiority of the partial hospitalization program in terms of the number of self-mutilating acts, suicide attempts, the number of patients who remained parasuicidal, the need for medication, self-reported state and trait anxiety scores, the Beck Depression Inventory scores, the global security index scale of the SCL-90-R, and the total Social Adjustment Scale self-score.

Bateman and Fonagy (1999) noted that only two earlier studies were controlled trials of intensive outpatient treatment for individuals with borderline or other severe personality disorder. One was by Linehan and her colleagues (Linehan, 1993; Linehan, Armstrong, Suarez, Allmon, & Heard, 1991) using dialectical behaviour therapy. The other was by (Piper et al., 1996), which utilized similar self-report measures to the Bateman and Fonagy (1999) study and documented the superiority of the treatment offered in comparison to a wait list control group.

There are a number of other notable similarities between the Bateman and Fonagy (1999) study and the Piper et al. (1996) study. For example, although the Piper et al. study chose the more modest designation of psychodynamic orientation, one of the three program psychiatrists in this study had been a practicing psychoanalyst and a leader of day and evening hospitalization programs for over two decades, another had a diploma in psychotherapy, and the third was chosen for his proven track record as a psychodynamic psychotherapist. The three psychiatrists had led more than one third of the groups. The program employed as well several highly skilled psychotherapists (nurses, social workers, occupational therapists, and psychologists) with an average tenure in the program of over ten years. They received regular in-service

training, individual family and group therapy supervision, and co-led the groups and the management of all patients with the psychiatrists. In the Bateman and Fonagy program, however, all therapy was provided by "psychiatrically trained nurses who were members of partial hospitalization program's team but who had not formal psychotherapy qualifications" (p. 1565).

Furthermore, the estimated number of hours of therapy received by each patient in both studies was almost identical: in Bateman and Fonagy's program, the average length of stay was about 75 weeks and the number of treatment hours was about seven per week for a total of 525 hours, while in the Piper study, the length of stay was 18 weeks and the number of hours of therapy per week was 30, for a total of 546 hours. There has been accumulating evidence in the literature indicating that the total number of sessions, regardless of the duration of therapy, correlates with outcome (Banon et al., 1995).

At the time of writing, the Bateman and Fonagy (1999) investigation and the Piper et al. (1996) are the only two randomized controlled studies of the effectiveness of psychoanalytically oriented treatment of the severe and persistent personality disordered, including the borderline personality disordered.

All the above research results suggest that more partial hospitalization programs dedicated to the personality-disordered patients should become available and that more rigorous studies need to be conducted in the future.

REFERENCES

American Psychiatric Association. (1987). *Diagnostic and statistical manual of mental disorders* (3rd ed., rev.). Washington, DC: Author.

Azim, H. F. A. (1993). Group psychotherapy in the day hospital. In H. I. Kaplan & B. J. Sadock (Eds.), *Comprehensive group psychotherapy* (3rd ed., pp. 619–634). Baltimore: Williams & Wilkins.

Azim, H. F. A., Piper, W. E., Segal, P. M., Nixon, G. W.

H., & Duncan, S. (1991). The quality of object relations scale. *Bulletin of the Menninger Clinic, 55,* 323–343.

Banon, E., Perry, J. C., & Ianni, F. (1995). *The effectiveness of psychotherapy for personality disorders.* Paper presented at the meeting of the International Society for the Study of Personality Disorders, Dublin, Ireland.

Bateman, A. W., & Fonagy, P. (1999). Effectiveness of partial hospitalization in the treatment of borderline personality disorder: A randomized controlled trial. *American Journal of Psychiatry, 156*(10), 1563–1569.

Bowman, E. P., Shelley, R. K., Sheehy-Skeffington, A., & Sinanan, K. (1983). Day patient versus inpatient: Factors determining selection of acutely ill patients for hospital treatment. *British Journal of Psychiatry, 142,* 584–587.

Buckley, W. F. (1967). Social control: Deviance, power and feedback processes. In W. F. Buckley (Ed.), *Sociology and modern systems theory* (pp. 163–207). Englewood Cliffs, NJ: Prentice Hall.

Cameron, D. E. (1947). The day hospital: An experimental form of hospitalization for psychiatric patients. *The Modern Hospital, 68,* 60–62.

The compact edtion of the Oxford English dictionary (1971). Oxford, UK: Oxford University Press.

Creed, F., Black, D., & Anthony, P. (1989). Day hospital and community treatment for acute psychiatric illness: A critical appraisal. *British Journal of Psychiatry, 154,* 300–310.

Dick, P. H., Sweeney, M. L., & Crombie, I. K. (1991). Controlled comparison of day-patient and out-patient treatment for persistent anxiety and depression. *British Journal of Psychiatry, 158,* 24–27.

Dickey, B., Berren, M., Santiago, J., Breslau, J. A. (1990). Patterns of service use and costs in model day hospital: In programs in Boston and Tucson. *Psychiatric Services, 41,* 419.

Dulit, R. A., Fyer, M. R., Haas, G. L., Sullivan, T., & Frances, A. J. (1990). Substance use in borderline personality disorder. *American Journal of Psychiatry, 147,* 1002–1007.

Fink, E. B., Longabaugh, R., & Stout, R. (1978). The paradoxical underutilization of partial hospitalization. *American Journal of Psychiatry, 135,* 713–716.

Frederickson, J. (1990). Hate in the countertransference as an empathic position. *Contemporary Psychoanalysis, 26,* 479–496.

Geagea, K. (1999, January). Managing difficult cases of depression. *Canadian Journal of CME, 11*(1), 45–58.

Glenner, J., & Glenner, G. G. (1989). The crucible—family dilemmas in Alzheimer's disease: Day care—an alternative. *Activities, Adaptation, and Aging, 13,* 1–23.

Groves, J. (1978). Treating the hateful patient. *New England Journal of Medicine, 298,* 883–887.

Herz, M. I., Ferman, J., & Cohen, M. (1985). Increasing utilization of day hospitals. *Psychiatric Quarterly, 57,* 187–192.

Karterud, S.W. (1993). Community meetings in the therapeutic community. In H. I. Kaplan & B. J. Sadock (Eds.), *Comprehensive group psychotherapy*

(3rd ed., pp. 598–606). Baltimore: Williams & Wilkins.

Karterud S., Vaglum, S., Friis, S., Irion, T., Johns, S., & Vaglum, P. (1992). Day hospital therapeutic community treatment for patients with personality disorders: An empirical evaluation of the containment function. *Journal of Nervous and Mental Disease, 180,* 238–243.

Kiesler, C. A. (1982). Public and professional myths about mental hospitalization: An empirical reassessment of policy-related beliefs. *American Psychologist, 37,* 1323–1329.

Klein, J. R. (1974). The day treatment center for chronic patients: The politics of despair. *Massachusetts Journal of Mental Health, 4,* 10–31.

Klein, R. H. (1981). The patient–staff community meeting: A tea party with the mad hatter. *International Journal of Group Psychotherapy, 31,* 205–222.

Koenigsberg, H. W. (1993). Combining psychotherapy and pharmacotherapy in the treatment of borderline patients. In J. M. Oldham, M. B., Riba, & A. Tasman (Eds.), *American Psychiatric Press review of psychiatry* (Vol. 12). Washington, DC: American Psychiatric Press.

Kris, E. (1965). Day hospitals. *Current Therapeutic Research, 7,* 320–323.

Lin, K. M., Polaud, R. E., Smith, M. W., Strickland, T. L., & Mendosa, R. (1991). Pharmacokinetic and other related factors affecting psychotropic responses in Asians. *Psychopharmacololgy Bulletin, 27,* 427–439.

Linehan, M. M., Armstrong, H. E., Suarez, A., Allmon, D., & Heard, H. (1991). Cognitive-behavioral treatment of chronically parasuicidal borderline patients. *Archives of General Psychiatry; 48,* 1060–1064.

Linehan, M. M. (1993). *Cognitive-behavioral treatment of borderline personality disorder.* New York: Guilford Press.

Lystad, M. H. (1958). Day hospital care and changing family attitudes toward the mentally ill. *Journal of Nervous and Mental Disease, 127,* 145–152.

Main, T. F. (1946). The hospital as a therapeutic institution. *Bulletin of the Menninger Clinic, 10,* 66–70.

Main, T. F. (1975). Some psychodynamics of large groups. In L. Kreeger (Ed.), *The large group: Dyanmics and therapy* (pp. 57–86). London Constable.

MacKenzie, K., & Pilling, L. (1972). An intensive-therapy day clinic for out-of-town patients with neurotic and psychosomatic problems. *International Journal of Group Psychotherapy, 22,* 352–363.

Misunis, R., Feist, B., Thorkelsson, J., & McAuley, L. (1990, Summer). Outpatient groups for chronic psychiatric patients. *Group,* pp. 111–120.

Odenheimer, J. (1965). Day hospital as an alternative to the psychiatric ward: Attitudes and responses of relatives. *Archives of General Psychiatry, 13,* 46–53.

O'Kelly, J. G., & Azim, H. F. A. (1993). Staff–staff relations group. *International Journal of Group Psychotherapy, 43,* 469–483.

Penk, W. E., Charles, H. L., Van Hoose, T. A. (1978). Comparative effectiveness of day hospital and inpatient psychiatric treatment. *Journal of Consulting and Clinical Psychology, 46,* 94–101.

Perry, J. C. (1993, Spring). Longitudinal studies of personality disorders. *Journal of Personality Disorders* (Suppl.), 63–85.

Piper, W. E., Joyce, A. S., McCallum, M., & Azim, H. F. (1998). Interpretive and supportive forms of psychotherapy and patient personality variables. *Journal of Consulting and Clinical Psychology, 66.*

Piper, W. E., McCallum, M., Joyce, A. S., Azim, H. F., & Ogrodniczuk, J. S. (in press). *Interpretive and supportive psychotherapies: Matching therapy and patient.* Washington, DC: American Psychological Association.

Piper, W. E., Rosie, J. S., Azim, H. F., & Joyce, A. S. (1993). A randomized trial of psychiatric day treatment. *Hospital and Community Psychiatry, 44,* 757–763.

Piper, W. E., Rosie, J. S., Joyce, A. S., & Azim, H. F. (1996). *Time-limited treatment for personality disorders: Integration of research and practice in a group program.* Washington, DC: American Psychological Association.

Rapoport, R. N. (1980). *Community as doctor.* New York: Arno.

Rockland, L. H., (1989). *Supportive therapy: A psychodynamic approach.* New York: Basic Books.

Rosie, J. S. (1987). Partial hospitalization: A review of the recent literature. *Hospital and Community Psychiatry, 38,* 1291–1299.

Rosie, J. S., & Azim, H. F. A. (1990). Large group psychotherapy in a day treatment program. *International Journal of Group Psychotherapy, 40,* 305–321.

Rosie, J. S., Azim, H. F. A., Piper, W. E., & Joyce, A. S. (1995). Effective psychiatric day treatment: Historical lessons. *Psychiatric Services, 45,* 1019–1026.

Schene, A. H., & Gensons, B. P. R. (1986). Effectiveness and application of partial hospitalization. *Acta Psychiatrica Scandinavica, 74,* 335–340.

Schene, A. H., van Lieshout, P. A., & Mastboom, J. C. (1988) Development and current status of partial hospitalization in the Netherlands. *International Journal of Partial Hospitalization, 3,* 237–246.

Skodol, A. E., Oldham, J. M., & Gallaher, P. E. (1999). Axis II comorbidity of substance use disorders among patients referred for treatment of personality disorders. *American Journal of Psychiatry, 156*(5), 733–738.

Stefansson, S. B., & Petursson, H. (1989). Psychiatric day hospital versus inpatient treatment. *Nordisk Psykiatrisk Tidsskrift, 43,* 387–393.

Stein, L. I., & Test, M. A. (1980). Alternatives to mental hospital treatment: I. Conceptual model, treatment program and clinical evaluation. *Archives of General Psychiatry, 37,* 392–397.

Steiner, J. (1993). *Psychic retreats: Pathological organizations in psychotic, neurotic and borderline patients.* London: Routledge.

Sternquist, E. F. (1991). An afterschool day treatment program. In G. K. Farley & S. G. Zimet (Eds.), *Day treatment for children with emotional disorders* (vol. 2, pp. 153–170). New York: Plenum.

Wallerstein, R. S. (1986). *Forty-two lives in treatment: A study of psychoanalysis and psychotherapy.* New York: Guilford Press.

Washburn, S., Vannicelli, M., Longabaugh, R., & Scheff, B. (1976). A controlled comparison of psychiatric day treatment and inpatient hospitalization. *Journal of Consulting and Clinical Psychology, 44,* 665–675.

Whitelaw, C. A., & Perez, E. L. (1987). Utilization review of psychiatric day hospital in a Canadian urban region: I. The service profile. *International Journal of Partial Hospitalization, 4,* 209–215.

Zwerling, I., & Wilder, J. (1964). An evaluation of the applicability of the day hospital in the treatment of acutely disturbed patients. *Israel Annals of Psychiatry, 2,* 162–185.

CHAPTER 26

Treatment of Personality Disorders in Association with Symptom Disorders

PAUL A. PILKONIS

The treatment of personality disorders in the context of symptom disorders is an important topic because of the clinical epidemiology of personality disorders. It is the rare patient in most clinical settings who presents with a personality disorder without an associated symptom disorder. Fabrega, Ulrich, Pilkonis, and Mezzich (1992) documented that in a group of more than 18,000 patients presenting for evaluation at an academic medical center, only 2.8% received an Axis II diagnosis as their sole definite diagnosis. The DSM system also allows an Axis II personality disorder to be designated the "principal diagnosis," superseding an Axis I symptom disorder, but despite its potential for conveying important clinical information, this alternative is not often used. Outside tertiary care settings, it seems plausible that an Axis II disorder might be the sole or primary diagnosis for a proportion of patients who present with interpersonal problems as major complaints (e.g., marital distress, interpersonal conflicts, interpersonal deficits, loneliness, and other V-codes in the DSM system). Unfortunately, we have no good data on the size of this proportion.

Despite these exceptions, however, comorbidity between Axis I and II disorders is common and has conceptual and clinical implications. Conceptual clarity requires that principles for treatment be guided by an underlying formulation of how Axis I and II disorders

could be linked. Regardless of the details of any specific model, however, the most important implication for treatment is the need for a longitudinal perspective, that is, the use of a chronic (rather than an acute or "infectious") illness model. Consistent with this perspective is the potential value of thinking in developmental terms, that is, organizing one's approach to the patient around normative issues in adult development and setting as goals not only symptomatic relief and improvement in clinical status but also improved adaptation in the areas of attachment and interpersonal relationships; autonomy, accomplishment, and self-definition; and generativity on behalf of others.

CONCEPTUAL ISSUES

Lyons, Tyrer, Gunderson, and Tohen (1997) describe six models of the co-occurrence of Axis I and II disorders (see also Dolan, Krueger, & Shea, Chapter 4, this volume). The first model is the "null hypothesis" model, a model that contends that disorders on the two axes are independent, occurring together only by chance. The second model is the "overlapping" model, which proposes that two syndromes (e.g., an Axis I disorder such as social phobia and an Axis II disorder such as avoidant personality disorder) arise from the same pathophysiology and etiology (genetic, environmental, or both) and simply represent alternative phenotypes. Tyrer (1996) has used the term "consanguinity" to describe the same phenomenon: "The major problem is that what is true comorbidity (separate diseases) and what is false comorbidity (consanguinity, or such an intimate relationship between the disorders that they are one and the same) is difficult to determine and certainly can not be confirmed in simple cross-sectional studies" (p. 669). The third model, labeled the "subsumed" model, introduces greater complexity by positing that some comorbid cases reflect consanguinity, whereas others may actually be independent. The fourth model is the "nonspecific symptom" model, which suggests that some disorders appear to be comorbid in descriptive terms because some symptoms are a final common pathway shared by multiple disorders. Unraveling this possibility requires considerable thoughtfulness about distinguishing final-common-pathway symptoms from other symptoms, signs, and indicators that are pathognomonic for specific disorders.

The fifth model is the "spectrum of severity" model, which hypothesizes that different individuals may share qualitatively similar etiological and pathophysiological mechanisms but may differ quantitatively on the burden of each, leading to different phenotypical presentations (e.g., schizophrenia vs. schizotypal personality disorder). It is also possible to propose spectrum models that focus less on the dimension of severity and more on the issue of alternative phenotypical presentations, for example, "one stem, many branches," or the idea that "the multitude of disorders or psychopathological syndromes or parts of syndromes observed in an individual patient reflect the various manifestations of a single biological abnormality. In other words, the disorders/syndromes are interdependent . . . not in a hierarchical fashion . . . but horizontally" (Van Praag, 1996, p. 131). The sixth model is the "predisposing" model in which two disorders are assumed to have different roots and one disorder (typically the personality disorder) is temporally prior and represents a risk factor for the second disorder, which has its own separate causes.

Two other possibilities about relationships between Axis I and II disorders, growing out of the literature on relationships between personality and depression (Akiskal, Hirschfeld, & Yerevanian, 1983), also deserve comment. The "pathoplasty" model assumes that personality influences the expression, clinical presentation, and course of an Axis I disorder. The "complication" or "scarring" model (Shea et al., 1996) assumes that the emergence of an Axis I disorder such as depression influences personality (rather than the opposite) and that personality traits and interpersonal functioning may change as a result of developing a major Axis I disorder, especially if the symptom disorder has an early onset and a chronic course.

With all these hypotheses about alternative models (some of which are not mutually exclusive), the conceptual possibilities become complex and are often too confusing to serve their intended heuristic purposes. At the risk of being arbitrary, but in the spirit of being pragmatic, I propose that the most useful approaches from a treatment perspective are the spectrum models and predisposition models.

Spectrum Models

Spectrum models hypothesize that Axis I and II disorders are caused by the same underlying third variables, frequently understood as genetically determined, biologically based, temperamental variables. There are two variants of these models: (1) continuum-of-severity models, in which the disorders take different forms because of a lesser or greater "burden" of the presumed underlying etiology; and (2) interdependent "family" models, in which the disorders are assumed to be linked in horizontal but not necessarily hierarchical fashion (cf. Van Praag's, 1996, "one stem, many branches" alternative).

Battaglia, Przybeck, Bellodi, and Cloninger (1996) assert a strong version of the spectrum position, arguing that the temperament dimensions in the Cloninger model of the psychobiology of personality (Cloninger, 1987; Cloninger, Svrakic, & Przybeck, 1993) underlie the "liability for both personality disorders and clinical syndromes" and that the "joint relations of these [Axis I and II] disorders to multiple temperament dimensions accounted for their characteristic patterns of comorbidity" (p. 292). These investigators studied a sample of 164 outpatients and 36 controls who were assessed with structured Axis I and II interviews and the Tridimensional Personality Questionnaire (TPQ), with this last measure administered during a state of "at least moderate remission." Novelty seeking and harm avoidance were the two temperament dimensions with the strongest associations to the presence versus absence of various Axis I and II disorders, but the larger point is the assertion that "psychiatric comorbidity arises from predictable patterns of interaction among specific temperament dimensions" (p. 297).

A similar but less pronounced position is proposed by Mulder, Joyce, and Cloninger (1994), who investigated the joint influences of temperament and retrospective reports about early experience (using the Parental Bonding Instrument; PBI) to understand better the comorbidity between depression, other Axis I disorders, and Axis II disorders. Their major finding was that "temperament measures do not simply reflect higher levels of psychopathology, but appear to display a unique profile of correlations with specific comorbid disorders. . . . Personality disorder was associated with low RD [reward dependence]" (p. 230). In a similar vein, Mulder and Joyce (1997) factor-analyzed reports of personality disorder symptoms in a sample of 148 psychiatric patients and interpreted four factors from their solution: a factor capturing the Cluster B (dramatic, expressive) personality disorders, along with passive–aggressive and paranoid features; a factor for schizoid personality; a factor for avoidant, dependent, and self-defeating features; and a factor for obsessive–compulsive features. They correlated these four factor scores with the temperament dimensions from the TPQ, noting positive correlations between novelty seeking and the Cluster B factor, harm avoidance and the avoidant–dependent factor, and persistence and the obsessive–compulsive factor, and negative correlations between reward–dependence and the schizoid and obsessive–compulsive factors. Their conclusion is that a "model of personality disorders using four categories which are related to extremes of normally distributed human temperament measures is feasible" (p. 103).

Akiskal (1983; Akiskal et al., 1980) has discussed affective and personality disorders largely in the context of models of temperament. He made a fundamental distinction between "subaffective dysthymias" (temperamentally based chronic depressions linked to the occurrence of major depressive disorder) and "character spectrum disorders" (also linked to chronic depression, but largely as a result of personality features characterized by interpersonal turmoil and molded by developmental adversity). The former presentation fits the notion of a spectrum model linking depressive personality, dysthymia, and major depression, whereas the latter presentation fits better a predisposition or risk-factor model, with the underlying personality issues being primary and the chronic depression being secondary.

Anderson et al. (1996) found "mixed support" for Akiskal's typology in a study of 97 dysthymic patients, 41 of whom were classified as subaffective and 56 as character spectrum. In support of the typology, subaffective patients had higher rates of major depressive disorder and general depressive symptoms and cognitions. Character spectrum patients had higher rates of alcoholism among their relatives. Contrary to prediction, however, the groups were not different with regard to sex, Cluster B personality disorders, family history of mood disorders, or retrospective accounts of early home environments.

Clark (2000) is also helpful in elucidating links between emotion-based aspects of personality (presumably due to temperament) and personality disorders. She makes the clear argument that at least for "emotion-based" aspects of personality, there is an underlying biological substrate and a continuum of affective experience, especially in the realms of positive and negative affectivity (understood as separate, orthogonal constructs), that inform both state and trait assessments. In this context, she also proposes connections across the psychobiological dimensions described by Siever and Davis (1991) and Gray (1982, 1987), the five-factor model (FFM) of personality (Costa & McCrae, 1992; Goldberg, 1993), and the Watson and Tellegen (1985) model of affectivity. This "cross-walk" is useful for organizing our thinking about possible connections between personality disorders and symptom disorders. Two themes map especially well across these models: a dimension of positive affect (Watson & Tellegen, 1985), extraversion (FFM), behavioral activation (Gray, 1982, 1987), and affective instability (Siever & Davis, 1991), and a dimension of negative affect, neuroticism, behavioral inhibition, and anxiety/inhibition, respectively. Describing a third consensual dimension is more difficult, but Clark makes the case that the major candidate would be hostility, lack of agreeableness and lack of conscientiousness, reactive fight/flight responses, and impulsivity and aggression.

To provide some empirical support for her assertions, Clark reports that more than half the variance in interview diagnoses of antisocial, borderline, paranoid, and dependent personality disorders was predicted in multiple regression equations from self-reports, with "approximately 40–70% of the predictable variance . . . accounted for by the three temperament scales [negative temperament, positive temperament, and disinhibition]" (p. 195). For other disorders, however, less than a third of the variance in interview-based assessments was predicted from self-reports, including reports of temperament, prompting Clark to suggest "that scales assessing the quality and quantity of interpersonal engagement is as or more important as affective temperament in some personality pathology" (p. 196). This comment suggests not a spectrum model but, rather, a predisposition model in which interpersonal relations may play a leading role, a possibility that is addressed later.

Clark has made general contributions to the dimensional assessment of personality disorders, whether or not understood as spectrum/temperamental disorders, with her Schedule for Nonadaptive and Adaptive Personality (SNAP; Clark, McEwen, Collard, & Hickok, 1993). The SNAP includes 15 scales: 3 reflecting higher-order temperamental variables (negative temperament, positive temperament, disinhibition) and 12 reflecting lower-order personality disorder themes (mistrust, manipulativeness, aggression, self-harm, eccentric perceptions, dependency, detachment, exhibitionism, entitlement, impulsivity, propriety, and workaholism). Livesley and his colleagues (Livesley, 1990; Livesley, Jackson, & Schroeder, 1992) have developed a similar instrument, the Dimensional Assessment of Personality Pathology (DAPP), which incorporates 18 dimensions retained from analyses of personality pathology reflected in 100 different personality scales completed by both a clinical and a general population sample. These dimensions include affective lability, anxiousness, callousness, cognitive distortion, compulsivity, conduct problems, identity problems, insecure attachment, intimacy problems, narcissism, oppositionality, rejection, restricted expression, self-harm, social avoidance, stimulus seeking, submissiveness, and suspiciousness.

Jang, Livesley, Vernon, and Jackson (1996) investigated the heritability of these dimensions in a sample of 483 twins. Their results were similar to those of studies of the genetic and environmental influences on normal personality traits. The dimensions had heritabilities in the range from 35% to 56% (with a median of 47%), almost all of which could be modeled by additive genetic influences. Shared environment contributed relatively little, with most of the environmental influence captured by non-shared environmental factors. Nigg and Goldsmith (1994) provide an overview and summary of the evidence about the genetics of personality disorders. They make the point that dimensional assessments of features cutting across current personality disorder categories may be particularly useful and that the heritability of these dimensions may be most informative. Belmaker and Biederman (1994) draw a similar conclusion. Their assumption is that genes underlie general temperaments and that it may be more profitable to look for genetic linkages at this level rather than at the level of family pedigrees and specific disorders.

One associated but unresolved problem is the selection of the level of the trait hierarchy at which to investigate such issues. Harkness (1992) points out that the "number of dimensions depends on the level at which one slices through the hierarchy," creating the inevitable trade-off between "bandwidth" and "fidelity" that such a decision entails (p. 251). Most approaches to this problem have focused on higher levels of the trait hierarchy (e.g., the FFM). Examples of informative but different levels of the hierarchy would be the Big Five factors, followed by the 12–18 first-order domains described by Clark and Livesley and colleagues, followed by the 39 "narrow" traits described by Harkness. The important point here is that one must be clear about the level of the trait hierarchy at which one is working for conceptual, assessment, or treatment purposes and that one must be prepared for different levels to have different utilities. For example, it may be possible to screen for personality disorders at a global level, but most clinical work is likely to proceed at a middle to lower level, addressing problems of anger, attachment, impulsivity, and so on.

Relevant to a discussion of spectrum models are data on behavioral genetics at the higher levels of the trait hierarchy. Viken, Rose, Kaprio, and Koskenvuo (1994) document that there are age-variant (and sex-related) changes in the influence of genetic and environmental factors on the major personality traits of neuroticism and extraversion. Genetic influences appear to be stronger earlier in life, with new environmental contributions appearing throughout life, presumably as a function of nonshared environmental influences: "There was little evidence of new genetic contributions to individual differences after age 30; in contrast, significant new environmental effects emerged at every age" (p. 722) in a cross-sequential design in which almost 15,000 Finnish twins were assessed initially at ages 18 to 53 and then reassessed 6 years later. McGue, Bacon, and Lykken (1993) reached a similar conclusion in a study of 127 twin pairs who completed the Multidimensional Personality Questionnaire (MPQ) at age 20 and 30: "It is concluded that the stable core of personality is strongly associated with genetic factors but that personality change largely reflects environmental factors" (p. 96).

These inferences about the changing impact of genetics and experience across the lifespan and the role of environmental influences on personality *change* (regardless of the original genetic substrate) echo Parker's (1997) reservations about whether extremes in temperament alone can account for ultimate membership in some personality disorder class. His argument is that there may be a separate component of functional impairment, with a distinct trajectory, that also needs to be conceptualized and investigated empirically. These questions lead us to predisposition and risk-factor models rather than pure spectrum approaches.

Predisposition Models

The second group of models that deserve close attention is predisposition models in which Axis II risk factors are linked to Axis I symptom disorders through various developmental pathways (see Holmbeck, 1997, and Kraemer et al., 1997, for helpful discussions of conceptualizing risk, moderating, and mediating factors). Strong versions of such models hypothesize causal risk factors and point to direct etiology. Weaker versions include diathesis–stress models (only in interaction with certain life stresses or developmental challenges do personality features and disorders produce negative outcomes) and pathoplasty models (regardless of causality, personality influences the phenotypical expression and clinical characteristics of symptom disorders).

Examples of risk factors that reflect stable personality vulnerabilities (if not always diagnosable personality disorders in categorical terms) include the "general neurotic syndrome" (i.e., high arousability and low inhibition), affective dysregulation in general, and attachment disturbances. In describing the first factor, Tyrer, Seivewright, Ferguson, and Tyrer (1992) argue that features of dependent, avoidant, and obsessive–compulsive personality disorders associated with intermittent exacerbations of anxiety and depression constitute a single entity called the general neurotic syndrome (GNS), best understood as "a personality diathesis that makes the individual more vulnerable to both anxiety and depressive symptoms" (p. 201). In their report, the presence versus absence of GNS and initial levels of psychopathology were the best predictors of symptomatic outcome following treatment, suggesting that the presence of GNS "could be an explanation for the finding that a significant minority of patients with anxiety and depressive disorders fare badly in long-term follow-up studies" (p. 204).

Andrews (1996) characterizes this general vulnerability factor as a combination of high trait anxiety and poor coping and uses it to account for the substantial comorbidity among depressive and anxiety disorders: "In the model we espouse. . . , adversity is regarded as a trigger stimulus for symptoms; trait anxiety as a powerful moderating variable on the extent of arousal produced by the adversity; and reality-focused and emotion-focused coping as trait-like attributes that the person uses to focus attention on resolving the adversity or on preventing the anxiety from becoming debilitating" (p. 77). Much of this vulnerability, given its temperamental cast, is genetically and biologically mediated, whether measured at the level of symptoms or at the level of "antecedent constructs" such as neuroticism, trait anxiety, and coping style. The clear implication is that treatment should be aimed not only at resolving symptoms but also at diminishing the vulnerability through strategies for improving reality-based coping, lessening arousal, or both.

An inability to regulate emotional experience may itself may be a risk factor best understood as a personality vulnerability often associated with symptom disorders, especially affective disorders. Mood has a variety of second-order, as well as first-order, components that are likely to have important clinical implications. The most obvious first-order component is the general level of positive and negative mood (as we have seen previously in discussing spectrum models), but various second-order features have also been identified as relevant: for example, differences in (1) the ability to modulate affect regardless of its absolute level, (2) the importance of the intensity versus frequency of affective experiences, (3) a focus on the arousal versus valence components of mood, (4) the intrapersonal variability of mood, (5) the circadian experience of mood, and (6) the amount of attention devoted to moods and related perceptions, beliefs, and attitudes about emotion.

Linehan (1993), for example, has proposed a "biosocial" theory of borderline personality disorder that focuses on a predisposition to affective dysregulation that is then amplified by the developmental influences of an emotionally "invalidating" environment. Affective dysregulation is described in terms similar to the Thomas and Chess (1977) definition of a "difficult" temperament (i.e., proneness to negative affect, proneness to intense affect, and a slow return to baseline once negatively aroused). Although emphasizing temperament, Linehan's model is not a pure spectrum model. It requires some interaction with an "invalidating" environment to produce the clinical disorder of borderline personality disorder, which then predisposes to a host of symptom disorders—depression, panic disorder, substance abuse, eating disorders, somatoform disorders, and others.

Diener, Colvin, Pavot, and Allman (1991) have commented on the costs of intense positive affect that may counterbalance its intuitive appeal, pointing out that measures of subjective well-being are more heavily influenced by the frequency of positive versus negative emotional experiences than by the occurrence of intense positive affect. Feldman (1995) has investigated the relative importance of the valence versus arousal components of moods. She hypothesizes individual differences in the degree to which people attend to these aspects of mood experience: "Degree of valence focus is defined as individual differences in the tendency to attend to and report the pleasant or unpleasant aspects of emotional experience. . . . Degree of arousal focus is defined as individual differences in the tendency to attend to and report the physiological arousal associated with affective states" (pp. 153–154). Feldman presents some preliminary evidence that relationships between reports of anxiety and depression and between positive and negative affectivity vary as a function of these individual differ-

ences, making the point that there are "potentially important differences between cross-sectional and within-subject measurements of mood" (p. 165).

Penner, Shiffman, Paty, and Fritzsche (1994) used a direct experience-sampling methodology over a 12–14-day period to document that mood variability was both stable across time and over situations and that it could be distinguished from item valences, response biases, or response errors. They drew the conclusion "that intraperson mood variability appears to be as stable and reliable across time and across situations as mood level, and its stability approximates that of other personality characteristics. . . ." (p. 718). Also on the theme of mood variability, Rusting and Larsen (1998) provide data showing that an "evening-worse" pattern of diurnal variation in negative mood "was associated with many neurotic features, with scores on depression and anxiety measures, and with a cognitive style indicative of hopelessness" (pp. 85–86).

The literature on the meta-experience of mood points to the importance of the differential deployment of attention to mood and the differing attitudes and expectations that people have about emotional experience. Salovey, Mayer, Goldman, Turvey, and Palfai (1995) developed a measure called the Trait Meta-Mood Scale (TMMS), with three subscales—the attention to mood subscale, which focuses on attitudes regarding the importance of attending to mood and the amount of attention devoted to affective experience; the clarity in discrimination of feelings subscale, which reflects how distinctly and clearly people report experiencing moods; and the mood repair subscale, which reflects a person's attempts to counteract negative affectivity in order to maintain a more positive emotional tone. In later studies, they pointed out that such second-order attitudes and relationships to moods may be important moderators of "the relation between distress and symptom and illness reporting" (Goldman, Kraemer, & Salovey, 1996, p. 115).

Izard (1993) has described a model designed to integrate an understanding of emotional activation across various "levels" of experience. He describes four systems for the activation of emotions: neural systems, sensorimotor systems, motivational systems, and cognitive systems. He suggests that these systems are arranged hierarchically (in the order just listed), with "continuously active" neural systems at the bottom of the hierarchy and cognitions at the top of the hierarchy. He also acknowledges that these systems for activating emotions are also influenced by at least three kinds of constraints: individual differences (some of which are genetically and biologically mediated), social and interpersonal factors (including the impact of early attachment relationships), and situational factors.

The point of focusing on the second-order components of emotional experience is to alert us to the clinical possibilities that these features suggest. As clinicians, we must attend to the general level of negative and positive mood that our patients describe, but also relevant are their reports of other attributes of their emotions (e.g., intensity, variability, and circadian rhythms) and their attitudes toward moods and their vicissitudes. If we assume that general levels of negative and positive mood operate within certain, relatively stable temperamental constraints, then trying to alter these general levels assumes less clinical priority than changing a patient's relationship to his or her own affective experience (e.g., by providing understanding about the parameters of expectable mood, by providing skills for better modulation of mood, and in general, by enhancing self-efficacy in relation to affective experience).

A third risk factor that can be understood in personality terms and that has received much attention in relation to symptom disorders is attachment disturbances. The variants of insecure attachment are most often described, on the one hand, as anxious/ambivalent, sociotropic, anaclitic, and dependent, and on the other hand, as anxious/avoidant, autonomous, introjective, and self-critical. There is a rich literature focusing on relationships between these attachment styles and depression in particular (Nietzel & Harris, 1990). Blatt and Shichman (1983) have contended that these themes can be used as a general conceptual framework for understanding developmental psychopathology.

Ouimette, Klein, Anderson, Riso, and Lizardi (1994) have also made the case for "extending the range of psychopathology associated with the dimensions of sociotropy/dependency and autonomy/self-criticism to the personality disorders" (p. 748). They reported data showing the convergence between these themes and the assessment of DSM personality disorders in a way that is theoretically meaningful and clinically useful. By contrast, Coyne and Whiffen (1995) offer an extensive critique of this litera-

ture. They are quite critical of some attempts to measure these constructs, they point to the confounding of personality styles and the signs and symptoms of depression in particular, and they discuss the difficulty of separating the influence of personality from that of the social context, especially when stable environmental pressures and serious life events may be linked to depression.

TREATMENT ISSUES

The usual conclusion, in psychiatric samples, is that personality disorders complicate first-line treatments, producing slower response, less complete response, or both (Pilkonis & Frank, 1988; Shea, Widiger, & Klein, 1992). In particular, the impact of a comorbid personality disorder on the course and treatment of affective disorders has received considerable attention. Comorbidity rates have been found to be high, with studies estimating the prevalence of personality disorders among depressed patients to range from 30% to 81% (Alnaes & Torgersen, 1988; Charney, Nelson, & Quinlan, 1981; Farmer & Nelson-Gray, 1990; Pilkonis & Frank, 1988; Shea, Glass, Pilkonis, Watkins, & Docherty, 1987). In general, the literature indicates that a comorbid personality disorder leads to a worse prognosis for patients with depressive disorders (Frances, Fyer, & Clarkin, 1986; Shea et al., 1992), with an earlier onset of depression (Charney et al., 1981; Pfohl, Stangl, & Zimmerman, 1984), more suicide attempts and ideation (Black, Bell, Hulbert, & Nasrallah, 1988; Shea et al., 1987), and worse treatment outcome (Charney et al., 1981; Pilkonis & Frank, 1988; Shea et al., 1990; Zimmerman, Coryell, Pfohl, Corenthal, & Stangl, 1986). In particular, borderline personality disorder has been associated with an increased risk of suicide attempts in depressed patients (Friedman, Aronoff, Clarkin, Corn, & Hurt, 1983; McGlashan, 1987; Pfohl et al., 1984), although the judged lethality of such attempts has varied across studies.

Some studies have found that comorbid personality disorders are equally or even more common with anxiety, somatoform, and substance abuse disorders than with affective disorders (Alnaes & Torgersen, 1988; Koenigsberg, Kaplan, Gilmore, & Cooper, 1985; Nace, Davis, & Gaspari, 1991; Ross, Glaser, & Germanson, 1988). The presence of personality disorders has also been found to affect adversely the treatment outcome of these other Axis I disorders (Reich & Vasile, 1993; Stein, Hollander, & Skodol, 1993). Despite this consensus, Tyrer, Gunderson, Lyons, and Tohen (1997) caution that certain of these conclusions may be overstated, and they provide some counterexamples in which a comorbid personality disorder had no effect, or even a positive effect, on treatment outcome (pp. 252–254).

Developing Optimal Treatment Strategies

The goal of increased focus on Axis II disorders in the context of symptom disorders is to promote greater clinical effectiveness and, thus, to improve outcome for patients. Adaptations required include increased attention to temperaments and vulnerabilities, whether understood as spectrum phenomena or predisposing risk factors; improved case formulation, with greater emphasis on longitudinal profiles, life charts, and similar tools; greater attention to prodromal features that signal the onset or exacerbation of a symptom disorder; and the use of a chronic illness model and strategies for "maintenance" treatment with the goal of decreasing the probability of relapse or recurrence (cf. Frank et al., 1990).

Key Role of Formulation

The first challenge is case formulation. One must gather and integrate all relevant information across the two (Axis I and II) domains in a way that is conceptually meaningful *and* actually informs clinical technique. Harkness and Lilienfeld (1997) make a strong plea for incorporating an awareness of the current science of personality psychology and individual differences, including work on behavioral genetics, into any treatment plan. They point to several advantages for such an approach, including focusing efforts at change on "characteristic adaptations" rather than "basic tendencies" in temperament and personality (which are less likely to change), matching personality to treatment, and promoting the development of the patient's sense of self by articulating more clearly the "basic tendencies" of the self and by devising more adaptive ways of coping. The broad goal is to create realistic expectations about the changes possible in psychotherapy: "[W]e will hazard a proposal: The single great-

est misconception that patients (and perhaps some therapists) hold about therapy is the expectation that a high-NE [negative emotionality] person can be turned into a low-NE person" (Harkness & Lilienfeld, 1997, p. 356).

With spectrum models, the focus is on temperamental extremes, exaggerations, or blends. The goal is to help patients develop a better recognition of and relationship with their own temperament. Therefore, the focus of treatment is on modulation of characteristic temperamental extremes, recognition of prodromal signs of symptomatic exacerbations that may cross the threshold into diagnosable Axis I problems, and interruption of such processes of amplification and escalation.

Cassano et al. (1997) describe a clinically oriented approach to understanding and treating the panic–agoraphobia spectrum. These investigators have created an interview to assess 144 behaviors and experiences in seven domains that they regard as parts of a single spectrum with a "unitary pathophysiology" (p. 27). For panic–agoraphobia, the domains are panic symptoms, anxious expectation (both anticipatory anxiety about panic symptoms and a heightened vigilance in general), phobic features, sensitivity to reassurance, sensitivity to substances, sensitivity to general stress, and sensitivity to separation. Cassano et al. (1997) argue for the clinical utility of a spectrum approach on several grounds: improved formulation of patients' problems because more subtle and subthreshold phenomena are included, the use of such formulation to guide treatment selection (they hypothesize, for example, that a depressed patient with a spectrum liability of panic/agoraphobia/anxiety will benefit from different treatments than a depressed patient with another spectrum comorbidity such as eating spectrum problems), and the enhancement of the therapeutic relationship, which results in greater treatment compliance and efficacy—patients will feel better understood and will be more motivated and collaborative as a result.

With predisposition and risk-factor models, the challenge is to specify the mechanisms that moderate and mediate risk. The three risk factors discussed previously fit best within a diathesis–stress framework in which the risk factor serves as a moderator that interacts with environmental and situational stressors to produce symptom disorders. Hypotheses regarding the general neurotic syndrome or affective dysregulation in general propose that there are people with vulnerable temperaments who, when confronted with various challenges, become hyperaroused, often without adequate tools for coping with such arousal. Hypotheses regarding attachment disturbances focus less on issues of temperament and arousal and more on the interpersonal processes and cognitive appraisals instigated by life events and developmental challenges; thus, people who are preoccupied with attachment (anxious/ambivalent) are most vulnerable in the face of loss and separation, whereas people who are dismissive (anxious/avoidant) are vulnerable in the face of experiences that compromise their sense of mastery, control, and autonomy. In either case, treatment must focus on the identification and management of stressors or triggers that interact with vulnerability, whether those vulnerabilities are based in temperament or in relationship issues.

In the area of mood specifically, spectrum models, with a heavier emphasis on temperament per se, are more likely to focus on strategies for up- and downregulating mood (e.g., heightening positive affect and lessening negative affect). Risk-factor models are more likely to focus on second-order characteristics of mood experience and regulation (e.g., attitudes about affect, self-efficacy regarding the ability to manage moods, and modulating the variability of moods), regardless of their valence.

Need for Innovative Treatment Development

By definition, personality disorders are chronic. Thus, we need innovation and efforts at treatment development that incorporate state-of-the-art principles of chronic illness management, including concerns about cost-effectiveness (but not simply attempts at cost containment). There are at least three "families" of treatment alternatives: (1) continuous treatment, at different intensities; (2) acute treatment, followed by maintenance strategies; and (3) primary care models (i.e., brief acute treatments at the patient's discretion, provided in the context of a stable relationship over time and a willingness to treat many different kinds of problems). There are suggestions in the literature on somatoform disorders (Bass & Benjamin, 1993), however, that being proactive, even without highly intensive outpatient treatments, can be beneficial (e.g., scheduling regular brief appointments in advance rather than relying on requests for care initiated by patients). We also need "dosage" guidelines for all these possibilities, and the work of Howard and his colleagues (Howard, Kopta, Krause, & Orlinsky, 1986; Kopta, Howard, Lowry, & Beutler, 1994) has been seminal in this regard.

A potential compromise between continuous and intermittent models of care could be "staged" models of treatment, in which different stages or sequences are identified, operationalized, and offered in flexible ways (either consecutively or separated in time). Such models are conceptually appealing, but a critical empirical issue is the ability to identify "milestones" that have sufficient predictive validity to drive decisions about the course, sequencing, and interruption of care. Thus, it may be useful to develop models of sequential changes in treatment that can be measured reliably and that signal positive long-term outcomes; in such models, the ability of patients to move from stages 1 to 2 to 3 would be an important outcome in itself. For patients with severe personality disorders, such stages are likely to involve (1) the achievement of physical safety and evidence of day-to-day emotional stability, (2) articulation and emotional processing of adverse concurrent and historical circumstances, and (3) efforts at personal growth and improvements in the quality of life.

Examples of attempts at such models include dialectical behavior therapy (DBT; Linehan, 1993) for patients with borderline personality disorder, where Stage I is focused on life-threatening and treatment-interfering behavior; Stage II can then involve emotional processing of earlier developmental adversity, and Stage III focuses on quality-of-life issues. There are similar suggestions in the literature on the treatment of trauma and early abuse (Herman, 1992) where the first stage is stabilization of the patient, the second is the "working through" of the trauma, and the third is promotion of greater involvement with current life circumstances and relationships.

A staged model has also been implemented by Hogarty et al. (1997) in their personal therapy for schizophrenia, that is, a "graduated, three-stage, systemic approach" (p. 1506). The first, basic phase aims at establishing a treatment alliance and stabilizing the patient's clinical state; the intermediate phase focuses on more advanced psychoeducation, internal coping strategies to manage stress, and skills training to remediate deficits in social behavior; the advanced phase focuses on increased social and vocational initiatives in the community. The approach is purposely designed to be flexible: "[T]he many strategies embodied in personal therapy were not applied in equal 'doses' to every patient. Rather, selected principles of personal therapy were tailored to patients' individual needs" (p. 1507).

Incorporation of Adult Developmental Tasks into an Optimal Treatment Framework

Given a longitudinal perspective on the etiology, pathogenesis, and treatment of personality disorders, it is often useful to frame treatment goals in a developmental context. Thus, the aims of treatment are not only to relieve symptomatic distress and to try to prevent future symptoms but also to ensure engagement with the developmental tasks of adulthood (cf. Erikson, 1978): the establishment of satisfying interpersonal attachments; the development of a consistent and positive sense of self, personal competencies, autonomy, and accomplishments; and the development of generativity (i.e., the capacity to "give back" to others and to foster their own development). Seen in these terms, state-related and symptomatic concerns (e.g., whether one is happy or sad) are important, but equally important is the experience of being "engaged," whether happy or sad, in the genuine tasks of adulthood and of feeling "vital" and alive as a result. A painful realization for some patients with Axis II disorders is the awareness that they have defaulted on the developmental challenges of life, regardless of the waxing and waning of their symptom disorders.

With many patients, the ability to take on these developmental tasks in vigorous ways will depend on the stability and comfort they feel with the therapist as a primary attachment figure. Thus, successful treatments may require certain common features: the provision of psychoeducation regarding the consequences of early attachment adversity, abuse, or neglect; a functional analysis of different styles of interpersonal coping and defense, with suggestions about possible alternatives; and an explanation of the importance of developing a secure interpersonal base that is respectful of needs for both attachment and autonomy. Thus it is often necessary to monitor patients' expectation about the current therapeutic relationship, to be flexible in deploying various relationship-building techniques, to identify the inevitable "ruptures" (sometimes subtle and private) that occur in any therapeutic context, and to work to repair such ruptures when they do occur.

Because of increased interest in blending work on developmental themes with the treatment of symptom disorders, the literature on applications of attachment theory to psychotherapy is growing. Holmes (1993, 1996) has described the importance of attachment and the perception of a "secure base" in therapy; the impact of emotional processing focused on issues of loss, separation, and other forms of trauma; and the process of reworking of internal representational models of attachment relationships. Such a discussion points to the need to do an attachment "diagnosis" and then to alter one's relationship repertoire to fit the particular patient's attachment style. Thus, Holmes (1993, Table 8.1, p. 163) suggests that the avoidant person is initially frightened of close contact with the therapist, who must allow the relationship to develop at an arm's length while remaining friendly and engaged and avoiding the temptation to "intrude" excessively on the patient. The ambivalent person is more frightened of separation and needs a combination of "absolute reliability and firm limit setting to help with secure attachment, combined with a push towards exploration" (p. 154).

Dolan, Arnkoff, and Glass (1993) describe another example of this combination of assessment of attachment style and an attempt on the part of the therapist to match that style. In their study, attachment style was related to symptomatology and perceptions of the working alliance on the part of the therapist. Dozier, Cue, and Barnett (1994) provide evidence that clinicians' own attachment styles influence their work: "Compared with secure case managers, insecure case managers attended more to dependency needs and intervened in greater depth with preoccupied clients than they did with dismissing clients. Case managers who were more preoccupied intervened with their clients in greater depth than did case managers who were more dismissing" (p. 793). Finally, West, Sheldon, and Reiffer (1989) discuss the use of attachment themes in brief psychotherapy where the focus is on "undoing of the denied impact of 'losses,' the expression of disavowed feelings, principally anger and sorrowful yearning, and the integration of dissociated information relevant to attachment" (p. 373).

Use of a Treatment Team

For work with patients with severe personality disorders, the use of a treatment team is indicated. Such "teams" might vary from a collection of individual therapists providing peer supervision, all of whom are committed to working with a "difficult-to-treat" population, to integrated teams where members play defined roles within the model of care being provided (e.g., DBT, with its collection of individual therapists, group skills leaders, and pharmcotherapists when needed). In any case, the emotional burden of treating patients with severe personality disorders and socially disruptive behaviors, whether directed at self (e.g., parasuicide) or others (e.g., verbal and physical aggression), is often too great for an individual therapist alone. A team helps to "metabolize" intense affect and to provide support to continue the work in the face of discouragement, slow progress, and incentives to simply give up the treatment. Most patients of this sort have experienced an iatrogenic pattern of initial willingness on the part of therapists to work with them, only to be followed by rejection when therapists become hopeless and discouraged (cf. Maltsberger & Buie, 1974, on negative reactions experienced by the therapist, their dual elements of malice and aversion, and their assertion that it is aversion [i.e., "abandoning" a patient], not malice [i.e., "hating" a patient], that constitutes a greater risk factor for those we treat). The use of a treatment team can also foster a "group" attachment and a sense of social integration that many patients find sustaining ("there is a group of people out there caring for me, working with my therapist, and monitoring how I am doing").

Need for the Application of More Powerful Research Designs and Quantitative Tools

A comment on the need for evaluation of treatment outcome and appropriate models for evaluation can provide a closing note. Regardless of the treatment modalities used, we need more data-intensive research designs to evaluate them and the use of more sophisticated tools to model longitudinal data rather than the traditional reliance on group averages and pre–post analyses. Longitudinal designs, of course, involve repeated measurements, and repeated measurements introduce certain statistical complexities (e.g., correlated measurement error). In addition, longitudinal designs can be compromised by attrition or missing data at various assessment points, even if subjects are not lost completely. Kraemer and Thiemann (1989) have provided useful suggestions about the analysis of data from such "intensive designs." In a similar vein, Gibbons et al. (1993) and Lavori (1990) surveyed several competing methods for analyzing longitudinal data, including repeated-measures analysis of variance, multivariate analysis of variance, and random regression models. This last approach is especially useful because it can accommodate most kinds of missing data, irregularly spaced measurements, correlated errors of measurement, time-varying and time-invariant covariates, and individual deviations from an aggregate response trend. The general point is that such techniques should become first-line approaches to treatment outcome data. Such models provide more understanding of individual differences among patients and allow inspection of alternative trajectories of change. The rate at which different treatments achieve their effects is a significant concern, especially if we are to investigate modalities of extended care for chronic disorders.

REFERENCES

Akiskal, H. S. (1983). Dysthymic disorder: Psychopathology of proposed chronic depressive subtypes. *American Journal of Psychiatry, 140,* 11–20.

Akiskal, H. S., Hirschfeld, R. M. A., & Yerevanian, B. I. (1983). The relationship of personality to affective disorders: A critical review. *Archives of General Psychiatry, 40,* 801–810.

Akiskal, H. S., Rosenthal, T. L., Haykal, R. F., Lemmi, H., Rosenthal, R. H., & Scott-Strauss, A. (1980). Characterological depressions: Clinical and sleep EEG findings separating "subaffective dysthymias" from "character spectrum disorders." *Archives of General Psychiatry, 37,* 777–783.

Alnaes, R., & Torgersen, S. (1988). DSM-III symptom disorders (Axis I) and personality disorders (Axis II) in an outpatient population. *Acta Psychiatrica Scandinavica, 78,* 348–355.

Anderson, R. L., Klein, D. N., Riso, L. P., Ouimette, P. C., Lizardi, H., & Schwartz, J. E. (1996). The subaffective-character spectrum subtyping distinction in primary early-onset dysthymia: A clinical and family study. *Journal of Affective Disorders, 38,* 13–22.

Andrews, G. (1996). Comorbidity and the general neurotic syndrome. *British Journal of Psychiatry, 168*(Suppl. 30), 76–84.

Bass, C., & Benjamin, S. (1993). The management of chronic somatisation. *British Journal of Psychiatry, 162,* 472–480.

Battaglia, M., Przybeck, T. R., Bellodi, L., & Cloninger, C. R. (1996). Temperament dimensions explain the comorbidity of psychiatric disorders. *Comprehensive Psychiatry, 37,* 292–298.

Belmaker, R. H., & Biederman, J. (1994). Genetic markers, temperament, and psychopathology. *Biological Psychiatry, 36,* 71–72.

Black, D. W., Bell, S., Hulbert, J., & Nasrallah, A. (1988). The importance of Axis II in patients with major depression. *Journal of Affective Disorders, 14,* 115–122.

Blatt, S. J., & Shichman, S. (1983). Two primary configurations of psychopathology. *Psychoanalysis and Contemporary Thought, 6,* 187–254.

Cassano, G. B., Michelini, S., Shear, M. K., Coli, E., Maser, J. D., & Frank, E. (1997, June). The panic-agoraphobic spectrum: A descriptive approach to the assessment and treatment of subtle symptoms. *American Journal of Psychiatry, 154* (Festschrift Suppl.) 27–38.

Charney, D. S., Nelson, J. C., & Quinlan, D. M. (1981). Personality traits and disorder in depression. *American Journal of Psychiatry, 138,* 1601–1604.

Clark, L. A. (2000). Mood, personality, and personality disorder. In R. Davidson (Ed.), *Anxiety, depression and emotion* (pp. 171–200). New York: Oxford University Press.

Clark, L. A., McEwen, J. L., Collard, L. M., & Hickok, L. G. (1993). Symptoms and traits of personality disorder: Two new methods for their assessment. *Psychological Assessment, 5,* 81–91.

Cloninger, C. R. (1987). A systematic method for clinical description and classification of personality variants: A proposal. *Archives of General Psychiatry, 44,* 573–588.

Cloninger, C. R., Svrakic, D. M., & Przybeck, T. R. (1993). A psychobiological model of temperament and character. *Archives of General Psychiatry, 50,* 975–990.

Costa, P. T., Jr., & McCrae, R. R. (1992). The five-factor model of personality and its relevance to personality disorders. *Journal of Personality Disorders, 6,* 343–359.

Coyne, J. C., & Whiffen, V. E. (1995). Issues in personality as diathesis for depression: The case of sociotropy–dependency and autonomy–self-criticism. *Psychological Bulletin, 118,* 358–378.

Diener, E., Colvin, C. R., Pavot, W. G., & Allman, A. (1991). The psychic costs of intense positive affect. *Journal of Personality and Social Psychology, 61,* 492–503.

Dolan, R. T., Arnkoff, D. B., & Glass, C. R. (1993). Client attachment style and the psychotherapist's interpersonal stance. *Psychotherapy, 30,* 408–412.

Dozier, M., Cue, K. L., & Barnett, L. (1994). Clinicians as caregivers: Role of attachment organization in treatment. *Journal of Consulting and Clinical Psychology, 62,* 793–800.

Erikson, E. H. (Ed.). (1978). *Adulthood.* New York: Norton.

Fabrega, H., Jr., Ulrich, R., Pilkonis, P. A., & Mezzich, J. E. (1992). Pure personality disorders in an intake psychiatric setting. *Journal of Personality Disorders, 6,* 153–161.

Farmer, R., & Nelson-Gray, R. O. (1990). Personality disorders and depression: Hypothetical relations, empirical findings, and methodological considerations. *Clinical Psychology Review, 10,* 453–476.

Feldman, L. A. (1995). Valence focus and arousal focus: Individual differences in the structure of affective experience. *Journal of Personality and Social Psychology, 69,* 153–166.

Frances, A., Fyer, M., & Clarkin, J. (1986). Personality and suicide. *Annals of the New York Academy of Sciences, 487,* 281–293.

Frank, E., Kupfer, D. J., Perel, J. M., Cornes, C., Jarrett, D. B., Mallinger, A. G., Thase, M. E., McEachran, A. B., & Grochocinski, V. J. (1990). Three-year outcomes for maintenance therapies in recurrent depression. *Archives of General Psychiatry, 47,* 1093–1099.

Friedman, R. C., Aronoff, M. S., Clarkin, J. F., Corn, R., & Hurt, S. W. (1983). History of suicidal behavior in depressed borderline inpatients. *American Journal of Psychiatry, 140,* 1023–1026.

Gibbons, R. D., Hedeker, D., Elkin, I., Waternaux, C., Kraemer, H. C., Greenhouse, J. B., Shea, M. T., Imber, S. D., Sotsky, S. M., & Watkins, J. T. (1993). Some conceptual and statistical issues in the analysis of longitudinal psychiatric data: Application to the NIMH Treatment of Depression Collaborative Research Program dataset. *Archives of General Psychiatry, 50,* 739–750.

Goldberg, L. R. (1993). The structure of phenotypic personality traits. *American Psychologist, 48,* 26–34.

Goldman, S. L., Kraemer, D. T., & Salovey, P. (1996). Beliefs about mood moderate the relationship of stress to illness and symptom reporting. *Journal of Psychosomatic Research, 41,* 115–128.

Gray, J. A. (1982). *The neuropsychology of anxiety: An enquiry into the functions of the septo-hippocampal system.* Oxford, UK: Oxford University Press.

Gray, J. A. (1987). *The psychology of fear and stress* (2nd ed.). Cambridge, UK: Cambridge University Press.

Harkness, A. R. (1992). Fundamental topics in the personality disorders: Candidate trait dimensions from lower regions of the hierarchy. *Psychological Assessment, 4,* 251–259.

Harkness, A. R., & Lilienfeld, S. O. (1997). Individual differences science for treatment planning: Personality traits. *Psychological Assessment, 9,* 349–360.

Herman, J. L. (1992). *Trauma and recovery.* New York: Basic Books.

Hogarty, G. E., Kornblith, S. J., Greenwald, D., DiBarry, A. L., Cooley, S., Ulrich, R., Carter, M., & Flesher, S. (1997). Three-year trials of personal therapy among schizophrenic patients living with or independent of family: I. Description of study and effects on relapse rates. *American Journal of Psychiatry, 154,* 1504–1513.

Holmbeck, G. N. (1997). Toward terminological, conceptual, and statistical clarity in the study of mediators and moderators: Examples from the child–clinical and pediatric psychology literatures. *Journal of Consulting and Clinical Psychology, 65,* 599–610.

Holmes, J. (1993). *John Bowlby and attachment theory.* New York: Routledge.

Holmes, J. (1996). *Attachment, intimacy, autonomy: Using attachment in adult psychotherapy.* Northvale, NJ: Jason Aronson.

Howard, K. I., Kopta, S. M., Krause, M. S., & Orlinsky, D. E. (1986). The dose–effect relationship in psychotherapy. *American Psychologist, 41,* 159–164.

Izard, C. E. (1993). Four systems for emotion activation: Cognitive and noncognitive processes. *Psychological Review, 100,* 68–90.

Jang, K. L., Livesley, W. J., Vernon, P. A., & Jackson, D. N. (1996). Heritability of personality disorder traits: A twin study. *Acta Psychiatrica Scandinavica, 94,* 438–444.

Koenigsberg, H. W., Kaplan, R. D., Gilmore, M. M., & Cooper, A. M. (1985). The relationship between syndrome and personality disorder in DSM-III: Experience with 2,462 patients. *American Journal of Psychiatry, 142,* 207–212.

Kopta, S. M., Howard, K. I., Lowry, J. L., & Beutler, L. E. (1994). Patterns of symptomatic recovery in psychotherapy. *Journal of Consulting and Clinical Psychology, 62,* 1009–1016.

Kraemer, H. C., Kazdin, A. E., Offord, D. R., Kessler, R. C., Jensen, P. S., & Kupfer, D. J. (1997). Coming to terms with the terms of risk. *Archives of General Psychiatry, 54,* 337–343.

Kraemer, H. C., & Thiemann, S. (1989). A strategy to use soft data effectively in randomized controlled clinical trials. *Journal of Consulting and Clinical Psychology, 57,* 148–154.

Lavori, P. (1990). ANOVA, MANOVA, my black hen. *Archives of General Psychiatry, 47,* 775–778.

Linehan, M. M. (1993). *Cognitive-behavioral treatment of borderline personality disorder.* New York: Guilford Press.

Livesley, W. J. (1990). *Dimensional Assessment of Personality Pathology—Basic Questionnaire.* Department of Psychiatry, University of British Columbia.

Livesley, W. J., Jackson, D. N., & Schroeder, M. L. (1992). Factorial structure of traits delineating personality disorders in clinical and general population samples. *Journal of Abnormal Psychology, 101,* 432–440.

Lyons, M. J., Tyrer, P., Gunderson, J., & Tohen, M. (1997). Heuristic models of comorbidity of Axis I and Axis II disorders. *Journal of Personality Disorders, 11,* 260–269.

Maltsberger, J. T., & Buie, D. H. (1974). Countertransference hate in the treatment of suicidal patients. *Archives of General Psychiatry, 30,* 625–633.

McGlashan, T. (1987). Borderline personality disorder and unipolar affective disorder. *Journal of Nervous and Mental Disease, 175,* 467–473.

McGue, M., Bacon, S., & Lykken, D. T. (1993). Personality stability and change in early adulthood: A behavioral genetic analysis. *Developmental Psychology, 29,* 96–109.

Mulder, R. T., & Joyce, P. R. (1997). Temperament and the structure of personality disorder symptoms. *Psychological Medicine, 27,* 99–106.

Mulder, R. T., Joyce, P. R., & Cloninger, C. R. (1994). Temperament and early environment influence comorbidity and personality disorders in major depression. *Comprehensive Psychiatry, 35,* 225–233.

Nace, E. P., Davis, C. W., & Gaspari, J. (1991). Axis II comorbidity in substance abusers. *American Journal of Psychiatry, 148,* 118–120.

Nietzel, M. T., & Harris, M. J. (1990). Relationship of dependency and achievement/autonomy to depression. *Clinical Psychology Review, 10,* 279–297.

Nigg, J. T., & Goldsmith, H. H. (1994). Genetics of personality disorders: Perspectives from personality and psychopathology research. *Psychological Bulletin, 115,* 346–380.

Ouimette, P. C., Klein, D. N., Anderson, R., Riso, L. P., & Lizardi, H. (1994). Relationship of sociotropy/autonomy and dependency/self-criticism to DSM-III-R personality disorders. *Journal of Abnormal Psychology, 103,* 743–749.

Parker, G. (1997). The etiology of personality disorders: A review and consideration of research models. *Journal of Personality Disorders, 11,* 345–369.

Penner, L. A., Shiffman, S., Paty, J. A., & Fritzsche, B. A. (1994). Individual differences in intraperson variability in mood. *Journal of Personality and Social Psychology, 66,* 712–721.

Pfohl, B., Stangl, D., & Zimmerman, M. (1984). The implications of DSM-III personality disorders for patients with major depression. *Journal of Affective Disorders, 7,* 309–318.

Pilkonis, P. A., & Frank, E. (1988). Personality pathology in recurrent depression: Nature, prevalence, and relationship to treatment response. *American Journal of Psychiatry, 145,* 435–441.

Reich, J. H., & Vasile, R. G. (1993). Effect of personality disorders on the treatment outcome of Axis I conditions: An update. *Journal of Nervous and Mental Disease, 181,* 475–484.

Ross, H. E., Glaser, F. B., & Germanson, T. (1988). The prevalence of psychiatric disorders in patients with alcohol and other drug problems. *Archives of General Psychiatry, 45,* 1023–1031.

Rusting, C. L., & Larsen, R. J. (1998). Diurnal patterns of unpleasant mood: Associations with neuroticism, depression, and anxiety. *Journal of Personality, 66,* 85–103.

Salovey, P., Mayer, J. D., Goldman, S. L., Turvey, C., & Palfai, T. (1995). Emotional attention, clarity, and repair: Exploring emotional intelligence using the trait meta-mood scale. In J. Pennebaker (Ed.), *Emotion, disclosure, and health* (pp. 125–154). Washington, DC: American Psychological Association Press.

Shea, M. T., Glass, D. R., Pilkonis, P. A., Watkins, J., & Docherty, J. P. (1987). Frequency and implications of personality disorders in a sample of depressed outpatients. *Journal of Personality Disorders, 1,* 27–42.

Shea, M. T., Leon, A. C., Mueller, T. I., Solomon, D. A., Warshaw, M. G., & Keller, M. B. (1996). Does major depression result in lasting personality change? *American Journal of Psychiatry, 153,* 1404–1410.

Shea, M. T., Pilkonis, P. A., Beckham, E., Collins, J. F., Elkin, I., Sotsky, S. M., & Docherty, J. P. (1990). Personality disorders and treatment outcome in the NIMH Treatment of Depression Collaborative Research Program. *American Journal of Psychiatry, 147,* 711–718.

Shea, M. T., Widiger, T. A., & Klein, M. H. (1992). Comorbidity of personality disorders and depression: Implications for treatment. *Journal of Consulting and Clinical Psychology, 60,* 857–868.

Siever, L. J., & Davis, K. L. (1991). A psychobiological perspective on the personality disorders. *American Journal of Psychiatry, 148,* 1647–1658.

Stein, D. J., Hollander, E., & Skodol, A. E. (1993). Anxiety disorders and personality disorders: A review. *Journal of Personality Disorders, 7,* 87–104.

Thomas, A., & Chess, S. (1977). *Temperament and development.* New York: Brunner/Mazel.

Tyrer, P. (1996). Comorbidity or consanguinity. *British Journal of Psychiatry, 168,* 669–671.

Tyrer, P., Gunderson, J., Lyons, M., & Tohen, M. (1997). Extent of comorbidity between mental state and personality disorders. *Journal of Personality Disorders, 11,* 242–259.

Tyrer, P., Seivewright, N., Ferguson, B., & Tyrer, J. (1992). The general neurotic syndrome: A coaxial diagnosis of anxiety, depression and personality disorder. *Acta Psychiatrica Scandinavica, 85,* 201–206.

Van Praag, H. M. (1996). Comorbidity (psycho) analysed. *British Journal of Psychiatry, 168*(Suppl. 30), 129–134.

Viken, R. J., Rose, R. J., Kaprio, J., & Koskenvuo, M. (1994). A developmental genetic analysis of adult personality: Extraversion and neuroticism from 18 to 59 years of age. *Journal of Personality and Social Psychology, 66,* 722–730.

Watson, D., & Tellegen, A. (1985). Toward a consensual structure of mood. *Psychological Bulletin, 98,* 219–235.

West, M., Sheldon, A., & Reiffer, L. (1989). Attachment theory and brief psychotherapy: Applying current research to clinical interventions. *Canadian Journal of Psychiatry, 34,* 369–374.

Zimmerman, M., Coryell, W., Pfohl, B., Corenthal, C., & Stangl, D. (1986). ECT response in depressed patients with and without a DSM-III personality disorder. *American Journal of Psychiatry, 143,* 1030–1032.

CHAPTER 27

≈—◆—≈

Forensic Issues

STEPHEN D. HART

Personality disorder as a form of mental abnormality has been recognized in Anglo-American law for the past 200 years or so, and over the past century it has become an important concept in several distinct areas of law.[1] The first part of this chapter outlines the law's understanding of personality disorder and attempts to explain its relevance in forensic decision making. This section is general and will be of interest primarily to clinical psychiatrists and psychologists who make occasional forays into the forensic realm. The second part discusses ethical, professional, and clinical issues in the assessment of personality disorder as part of forensic mental health evaluations. This section is targeted primarily at forensic psychiatrists and psychologists, as well as lawyers, whose familiarity with the scientific and professional literature on personality disorder is limited. The conclusion sets out recommendations for best practice.

PERSONALITY DISORDER AND THE LAW

Law and the Mental Health Professions

Law, generally, is a set of rules and procedures designed to regulate the behavior of people (Melton, 1985). The fundamental goal of the law is to prevent and resolve, in a principled manner, conflicts among people. When people think about the law, they typically imagine lawyers arguing in front of a judge or jury in criminal court, yet people's encounters with the law take place, for the most part, outside court. Indeed, the law is so much a part of day-to-day life in our society that we rarely are conscious of the extent to which it influences our actions. Even our formal contacts with the law are less likely to occur in criminal court than in civil court or in front of quasi-judicial bodies such as administrative boards and tribunals. The umbrella term "forensic" (from the Latin *forensis,* meaning *forum*) is used to describe legal proceedings of all kinds.

The law assumes that people think and act in a reasoned, deliberate manner. People may be treated differently under the law when it is demonstrated that their behavior is involuntary or irrational—that is, when they suffer from some kind of volitional[2] or cognitive impairment. Mental disorder is one factor that may cause cognitive or volitional impairment. Courts and tribunals often call on mental health professionals to render opinions concerning the existence and impact of mental disorder in a given case, recognizing the special expertise that psychiatrists and psychologists have in evaluating people and understanding human behavior, especially abnormal behavior.

555

It is important for mental health professionals to understand that, in forensic decision making, mental disorder is a legal rather than a scientific, medical, or psychological concept. The trier of fact (judge, jury, tribunal) is responsible for defining mental disorder and for deciding whether or not the person has a mental disorder, in accord with relevant statutory and case law. Mental health professionals act merely as consultants to the trier of fact, providing expert observations and opinions. It is irksome to mental health professionals, but a fact of life, that their opinions may be accorded relatively little weight or even disregarded entirely.

Mental Disorder and the Law

Mental disorder in Anglo-American law often is conceptualized broadly to include any impairment of psychological functioning that is internal, stable, and involuntary in nature—that is, not a reflection of situational or contextual factors, not an ephemeral or transient state, and not a self-induced condition (Verdun-Jones, 1989). As do the mental health professions, however, the law often distinguishes between mental illness and personality disorder. Mental illness can be defined as acute and severe disturbances in psychological functioning—that is, disorders falling on Axis I of the fourth edition of the *Diagnostic and Statistical Manual of Mental Disorders* (DSM-IV; American Psychiatric Association, 1994). In contrast, personality disorder can be defined as a chronic disturbance of character or social relations, disorders falling on Axis II of DSM-IV.

Mental illness has been recognized in medicine—and law—for millennia. If a mental illness causes substantial cognitive or volitional impairment, the law may deem the person incapable of making rational choices and therefore nonculpable (i.e., not responsible and undeserving of punishment) for past, current, or future acts (Verdun-Jones, 1989). In other words, mental illness may be considered a mitigating factor in forensic arenas. The fact that people are no longer considered agents, exercising free will, may be used to justify decisions to detain or incapacitate them for their own safety or for the safety of the general public. There are, however, reasonable grounds to believe that mental illnesses may remit (they are, after all, acute in nature) and if this happens it is generally the case that people's full rights and freedoms are returned to them.

Personality disorder came to be recognized in psychiatry only recently, in the late 19th and early 20th centuries (Berrios, 1996). It was defined as a chronic disturbance of emotion or volition, or a disturbance of their integration with intellectual functions, that was distinct from both psychotic and neurotic illness and that resulted in socially disruptive behavior. Although there was little agreement among alienists in the specific variants of personality disorder they identified, or in the names given to these disorders, there was general consensus that one important cluster was characterized by impulsive, aggressive, and antisocial behavior (Berrios, 1996). For example, Schneider described "labile," "explosive," and "wicked" psychopaths; Kahn described a cluster of "impulsive," "weak," and "sexual" psychopaths; and Henderson described a cluster of psychopaths with "predominantly aggressive" features.

The law quickly accepted the idea that personality disorder also can influence cognition and volition.[3] For example, people suffering from personality disorder appear to be at increased risk for engaging in violent and other criminal behavior. Personality disorder is, however, unlikely to impair cognition and volition substantially, and therefore people with personality disorders rarely are considered nonculpable for their acts (as discussed below). This is particularly true when the personality disorder is psychopathy (also commonly referred to as antisocial or dissocial personality disorder), reflecting characteristics such as impulsivity, irresponsibility, lack of empathy and remorse, and so forth (e.g., Hare, 1996). A related concern is that personality disorder is, by definition, not likely to remit. If the personality disorder is not severe enough to be a mitigating factor in forensic decision making it may be considered, somewhat ironically, an aggravating factor, something that can be used to argue for harsher punishment or imposition of long-term social controls.

In summary, both forms of mental disorder—mental illness and personality disorder—are relevant under the law. Both are believed to play a role in influencing people's choices and actions. But whereas mental illness generally is considered a mitigating factor in forensic decision making, personality disorder generally is considered to be an aggravating factor. Note that although this is the rule, there are many exceptions to it; I discuss some of the exceptions later.

How Might Personality Disorder Impair Functioning?

As discussed earlier, personality disorder can influence cognition or volition, and of special concern to the law is the increased risk for violence and criminality associated with personality disorder. If one considers the diverse nature of personality disorder symptomatology, there are several potential ways in which personality disorder may influence cognition and volition. The task is easier when one considers these symptoms in terms of broad factors that cut across specific diagnostic categories (e.g., Clark, Vorhies, & McEwen, 1994; Costa & Widiger, 1994; Schroeder, Wormworth, & Livesley, 1994). Let us consider two such factors: neuroticism, which includes symptom dimensions such as insecure attachment, anxiousness, depression, and affective lability, and antagonism, which includes dimensions such as suspiciousness and lack of empathy.

Neuroticism is the tendency to experience intense and labile negative affect. Insecure attachment is the tendency to have intense and unstable relationships with family, close friends, and intimate partners. This symptom may lead to increased interpersonal stress and conflict, which may in turn lead to increased likelihood of aggression on the part of self or others. Anxiety may cause people to misperceive threat or danger around them, leading them to act impulsively or even aggressively in "self-defense." Affective lability may lead people to overreact to real or perceived provocation by others in an impulsive or aggressive manner. Both anxiety and affective lability may lead to intense dysthymia that interferes with a person's natural tendency toward self-interest, at the extreme resulting in deliberate self-punishment or self-harm.

Antagonism is the tendency to be arrogant and calculating in interactions with others. Suspiciousness is the tendency to infer maleficent motives underlying the behavior of others. Like anxiety, it may lead people to misperceive threat or danger around them and aggressive actions in self-defense. Lack of empathy is the tendency to be uncaring of others, or the tendency not to appreciate others' feelings, especially the impact of one's own behavior on them. Lack of empathy may result in an increased likelihood of violent or criminal behavior—both impulsive (reactive) and planned (instrumental)—because it reduces the psycho-logical cost to the individual of committing such acts or getting caught doing so.

Let us now turn to a discussion of the relevance of personality disorder to some specific legal issues. The purpose of this discussion is to provide readers with a sense of the wide range of matters in which personality disorder must be considered and the manner in which the law views personality disorder. A full discussion of any of the legal issues is beyond the scope of this chapter; readers interested in more detail should consult a comprehensive textbook of forensic mental health (e.g., Blackburn, 1993; Bull & Carson, 1995; Hess & Wiener, 1999; Melton, Petrila, Poythress, & Slobogin, 1997) and the relevant civil or criminal codes of the jurisdiction in which they practice.

Personality Disorder and "Character"

Character is an important, if somewhat vague, concept in the law. For example, Anglo-American law holds that criminal proceedings should be reserved for situations in which there is no other way to express public condemnation or ensure public safety (Verdun-Jones, 1989). A person who is charged with a relatively minor criminal offense but who is otherwise of "good character" may be diverted out of the criminal justice system. This is especially true in the case of young people (i.e., juveniles; Melton et al., 1997). People with "bad character," contrariwise, are not seen as appropriate candidates for diversion. Similarly, evidence of "bad character" may be entered in criminal or civil proceedings to call into question the credibility of a person's statements or testimony, or in family law disputes to argue that a person may be an unfit parent (Lyon & Ogloff, 2000). Bad character generally is defined as a tendency toward deceitfulness, minimization or denial of responsibility and lack of remorse for past misdeeds, lack of empathy, irresponsibility, and a history of committing antisocial and aggressive acts. At least at the extremes, then, bad character clearly resembles personality disorder, especially psychopathic (antisocial, dissocial) personality disorder.

Personality Disorder and Decision-Making Capacity

Adjudicative Competency

Consideration of accuracy and fairness in criminal proceedings requires that defendants are able to communicate about and appreciate, at least to a limited extent, the nature and the possible consequences of the charges against them when dealing with police and courts (Melton et al., 1997; Roesch, Zapf, Golding, & Skeem, 1999; Roesch, Hart, & Zapf, 1996). In some jurisdictions, the law further requires that people are capable of using this understanding to make a rational decision (Roesch et al., 1996). People who are judged to have a mental illness that renders them incompetent to make decisions about their legal defense may be hospitalized and treated involuntarily until they become competent, or if the charges are relatively minor and they present no undue risk to public safety, they may be diverted out of the criminal justice system altogether.

In most Anglo-American jurisdictions, courts have considered personality disorder and determined that, as a general rule, it does not sufficiently impair adjudicative competence so as to render people incompetent (Melton et al., 1997; Verdun-Jones, 1989). This is because symptoms of personality disorder are unlikely to result in gross impairments of thought and speech or in grossly irrational perceptions of and beliefs about the external world. Only substantial impairment is likely to result in adjudicative incompetence, in part because the law expects that people can be represented by attorneys who are, of course, expert in criminal proceedings and who will spend considerable time and effort working on behalf of their clients (Roesch et al., 1996).

Criminal Responsibility

In Anglo-American law, a criminal offense comprises two elements: commission of a forbidden act (the *actus reus*) with negligent, reckless, or maleficent intent (the *mens rea*). Both elements must be proven in court to convict a defendant (Blackburn, 1993; Carson, 1995; Golding, Skeem, Roesch, & Zapf, 1999; Verdun-Jones, 1989). When deciding whether the *actus reus* element exists, the law presumes that a person who acts has done so freely and voluntarily, with the opportunity to have considered the consequences of the act. This presumption is rebuttable, however. The law acknowledges that mental disorder (e.g., delirium and severe dissociative states) may lead people to act when not in a state of full consciousness or in an involuntary manner, a condition sometimes referred to as automatism. When deciding whether *mens rea* exists, the law presumes that a person had the ability to understand the nature and consequences of the act and that the act was wrong (Golding et al., 1999; Verdun-Jones, 1989). This presumption is also rebuttable. The law acknowledges that mental disorder (e.g., psychosis and dementia) may lead people to have beliefs or perceptions so irrational that they did not understand what they were doing or that what they were doing was wrong. (Attempting to rebut this presumption often is called "raising the insanity defense.") When defendants are found not guilty on account of mental disorder, they usually are hospitalized until they are no longer mentally ill or no longer present a risk to public safety (Golding et al., 1999).

Defining the nature and degree of the impairment that must exist before a person is found not criminally responsible on account of mental disorder has proved difficult. The legal definition varies across jurisdictions and even within jurisdictions over time, partly in reaction to governmental and public concerns that mentally ill people should not escape sanctions for criminal behavior. What seems clear from research (Steadman et al., 1993) is that the insanity defense is raised in only a tiny fraction of criminal cases—somewhere between about 1 in 100 and 1 in 1,000 cases in which people are charged with serious crimes. As many as half of these cases never go to trial because the prosecution and defense agree that defendants were not responsible when they committed the acts. Furthermore, people found not guilty on account of mental disorder often spend more time in the hospital than they would have spent in prison had they been found guilty. There seems little reason for concern that large numbers of mentally ill people are "getting away with murder."

Although the law (somewhat grudgingly) accepts that a small number of people with mental illness—primarily those with psychoses—will be found not criminally responsible on account of mental disorder, it is loath to accept this for people with personality disorders. Yet people with personality disorders have, on occasion, successfully raised the insanity defense (Golding et al., 1999; Melton et al., 1997; Steadman et al., 1993). In an effort to prevent this, the law has tried to narrow the scope of the legal test for criminal responsibility in two ways: (1) by restricting the legal definition of mental disorder, and (2) by increasing the severity of the cognitive or volitional impairments required. The first strategy involves specifying certain psychiatric symptoms that must be present for the insanity defense to be raised. For example, the U. S. federal penal code requires that the diagnosis of mental disorder must be based on something more than merely repeated antisocial behavior—a sort of "no psychopaths" clause (Melton et al., 1997). The second strategy involves specifying that the mental disorder must result in cognitive (as opposed to emotional or volitional) impairment, and that the impairment must be severe (Verdun-Jones, 1989). It is relatively easy for people with personality disorders to argue that their mental disorder results in emotional impairment (e.g., the intense and labile affect characteristic of borderline personal disorder, or the generalized affective deficits characteristic of psychopathy) or in volitional impairment (e.g., the impulsivity characteristic of borderline and psychopathic personality disorder) but difficult to argue that their mental disorder results in severe cognitive impairment (except, perhaps, the persecutory ideation or perceptual disturbances found in some cases of schizotypal personality disorder). Of these two strategies, the second seems preferable. It seems arbitrary simply to decree that certain mental disorders recognized in psychiatry just "don't count" in the law. Also, it should be relatively easy to argue successfully that personality disorders are not diagnosed solely on the basis of repeated antisocial behavior.[4]

Competency to Consent to Treatment

Competency to consent to medical or psychological treatment is, in many respects, parallel to adjudicative competency (Applebaum & Grisso, 1995; Roesch et al., 1996). The law requires that people are able to communicate about the decision and have at least a basic understanding of the possible risks and benefits of treatment options. Once again, in some jurisdictions, there may be a further requirement that people be able to use this understanding to make a rational decision (Roesch et al., 1996). People who are judged to have a mental illness that renders them incompetent to make decisions about treatment may be treated or hospitalized involuntarily, with their decision-mak-

ing powers transferred to family members, guardians, or health care professionals. Only a substantial impairment of cognition will result in a finding of incompetence, in part because the law expects that people's welfare typically is protected by physicians or other professionals who are expert in health care and who are bound by professional ethics to act in the best interests of their patients (Applebaum & Grisso, 1995). Symptoms of personality disorder, however, are unlikely to result in such severe impairment.

Other Issues

There are literally dozens of specific decision-making competencies recognized in law. These include such things as testamentary competency (competency to make a will) and competency to enter into contractual obligations (Melton et al., 1997; Slovenko, 1999). As is the case with adjudicative and treatment competency, however, personality disorder generally is not relevant in such matters because it is unlikely to substantially impair cognition.

Personality disorder may also be relevant to determining culpability for harm in civil matters. For example, it has been argued (albeit with little success) that the impulsivity associated with antisocial personality disorder may mitigate responsibility for apparently reckless or negligent behavior (Lyon & Ogloff, 2000). Also, in employment law, mental disorder—including personality disorder—may be considered a mitigating factor when deciding how to discipline people who engage in isolated acts of violence or disruptive behavior in the workplace. Mental disorder that results in continuing or long-term risk for violence, however, is an aggravating factor that may be used to justify dismissal (Melton et al., 1997).

Personality Disorder and Risk for Criminality and Violence

General Sentencing Issues

As discussed earlier, mental disorder that influences cognition or volition but does not substantially impair them may be considered an aggravating factor in sentencing for criminal offenses. There are two possible rationales for this. One is based on the notion of *specific deterrence,* which refers to the idea that criminal sentences are punishments meted out against specific individuals that can be used to change their future behavior. People with personality disorders, it could be argued, have demonstrated that they were not deterred by the usual social mechanisms and therefore may be in need of a special warning or reminder that criminal behavior will not be tolerated by the courts. The second rationale is to ensure the protection of public safety. People with personality disorders may require special controls—ranging from intensive supervision in the community to electronic monitoring to incarceration—to manage effectively their increased risk for future crime and violence.

Indeterminate Sentencing

Some jurisdictions allow for the indeterminate (i.e., indefinite) commitment of people found guilty of repeated and serious criminal offenses, especially sexual offenses, who also are believed to be at high risk for future violence (Griffiths & Verdun-Jones, 1994; Melton et al., 1997). Such laws are based primarily on the principle of protection of public safety. Personality disorders (such as psychopathy) or symptoms of personality disorder (such as impulsivity, callousness, or lack of remorse) often are considered to be *prima facie* grounds for determining that an individual presents a high risk for violence (MacLean, 2000).

Capital Sentencing

The United States is the only Anglo-American legal jurisdiction that still routinely practices capital punishment. Capital sentences can be imposed only after consideration of relevant aggravating and mitigating factors (Melton et al., 1997). Two such factors include the character of the offender and risk for future violence. Evidence that an offender suffers from a personality disorder—especially psychopathic or antisocial personality disorder—may be relevant to both these factors, suggesting the absence of good character in the offender (a mitigating factor) and the offender's elevated risk for violence (an aggravating factor).

Civil Commitment

Civil commitment allows for the involuntary hospitalization and/or treatment of people who suffer from a mental disorder that impairs their ability to care for themselves (e.g., to meet their nutritional, hygiene, or health needs) or that causes them to be a high risk for suicide or violence. The most common statutes provide for the short-term (several weeks to several months) commitment of individuals who present an imminent risk (Melton et al., 1997). The expectation is that people will receive treatment and be released either to the least restrictive alternative or altogether as soon as their mental disorder is in remission, or as soon as they no longer present an imminent risk. It is usually the case in law or, if not, in practice that the only people subject to civil commitment of this sort are those suffering from a severe mental illness (Melton et al., 1997). Personality disorder may be explicitly excluded from the legal definition of mental disorder; but even if it is not, it is unlikely to be considered a factor that results in imminent risk.

Another type of civil commitment that is becoming increasingly common is one designed for the indeterminate (several years to lifetime) commitment of people with mental disorder that makes them a long-term risk for violence—specifically, in some jurisdictions, sexual violence (Janus, 2000; MacLean, 2000; Schlank & Cohen, 1999). Given the focus on long-term risk, it is not surprising that personality disorder is a major focus of indeterminate commitment laws.[5] People committed in this manner are subject to or may request periodic reviews (typically at least once per year) to determine whether they may be released to a less restrictive alternative or freed altogether due to remission of the mental disorder or reduction in violence risk. Indeterminate civil commitment laws are controversial because they often are targeted at prison inmates who are completing a lengthy sentence and nearing their time for release into the community; thus, it is argued, they constitute a second punishment for offenses committed many years previously (Janus, 2000).

Other Issues

Personality disorder, insofar as it is related to risk for criminality and violence, may be relevant in a host of other, less common legal issues, including immigration (e.g., deportation) decisions and the imposition of civil or criminal restraining orders, which are intended to restrict specific liberties of people to prevent them from causing some harm (Lyon & Ogloff, 2000; Melton et al., 1997).

THE FORENSIC ASSESSMENT OF PERSONALITY DISORDER

Professional Issues

Ethics

Forensic psychologists and forensic psychiatrists assess or treat people in legal contexts (Hess, 1999; Melton et al., 1997). One important aspect of forensic practice is that professionals know there is a likelihood that their opinions will be solicited for use in legal decision making (e.g., decisions to detain or release people according to various statutes). The practice of forensic mental health requires specialized knowledge of the law. For their opinions to be useful, professionals need to know the nature of the decision being made, the types of opinions that may be expressed, and any limits concerning the type of information that can be considered or discussed by the professional. Professionals also must learn how to communicate their opinions in a manner that is comprehensible to people who are not mental health experts. Professionals who lack special knowledge of the law or who communicate information poorly risk having their opinions misunderstood or ignored altogether.

Depending on the jurisdiction in which they practice and the professional and regulatory bodies that govern them, forensic psychiatrists and psychologists may be bound by both general and specialized ethical codes. Examples of specialized ethical codes in North America are those of the American Academy of Psychiatry and the Law (1995) and the joint guidelines of the American Academy of Forensic Psychology and the American Psychology–Law Society (Committee on Ethical Guidelines for Forensic Psychologists, 1991). Professionals are sometimes surprised to learn that procedures deemed acceptable or even good practice in general clinical settings may be unacceptable in forensic settings. For example, it is not considered sound practice in forensic mental health to accept at face value the uncorroborated statements made by a person, especially someone who is the subject of an evaluation. This means one should not rely solely on a clinical interview to gather information concerning past or current psychosocial functioning; efforts must

be made to corroborate important claims by reviewing documentary evidence or interviewing collateral informants. Another example is that reports by third parties concerning a person's statements to them (hearsay—for example, a wife's reports of what her husband said to her) may be inadmissible as evidence, and they may even be considered unsuitable as the basis for a clinical opinion. Professionals who form opinions on the basis of clinical interviews or hearsay reports may be presented with new information, asked to ignore old information and to reformulate their opinions, or they may have their opinions deemed "tainted" and excluded from the proceedings.

Admissibility

Psychiatrists and psychologists should not assume that their professional credentials are sufficient for them to be guaranteed entry into forensic arenas. Every time an expert opinion is tendered before a court or tribunal, the trier of fact must determine whether it is admissible as evidence. The legal criteria for admissibility vary according to the issue being considered and the jurisdiction (Melton et al., 1997), but generally include the following. First, experts must have some kind of specialized knowledge. Education and training are helpful in establishing specialized knowledge, but so are experience and evidence that professionals have kept their knowledge up-to-date (e.g., through continuing education workshops and reading scientific journals). Second, expert opinions must be relevant, that is, they must address a pertinent legal issue and therefore be (potentially) helpful to the trier of fact in reaching a decision. Third, expert opinions must not be prejudicial, or at least the probative value (usefulness) of the opinions must outweigh their prejudicial impact. Additional criteria may apply, especially when an expert opinion is based on novel scientific findings or principles.[6] For example, courts may require that the scientific findings or principles are generally accepted within the field of study, and that the theoretical and empirical support for them meets certain standards of reliability or accuracy.

Common Problems

Perhaps the most basic mistake a professional can make is to be unfamiliar with the law relevant to the issue being decided. Ignorance of the law can lead to a variety of errors. One example is reliance by the professional on inadmissible evidence (such as hearsay statements) to form an opinion. This can render the opinion itself inadmissible because it is deemed unreliable or prejudicial. How does one avoid the problem of legal ignorance? Mental health professionals are not lawyers, of course, but they are capable of learning (and, indeed, ethically obliged to learn) the basics of the law as it relates to their professional practice. The best ways to do this are to read introductory or reference texts and to talk with lawyers working in the field.

A second common mistake is for psychiatrists or psychologists who are involved in treating a patient to offer an opinion to that person in the role of a forensic evaluator. Ethical codes, both general and specialized, warn about the possible problems resulting from conflicts of interest, also known as "dual role relationships," and the law is sensitive to the bias that may result from such conflicts. It is difficult, if not impossible, to switch from the role of treatment provider, in which the professional works for a patient and advocates for that person's well-being and best interests, to that of neutral evaluator, in which the professional is duty-bound to tender an objective opinion regardless of who is paying the bill. Forensic professionals should avoid dual role relationships whenever possible. When they are unavoidable, conflicts of interest should be declared a potential limitation on the professional's opinion.

A third common mistake is the failure to use, or the misuse of, accepted assessment procedures. Forensic professionals who testify about the assessment of personality disorder should expect to be confronted with opinions from other experts or with authoritative treatises regarding recommended practice. For example, it would be easy for a competent lawyer to attack the credibility of an expert who assessed personality disorder in a criminal defendant relying solely on self-report inventories. There are at least three concerns here. One is that a clinical interview is the basic method for assessing any form of mental disorder and triers of fact may be justifiably concerned by diagnoses that are not based on standard procedures. The second is that, arguably, self-report inventories constitute a series of uncorroborated statements made by the accused. The scales designed to detect response distortion incorporated in most self-report inventories do not obviate this fact. Finally, there is no body of research supporting the concurrent validity of self-report inventories with respect to clinical diagnoses of personality disorder in forensic settings. The little evidence that does exist suggests that the concurrent validity is low to moderate at best (Rogers, 1995; Zimmerman, 1994).

A fourth and final common problem is the failure to cite or the improper citation of relevant scientific literature when forming an opinion. For example, a substantial body of research supports the predictive validity of psychopathic personality disorder, as measured by the PCL-R, with respect to future criminal and violent behavior, response to some kinds of institutional treatment programs, and so forth (Hemphill, Hare, & Wong, 1998; Salekin, Rogers, & Sewell, 1996). Research also indicates that the correspondence of self-report measures of psychopathy or even DSM-IV diagnoses of antisocial personality with the PCL-R is limited (Hart & Hare, 1997). It is therefore inappropriate to cite research based on the PCL-R to support a professional opinion in which the patient was assessed using some other measure or set of diagnostic criteria (Hare, 1998).

Clinical Issues

Categorical versus Dimensional Models of Personality Disorder

There is, as readers will be aware from discussions in other chapters, considerable debate in the scientific literature concerning the appropriateness of categorical versus dimensional models of personality disorder (Widiger & Sanderson, 1995). To summarize, the categorical model assumes that personality disorder symptomatology can be defined in terms of a small number of types that are more or less independent of each other. Each type is characterized by a specific set of symptoms, and people with a given type of personality disorder are assumed to be a relatively homogeneous group. Both the DSM-IV and the 10th edition of the World Health Organization's (1992) diagnostic manual, the *International Classification of Diseases and Causes of Death* (ICD-10), rely on a categorical model for the diagnosis of personality disorder. In contrast, the dimensional model assumes that personality disorder symptomatology can be well described in terms of a small number of global traits that are orthogonal (i.e., uncorrelated) and comprise several specific traits. These traits typically are believed to be bipolar and normally distributed, with most people having average levels of the trait and people with extreme levels at either end of the continuum exhibiting impairment. Several dimensional models exist; examples include the five-factor model (FFM), which originally was developed to describe normal personality but more recently has been applied to personality disorder (e.g., Costa & McCrae, 1992; Costa & Widiger, 1994) and the Dimensional Assessment of Personality Pathology (e.g., Livesley, Jackson, & Schroeder, 1989, 1992; Schroeder et al., 1994).

Forensic mental health professionals should be prepared to acknowledge both the strengths and limitations of the measurement models on which their assessments of personality disorder are based and the consequent impact on their opinions. A full discussion of the two approaches is beyond the scope of this chapter. It may suffice for the present purposes, however, to note that of primary forensic importance is the fact that the categorical model is commonly used in clinical practice and has been a focus of considerable research. The widespread acceptance of this model is compelling to laypeople when they attempt to judge the credibility of a professional opinion, even if it is considered weak evidence of credibility in the scientific community. As a consequence, forensic professionals whose opinions regarding personality disorder are based on dimensional models should be prepared to defend their "unusual" practice by outlining the clear advantages of the dimensional approach.

The High Prevalence of Personality Disorder

Regardless of whether mental health professionals adopt a categorical or a dimensional model, their assessments are complicated by the high prevalence of personality disorder. According to epidemiological research about 10% of community resident adults suffer from some form of personality disorder (Weissman, 1993). In forensic settings, the rate is even higher (Trestman, 2000). For example, between 50% and 80% of all incarcerated adult offenders meet the diagnostic criteria for antisocial personality disorder (Hare, 1983; Robins, Tipp, & Przybeck, 1991); if one considers all the personality disorders contained in the DSM-IV or

ICD-10, then the prevalence rate may be as high as 90% (Neighbors, 1987). Of course, from the dimensional perspective things are even worse: Every offender has traits of personality disorder; the only question is, how severe are the traits?

Triers of fact may be unaware that personality disorder is pandemic in forensic settings and place undue weight on or draw unwarranted conclusions from the diagnosis. Accordingly, forensic mental health professionals should attempt to provide a context for diagnoses of personality disorder in three ways. First, they should explicitly acknowledge its high prevalence (e.g., "Mr. X meets the DSM-IV diagnostic criteria for antisocial personality disorder, which is found in about 50% to 80% of all incarcerated adult offenders"). Second, they should characterize it in terms of relative severity (e.g., "My assessment of Mr. X using the PCL-R indicates that he has traits of psychopathic personality disorder much higher than those found in healthy adults, but only average in severity relative to incarcerated adult male offenders"). Third, they should explain what they believe to be the personality disorder's legal relevance in the case at hand (e.g., "In my opinion Mr. X poses a high risk for future sexual violence relative to other sexual offenders that is due at least in part to a mental disorder, specifically a severe antisocial personality disorder characterized by extreme impulsivity and lack of empathy."). This latter point is discussed in more detail later.

Complexity of Personality Disorder Symptomatology

It is difficult to describe in simple terms a person's functioning with respect to a domain as broad as personality. Forensic professionals who rely on categorical models will be forced to grapple with the issue of comorbidity (Zimmerman, 1994). Research indicates that people who meet the diagnostic criteria for a given DSM-IV or ICD-10 personality disorder also typically meet the criteria for two or three other personality disorders (e.g., Stuart et al., 1998). Even people with the same singleton personality disorder diagnosis vary considerably with respect to the number and severity of symptoms they exhibit. Professionals who rely on dimensional models are no better off, as the same level of trait severity can be manifested at the behavioral level in many different ways. Regardless of which model they use, professionals have to rely on information provided by the patient or from other sources to reach a judgment regarding the presence or absence of symptomatology, a judgment that is inherently subjective.

Forensic professionals should be prepared to admit—without making a personal apology for the limitations of scientific knowledge—that assessing personality can be a messy business; the types or dimensions used in assessment are somewhat fuzzy and imprecise concepts. Of course, this does not necessarily render invalid the inferences professionals can draw from the assessment of personality disorder. Also, it should be remembered that acknowledging the limitations of one's opinions might help to establish the credibility of those opinions in the eyes of the trier of fact.

Comorbidity with Acute Mental Disorder

In forensic settings, personality disorder frequently is comorbid with acute mental disorders such as substance use, mood, and anxiety disorders (e.g., Trestman, 2000). Acute mental disorders can complicate the assessment of personality disorder, leading to uncertain or even incorrect inferences about personality (e.g., poverty of affect in a person with schizophrenia mimicking the shallow emotion often associated with psychopathic personality disorder). Also, the existence of acute mental disorder can be obscured by comorbid personality disorder. If the acute mental disorder has an impact on psychological functioning or behavior that is independent of but mistakenly attributed to personality disorder, the evaluator may reach inaccurate conclusions regarding the severity and forensic relevance of the personality disorder.

Forensic mental health professionals should conduct comprehensive assessments of acute mental disorder before making diagnoses of personality disorder. They should also clearly indicate the existence of any acute mental disorder and discuss the extent to which it may have influenced any opinions related to personality disorder.

Inchoate Diagnoses

A special issue here concerns diagnosis in cases where the individual being evaluated manifests symptoms of personality disorder but does not meet the criteria for any specific disorder. It

is common for clinicians to diagnose such patients as suffering from traits of one or more personality disorder (e.g., "Axis II: histrionic and narcissistic traits, moderate severity") or from a rare or unspecified personality disorder (e.g., "Axis II: personality disorder, not otherwise specified").[7] In civil settings, this practice makes sense. Alerting others to the possibility that a patient suffers from personality disorder may help them to plan or deliver treatments more effectively. The costs of false positive and false negative diagnoses are relatively small and roughly equal. In forensic settings, though, the routine diagnosis of personality disorder traits or unspecified personality disorders can have serious repercussions. Triers of fact may not realize that such diagnoses may reflect relatively minor adjustment problems on the part of the patient (especially in light of the high prevalence of personality disorder in forensic settings, as discussed previously) or significant uncertainty on the part of the evaluator. They may also not be aware that the reliability and validity of these diagnoses is highly questionable.

Forensic professionals should keep in mind that what to them may be a rather minor part of their overall diagnostic formulation may be used in forensic decision making as grounds for something as serious as indeterminate commitment or capital sentencing. Accordingly, forensic professionals should be very cautious—or even avoid altogether—making diagnoses of personality disorder traits or unspecified personality disorders. Those who do so should be prepared to justify their diagnoses in light of the general definition of personality disorders (e.g., American Psychiatric Association, 1994; World Health Organization, 1992) and in light of the specific symptoms present in the case at hand. Forensic professionals also should acknowledge the uncertain reliability and validity of their diagnoses.

Causal Role of Personality Disorder

An evaluator's opinion that a person suffers from personality disorder is, in itself, not of much interest in forensic decision making. As noted previously, the personality disorder is relevant only if the evaluator's opinion is that it *causes,* at least in part, some impairment of competency or elevated risk for criminality and violence *in this individual.* The unwarranted assumption of causality may render an opinion inadmissible because it is deemed to be irrelevant, not probative, or more prejudicial than probative.

Forensic mental health professionals should make explicit their opinions regarding the causal role played by personality disorder with respect to the relevant legal issue, whether impairment or risk. They should also acknowledge that such opinions are, ultimately, professional rather than scientific in nature—that is, based on inference and speculation, not on the direct application of scientific principle or procedures.

The Diagnostic Significance of Antisocial Behavior

A history of antisocial behavior may be of considerable diagnostic significance in civil psychiatric settings, where only a minority of patients has been charged with or convicted of criminal offenses. In the DSM-IV, the diagnostic criteria for antisocial personality disorder are based largely on such a history. Obviously, antisocial behavior is of little diagnostic significance in many forensic settings, where virtually everyone has record of arrests (American Psychiatric Association, 1994).

Forensic professionals should be careful not to overfocus on antisocial behavior—especially on isolated criminal acts—when diagnosing personality disorders. By definition, personality disorders should be manifested across various domains of psychosocial functioning, across time, and across important personal relationships (American Psychiatric Association, 1994; World Health Organization, 1992). A person who engages in antisocial behavior only of a specific type, only against a specific person, or only at specific times may not suffer from a personality disorder at all. For example, consider a 50-year-old man who suffers from a sexual deviation and exposes his genitals to teenage girls in public places several times per year, but who is otherwise well adjusted—has a relatively stable marriage, holds a steady job, has good peer relationships, and so forth. In this case, the sexual deviation accounts for all the patient's antisocial behavior; there is no need to infer the presence of a personality disorder or even traits of personality disorder. Other mental disorders commonly associated with specific patterns of antisocial behavior include impulse control disorder such as kleptomania (stealing) and pyromania (fire setting).

Reliability of Assessments

Reliability refers to the consistency or stability of information derived from the assessment procedure. Information concerning reliability is important in legal proceedings because it helps the trier of fact to have confidence that other evaluators using similar procedures would have reached similar opinions. Two key types of reliability with respect to personality disorder are interrater reliability (i.e., diagnostic agreement) and test–retest reliability (i.e., temporal stability). Interrater reliability is the extent to which different professionals, using the same procedures to evaluate the same subject at about the same time, reach the same conclusions regarding the presence or severity of personality disorder. Test–retest reliability is the extent to which the same or different professionals, using the same procedures to evaluate the same subject but at different points in time, reach the same conclusions regarding the presence or severity of personality disorder. Both forms of reliability typically are indexed using Cohen's kappa or the intraclass correlation. Both reflect chance-corrected agreement, but the former is used for categorical variables (i.e., diagnoses) and the latter for continuous variables (i.e., severity ratings). A third form of reliability, internal consistency, is relevant only to multi-item scales and reflects the coherency of (average association among) the items. It typically is indexed using Cronbach's alpha. Information concerning the reliability of assessment procedures, if it exists, generally can be found in narrative or quantitative reviews published in scientific journals.

Reviews indicate that personality disorder can be assessed with moderate levels of reliability on the basis of structured or semistructured clinical interviews and a review of case history information (Rogers, 1995). In general, interrater reliability seems to be slightly higher than test–retest reliability, with the former best characterized as "moderate or moderate-to-high" and the latter as "moderate or moderate-to-low." These findings are true for both categorical diagnoses (presence vs. absence) and dimensional assessments (severity ratings or symptoms counts) made according to DSM-IV or ICD-10 criteria (First et al., 1995; Loranger et al., 1994) or according to alternative criteria for specific personality disorders such as psychopathic, borderline, and narcissistic personality disorder (e.g., Hare, 1991).

The evidence supporting the reliability of self-report scales or inventories of personality disorder is perhaps slightly weaker. Test–retest reliability of these measures typically is moderate or moderate-to-low; their internal consistency reliability, however, usually is low or low-to-moderate (Zimmerman, 1994).

There is little evidence supporting the reliability of personality disorder assessments made using other methods. In particular, unstructured clinical assessments of specific personality disorders appear to have low interrater reliability (Zimmerman, 1994).

Validity of Assessments

Validity refers to the meaningfulness of information derived from an assessment procedure (i.e., its accuracy for making descriptive or prognostic statements). Information concerning validity is important in legal proceedings because it helps the trier of fact to have confidence that other evaluators would have reached the same conclusion based on the same assessment data. Two key types of reliability with respect to personality disorder are *concurrent validity,* or the extent to which a measure is associated with other measures of the same personality disorder symptomatology, and *predictive validity,* or the extent to which the measure predicts behavior or other outcomes of interest.

Research indicates that personality disorder assessments made on the basis of a particular structured clinical method (e.g., structured clinical interviews and a review of case history information) have moderate concurrent validity with respect to other such methods (Zimmerman, 1994). This is true for both categorical diagnoses (presence vs. absence) and dimensional assessments (severity ratings or symptoms counts). There is considerable evidence supporting the predictive validity of psychopathy diagnoses and dimensional ratings with respect to violent and other criminal behavior in correctional, forensic psychiatric, and civil psychiatric settings. There is even some research on the predictive validity of psychopathic personality traits in "normal" people (e.g., community residents such as employees of large corporations or university students; see Babiak, 1995; Forth, Brown, Hart, & Hare, 1996). Research on response to treatment is limited but suggests that psychopathy predicts treatment dropout, problematic behavior during treatment, and posttreatment criminality and violence (Hart &

Hare, 1997). Compared to psychopathy, research on other forms of personality disorder—assessed using structured methods—is limited, although it is still possible to draw some conclusions based on individual studies or focused reviews on specific issues (Dutton, Bodnarchuk, Kropp, Hart, & Ogloff, 1997; Widiger & Trull, 1994).

The validity of personality disorder assessments based on self-report or other methods (e.g., unstructured clinical assessment) is low to moderate (Edens, Hart, Johnson, Johnson, & Olver, 2000; Hart, Forth, & Hare, 1991; Rogers, 1995; Zimmerman, 1994).

CONCLUSIONS

Summary

Personality disorder—like other forms of mental disorder—can play an important role in forensic decision making with respect to a wide range of civil and criminal issues. Evidence concerning personality disorder is likely to be of the greatest relevance when questions are raised regarding a person's character or risk for criminality and violence. It is less likely to be relevant, however, when the question concerns a person's competency to make decisions. Unlike other forms of mental disorder, personality disorder typically is considered in law to be an aggravating factor, the presence of which can be used to justify the imposition of long-term social controls or harsher punishments.

Professionals who venture into forensic arenas should be aware of the general and specialized ethical guidelines that apply to their practice, as well as the basics of the law insofar as it relates to the issues under consideration. They should also be familiar with important clinical issues, including the categorical–dimensional measurement model debate, the complexity of personality disorder symptomatology, and research on the reliability and validity of personality disorder assessments. This awareness should help professionals to avoid making common mistakes that jeopardize the admissibility, credibility, and perceived importance of their testimony.

Recommendations

To conclude, following is a list of specific recommendations for best practice regarding the clinical–forensic assessment of personality disorder. The recommendations are intended to improve the usefulness of expert testimony by clarifying the foundation of professional opinions, increasing the richness of information provided to decision makers, and facilitating discussion of the limitations of the testimony.

- Personality disorder symptomatology should be assessed using methods that integrate information obtained from collateral sources with (whenever possible) information from direct interviews; methods based solely on oral or written self-report should not be used.
- Personality disorder symptomatology should be assessed using methods that provide dimensional information regarding symptoms and/or symptom dimensions (e.g., severity ratings and symptom counts), either in addition to or instead of categorical diagnoses made according to established or accepted criteria.
- When communicating their opinions, professionals should acknowledge the weaknesses of the assessment methods they used and the information on which the assessment was based and discuss the likely impact of these limitations on their conclusions.
- Professionals should conduct comprehensive assessments of acute mental disorder before making diagnoses of personality disorder.
- Professionals should provide a context for diagnoses of personality disorder by discussing its prevalence in forensic settings.
- Whenever possible, forensic professionals should avoid diagnosing personality disorder traits or unspecified personality disorders. In cases where such diagnoses are warranted, professionals should justify their opinions in light of the general clinical definition of personality disorder and the symptom pattern present in the case at hand, and also should acknowledge the unknown reliability and validity of their diagnoses.
- When communicating their opinions, professionals should outline the (putative) causal connection between personality disorder symptomatology and any legally relevant impairment from which the person suffers or risk the person presents.
- Professionals should avoid overestimating the significance of antisocial behavior in the assessment of personality disorder.

- Professionals should be prepared to discuss the scientific and professional literature as it relates to the legal issues at hand; in particular, professionals should be prepared to admit when their opinions lack a strong foundation, are controversial, or reflect a minority view.

NOTES

1. By Anglo-American law, I refer to the adversarial legal system based on English common law. It is the dominant legal system in countries including England and Wales, the United States, Canada, Australia, and New Zealand. Although this chapter focuses on Anglo-American law, many of the major points are consistent with other legal traditions, especially the inquisitorial systems of many Western European countries.
2. "Volition" is a term not used widely in modern psychiatry and psychology. In the law, the term refers to the ability to exercise control over one's behavior, including the control over the affective and motivational precursors of behavior.
3. It is interesting that part of the motivation for developing the psychiatric concept of volitional disturbance, and more specifically the notion of *impulsion*—a disturbance characterized by unreflective or involuntary aggression and the absence of other symptoms which, according to Berrios (1996), "provided the kernel around which the notion of psychopathic personality was eventually to become organised" (p. 428)—was forensic. For their testimony to be relevant, the expertise of alienists in that era had to extend beyond the realm of "total insanity" (i.e., major mental illness; Berrios, 1996).
4. Although the DSM-IV criteria for antisocial personality disorder focus primarily on antisocial behavior, the focus is not exclusive. Also alternative diagnostic criteria, such as those in the Hare Psychopathy Checklist—Revised (PCL-R; Hare, 1991), focus as much on interpersonal and affective symptoms as they do on symptoms related to antisocial behavior.
5. Other chronic conditions, such as sexual deviation, organic mental disorders, and mental retardation are also relevant in some jurisdictions.
6. Because an opinion based on science is likely to be accorded more weight than one based merely on experience, the scientific basis of the opinion must be scrutinized more closely.
7. This practice is, in fact, encouraged in the DSM-IV.

REFERENCES

American Academy of Psychiatry and the Law. (1995). *American Academy of Psychiatry and the Law ethical guidelines for the practice of forensic psychiatry* [Online]. Internet: http://aapl.org/ethics.htm

American Psychiatric Association. (1994). *Diagnostic*

and statistical manual of mental disorders (4th ed.). Washington, DC: Author.

Applebaum, P., & Grisso, T. (1995). The MacArthur Treatment Competence Study (1): Mental illness and competence to consent to treatment. *Law and Human Behavior, 19,* 105–126.

Babiak, P. (1995). When psychopaths go to work: A case study of an industrial psychopath. *Applied Psychology: An International Review, 44,* 171–178.

Berrios, G. E. (1996). *The history of mental symptoms: Descriptive psychopathology since the nineteenth century.* Cambridge, UK: Cambridge University Press.

Blackburn, R. (1993). *The psychology of criminal conduct: Theory, research and practice.* Chichester, UK: Wiley.

Bull, R., & Carson, D. C. (Eds.). (1995). *Handbook of psychology in legal contexts.* Chichester, UK: Wiley.

Carson, D. C. (1995). Criminal responsibility. In R. Bull & D. C. Carson (Eds.), *Handbook of psychology in legal contexts* (pp. 277–289). Chichester, UK: Wiley.

Clark, L. A., Vorhies, L., & McEwen, J. L. (1994). Personality disorder symptomatology from the five-factor model perspective. In P. T. Costa & T. A. Widiger (Eds.), *Personality disorders and the five-factor model of personality* (pp. 95–116). Washington, DC: American Psychological Association.

Committee on Ethical Guidelines for Forensic Psychologists. (1991). Specialty guidelines for forensic psychologists. *Law and Human Behavior, 15,* 655–665.

Costa, P. T., Jr., & McCrae, R. R. (1992). *Revised NEO Personality Inventory (NEO-PI-R) and NEO Five-Factor Inventory (NEO-FFI): Professional manual.* Odessa, FL: Psychological Assessment Resources.

Costa, P. T., & Widiger, T. A. (1994). Introduction: Personality disorders and the five-factor model of personality. In P. T. Costa & T. A. Widiger (Eds.), *Personality disorders and the five-factor model of personality* (pp. 1–12). Washington, DC: American Psychological Association.

Dutton, D. G., Bodnarchuk, M. A., Kropp, P. R., Hart, S. D., & Ogloff, J. R. P. (1997). Client personality disorders affecting wife assault post-treatment recidivism. *Violence and Victims, 12,* 37–50.

Edens, J. F., Hart, S. D., Johnson, D. W., Johnson, J. K., & Olver, M. E. (2000). Use of the personality assessment inventory to assess psychopathy in offender populations. *Psychological Assessment, 12,* 132–139.

First, M. B., Spitzer, R. L., Gibbon, M., Williams, J. B. W., Davies, M., Borus, J., Howes, M. J., Kane, J., Pope, H. G., & Rounsaville, B. J. (1995). The Structured Clinical Interview for DSM-III-R personality disorders (SCID-II): II. Multi-site test–retest reliability study. *Journal of Personality Disorders, 9,* 92–104.

Forth, A. E., Brown, S. L., Hart, S. D., & Hare, R. D. (1996). The assessment of psychopathy in male and female noncriminals: Reliability and validity. *Personality and Individual Differences, 20,* 531–543.

Golding, S., Skeem, J., Roesch, R., & Zapf, P. (1999). The assessment of criminal responsibility: Current controversies. In A. K. Hess & I. B. Wiener (Eds.), *Handbook of forensic psychology* (2nd ed., pp. 379–408). New York: Wiley.

Griffiths, C. T., & Verdun-Jones, S. N. (1994). *Canadi-*

an criminal justice. (2nd ed.). Toronto: Harcourt Brace.

Hare, R. D. (1983). Diagnosis of antisocial personality disorder in two prison populations. *American Journal of Psychiatry, 140,* 887–890.

Hare, R. D. (1991). *The Hare Psychopathy Checklist—Revised.* Toronto, Ontario: Multi-Health Systems.

Hare, R. D. (1996). Psychopathy: A clinical construct whose time has come. *Criminal Justice and Behavior, 23,* 25–54.

Hare, R. D. (1998). The Hare PCL-R: Some issues concerning its use and misuse. *Legal and Criminological Psychology, 3,* 101–122.

Hart, S. D., Forth, A. E., & Hare, R. D. (1991). The MCMI-II as a measure of psychopathy. *Journal of Personality Disorders, 5,* 318–327.

Hart, S. D., & Hare, R. D. (1997). Psychopathy: Assessment and association with criminal conduct. In D. M. Stoff, J. Brieling, & J. Maser (Eds.), *Handbook of antisocial behavior* (pp. 22–35). New York: Wiley.

Hemphill, J. F., Hare, R. D., & Wong, S. (1998). Psychopathy and recidivism: A review. *Legal and Criminological Psychology, 3,* 141–172.

Hess, A. K. (1999). Practicing principled forensic psychology: Legal, ethical, and moral considerations. In A. K. Hess & I. B. Wiener (Eds.), *Handbook of forensic psychology* (2nd ed., pp. 673–699). New York: Wiley.

Hess, A. K., & Wiener, I. B. (Eds.) (1999). *Handbook of forensic psychology* (2nd ed.). New York: Wiley.

Janus, E. S. (2000). Sexual predator commitment laws: Lessons for law and the behavioral sciences. *Behavioral Sciences and the Law, 18,* 5–21.

Livesley, W. J., Jackson, D., & Schroeder, M. L. (1989). A study of the factorial structure of personality pathology. *Journal of Personality Disorders, 3,* 292–306.

Livesley, W. J., Jackson, D., & Schroeder, M. L. (1992). Factorial structure of traits delineating personality disorders in clinical and general population samples. *Journal of Abnormal Psychology, 101,* 432–440.

Loranger, A. W., Sartorius, N., Andreoli, A., Berger, P., Buchheim, P., Channabasavanna, S. M., Coid, B., Dahl, A., Diekstra, R. F. W., Ferguson, B., Jacobsberg, L. B., Mombour, W., Pull, C., Ono, Y., & Regier, D. (1994). The International Personality Disorder Examination: The World Health Organization/Alcohol, Drug Abuse, and Mental Health Administration international pilot study of personality disorders. *Archives of General Psychiatry, 51,* 215–224.

Lyon, D., & Ogloff, J. R. P. (2000). Legal and ethical issues in psychopathy assessment. In C. Gacono (Ed.), *The clinical and forensic assessment of psychopathy: A practitioner's guide* (pp. 139–173). Mahwah, NJ: Lawrence Erlbaum.

MacLean, R. (Chairman) (2000). *Report of the Committee on Serious Violence and Sexual Offenders.* Edinburgh: Scottish Executive.

Melton, G. B. (Ed.) (1985). *Nebraska symposium on motivation: Vol. 33. The law as a behavioral instrument.* Lincoln: University of Nebraska Press.

Melton, G. B., Petrila, J., Poythress, N. G., & Slobogin, C. (1997). *Psychological evaluations for the courts: A handbook for mental health professionals and lawyers* (2nd ed.). New York: Guilford Press.

Neighbors, H. (1987). The prevalence of mental disorder in Michigan prisons. *DIS Newsletter, 4,* 8–11.

Robins, L. N., Tipp, J., & Przybeck, T. (1991). Antisocial personality. In L. N. Robins & D. Regier (Eds.), *Psychiatric disorders in America: The Epidemiologic Catchment Area study* (pp. 258–290). New York: Free Press.

Roesch, R., Hart, S. D., & Zapf, P. (1996). Conceptualizing and assessing competency to stand trial: Implications and applications of the MacArthur treatment competence model. *Psychology, Law, and Public Policy, 2,* 96–113.

Roesch, R., Zapf, P., Golding, S., & Skeem, J. (1999). Defining and assessing competency to stand trial. In A. K. Hess & I. B. Wiener (Eds.), *Handbook of forensic psychology* (2nd ed., pp. 327–349). New York: Wiley.

Rogers, R. (1995). *Diagnostic and structured interviewing: A handbook for psychologists.* Odessa, FL: Psychological Assessment Resources.

Salekin, R., Rogers, R., & Sewell, K. (1996). A review and meta-analysis of the Psychopathy Checklist and Psychopathy Checklist—Revised: Predictive validity of dangerousness. *Clinical Psychology: Science and Practice, 3,* 203–215.

Schlank, A., & Cohen, F. (Eds.). (1999). *The sexual predator: Law, policy, evaluation, and treatment.* Kingston, NJ: Civic Research Press.

Schroeder, M. L., Wormworth, J. A., & Livesley, W. J. (1994). Dimensions of personality disorder and the five-factor model of personality. In P. T. Costa & T. A. Widiger (Eds.), *Personality disorders and the five-factor model of personality* (pp. 1–12). Washington, DC: American Psychological Association.

Slovenko, R. (1999). Civil competency. In A. K. Hess & I. B. Wiener (Eds.), *Handbook of forensic psychology* (2nd ed., pp. 151–167). New York: Wiley.

Steadman, H. J., McGreevy, M. A., Morrissey, J. P., Callahan, L. A., Robbins, P. C., & Cirincione, C. (1993). *Before and after Hinckley: Evaluating insanity defense reform.* New York: Guilford Press.

Stuart, S., Pfhol, B., Battaglia, M., Bellodi, L., Grove, W., & Cadoret, R. (1998). The co-occurrence of DSM-III-R personality disorders. *Journal of Personality Disorders, 12,* 302–315.

Trestman, R. L. (2000). Behind bars: Personality disorders. *Journal of the American Academy of Psychiatry and the Law, 28,* 232–235.

Verdun-Jones, S. N. (1989). *Criminal law in Canada: Cases, questions and the code.* Toronto: Harcourt Brace Jovanovich.

Weissman, M. M. (1993). The epidemiology of personality disorders: A 1990 update. *Journal of Personality Disorders, 7,* 44–62.

Widiger, T. A., & Sanderson, C. J. (1995). Toward a dimensional model of personality disorders. In W. J. Livesley (Ed.), *The DSM-IV personality disorders* (pp. 433–458). New York: Guilford Press.

Widiger, T. A., & Trull, T. J. (1994). Personality disorders and violence. In J. Monahan & H. J. Steadman (Eds.), *Mental disorder and violence: Developments in risk assessment.* Chicago: University of Chicago Press.

World Health Organization (1992). *International classification of diseases and causes of death* (10th ed.). Geneva: Author.

Zimmerman, M. (1994). Diagnosing personality disorders: A review of issues and research methods. *Archives of General Psychiatry, 51,* 225–245.

CHAPTER 28

———⟢✦⟣———

A Framework for an Integrated Approach to Treatment

W. JOHN LIVESLEY

The wide range interventions and theoretical positions described in the chapters on treatment calls to mind the medical adage that when multiple treatments are proposed to treat a condition, none is very effective. Yet, as reviews of psychosocial interventions (Piper & Joyce, Chapter 15, this volume) and pharmacological treatments (Markovitz, Chapter 23, this volume) show, personality disorder responds to treatment. It does not appear, however, that any single approach or theory has a monopoly. Instead, many interventions are effective in changing at least some components of personality disorder. This suggests that an integrated approach using a combination of interventions drawn from different approaches, and selected whenever possible on the basis of efficacy, may be the optimal treatment strategy. The challenge is to deliver diverse interventions in an integrated way when managing individual patients. Ideally, this requires a comprehensive, evidence-based theory of personality disorder. As Benjamin and Pugh (Chapter 20, this volume) pointed out, effective interventions ultimately depend on understanding etiological and developmental mechanisms. Unfortunately, current knowledge is probably too rudimentary for such a theory to emerge in the near future. An alternative is to develop a general framework based on what is known personality disorder

that can be used to organize treatment and select interventions to treat specific problems. Actual interventions could be selected on the basis of demonstrated efficacy, or, if such information is not available, on the basis of a rational consideration of the interventions likely to be effective for a given problem.

This chapter argues that a descriptive analysis of personality disorder and a review of effective interventions dictate the broad outlines of a comprehensive approach. The result is not a theoretical model for treating personality disorder but something less complex: a general framework that can be used flexibility to tailor therapy to the needs of individual patients. As we consider a suitable framework it is useful to begin by examining ideas about psychotherapy integration.

PSYCHOTHERAPY INTEGRATON

Three forms of integration are often recognized: technical eclecticism, theoretical integration, and a common factors approach (Arkowitz, 1989; Norcross & Grencavage, 1989). *Technical eclecticism* involves selecting the best intervention or combination of interventions to treat a person or problem. Given Piper and Joyce's conclusion that interventions ranging from skills training to psychodynamic therapy are effective and evidence that medication may modify some behaviors, technical eclecticism appears to be necessary component of an evidence-based approach. Technical eclecticism alone, however, is unlikely to be sufficient because personality disorder involves more than dysfunctional behaviors. It also involves problems with the organization and integration of the personality system (see Livesley, Chapter 1, this volume). For this reason, consideration has to be given to the interventions required to achieve more integrated personality functioning (Ryle, 1997, Chapter 19, this volume). This suggests that the combination of interventions required for optimal treatment needs to be delivered in ways that facilitate integration.

Theoretical integration involves the synthesis of different approaches and the theories underlying them. This appears difficult to achieve given the fundamental and perhaps irreconcilable distinctions among theories of personality disorder. In the long run, this may not be important because most contemporary theories have too limited a focus to account for the diverse pathology of personality disorder. They also fail to provide a coherent explanation of the interaction between biological and psychosocial factors in the development of personality pathology. Nevertheless, there are avenues for integration that may be profitably explored. The concept of cognitive structure is one potentially integrating idea (Eells, 1997; Gold, 1996) because most therapies share the idea that representations of the self and others are an important components of personality (Holt, 1989). The terms used to describe these representations include "object relationships" as used in psychoanalytic theories, "cognitive schemata" (Beck, Freeman, & Associates, 1990); "self" or "interpersonal schemata" (Guidano, 1987, 1991; Horowitz, 1998), "self" and "object representations" (Gold, 1996), and "working models" (Bowlby, 1980). Despite this variety, all therapies share the idea that change in these structures is the goal of therapy.

A *common factors approach* to integration arises from the finding that different forms of therapy are equally effective (Beutler, 1991; Luborsky, Singer, & Luborsky, 1975). This prompted the search for change mechanisms common to all therapies. Two sets of factors seem important. Relationship and supportive factors arising from the therapeutic relationship, and technical factors involving opportunities to learn and test new skills (Lambert, 1992; Lambert & Bergin, 1994). Although common factors are important, specific interventions related to particular therapies also appear to be effective with specific disorders. For example, differential effectiveness has been established for cognitive therapy for panic disorder and behavior therapy for child conduct disorder (Lambert & Bergin, 1994). Differential effectiveness has not been established conclusively for personality disorder. However, as noted previously, the limited evidence available and rational considerations suggest that some components of personality pathology are likely to show differential responsiveness to some interventions. Nevertheless, the implications of these findings are clear: *Evidence-based treatment of personality disorder should seek to maximize the effects of common factors.*

This brief overview of different approaches to integration reveals some of the essential features of an integrated approach. It suggests that it may be possible to develop an approach to treatment that combines technical eclecticism and a common factors approach and also has the potential to lead to theoretical integration. The framework proposed has three elements: a theoretical foundation based on a descriptive account of the nature and etiology of personality disorder, a framework for describing therapeutic change, and a set of therapeutic strategies divided into general strategies based on the common factors model and used to manage and treat core pathology and specific strategies to treat those features of personality pathology that differ across individuals (Livesley, 2000).

THEORETICAL FOUNDATIONS

An evidence-based approach to treatment should rest on empirical knowledge about personality disorder and studies of treatment outcome. Although our knowledge has increased substantially in recent years, it remains fragmented and rudimentary. Nevertheless, a new picture of personality disorder is emerging that differs from that assumed by some contemporary approaches to treatment. This section does not review such work in detail but, rather, seeks to identify some general facts about personality disorder that have implications for treatment.

Principle 1: Personality Disorder Involves Multiple Domains of Psychopathology

Implication: Comprehensive treatment requires a combination of interventions tailored to the problems of individual patients.

Personality disorder involves all regions of the personality system rather than a circumscribed set of problems. Typical problems include symptoms such as anxiety, dysphoria, self-harming acts and transient psychotic features; situational problems, difficulty regulating affects and impulses; maladaptive expression of basic traits such as dependency and social avoidance; dysfunctional interpersonal relationships; problems forming integrated representations of self and others; and failure to develop a cohesive self and the capacity for intimacy and mature attachment. Not all problems are found in every case. Instead, considerable individual differences are observed, hence the need for a tailored approach.

This range of psychopathology suggests that a single intervention or treatment model is unlikely to be effective for treating all problems. The evidence reviewed in Chapters 15 (Piper & Joyce) and 23 (Markovitz) suggested that symptomatic features are likely to respond to cognitive behavioral interventions and medication. Linehan's (1993, Chapter 21, this volume) cognitive-behavioral approach reduces parasuicidal behavior and feelings of hopelessness. Low-dose neuroleptics are helpful in managing cognitive disorganization and transient psychotic episodes whereas the selective serotonin reuptake inhibitors are often useful in treating impulsivity (Soloff, 1998, 2000). However, there is little evidence at present that either dialectical behavior therapy or medication changes core self and interpersonal pathology. Nor should either be expected to lead to such changes. Dialectical behavior therapy, for example, does not include interventions that address maladaptive interpersonal schemata and behavior directly. On the other hand, Benjamin's interpersonal therapy (Benjamin, 1993; Benjamin & Pugh, Chapter 20, this volume) and cognitive therapy (Beck et al., 1990; Cottraux & Blackburn, Chapter 18, this volume) may be expected to produce changes in these areas because they use of strategies that directly address these problems. Similarly, the psychodynamic therapies including self psychology may be expected to be more successful in

changing dysfunctional relationship patterns and self-pathology. These considerations suggest that a comprehensive approach should include interventions from at least cognitive-behavioral therapy, interpersonal therapy, psychodynamic therapy and self psychology, and pharmacotherapy.

Principle 2: Personality Disorder Involves General or Core Features Common to All Cases and All Forms of Disorder, and Specific Features Observed in Some Cases but Not Others

Implication: A comprehensive treatment model requires two components: general strategies to manage and treat general psychopathology and specific interventions tailored to the specific features of individual cases.

Although DSM-IV lists general criteria for diagnosing personality disorder, few treatments emphasize the strategies required to treat the universal features of personality pathology. Nevertheless, the DSM-IV approach has important implications for treatment. It implies a model of personality disorder that consists of core or general features observed in all cases and specific features found in some cases but not others. A corresponding model of therapy would consist of general strategies and specific interventions.

To identify appropriate therapeutic strategies we need to explicate the core features of personality disorder. Chapter 1 argued that personality disorder could be defined as the failure to solve life tasks related to the establishment of stable and integrated representations of self and others; the capacity for intimacy, attachment, and affiliation; and the capacity for prosocial behavior and cooperative relationships. In essence, it involves chronic interpersonal problems and self-pathology (Livesley, 1998). Although all cases share the failure to form adaptive self and interpersonal systems, the problems arising from these failures may be expressed differently according to the other personality features that are present. For example, an inhibited–withdrawn (schizoid) person may express core interpersonal pathology as an inability to relate to others, whereas the emotionally dysregulated (borderline) person may show the same pathology through a tendency to move in and out of relationships quickly and difficulty tolerating closeness. The key issue is that both lack the ability to form close, intimate attachments.

Core deficits have major implications for treatment. Self-pathology involves problems with interpersonal boundaries, unstable self-representations, a poorly integrated sense of self, fragmented representations of other people, and problems with self-regulation. Interpersonal deficits lead to maladaptive interpersonal patterns, difficulty in tolerating closeness and intimacy, and problems with collaborative and cooperative relationships. In treatment, core pathology leads to difficulty establishing a treatment alliance and maintaining a collaborative working relationship, adhering to the frame of therapy, and maintaining a consistent therapeutic process. These are the key ingredients of a common factors approach. This suggests that the common factors approach could form the basis for the general strategies required to manage and treat core pathology. That is, these strategies should emphasize establishing and maintaining the therapeutic relationship, the treatment alliance, validation, and a consistent therapeutic process.

The importance of the therapeutic relationship was noted in most of the chapters on treatment. Even the more structured interventions such as cognitive therapy that typically assume patient participation acknowledge that this does not occur with the personality-disordered patient and that considerable attention has to be paid to relationship factors (Young, 1990; Cottraux & Blackburn, Chapter 18, this volume). There is also general recognition that a more supportive and empathic approach represents the most effective way to manage severe personality disorder (Buie & Adler, 1982; Gabbard, Chapter 17, this volume) An alternative approach is that of Kernberg (Clarkin, Yeomans, & Kernberg, 1999), which makes greater use of a more confrontational and interpretive approach. However, there appears to be support for an approach that provides support, validation, and empathy. This combination incorporates Rogerian dimensions and the emphasis that self psychology places on empathic validation in the treatment of deficit pathology.

The general strategies form a therapeutic structure to which more specific interventions may be added as required to treat the problems of the individual patient. Thus, the proposed framework is isomorphic with the underlying model of personality disorder. This approach has the additional advantage of introducing economy into the organization of treatment programs—the same conceptual approach may be used to treat all forms of disorder in all settings. The approach also affords the opportunity to foster the integration required to promote the synthesis of more cohesive interpersonal and self-systems. What is proposed here is not a one-model-fits-all approach to treatment but rather a general framework that can be tailored to the individual and the treatment situation.

Principle 3: Personality Disorder Is a Biopsychological Condition with a Complex Biological and Psychosocial Etiology

Implications: (1) Both biological and psychological interventions may have a role to play in treating individual cases. (2) Biological and developmental factors may place limits on the extent to which some features of personality disorder are amenable to change. (3) A major goal of treatment is to enhance adaptation.

Although psychosocial and biological factors are involved in the development of personality disorder, most treatments assign a primary etiological role to psychosocial adversity and focus on ameliorating the consequences of trauma, abuse, and deprivation. The role of biological factors is usually recognized, but this recognition is rarely translated into treatment strategies. An integrated approach, however, requires that the contribution of biological factors to personality disorder is incorporated into both the theoretical framework on which treatment is based and the interventions that are used. At the simplest level this means that medication is often part of integrated treatment. Yet despite evidence of the value of medication (Markovitz, Chapter 23, this volume) some clinicians are still reluctant to combine medication and psychotherapy. Within the framework proposed here, however, medication is merely another form of specific intervention to be delivered in the context of generic interventions

An understanding of the biological contributions to personality disorder has wider and perhaps more profound implications for treatment than simply acknowledging that medication may have a role. It also has a bearing on ideas about therapeutic change and the overall goals of therapy. The traits that form critical elements of personality structure are highly heritable (see Jang & Vernon, Chapter 8, this volume). This raises the question whether it is possible to change traits such as impulsivity, affective lability, submissiveness, and social avoidance that are important features of clinical presentations. The fact that a trait is heritable does not mean that it cannot be changed. Genetically determined traits can be modified with appropriate intervention. For example, the outcome of phenylketonuria, a recessive disorder that leads to mental retardation, can be changed if the diet of affected individuals is deficient in phenylalanine. In this case, modification of the environment modifies the expression of the genetic trait. The question of interest is whether similar considerations apply to personality traits.

Unfortunately, personality traits present a more complex problem. During development, genetic predispositions interact with environmental factors to form the biopsychological structures that underlie trait-based behavior. These structures may be described biologically in terms of neural networks and associated transmitter systems (see Coccaro, Chapter 6, this volume), and psychologically in terms of the cognitive processes and schemata that initiate trait-based behavior. As these structures emerge they influence the way the individual reacts to the environment, the way information is interpreted, and the environments that the individual seeks out. Thus, the environment is not independent of the person but rather a product of the interaction between previous environments and genetic predisposition. In an important sense, individuals create the environments to which they respond. This leads to considerable behavioral stability. At the same time, the biological, cognitive, affective, and behavioral components of traits form a mutually supporting system that resists change.

It seems improbable, therefore, that currently available interventions will lead to substantial change in basic personality traits. To take an extreme example, it is unlikely that the highly inhibited or schizoid individual will be able to change substantially in the direction of becoming highly sociable. Thus it should be expected that individuals with strong propensities toward affective lability, impulsivity, and stimulus seeking will continue to show these tendencies throughout life. For these reasons, treatment should focus on helping patients to adapt to their basic traits and to express them more adaptively rather than attempting to change the trait structure of personality. With this approach, *the goal of integrated treatment is to enhance adaptation by building competence.*

Principle 4: Psychosocial Adversity Influences the Contents, Processes, and Organization of the Personality System

Implication: Treatment should incorporate strategies to address all consequences of adversity.

Implementation of effective interventions to manage the consequences of adversity requires an understanding of the way psychosocial adversity influences personality development and the mechanisms through which it exerts a lasting influence on adaptive behavior. Several factors seem to be involved. First, memories of traumatic events lead to rumination, numbing, flashbacks, depersonalization and derealization, negative affects, and other recognized consequences of trauma. These symptoms can be addressed using established interventions for managing trauma. Second, repetitive adverse experiences give rise to schemata, beliefs, and expectancies that influence the way self, others, and the world are experienced. Because abuse and trauma usually occur in the context of unpredictable relationships, they give rise to expectations that people are untrustworthy, unreliable, unhelpful, and unpredictable. The child experiencing abuse and trauma often feels unable to control or influence events. Over time, feelings of powerlessness crystallize into doubts about competence and self-efficacy. They also contribute to dependency, submissiveness, passivity, and the conviction that there is little one can do to change things. Third, adversity influences the information-processing structures that are basic to personality functioning and the maintenance of self-esteem. For example, invalidating experiences lead to self-invalidating ways of thinking in which people continually question the authenticity of their experience and decisions, thereby undermining their sense of self. Finally, adversity can also affect the structure of the personality, culminating in poorly defined self and interpersonal boundaries, poorly integrated self-states, and a self-system that lacks integration and cohesion.

Interventions are required to treat the effects of traumatic memories and the cognitive and structural consequences of adversity. Treatments that only deal with traumatic experiences are unlikely to be sufficient. Supportive and validating interventions need to be emphasized to offer new experiences to counter the consequences of adversity. Distrust and problems with cooperation can be addressed through empathic interventions that focus on building and maintaining a collaborative treatment alliance, and by establishing a consistent therapeutic process. These problems are also addressed through a therapeutic process that emphasizes collaboration in understanding and solving problems. Invalidation and self-invalidating styles of thinking can be countered by validating interventions; unpredictability is countered by establishing and maintaining a consistent therapeutic process; and powerlessness is countered by promoting autonomy and by building competency and by interventions designed to build and maintain the motivation for change.

This brief analysis of the effects of psychosocial adversity identifies some broad strategies required to effect change. To establish a treatment process that can effectively address these issues it is necessary to adopt interventions drawn from several approaches. Change in maladaptive cognitions is most likely to be achieved through interventions based on cognitive and interpersonal therapy. It is also apparent that considerable attention has to be paid to maintaining a consistent and supportive process that may require the therapist to draw on the ideas and concepts of psychodynamic and generic approaches.

A FRAMEWORK FOR UNDERSTANDING CHANGE

A key element of any approach to treatment is a conception of therapeutic change: What changes, why it changes, and how it changes. This section examines the way the work of therapy can be understood using a generic approach, and the process through which change in personality pathology may be achieved.

Therapeutic Work

Different therapies offer alternative conceptualizations of the therapeutic process. Psychoanalysis emphasizes emphases clarification, confrontation, and interpretation of the patient's free associations and the working through of this interpretive work in the transference. Cognitive therapy adopts collaborative empiricism and a more didactic process. Several authors have suggested that the work of therapy with personality-disordered patients is best understood as one of engaging the patient in a process of *collaborative description* (Ryle, 1997; Livesley, 2000, in press). This suggestion is similar to the constructivist idea that therapy may be thought to involve "conversational elaboration" (Neimeyer, 1995). With this approach, the therapeutic task is to engage patients in a collaborative process of describing and understanding their problems and the way these problems affect their lives and relationships. As the patient's descriptions are elaborated and reframed, a new understanding emerges that inevitably leads the patient to contemplate change. The therapist's role is that of guide and consultant. Important issues are highlighted and selected for more detailed description. Details are sought when descriptions are too general. Clarification is requested when descriptions are unclear. Through this process, understanding does not simply emerge during therapy but, rather, it is shaped by the active collaboration of patient and therapist.

This approach to the work of therapy is consistent with generic interventions emphasizing support, empathy, and validation. The process facilitates the development of more cooperative ways of relating by engaging the patient in a collaborative process from the beginning of treatment. Through this process patients learn to reframe images of themselves, their lives, and their problems in ways that are less distressing and more adaptive (Ryle, 1997). At the same time, the approach reduces the tendency for reactive and maladaptive behaviors to become activated in ways the impede therapy.

Process of Change

The next step in developing a framework for understanding change is to consider the steps through which change occurs. Prochaska and DiClemente's naturalistic description of changes in addictive behavior is useful for this purpose (DiClemente, 1994; Prochaska & DiClemente, 1983, 1992; Prochaska, DiClemente, & Norcross, 1992). They described a six-stage process. The initial stage is *precontemplation,* in which there is no clearly defined intention to change. The stage of *contemplation* emerges when the person becomes aware of an addiction problem and begins to think seriously about dealing with it. *Preparation* is the stage that combines an intentional decision to change with actual steps that lead to action. The *action* stage involves serious efforts to change behaviors and experiences that maintain the addiction. *Maintenance* is the stage in which gains are consolidated. The final stage is *termination,* which occurs when change is well-established without fear of relapse.

Each stage involves a set of tasks that need to be accomplished before treatment can proceed to the next stage (Prochaska & DiClemente, 1992). For example, during the first stage of problem recognition, the patient's task is to describe and acknowledge problems and to commit to change, whereas the therapist's task is to help the patient to feel sufficiently secure to recognize problems. Interventions should be appropriate to the stage that the patient is currently in with respect to a given problem. There is little value, for example, in encouraging alternative actions before the need to change is acknowledged. The model introduces order into the change process. It also forms a framework that can be modified to understand therapeutic change in personality disorder. A four-stage process can be derived from the model: problem recognition, exploration, acquisition of alternatives, and generalization and maintenance.

Problem Recognition

Change can only begin when problems are recognized and there is a commitment to work toward changing them. Problem recognition takes time because many problems are ego syntonic and patients with personality problems tend to externalize responsibility. For the therapist, the task is to create the safety needed to acknowledge problems, and to provide sufficient explanation to enable patients to understand how these behaviors contribute to their other difficulties. For patients, the task is to recognize and accept their problems and commit to change.

Problem recognition often involves some degree of reframing to help patients to understand how a given behavior affects their lives. For those who are unable to acknowledge their problems, the best course of action is to continue to provide support and encouragement without pressuring the patient to change. Although some therapists believe that denial can be dealt with through active confrontation, the evidence suggests that it does not work (Miller & Rollnick, 1991). What is required instead is a supportive confrontation that raises doubts in patients' minds about their denial. Unless done supportively with an emphasis on observing and describing behavior rather than prematurely changing behavior, there is the danger that the therapist will be seen as critical or not understanding—perceptions that tend to activate reactive and oppositional patterns. This degree of tolerance and acceptance often reduces the pressure on the patient sufficiently to allow him or her to move on. Similarly, patiently and casually inquiring about a problem behavior and the effect that it has on the patient's life and other people, and whether it has caused difficulty, is often sufficient to enable the patient to recognize and own the problem.

Exploration

The patient's task during this stage is to be open to self-exploration and to collaborate in the process. This is often difficult because many behaviors that are the target of change are experienced as arising spontaneously without apparent cause. Thus, exploration often begins by helping patients recognize events that trigger problem behaviors. The therapist's role is to help patients to understand the sequence of events leading to these behaviors and the consequences of their actions. This involves managing the process to ensure that it proceeds at an appropriate pace and dealing with obstacles to self-exploration. In the process, the therapist models openness and an inquiring mind. The continuous product of exploration is increased self-knowledge. This eventually leads to the realization that alternatives are available and solutions exist.

Creating Connections within Descriptions

To have self-knowledge is to understand intuitively the relationship between events, what one experiences, and one's actions. This understanding creates a sense of consistency and stability. Thus a key component of exploration is to help patients to recognize patterns to their behavior and experience. This is achieved by *linking and connecting* the different elements of their experience and behavior. The antecedents–behavior–consequences model (A–B–C model) used in behavioral and cognitive therapy provides a useful structure for organizing this process regardless of the theoretical orientation of the therapist. Linking is not confined to the temporal sequence of antecedents, behavior, and consequences. It is also important to connect feelings, cognitions, and action. As Ryle (Chapter 19, this volume) noted, major discontinuities exist within experience for most personality-disordered patients. Connecting events, experiences, actions, and consequences brings meaning and order to experience that builds a sense of mastery and control and promotes integration.

A focus on the interpersonal factors that contribute to the targeted problem is a key element that helps patients recognize cyclical maladaptive patterns. With this approach emphasis is placed on understanding the cognitions associated with these patterns. Description and exploration of these beliefs lead naturally to a consideration of alternative ways of thinking about the issue in question, and hence to alternative ways of responding.

The interventions used to generate understanding will vary with the orientation of the therapist. Those comfortable with a psychodynamic approach will want to avoid or minimize structured interventions and rely on the analysis of defenses and the exploration of current and past relationships. Those with a more cognitive-behavioral orientation will probably make greater use of structured procedures such as diaries and reports of specific incidents to generate self-understanding. Those adopting a more integrated approach will probably use a combination of interventions according to the nature of the problem and the personality style of the patient. With many severely disturbed patients, structured methods are often useful. Diaries and daily records of problem behaviors help to engage patients in the treatment process. They are also relatively neutral ways of helping patients to identify events that trigger problem behaviors and encouraging them to reflect on their problems between sessions.

Descriptive Reframing

A second key element of descriptive exploration is to reframe the meanings and explanations attributed to experience. Reframing statements may be simple responses to a specific event. For example, a patient who considers herself to be a bad person because she self-mutilates may be helped to be less critical by a reframe that allows her to understand that these acts are the only way that she can cope with painful feelings. Other reframes may be more complex interventions that are offered after lengthy descriptive exploration. Such reframes help patients to reformulate their understanding of major areas of their life experience. For example, a patient who was unable to decide on a direction for his life, including a career, attributed this to the fact that he was a weak and inadequate person. This exacerbated problems by increasing feelings of hopelessness and passivity. He was helped to reformulate his understanding of his life in ways that opened up the possibility for change by a reframing intervention that linked his lack of achievement to a fear of surpassing a parent who was treated by everyone as extremely vulnerable. This fear had led the patient to devalue his own beliefs and aspirations and to sacrifice his own ideas in favor of those of others.

Reframing statements offer a new perspective that changes the way events are perceived and alters their significance for the self. For this reason they can be unsettling. They seem to be most effective when they arise from the immediate contents of therapy and when they are not affectively or cognitively overwhelming. They are also extensions of collaborative description. Rather than attempting to interpret unconscious material, the goal is to reorganize the patient's descriptive material to create a new understanding that is less distressing and facilitates more adaptive action.

Focus on the General and Specific Components of Maladaptive Patterns

An aspect of descriptive exploration that requires additional comment is the need to ensure recognition of repetitive maladaptive patterns and the specific behaviors through which these patterns are expressed. This requires the integration of psychodynamic and behavioral interventions. The psychodynamic tradition focuses on understanding broad maladaptive interpersonal patterns. In contrast, the behavior therapy tradition emphasizes behavioral analysis to identify specific behaviors for change, triggering stimuli, causal chains leading to problem behaviors, and environmental contingencies that reinforce and maintain these patterns.

Both strategies are important. The psychodynamic approach contributes to change by helping patients to recognize the global themes that characterize their lives. This integrates a range of behaviors, thoughts, and feelings and begins to change the way events are experienced. Pattern recognition enables the patient to exercise more control over these behaviors and promotes the integration that is one of the goals of long-term treatment. But change lies in the details. It is difficult to change broad patterns such as extreme submissiveness directly. Change depends on recognizing the specific instances in which the person behaved in an inappropriately submissive manner in the microevents of everyday life. By recognizing concrete instances of these patterns it is often possible for people to challenge and question their behavior. Over time these small changes consolidate into more global change.

Promoting Self-Observation

An important objective of descriptive exploration is to improve skills in self-observation and self-monitoring. Most therapies promote self-observation as a core skill that is required for change, whether this is expressed in the psychodynamic terms of facilitating the observer ego or in the behavioral sense of enhancing self-monitoring. Self-monitoring and self-awwareness are not the same. Self-awareness refers to the focusing of attention on an aspect of the self (Wicklund, 1975; Wicklund & Duval, 1971). Self-monitoring refers to *awareness* of an aspect of the self and an *evaluation* of the experience. This involves objective appraisal of the self, including attention to the causes and consequences of this aspect of the self.

This distinction between self-awareness and self-monitoring is especially pertinent to personality disorder. Most personality-disordered individuals are exquisitely self-aware and experience things intensely. However, they often have difficulty in reflecting on this experience and need assistance in developing self-monitoring skills. The challenge is to encourage patients to take an interest in their own minds so that they learn to reflect on the nature, causes, and consequences of their experiences rather than simply reacting to them.

Self-monitoring skills are promoted by encouraging patients to reflect on their experiences during treatment. Often it is also useful to encourage patients to keep a journal that records thoughts, feelings, and actions associated with everyday events. To be effective in encouraging self-monitoring, such a journal should be used not merely to emote but also as a vehicle for reflecting on experience.

Identifying Maintenance Factors

An important part of exploration is to identify those aspects of the person and environment that maintain problems. People seek out situations and relationships that are congenial to their personality even when these contribute to their difficulties. For this reason, it is useful to help patients to recognize how other people's reactions can confirm maladaptive cognitions and maintain problem behaviors. Under most circumstances, patients do not recognize these factors and are unaware of the way their actions are reinforced by the actions of others. In some cases, patients may need assistance in acquiring the assertiveness and communication skills required to change the interpersonal situations that contribute to their problems (Linehan, 1993; Robins, Ivanoff, & Linehan, Chapter 21, this volume).

Obstacles to Exploration

The path to self-knowledge is often blocked by a variety of self-deception strategies. Suppression, avoidance, and distraction are among the many strategies used to limit self-understanding because of the fear, shame, guilt, or pain that patients believe will result from acknowledging, thinking about, and revealing avoided experiences, feelings, or impulses. Patients often say, "I don't want to think about that," or "I don't want to talk about that." These problems may be managed using the classical defense interpretation of psychodynamic therapy (Malan, 1979) or a less interpretive approach that encourages the patient to describe these strategies and their effect. With some short-term therapies, the defense (or self-deception strategy) is actively addressed using confrontation and interpretation of the hidden feelings and impulses. This *anxiety-provoking approach* tends to cause problems when treating personality disorder. With more emotionally dysregulated (borderline) patients, the anxiety provoked increases behavioral disorganization. At the same time, interpretations are often experienced as confrontational, leading to an increase in reactive patterns. With the more inhibited (schizoid) patient, these interventions are often felt to be intrusive, leading to further withdrawal. For these reasons an *affect-regulating approach* is more effective in helping patients to face the fear, pain, or shame associated with the warded-off experience in amounts that are bearable (McCullough Vaillant, 1997). This may be achieved by noting the avoidance and inviting the patient to join the therapist in observing his or her own behavior. For example, "I have noticed that whenever we begin to discuss your anger toward your parents, you quickly start talking about something else. Have you noticed this?" Such interventions invite collaboration in self-observation. This can then be extended by asking about the worse aspects of the patient's fears, shame, or pain (McCullough Vaillant, 1997). This provides support while encouraging exploration of the most feared consequences of disclosure.

Other personality structures and processes may also obstruct the growth of self-knowledge. Affective lability, for example, may produce an intense and volatile affective climate that is not conducive to exploration and reflection. The cognitive styles associated with some personality patterns are a further obstacle. For example, the global and diffuse way of thinking that characterizes the hysterical cognitive style (Shapiro, 1965) limits self-understanding by avoiding the details of experience. Similarly, self-invalidating ways of thinking limits self-understanding by making the person uncertain about his or her actual experience.

Acquisition of Alternative Behaviors

This is a critical stage of change that warrants more attention than it typically receives from most therapies. The patient's task is to be open to change, to identify alternative ways of behaving, and to test out new behaviors in therapy and everyday life. The therapist's task is to ensure that understanding gets translated into behavioral change.

Change has attitudinal and behavioral components. The attitudinal component is represented by a fear of change and anxieties about the consequences of behaving differently. The behavioral component involves acquiring new responses and skills and learning to inhibit old behavioral patterns (Benjamin, 1993; Benjamin & Pugh, Chapter 20, this volume). Considerable therapist activity is often required to support and validate new ways of understanding self and others, new feelings, and new ways of behaving. This role is readily accepted by therapists of more eclectic, cognitive, or behavioral orientations. Psychodynamic therapists have also noted that many aspects of personality disorder are best modified by a noninterpretive stance that supports new experiences and actions (Buie & Adler, 1982; Gunderson, 1984; Masterson, 1976).

Generating Alternatives

This is a *problem-solving stage* that is managed through careful attention to process. The objective is to encourage the patient to use the same problem-solving skills that the therapist uses to understand and resolve problems. Problem solving can often be handled in a direct way, but sometimes it is necessary to encourage the patient to "play" with the idea of doing things differently to reduce the feeling of being pressured to change. It is interesting to note that many patients have difficulty playing and there is little sense of fun or joy in their lives. Hence this stage provides an opportunity for patients to explore more spontaneity, to try things out, and to enjoy the idea of doing things differently.

Maintaining Motivation to Change

For many patients, frustration caused by difficulty experienced in implementing change decreases self-esteem and reactivates maladaptive patterns. The challenge for the therapist is to acknowledge and validate the patient's fears and frustration while maintaining hope and the commitment of change. As patients weigh the costs of staying the same versus the costs of changing, their ambivalence may lead them to express the desire to change at one moment and disinterest at another. The danger is that this situation may lead to the therapist promoting change and the patient steadfastly defending the status quo (Miller & Rollnick, 1991). Obstacles to change are probably best managed using the descriptive approach applied to any behavior. This approach helps the patient to recognize that this situation is a natural reaction to change and can be dealt with using the same matter-of-fact descriptive approach that was used with other problems. This avoids the polarization of patient and therapist into complementary positions. It also leads to a discussion of the way treatment has created choice.

Encouraging New Behaviors

When working on encouraging behavioral change it is useful to recall that the general goal is to increase competency in the targeted area. This competency may be achieved by sudden change or through the *gradual substitution of progressively more adaptive behaviors*. Gradual change is often an effective way to modify self-harming behaviors and care-demanding actions and to change maladaptive traits. For example, early in treatment patients may have difficulty changing self-harming behaviors because these actions reduce distress and elicit care and support. It is difficult to relinquish these behaviors until alternatives are available. Consequently, it may be easier to change some behaviors by gradually substituting more adaptive ways of handling distress and associated needs. For example, patients may initially be encouraged to seek help from a crisis clinic or an emergency room without engaging in self-harming behaviors. The next step would be to promote alternative ways of dealing with their distress and postpone contact with the health care system until the next appointment. In this way, more adaptive responses to crises are gradually adopted until skills are acquired to manage and tolerate distress without engaging in self-harm. With a gradual approach, change does not appear overwhelming or impossible.

Inhibiting Old Patterns

Change also requires that the patient learn to inhibit old patterns (Benjamin, 1993). Within transference-focused therapy this inhibition is achieved by contracting and limit setting (Clarkin et al., 1999). Perhaps the simplest way to inhibit old patterns is for the therapist to rely on his or her authority to inhibit an action. Although this may create problems for the alliance, the approach may help when the patient is engaged in serious self-harming behaviors. Other simple interventions may be to encourage the use of distracting activities such as exercise, seeking the company of a friend, or watching a movie, to reduce self-harming acts especially during the early stages of treatment. Many maladaptive behaviors are activated so rapidly and automatically that it is difficult to apply new learning. Hence strategies are required to inhibit these habitual responses and to build a delay between the triggering stimulus and the resulting response. These strategies apply to a wide range of problems including automatic thoughts (Beck et al., 1990), impulsive responses to dysphoric affects, and tendencies to react rapidly and automatically to interpersonal situations with maladaptive responses such as inappropriate anger or withdrawal that lead to further interpersonal problems.

The need to inhibit old behaviors is most apparent with emotionally dysregulated or borderline patients who move rapidly from affect to action so that it is necessary to build steps between affect and action that slow down their responses (Kroll, 1988). This may require multiple techniques such as cognitive strategies to help patients to reflect on the thoughts and feelings that precede action, and affect regulating techniques that promote affect tolerance and increase affective control. Old responses can also be inhibited by encouraging patients to think about the consequences of their actions.

Teaching New Skills

Change often depends on skills that the individual is uncomfortable using or skills that are not part of the individual's repertoire, so that skill learning and strengthening are important therapeutic tasks (Linehan, 1993; Robins, Ivanoff, & Linehan, Chapter 21, this volume). Common skill deficits include poor assertiveness, social, and communication skills. These deficiencies often make it difficult for patients to change interpersonal relationships that contribute to their problems or reinforce maladaptive patterns. These deficits can usually be remedied by skill training. These instrumental deficits, however, often involve problems of a procedural nature that are more difficult to treat. Many patients lack an intuitive understanding of what behaviors are appropriate or expected in given situations. This difficulty is part of core pathology that does not always respond to skill training.

Consolidation and Generalization

Many features of personality disorder that are targets for change are acquired in repetitive interactions with significant others and consolidated through consistent patterns of internal and external reinforcement. It takes time to change such enduring patterns. Behaviors fluctuate and dysfunctional patterns return, especially at times of stress. Thus, an important part of therapy is to ensure that new behaviors become habitual patterns of action that are generalized to everyday situations. The patient's task during this stage is to apply learning acquired in treatment to everyday life and to acquire skills such as self-monitoring, self-validation, and self-motivation that are required to maintain change. The therapist's task is to ensure that these skills are learned and applied to everyday situations and to deal with obstacles that impede the process. Therapists also need to help patients to anticipate problems that are likely to occur in the future and to explore strategies that the patient might use to deal with these problems should they arise.

Applying New Learning to Specific Situations

Generalization is facilitated by encouraging patients to apply new learning to specific situations. Successful outcomes reinforce new behaviors and build self-esteem and self-efficacy. It is often helpful to rehearse these scenarios either in imagination or in actual role plays in therapy. This rehearsal enables the patient to fine-tune his or her behavior. If treatment is conducted using a group therapy format, the possibilities for role playing are even greater. Rehearsal also provides an opportunity to discuss the patient's reactions if the desired outcome is not achieved. This is important because an unfavorable outcome may be devastating and may reinforce old beliefs. Once a new course of action has been implemented it is helpful to work through the patient's experience of acting differently again in therapy to consolidate changes and to strengthen feelings of self-efficacy.

Developing Maintenance Strategies

Throughout therapy patients are provided with an opportunity to learn the methods that the therapist uses to understand and solve therapeutic problems and to apply these skills for themselves. These skills are critical to the maintenance of change after termination. As therapy moves into the later stages, skills in self-understanding and problem analysis, affect and impulse regulation, self-monitoring, self-validation, problem solving, and so on, should be explicitly reviewed and ways in which they may be used in the future should be discussed. This process should also include a discussion of the self-deception mechanisms that the person habitually uses and the way these contribute to problems. Coping mechanisms that are critical for the individual can be highlighted and problems in their application can be discussed.

Attribution of Change

Beliefs about the factors that contributed to change influence the stability of change. Research on normal subjects showed that change attributed to internal rather than external factors is more likely to last (Schoeneman & Curry, 1990; Sonne & Janoff, 1979). In addition, subjects who reported successful change are more likely to refer to internal control over be-

havior and are less likely to refer to external obstacles (Heatherton & Nichols, 1994). This suggests that attributing change to personal effectiveness, agency, and internal control may help to maintain changes (Weiner, 1985). These studies were conducted on nonclinical subjects; nevertheless, there is no reason to believe that these attributions are less important in maintaining changes in personality disorder.

Attributing of change to one's own effort may create a self-fulfilling prophecy that helps to maintain the change (Heatherton & Nichols, 1994), which suggests that therapists should help patients take realistic credit for any changes they make—something many patients resist. Taking credit should promote a sense of mastery and help patients to "own" the changes they have made (Horvath & Greenberg, 1994). It is also helpful for the patient to acknowledge the therapist's contribution. This consolidates cooperative behavior—an objective of therapy—and offsets the danger of perpetuating maladaptive beliefs because the patient believes that "I had to do it all by myself" (Horvath & Greenberg, 1994, p. 4).

This description of change shows how collaborative description may be applied throughout the change process and the way interventions from different models of therapy may be applied in a synergistic way. The stage model is not an invariant sequence of events but, rather, a general framework that makes the process understandable and manageable. Each problem that is a target for change can be dealt with using this approach. Because any treatment typically addresses multiple problems, at any moment several problems may be the focus of attention, each at a different stage of change. The approach emphasizes generic mechanisms such as the therapeutic relationship, the provision of new experiences and ways of relating, increasing self-knowledge, and the development of new behaviors. It also emphasizes cognitive processes and the use of multiple interventions to target specific problems.

GENERAL THERAPEUTIC STRATEGIES

A descriptive analysis of the nature of personality disorder and evidence of the importance of generic interventions lead to proposals that treatment be organized around generic interventions designed to manage and treat core pathology. Four general therapeutic strategies are proposed: building and maintaining a collaborative working relationship, maintaining a consistent therapeutic process, validation strategies, and building a commitment to change and maintaining motivation. Together these strategies provide the support required for change. They also establish the conditions for effective application of specific interventions while addressing key aspects of core pathology.

Strategy 1: Build and Maintain a Collaborative Relationship

Priority is given to establishing and maintaining a treatment alliance because patients have difficulty establishing the kind of working relationship that is critical to the change process. Most current formulations of the alliance emphasize the idea of collaboration (Horvath & Greenberg, 1994). This idea is central to treating personality disorder because therapists, regardless of their theoretical orientation, agree that a collaborative working relationship is difficult to establish and that considerable effort must be invested in building, maintaining, and repairing the alliance.

Luborsky (1984) suggested that the alliance has two components: (1) a perceptual component in which the patient sees the therapy and the therapist as helpful and him- or herself as accepting help and (2) a relationship component in which the patient and therapist work collaboratively to help the patient. This description is particularly useful in translating ideas about the alliance into a set of interventions because the two components are described using concrete behaviors that are easily translated into specific interventions. The *perceptual and attitudinal component* is marked by feelings that the therapist is warm and supportive, beliefs that therapy is helping, feelings of rapport with the therapist, beliefs that the therapist values and respects the patient, and beliefs in the value of the treatment process. The therapist's task, therefore, is to help the patient see that his or her condition can be treated and that therapy and the therapist are credible and to encourage the patient to accept help. The *relationship component* is marked by the patient experiencing working with the therapist in a collaborative way, the patient giving the therapist ideas about the cause of problems, the patient expressing the idea that it is increasingly possible to work

cooperatively with the therapist; and the patient showing the ability to use the same skills and tools that the therapist uses to understand problems.

Building Credibility: The Perceptual and Attitudinal Component

An effective alliance depends on patients believing that treatment and the therapist are credible. Luborsky's (1984) description of the behavioral markers of this component suggest that the following interventions contribute to developing the alliance.

Generate Optimism. The foundations for credibility and optimism are probably established at the outset of treatment by the professional manner of the therapist, which conveys respect, understanding, and support, and by educating patients about their problems and the ways that therapy can help them to attain treatment goals. The alliance is also enhanced by instilling confidence and hope. Even during assessment, the clinician should be mindful of the importance of hope because pretherapy expectations of success are associated with a favorable outcome (Goldstein, 1962). Early exploration of the patient's doubts or reservations about therapy or the therapist may help to resolve problems of confidence and credibility and help reduce premature termination—a major problem in treating personality disorder (Gunderson et al., 1989; Skodol, Buckley, & Charles, 1983; Waldinger & Gunderson, 1984).

Communicate Understanding and Acceptance. Listening carefully and responding sensitively create a sense of understanding and acceptance that establishes the rapport on which the alliance is built. Understanding and acceptance are conveyed by reflecting the patient's statements and by providing regular summaries of the impressions that the therapist has formed of the patient's difficulties, beginning during the assessment interviews. The provision of such summaries also provides an opportunity for patients to correct impressions that they believe are wrong. In the process, the idea of collaboration is established and fears are addressed that the therapist will not listen or has preconceptions about what is wrong.

Indicate Support for the Goals of Therapy. A focus on goals tends to be associated with patients' ratings of progress and the quality of the treatment relationship. Similarly, collaborative goal setting between therapist and patient contributes to the working relationship and the quality of the therapeutic bond (Bordin, 1994). Consequently, the relationship is consolidated by summarizing the joint understanding of goals, and by the therapist indicating a desire to work with the patient to achieve these goals. Support of patients' goals is also provided by encouraging patients to talk about their goals, how important they are, and about the progress they think they are making toward achieving their goals. Reminding the patient of these goals from time to time maintains the patient's focus on change and conveys the idea that the patient's beliefs and wants are important—a process that helps the patient develop self-esteem.

Recognize Progress. The working relationship is ultimately consolidated by progress. Many patients, however, are reluctant to acknowledge progress even to themselves. For this reason, it is useful for therapists to highlight even small changes as they occur. For example, if a goal is to reduce anxiety, occasions when the patient feels that he or she has not overreacted and has managed to contain his or her sense of panic should be acknowledged. Recognition of progress changes patients' perception of therapy, modifies beliefs of self-efficacy, builds competence, and begins to contribute to a sense of self-esteem.

Building Cooperation and Collaboration: The Relationship Component

The relationship component of the therapeutic alliance involves the translation of attitudinal and perceptual changes into behavioral change within therapy. Although it is convenient to think of this component as being built on the perceptual component, in practice the two are interwoven and many interventions incorporate both components. Luborsky's description suggests the following interventions.

Acknowledge the Use of Skills and Knowledge Learned in Therapy. A goal of therapy is to teach skills that subsequently can be used. Acknowledging that the patient has applied methods that the therapist and patient used in therapy to a specific situation builds the therapeutic bond by helping the patient to realize

that he or she used skills learned in therapy and that therapist and patient now have skills in common.

Use Relationship Language. Most conceptions of the alliance emphasize the bond or attachment formed by the patient with the therapist and the degree to which the patient feels secure enough to discuss problems (Allen, Newsom, Gabbard, & Coyne, 1984; Luborsky, 1984; Orlinsky, Grawe, & Parks, 1994; Orlinsky & Howard, 1986). This attachment is experienced and expressed in terms of liking, trust, mutual respect, shared commitment to the process, and a shared understanding of the treatment process and goals (Bordin, 1994). Attachment and trust form the basis for cooperation and enable the alliance to withstand the inevitable strains of therapy. The bond is fostered by a therapeutic style that conveys respect and collaboration. It can also be fostered by the words used. As Luborsky (1984) noted, the use of words such as "we" and "together" are simple ways to cement the relationship. Acknowledging that "we were able to make some progress with that problem . . ." or "In the past we were able to work this out together" promotes cooperation. Used judiciously, such statements begin to create a bond and to move patients away from perceiving relationships in a polarized way in terms of status or control.

Refer to Shared Experiences During Treatment. An important aspect of any relationship is the sense of shared history. This shared history creates a sense of continuity on which trust can be built. It also helps to form the idea that relationships are stable, a conviction lacking in many patients. A sense of shared history is established by recalling times when the patient and therapist worked together to find a solution to a given problem. Comments such as "we spent a lot of time working on those sort of problems in the past, so you must be pleased that the effort is really beginning to pay dividends" deepen the alliance. As therapy progresses, more opportunities arise to refer to past experiences together. Toward the end of therapy, such discussions help to consolidate change. It is also important to recall how things have changed and to note that the patient's and therapist's interaction was very different in the past.

Engage in a Collaborative Search for Understanding. The development of understanding is an important component of therapeutic work (Strupp & Binder, 1984). Understanding occurs at different levels, and it may not necessarily mean deep insight. With the integrated, tailored approach discussed here, less emphasis is placed on developing deep insights by reconstructing early development. Instead, the goal is to develop an understanding of the contemporary processes that underlie maladaptive patterns and to help patients make sense of their experiences.

Monitoring the Alliance and Managing Ruptures

The crucial role of the alliance in the change process means that the state of the alliance needs to be monitored throughout treatment. In this connection, it is helpful to differentiate problems in establishing an alliance at the beginning of treatment from strains or ruptures to the alliance that occur during treatment (Bordin, 1994). Protracted alliance formation is a common problem that reflects patients' relationship problems. This is not necessarily a disadvantage, nor should it be viewed as "pretherapy." Instead, it offers an opportunity to address important interpersonal schemata, to model tolerance and empathy, and to offer new relationship experiences. Difficulty in forming an alliance is best dealt with by using an empathic approach rather than confrontation and interpretation, which usually exacerbate problems and may precipitate termination.

Besides the effect of psychopathology, difficulty in forming an alliance may reflect lack of clarity or disagreement between patient and therapist about the goals of therapy. For this reason, particular attention should be paid to alliance formation when discussing collaborative treatment goals. Problems may also arise because the patient is confused about the way therapy works and his or her role in the process. Thus it is important to educate the patient about these issues when discussing treatment and establishing the treatment contract. Although these steps do not eliminate all obstacles to alliance formation, they reduce some of the factors that may exacerbate the problem.

Once the alliance develops, careful monitoring is required to identify strains or ruptures as soon as they occur. When monitoring the alliance, it is important to note that it is the patient's opinion about the alliance, not the therapist's, that predicts outcome. Any deterioration in the therapeutic relationship should be dealt with promptly. As with failure to form an alliance, ruptures should be approached in an empathic rather than a confrontational and interpretive manner. This usually means dealing with the problem in the here and now rather than interpreting the problem as resistance originating in past relationship problems. Safran and colleagues (Safran, Crocker, McMain, & Murray, 1990; Safran, Muran, & Samstag, 1994) have investigated the process of rupture and ways to repair ruptures. Their emphasis on alliance ruptures as opportunities to change dysfunctional interpersonal schemata is particularly relevant to treating personality disorder. They suggest that ruptures should be dealt with in four steps. The first step is to notice changes in the alliance—what they call "rupture markers." These include affect changes, decreased involvement, irritation, and so on. The second step is to explore the reasons for the rupture by focusing the patient's attention on the event and exploring the way it was experienced. The intent is to encourage the patient to express any negative feelings associated with the rupture. Third, the patient describes his or her experience, which is validated by the therapist. Validation is an important part of the process. If these steps are not effective, an additional step is to explore the way in which the patient avoids recognizing and exploring the rupture.

This sequence provides an opportunity to apply several change processes. By noticing and discussing the rupture, the therapist demonstrates empathy, models cooperation, teaches interpersonal problem-solving skills, and communicates the idea that interpersonal problems can be understood and resolved. Successful outcome depends on the therapist acknowledging the way he or she contributed to the rupture. Although patients with personality disorder are often hypercritical of their therapists, there is often a grain of truth to their criticisms (Vaillant, 1992). Therapists should always acknowledge their mistakes. For patients with severe personality disorder, such an acknowledgment can be a powerful experience. The ability to acknowledge error appears to help patients to be less defensive and to reflect on their behavior.

Strategy 2: Establish and Maintain a Consistent Treatment Process

The establishment of an agreed arrangement for therapy is an important part of generic approaches. The issue is especially important with personality disorder because many aspects of personality pathology mitigate against a stable therapeutic process. Difficulty with cooperation, mistrust, avoidance of intimacy, intense dependency, volatile affects, and impulsivity are among the many features that make it hard for patients to maintain stable relationships. Reviews of intensive psychodynamic treatment note that virtually all clinicians advocating this approach emphasize the importance of a consistent frame (Waldinger & Gunderson, 1989). Consistency provides the stability required for the effective implementation of interventions and offers the opportunity to learn new ways of relating. It is helpful to consider both the conditions required for a consistent therapeutic process and the interventions required to maintain consistency.

Establishing a Consistent Frame

Consistency is only possible if an explicit and clearly defined frame is established to contain the therapeutic process. The frame can be described in terms of three components: (1) the therapeutic contract; (2) the therapeutic stance—the therapist's approach to treatment; and (3) the treatment situation. This framework establishes therapeutic boundaries and creates a context for therapeutic interactions.

Treatment Contract. Most treatments advocate an explicit therapeutic contract that specifies the goals and conditions of therapy. Goals organize treatment by defining therapeutic tasks and hence delineate treatment boundaries; the treatment agreement defines the spatial and temporal aspects of these boundaries by specifying the practical arrangements for treatment. Borden (1994) suggested that the strength of the alliance depends on the level of agreement between patient and therapist on the goals and tasks of therapy.

The first step in developing a treatment contract is to agree on treatment goals. The general goal of improving adaptation by building competency noted earlier provides a context for discussing with the patient collaborative goals that are specific and attainable. Goal identification begins during assessment regardless of the type or duration of treatment, and it is finalized toward the end of the assessment process when the treatment contract is discussed. The next step is to reach an agreement on the practical arrange-

ments for therapy, including frequency and duration of sessions, and the duration of therapy.

Contract setting often requires that patients be educated about personality problems, the way therapy works, and the roles of patient and therapist in the process. This ensures that patients understand what to expect from treatment and the steps they need to take to reach their goals. Although psychoeducation has a well-recognized role in treating conditions such as eating disorders and schizophrenia, it is used less often in the treatment of personality disorder (Ruiz-Sancho, Smith, & Gunderson, Chapter 22, this volume). Psychoeducation is important, however, because many patients and their significant others do not understand the nature of the patient's personality problems and interpersonal difficulties.

Therapeutic Stance. The stance refers to "the interpersonal positions, in responsibilities, and activities that define the frame or the interaction between patient and therapist" (Gold, 1996, p.72). The stance contributes to consistency because it determines the therapist's approach to treatment, influences the therapeutic climate, and helps to shape therapeutic strategies. Because the stance acts as an anchor to treatment, it is important that therapists are clear about the most appropriate stance for treating personality disorder. Lack of clarity leaves the therapeutic process open to the influence of a range of pressures. As noted earlier, clinical observation and a consideration of etiology suggest that the most appropriate stance is an empathic, supportive, and validating approach that fosters the patients' involvement in a collaborative description and exploration of problems.

Treatment Context. The contribution of the treatment setting to consistency is easily overlooked. Patients are often acutely aware of the context in which treatment is offered and contextual events often influence treatment. Consequently, all staff members who come into contact with patients should understand personality disorder sufficiently to ensure that their interactions with patients are consistent with the therapeutic approach. In private offices little is needed other than advice to receptionists on how to respond to patients and their demands in a professional and nonconfrontational way. In hospitals and clinics, where contact with other staff is common, more systematic attention needs to be given to ensuring that everyone understands the treatment approach so that therapeutic endeavors are not inadvertently undermined by other staff.

Another organizational contribution to consistency is the provision of support and consultation to therapists. Personality disorder is difficult and demanding to treat. The provision of support or consultation helps to reduce problems and maintain consistency. The proponents of dialectic behavior therapy (DBT) go as far as suggesting that all therapists conducting DBT work only as part of a team (Robins, Ivanoff, & Linehan, Chapter 21, this volume). Although this requirement is too stringent, the principle is important. The ideal situation is for regular discussions with a consultant. If this is not possible peer supervision is a useful alternative.

Maintaining Consistency

Consistency may be defined simply as adherence to the therapeutic frame. It requires meticulous compliance by the therapist and prompt intervention when patient behavior threatens to alter the frame. Consistency is a major challenge throughout treatment because personality pathology inevitability leads to attempts to change the frame and challenges of the therapist's resolve to maintain stability. In addition, recurrent crises and episodes of intense distress often appear to make it difficult to adhere to a treatment plan without disturbing the alliance. These pressures are best dealt with through a supportive approach that acknowledges the pressures that initiated attempts to change the frame while also pointing out and exploring the consequences of such violations. This means that limit setting is an essential part of treatment. Often treatment failures can be traced to a failure to set limits promptly and supportively.

A common error is the failure to act when deviations from the frame are either threatened or first occur. Therapists often wait until therapy is disrupted before taking action because they do not recognize that supportive limit setting helps to contain aggressive and self-destructive behaviors or because they are afraid of harming the alliance. The patient's personality pattern may also contribute to therapists' difficulties. Therapists are often cautious with emotionally dysregulated and dissocial patients due to fear of activating anger and triggering termination. With inhibited patients, therapists are prone to accommodate frame violations in an attempt to build a relationship. Often the failure to act occurs because therapists hope that problems will resolve themselves without action on their part. Unfortunately this rarely works. Instead, the failure to act often leads to further acting out until the therapist is forced to set limits. By this time, however, the severity of frame violations and the intensity of countertransference reactions often make it difficult to deal with the problem constructively.

Strategy 3: Validation

Validation is a key ingredient of the common factors approach and therapies ranging from self psychology (Kohut, 1971) to cognitive-behavioral therapy (Linehan, 1993). Validation may be defined as an active strategy using interventions that recognize the legitimacy of the patient's experience (Livesley, 2000, in press). Emphasis is placed on nonevaluative acceptance and acknowledgement of the patient's reality and the authenticity of his or her experience. Validating interventions support and strengthen the alliance and contribute to changing the self-invalidating ways of thinking that are the hallmark of many forms of personality disorder.

Recognize, Acknowledge, and Accept Behavior and Experience

An important source of validation is the attitude with which the therapist approaches treatment. An attentive, empathic, and nonjudgmental attitude is often a more effective source of validation than the actual words communicated to the patient. Validation also depends on the therapist allowing an adequate opportunity to express affects and describe experiences. In most instances, validation is a matter of avoiding interventions that are likely to be experienced as invalidating. Common therapist behaviors that may be experienced as invalidating include prematurely focusing on the positive, dismissing and criticizing experiences and actions, giving the impression that problems and feelings are not being taken seriously, insisting that an intervention or interpretation is correct when the patient disagrees, communicating unreasonable expectations of change such as rapid change in self-harming behaviors, not acknowledging mistakes, and using inappropriate reassurance that trivializes patients' concerns.

Search for Meaning

The general purpose of validation is to help patients to understand their experiences and responses (Linehan, 1993; see Robins, Ivanoff, & Linehan, Chapter 21, this volume). Linehan described three steps leading to validation: (1) listening and observing actively and attentively; (2) accurately reflecting back to the patient his or her feelings, thoughts, and behaviors; and (3) direct validation. The first two steps are part of most forms of therapy. Linehan considers the third step, direct validation, to be specific to her approach. Here the therapist communicates to the patient that his or her responses make sense within the context in which they occur. Linehan recommends that therapists search for the adaptive and coping significance of behavior, and then communicate this understanding to their patients. These interventions may be considered part of a more general strategy involving a search for meaning that Yalom (1975, 1985) considered an important therapeutic factor.

The search for meaning is especially relevant to treating personality disorder because most patients find their lives and experiences inexplicable. For some patients, this causes intense distress and is a further reason for them to berate themselves. Thus it is helpful to explain how the patient's behavior is understandable in terms of his or her history and basic physiological and psychological mechanisms. For example, patients who blame themselves for not coping better because they dissociate or because their thinking becomes confused at times of stress can be offered information about the way intense anxiety affects performance. Emotionally dysregulated patients who are puzzled by their emotional lability and inability to control their feelings may find it useful to understand the biological and cognitive factors involved in regulating emotions. Interventions of this type help patients to make sense of their problems and symptoms without being overwhelmed or undermining the assumption of personal responsibility for change. Inevitably such explanations vary in depth according to the individual patient's ability to process and tolerate the information, as well as his or her current stage of therapy.

The specific component of the search for meaning that Linehan emphasizes is *to help the patient recognize that problem behaviors may be adaptive.* That is, actions that were previously considered to be either inexplicable or merely manifestations of pathology may represent the only way to cope with the problem available to the patient, given his or her life experiences and situation. Although not all behavior is explicable in this way, this is a useful form of validation for behaviors that make adaptive sense. For example, patients who self-mutilate when faced with intolerable feelings find it helpful to recognize that such acts may be the only way to terminate intolerable feelings that they had available at the time. It is important, however, that this recognition is achieved in ways that do not reinforce these behaviors or prevent patients from recognizing that there are alternative ways to handle distress.

Counteract Self-Invalidation

Earlier it was suggested that one way that adversity exerts a lasting influence is through the development of a self-invalidating cognitive style. Most patients do not realize the extent to which they question their experiences and ideas or how this way of thinking undermines their self-esteem and their sense of self. It also takes time for patients to recognize the many subtle ways this style of thinking manifests itself in everyday life. For this reason it is useful not only to identify the broad theme but also to focus repeatedly on specific examples that occur during treatment. Once patients begin to recognize their self-invalidating style, the benefits of this awareness can be extended by explaining the effects of this way of thinking on other mental processes, including feelings of confusion and poor self-esteem.

Acknowledge Areas of Competence

A useful form of validation is to recognize and support strengths and areas of competence such as recognizing that a patient manages to attend regularly despite a chaotic lifestyle or manages to hold down a part-time job despite severe problems. This approach seems to be most effective if areas of successful coping are not examined in detail but, rather, recognized as achievements that can be built on.

Acknowledging competence must be approached carefully. Patients can interpret such interventions as an indication that the therapist is insensitive to their pain or minimizes their distress. Nevertheless, recognition of areas of competence can be beneficial for patients who feel badly about their inability to organize their lives effectively. Such acknowledgement often enables patients to talk more freely about their problems because their assets are recognized.

Reduce Self-Derogation

Linked to interventions focusing on self-invalidating modes of thinking are interventions to reduce self-criticism—a common mode of thinking that contributes to dysphoria and self-harming acts. Given the pervasiveness of this style, it is useful for therapists to develop a repertoire of interventions that reduce self-criticism by validating actions that evoke self-criticism in ways that do not imply that change is unnecessary—for example, "Of course you behaved in that way; what choice did you have? It was the only way you could survive as a child"; "It is not surprising that you avoid showing your feelings because you were criticized if you did." Such interventions help the patient to see that his or her behavior was understandable given the circumstances in which it developed, while at the same time holding open the possibility of change.

On other occasions, self-blaming responses can be addressed directly. Sometimes patients can change this style by being helped to recognize that they blame themselves rather than trying to understand themselves. Change may also be facilitated by helping patients to recognize that they use insights gained in treatment to blame themselves further, and to contrast their own responses with those of the therapist, who seeks only to understand. Often this contrast gives the patient sufficient distance to begin to recognize how he or she runs an inner commentary of self-criticism.

Managing Validation Ruptures

Invalidating interventions are almost unavoidable when treating personality problems because patients are hypersensitive to invalidation and the nature of personality pathology makes it easy for therapists to invalidate inadvertently. Modest failures of validation are nodal points in therapy that afford the opportunity for useful work. When these events occur, it is important that they are handled in ways that do not lead to further invalidation. The sequence of interventions for managing alliance ruptures suggested by Safran and colleagues can readily be applied to validation failures. The first step of acknowledging the event is often sufficient. Such a response differs from patients' expectations and previous experiences. Indications of the failure of validation are varied. With the more emotionally dysregulated person the responses include anger and hostility, direct criticism, or angry withdrawal. The inhibited individual, in contrast, is more likely to internalize the response so that it is less discernible. The second step is to explore reactions to invalidation, including ideas about its causes. The final step is to validate the patient's responses and for the therapist to acknowledge any error.

Strategy 4: Build and Maintain Motivation

Motivation is a complex issue in the treatment of personality disorder. On the one hand, motivation is essential to bring patients to treatment and to keep them in treatment. Change is difficult and painful; hence patients need to be motivated to stay the course. On the other hand, many patients are poorly motivated for change because of feelings of passivity and beliefs that change is not possible and by the lack of resources to effect change. Because low motivation is inherent to personality disorder, therapists need to monitor motivation throughout therapy and hone skills in building motivation. Unfortunately, empirical analyses of motivating interventions are sparse. One of the most useful clinical discussions of motivation is the volume *Motivational Interviewing* (Miller & Rollnick, 1991). Although written specifically about the treatment of addictive behavior, these ideas have wider currency. Miller and Rollnick characterize motivation as "the probability that a person will enter into, continue, and adhere to a specific change strategy" (p.19). This probability is not constant—that is, motivation is not a trait—rather, motivation consists of "a state of readiness or eagerness to change, which may fluctuate from one time or situation to another" (p.14). Whereas sufficient motivation is required to attend therapy, subsequent levels of motivation are influenced by therapist behavior. Effective therapists are successful in increasing patient motivation (Meichenbaum & Turk, 1987). Nevertheless, therapists often seem to regard motivation as the sole responsibility of their patients.

Miller and Rollnick (1991) described eight general interventions for building motivation that are pertinent to treating personality disorder: giving advice, removing barriers, providing choice and creating options, decreasing desirability of maladaptive behaviors, practicing empathy, providing feedback, clarifying goals, and active helping. Beyond these interventions, the evidence suggests that general aspects of therapeutic style influence patient motivation. Some therapists seem to believe that a lack of motivation should be countered by active confrontation. Confrontational styles, however, often increase resistance and evoke adverse reactions. Miller, Benefield, and Tonigan (1993), for example, in a study of problem drinkers that compared a confrontational approach, a client-centered approach, and a wait-list control group, found that clients in the confrontational group showed more arguing, interrupting, ignoring, and denial of problems. Moreover, the more confrontation the therapist used the more the patient drank at 1-year follow-up. Confrontation, therefore, seems to be counterproductive, whereas a more supportive, encouraging, and validating style seems to facilitate a commitment to change. This suggests that the general alliance building and validating strategies will also enhance motivation, and that these strategies should be used whenever motivational problems arise. Supporting patients when they feel stuck, recognizing and thereby validating their fears of change, and encouraging a discussion of the options available are likely to be more effective than a more aggressive confrontation of "resistance."

Using Discontentment

A commitment to change is often stimulated by the discontentment that frequently accompanies problem recognition. As Baumeister (1991, 1994) noted, "discontent is a powerful motivator." Studies of successful and unsuccessful changes in lifestyles, relationships, and personality among students indicated that those who reported major changes also reported much stronger negative affects and suffering than those who did not change or changed less (Heatherton & Nichols, 1994). It appears that the pain associated with the targeted problem is important in bringing about change. Baumeister (1991) refers to this phenomenon as the "crystallization of discontent."

The way that people perceive their lives and themselves helps to maintain the stability of their behavior and personality. Change is avoided by perceiving themselves and their lives in a positive way. When people are content they have

little incentive to change. As long as personality-disordered persons see their self-destructive, self-harming behaviors as unavoidable ways of dealing with distress; as long as they believe that their dysfunctional relationships are positive, fun, or exciting; and as long as they perceive their maladaptive life styles to be normal ways of being, they have little incentive to change. Many patients maintain these perceptions despite seeking treatment. They see the different parts of their lives as separate and unrelated. Mobilization of the commitment to change requires a reframing of these subjective assessments. It is here that the crystallization of discontent is a helpful concept. In his explication of the crystallization of discontent, Baumeister discusses situations in which a critical incident triggers a sudden shift in the way individuals see themselves and their lives. As a result, discontentment with the way things are suddenly emerges as the factor that integrates experiences, behavior, and circumstances that were previously believed to be unrelated. It is this sudden perceptual shift that motivates change. In treatment, the therapist can sometimes seize the opportunity afforded by relatively minor incidents to build motivation by focusing on the discrepancy between the way the person is and the way that he or she would like to be. Discontentment may be amplified simply by noting and thereby underlining the patient's frustration with the way he or she behaves. On other occasions it may be helpful to take this a step further by exploring the dissatisfaction through a detailed discussion of the effects of the problem behavior on everyday life. Such a focus on the negative affects associated with these behaviors challenges any underlying passivity and the ego-syntonic nature of such actions.

Building a sense of hope that change is possible can also increase the motivating effects of discontentment. The danger of focusing on discontentment is that it may become chronic or adversely affect self-esteem. Sufficient discontentment is needed for the patient to contemplate change without increasing demoralization and ruminative guilt. Hope helps to prevent discontentment from spiraling into despair. The challenge is to balance discontentment and realistic hope to enhance the commitment to change.

Creating Options

For many patients, motivation is limited by their inability to identify an alternative course of action, and by beliefs that change is not possible. Change is therefore a daunting prospect because it is difficult to relinquish familiar ways, even if they are maladaptive, unless alternatives are available. To promote motivation for change it is often necessary to help patients to recognize that they are free to choose alternative paths. This sense of choice helps to reduce feelings of pressure and constraint. Active work on these issues is often required if patients have especially strong beliefs that choice does not exist. The absolute quality of some of these beliefs needs to be challenged. Cognitive therapy techniques for changing schemata are often useful for this purpose (see Cottraux & Blackburn, Chapter 18, this volume).

Focus on Small Steps

For many patients change seems overwhelming because they confront themselves with all their problems at once and focus on global problems rather than breaking each problem into manageable components. Information about goals and the way goals are organized into a hierarchy with more general goals subdividing into more specific goals (Carver & Scheier, 1998) is often helpful. Patients often focus on broad goals such as developing a sense of identity but neglect the more specific goals that contribute to such general goals (e.g., defining leisure activities they enjoy, establishing career goals, and defining their major characteristics). Each of these goals can in turn be subdivided into even more specific goals. It is at the more specific level that change becomes possible. Motivation is increased by identifying small steps that can be tackled sequentially.

This idea is similar to the means–end analysis employed in problem solving in which a problem is divided into concrete components in order to facilitate its solution (Newell & Simon, 1972). Time spent on teaching problem analysis is worthwhile because it is a skill that will help the patient to deal with problems when treatment ends.

Identifying Incentives for Not Changing

All actions are associated with perceived costs and benefits. Nevertheless, patients rarely examine the costs and benefits of their actions, even when these actions are obviously harmful and even life threatening. Self-mutilating and parasuicidal acts may be considered unavoidable, and the costs involved may be dismissed as inconsequential. As captured by the idea of secondary gain, many maladaptive behaviors benefit the patient in ways that are not always apparent. Thus, as Miller and Rollnick (1991) noted, it is important to identify incentives for not changing. These incentives may include relief from emotional distress, as illustrated by many self-harming behaviors, or gratification of a wide range of interpersonal needs, such as care and attention. What matters is the person's perception of the costs involved, rather than the actual costs in an objective sense. Thus, therapists need to recall that their appraisal may be different from that of their patients.

Managing Ambivalence

A common problem is the patient's ambivalence about change. Change is recognized as desirable and even necessary, but at the same time the idea of change often evokes fear and even resentment that change is necessary. Miller and Rollnick (1991) suggested that for many patients, change represents an approach–avoidance conflict. Change is desirable because it means relinquishing painful patterns, but it also has negative aspects because it means exchanging familiar patterns for unfamiliar ones with unknown consequences. Moreover, there are often concerns about the impact of change on others. As the costs and benefits of changing versus staying the same are evaluated, patients frequently experience ambivalence about treatment due to frustration at feeling stuck and fear stemming from uncertainty. The danger is that this dilemma will activate old reactive patterns.

Besides maintaining motivation using techniques such as building hope, providing support, and encouraging the application of new behaviors, therapists can also intervene to change the relative strengths of the positive and negative aspects of change. One approach is to increase the discrepancy between the way one is and the way one would like to be (Miller & Rollnick, 1991). Encouraging individuals to consider the benefits of change and stimulating their desire to relinquish old patterns can increase the value of the positive side of this conflict. At the same time, exploring the fear of change and addressing the concerns raised can reduce the negative aspects of the conflict. This may involve helping patients acquire the specific new skills that are required to change.

General Therapeutic Strategies: An Overview

The general strategies organize the therapeutic process and establish a context for implementing any specific interventions that may be required to treat the problems of individual cases. They form the basic framework of therapy regardless of the specific problems of individual patient, the type and duration of therapy, and the stage of treatment. The strategies form an approximate hierarchy of priority and importance. Priority is given to interventions that ensure patient and therapist safety. Next are the general strategies with the alliance building and validating interventions taking priority over consistency maintaining and motivating interventions. Finally, specific interventions are used when other conditions have been meet.

The general strategies not only establish the conditions for change but also bring about change directly and indirectly by their effects on core pathology. Interventions based on general strategies provide new relationship experiences that counter the more maladaptive relationships experiences of the past. They also facilitate the development of cooperation and collaboration, the capacity for closeness, and effective interpersonal boundaries.

SPECIFIC THERAPEUTIC STRATEGIES

The extent to which specific interventions are used to treat the individual case depends on the goals of therapy, the treatment setting, and the duration of treatment. With longer-term cases a wide variety of interventions may be used, whereas short-term crisis management may involve a more limited repertoire. The numerous kinds of specific problems presented by individual patients inevitably means that therapists using an integrated approach should be prepared to employ an extensive array of interventions and expect to change intervention strategies during the course of treatment. It is not possible to consider all possible specific treatment strategies; therefore, discussion will focus on the broader principles involved in managing symptoms and crises, maladaptive expressions of personality traits, and self- and interpersonal pathology.

Symptoms and Crises

The management of crises and symptom states provides an excellent illustration of the importance of combining psychosocial and pharmacological interventions (Gabbard, 1998). Crisis states usually involve dysphoric and impulsive symptoms including self-harming acts. Often management is complicated by features of cognitive dysregulation, such as confused thought processes, difficulty processing information, and, in a small percentage of patients, paranoid ideation, schizotypal cognition, and the symptoms of a brief psychotic episode. Under these circumstances the patient's ability to process information is severely compromised. The evidence suggests that management of acute symptoms may include a combination of medication (Soloff, 1998, 2000) and containment interventions until the acute behavioral disorganization settles followed by medication and cognitive-behavioral interventions (Beck et al., 1990; Linehan, 1993) to treat ongoing symptoms.

Containment

The immediate requirements of crisis management are to assess suicidal potential, ensure safety, and contain emotions and impulses. In these states, the patient's priority is usually to obtain relief from his or her distress. This usually comes from feeling understood (Joseph, 1983; Steiner, 1993). This helps to contain the emotional turmoil and behavioral disorganization. Failure to achieve containment almost invariably leads to an escalation of dyscontrol. Containment is achieved by the therapist communicating that he or she understands the patient's feelings and concerns. Containment is weakened by the failure to acknowledge distress and by attempts to interpret the patient's thoughts, feelings, or impulses. In these states, a common problem is that therapists attempt to achieve too much which overwhelms that patient's capacity to handle information. All that is needed are concrete statements that recognize the current situation. Attempts to interpret the distress are easily experienced as invalidating and as evidence that the therapist does not understand or care.

Medication

Medication is useful in treating three important symptom clusters that are common in these states: emotional dysregulation, impulsivity, and cognitive dysregulation. The selective serotonin reuptake inhibitors appear to be especially useful in managing emotional dysregulation and impulsivity (Markovitz, 1995, Chapter 23, this volume; Soloff, 1998, 2000). These agents contribute to a reduction in affective lability, including anger and rage and impulsivity, thereby increasing control and providing an opportunity for patients to reflect on their experiences and their situation rather than simply reacting to them. Similarly, there is evidence for the value of low dosages of typical and atypical neuroleptics in the management of cognitive dysregulation and quasi-psychotic features (Goldberg et al., 1986; Soloff, 1998, 2000).

With this approach, medications are considered a form of specific intervention, and like other specific interventions, they should be delivered in the context of the general therapeutic strategies. Care should be taken to ensure that the patient understands the role of medication within the overall treatment plan and that the medications are being used to treat specific features and should not be expected to resolve all problems. In many cases it is also useful to involve significant others and make them aware of the reasons for prescribing medication and the likely benefits. This prevents unreasonable expectations by patients and their families. Used in this way, medications act synergistically with generic interventions to contain the distress, reduce symptoms, and minimize the escalation that occurs so easily with these patients in crisis situations. If effective, medications also help to foster the alliance by increasing therapist and treatment credibility.

Cognitive-Behavioral Interventions

A variety of cognitive-behavioral interventions have an important role in managing parasuicidal and self-harming behavior (Linehan, Armstrong, Suarez, Allnon, & Heard, 1991; Robins, Ivanoff, & Linehan, Chapter 21, this volume). Such an approach lends itself readily to the stages-of-change model discussed earlier. As containment is achieved, interventions can begin to focus on developing a commitment to make self-harming behaviors targets for change. Subsequently attention can focus on understanding these behaviors, the events that trigger them, and the factors that maintain them. This exploratory process can be supplemented through the use of diaries and rating scales to monitor these behaviors. These methods establish a baseline against which progress can be evaluated and helps the patient to recognize internal and external triggers. They also begin the process of helping the patient to acquire skills in self-observation. Over time, attention is paid to analyzing and understanding the problem behavior, the immediate and distal triggers and antecedents, and the short- and long-term consequences of these acts. As an understanding of the sequence of events that trigger problem behaviors becomes apparent, alternative ways of dealing with problems are automatically considered.

While this process unfolds, it may be necessary to use a variety of interventions to reduce self-harm and manage dysphoric affects. The frequency of self-harming acts can often be reduced through nonspecific interventions, including a focus on the effects of these acts on the treatment process (Clarkin et al., 1999). Simple behavioral interventions based on avoidance and distraction may also promote control. These steps rarely seem to achieve lasting change, but they often create a respite that makes it possible to implement more definitive interventions such as affect regulation strategies, including affect tolerance, problem-solving skills, and the identification of alternative sources of reinforcement. As with all specific interventions, this combination of behavioral and cognitive techniques should be delivered with considerable attention to the therapeutic process and the treatment relationship.

Promoting More Adaptive Expression of Basic Traits

Although maladaptive expressions of traits are a feature of most clinical presentations and DSM-IV defines personality disorder as inflexible and maladaptive traits, most treatments do not discuss specific interventions for treating maladaptive traits (Paris, 1998; Livesley, 1999, 2000, in press). There are several reasons for this omission. First, most therapies concentrate on the consequences of developmental adversity such as interpersonal conflicts, maladaptive relationships, and dysfunctional cognitions. When behaviors that are influenced by basic traits are the focus of therapeutic effort they are treated in the same way. Second, some therapies assume that trait constellations, like other components of personality, are the products of developmental conflict, and hence it is also assumed that they can be modified using traditional psychotherapeutic techniques. It is apparent, however, from behavioral genetic studies that such explanations are at best only partly correct. It seems unlikely, therefore, that fundamental changes can be made to the basic trait structure of personality disorder. This unlikelihood creates something of a dilemma because maladaptive expressions of basic traits are important features of personality disorder and effective treatment requires that these maladaptive expressions change. The solution to this problem becomes apparent when we examine the structure of traits and way environmental factors influence their development.

Traits are complex structures that develop from the interaction of genetic predisposition and environmental influences. This interaction gives rise to relatively stable structures consisting of an underlying behavioral tendency and associated cognitions and affects that give rise to trait-based behavior. This tripartite structure of behaviors, cognitions, and affects tends to be highly stable because the different components are mutually supportive.

Twin studies show that environmental factors contribute approximately 50% of the variance in a given trait. Although it is unlikely that environment factors can totally modify trait expression, they exert an important influence. They appear to operate by modifying the level of trait expression, either dampening or amplifying the effects of genetic predispositions. They also influence the behaviors through which a given trait is expressed. For example, not everyone who has a high score on sensation seeking will express this tendency in the same way, nor are all these expressions equally maladaptive. Maladaptive expressions may include the excitement that some personality-disordered persons get from taking an overdose and calling the paramedics or from their crisis-ridden lifestyle. Somewhat more adaptive expressions may include engaging in high-risk sports or high-risk speculation on the financial markets. Within the limits imposed by both genetic and environmental influences, therefore, some degree of change seems possible. This suggests three general strategies: (1) increase tolerance and acceptance; (2) attenuate trait expression; and (3) progressively substitute more adaptive responses.

Strategy 1: Increase Tolerance and Acceptance

The assumption behind this strategy is that the trait structure of personality is relatively fixed and hence individuals need to be helped to accept their basic traits and use them adaptively. Patients with personality problems often attack themselves for having certain characteristics. This internal conflict increases distress and hinders adaptive use of these qualities. Self-blame may be reduced by helping individuals to understand that their personality traits are part of their biological heritage and to recognize the potential benefits of these traits. Reduction of self-blame often allows patients to reflect on their qualities and to focus their efforts on finding productive ways of using their traits as opposed to trying to change them abruptly.

Most traits are adaptive in some way and it is often validating to help patients to recognize the value of their traits. The challenge is to identify social niches in which the patient's basic traits may be used adaptively. For traits such as compulsivity that are often viewed as desirable in our society, this is not difficult. For other traits, especially affective traits, this may be more difficult. However, reducing self-blame and other cognitive strategies that amplify the expression of these traits often reduces their intensity a little to permit the patient to develop other ways of looking at these qualities. For example, the development of more tolerance of affective lability in one patient reduced the intensity of her frequent episodes of self-blame. This led to a modest reduction in affective instability, which in turn allowed her to recognize that her mood changes were an importance source of creativity that she valued. This recognition made affective changes less anxiety provoking.

Strategy 2: Attenuate Trait Expression

This approach involves learning skills to regulate and control trait-based behavior. This is achieved most eeffectively by focusing on the cognitive component. For example, traits that characterize emotional dysregulation often involve such schemata as feelings cannot be tolerated, inability to control and regulate affects, and catastrophic thinking. These schemata may be expressed through statements such as "I cannot tolerate the way I feel," "It would be unbearable if these feelings," "There is nothing I can do to control or change the way I feel," and "My feelings are unpredictable." The cognitive component of traits is probably the most open to exploration, reframing, and change. Hence, standard cognitive interventions (see Cottraux & Blackburn, Chapter 18, this volume) may help to modify these traits.

In addition, many patients use cognitive strategies that amplify the expression of affective traits. They ruminate on their experiences in ways that amplify their distress rather than use coping strategies that reduce affect. In these cases, it is often possible to help patients to acquire affect regulating skills. Medication may be useful in attenuating affective lability, impulsivity, and cognitive dysregulation.

With nonaffective traits it may be possible to help the patient to acquire skills that are complementary or incompatible with trait-based behavior. For example, those who are excessively submissive can be taught assertiveness skills, and those who are socially apprehensive may be helped to develop strategies to enable them to deal with others. Again the avenue to change involves a focus on the cognitions associated with these behaviors accompanied with interventions that teach new behaviors.

Strategy 3: Progressively Substitute More Adaptive Trait Expression

With this strategy, maladaptive expressions are gradually replaced by more adaptive behaviors. For example, patients at the extremes of dependency dimensions often report that self-harming and parasuicidal behaviors are gratifying because they elicit care and attention. These patients can be helped by exploring more adaptive ways to express these traits and meet these needs. Others find that such behaviors satisfy their need for stimulation. Such individuals may be encouraged to identify more adaptive activities that they find exciting as opposed to more destructive behaviors that bring them into contact with the mental health system.

These strategies can be implemented through a wide range of interventions selected according to the therapist's orientation and tailored to the patient's preferred approach. The important feature of the approach is that it involves a change from the usual way in which therapists approach the management of trait-based behavior. Those who are more familiar with attempting to change these behaviors in more fundamental ways may find such ideas uncomfortable. However, the idea that radical change in traits is possible is a common misconception that leads to less than optimal ways of managing these problems.

Self and Interpersonal Problems

Maladaptive self-structures and interpersonal patterns are the hallmark of personality disorder, and change in these characteristics is the focus of most treatments that extend beyond immediate crisis management. The major goals are (1) to change dysfunctional self and interpersonal schemata and associated maladaptive interpersonal patterns and (2) to promote the development of a more cohesive self-system and integrated representations of others. The first goal involves changing cognitions used to understand self and others and maladaptive behaviors. This is standard psychotherapy that may be approached using cognitive, interpersonal, and psychodynamic interventions. The second goal is more difficult to achieve. It involves the synthesis of a more stable and cohesive self system and integrated representations of other people. Most therapies recognize that this is the central challenge in more definitive treatments but offer few strategies or specific interventions to achieve this outcome. The exception is the work of Ryle (1997; see Chapter 19, this volume) who discusses ways to explore and integrate the poorly integrated self states associated with borderline personality disorder. Most approaches appear to assume that integration is accomplished indirectly through other interventions. There is some justification for this assumption because general interventions that offer support and validation are likely to encourage self development by confirming the authenticity of self-experience and changing self-invalidating modes of thought that hinder the formation of an adaptive self system. Nevertheless, as Ryle's cognitive analytic therapy makes clear, it is also important to use interventions that address this problem more directly.

Repetitive Maladaptive Interpersonal Behavior Patterns

An important step toward attaining both goals is to enable the patient to recognize and change *repetitive maladaptive behavior patterns.* Because change depends on the recognition of patterns in emotional reactions, ways of thinking, and behavioral reactions, *pattern recognition* is an important part of the change process. The idea that there is a "pattern" to their behavior and experience is readily accepted by most patients, although most are not aware of these characteristics. The idea introduces order and meaning to experience. At the same time, the word is benign and free from negative connotations. Descriptions of patterns often help patients to gain some distance from events in their lives rather than simply reacting to them. Self-observation is enhanced and the pattern becomes the focus of change. At the same time, pattern recognition promotes integration by establishing connections among events, behaviors, and feelings that were experienced as unrelated.

Interpersonal Schemata. As noted earlier, the concept of schema provides a potentially integrating concept that links diverse therapies. As used in cognitive psychology, the term was first used by Piaget (1926) and Bartlett (1932). According to Rumelhart (1980), theories using the schema concept propose that knowledge is organized in units consisting of attributes (items of knowledge) and an explanation of how these attributes are connected. In this sense the term can be applied to the person's images of self and others and the clusters of ideas and beliefs that the person has about him- or herself, other people, and the world. The concept forms the cornerstone for understanding and changing repetitive maladaptive patterns.

Schemata not only organize information and experience but also influence the acquisition of information. They influence what is noticed, what becomes the focus of attention, and what is discounted or ignored. For example, suspicious individuals who believe that the world is hostile and that other people are likely to trick or harm them are hypervigilant. They notice anything that confirms these beliefs. Hence they readily notice minor slights or expressions of hostility. Equally important, they ignore or discount behaviors such as expressions of concern or altruism that are inconsistent with this idea. Because such individuals are highly selective in the way they perceive and process information, the schema is continually confirmed. Suspicious individuals also behave toward others in a wary and even hostile way that tends to elicit hostile or distancing responses. These responses are then taken as evidence that the underlying beliefs are valid. Thus, schemata are maintained because they give rise to cognitive processes and behavioral responses that tend to confirm the core beliefs (Young, 1990).

An important part of treatment is to help patients to identify core schemata and to understand the role they play in repetitive maladaptive patterns. Schemata are usually identified in the normal course of therapy when the patient describes scenarios with other people. In addition, specific techniques may be used to identify schemata such as the questionnaire methods and other procedures discussed in the chapter on cognitive therapy (Cottraux & Blackburn, Chapter 18, this volume). Structured methods to assess interpersonal behavior may also be used to identify associated interpersonal patterns (MacKenzie, Chapter 14; Benjamin & Pugh, Chapter 20, this volume).

As schemata become the focus of therapeutic efforts, it is often helpful to represent core schemata in the form of a diagram that show how the schema influences interpersonal behavior with specific individuals and how the schema influences perception and action in ways that confirm the belief. Diagrams are useful because they capture the patient's experiences and behaviors in a concrete form that is readily understood. The use of a diagram forces therapists and patients to clarify the details of these patterns and to engage in a collaborative exercise to elaborate on the details of the different components of the pattern. A diagram also helps patients to distance themselves from their own reactions and enables them to process information more effectively. Often such diagrams are an important intermediate step toward internalizing a full recognition and understanding of their patterns. Besides working collaboratively on diagramming key schemata it is often useful to encourage patients to work on other schemata on their own between therapy sessions. This helps to consolidate their understanding of the ideas involved and to generalize them to everyday life.

Changing Schemata. Schema change can be approached using the sequence of recognition, exploration, acquisition of alternatives, and generalization and maintenance described in the stages-of-change model discussed earlier. The first stage, schema recognition, is often time-consuming because many schemata that are central to the pathology of personality disorder are applied automatically, often without awareness. Recognition is frequently a two-step process. The first is to identify the pattern during treatment and to help the patient to understand how the pattern contributes to his or her problems. This is usually a relatively straightforward step. The next step is for the patient to apply this understanding outside therapy and to recognize the pattern in all its manifestations both in therapy and, more important, in everyday life. This is usually a more time-consuming process. The automatic nature of these thoughts makes them difficult to recognize. At the same time, the associated affects are often aroused so quickly that these and not the thoughts that triggered them become the focus of attention. When this happens, other schemata and thoughts become active, such as "I can't cope," and "These feelings are intolerable." These thoughts often lead to further increases in affect.

Usually repeated recognition of the schema is required to reduce automatic thoughts and reactions. As patients reflect on these patterns in everyday life, they inevitably begin to wonder whether their perceptions are correct, whether they could behave differently, and whether they do not notice things that disconfirm their beliefs. This process is readily supplemented by the techniques developed by cognitive therapists to effect schema change. In applying these techniques it is useful to bear in mind the importance of the therapeutic process and the therapeutic context in which these specific interventions an placed to avoid the adverse consequences of activating reactive and maladaptive patterns that readily occurs when more didactic interventions are used.

Self-Pathology

Self-pathology includes problems with the contents of the self—dysfunctional thoughts, beliefs, and feelings about the self—and the structure and organization of the self. Dysfunctional cognitions may be managed using methods for changing schemata discussed earlier (see Cottraux & Blackburn, Chapter 18). Structural problems are more difficult to define and change. These problems are often described using terms such as a "lack of cohesiveness to the self" (Kohut, 1971) and "identify diffusion" (Akhtar, 1992; Kernberg, 1984). The develop-

ment of a set of interventions would be facilitated by a more operational definition. Again the concept of schema is useful for this purpose. Using this concept, the self may be conceptualized as a set of schemata that are used to organize information about the self. These schemata are not distinct but rather organized into clusters that represent different facets of the self or different self-images. Self-schemata form a hierarchy with the different levels representing increasingly general images of the self (Horowitz, 1998). At the highest level is a global schemata that represents the individual's understanding of the self—what Epstein (1973, 1990) referred to as a theory of the self. Epstein maintained that the self is really a theory about the self. It consists of an account that makes sense of one's life by explaining who one is and how one came to be that way.

With this model, cohesiveness or integration arises from the links or connections among self-schemata. The more extensive these links are, the greater the sense of coherence. These links may take several forms. Some will depend on images and feelings that connect different aspects of self-knowledge. Different experiences of being accepted and cared for or being recognized as competent may be linked by feelings of satisfaction and pleasure. Over time these linkages may crystallize respectively into a sense of self as loved and lovable and competent. As cognitive functions develop, these links are likely to become increasingly cognitive and verbally mediated. Ultimately integration is also achieved through the development of a theory of the self. This global, overarching schema is the ultimate expression of the links within self-knowledge. This model suggests two kinds of intervention: interventions that promote integration by building links within self-knowledge, and more global interventions that help the person to construct a new "theory of the self."

Even in well-adapted individuals, integration of the self is never complete. The self always involves different representations of the self. Some of these representations persist when activated, creating states of mind or self-states that last for variable lengths of time (Horowitz, 1979, 1998; Ryle, 1997). These recurrent experiential states are characterized by a constellation of qualities (schemata) attributed to the self, feelings, and moods ranging from pleasant to unpleasant according to the state, ways of experiencing the self and the world, and associated behaviors and ways of relating. The basic schema or schemata defining a self-state may be triggered by specific situations (usually interpersonal) or mood changes that arise primarily from biological factors. These states are important in understanding the structure of experience and the flow of interpersonal behavior. They define characteristic ways of experiencing the world and relating to other people. Interpersonal behaviors associated with a self-state tend to evoke responses from others that confirm the triggering beliefs and hence the self-state (Ryle, 1997). Thus the cycle is maintained. The sequence of triggering situation, basic schema, experiential state, behavioral response, reciprocating responses, and evaluation of outcome leading to confirmation of the basic belief creates cyclical patterns that tend to be self-maintaining and difficult to break.

With normal personality self-states are not widely divergent and the transition from one state to another is usually gradual. Moreover, the existence of multiple states does not impair the subjective experience of the cohesiveness of the self. With personality disorder integration of the different states is limited, transitions are often more abrupt, and marked disjunctions exist with experience of the self. As Ryle (1997) noted, multiple self-states are most apparent with borderline or emotionally dysregulated persons because the intense affects associated with each state increase the differences between states. Sometimes the discrepancy between states is so great that the patient has difficulty recalling experiences in one state when in another. Thus many patients in intensely dysphoric states find it difficult to recall how they felt in a more pleasant state even when it was only a short time ago. The state-dependent quality of experience and recall deepens the despair of dsyphoric states and contributes to the fragmentation of the self and the sense that the patient's life is "lived in pieces" (Pfeiffer, 1974).

With other forms of personality disorder, multiple self-states are often associated with less intense affects. Patients with schizoid–avoidant or inhibited traits often have self-states organized around discrepant self-perceptions rather than affects. For example, one man described self-states that included the self as sensitive, caring, and understanding and the self as ruthless and aggressive in pursuit of his own interests. The apparently inconsistent traits were the source of considerable identity confusion (Ahktar, 1992) because he was unable to integrate and reconcile these qualities. Some of these patients experience a second form of disjunction, a disconnection between the real self and the false self. They feel that the self that is presented to the world is false, a façade that masks or hides the real self which is hidden inside and cannot be shown. This gives rise to a lack of authenticity, the feeling that experiences are not genuine or real. Because experience feels unreal, the person feels like a detached observer who is alienated from the world. This discontinuity appears to arise because feelings are divorced from cognitions. Feelings are rarely expressed or integrated with thoughts.

Treating Self-Disjunctions. Integration is developed by strengthening self-experiences, establishing interpersonal boundaries, establishing links within self-knowledge, and promoting the synthesis of a new and more adaptive understanding of the self. General validating interventions strengthen the self, and collaborative description builds connections within self-experience. Specific interventions can also facilitate this process. Recognition of broad patterns of interpersonal behavior produces a sense of integration by linking events that were previously experienced as unrelated. At the same time, encouraging the patient to describe different self-states helps him or her to recognize the triggers for these states and the connections among them. Patients often report states in which they feel totally inadequate so that they withdraw from the world. At other times they may feel filled with anger and rage so that they are unable to function effectively. Often the experiences are confusing and difficult to explain. Detailed descriptions of the different states and the beliefs and feelings associated with each help to impose meaning and structure on their experience. This itself often helps to create the feeling that these experiences are not inexplicable and that control and change is possible. As the descriptive process continues, patients come to recognize how their behavior affects others and how they often precipitate the very reactions in others that they fear. Over time the schemata and affects associated with each state become clear, typical behaviors are understood, and others' reactions are clarified. This process integrates a wide range of information and sets the groundwork for questioning and changing specific components of the pattern.

Ryle (1997; see Chapter 19, this volume) suggested that the therapist works with the patient to develop diagrammatic representations of self-states, the relationships among them, and associated interpersonal behaviors. In this way the patient can see the connections among different aspects of self-experience and how these states lead to actions that tend to elicit from others responses that confirm and perpetuate these states. This idea incorporates the social environment into therapy and enables patients to recognize the nature of their interactions with others. A diagram also provides something concrete for patients to take from therapy that they can refer to later and begin to apply to understanding the ways these patterns unfold in everyday interactions. The process also involves an active collaboration that gives the patient an opportunity to work in a focused way with the therapist to elaborate his or her understanding of each state. This process illustrates the idea discussed earlier that change in entrenched maladaptive patterns requires that the patient recognize broad patterns and then work on understanding the detailed way that these patterns unfold in everyday experience.

Real self–false self disjunctions do not lend themselves as readily to such a systematic approach. Usually change is dependent on more indirect interventions and the opportunities that emerge to address these problems when dealing with other problems. Perhaps even more than with other problems, change requires a safe therapeutic environment that allows the patient to experience and express affect. Given that the problems with affect expression are closely intertwined with avoidant and inhibited traits, change is gradual and attempts to press for affective expression are likely to evoke further withdrawal. An important step in the change process is to identify situations in which the patient feels as if he or she is "really himself or herself." One patient, for example, only felt real when reading poetry; another when playing with a pet. Patients are usually comfortable talking about these experiences because they are nonthreatening and felt to be nonpersonal. Nevertheless, the process begins to create ideas that "I can be me," or "I can be real" and it is "safe to be myself." These discussions can then be extended to explore the emotions experienced on such occasions. This begins the process of tolerating and integrating affect. For many patient's this process is often aided by explanations that make the experience of "hiding the real self" understandable in developmental terms.

Construct a New "Theory of the Self." Besides promoting integration by linking related schemata and connecting them to interpersonal behaviors and experiences, it is also useful to help the patient to develop a new higher-order understanding or theory of self that is more adaptive than his or her previous theory. The ultimate task of longer-term treatment is to help individuals to construct a new understanding of themselves and their experiences that integrates different aspects of self-knowledge. Throughout therapy periodic summaries that offer broad summaries of the therapist's understanding help patients to synthesize a new theory of themselves. These accounts integrate a wide range of events, experiences, and actions that were previously seen as unrelated and hence promote the connections within self-knowledge that form the matrix of the self.

REFERENCES

Allen, J. G., Newsom, G. E., Gabbard, G. O., & Coyne, L. (1984). Scales to assess the therapeutic alliance from a psychoanalytic perspective. *Bulletin of the Menninger Clinic, 48,* 383–400.

Akhtar, S. (1992). *Broken structures: Severe personality disorders and their treatment.* Northvale, NJ: Aronson.

Arkowitz, H. (1989). The role of theory in psychotherapy integration. *Journal of Integrative and Eclectic Psychotherapy, 8,* 8–16.

Bartlett, F. C. (1932). *Remembering: A study in experimental and social psychology.* New York: Cambridge University Press. (Reprinted in 1995)

Baumeister, R. F. (1991). *Meanings of life.* New York: Guilford Press.

Baumeister, R. F. (1994). The crystallization of discontent in the process of major life change. In T. F. Heatherton & J. L. Weinberger (Eds.), *Can personality change?* (pp. 281–297). Wasington, DC: American Psychological Association.

Beck, A. T., Freeman A., & Associates. (1990). *Cognitive therapy of personality disorders.* New York: Guilford Press.

Benjamin, L. S. (1993). *Interpersonal diagnosis and treatment of personality disorders.* New York: Guilford Press.

Beutler, L. E. (1991). Have all won and must all have prizes? Revisiting Luborsky et al's verdict. *Journal of Consulting and Clinical Psychology, 59,* 226–232.

Bordin, E. S. (1994). Theory and research in the therapeutic working alliance: New directions. In A. Horvath, & L. S. Greenberg (Eds.), *The working alliance* (pp. 13–37). New York: Wiley.

Bowlby, J. (1980). *Attachment and loss: Vol. 3.* New York: Basic Books

Buie, D. H., & Adler, G. (1982). The definitive treatment of the borderline personality. *International Journal of Psychoanalytical Psychotherapy, 9,* 51–87.

Carver, C. S., & Scheier, M. F. (1998). *On the self-regulation of behavior.* Cambridge, UK: Cambridge University Press.

Clarkin J. F., Yeomans, F.E., & Kernberg, O. (1999). *Psychotherapy for borderline personality.* New York: Wiley.

DiClemente, C. C. (1994). If behaviours change, can personality be far behind? In T. F. Heatherton, & J. L. Weinberger (Eds.), *Can personality change?* (pp. 175–198). Washington, DC: American Psychological Association.

Eells, T. D. (1997). Psychotherapy case formulation: History and current status. In T. D. Eells (Ed.), *Handbook of psychotherapy case formulation.* New York: Guilford Press.

Epstein, S. (1973). The self-concept revisited, or a theory of a theory. *American Psychologist, 28,* 404–416.

Epstein, S. (1990). Cognitive-experiential self-theory. In L. A. Pervin (Ed.), *Handbook of personality: Theory and research* (pp. 165–192). New York: Guilford Press.

Gabbard, G. O. (1998). Treatment-resistant borderline personality disorder. *Psychiatric Annals, 28,* 651.

Gold, J. R. (1996). *Key concepts in psychotherapy integration.* New York, Plenum.

Goldberg, S. C., Schulz, S. C., Schulz, P. M., Resnick, R. J., Hamer, R. M., & Friedel, R. O. (1986). Borderline and schizotypal personality disorders treated with low-dose thiothixine vs. placebo. *Archives of General Psychiatry, 43,* 680–686.

Goldstein, A. P. (1962). *Therapist patient expectancies in psychotherapy.* New York: Pergamon Press.

Gunderson, J. G. (1984). *Borderline personality disorder.* Washington, DC: American Psychiatric Association.

Gunderson, J. G., Frank, A. F., Ronningstam, E. F., Wachter, S., Lynch, V. J., & Wolf, P. J. (1989). Early discontinuance of borderline patients from psychotherapy. *Journal of Nervous and Mental Disease, 177,* 38–42.

Guidano, V. F. (1987). *Complexity of the self: A developmental approach to psychopathology and therapy.* New York: Guilford Press.

Guidano, V. F. (1991). *The self in process: Toward a post-rationalist cognitive therapy.* New York: Guilford Press.

Heatherton, T. F., & Nichols, P. A. (1994). Personal accounts of successful versus failed attempts at life change. *Personality and Social Psychology Bulletin, 20,* 664–675.

Holt, R. R. (1989). *Freud reappraised: A fresh look at psychoanalytic theory.* New York: Guilford Press.

Horowitz, M. J. (1979). *States of mind.* New York: Plenum.

Horowitz, M. J. (1998). *Cognitive psychodynamics.* New York: Wiley.

Horvath, A., & Greenberg, L. S. (1994). Introduction. In J. Horvath & L. S. Greenberg (Eds.), *The working alliance* (pp. 1–9). New York: Wiley.

Joseph, B. (1983). On understanding and not understanding: Some technical issues. *International Journal of Psychoanalysis, 64,* 291–298.

Kernberg, O. F. (1984). *Severe personality disorders.* New Haven, CT: Yale University Press.

Kohut, H. (1971). *Analysis of the self.* New York: International Universities Press.

Kroll, J. (1988). *The challenge of the borderline patient.* New York: Basic Books.

Lambert, M. J. (1992). Psychotherapy outcome research: Implications for integrative and eclectic therapists. In J. C. Norcroft & M. R. Goldfried (Eds.), *Handbook of psychotherapy integration* (pp. 94–129). New York: Basic Books.

Lambert, M. J., & Bergin, A. E. (1994). The effectiveness of psychotherapy. In A. E. Bergin & S. L. Garfield (Eds.), *Handbook of psychotherapy and behavior change* (4th ed., pp. 143–189). New York: Wiley.

Linehan, M. M. (1993). *Cognitive-behavioral treatment of borderline personality disorder.* New York: Guilford Press.

Linehan, M. M., Armstrong, H. E., Suarez, A., Allmon, D., & Heard, H. L. (1991). Cognitive-behavioral treatment of chronically parasuicidal borderline patients. *Archives of General Psychiatry, 48,* 1060–1064.

Livesley, W. J. (1998). Suggestions for a framework for an empirically based classification of personality disorder. *Canadian Journal of Psychiatry, 43,* 137 147.

Livesley, W. J. (1999). The implications of recent research on the etiology and stability of personality and personality disorder for treatment. In J. Derksen, C. Maffei, & H. Groen (Eds.), *The treatment of personality disorders.* New York: Plenum.

Livesley, W. J. (2000). A practical approach to the treatment of patients with borderline personality disorder. *Psychiatric Clinics of North America, 23,* 211–232.

Livesley, W. J. (in press). *The practical management of personality disorder.* New York: Guilford Press.

Luborsky, L. (1984). *Principles of psychoanalytical psychotherapy.* New York: Basic Books.

Luborsky, L., Singer, B., & Luborsky, L. (1975). Comparative studies of psychotherapies. *Archives of General Psychiatry, 32,* 995–1008.

Malan, D. H. (1979). *Individual psychotherapy and the science of psychodynamics.* London: Butterworth's.

Masterson, J. (1976). *Psychotherapy of the borderline adult.* New York: Brunner/Mazel.

Markovitz, T. (1995). Pharmacotherapy of impulsivity, aggression, and related disorders. In E. Hollinger & D. G. Stein (Eds.), *Impulsivity and aggression* (pp. 263–287). New York: Wiley.

McCullough Vaillant, L. (1997). *Changing character.* New York: Basic Books.

Meichenbaum, D., & Turk, D. C. (1987). *Facilitating treatment adherence: A practitioner's guidebook.* New York: Plenum.

Miller, W. R., Benefield, R. G., & Tonigan, J. S. (1993). Enhancing motivation for change in problem drinking: Comparison of two therapist styles. *Journal of Consulting and Clinical Psychology, 61,* 455–461.

Miller, W. R., & Rollnick, S. (1991). *Motivational interviewing: Preparing people to change addictive behavior.* New York: Guilford Press.

Neimeyer, R. A. (1995). Constructivist psychotherapies: Features, foundations, and future directions. In R. A.

Neimeyer & M. J. Mahoney, *Constructivism in psychotherapy* (pp. 11–38). Washington, DC: American Psychological Association.

Newell, A., & Simon, H. A. (1972). *Human problem solving.* Englewood Cliffs, NJ: Prentice Hall.

Norcross, J. C., & Grencavage, L. M. (1989). Eclecticism and integration in counseling and psychotherapy: Major themes and obstacles. *British Journal of Guidance and Counseling, 17,* 117–247.

Orlinsky, D. E., Grawe, K., & Parks, B. K. (1994). Process and outcome in psychotherapy—Noch einmel. In A. E. Bergin & S. L. Garfield (Eds.), *Handbook of psychotherapy and behavior change* (3rd ed., pp. 270–376). New York: Wiley.

Orlinsky, D. E., & Howard, K. I. (1986). Process and outcome in psychotherapy. In A. E. Bergin & S. L. Garfield (Eds.), *Handbook of psychotherapy and behavior change* (3rd ed., pp. 311–381). New York: Wiley.

Paris, J. (1998). *Working with traits.* Northdale, NJ, Jason Aronson.

Pfeiffer, E. (1974). Borderline states. *Diseases of the Nervous System, 35,* 212–219.

Piaget, J. (1926). *Language and thought of the child.* New York: Harcourt Brace.

Prochaska, J. O., & DiClemente, C. (1983). Stages and processes of self change of smoking: Toward an integrative model of change. *Journal of Consuling and Clinical Psychology 51,* 390–395.

Prochaska, J. O., & DiClemente, C. (1992). The transtheoretical approach. In J. C. Norcross & M. R. Goldfried (Eds.), *Handbook of psychotherapy integration* (pp. 300–334). New York, Basic Books.

Prochaska, J. O., DiClemente, C. C., & Norcross, J. C. (1992). In search of how people change. *American Psychologist 47,* 1102–1114.

Rumelhart, D. E. (1980). On evaluating story grammars. *Cognitive Science, 4,* 313–316.

Ryle, A. (1997). *Cognitive-analytic therapy and borderline personality disorder.* Chichester, UK: Wiley.

Safran, J. D., Crocker, P., McMain, S., & Murray, P. (1990). Therapeutic alliance rupture as a therapy event for empirical investigation. *Psychotherapy, 27,* 154–165.

Safran, J. D., Muran, J. C., & Samstag, L. W. (1994). Resolving therapeutic alliance ruptures: A task-analytic investigation. In O. A. Horvath & L. S. Greenberg (Eds.), *The working alliance* (pp. 225–255). New York: Wiley.

Schoeneman, T. J., & Curry, S. (1990). Attributions for successful and unsuccessful health behavior change. *Basic and Applied Social Psychology, 11,* 421–431.

Shapiro, D. (1965). *Neurotic styles.* New York: Basic Books.

Skodol, A. E., Buckley, P., & Charles, E. (1983). Is there a characteristic pattern to the treatment history of clinic outpatients with borderline personality? *Journal of Nervous and Mental Disease, 171,* 405–410.

Soloff, P. H. (1998). Algorithms for pharmacological treatment of personality dimensions: Symptom specific treatments for cognitive–perceptual, affective, and impulsive–behavioral dysregulation. *Bulletin of the Menninger Clinic, 62,* 195–214.

Soloff, P.H. (2000). Psychopharmacology of borderline personality disorder. *Psychiatric Clinics of North America, 23,* 169–192.

Sonne, J. L., & Janoff, D. S. (1979). The effect of treatment attributions on the maintenance of weight reduction: A replication and extension. *Cognitive Therapy and Research, 3,* 389–387.

Steiner, J. (1993). *Psychic retreats: Pathological organizations in psychotic, neurotic and borderline patients.* London: Routledge.

Strupp, H. H., & Binder, J. (1984). *Psychotherapy in a new way: A guide to time-limited dynamic \psychotherapy.* New York: Basic Books.

Vaillant, G. E. (1992). The beginning of wisdom is never calling a patient a borderline. *Journal of Psychotherapy Practice and Research, 1,* 117–134.

Waldinger, R. J., & Gunderson, J. G. (1984). Completed psychotherapies with borderline patients. *American Journal of Psychotherapy, 38,* 190–202.

Waldinger, R. J., & Gunderson, J. G. (1989). *Effective psychotherapy with borderline patients.* Washington, DC: American Psychiatric Association.

Weiner, B. (1985). An attributional model of achievement theory and emotion. *Psychological Review, 92,* 548–573.

Wicklund, R. A. (1975). Objective self-awareness. In L. Berkowitz (Ed.), *Advances in experimental social psychology* (Vol. 8, pp. 233–275). New York: Academic Press.

Wicklund, R. A., & Duval, S. (1971). Opinion change and performance facilitation as a result of objective self-awareness. *Journal of Experimental Social Psychology, 7,* 319–342.

Yalom, I. D. (1975). *The principles and practice of group psychotherapy.* New York: Basic Books.

Yalom, I. D. (1985). *The theory and practice of group psychotherapy* (3rd ed.). New York: Basic Books.

Young, J. E. (1990). *Cognitive therapy for personality disorders: A schema-focused approach.* Sarasota, FL: Professional Resource Exchange.

Author Index

Subject Index